Respiratory Care

Respiratory Care

Respiratory Care
A Guide to Clinical Practice
Third Edition

Edited by

George G. Burton, M.D.
Medical Director, Respiratory Services
Kettering Medical Center, Kettering, Ohio
Clinical Professor of Medicine and Anesthesiology
Wright State University School of Medicine
Dayton, Ohio

John E. Hodgkin, M.D.
Clinical Professor of Medicine
University of California, Davis
Medical Director, Center for Health Promotion and Rehabilitation
Medical Director, Respiratory Care and Pulmonary Rehabilitation
St. Helena Hospital and Health Center
Deer Park, California

Jeffrey J. Ward, M.Ed., R.R.T.
Program Director
Rochester Community College/Mayo
Respiratory Therapy Program
Assistant Professor, Mayo Medical School
Department of Anesthesia
Rochester, Minnesota

J. B. Lippincott Company
Philadelphia
New York   St. Louis   London   Sydney   Tokyo

Acquisitions Editor: Charles McCormick
Developmental Editor: Kimberley Cox
Project Editor: Tom Gibbons
Indexer: Katherine Pitcoff
Cover and Interior Designer: Anita Curry
Design Coordinator: Kathy Kelley-Luedtke
Production Manager: Helen Ewan
Production Coordinator: Pamela Milcos/William F. Hallman
Compositor: Bi-Comp, Inc
Printer/Binder: Murray Printing Company

3rd Edition

1   3   5   6   4   2

Library of Congress Cataloging-in-Publication Data

Respiratory care: a guide to clinical practice/edited by George
    G. Burton, John E. Hodgkin, Jeffrey J. Ward. -- 3rd ed.
        p.   cm.
    Includes bibliographical references.
    Includes index.
    ISBN 0-397-50909-X
    1. Respiratory therapy.   I. Burton, George G., 1934–

II. Hodgkin, John E. (John Elliott), 1939–   . III. Ward,
    Jeffrey J., 1948–
    [DNLM: 1. Respiratory Therapy.   2. Respiratory Tract
    Diseases-therapy.   WF 145 R434]
    RC735.I5R47   1991
    616.2'0046--dc20
    DNLM/DLC
    for Library of Congress   90-6616
                                                          CIP

The authors and publisher have exerted every effort to ensure
that drug selection and dosage set forth in this text are in
accord with current recommendations and practice at the time
of publication. However, in view of ongoing research, changes
in government regulations, and the constant flow of information relating to drug therapy and drug reactions, the reader is
urged to check the package insert for each drug for any change
in indications and dosage and for added warnings and precautions. This is particularly important when the recommended
agent is a new or infrequently employed drug.

This book is dedicated to our parents and to our children, who gladden the hours and days of our lives.

Joan Rubino, David, Kevin, Janelle, and Jon Burton
Steven, Kathyrn, Carolyn, Jonathan, and Jamie Hodgkin
Caryn Ward

■ Contributors

Harry Linne Anderson III, M.D.
Chief Resident in General Surgery, University of Michigan Medical Center, Ann Arbor, Michigan (Chapter 30)

Robert A. Balk, M.D.
Associate Professor of Medicine, Rush Medical College of Rush University; Director of Medical Intensive Care Unit, Director of Respiratory Therapy, Rush-Presbyterian–St. Luke's Medical Center, Chicago, Illinois (Chapter 27)

Robert H. Bartlett, M.D.
Professor of Surgery, University of Michigan School of Medicine, Ann Arbor, Michigan (Chapter 30)

Clifford E. Bickford, R.R.T., R. PSG.T., C.P.F.T.
Assistant Director, Cardiopulmonary Department, St. Helena Hospital and Health Center, Deer Park, California (Appendix A)

Lia S. Bickford, B.A., R.C.P.
Deer Park, California (Appendix A)

Paul B. Blanch, B.A., R.R.T.
Instructor in Respiratory Therapy, Santa Fe Community College; Equipment Supervisor (Biomedical Engineer), Shands Hospital at the University of Florida, Gainesville, Florida (Chapter 21)

A. Jay Block, M.D.
Professor of Medicine and Anesthesiology, University of Florida College of Medicine; Chief, Pulmonary Division, J. Hillis Miller Health Center; Pulmonary Staff Physician, Veterans Administration Medical Center, Gainesville, Florida (Chapter 15)

Roger C. Bone, M.D.
Professor and Chairman, Department of Internal Medicine, and Chief, Section of Pulmonary and Critical Care Medicine, Rush-Presbyterian–St. Luke's Medical Center, Chicago, Illinois (Chapters 27, 31)

Richard D. Branson, R.R.T.
Clinical Instructor, Department of Surgery, University of Cincinnati/Pritzker School of Medicine, Cincinnati, Ohio (Chapter 34)

W. Mark Brutinel, M.D.
Assistant Professor of Medicine, Mayo Graduate School of Medicine, Rochester, Minnesota (Chapter 26)

George G. Burton, M.D.
Medical Director, Respiratory Services, Kettering Medical Center, Kettering, Ohio, Clinical Professor of Medicine and Anesthesiology, Wright State University School of Medicine, Dayton, Ohio (Chapter 22, Appendix E)

Clarence A. Collier, M.D.
Professor Emeritus of Medicine and Physiology and Biophysics, School of Medicine, University of Southern California, Los Angeles, California (Chapter 10)

Gerilynn A. Connors, B.S., R.C.P., R.R.T.
Director, Pulmonary Rehabilitation, St. Helena Hospital and Health Center, Deer Park, California (Chapter 24)

Denis A. Cortese, M.D.
Professor of Medicine, Mayo Medical School, Rochester, Minnesota (Chapter 26)

Kenneth Davis, Jr., M.D.
Assistant Professor of Surgery, University of Cincinnati Medical Center, Cincinnati, Ohio (Chapter 34)

Thomas J. DeKornfeld, M.D.
Professor of Anesthesiology (Emeritus), University of Michigan Medical School, Ann Arbor, Michigan (Chapter 5)

David A. Desautels, M.P.A., R.R.T.
Instructor, Respiratory Care Program Santa Fe Community College; Technical Director, Hyperbaric Medicine Program, Shands Hospital at the University of Florida, Gainesville, Florida (Chapters 16, 21)

Gerald K. Dolan, M.S., R.R.T.
Associate Professor and Director, Respiratory Therapy Program, Ferris State University School of Allied Health, Big Rapids, Michigan (Chapter 1)

F. Herbert Douce, M.S., R.R.T., R.P.F.T.
Assistant Professor and Director, School of Allied Health Professions, Ohio State University, Columbus, Ohio (Chapter 8)

Paul L. Enright, M.D.
Instructor, Department of Medicine, Mayo Medical School; Staff Consultant, Division of Thoracic Diseases, Mayo Clinic, Rochester, Minnesota (Chapter 9)

L. Jack Faling, M.D.
Associate Professor of Medicine, Tufts University School of Medicine; Associate Chief of Medicine and Pulmonary Section, Medical Director Respiratory Therapy, Boston Veterans Administration Medical Center, Boston, Massachusetts (Chapter 23)

John M. Fiascone, M.D.
Assistant Professor of Pediatrics, Tufts University School of Medicine; Assistant Neonatologist, Floating Hospital for Infants and Children, New England Medical Center, Boston, Massachusetts (Chapter 28)

Ivan D. Frantz III, M.D.
Professor of Pediatrics, Tufts University School of Medicine; Chief, Division of Newborn Medicine, Floating Hospital for Infants and Children, New England Medical Center; Director, Boston Perinatal Center, Boston, Massachusetts (Chapter 28)

Mary E. Gilmartin, R.N., R.R.T.
National Jewish Center for Immunology and Respiratory Medicine, Denver, Colorado (Chapter 25)

Allen I. Goldberg, M.D.
Assistant Professor of Anesthesia and Pediatrics, Northwestern University Medical School; Medical Director, Department of Respiratory Care, Children's Memorial Hospital, Chicago, Illinois (Chapter 29)

Douglas R. Gracey, M.D.
Professor of Medicine, Mayo Medical School; Vice-Chairman for Practice, Department of Medicine, Mayo Medical Center, Rochester, Minnesota (Chapters 33, 35)

Susan Rickey Hatfield, Ph.D.
Associate Professor, Speech Communication, Winona (Minnesota) State University, Winona, Minnesota (Chapter 3)

Timothy A. Hatfield, Ph.D.
Professor, Counselor Education, Winona (Minnesota) State University, Winona, Minnesota (Chapter 3)

H. Frederic Helmholz, Jr., M.D.
Associate Professor (Emeritus), Physiology, Mayo Clinic and Mayo Graduate School of Medicine, Rochester, Minnesota (Chapter 17, Appendix E)

Dean R. Hess, M.S., R.R.T.
Instructor, Respiratory Therapy Program, York College of Pennsylvania; Assistant Director of Clinical Research, York Hospital, York, Pennsylvania (Chapters 7, 22)

John E. Hodgkin, M.D.
Clinical Professor of Medicine, University of California, Davis; Medical Director, Center for Health Promotion and Rehabilitation, and Medical Director, Respiratory Care and Pulmonary Rehabilitation, St. Helena Hospital and Health Center, Deer Park, California (Chapters 9, 10, 11, 22, 24, Appendices A, B, C, D, F)

Leonard D. Hudson, M.D.
Professor of Medicine and Head, Division of Pulmonary and Critical Care Medicine, University of Washington; Chief, Division of Pulmonary and Critical Care Medicine, Harborview Medical Center, Seattle, Washington (Chapter 32)

James M. Hurst, M.D.
Associate Professor of Surgery and Anesthesia, University of Cincinnati College of Medicine; Director, Division of Trauma and Critical Care, University of Cincinnati Medical Center, Cincinnati, Ohio (Chapter 34)

Jay A. Johannigman, M.D.
Fellow, Division of Trauma and Critical Care, University of Cincinnati College of Medicine, Cincinnati, Ohio (Chapter 34)

Joseph Kaplan, M.D.
Assistant Professor of Medicine, Mayo Medical School, Jacksonville, Florida (Chapter 13)

Gary W. Kaufman, M.P.A., R.R.T.
Adjunct Faculty, Millersville University Program in Respiratory Therapy, Millersville, Pennsylvania; Director, Therapeutics and OAS, St. Joseph Hospital and Health Care Center, Lancaster, Pennsylvania (Chapter 7)

J. Robert Kinker, Jr., Ph.D., R.R.T.
Cardio-Pulmonary and Vascular Services, Exercise Physiologist, Mansfield General Hospital, Columbus, Ohio (Chapter 8)

Steven E. Levy, M.D.
Clinical Professor of Medicine, School of Medicine, University of California, Los Angeles; Co-Director, Pulmonary Department, Brotman Medical Center, Culver City, California (Chapter 36)

Robert M. Lewis, B.A., R.R.T.
Clinical Instructor, Respiratory Care Department, The Children's Memorial Hospital, Chicago, Illinois (Chapter 29)

Glen A. Lillington, M.D.
Professor of Medicine, Pulmonary/Critical Care Division, University of California, Davis, School of Medicine, Sacramento, California (Chapter 12)

James M. Maguire, Ph.D., R.C.P.
Pall Biomedical, Glen Cove, New York (Chapter 14)

Barry J. Make, M.D.
Associate Professor of Medicine, Pulmonary Section, University of Colorado School of Medicine; Director, Pulmonary Rehabilitation, National Jewish Center for Immunology and Respiratory Medicine, Denver, Colorado (Chapter 25)

Ray Masferrer, R.R.T.
Associate Executive Director, American Association for Respiratory Care, Dallas, Texas (Chapter 1)

James A. Peters, M.D.
Associate Professor, School of Allied Health Professions, Loma Linda University, Associate Medical Director, Department of Respiratory Care, St. Helena Hospital and Health Center, Deer Park, California (Chapter 10)

Steve G. Peters, M.D.
Assistant Professor of Medicine, Mayo Medical School, Rochester, Minnesota (Chapter 33)

Thomas L. Petty, M.D.
Professor of Medicine, University of Colorado School of Medicine; President, Presbyterian/St. Luke's Center for Health Sciences Education, Denver, Colorado (Chapter 37)

David Joseph Plevak, M.D.
Assistant Professor of Anesthesiology, Mayo Medical School; Consultant in Critical Care Medicine, Mayo Clinic, Rochester, Minnesota (Chapter 20)

Alan L. Plummer, M.D.
Associate Professor of Medicine, Pulmonary Diseases and Critical Care, Emory University School of Medicine; Medical Director, Respiratory Care Department, Emory University Hospital, Atlanta, Georgia (Chapter 4)

Ray H. Ritz, B.A., R.R.T.
Assistant Director of Clinical Services, Respiratory Care, Massachusetts General Hospital, Boston, Massachusetts (Chapter 6)

Eugene G. Ryerson, M.D.
Assistant Professor of Medicine, College of Medicine, University of Florida; Director, Medical Intensive Care Facilities, Veterans Administration Hospital, Gainesville, Florida (Chapter 15)

Myron M. Stein, M.D.
Clinical Professor of Medicine, University of California, Los Angeles, School of Medicine; Co-Director, Department of Pulmonary Medicine, Brotman Medical Center, Culver City, California (Chapter 36)

Thomas E. Sych, C.R.T.T.
Manager for Supply and Equipment for Respiratory Services, Kettering Medical Center, Kettering, Ohio (Chapter 14)

Stephen L. Thompson, M.S., R.R.T.
Educational Director, Respiratory Care Services, University of Illinois College of Medicine, Chicago, Illinois (Chapter 29)

Philip A. von der Heydt, M.Ed., R.R.T.
Executive Director, Joint Review Committee for Respiratory Therapy Education, Euless, Texas (Chapter 2)

Patricia N. Vreeland, C.R.T.T.
Respiratory Therapist/Research Technician, Floating Hospital for Infants and Children, New England Medical Center, Boston, Massachusetts (Chapter 28)

Jeffrey J. Ward, M.Ed., R.R.T.
Program Director, Rochester Community College/Mayo Respiratory Therapy Program; Assistant Professor, Mayo Medical School, Department of Anesthesia, Rochester, Minnesota (Chapters 1, 17, 20)

John A. Washington, M.D.
Chairman, Department of Microbiology, The Cleveland Clinic Foundation, Cleveland, Ohio (Chapter 18)

James M. Webb, B.S., R.R.T.
Director, Respiratory Care Services, Florida Hospital, Orlando, Florida (Chapter 14)

John T. Wheeler, R.R.T.
Instructor, Respiratory Therapy Program, Rochester Community College; Supervisor, Respiratory Care, Mayo Foundation, Rochester, Minnesota (Chapter 33)

Robert L. Wilkins, M.A., R.R.T.
Associate Chairman/Associate Professor and Program Director, Associate in Science, Department of Respiratory Therapy, School of Allied Health Professions, Loma Linda, California (Chapter 11)

Irwin Ziment, M.D.
Chief of Medicine, Olive View Medical Center, Sylmar, California; Professor of Medicine, University of California, Los Angeles, School of Medicine, Los Angeles, California (Chapter 19)

■ Preface to the Third Edition

As this introduction to the third edition of *Respiratory Care: A Guide to Clinical Practice* is being written, the American Association for Respiratory Care (AARC) is holding its 35th Annual Meeting in Anaheim, California. Some 8,000 respiratory care practitioners (RCPs) attending heard exciting presentations regarding new scientific concepts and approaches to the assessment and treatment of patients with pulmonary disorders. They viewed an exhibition hall filled with remarkable devices, whose technology was unheard of when the first edition of this volume appeared sixteen years ago.

While scientific presentations at the AARC Annual Meeting cover a spectrum of respiratory care activities, from disease prevention to intra-uterine respiratory care to ethical considerations regarding the initiation and withdrawal of life support in the aged, a Select Committee of the AARC sits in deliberation to discuss the future of respiratory care as a profession, reexamining the roles and functions of RCPs in many diverse areas. The professionalism of RCPs is evident in the current licensure/credentialing activity in nearly every state, in the well-developed specific professional efforts of the organization itself (NBRC), in the stature of the national organization (AARC), and, most importantly, in the continuous display of caring, concerned patient care activities by the vast majority of our respiratory care colleagues.

The respiratory care student entering the field today finds a dazzling array of job opportunities to choose from; entry-level job openings exist in nearly every hospital in the country. Though regional differences may exist, the tasks performed by the new respiratory care practitioners range from routine, repetitive, "low-tech, low-touch" procedures to those demanding more complex psychomotor and interpersonal skills and relationships. Indeed, it has recently been suggested that it is the very diversity of such work that correlates best with job satisfaction in RCPs.[1] This diversity of tasks has been reviewed by the NBRC and is being incorporated into their certification (CRTT) and registered therapist (RRT) examination matrices. The reader will note that a large number of respiratory care educators have contributed to the current edition in an attempt to make the volume practical as well as timely.

An increasing volume of pertinent background information and applied technology fills the curricula of accredited respiratory care training programs, where the emphasis has shifted from "process" compliance to "outcome" measures, in the newest version of JRCRTE "Essentials."

The exponential growth of device technology is well demonstrated by the proliferation of types, and the sophistication (and cost) of various ventilators, from multiple units of a basically simple design (see Figure) first used in 1928[2] to the numerous units described by Desautels and Blanch in Chapter 21 of this volume. However, with cost-containment concerns determining many care delivery priorities and strategies, there appears to be no clear perception that these more complex technologies translate into better, let alone safer, patient outcome.

A recent AARC Task Force on Professional Development[3] of RCPs has noted an increasingly wide service base for respiratory care activities and a branching out of competencies into other avenues, including cardiopulmonary diagnostics. In this spirit we have added chapters on home care, sleep-disordered breathing, hyperbaric oxygen therapy, and fiberoptic bronchoscopy. We believe that these activities contribute a reasonable, desirable part of the RCP's domain and are likely to remain so in the foreseeable future. Other, yet to be determined areas of expertise, not covered intensively in this textbook, may be required of respiratory care prac-titioners in the future. It is for this reason, as well as to provide new concepts and to delete information shown to be no longer valid, that new editions of books are prepared and published.

It is our belief that respiratory care will become increasingly therapist-driven, with preoperative respiratory care protocols, ventilator weaning protocols, daily change in bronchial hygiene programs, and variable-assist home-care and pulmonary rehabilitation programs representing but a tip of the iceberg. In the "sicker-in, quicker out" milieu of the 90s, in-hospital respiratory care will need to become still more efficient. The need for RCPs in the outpatient setting will become increasingly more obvious.[4] Comprehensively trained, flexible, and innovative RCPs will do well in the new environment.

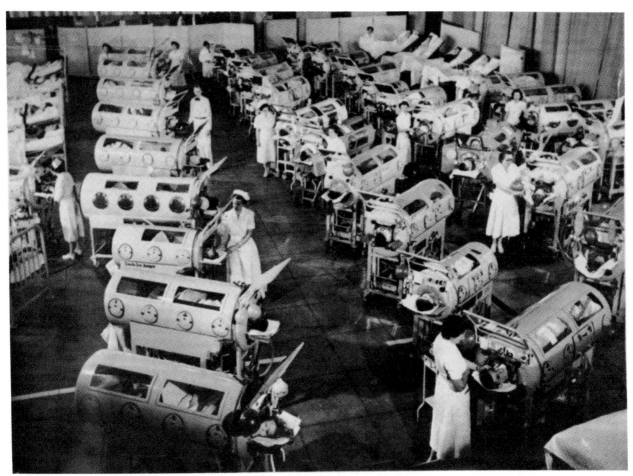

Iron lungs in use during the polio epidemics at Los Angeles County Hospital, ca. 1951-53. (Reprinted with permission of the author, W.E. Collins, Inc., and the Journal of the American Medical Association)

The format of this volume remains unchanged from previous editions. We have tried to group the material in a way that will integrate well into classroom teaching, student review, RCP and department reference, and—most of all—RCP practice.

Our appreciation is again extended to our secretaries, Flossie Hodgson and Carol Lewis, who tolerated our forays into the ordered world of their word processors to allow us to reword, rearrange, and otherwise interfere with their already busy lives. Again, our thanks to the 67 contributors to this volume: their timely responses to our pleas for manuscript and illustration material have kept this volume from being later than it could be. All are busy clinicians, educators, and researchers who have found that evaluative, summative, and cognitive writing is even more challenging than in times past.

Finally, our thanks to Kim Cox, our editor at J. B. Lippincott Company, for her long-suffering patience, assistance, and encouragement.

We hope that our readers will find this new edition refreshing and pertinent to their practice, and that their satisfaction in the field will be as great and enduring as has ours. As new and old students alike, who critically read or only peruse this material, we hope memory will speak to those who listen, and that the lessons of the past will reach out to transform the present into an exciting, professional future.

REFERENCES

1. Hmelo C, Aston KL Jr: Job satisfaction and task complexity among respiratory care practitioners. Respir Care 34:1129, 1989
2. Drinker E, McKhann CF: The use of new apparatus for the prolonged administration of artificial respiration. I. A fatal case of poliomyelitis. JAMA 92:1658, 1929
3. Bunch D: Task force update. AARC Times 11:17, 1987
4. Wissing DR, George RB: The coming decade. Respir Care Management 19:149, 1989

▮ Contents

SECTION THREE
RESPIRATORY CARE IN CRITICAL ILLNESSES

APPENDICES

Respiratory Care

Respiratory Care Service and Education in the Modern Hospital

ONE

History of the Respiratory Care Profession

Ray Masferrer
Gerald K. Dolan
Jeffrey J. Ward

The development of clinical respiratory care and the respiratory care profession involves a diverse historical record. There is the history of biology unraveling the "secrets" of the anatomy and function of the cardiopulmonary system. Concurrently, discovery of physiologic gases was made, and their chemistry, physics, and roles in body function were elicited. In addition, there has been an ongoing evolution of clinical pulmonary medicine, with key technical advancements in areas of gas therapy, resuscitation, mechanical ventilation, and cardiopulmonary diagnostics and monitoring. Coupled with the history of medical science and technology, there is also a legacy of an evolving organized profession. The purpose of this chapter is to briefly review highlights in the history of respiratory care and the structure of the respiratory care profession.

The story of the search for knowledge about respiration goes back to ancient times.

> And he put his mouth upon his mouth . . . and the flesh of the child became warm.
>
> II Kings 4:34

Twenty-eight centuries ago, the biblical story of the prophet Elisha recounted the restoration to life of the son of a Shunammite woman. In this account, the principle that respirable air was necessary for human life was recognized. This early con-cept fit into the practical medicine of the Egyptians and Babylonians. About 3000 B.C., ancient Egyptian science had reached its zenith. The Chinese had a part-philosophic and part-physiologic concept of breathing; in which breath from the air was transmitted into the soul. Earlier, about 2000 B.C., they had developed acupuncture points, elaborate rituals for taking pulse and used moxibustion (burning substances on the skin).[1]

An important portion of our scientific heritage began with the Greeks, who sought knowledge for its own sake, without need for practical application. Pythagoras (580–489 B.C.) defined life and matter as comprising four basic elements: earth, fire, water, and air. Hippocrates (460–370 B.C.) developed the doctrine of "essential humors." He attributed all diseases to humoral disorders within body fluids and taught than an essential, yet undefined, material derived from the inspired air, entered the heart and was then distributed throughout the body systems. Hippocrates and his contemporaries promoted examination and identification of signs of diseases. Aristotle (384–322 B.C.) recorded the first probable scientific experiment in respiratory physiology when he observed that animals kept in air-tight chambers soon died. He ascribed their deaths to the animals' inability to cool themselves by secretion of "phlegm." He also identified the heart as the source of the body's heat and nervous center.[1,2]

Erasistratus worked in Alexandria (about 304 B.C.) and founded the "pneumatic" theory of respiration. He felt that the lungs passed air to the left ventricle, which used air-filled arteries for transport to the body tissues. He apparently understood that heart valves provided one-way flow.

In Asia Minor, Galen (130–199 A.D.) dominated the study of respiration longer than any previous scholars. He felt that "pneuma" or "world spirit" from inspired air passed through invisible pores in the heart's intraventricular septum. There blood became charged with this vital spirit. Against popular thought, Galen believed that blood, not air, was carried by the arterial circulation, and that there were pulmonary and systemic capillaries. By dissection he disproved Aristotle's theories by showing that nerves originate in the brain and spinal cord, not the heart. He worked out the effects of cord transections and hemisection while serving as a physician to gladiators.

Little new "physiologic" investigation was done after Galen until the 11th century.[1,2] Antisecular and antiscientific feeling during the medieval period resulted in a gap in progress and the loss of many priceless written documents. Bright lights of this period were naturalists Albertus Magnus (1192–1280) and physicist and mathematician Roger Bacon (1214–1294). The Renaissance brought a renewed interest in the sciences. In Italy, Leonardo da Vinci (1452–1519) took up human dissection and physiologic experiments on animals. He concluded that subatmospheric (intrapleural) pressure inflated the lungs. Da Vinci observed that fire consumed a component in air, and that animals could not live in an atmosphere that could not support flames. In 1542, Andreas Vesalius (Fig. 1–1) performed a thoracotomy on a pig and observed the effect of pneumothorax. The pig exhibited "wavelike pulsations of the heart and arteries," which probably was ventricular fibrillation. Vesalius reported that the heart returned to normal after ventilation through a tracheostomy tube made from a reed. He published his great work on anatomy in 1543, contradicting some of Galen's earlier observations. This manuscript and "a cardiac resuscitation" during the autopsy of a "just expired" Spanish nobleman brought on the wrath of the Inquisition. The Spanish anatomist Michael Servetus (1509–1553) was the first to discover that the blood in the pulmonary circulation, after mixing with the air in the lungs, returned to the left side of the heart. Servetus' "heretical" anatomy text resulted in his being burned at the stake.[1,2]

It required 75 years before the physiology of the circulation could be correctly clarified. In 1628, William Harvey (1578–1657; Fig. 1–2) described

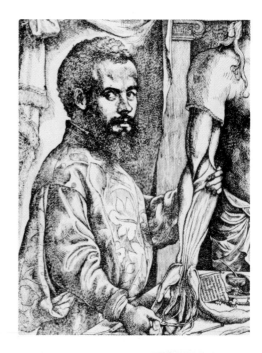

Figure 1–1. Andreas Vesalius, founder of "modern" human anatomy. (Courtesy of History of Medicine Library, Mayo Foundation, Rochester, Minnesota)

Figure 1–2. William Harvey described the circulatory system. (Courtesy of the Wellcome Historical Medical Museum, London)

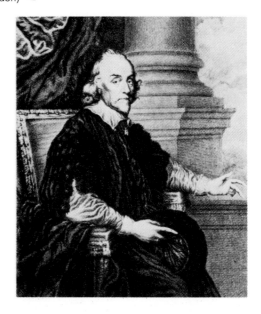

the heart as a muscular pump propelling the blood to the body through the arterial circulation, with return through the venous system.

In Italy, Evangelista Torricelli (1608–1647) and associates made the first barometer in the 1640s. Blaise Pascal (1623–1662) in France, confirmed the relationship between barometric pressure and altitude. In 1666, England's Robert Boyle (1627–1691) speculated that there must be within air:

> . . . numberless exhalations of the terraqueous globe . . . The difficulty we find in keeping flame and fire alive . . . without air renders it suspicious that there may be disbursed throughout the rest of the atmosphere some odd substance, either solar, astral, or other foreign nature: on account whereof the air is so necessary to flame.

This note from Boyle's *Philosophical Transactions* (1670) surmises that the lack of oxygen, or a similar substance, was also a destructive factor. He recorded the production of aeroembolism by subjecting animals to low pressure. Boyle also developed Torricelli's barometer into the U-shaped form we know today and proposed the relationship between volume and pressure, which we know as Boyle's law.[1,2]

In 1771, Swedish apothecary Carl Scheele (1742–1786; Fig. 1–3) made oxygen by heating magnesium oxide (MgO_2) with concentrated sulfuric acid (H_2SO_4). He communicated his findings on this "fire air" to others, and a summary of Scheele's findings was published in June 1774. However, the Englishman Joseph Priestley (1733–1804; Fig. 1–4) was credited with the discovery of oxygen, although his work was published 3 months later. Priestley described his response to breathing pure oxygen, "phlogisticated air," as follows:

> . . . my breath felt peculiarly light and easy for some time afterward. Who can tell but that in time this pure air may become a fashionable luxury. Hitherto, only two mice and myself have had the privilege of breathing it.

Both Scheele and Priestley followed the phlogiston theory proposed by the German George Stahl. This theory stated that combustible objects use up phlogiston when burned. In France, Antoine Lavoisier (1743–1794; Fig. 1–5) published details of his findings on oxygen in 1775. He renamed the gas "oxygen" or "acid maker." It was Lavoisier who appeared to have truly understood the physiologic relationships of oxygen and carbon dioxide. Be-

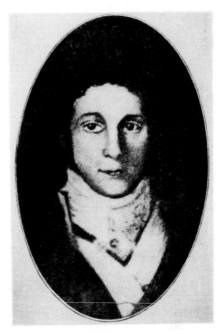

Figure 1—3. Carl Wilhelm Scheele, a Swedish apothecary, who was the first to synthesize oxygen. (Amer Pharm Soc J 20:1061, 1931, with permission)

Figure 1—4. Joseph Priestley is credited as the "discoverer" of oxygen. (Courtesy of Wellcome Historical Medical Museum, London)

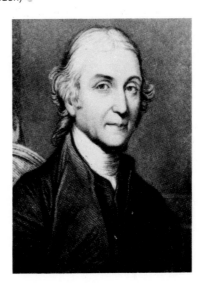

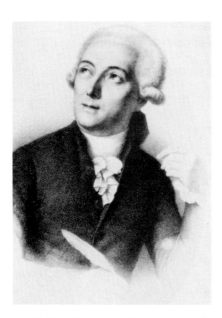

Figure 1–5. Antoine-Laurent Lavoisier described the relationship of oxygen utilization and carbon dioxide elimination as respiration. (Courtesy of Wellcome Historical Medical Museum, London)

tween 1775 and 1794, his experiments showed that oxygen was absorbed by the lungs and consumed by the body. He further confirmed that carbon dioxide and water vapor were primary components of exhalation and that an inert gas (nitrogen) was essentially unchanged in the process. This work destroyed acceptance of the phlogiston theory. Unfortunately, the knowledge that Lavoisier's laboratory was supported by the French royalty resulted in his death by the guillotine in the prime of his career.[1,2]

Joseph Black (1728–1799; Fig. 1–6) is credited with the discovery of carbon dioxide gas, dephlogisticated "fixed air," which he produced by heating limestone. Actually, Black only rediscovered work done by Jean Baptiste van Helmont 100 years earlier.

During the late 1700s and early 1800s, several scientists provided significant discoveries in essential background physics that applied to pulmonary physiology. Jacques-Alexandre-Cesar Charles (1746–1823), Joseph Louis Gay-Lussac (1778–1850), John Dalton (1766–1844), William Henry (1774–1836), and Pierre-Simon de Laplace (1749–1827) provided essential discoveries.[1,2]

Early clinical application of lung physiology began to take place in the late 1700s in the form of cardiopulmonary resuscitation. Societies for rescu-

ing drowning victims were set up in Denmark, England, and Europe. Several techniques were used: fumigation (blowing smoke into the rectum), chest–belly compression, blood letting, and administration of stimulants. Reports of successful resuscitation (by now through the airway!) began in 1744 with John Fothergill of England. In 1776, John Hunter advocated the use of fireplace bellows with oxygen. Later the bellows was abandoned because of cases of complications such as pneumothorax. Tracheal intubation and electrical stimulation of the heart were suggested but either overlooked or forgotten until years later.[3]

Lazzaro Spallazani (1729–1799) was the first scientist to measure oxygen consumption and carbon dioxide production of laboratory animals. By 1837, Heinrich Magnus (1802–1870) made the first quantitative analyses of arterial and venous oxygen and carbon dioxide content. In England, John Hutchinson (1811–1861) developed the spirometer and measured the vital capacity of over 2000 subjects. Eduard Pfluger (1829–1910) provided evidence that oxidation occurs in tissues proportional to their needs, and devised the term *respiratory quotient*. In 1878, Paul Bert (1833–1886) demonstrated that reduced inspired oxygen tension caused hyperventilation and, in 1885, F. Miescher-Rusch provided evidence that carbon dioxide was

Figure 1–6. Joseph Black is credited with the discovery of carbon dioxide. (Courtesy of the University of Edinburgh, Edinburgh, Scotland)

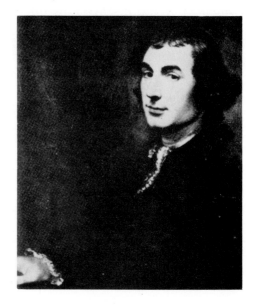

the primary stimulus for ventilation. Christian Bohr (1855–1911; Fig. 1–7) constructed the oxyhemoglobin dissociation curve for purified hemoglobin in 1886. In 1904, Bohr, K. A. Hasselbalch, and August Krogh (1874–1949) linked the process of oxygen and carbon dioxide transport.[1,2]

John Scott Haldane (1860–1936; Fig. 1–8), John Gillies Priestly (1880–1941), and Yandell Henderson (1873–1944) demonstrated that carbon dioxide is primarily responsible for maintaining ventilation. Joseph Barcroft (1872–1947) contributed to the understanding of the oxyhemoglobin dissociation curve, and his high-altitude experiments proved that pulmonary alveolocapillary oxygen transfer involves only the simple process of diffusion. Lawrence J. Henderson (1878–1942; Fig. 1–9) calculated the oxygen dissociation constants for oxygenated and reduced hemoglobin. He also applied the law of mass action to the $CO_2/[HCO_3^-]$ system. In 1917, Hasselbach introduced the logarithmic version, interrelating blood pH, carbon dioxide tension, and bicarbonate ion concentration. The study of acid–base chemistry became intense in the 1920s and 1930s. Wallace O. Fenn (1893–1917) contributed primary research in understanding the

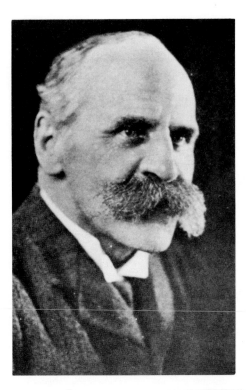

Figure 1–8. John Scott Haldane demonstrated that carbon dioxide provides the primary respiratory stimulus and developed oxygen administration devices. (Courtesy Wellcome Historical Medical Museum, London)

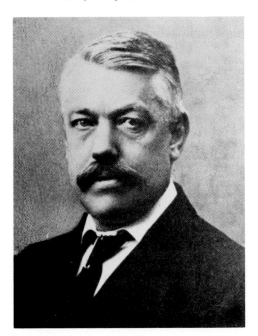

Figure 1–7. Christian Bohr established the oxyhemoglobin dissociation curve and oxygen and carbon dioxide's loading–unloading relationship. (Courtesy of Universitets Medicinsk-Historiske Museum, Copenhagen)

mechanics of breathing. He and Herman Rahn developed a diagram for displaying alveolar gas information. Werner Forssmann performed the first human cardiac catheterization on himself in 1928, offering a technique to study the cardiovascular system in vivo. Application of this technique resulted in Andre Cournand, Dickinson Richards, and Forssmann receiving the Nobel Prize for medicine–physiology in 1956. The Nobel Prize was also awarded to Linus Pauling for his discovery of sickle cell hemoglobin and other hemoglobinopathies.[1,4]

Clinical medicine entered the "antibiotic era," and corticosteroids were synthesized in the 1940–1950s. Cardiac surgery advanced into more involved procedures, with the use of cardiopulmonary bypass. Experience gained during the Korean and Vietnam wars added to the knowledge base in critical care and developed technology. Mouth-to-mouth resuscitation and external cardiac compression replaced older protocols. The emergency medical care system became organized and more sophisticated during the 1970s. The adult respira-

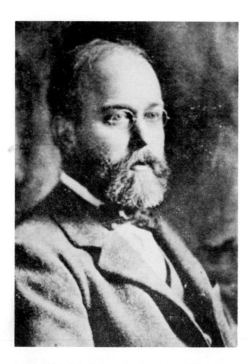

Figure 1—9. Lawrence J. Henderson described the inter-relationships among carbon dioxide, bicarbonate ion, and pH. (Courtesy of the New York Academy of Medicine, New York, NY)

tory distress syndrome (ARDS) was identified in 1967, and therapy was developed consisting of ventilation with positive end-expiratory pressure (PEEP).[5] In 1970, Swan and Ganz developed the flow-directed pulmonary artery catheter, providing a clinical intensive care unit (ICU) tool for hemodynamic monitoring.[6] Perinatal critical care advanced in the 1970s as the etiology of "idiopathic respiratory distress syndrome" (IRDS) was elucidated as a pulmonary surfactant deficiency. In 1971, Gregory described the therapeutic use of constant positive-airway pressure (CPAP) for neonates with IRDS.[7] Ventilators designed to match newborn physiology were soon made available.[8]

The 1980s have seen a growth in transplantation medicine with development of pharmacologic agents and radiation that suppress the immune system. Other major factors in medicine since the mid-1980s have been the acquired immunodeficiency syndrome (AIDS) "epidemic," and the escalating cost of health care. Legislation and public sentiment regarding ethical questions of withholding or withdrawing life support technology remain difficult issues.

CLINICAL USE OF OXYGEN THERAPY

In 1880, Thomas Beddoes established the Pneumatic Institute in Bristol, England. There he began the use of oxygen to treat heart disease, asthma, and opium poisoning. Beddoes is generally regarded as the "father" of inhalation therapy. However, he used supplemental oxygen as a panacea for medical problems. It was not until 1920 that a firm physiologic basis for oxygen therapy was established.[2,4,9]

It was the scientific studies of John Scott Haldane and Joseph Barcroft on oxygen deficiency in humans that defined the benefits of oxygen therapy. In a pioneering study conducted in 1920, Barcroft remained for 5 days in a chamber filled with 15% oxygen. In describing the symptoms associated with simulated high-altitude breathing he noted nausea, headache, visual disturbances, rapid pulse, and lassitude. Haldane subjected himself to even lower partial pressures of oxygen and became disoriented. He might have died had his assistants not removed him from the chamber.[1,4]

The development of oxygen administration devices (face mask, metal/rubber catheters, oxygen chambers) facilitated clinical studies that clarified the role of oxygen in the management of hypoxemia. As early as 1907, Sir Arbuthnot Lane advocated the administration of oxygen by a nasal catheter. Haldane perfected an oxygen mask in 1918, which was used to treat patients with combat gas–induced pulmonary edema. During 1920, Sir Leonard Hill developed an oxygen tent used to treat leg ulcers. Although this apparatus had no method for the removal of heat or moisture, it led others to further refine and expand upon this mode of therapy. In 1926, Alvan L. Barach developed an oxygen tent capable of carbon dioxide removal with soda lime, water vapor extraction using calcium chloride, and thermal control maintained by passing oxygen over a chunk ice refrigeration unit (Fig. 1—10).[9]

Large oxygen chambers were also developed by Barcroft in England and W. C. Stadie in the United States. Barach went on to design entire rooms in which patients could be treated with oxygen.

During this same period, J. S. Haldane developed a method to dilute gases with room air, used in the therapeutic administration of carbon dioxide. Barach expanded on this concept to develop a "meter mask" for diluting oxygen with room air. He also devised a positive-pressure breathing (CPPB or CPAP) mask capable of developing up to 4 cm H_2O on exhalation.[9,10]

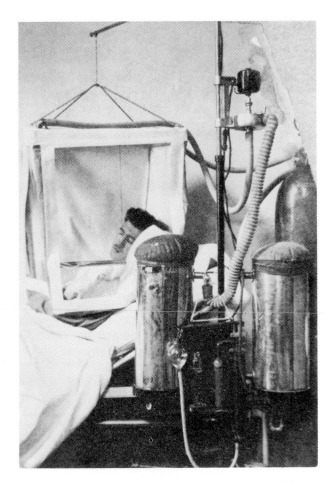

In 1938, William Boothby, W. Randolf Lovelace, and Arther Bulbulian devised the BLB mask at the Mayo Clinic. This mask allowed a high oxygen concentration (80–100%) with minimal rebreathing. It was developed to provide pilots oxygen while flying at high altitudes in World War II (Fig. 1–11).[4,11]

In the late 1940s, the somewhat indiscriminate use of oxygen in premature newborns resulted in a large number of cases of retrolental fibroplasia.[12] By the mid-1960s, the Clark and Severinghaus electrodes allowed clinical blood gas analysis. The ear oximeter was clinically available by 1974. During the late 1970s and early 1980s transcutaneous oxygen and pulse oximetric analysis became part of clinical measurement in the operating room and intensive care unit.[13] The mass spectrometer became a clinical and diagnostic tool.

In 1960, E. J. Moran Campbell developed the "Venti-mask" in response to the need for a high-flow, controlled F_{IO_2} appliance. This device had the ability to meet tachypneic patients' inspiratory flow demands while reducing the risk of carbon dioxide retention.[5] During the 1970s long-term oxygen therapy was shown to reduce mortality in patients requiring supplemental oxygen.[14] Conserving devices such as reservoirs, demand pulse units, and tracheal catheters were developed in the 1980s to attempt cost savings in long-term oxygen therapy.[14,15]

Figure 1–10. Oxygen tent, circa 1926, developed by Alvan Barach (shown in tent). (Barach AL: Inhalation therapy: historical background. Anesthesiology 23:407, 1962, with permission)

Figure 1–11. (A) Researchers wearing BLB oxygen masks developed for aviation application during World War II. (B) Aviator wearing BLB mask. (Courtesy H. F. Helmholz, Jr., MD)

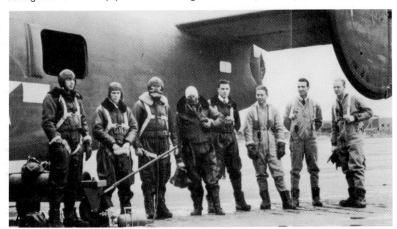

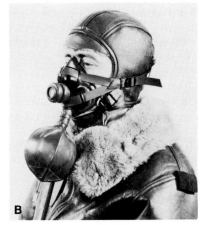

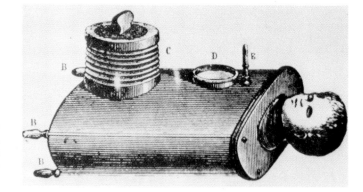

Figure 1—12. Woillez's "Spirophore" negative-pressure ventilator circa 1876. (Mushin WW, Rendell-Baker L, Thompson PW, Mapleson WW: Automatic Ventilation of the Lungs, 3rd ed. London, Blackwell Scientific, 1980, with permission)

CLINICAL USE OF MECHANICAL VENTILATION

A complete historical review of mechanical ventilators is beyond the scope of this introductory chapter. The reader is referred to Chapter 22 for a more detailed discussion and to other sources for a definitive presentation.[3,16] Mechanical-ventilating devices that were more involved than a "fireplace bellows" began appearing in the mid-1800s. Most early devices used a body-enclosing iron lung with a large bellows to create subatmospheric pressure, such as Woillez's 1876 "Spirophore" (Fig. 1—12). Other devices resembled steam cabinets or phone booths. The negative-pressure scheme was considered physiologic, and tracheal intubation was not attempted until the 1890s. Surgeons were eager to use their advancing techniques on the chest but were aware of the problems of pneumothorax. To deal with this perioperative problem, some considered positive-pressure ventilation. To accomplish this, an artificial airway was required. By 1900 flexible metallic tubes were available, and Meltzer introduced oral intubation in 1909.

However, in 1904, the German surgeon Sauerbruch developed a negative-pressure operating chamber (Fig. 1—13). This differential (positive–negative) pressure method caught on and continued to be popular in Europe. In contrast, most American surgeons and anesthetists turned to endotracheal intubation and direct introduction of air into the lungs. By 1913, Chevalier Jackson had developed the laryngoscope and intratracheal catheters in Pittsburgh. However, positive-pressure ventilation by mask continued until the mystique enshrouding intubation technique lessened. This occurred largely because of the work of Ivan Magill and coworkers during World War I.[16–18]

A number of positive-pressure devices were developed for surgery or resuscitation. The 1888 Fell-O'Dwyer apparatus combined a laryngeal tube and foot-operated bellows (Fig. 1—14). In 1907 Heinrich Drager developed his "Pulmotor" in Germany, and in 1910 American Henry Janeway constructed his anesthesia machine.

One of the first poliomyelitis epidemics was in New York, in 1916. By 1928, Philip Drinker,

Figure 1—13. Ernest Ferdinand Sauerbruch developed a differential-pressure chamber for surgical application, circa 1904. (Mörch ET: History of mechanical ventilation. In Kirby RR, Banner MJ, Downs JB (eds): Clinical Applications of Ventilatory Support. New York, Churchill Livingstone, 1990, with permission)

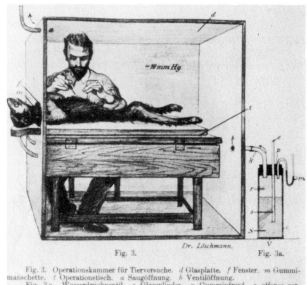

Fig. 3. Operationskammer für Tierversuche. d Glasplatte. f Fenster. m Gummimanschette. f Operationstisch. a Saugöffnung. b Ventilöffnung.
Fig. 3 a. Wasserdruckventil. c Glascylinder. p Gummipfropf. e offenes verschiebliches Glasrohr. k Glasrohr. m Manometer. r Ventilraum. s Wassersäule in c. s Wassersäule im Cylinder. V Ventil.

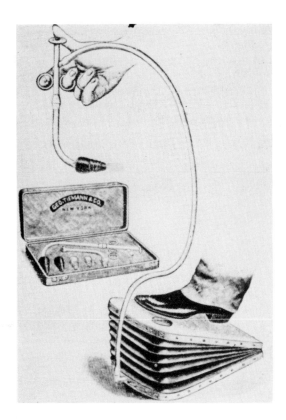

Figure 1—14. Fell-O'Dwyer bellows and endotracheal intubating device, circa 1899. (Mörch ET: History of mechanical ventilation. In Kirby RR, Banner MJ, Downs JB (eds): Clinical Applications of Ventilatory Support. New York, Churchill Livingstone, 1985, with permission)

Charles McKhann, and Louis Shaw developed the first iron lung at Harvard, and it was widely used. In 1932 J. H. Emerson developed his iron lung, which improved access to the patient and had a transparent dome to provide positive-pressure ventilation while the tank was opened (Fig. 1—15). The poliomyelitis epidemic surfaced in England about 1938, and there was an inadequate supply of iron lungs. Epidemics flared in Scandinavia, Europe, and America into the 1950s (see Preface). This "catastrophic" need for mechanical ventilation, as well as the increasing need for anesthesia ventilators, prompted a surge of international development. Manufacturers looked to the poliomyelitis centers to guide improved designs.[16–18]

During the catastrophic 1952 poliomyelitis epidemic in Copenhagen, Dr. Bjørn Ibsen effected a change from the iron lung to the use of tracheostomy and positive pressure ventilators. With limited numbers of machines, vast numbers of medical students (1400) provided manual ventilation. The Ambu-bag (adult manual breathing unit) was developed by Henning Ruben in 1954. The Scandinavians produced positive-pressure devices, such as the Aga Pulmospirator, Engstrom, and Mörch (Fig. 1—16). Mörch's prototype was constructed using a cylinder made from a sewer pipe in German-occupied Copenhagen. British anesthesiologists produced the Beaver, Blease Pulmoflator, and Barnet. In Germany, the Drager Company developed the Poliomat. This experience with long-term positive-pressure ventilation led to its application during thoracic and cardiac surgery, as well as postopera-

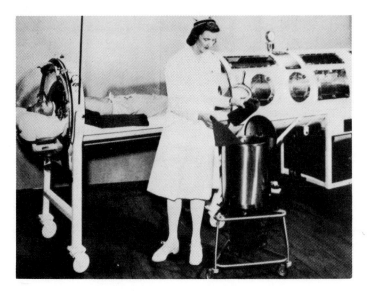

Figure 1—15. Emerson iron lung with head canopy for ventilation when the body chamber was opened. (Courtesy J. H. Emerson, Cambridge MA)

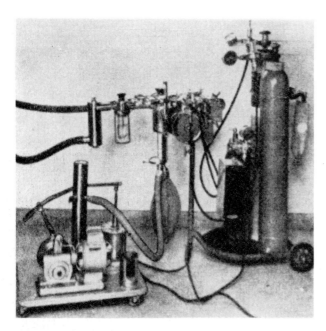

Figure 1—16. First piston ventilator designed by Ernst Trier Mörch in 1940. (Mörch ET: History of mechanical ventilation. In Kirby RR, Banner MJ, Downs JB (eds): Clinical Applications of Ventilatory Support. New York, Churchill Livingstone, 1990, with permission)

tively. Swedish surgeons Bjork and Engstrom led the way in addition to Britishers Macintosh and Mushin.[3,16,17]

Although Europeans largely abandoned the iron lung, poliomyelitis patients continued to be treated with tank respirators in the United States into the mid-1950s. The National Foundation for Infantile Paralysis was the major force in the effort to eradicate poliomyelitis. As the epidemic of this disease eased in the United States with the introduction of the Salk and, later, Sabin vaccines, the former poliomyelitis facilities expertise evolved into centers for development of intensive care. The United States then followed the Scandinavians and British in postoperative controlled ventilation. During this time, V. Ray Bennett introduced the TV-2P "assister" in 1948, and Forrest Bird developed his "clinical magnetic respirator" in 1951. By the mid-1950s E. Trier Mörch's piston ventilator was clinically available in the United States' Midwest. First-generation pressure-limited ventilators, such as the Bird Mark 7 and Bennett PR-1, were in large-scale production by 1958 and 1961, respectively. Jack Emerson took the lead with his volume/time-limited "Post-Op" or 3-PV ventilator in 1964. Over the next 10 years the second-generation volume ventilators followed with the Puritan-Bennett MA-1, Ohio 560, Bear I, and Siemens 900B. These

ventilators became ICU "workhorses" in the United States. Table 1–1 lists the chronologic development of modern critical care ventilators.

Breathing modes and methods of controlling ventilator function have also evolved. Early ventilators used pneumatic or basic mechanical switches. These were updated by fluidics, and the

Table 1—1 "Modern" Acute Care Mechanical Ventilators

YEAR	BRAND/MODEL
1948	Bennett TV-2P
1950	Engstrom 150
1954	Drager Poliomat
1954	Thompson Portable Respirator
1955	Morch "Piston"
1955	Bird Mark 7
1955	Emerson High-Frequency Ventilator
1958	Emerson Assistor/controller
1963	Air-Shields 1000
1963	Puritain-Bennett PR-2
1964	Emerson "Post-Op" 3-PV
1964	Bourns LS-104-150
1967	Puritain-Bennett MA-1
1968	Ohio/Monaghan 560
1968	Drager Spiromat
1968	Loos Co. Amsterdam
1968	Engstrom 300
1970	Veriflo CV 2000
1970	Hamilton Standard PAD 1
1972	Monaghan 225, 225-SIMV
1972	Bird-Baby Bird
1972	Bird-IMV Bird
1972	Siemens Servo 900/900B
1973	Chemtron Gill 1
1974	Emerson IMV
1974	Searle VVA
1974	Ohio 550
1975	Bourns Bear 1
1976	Forreger 210
1978	Puritan Bennett MA-II; 2 + 2
1980	Engstrom Erica
1982	Siemens Servo 900C
1983	Biomed IC-5
1984	Puritan-Bennett 7200
1984	Sechrist Adult
1985	Bear Medical Bear 5
1985	Ohmeda CPU
1986	Hamilton Veolar
1986	Bird 6400 ST
1986	Infrasonics Infant Star
1988	Bear 3
1988	Hamilton Amadeus
1988	Siemens E
1989	Bunnell Life Pulse
1989	PPG (Drager) IRISA

transistor with printed circuit boards in the 1970s. Currently, the microprocessor is today's technology for the third-generation ventilators. The variety of monitoring and breathing modes has expanded from control and assist/control, to intermittent mandatory ventilation (IMV), pressure support (PS), airway pressure-release ventilation (APRV), inverse ratio ventilation (IRV), and a variety of styles of high-frequency ventilation.[19–22]

The use of ventilators for long-term nonhospital (i.e., home) use has increased since Thompson introduced their portable wheelchair unit in 1954.[23] In recent years, there has been a proliferation of similar devices with DC battery capabilities. Although the negative-pressure ventilators such as the iron lung are rarely used today in the ICU, cuirass type chest devices are still used for long-term ventilation in certain patients to avoid tracheostomy.

CLINICAL USE OF INTERMITTENT POSITIVE-PRESSURE BREATHING

During the 1930s, research found intermittent positive-pressure breathing (IPPB) devices less effective than constant positive-pressure breathing (CPPB) in increasing the altitude tolerance of pilots.[13] Clinical use of IPPB was first described by Guedel in 1934 for treatment of apnea following deep ether anesthesia. Three years later Barach used IPPB to treat pulmonary edema and other pulmonary disease. By 1945, Motley and associates suggested that it be used for a variety of medical problems, including carbon monoxide poisoning, asthmatic attacks, and postoperative thoracic surgery.[18] A vast enterprise followed, providing IPPB therapy without scientific basis until the early 1970s.[24] Currently, this therapy is used for specific clinical situations, including atelectasis resistant to more conservative therapy, neuromuscular disease (e.g., kyphoscoliosis), and for administration of aerosolized drugs to patients incapable of deep breathing.[17,25–28]

ORGANIZATION AND INCORPORATION OF THE INHALATION THERAPY ASSOCIATION

With major advances being made in the clinical techniques used to administer oxygen and "inhalation therapy" to an increasing diversity of patients, during the 1940s a group of interested physicians and "oxygen technicians" in the Chicago area began to meet and discuss oxygen therapy, its rationale, and means to improve the care of patients.[29] The physicians Albert Andrews, Edwin Levine, and Max Sadov were the prime movers in recognizing the need for an organization the mission of which would be to promote the education of those involved in the administration of therapeutic gases to patients. Following an organizational meeting at the University of Chicago in 1946, the Inhalational Therapy Association (ITA) was chartered as a nonprofit organization in the State of Illinois on April 15, 1947. There were 59 members of this new association. The vision, enthusiasm, and commitment of this group cannot be underestimated. From this humble beginning has arisen an entire profession whose members, then and now, have a significant impact on clinical provision of respiratory care.[17]

The emphasis of the ITA was on member education. The fostering of cooperative dialogues with physicians and other allied health professions, and the advancement of the art and science of respiratory care, set the foundation for the philosophy that continues to drive this profession and its practitioners to this day.

In 1948, the name of the association was changed to the Inhalation Therapy Association. Beginning in 1950, the ITA began to publish a quarterly journal titled the *Bulletin*, which was sent without charge to 1500 hospitals in the United States. Throughout that same year the ITA sponsored a series of lectures and educational workshops. In December 1950, 31 certificates were awarded to those who had attended 16 of those workshops. This was clearly a monumental occasion, for it signaled the legitimacy of the ITA's commitment to education and those who shared its goals. In 1951, at only 4 years of professional age, the ITA and the American College of Chest Physicians (ACCP) cosponsored a 5-day workshop. This too was significant, for it indicated the importance the prestigious ACCP placed on those providing respiratory care and represented a true and cooperative relationship between the two groups. Two years after this workshop, the ACCP became an official sponsor of the ITA. The expansion of the membership, now representing 14 states, led to a third name change in 1954, when the ITA officially became the American Association of Inhalation Therapists (AAIT).

THE AMERICAN ASSOCIATION FOR RESPIRATORY CARE

Since the formation of the Inahalational Therapy Association, the profession has matured and undergone profound changes. The growth of any profession is dependent upon much more than circumstances or windows of opportunity. Respiratory care is indeed a profession of individuals with a collective intellect, curiosity, ambition, resourcefulness, and competence. It is these characteristics that have assured the growth of the profession, its practitioners, and the organization representing them.

After the formation of the AAIT, the development of more sophisticated equipment and procedures enhanced the importance of qualified practitioners. It was during this time that many were called, or called themselves, *inhalation therapists.* The need for greater professional identity and interaction further increased the membership of these therapists in the AAIT. In 1960, there were 21 state affiliates of the AAIT; this increased to 31 by 1966. In 1982 the organization again changed its name to the American Association for Respiratory Care (AARC). This name was felt to better reflect the scope of practitioner involvement in diagnostic pulmonary function testing as well as cardiovascular diagnostics.[30] Today there are 48 state affiliates of the AARC and two international affiliates.

CURRENT ORGANIZATIONAL STRUCTURE OF THE AARC

The AARC is a professional association whose members directly elicit its leadership. The leadership of the association is vested in a Board of Directors consisting of six officers (President, President-Elect, Past President, Vice-President, Secretary, and Treasurer) and nine directors. The Executive Committee of the AARC comprises the AARC's elected officers and is responsible for the day-to-day operations of the Executive Director and the Executive Office, which is located in Dallas, Texas. The Board of Directors are responsible for all actions of the Executive Committee and the overall operations of the association. These include the establishment and review of association goals, budgetary planning and control, committee appointments and monitoring, revising, upgrading, and approving membership benefits, and assuring association compliance with its bylaws and charter.

Of great importance to the operation of the AARC is its House of Delegates. The active membership in each of the 48 chartered affiliates elects one delegate and one alternate delegate to the House of Delegates. The House of Delegates is responsible for approving the annual budget of the AARC, changes in the AARC's bylaws, and the an-

nual slate of officers and directors. In other capacities, it is advisory to the Board of Directors and routinely forwards recommendations for action to the Board.

THE BOARD OF MEDICAL ADVISORS

The extraordinary growth of the AARC and the profession is in great measure the result of the relationship both have shared with physicians involved in respiratory care. The pivotal role that physicians played in the development of the ITA helped to set the stage for decades of collegial relationships between respiratory care practitioners and physicians. The mutual dependence of physicians and therapists has fostered a peer relationship and understanding. In recognition of the valued support of physician groups, the AARC has maintained since its inception a Board of Medical Advisors (BOMA). Initially the BOMA comprised six physicians appointed by the American College of Chest Physicians (ACCP) and the American Society of Anesthesiologists (ASA). By 1966, BOMA membership had increased to five medical specialty groups representing the ACCP, the ASA, the American Thoracic Society (ATS), the American Academy of Pediatrics (ACP), and the American Academy of Allergists (AAA). Today those groups, in addition to the Society for Critical Care Medicine (SCCM), continue to maintain their membership on the BOMA.

The BOMA meets twice a year and provides advice and council to the AARC's Board of Directors. In addition, AARC bylaws require BOMA approval of any position statement or other association-approved documents that impinge on or refer to any aspect of medical practice. In recognition of the importance of the BOMA and its sponsors, the Chairman of that body sits with voice at all meetings of the association's BOD. He or she also serves as a member of the AARC's Executive and Budget Committees.

AARC ACTIVITIES

From an original membership of 59 in 1947, the AARC now has a membership of over 27,000 practitioners. Each state, plus Puerto Rico, is represented in the AARC's House of Delegates. The AARC has over 400 international members. In addition, two international affiliates (Central America and Mexico) have joined the AARC since 1987.[30]

The AARC continues with its primary mission as a source of education, research, and responsiveness to practitioner needs. Three monthly publica-

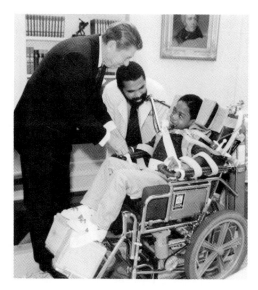

Figure 1–17. President Reagan acknowledges Respiratory Therapy Week with respiratory therapist Dean Sterling and paralyzed patient John Magbie. (AARC Times, 6:12, 1982, with permission)

tions, including the scientific journal *Respiratory Care*, continue the strong membership service philosophy that began with the ITA's original *Bulletin*. Eight specialty sections provide for information exchange in a fourth publication among those with particular interests in specific areas of practice.

The association sponsors a national convention in the fall of each year. The largest convention of its type in the nation, its attendance has risen from some 400 in 1963 to over 6500 in 1989. In addition, each year the AARC sponsors a second major meeting, its Summer Forum, as well as an annual Washington Symposium, which is directed at legislative and regulatory issues. The AARC has increased its political awareness and representation in national matters of health care. The association continues to monitor legislation that may affect its members, such as antismoking laws, licensure, and medical care reimbursement. There is national, state, chapter, and individual support for a number of charitable, philanthropic, and humanitarian activities (Fig. 1–17).

CREDENTIALING OF RESPIRATORY CARE PRACTITIONERS

As educational requirements and accreditation began to develop under the original Board of Schools for Inhalation Therapy (detailed in Chap. 2), it was also recognized that a system to credential individual practitioners was warranted. The growth in the number of technicians and therapists nationwide and the absence (at the time) of any state credentialing that assured practitioner competence led to the development of a voluntary national credentialing system. In 1960 the American Registry of Inhalation Therapists (ARIT) was incorporated in the State of Illinois. Among several purposes of this new organization were two of particular importance:

1. To encourage the establishment of high standards by which the competency of inhalation therapists . . . could be determined
2. To prepare, conduct, and control investigations and examinations to test the qualifications of voluntary candidates

In 1961, 12 examinees were the first to receive their registry credential. In the years that followed, the then ARRT continually improved its examination process and qualifications. Today there are more than 34,000 registered respiratory therapists.

The registration awarded by the ARIT was intended to recognize knowledge and competence beyond that expected of those just entering the profession. Although the credential was prized, large numbers of those not satisfying ARIT admission requirements continued to practice without the benefit of any credential. In recognition of the need to examine and certify those with entry-level skills, the AAIT established the Technician Certification Board (TCB) in 1969. The AAIT continued to administer the examination and awarded the Certified Inhalation Therapy Technician (CRIT) credential through 1974. Beginning in 1972, discussions between the American Association for Respiratory Therapy (ARRT) and the ARIT recognized the benefits of a single national credentialing organization for the respiratory care profession. In 1974 the ARIT was reorganized as the National Board for Respiratory Therapy (NBRT), now known as the National Board for Respiratory Care (NBRC).[3,31] Concurrent with this reorganization, the AART transferred the certification system to the NBRT. Currently, more than 50,000 practitioners hold the entry level CRTT credential. The NBRC remains the only nationally recognized credentialing body in respiratory care.

In recognition of the critical role respiratory

care practitioners play in the health care system, many states have instituted some form of state credentialing. In the early 1970s Louisiana became the first state to credential respiratory therapists. Since 1980 the number of states requiring some form (licensure or registration) of state credential has increased to 26. The activity occurring in the remaining states suggests that this number should greatly increase within the next few years.

THE RESPIRATORY CARE PRACTITIONER

Unfortunately, statistical data on the growth of the profession over the past 40 years are lacking. However, we do know the human resource characteristics of the profession today. In 1986, 5368 acute care hospitals reported an organized respiratory care service. Respiratory care practitioners of today are a breed apart from their counterparts of even a decade ago. In the past, much of the growth of the profession was the result of the need for practitioners in acute care hospitals. This growth was stimulated by significant advances in the technology and medical management of patients with cardiopulmonary disorders. Hospital departments have broadend their scope of clinical activities. The list might include noninvasive and invasive cardiopulmonary diagnostics, sleep disorders monitoring, hyperbaric oxygen therapy, bedside hemodynamic monitoring, air transport of critical or ventilator-dependent patients, and patient education, including smoking cessation.[32]

The increasing technology, sophistication in documentation and quality assurance, and increased acuity of pulmonary patients combined to stimulate the demand for more and better-qualified technicians and therapists. Among the members of the health care team, the respiratory care practitioners' knowledge base and skills appear to have prepared them to assume more diverse and complex responsibilities. As has been the character of the profession, this expansion of roles has been viewed as a challenge and opportunity rather than an additional burden.

Multicompetency within cardiopulmonary care is becoming more common in medium-sized and smaller community hospitals. There is also a growing number of respiratory therapy practitioners who are also competent and credentialed as nurses, radiographers, perfusionists, polysomnographers, and nurse anesthetists.

Acute care hospitals remain the principal sites of respiratory care employment. According to the Human Resources Survey conducted by the AARC in 1987, nearly 70,000 respiratory care practitioners are employed in the nation's acute care hospitals. Although this represents a decrease in hospital-employed respiratory care practitioners when compared with projections in a similar survey completed in 1982, the proportions of registered therapists and certified technicians increased from 38.7% in 1982 to 65.3% in 1987. In addition, the percentage of practitioners with 2 or more years of college education increased by 28.6% over the same period.[32]

The past decade has witnessed substantial changes in the types of health care facilities providing respiratory care. Changes in health care reimbursement policies, the aging of the American population, and advances in health promotion and medical technology, all have influenced a dramatic shift to the provision of health care in sites other than the acute care hospital. These "alternative" sites, such as skilled nursing facilities, patients' homes, and hospices, have introduced a whole new dimension to the role of the respiratory care practitioner.

The diversity of skills—clinical, theoretical, and interpersonal—now required of respiratory care practitioners clearly equips them with a potential not imagined in 1947. Few, if any, allied health professions have witnessed professional growth equaling that of respiratory care. Continued AARC-sponsored study of changing patterns in health care delivery should provide guidance for the growth and maturation of the profession.

The contributions each practitioner makes each day, the curiosity characteristic of the profession, the acceptance of challenges, and the creation of opportunities so typical of this profession assure a dynamic and rewarding career. Yet a growth-oriented profession is constituted of individuals who collectively define its character. Although the work is technical and science oriented, it is distinguished as a profession by its human service, ethical standards, and each practitioner's obligation to provide the best patient care possible. This purpose of this chapter has been to review this outstanding and unique heritage.[33,34]

REFERENCES

1. Perkins JF: Historical development of respiratory physiology. In Fenn WO, Rahn H (eds): Handbook of Physiology: Respiration (section 3). Washington, DC, American Physiological Society, 1964

2. Helmholz HF: Early foundations. In Smith GA (ed): Respiratory Care: Evolution of a Profession. Lexena, Kan, Applied Measurement Professionals, 1989, p 15

3. Mörch ET: History of mechanical ventilation. In Kirby RR, Banner MJ, Downs JB (eds): Clinical Applications of Ventilatory Support. New York, Churchill Livingstone, 1990

4. Helmholz HF: Professional champions (1900–1940). In Smith GA (ed): Respiratory Care: Evolution of a Profession. Lexena, Kan, Applied Measurement Professionals, 1989, p 22

5. Ashbaugh DG, Bigelow DB, Petty TL: Acute respiratory distress in adults. Lancet 1:319, 1967

6. Swan HJ, Ganz W, Forrester JS et al: Catheterization of the heart in man with the use of a flow directed balloon-tipped catheter. N Engl J Med 283:447, 1970

7. Gregory GA, Kitterman JA, Phibbs RH et al: Treatment of the idiopathic respiratory distress syndrome with continuous positive airway pressure. N Engl J Med 284:1333, 1971

8. Kirby RR, Robinson EJ, Schultz et al: A new pediatric volume ventilator. Anesth Analg 50:533, 1971

9. Barach AL: Inhalation therapy: historical background. Anesthesiology 23:407, 1962

10. Barach AL: Perspectives in pressure breathing. Respir Care 18:677, 1973

11. Boothby WM: Effects of high altitude on the composition of alveolar air: introductory remarks. Proc Staff Meet Mayo Clin 20:209, 1945

12. Silverman WA: The lesson of retrolental fibroplasia. Sci Am 236(6):100, 1977

13. Harris K: Noninvasive monitoring of gas exchange. Respir Care 32:544, 1987

14. Nocturnal Oxygen Therapy Trial Group: Continuous or nocturnal oxygen therapy in hypoxemic chronic obstructive lung disease: a clinical trial. Ann Intern Med 93:391, 1980

15. O'Donohue WJ: Oxygen conserving devices. Respir Care 32:37, 1987

16. Mushin WW, Rendell-Baker L, Thompson PW, Mapleson WW: Automatic Ventilation of the Lungs, 3rd ed. London, Blackwell Scientific, 1980

17. Helmholz HF: Oxygen/inhalation therapy in the 50's: clinical developments. In Smith GA (ed): Respiratory Care: Evolution of a Profession. Lexena, Kan, Applied Measurement Professionals, 1989, p 41

18. Motley HL: Observations on the use of positive pressure. J Aviat Med 18:417, 1947

19. Downs JB, Klein EF, Desautels D: Intermittent mandatory ventilation: a new approach to weaning patients from mechanical ventilation. Chest 64:331, 1973

20. Froese AB, Bryan AC: High frequency ventilation: state of the art. Am Rev Respir Dis 135:1363, 1987

21. MacIntrye NR: Respiratory function during pressure support ventilation. Chest 89:677, 1986

22. Stock MC, Downs JB, Frolicher DA: Airway pressure release ventilation. Crit Care Med 15:462, 1987

23. Prentice WS: Placement alternatives for long-term ventilator care. Respir Care 31:288, 1986

24. Murray JF: Review of the state of the art in intermittent positive pressure breathing therapy. Am Rev Respir Dis 110:193, 1974

25. Intermittent Positive Pressure Breathing Trial Group: Intermittent positive pressure breathing therapy of chronic obstructive pulmonary diseases: a clinical trial. Ann Intern Med 99:612, 1983

26. O'Donohue WJ: IPPB past and present. Respir Care 27:588, 1982

27. Ziment I: Intermittent positive pressure breathing. In Burton GG, Hodgkin JE (eds): Respiratory Care: A Guide to Clinical Practice, 2nd ed. Philadelphia, JB Lippincott, 1984, p 529

28. Respiratory Care Committee of the American Thoracic Society: Intermittent positive pressure breathing (IPPB). Clin Notes Respir Dis 18:3, 1979

29. Hinshaw HC: Clinical applications of oxygen therapy. Arch Phys Ther 23:598, 1942

30. Smith GA: The 1980's—banner years and trying times. In Smith GA (ed): Respiratory Care: Evolution of a Profession. Lexena, Kan, Applied Measurement Professionals, 1989, p 147

31. Tomashefski JF: The National Board for Respiratory Therapy. Bull Am Coll Chest Phys 14:9, 1975

32. Bunch D: Task force update. AARC Times 11:17, 1987

33. Allen JS: Ethics and professional adjustment. Respir Care 18:376, 1973

34. Pierson DJ: Respiratory care as a science. Respir Care 33:27, 1988

TWO

Education of Respiratory Care Personnel

Philip A. von der Heydt
Gilbert D. Grossman

The education of respiratory care personnel, like that of any professional, extends over the entire career of the learner. It begins with the entering student, whether a recent high school graduate or an adult learner returning to school seeking a more rewarding career. Education continues with training the therapist as a sophisticated practitioner who exercises clinical judgment and deals with critically ill patients. In this era of challenge to provide high-quality yet economical health care, the educational system increasingly is expected to produce a multicompetent graduate, one whose professional expertise extends beyond the traditional boundaries of respiratory care. Finally, the system for respiratory care education must provide for the postgraduate education of those practitioners who wish to specialize, teach, or simply keep abreast of current trends in this rapidly evolving profession.

Because the respiratory care practitioner is increasingly called upon to assist in the management of life-threatening disease and will increasingly serve as a bedside biomedical technology provider, the quality of respiratory care education and, thereby, practice has an important impact on community health. Thus it is incumbent on the educational system to provide respiratory care students, at all levels, the tools to deal with health care learning into the next century and to assure that the system is constantly adaptive to community needs.

In this chapter we will focus individually on the major issues leading to respiratory care educa-

tion, including history, philosophy, quality assurance, and future perspectives. Recognizing the interrelationship of these topics will help clarify some matters while further explaining the complexity of the educational aspects of respiratory care as a health profession.

BACKGROUND

The development of formal education in the profession of respiratory care has followed the same pattern as many other professions. Individuals working in hospitals began to specialize in an area of need, in this case inhalation therapy. Soon a cluster of individuals became a department, and this department developed its own internal or in-service educational system. Formal programs of education were commonly developed through the leadership of departmental medical directors. These physicians supplied credibility to the educational program and the professional importance needed to gain institutional support for additional formal programs. What is unique about the profession of respiratory care and its formal education system is that it grew in direct parallel with the community college system throughout the United States.

It was, in fact, the community college that provided a formal educational structure for inhalation therapy, as it was known in the early years. Program curricula were integrated into the 2-year model, consistent with the terminal educational goal of the emerging college. The academic home that these institutions gave to inhalation therapy across the country legitimatized the profession more quickly than if the profession had emerged in a different period in the history of higher education in the United States.

The relationship between respiratory care education and the community college may also prove to be an obstruction to the continued academic growth of the profession. Although the curriculum content necessary for full technical education fits well into the associate degree pattern of the early 1970s, the fund of medical knowledge within the scope of the profession has expanded exponentially over the last 2 decades. Thus, programs encounter substantial difficulty incorporating into an associate degree curriculum enough technical knowledge for entry skill at the therapist level. Conflict begins to emerge between the sponsoring institution's mission and the needs of the profession for level knowledge and technical skill.

The goal of the educational process in respiratory care, as indeed in all health professions, is to take an amorphous pool of human raw material and, in a brief time, transform it into learned, competent, concerned, dedicated health professionals. The highest praise that can be bestowed on the present system is that it succeeds in accomplishing this goal in a remarkable number of instances.

Medical and nursing education, once formally established, developed very slowly and were hampered by tradition and by the massive conversion of organized medicine. In fact, medical education was a morass until its weaknesses were demonstrated by Abraham Flexner in the first years of the 20th century. Following the appearance and acceptance of the Flexner Report, medical education assumed the shape that we see today. The apprentice system was abandoned except as part of a structured curriculum, science education became an integral part of medical education, and medical educators became academicians, both in the basic and clinical sciences. This era was also characterized by an explosive growth in research and an exponential increase in medical information.

Nursing education lagged somewhat behind medical education, remaining a largely hospital-based apprenticeship training function until the 1950s to 1960s, when the proliferation of 4-year baccalaureate programs and the gradual development of graduate programs changed this major branch of health education into a modern educational system.

It is both interesting and pertinent that the general acceptance of formal undergraduate education for nurses was rapidly followed by the development of a lower-level, formal educational system based in community colleges and culminating in an Associate in Arts degree. Thus, currently, nursing training still takes place at three levels, although hospital-based 3-year programs have become fewer.

The educational systems in the other health professions followed similar patterns, practically without exception. Recognition of a need for specialized knowledge and skills was followed by the emergence of small numbers of interested people who may or may not have had hospital experience in another field. If the validity of the "new" profession could be demonstrated, training programs emerged. A purely apprenticeship-level training was followed rapidly by the establishment of more formal systems, first based in hospitals and, later, in educational institutions. The accreditation of the programs and the credentialing of the graduates followed as a matter of course. The next step in almost all the allied health professions was a fragmentation of the educational system and the establishment of two or more levels of training and formal recognition. The results of these developments are too recent to be fully tested, although this has not prevented a continued drive for more and more formal education and subjective criticism of the existing system.

RESPIRATORY CARE EDUCATION

The foregoing developmental patterns outlined apply, with very minor modifications, to the history of respiratory care education.

The need for specially trained personnel to manage patients with respiratory problems was recognized in the years immediately after World War II. The formation of the Inhalation Therapy Association in 1947 was followed, very shortly, by the first formal educational program. In 1950, a 16-week course was presented in Chicago, and a total of 31 participants received a Certificate of Completion.

That same year two publications, originating in New York City, dealt with the standards required for the safe and effective administration of inhalation therapy. These two publications, by Barach and his associates and by the Committee on Public Health Relations of the New York Academy of Medicine, established the basis for most of the early educational activities in this field.[1,2]

In rapidly developing health fields, the supply of trained personnel often lagged behind the number of positions available in the major metropolitan and academic health centers. The only form of training was apprenticeship or on-the-job training (OJT). In effect, the technologists who entered the field, usually from the ranks of orderlies and aides or, rarely, from the ranks of nursing, were instructed by physicians interested in respiratory problems. This, of course, meant that the instruction was highly individualized and reflected the likes or dislikes, knowledge or ignorance, idiosyncrasies or prejudices of the individual mentors.

After several years of this method, a movement to standardize the educational process led to the formation of an advisory committee to the Council of Medical Education (CME) of the American Medical Association (AMA) in 1956. This advisory committee represented the three organizations most concerned with respiratory care education: the American Society of Inhalation Therapy, the American College of Chest Physicians, and the American Society of Anesthesiologists.

The next year the New York delegation to the House of Delegates of the AMA introduced, at the annual meeting, a resolution to develop schools of inhalation therapy. This resolution was referred for action to the CME, which in turn issued a document entitled *Essentials for an Approved School of Inhalation Therapy Technicians*. After a trial period of 3 years the CME formally endorsed these "Essentials" and submitted them to the House of Delegates of the AMA for formal approval. This was granted by the House in December 1962; the early development of respiratory care education had reached its initial plateau.

To assure implementation of and compliance with the Essentials, a group of "experts" was needed who would be willing to assume the responsibility for this task. Therefore, in January 1963, on invitation by the CME and under its auspices, the first Board of Schools of Inhalation Therapy was established. Its membership comprised four physicians (two representing the ASA and two representing the ACCP) and three therapists (representing the AAIT). The board was formally charged with the responsibility of reviewing applications, performing on-site evaluations, and making recommendations to the CME on the formal accreditation of programs in respiratory care.

The Essentials were revised in 1966, and the revision was approved by the House of Delegates of the AMA in June 1967. These Essentials were an improvement over the first set and required a training period of 18 months. The board officially still opposed academic orientation in respiratory care education and was unwilling to recommend accreditation for programs sponsored by post-secondary education institutions. This policy, reflecting the personal bias of the chairman, was not shared by most members. Therefore, in 1969, it was decided to disband the Board of Schools to establish immediately the Joint Review Committee for Inhalation Therapy Education under the chairmanship of H. F. Helmholz, Jr., M.D. and to give parity to the therapist members. Accordingly, and with AMA approval, the Joint Review Committee was incorporated under the laws of the state of Minnesota on January 15, 1970.

The new Joint Review Committee immediately undertook the revision of the Essentials, which were finally approved by the AMA in June 1972. The new Essentials made significant contributions to respiratory care education: They recommended academic sponsorship for the therapist-level programs, and for the first time recognized a second level of education in respiratory care. This was the result of the establishment of the Technician Certification Board by the AAIT and the formal recognition by the professional organization that the field of respiratory care required health professionals functioning at two levels—therapist and technician.

Also in 1972, the Joint Review Committee expanded by admitting the American Thoracic Society (ATS) as a sponsor. To maintain parity, the number of therapist members was increased to six. In 1974, in conformity with proper usage, the name of the committee was changed to the Joint Review Committee for Respiratory Therapy Education (JRCRTE). At the same time a public representative was added to the membership of the committee.

Because the field of respiratory care was changing rapidly, it was necessary to revise the Essentials again starting in 1975. These new Essentials mandated that therapist level programs be sponsored by the educational institutions and that technician programs, which for the first time had separate Essentials, be at least "affiliated" with educational institutions. These Essentials also made significant advances in recognizing the need for "advanced standing" for proper experience and training for the key personnel of the programs, for an expanded curriculum, and for relevant laboratory experience before clinical contact for the students.

In 1982, yet another revision of the Essentials was begun. Building on a set of standards, which by their design had excluded information concerning graduate success and focused on internal resources, the Joint Review Committee found its first attempts to revise the Essentials frustrating. Under the leadership of Craig L. Scanlan, the first therapist chairman of the committee, a new philosophical approach to program accreditation began. Drawing from academic literature and trends in public awareness of educational costs and institutional accountability, the Joint Review Committee developed a model of accreditation using programmatic plans for graduates as a basis for accreditation. After a long developmental period, final approval by all appropriate entities occurred in the fall of 1986, thus giving rise to the new "product-oriented Essentials." These standards have subsequently served as a model for other accreditation systems and for the first time combined Essentials for both technician and therapist programs.

The last few years have seen several changes in the formal structure of respiratory care education and its evaluation. Dr. Helmholz resigned as chairman of the Joint Review Committee in 1976. He had been instrumental in leading the Joint Review Committee into the era of modern health education—that is, from largely apprenticeship training in hospitals to the educational activities performed by educational institutions. Respiratory care education owes more to Dr. Helmholz than to any other person. The change in chairmanship brought a number of other changes, the most important of which were the establishment of an Executive Office, the selection of an Executive Director, the limitation of terms of office for officers, the establishment of an Executive Committee and a number of other subcommittees, and the establishment of a new process for handling applications.

The AMA has transferred final authority for their approval of Essentials from the House of Delegates to the CME. The CME, in turn, has established the Committee on Allied Health Education and Accreditation (CAHEA), which, in conjunction with the Joint Review Committee, has been recognized by the US Department of Education and by the Council on Postsecondary Accreditation as the official accrediting agency.

The responsibilities of CAHEA are derived from its original charge from the AMA Board of Trustees:

1. To evaluate and accredit allied health educational programs for which Essentials have been adopted by the collaborating organizations and by the AMA Council on Medical Education

2. To periodically review existing allied health educational Essentials and accreditation procedures

3. To maintain active liaison with the collaborating medical specialty and allied health associations in a consortium for the accreditation of allied health education programs and, in relation to allied health education, to maintain active liaison with the American Society of Allied Health Professions, the Association of Academic Health Centers, the National Health Council, and federal agencies such as the Department of Education, the Veterans Administration, and the Army, Navy, and Air Force

4. To establish and maintain liaison with technical and professional groups allied to medicine, but for which no Essentials have been adopted in collaboration with the AMA

5. To maintain liaison with institutions sponsoring accredited allied health education programs, such as community and junior colleges, 4-year colleges, universities, schools of allied health professions, hospitals and clinics, proprietary schools, and vocational and technical institutes

6. When new allied health occupations have been recognized by the AMA, to work with the most directly concerned medical specialty, allied health, and other national professional organizations to draft minimum standards as Essentials for an accredited allied health educational program and to establish collaborative relationships for the concerned organizations to accredit educational programs

As determined by the AMA Board of Trustees, the 14 members of CAHEA include persons with broad interest or competence in the allied health professions and services, including the following: members of the allied health professions, hospital administrators, practicing physicians, higher education administrators and educators, allied health students or recent graduates, and members of the public.

These 14 members work together with a Panel of Consultants and Special Advisors, the Assembly of Review Committee Chairpersons, and the Assembly of Institutional Administrators to formulate, review, and revise the basic policies and procedures for accreditation. The CAHEA works independently of these groups and the AMA in considering accreditation recommendations. An overview of the basic CAHEA accreditation process is shown in Figure 2–1.

The CAHEA, in cooperation with the review committees, is recognized nationally as an "umbrella" accrediting body by the US Department of Education and the Council on Postsecondary Accreditation for allied health educational programs in medical schools, junior and community colleges, senior colleges and universities, vocational and technical schools and institutions, consortia, proprietary schools, military training institutions, and hospitals, clinics, and other health care institutions.

The list of nationally recognized accrediting agencies published by the US Department of Education (ED) includes CAHEA, in cooperation with the review committees sponsored by the collaborating organizations. This continues the tradition established in 1952 when the AMA was one of 28 accrediting agencies on the initial list published by the commissioner. In cooperation with the review committees CAHEA is currently recognized by ED to accredit educational programs in 23 allied health occupational areas, as listed in Table 2–1.

The Council on Postsecondary Accreditation (COPA) recognizes CAHEA, in cooperation with the 19 review committees, as an accrediting agency for allied health education. In 1977, COPA granted CAHEA recognition for 23 occupational areas, in participation with 15 review committees sponsored by 27 collaborating organizations. This recognition for the appropriate occupational areas is renewed periodically.

The Council on Postsecondary Accreditation, formed from two predecessors' organizations—the

Table 2–1 Occupations for which CAHEA, in Cooperation with Review Committees, Is Recognized by the US Department of Education To Accredit Educational Programs

Cytotechnologist
Diagnostic Medical Sonographer
Electroencephalographic Technologist
Emergency Medical Technician–Paramedic
Histologic Technician/Technologist
Medical Assistant
Medical Laboratory Technician (Associate Degree)
Medical Laboratory Technician (Certificate)
Medical Record Administrator
Medical Record Technician
Medical Technologist
Nuclear Medicine Technologist
Occupational Therapist
Ophthalmic Medical Assistant
Perfusionist
Physician Assistant
Radiation Therapy Technologist
Radiographer
Respiratory Therapist
Respiratory Therapy Technician
Specialist in Blood Bank Technology
Surgeon's Assistant
Surgical Technologist

National Commission on Accreditation (NCA) and the Federation of Regional Accrediting Commissions of Higher Education (FRACHE)—began operations on January 1, 1975, As a national, non-governmental, nonprofit educational organization, COPA coordinates voluntary accrediting activities for institutions and programs at the postsecondary level. Thus, COPA stands as a "balance wheel" in relation to approximately 4100 institutions of higher education accredited through 50 national accrediting bodies that have met established standards for COPA recognition.[3]

CURRENT STATUS OF RESPIRATORY CARE EDUCATION

Respiratory therapy education currently represents the third largest allied health occupational category accredited under CAHEA (radiography and medical laboratory sciences being first and second in size, respectively). Some 430 accredited programs

Figure 2–1. Overview of the basic CAHEA accreditation process.

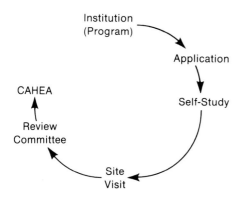

in 48 states enroll in excess of 10,000 students, graduating close to 5000 new respiratory therapy practitioners each year. About half of these graduates complete their education in respiratory technician programs and approximately one-third of these students graduate from so-called nontraditional programs. Since the adoption of Essentials for accredited educational programs for respiratory therapy technicians (1972), technician education has undergone remarkable growth and change. In the short period between 1974 and 1988, the number of accredited technician programs has increased more than 30-fold (Table 2–2). Although most of the early technician programs were hospital sponsored, most of those currently active now operate under the auspices of postsecondary educational institutions (junior colleges, community colleges, or vocational–technical schools). This trend in sponsorship changeover from hospital to college was due to the general change in health education and was catalyzed by the 1977 revision of the JRCRTE Essentials. These ensured that all students enrolled in technician programs are exposed to an academic milieu and receive at least some college credit for their educational experience. Approximately 15% of the current technician programs exceed 12 months in length; a small number of programs have curricula of 18 months or more. A few, however, provide an associate's degree or its equivalent. Most graduates receive a certificate of completion and are eligible to take the certification examination offered by the National Board of Respiratory Care (NBRC), provided all other criteria for eligibility are met. Successful completion of the entry-level examination results in credentialing as a Certified Respiratory Therapy Technician (CRTT).

The other respiratory therapy graduates complete their preparation for entry into the field through one of the approximately 250 accredited respiratory therapist educational programs. Technician and therapist programs must be sponsored by a properly accredited postsecondary vocational–technical school, college, university, or consortium. In this setting, students are granted full credit for both the academic and clinical components of their course work, receiving, upon completion of their education, both a certificate and a degree. The majority of therapist programs offer an associate's degree, although several provide for a baccalaureate degree. Graduate therapists are eligible for a two-level examination system offered by the NBRC. Upon successful completion of the advanced practitioner levels of the NBRC examination system, individuals are credentialed as Registered Respiratory Therapists (RRT).

PROGRAM RESOURCES

After having established a program mission that is focused on a particular level of knowledge and skill for each graduate, the educational program has the flexibility to dedicate appropriate resources for faculty, equipment, laboratory, and clinical experience, and curriculum length and structure consistent with the students' needs. Each program resource component has an identified purpose and, on an ongoing basis, is measured for its contribution to the overall success of the students as well as that of its individual purpose. As programs develop sophisticated evaluation systems to assure that resources are functioning appropriately, the need to adjust those resources will become apparent. This will make resource assignment by academic administration more defensible and will provide program personnel with an opportunity to defend expenditures because they will affect the overall success of the program; both in the number of students who can succeed in the program and in the ultimate attainment of the projected learning goals. It is predicted that most programs will identify the fact that expanding resources are necessary to increase program productivity as well as to increase the per-

Table 2–2 CAHEA Accredited Respiratory Therapy Programs

YEAR	TECHNICIAN	THERAPIST
1964	0	
1966	0	21
1968	0	44
1970	0	56
1972	0	125
1974	5	126
1976	55	147
1978	155	165
1980	193	192
1982	189	178
1984	194	234
1986	179	257
1988	163	263

centage of successful graduates who can demonstrate competency in all areas planned for their educational proficiency. With the expanding role and responsibility of respiratory care practitioners, additional technical knowledge is necessary for each graduate to attain the current state of the art for technical practice. Although time may not be the only determining factor in expanding resources, it certainly may be predicted as one that has the most significant influence on educational programs.

Under the flexible criteria presented in the 1986 Essentials, resources can be expanded or contracted in response to certain students' academic learning needs and personal schedules to appropriately assist this specific group of potential students to be served by an educational program. Because the program is held accountable for the success of its educational design and resource commitment, the flexibility that may have been construed as leniency at the inception stages of the Essentials has ultimately proved to be a strengthening of standards for program accountability and resource requirements. As time goes on, programs will become more and more individualized as they recognize the abilities of the student populations whom they serve and as they are driven by the communities of interest served by their programs.

QUALITY ASSURANCE

Quality assurance derives from a combination of regulatory mechanisms and procedures designed to hold the health professions accountable for the activities and practices of their members. Demands for accountability are based on the fundamental tenet that the public has the right to competently delivered health care and to practitioners proficient in the services they render.[8]

As in most other health professions, competency assurance in respiratory care is a joint venture. The educational and credentialing systems, and the individual practitioners who constitute the work force, must share the responsibility for demonstrating accountability for the public interest, safety, and welfare. Mechanisms that currently regulate the quality of practice in respiratory care include accreditation, certification, and legal recognition. Complementing these mechanisms, and designed to assure the continued competency of practitioners, is continuing the process of education.

ACCREDITATION

Accreditation is the process by which a private, nongovernmental agency or association grants public recognition to an institution or specialized program of study that meets certain established qualifications and educational standards. The primary purpose of the accreditation process in allied health care is to provide a professional judgment about the quality of the educational process and to encourage its continued improvement, thereby protecting the public against the professional or occupational incompetence of its graduates.

Institutional accreditation applies to a total institution and means that the organization, as a whole, is satisfactorily achieving its goals and objectives. *Programmatic accreditation* applies to specialized programs of study and means that the instructional resources and the learning experiences provided comply with the standards or criteria of accreditation.[3] Respiratory care educational accreditation is, appropriately, conducted at the program level, with institutional accreditation of program sponsors subsumed within the standards of accreditation.

Respiratory care programs are accredited by the Committee on Allied Health Education and Accreditation (CAHEA) in collaboration with the Joint Review Committee for Respiratory Therapy Education (JRCRTE). CAHEA is a quasi-independent, broadly representative agency responsible for accreditation of some 26 allied health occupations. It assumed the accreditation responsibilities, formerly held by the Council on Medical Education CME of the American Medical Association in January 1977 and has subsequently gained recognition as an umbrella accrediting agency for allied health educational programs by the US Department of Education (Office of Education) and the Council on Postsecondary Accreditation (COPA). CAHEA currently collaborates with about 46 organizations which, in turn, sponsor the discipline-specific accreditation review committees. Collaborating organizations also develop and adopt standards of accreditation or Essentials for their respective review committees. The AMA maintains its role as a collaborating organization in the accrediting of allied health educational programs through its CME. The CME is responsible for formal recognition of other collaborating organizations that sponsor review committees and adoption of Essentials, new or revised.

The JRCRTE is the agency responsible for the

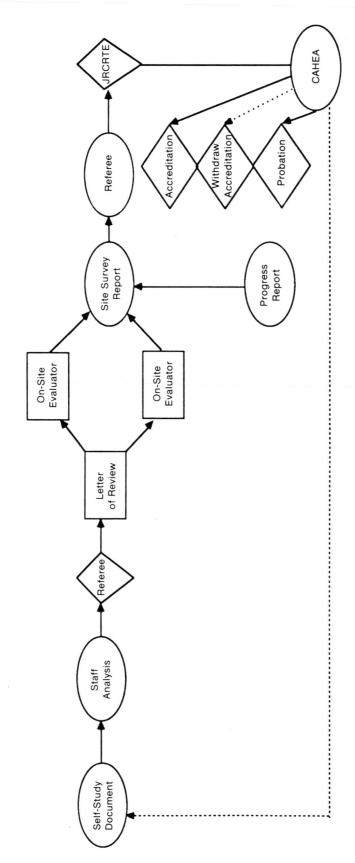

Figure 2–2. Joint Review Committee for Respiratory Therapy Education: Programmatic evaluation flowsheet.

logistics of the accreditation process and for the formulation of accreditation recommendations for all educational programs in respiratory care. It is sponsored by the American Association for Respiratory Care (AARC), the American College of Chest Physicians (ACCP), the American Society of Anesthesiologists (ASA), and the American Thoracic Society (ATS). The AARC appoints six representatives to the JRCRTE, and each physician sponsor organization appoints two representatives. One non–health-professional member represents the general public. The program review, evaluation, and accreditation processes are administered by an Executive Office staff consisting of an Executive Director, an Executive Secretary, and support personnel.

The accreditation process for respiratory care technician/therapist programs is identical. The process whereby a new program gains accreditation status is depicted in Figure 2–2. The reaccreditation process differs only in that established programs undergoing periodic reevaluation do not receive a letter of review.

As summarized in Figure 2–2, programs seeking accreditation voluntarily submit a self-study document to the JRCRTE. This document represents a detailed analysis of a program's goals and standards, instructional resources, and evaluation systems as they relate to the applicable Essentials. Normally, program faculty, administrative personnel, and students provide input to the analysis and assist in the identification of programmatic strengths and weaknesses.

Self-study documents, once submitted, are reviewed for completeness and clarity by the Executive Office staff. If staff analysis of the document indicates that all pertinent information has been included, the self-study is forwarded to a committee member serving as a referee. The referee is the program's ombudsman, communicating with the program's officials to clarify or correct potential deficiencies and working with the JRCRTE Executive Office and the committee as a whole to facilitate the program's progress through the accreditation process.

Once the referee is satisfied that the documentation provided by the program indicates substantial compliance with the Essentials, a Letter of Review is issued to the program by the Executive Office. The Letter of Review indicates that analysis of the written program documentation provides preliminary evidence of compliance with the Essentials. Upon issuance of a Letter of Review, the JRCRTE also communicates with the National Board for Respiratory Care, recommending that future program graduates be considered eligible for their respective credentialing examinations.

Following issuance of the Letter of Review, an on-site evaluation of the program is scheduled and a site-visit team selected. The site-visit team comprises two members: a physician qualified to be medical director of the program being evaluated, and a therapist with the experience and education necessary to fulfill the role of program director. The on-site evaluators confer with responsible members of the sponsoring institution's administration, the program faculty, staff, and students. Both the instructional resources of the program and the clinical resources of its affiliates are inspected, and all necessary documentation and records are reviewed. Finally, the team provides an overview of the perceived strengths and weaknesses of the program (in relation to the Essentials) and, when applicable, makes recommendations for improvement. A written report, summarizing the team's observations and conclusions, is subsequently forwarded to the JRCRTE Executive Office. The sponsoring institution receives a copy of the report and may respond to it with appropriate supplemental documentation. The display outlines the features considered for accreditation of an institution's educational program.

After the sponsoring institution has been given the opportunity to respond to the site-visit report, the referee presents the program to the full committee for an accreditation recommendation. For new programs, one of two recommendations can be made: full accreditation or withholding of accreditation. Accredited programs seeking reaccreditation may be recommended for full accreditation or probation. Programs coming before the committee with existing deficiencies that have not been remedied (or accredited programs with a significant number of serious deficiencies noted on reevaluation) may be recommended for probation. Programs holding probationary status and failing to remedy Essential violations in the allotted time are recommended for withdrawal of accreditation.

Recommendations for program accreditation status are forwarded from the JRCRTE to CAHEA; which has the final authority for accreditation action. Programs awarded full accreditation by CAHEA are those that have demonstrated substantial compliance with all the applicable Essentials. Probationary accreditation status indicates the existence of substantial deficiencies that threaten the program's ability to provide acceptable educational experiences for its students. Programs holding pro-

▪ CURRENT ESSENTIALS

PREAMBLE
  Objective
  Description of Program

REQUIREMENTS FOR ACCREDITATION
  I. Sponsorship
      A. Site of Educational Program
      B. Institutional Relationship
  II. Outline Orientation
      A. Program Goals and Standards
      B. Minimum Expectations
  III. Resources
      A. Personnel
          1. Key Personnel
          2. Number
          3. Qualifications
      B. Physical Resources
          1. Administrative and Instructional Resources
          2. Library Resources
      C. Clinical Resources
      D. Financial
  IV. Students
      A. Disclosure
      B. Admission
      C. Services
      D. Number
      E. Clinical experience
  V. Instructional plan
      A. Curriculum
          1. Basic sciences
          2. Clinical sciences
          3. Respiratory care content areas
      B. Length and credit
      C. Implementation
          1. Instructional methods
          2. Multiple program designs
          3. Integration
          4. Physician input
      D. Student evaluation
          1. Frequency and purpose
          2. Methods
          3. Documentation
  VI. Program evaluation

bationary status must normally submit a new self-analysis addressing the identified deficiencies, and may be required to undergo a new on-site evaluation to demonstrate compliance with the Essentials. Programs from which accreditation has been withheld are new programs that do not fulfill sev-eral major requirements of the Essentials, when such deficiencies are significant and not easily correctable. Programs that have their accreditation withheld may appeal directly to CAHEA or may, if they desire, reapply for accreditation later. Accreditation may be withdrawn voluntarily (at the request of the institutional sponsor) or may be mandated by failure of the program to provide evidence of compliance with the Essentials within the specified probationary period. Programs that have their accreditation involuntarily withdrawn may also appeal to CAHEA.

NATIONAL VOLUNTARY CREDENTIALING

Voluntary *credentialing*, or *certification*, is the process by which a nongovernmental agency or association grants recognition to a person who has met predetermined qualifications, including graduation from an accredited program, completion of a given amount of work experience, and acceptable performance on a qualifying examination or series of such examinations.[5] A similar term, *registration*, is often used synonymously with certification, although it more properly describes the process by which qualified persons are listed on an official roster maintained by a governmental or nongovernmental agency. The functions of certification and registration are commonly performed by a credentialing body or agency. The awards based on examination or recognition of qualified persons by such agencies are thus designated as credentials.

Respiratory care credentialing began in November 1960, when the National Board for Respiratory Care (NBRC) was called the American Registry of Inhalation Therapists (ARIT). The ARIT was formed through efforts by the American Association for Respiratory Therapy (AART), the American College of Chest Physicians (ACCP), and the American Society for Anesthesiologists (ASA). From 1960 to 1974, only one annual Written Registry Examination was given by the ARIT. In 1969, a group formed by the AART, the Technician Certification Board, began administering a certification examination for respiratory therapy technicians. In 1973, the ARIT and the AART began discussions on a merger of the two credentialing examination programs. Both organizations agreed to form a single, independent credentialing body in 1974, and the corporate structure for the ARIT was changed to form the National Board for Respiratory Therapy, Inc. (NBRT).

The NBRT's first national business office opened in July 1974 in Kansas City. At that time, one written registry examination was given in

March of each year; the second part of the registry examination, an oral examination, was offered twice yearly. To expand the opportunity for individuals to take the written registry examination, the NBRT began administering this examination twice annually in 1976. There were approximately 2400 RRTs and 8500 CRTTs when the NBRT was formed. Only 12 years later, the number of RRTs has increased over ten times, whereas the number of CRTTs has grown by nearly seven times.

In 1974 the three original sponsoring organizations, along with the American Thoracic Society (ATS), appointed 24 individuals to serve as members of the Board of Trustees. In 1983 the National Society for Cardiovascular and Pulmonary Technology (NSCPT) became the fifth sponsor. Today these five organizations continue to support the NBRC by appointing 30 representatives to serve on the board. In addition, a Public Advisor position was created in 1982, bringing the total membership of the board to 31.

Present-day students and recent graduates of respiratory therapy programs may not be aware of the many positive changes that have taken place since 1960. Today, the manner in which the NBRC's examinations are constructed and administered is remarkably different. In the early days, board members were not only asked to write the test questions but also to participate in administering the Registry Oral Examinations. These examinations were very costly to the candidates as well as time-consuming for the volunteer Board of Trustees and Associate Examiners. It was not unusual for a candidate to spend several hundred dollars to travel to the testing site to take the oral examination, after waiting 1 to 2 years for testing space to become available.

With the increasing candidate volume and the difficulty of standardizing the test procedure, the board recognized the need to develop an alternative method of examining candidates. In 1979 the Registry Oral Examination was replaced by the current Clinical Simulation Examination (CSE). With this decision, the waiting period to take the RRT examination was eliminated and the number of candidates who could be tested, close to their homes, was made unlimited. Costs to candidates fell from several hundred dollars per examination to 90 dollars, the current CSE fee.

Another major step forward in the history of the credentialing system occurred with the implementation of the Entry-Level Examination System in 1983. Beginning in 1978, the Board of Trustees developed a revised CRTT examination designed to test what a national job analysis study revealed was the common core of tasks required of all practitioners entering the profession. At the same time, the RRT examinations were revised to measure abilities required of advanced practitioners, testing job analysis tasks performed only after clinical experience or at higher levels of complexity than at entry. Identification of the advanced respiratory therapy practitioner by national job analysis effectively ended over 10 years of debate over whether there were actually two levels of practitioners in the field.

The entry-level CRTT examination also eliminated the group of "registry-eligible" individuals who had difficulty in passing the written registry examination, and thus had no credential, by providing them immediate access to the CRTT examination. It also helped set the stage for state licensure by providing an examination designed to measure beginning practice knowledge and skills.

In an effort to consolidate the credentialing process for the respiratory care community under one organization, the NBRT reached an agreement with the National Society for Cardiovascular and pulmonary technology (NSCPT) in 1983 to administer the Pulmonary Function Certification Examination (CPFT), the test administered by the National Board for Cardiovascular and Pulmonary Credentialing (NBCPC). This step led to the name change of the NBRT to the present National Board for Respiratory Care (NBRC) and the addition of the NSCPT as a sponsor of the board.

LEGAL CREDENTIALING

Nonvoluntary state credentialing or licensure is the process whereby an agency of the government grants permission to an individual to engage in a given occupation after verification that the applicant has demonstrated the minimum degree of competency necessary to protect the public health, safety, and welfare. Under constitutional law, licensure represents one of many powers delegated to the states; therefore, it is through state legislative processes that licensure laws are enacted.[6]

Medical practice acts were generally the first licensure laws adopted by the states to regulate health professionals. Subsequent legislative efforts to assure the minimal competency of other health occupational groups have tended to use the medical practice acts as models.[6] Typically, a licensing law defines the profession and delimits its scope of practice; it also describes the requirements and qualifications for obtaining a license and the grounds for revocation of the right to practice. Generally, the administrative mechanism by which the act has been implemented is detailed (including the formulation and responsibilities of a licensure board), and legal penalties for practicing without a license are specified.

Licensure laws may be either permissive or mandatory.[6] Permissive licensure laws permit unlicensed persons to work in the occupation as long as they do not use the title recognized by the state. Mandatory laws require that all persons engaged in the profession be licensed. Health professional licensure laws normally are mandatory, although exceptions do exist.

The respiratory care community, under its professional association leadership, vacillated between adamant opposition to state licensure laws and the current strong political thrust to support legal statutes recognizing the profession.[7,8]

Early opposition to licensure of respiratory care personnel was in concert with the 1971 US Department of Health, Education, and Welfare (HEW) recommendations for the states to observe a moratorium on the licensure of additional categories of health personnel. HEW's major concerns were related to the proliferation of health professional occupational categories and to the questionable efficacy of the existing mechanisms of assuring the competency of health care practitioners. The respiratory care national leadership was also concerned about regulation, since this was perceived to lead to the potential loss of peer control, dilution of standards of proficiency, and restrictions to practice.

Several changes combined to shift the position from opposition to support for respiratory care licensure. First, a general increase in the political awareness of the profession, as a whole, sensitized its leaders to the need for "legitimization" of the occupation in the eyes of state and federal government. Second, sporadic but disconcerting evidence of encroachment of other health professions on the "domain" of the respiratory care practitioner created, in the minds of many, the need to define legally an occupational scope of practice and thereby to protect the interests of the profession as a whole. Hand in hand with this "territorial imperative" was a continued effort toward professionalization of the work force and the concurrent desire to protect the public from the untrained, uncredentialed, or otherwise unqualified practitioner.

Licensure activity for respiratory care personnel has been particularly spirited since the withdrawal of the HEW moratorium in 1975. Thereafter, the federal government deferred the issue of nonvoluntary legal credentialing and any assessment of competency to the state level. Currently, 27 states have enacted licensure or legal credentialing acts for respiratory care. Active proposed legislation is under consideration in several other states. All serve to define the profession and scope of practice, set minimum standards for entry into practice, and mandate continuing education.

OTHER FORMS OF LEGAL RECOGNITION

Although licensure is by far the most common form of legal recognition, the state has several other avenues through which a health professional may gain legal recognition. These include the already mentioned noncompulsory licensure or "registration," institutional licensure, practice act modification, and certification by one of the state regulatory agencies.

Noncompulsory licensure is much less confining than regular licensure and is essentially a protection for the title of the health profession. In any state that has such recognition, only persons who meet the educational and other requirements of the statute may call themselves respiratory therapists or respiratory technicians. This form of regulation is nonrestrictive, that is, it does not prevent any person from performing the functions usually associated with respiratory care as long as they do not call themselves respiratory therapists or technicians. This form of regulation has merit because it is less expensive to administer and it provides both formal recognition of the professional and some protection to consumers.

Institutional licensure is another form of governmental regulation in which the state delegates the recognition process to the health care facility that employs the health professional. Under this regulation it becomes the responsibility of the hospital to assure the competence of its health care workers, and it is the institutional license that is in jeopardy if the hospital employs personnel who do not meet the prescribed standards.

Nonphysician health care practitioners may also be legally recognized by a statutory inclusion in the medical or nursing practice art. Under this scheme, the legislature amends the appropriate practice act and permits the medical or nursing board to establish and implement standards for the recognition (certification) of the new health care profession. Physicians' assistants have been recognized by this mechanism in several states.

Finally, the legislature may delegate this power to one of the state agencies, such as the Department of Licensing and Regulation or the Department of

Public Health. Under this system the state agency sets the standards and implements them.

CONTINUING EDUCATION

The competency assurance mechanisms thus far discussed (accreditation, certification, and licensure) share two major characteristics: they represent institutionalized approaches to the issue of professional accountability, and they are directed at demonstrating such accountability only on the practitioners' entry into practice.

Continuing education is an accountability mechanism based on individual responsibility, which, in theory, should assure the continued competency of practitioners after entry into the field and throughout a lifetime of practice. Continuing education may thus be broadly defined as any purposeful, systematic, and sustained effort conducted by professionals, after completion of their entry-level education, to update, maintain, or expand the proficiency, knowledge, skill, and sensitivity necessary to discharge their occupational roles effectively.[4]

Continuing education may be broadly divided into two major categories: that which is self-directed (individually planned and pursued) and that which is other-directed (formal activities planned and organized by an educational agent other than the learner). Evidence gleaned from other health disciplines indicates that all professionals regularly engage in some form of continuing education, with self-directed activity generally predominating. Other-directed continuing education (sponsored by professional associations, educational institutions, and health care agencies) generally attract only a portion of the active work force unless, of course, participation is mandated by licensure requirements. What is not generally appreciated is that professionals engage in organized, other-directed, continuing education activities for a variety of reasons. Such motives for participation may include professional advancement, learning for its own sake, acquisition of new credentials, compliance with formal requirements or expectations, escape from the routine of work and home, and social interaction.[4]

Although continuing professional education represents the fastest-growing segment of post-secondary education in the United States, it has generally failed to develop in a coordinated manner and has recently come under criticism for its questionable effectiveness in assuring the continued competency of its target population. Of particular concern

in health professions' continuing education is the general lack of empirical evidence demonstrating the effect of educational intervention on the quality of health care.[9] Respiratory care illustrates both the problems and the promise of continuing health profession education.

No one involved in respiratory care over the last decade can argue with the need for mechanisms to assist practitioners in updating and maintaining their clinical knowledge and skills. Changes in both theory and practice have been so dramatic that practitioners educated in 1970 would be functionally obsolete today without continued efforts to stay informed. There is, however, less agreement on exactly how the diverse learning needs of the respiratory care work force can best be met.

Organized, formal, other-directed continuing education opportunities for respiratory care personnel are generally provided through three organizational systems: professional associations, educational institutions, and health care agencies. By far the most active and visible component of the formal continuing-education delivery system has been the professional association (AARC). Through its national office and in conjunction with its chartered affiliates, the AARC has regularly provided formal continuing education activities for clinicians, educators, and management personnel in the field. The national convention annually attracts more than 5000 participants and offers a diversified fare of lectures, workshops, and related activities. A smaller but more highly focused activity is the annual Education Forum, also sponsored by the AARC. At the chartered affiliate level, activity is directed at serving regional, state, or local needs; monthly educational meetings and annual statewide or regional conferences are typical of such activity. Related formal learning opportunities are provided by other health professional associations, and cosponsorship arrangements are not uncommon.

Recognizing that such diverse activities were of variable educational quality and that no mechanism existed either to assure quality or to document participant learning activity, the AARC set out to establish a mechanism that could (1) guide the development of continuing education programs appropriate for respiratory care personnel, (2) approve and grant credit equivalents for participation in such programs, and (3) maintain cumulative records of continuing education activity for subscribers to the system. In 1982 the AARC initiated the Continuing Respiratory Care Education (CRCE) program, a membership service that reviews, receives, stores, and documents continuing education activities. The CRCE system consists of a provider component and a participant component, with a computer link to provide storage, retrieval, and documentation of activities. The provider component focuses on the process of sponsorship of continuing education activities and deals with the procedures by which programs are submitted, evaluated, and approved. The participant component focuses on the AARC membership and its use of continuing education activities.

The CRCE system consists of three distinct categories for reporting continuing education activities. Category I activities represent continuing respiratory care education programs or activities that meet specific requirements, including (1) educational objectives, (2) presentation content descriptions, (3) faculty descriptions, (4) exact program itinerary, and (5) evaluation instruments. Category II activities are "documented" CRCE experiences. These can include individual study activities, completion of self-assessment examinations, clinical conferences, patient rounds, and audiovisual programs. Participation or attendance is documented by a representative of the sponsoring institution. Signed certificates of attendance of continuing education activities are also acceptable. Category III activities represent college credit earned after final formal training in respiratory care that is germane to the individual's practice of respiratory care. This is also a self-reported activity, but all courses requested for approval must be verified by transcripts or grade reports, or both.[10]

FUTURE PERSPECTIVES

With more than three decades of combined experience in respiratory care and respiratory therapy education, we feel justified in speculating on the shape of things to come. Such prognostication is based on a firm belief that future events are the result of deliberate planning and not of fortuitous happenstance. We believe that careful consideration of alternative futures is a necessary and desirable means of controlling our collective destiny.

RESPIRATORY CARE PRACTICE

The future of respiratory therapy education is inextricably linked with the future of respiratory therapy practice. If past events portend future circumstances, as historians claim, tomorrow's practice of respiratory care will be very different from what we see today. Dramatic increases in knowledge and in its technologic application are a given. Concomitant with such changes, significant alterations in the nature of the health care delivery system are most likely. An aging population will require both institutional and ambulatory health care services of a different nature from those currently available. Chronic diseases will eventually largely supplant acute disorders, and increasing emphasis will be placed on ambulatory and domiciliary care and on patient education. Changing reimbursement mechanisms are likely to encourage this and will further deemphasize the role of the acute care facility in all but the most life-threatening maladies. High technology will continue to flourish, however, as the care of the acute illness becomes ever more sophisticated and concentrated in regionalized tertiary care facilities. In such facilities, specialized respiratory care practice will be commonplace. Although governmental intervention in cost/benefit and quality-of-care issues may decline, health care agencies and practitioners alike will be expected to demonstrate the efficacy and economy of their methods. The quality-of-care issue will intensify as the barriers to access decrease and the distributional problems are alleviated.

In such a context, the respiratory therapy practitioners of the future (if indeed that is what we will call ourselves) will find their role expanded outside the acute care institutions and will become increasingly responsible for extending the physician's role into the community and into the homes of health care consumers. Proficiency in patient education will become a necessary component of the respiratory care practitioner's repertoire of skills, as will sophisticated rehabilitation, health promotion, and health maintenance activities.

The acute care setting will continue, however, to remain the major focal point for most respiratory care practitioners. Within such a setting technology will have its greatest impact on both the nature and type of care provided and on the providers themselves. Foremost among the technologic changes will be the growth of noninvasive monitoring and diagnostic systems and the relentless increase of computer application in assessment and treatment. The "knob-turner" of the past will become the computer systems analyst of the future, as physiologic functions are monitored and controlled by sophisticated patient–machine interfaces. Such changes will demand that practitioners acquire technologic expertise well beyond the scope of what is currently required. Ironically, however, in such settings psychosocial skills will be at a premium.

The issues of quality and efficacy will be increasingly addressed by practitioners skilled in basic and applied research methods and working in conjunction with other members of the health care team. Such research will increasingly focus on less esoteric health care problems, and it is not inconceivable that the respiratory care researcher of the future may attempt to unravel the mysteries of the common cold and its attendant ailments! Research will extend beyond the pathophysiology and therapy of disease into investigation of the efficacy of various behavior-modification techniques dealing with the continued problems of our own improprieties.

RESPIRATORY CARE EDUCATION

Concomitant with changes in the scope and pattern of respiratory care practice will be changes in the nature of the educational systems that prepare people for entry into such practice. These changes will be evolutionary rather than revolutionary and, it is hoped, will be in tune with the needs of the health care system.

Settings and Levels

The advancing technology of the profession of respiratory care will create increasing pressure on the educational institutions that sponsor respiratory care programs because the growing technical content, consistent with the state of the art, may require more learning time than is typical for the mission of the sponsoring institutions, particularly community colleges and technical schools. Educational institutions may have to assess their ability to deliver all the content that may be necessary to develop a competent respiratory therapist within the 2-year curriculum designs inherent in their systems.

Alternative curriculum designs that may emerge in many community colleges might include entry-level training that is provided in conjunction with what are now perceived as associate degree–level programs leading to completion of the basic curriculum within a 2-academic-year model. Because there is little new interest at the baccalaureate institution level for respiratory care education models, it is projected that the continuing-education model for additional course work and skills

leading to therapist credential eligibility will be developed. Following an associate degree entry-level training program, modularized educational courses will be offered that, upon completion of enough specialized modules, will lead to eligibility for respiratory therapist credentialing examinations. This model of education will make it possible for 2-year academic institutions to continue to offer training at the level of respiratory therapist without conflicting with the mission statement of the sponsoring community college.

Additionally, educational programs will continue to be developed in conjunction with 4-year academic institutions, providing opportunity for baccalaureate credentials in association with specialty graduate training in respiratory care. Thus, dual credentials for the respiratory therapist graduate will be available with associated academic preparation in education, business administration, or specialty sciences such as cardiopulmonary diagnostics. Other advanced clinical skills may be available in academic health centers where the necessary clinical resources are available in sufficient quantity to support educational offerings in an economically feasible fashion.

Teaching–Learning Process

The teaching–learning process, not unlike clinical practice, will feel the impact of technology. As the cost of microprocessor hardware decreases and sophisticated instructional software becomes readily available, the laborious process of inculcating basic knowledge will be increasingly accomplished by computer-assisted instruction.[11] With cognitive testing, student progress monitoring, and instructional management efficiently handled by computer, educators will be better able to address the needs of clinical skill development and performance evaluation. Both cognitive and performance evaluations will become increasingly sophisticated, with computer and laboratory simulations providing reliable and valid measures of problem-solving ability and procedural expertise. The dream of true competency-based education will become a reality when standardized measures of proficiency become the criteria for unit, course, and program completion. With instructors freed from the more mundane and time-consuming elements of their role, such as transfer of knowledge, record-keeping, and cognitive testing, attention to individual student needs will be facilitated, and the creative side of the educational enterprise will be significantly enhanced.

Accreditation and Credentialing

With valid and continuously updated delineations of the roles and functions of both entry-level practitioners and specialists in respiratory care, the accreditation and credentialing systems will become fully integrated and mutually complementary.

The accreditation process for respiratory care educational programs will shift in emphasis from the assessment of input and process standards to the evaluation of the content validity of the curriculum—that is, the degree to which the curriculum content and organization coincides with the competencies requisite to entering practice and with criteria of student learning outcomes. The few input and process standards that remain will be those demonstrably related to achieving successful program outcomes and ensuring institutional probity and fair educational practices. The length of accreditation will be increased to 10 years, and the programmatic on-site evaluation process will become less frequent and substantially accomplished by paper review. Annual and interim report mechanisms will increasingly place the burden of responsibility and accountability on institutional sponsors and program personnel to provide empirical evidence of the quality and ongoing improvement of their program processes and outcomes. Accreditation mechanisms will be developed to ensure that specialized postgraduate experiences do indeed accomplish their goals.

Economic pressures will assure survival of the technician and technical training programs. The advanced generalist credential (RRT) will probably survive, but increasing emphasis will be placed on specialty credentialing examinations designed to assess competencies in discrete and focused domains of clinical practice (e.g., neonatal critical care). Licensure, in some form, will become a reality when and if the scope of respiratory care practice regularly extends outside the confines of the acute care setting. Such systems will initially mandate continuing education participation for renewal but will eventually require periodic proof of continued competence. Eventually, licensure or its equivalent will supplant voluntary credentialing at the entry level; such credentialing will, however, continue to recognize individuals in advanced and specialized areas of clinical practice.

REFERENCES

1. Barach AL, dela Scapelle E, Garthwaite B: Minimum standards for inhalation therapy. JAMA 144:25, 1950
2. Standards of effective administration of inhalation therapy. New York, NY Academy of Sciences, 1950
3. Committee on Allied Health Education and Accreditation: Allied Health Education Directory, 16th ed. Chicago, American Medical Association, 1988
4. Scanlan CL: Professional accountability and competency assurance. Respir Care 24(1):12, 1979
5. Report on Licensure and Relation Health Personnel Credentialing. Washington, DC, Department of Health, Education and Welfare, publication #(HSM) 72–11, 1971
6. Mishoe SC: Current and future credentialing in respiratory therapy. Respir Care 25(3):345, 1980
7. American Association for Respiratory Therapy, Ad Hoc Committee on Licensure Planning: Guidelines for writing a licensure bill for the practice of respiratory therapy. AARTimes 4(12):36, 1980
8. State licensure of inhalation therapy practice. Position paper of the ARIT Board of Directors, 13 Nov 1970. Respir Care 10:249, 1971
9. Scanlan CL: Encouraging professionals to continue their education. In Darkenwald GG, Larson GA (eds): Reaching the Hard to Reach Adult (New Direction for Continuing Education Series, no 8). San Francisco, Jossey-Bass, 1980
10. The CRCE System. Dallas, American Association for Respiratory Care, 1988
11. Rau JL: Computer-assisted instruction: a solid-state Socrates. Respir Care 22(6):581, 1977

Three

Effective Interpersonal Communication in Respiratory Care

Susan Rickey Hatfield
Timothy Hatfield

This chapter will review issues in interpersonal communication, a long overlooked area in texts for respiratory care professionals. By improving communication and by better understanding human relationships, the quality of patient care can be improved. Working to promote positive, effective communication can be difficult in a medical facility. Often relationships are complex and intense, and exist within a stratified milieu of workers. However, communication and coping skills can promote a more humane, supportive environment for professional growth.

We will present (1) a basic model of interpersonal communication that takes into account both the content and context of communications in respiratory care and (2) important communication, relationship, and coping skills and strategies that will help the reader maintain perspective, while meeting the ongoing demands of your work in respiratory care.

COMMUNICATION

We define *interpersonal communication* as two or more people involved in a transactional process of sending and receiving verbal and nonverbal messages with the goal of shared meaning. Several aspects of this definition deserve emphasis and explanation.

First, communication is a transactional process. The components of the process are interdependent, not independent. A message cannot be understood without some understanding of the message's sender, receiver, and situation. If one were to overhear a statement, but not see the communicators involved or understand their relationship, it would be unlikely that the message could be interpreted correctly.

Next, communication involves the simultaneous sending and receiving of messages. Even while we are talking, we are actively interpreting the verbal and nonverbal reactions of the person with whom we are talking, and tailoring our message accordingly. Effective teachers become very adept at interpreting their students' facial expressions to determine whether to expand upon a point, spell a word, or move on to something else.

Finally, the goal of communication is the creation of shared meaning. As Verderber pointed out, simply sharing ideas and feelings does not always result in effective communication.[1] Even though the person you are talking to may understand the individual words you are using, their understanding of your entire message might be different from the way you had intended your message to be understood.

THE COMMUNICATION PROCESS

In the last 25 years a number of theorists have advanced models of communication.[2,3] David Berlo's model is one of the most frequently cited and helps create an understanding of the four different elements of the communication process[4] (Fig. 3–1). Berlo's SMCR model defines four major variables of the communication process—source, message, channel, receiver—and describes several subcomponents of each variable.

Both the source (S) and receiver (R) of any message are affected by their written and verbal communication skills (for instance, some are better speakers and listeners than others), attitudes (how they feel about themselves, the other person in the interaction, and the situation itself), knowledge (what they have learned through education and experience), social system (the roles that they play and the roles that they are expected to perform), and their cultural system (dominant beliefs and values held by a specific culture, for instance, acceptable and unacceptable behaviors).

These individual characteristics of the speaker influence how that person makes choices concerning the elements and structure of the message, spe-cifically in terms of the message's content, treatment, and code. The content of the message refers to the information the speaker presents and any assertions or opinions that the speaker might make. The treatment of the message refers to the way in which the content is presented. For instance, information may be presented in a straightforward manner and be very direct, or it might be conveyed in some other way, making use of a hidden agenda. Finally the code of the message refers to the symbol used and its rules, for instance, English, Spanish, or American Sign Language for the deaf.

Once the speaker has made the choices pertaining to the message itself, the message must be sent to the receiver by using one or more of the five senses. It is very important to remember that nonverbal messages have just as much meaning as verbal messages.

Although Berlo emphasized the idea that communication is a process, this linear model does not accurately represent the complex nature of interpersonal communication. A better model for illus-

Figure 3–1. Berlo outlined factors under each element in the model that he believed were important to understand how communication operates. The skills, attitudes, knowledge, social system, and culture of the source were all seen as important to the communication process. The model also indicates the importance of the message's content, elements, treatment, and structure. Berlo acknowledged that all five senses were potential channels for sending and receiving information, and that the same individual factors that influenced the speaker also influenced the receiver. (Berlo D: The Process of Communication: An Introduction to Theory and Practice. New York, Holt, Rinehart and Winston, 1960, p 72, with permission)

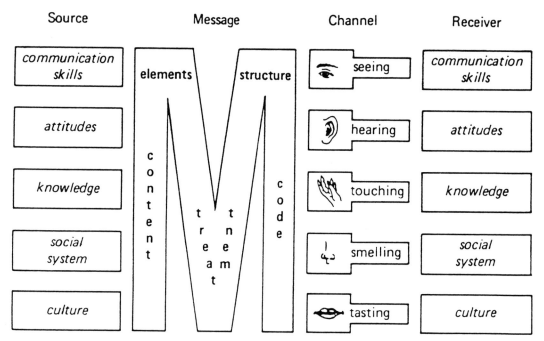

trating two-person communication is the model developed by James McCroskey, which appears in Figure 3–2.[5] The McCroskey model includes the same basic elements as the Berlo model (source, message, channel, and receiver) and adds the concepts of senders and receivers, encoding and decoding, and feedback.

Senders and Receivers

Each individual in the communication situation acts as both a sender and a receiver of information at the same time. As you speak to someone, you are likely to look at the receiver for responses indicating that they agree or disagree, understand or do not understand, approve or disapprove, are interested or bored. As you interpret these nonverbal messages, you are performing receiving functions, even as you continue to be sending messages. The Berlo model (see Fig. 3–1) outlined the individual factors that influence both the sender and the receiver. The importance of how individual variables, such as who you are, what you know, what you believe, how you live, what you value, and so on, cannot be overlooked. As DeVito pointed out, "who you are can never be divorced from the messages you send or the messages you perceive."[6]

Encoding and Decoding

Encoding is the transforming of ideas and perceptions into symbols that can be transmitted to the other person or persons in the communication situation.[6] The symbol system can be both verbal and nonverbal. For instance, a message may be encoded using a set of verbal symbols that are agreed upon by a certain culture (language), or a set of nonverbal gestures that have meaning to a specific audience (e.g., sign language for the deaf).

The choice of symbol systems is important, since it is the speaker's responsibility to select symbols that the receivers of the message are likely to understand. Obviously, a speaker would be unwise to encode a message with a symbol system that the receiver might not understand (e.g., Swahili). More subtle encoding errors are made when speakers overestimate the audience's level of knowledge or vocabulary, using words that the audience does not understand. Professional jargon is especially problematic. Many professionals are so used to encoding messages in the abbreviated jargon of their field that they have difficulty encoding messages for persons outside their field. As a respiratory care professional, you need to take special care in explaining treatment to patients or nurses and in answering their questions, always remembering that the goal of communication is *shared* meaning. As a communicator, you increase your patients' and coworkers' understanding by carefully encoding your messages.

Once encoded, messages are transmitted through one or more communication channels. Communication channels are the media through which the messages pass and involve any one or more of the five senses: visual, auditory, tactile, olfactory, gustatory. A message that has been encoded using language or words, can be transmitted verbally by speaking or singing (the auditory channel) or nonverbally through writing, using sign language, or pantomime (the visual channel). Perhaps a certain perfume or cologne would convey your message most effectively (olfactory channel), just as a reassuring hug (tactile channel) might express what is difficult to express using words. Finally, if

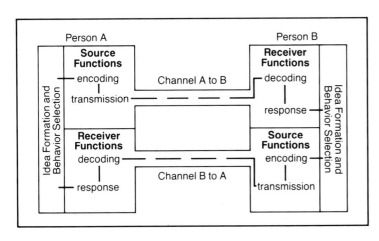

Figure 3–2. This model of interpersonal communication takes the four basic elements of the communication process (source, message, channel, and receiver) and adds the concepts of sender and receiver, encoding and decoding, and feedback. In McCroskey's model, an idea is formulated by the sender into a message through the process of encoding, and the message is transmitted (through one or more channels) to the receiver. The receiver "decodes" or makes sense of the message and then becomes a message source by formulating, encoding, and transmitting a response. (McCroskey JC. An Introduction to Rhetorical Communication, 4th ed. © 1982, p 15. Reprinted by permission of Prentice-Hall, Inc, Englewood Cliffs, NJ)

we believe the old saying, "The way to a man's heart is through his stomach," then we would probably want to focus on the gustatory channel.

Messages can—and often are—encoded by using more than one channel. For example, if you wanted to impress a friend with your cooking talents, you would want to make sure that the meal you created looked good, had a pleasant aroma and texture, and tasted great as well.

Once the message has been sent, it is up to the receiver to figure out what it means. This process of making sense out of the message is known as *decoding*. Decoding, as Berlo pointed out, is subject to the same personal variables specific to each receiver.[4]

Have you ever talked to someone about a movie you had both seen, only to find out that the other person had a totally different impression of the movie than you did? This is an example of how individual variables affect the manner in which a message might be interpreted. Some of these individual variables are the receiver's background, education, feelings, attitudes, and past experience with the sender. Let us go back to the food example mentioned earlier and assume that (for some reason) you selected escargots (snails) for the entree. Even cooking all day does not ensure that your friend is going to appreciate the meal. If your friend has never had escargots before, he or she might be hesitant to give them a try. Maybe your friend is not feeling too well that particular evening, and the sight of any food—especially snails—is unappealing. Perhaps your friend heard on the radio recently of a worldwide snail shortage and feels obligated to support a snail boycott. On the other hand, if your friend knows you are an excellent cook, he or she might dive right in, anticipating a new and exciting dining experience!

Feedback

Once the receiver has decoded or "made sense" of the message, the receiver is likely to provide some kind of indication of the interpretation of the message. This response is known as *feedback*. Feedback can directly address the message (The escargots are delicious!) or indirectly address the message (Could I have the recipe for this dish? I would like to serve it next week). Feedback can be either positive (complimentary), negative (critical), or ambiguous (This is very ... interesting.). It may be nonverbal as well. A dinner companion who has not said anything about the meal because she is eating is conveying just as strong a message as a companion who has not said anything and is just moving the escargots around on his plate.

Communication Breakdown

Although this process seems straightforward, we know from sometimes painful experience that the process does not always work as smoothly as we would like. Several factors can cause a "communication breakdown." Here are just a few of the factors that may cause the message to be interpreted differently than it was intended.

- The sender is using words that the receiver does not understand.
- The sender assumes that the listener has knowledge that the listener does not have.
- The sender is using words that the listener knows, but is using them in a way that the listener does not understand.
- Physical noise inhibits the listener from hearing the message.
- There is some kind of distraction in the environment that is disturbing to the receiver.
- The listener is not paying attention.
- The listener is paying attention but has been distracted by something that the sender has said.

Each of these examples involves some kind of *noise* in the channel. McCroskey defines noise as "any element that interferes with the generation of the intended meaning in the mind of the receiver."[5] Noise can occur in the sender, channel, or receiver. Although noise is not an essential part of the communication process, it is almost always present.

The most familiar type of noise is physical noise (sounds) in the environment. This category of noise, which involves the channel through which a message is sent, is known as *external noise*. For instance, physical noise intrudes upon the auditory channel, making it difficult for both the sender and the receiver to hear. A telephone connection that has a lot of static is a good example of physical noise. But noise in the channel is not limited to physical sounds. Messages using any of the five senses can be affected by some form of noise. For example, if your community were to experience a power outage while you are reading this, you might not be able to continue because it was too dark to see!

Noise can also be caused by the message sender. This form of noise is known as *semantic noise*, and is caused when a sender carelessly encodes a message. This carelessness can result in using words the receiver does not understand, using common words in a way that is unfamiliar to the audience, or using words that have so great an emotional impact on the audience that they overshadow the rest of the message. As an example, in the past few years, a number of political figures have suffered irreparable damage to their careers as a result of off-the-cuff remarks that involved inappropriate slang, obscenities, or stereotypes.

Finally, noise can also occur in the receiver. Have you ever found yourself rereading the same sentence of a book several times because you were not paying attention? Have you ever found yourself rereading the same sentence of a book several times because you were not paying attention? (No, you are paying attention; we just could not resist the visual joke!) Or have you ever found yourself daydreaming while listening to someone speak? This type of noise is a receiver issue, and is known as *internal noise*.

Consider some of the preceding issues and concepts as they apply to the following scenario.

▪ CASE STUDY: RESPIRATORY THERAPIST

You are the respiratory therapist, working on a Sunday afternoon, and are covering the intensive care unit of a 200-bed community hospital. A nurse calls you to the room of a 22-year-old asthmatic woman who is in increasing distress. The nurse is upset at the pulse oximeter monitor, which is sounding an alarm. Now the electrocardiograph (ECG) also sounds an alarm, as the patient's heart rate exceeds 140 beats per minute.

The woman is in profound distress, breathing rapidly, with obvious wheezing. She is perspiring and has a distressed appearance, showing the cosmetically distressing effects of chronic steroid therapy—acne, facial hair, "moon-faced" appearance, generally obese.

HISTORY

Repeated, prolonged admissions for severe asthma

Nonresponsive to conventional therapy

Unable to maintain employment

Very unsatisfying social life, with few social supports outside immediate family

Recent blood gas values suggest a worsening of her condition

Pulse oximeter readings are now below 85%

Patient now is using an oxygen mask

VISITORS

The patient's parents, who are "hovering," are pretty generally upset about everything (and saying so). They are especially upset that their daughter's regular doctor is unavailable. The patient's 12-year-old brother also is present, peering over the top of a comic book from time to time, but saying nothing.

DOCTOR

A surgeon, Dr. Power, is covering for the patient's physician, Dr. Gonzo, who left yesterday for a 2-week snorkeling vacation in Maui. Dr. Power is not familiar with the latest aerosol drugs to relieve bronchospasm and continues to prescribe a drug that is not the current "state of the art."

DISCUSSION QUESTIONS

1. What action do you take upon entering the room?
2. What kinds of "noise" may be present in this situation? For you? For the patient? For the parents? For the brother? For the nurse? For the doctor?
   External "noise"?
   Semantic "noise"?
   Internal "noise"?
3. With whom do you speak, and what do you say to them?
4. What statements will be *most* helpful for you to make to each of the persons you address?

THE COMMUNICATION CONTEXT

The communication process is inextricably linked to the context or situation in which it takes place.[1] The elements of the situation that affect the outcome of the communicative interaction are (1) the physical context, (2) the historical context, and (3) the social-psychological context.

Physical Context

The physical context involves the setting in which a conversation takes place. Elements of the physical situation include time of day, weather, and the room itself in terms of temperature, lighting, color, and furnishings.[7] Knapp noted that these physical characteristics of the setting give rise to perceptions of formality, familiarity, constraint, distance, warmth, and privacy—all of which influence the construction and interpretation of messages sent and received within that particular setting.[8]

For instance, you might be more guarded when talking about a critically ill patient with a doctor in a crowded public place (like a cafeteria) that is low in privacy and warmth than you would in the doctor's office, which is likely to afford more privacy. It is important to remember that your patients are likely to perceive the entire hospital setting differently than you do. Although the hospital might be familiar to you, it is probably an unfamiliar environment for your patient. This unfamiliarity, coupled with the patient's perceptions of hospitals as lacking warmth and privacy, in addition to being highly constraining, are very much likely to influence your interactions with the patient.

Historical Context

The historical context refers to the past relationship between the participants in the conversation. Each of us has probably had the uncomfortable experience of having to interact with someone with whom we have recently had an unpleasant experience, such as a disagreement or conflict. These previous encounters shape the tone of present and even future interactions. Although historical context certainly affects communication, in professional relationships it is important not to let history get in the way of offering responsible professional respiratory care.

Social-Psychological Context

The social-psychological context refers not only to the present emotional states of the persons communicating, but also to the social roles and rules operating in that situation. In terms of psychological context, it is a given that we all have "good" and "bad" days. It is important to recognize that how we are feeling influences the way we formulate messages, as well as the way we interpret them on those given days. It might be helpful to think in terms of giving and receiving constructive criticism. On a bad day, you might receive valid constructive criticism very defensively, whereas on a good day you are likely to be much more open— even receptive—to it. In addition, on those bad days you may find yourself being much more critical of others' performance (not to mention your own) than you would normally.

The social aspect of context concerns the social rules and roles that are operating in a situation. Status differences are likely to be clearly defined in the hospital setting and, with those differences come clear sets of communication rules. As DeVito

pointed out, communication rules are guidelines for communicative behavior.[9] Whereas some sets of rules are explicit (written down, as, for example, Robert's Rules of Order), most communication rules are implicit and learned as part of the socialization process of newcomers into an organization.[10] Common communication rules involve forms of address, who initiates conversations, topics permitted to be addressed, and length of conversation.

Respiratory therapists need to be aware of the effect that these different aspects of context have on communication, as well as how they are interrelated. As noted by DeVito, each aspect of context influences and is influenced by the others.[6] For example, a disagreement with a close friend last week (historical context) is likely to lead to a change in the "rules" of the relationship (social-psychological context), which in turn may lead to a change in plans for this week (physical context).

▪ CASE STUDY: THE CONTEXT CONTEST

DISCUSSION QUESTIONS

1. What are some of the important *physical context* issues for you to consider when working with the patient described earlier? Be sure to take into account *all* of the persons with whom you may be interacting.

2. What about *historical context* issues? (Feel free to speculate about some of the family issues, but pay primary attention to the kinds of historical context issues that may exist among the respiratory therapist and the other hospital staff.)

3. Concerning the *social-psychological context*, what kinds of *feelings* issues for all those present may be important for you to consider? How might you feel as the respiratory therapist walking into the room?

4. What are the unwritten "rules of the game" that need to be considered regarding the social context of the situation? Who is in charge? What role(s) are you expected to play? How do you communicate what you need to communicate? What do you do if you and the physician disagree about the most helpful course of treatment for the patient?

Although an understanding of the communication process is important, responsible respiratory care can best be delivered with the awareness and practice of specific communication skills.

COMMUNICATION SKILLS TO ENHANCE RESPIRATORY CARE

Basic Attending

Can you think back to a time, either in your respiratory care training or in your personal life, when you were attempting to communicate something to another person and had the other person say, "Yes, I'm listening," and *knew* that, in fact, the other person was *not* listening to you? Can you, just for a moment, recapture how you *felt* when this occurred? It was not a particularly positive feeling, was it?

Having a wealth of scientific and technological expertise does *not* guarantee that a respiratory care professional—or, we would maintain, *any* health care provider—will be either an effective practitioner or a good colleague. The kind of intensive helping implicit in respiratory care demands a real, unambiguous presence on the part of the helper; at the core of this presence, or in being there for another person, is the capacity and commitment to *attend to* the person.

Egan described the attending process as one that is conveyed, both verbally and nonverbally, and that can help to establish good rapport with a person.[11] The following skills, abbreviated by the acronym SOLER, can help communicate your positive presence both to patients and colleagues:

1. S: *Squarely* face the person, to communicate involvement by orienting yourself to them.
2. O: *Open* your posture to the person, thus communicating your availability and openness to them. Although crossing your legs or folding your arms does not per se close off effective attending, the key issue to consider is whether one's posture says, "I am open to what you have to say."
3. L: *Lean* slightly toward the person at times in appropriate ways, which conveys the nonverbal message, "I'm especially interested in what you're telling me now."
4. E. *Eye contact* is essential in telling the person that you are truly present in the conversation. Some happy medium between looking everywhere *but* at the person and fixing the person in a laserlike stare is the goal of good eye contact in our culture.
5. R: *Relaxed* presentation of all the foregoing attending skills in a natural way tells the person, "I am interested in what you have to say, and I am really here for you."

Egan went on to emphasize the importance of utilizing these skills in a nonrigid, nonabsolute way that is sensitive to a person's individual and cultural differences. The goal is to build connections between yourself and the other person because you *have* paid attention, attended to the person, not to assume that some "formula intimacy" will be equally effective with everyone.[11]

With practice, these kinds of basic attending skills can provide the foundation for even more effective listening and relationship-building—professional and collegial—in your ongoing work in respiratory care.

Listening: Nonverbals

Effective listening involves processing both verbal and nonverbal messages from a person, with the paramount goal of *understanding* what the person is communicating.

A variety of nonverbal cues—body movements and gestures, facial expressions, pitch and tone of voice, inflection, points of emphasis, rate of respiration, flushing or paleness of the skin, type of clothing—communicate messages when a person "listens" for them. Larson has noted, in fact, that important nonverbal messages also exist on The Far Side (Fig. 3–3).[12]

The communication and counseling literature makes it clear that nonverbal messages often convey more to the listener than do verbal ones.[8,11,13–15] In one very interesting line of research, Mehrabian and his colleagues report that when a person receives *inconsistent* verbal and nonverbal messages, it is the nonverbal message that is "heard" most strongly. In their work on expression of interpersonal liking, they reported: "If the facial expression is inconsistent with the words, the degree of liking conveyed by the facial expression will dominate and determine the impact of the total message."[16]

By extension, then, your asking about some of your work with a colleague can elicit verbal and nonverbal responses that are either consistent or inconsistent. Moreover, even if the *words* say that you are doing fine, a clear nonverbal message that

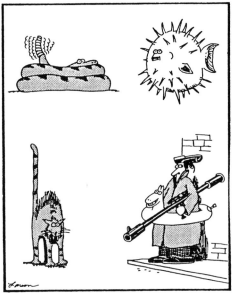

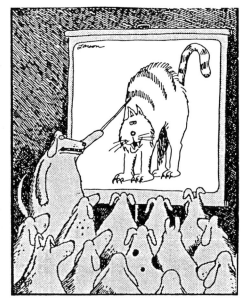

How nature says, "Do not touch."

"Now, in this slide we can see how the cornered cat has seemed to suddenly grow bigger.... Trickery! Trickery! Trickery!"

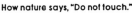

Figure 3–3. Nonverbal cues. (*The Far Side.* Copyright 1985, Universal Press Syndicate.

your work is flawed in some way will be what registers with you. Not checking out the response further could, then, leave you feeling confused about how well you are doing, if not absolutely certain that you have fallen short. You, your respiratory care colleagues, others on the health care team, and certainly your patients deserve clarity and consistency in the messages given and received.

■ CASE STUDY: THERE'S MORE TO BE "HEARD" THAN *WHAT* THEY SAY

DISCUSSION QUESTIONS

1. Discuss some of the important *nonverbal* cues that may be present in the situation.

2. How might the following *verbal* message (which could be stated by *anyone* present) convey very different meanings when a variety of body postures, gestures, facial expressions, tones of voice, and such, are taken into account? (As a class, brainstorm as many different possibilities as you can.)

"OK, let's do it."

Empathy

Another skill at the core of effective interpersonal relationships, as well as any kind of human helping, is the capacity to understand another person's experience from *his* or *her*—not your own—perspective. This involves listening carefully to the total verbal and nonverbal message in all its complexity, and communicating your understanding of the message back to the person. Called *empathy* or *empathic listening*, the skill involves a commitment to (1) immersing oneself in the perspective of another to understand the situation *in his or her terms*, and (2) communicating your understanding to the person so that he or she *knows* you understand. Carl Rogers' seminal work on empathy in counseling has had a profound effect on generations of skilled helpers.[17-19] He defined empathic listening as follows:

> Entering the private perceptual world of the other and becoming thoroughly at home in it. It involves being sensitive, moment by moment, to the changing felt meanings which flow in this other person . . . . It means temporarily living in the other's life, moving about in it delicately without making judgments . . . .[19]

It is the polar opposite of the situation cited earlier in this chapter, when someone says "I'm listening" and, in fact, is not. The basic message conveyed by the person who is not listening is one of disrespect. On the other hand, when a person knows that someone *has* listened empathically to them, their reaction is apt to be something like, "Yes, that's *it* exactly! You know what I'm talking about." They feel affirmed, respected, and empowered both to keep exploring their own issues and to allow you to accompany them in that process.

Empathic listening fosters respectful, supportive relationships among colleagues as well as between helper and patient. It exemplifies the essence of "being there" for someone else, and is a learnable skill that we feel must be a part of respiratory care professionals' repertoire, along with the myriad of technical skills for which they are responsible.

Even with the technology in place, it is clear that often what a patient needs *most* is someone to listen—carefully, sensitively, respectfully—to their own views about their situation. And often the people most available to listen are nurses, respiratory care personnel, or other specialists, other than the doctor or doctors in charge of the case. Burton has spoken to the important need for physicians to listen and communicate well with respiratory care professionals,[20] and Garber, like Burton a physician, addressed the benefits to physicians and patients alike if physicians were to have better training in basic attending and empathic listening skills.[21] The norm, however, is not in that direction, and vital "bedside manner" responsibilities likely will continue to rest with others, including you.

Rhetorical Sensitivity

Attending, listening, nonverbal awareness, and empathy skills help one to become a better communicator. These skills, taken collectively, help promote an *attitude* toward communication known as rhetorical sensitivity.

Consider for a moment how you would describe your activities last weekend to (1) your mother or father, (2) your grandmother, (3) your boss, (4) your best friend, and (5) a small child. Chances are that you would change both the structure and the content of the message for each person. Hart and Burks labeled this perspective as an attitude toward communication.[22] In other words, a person's attitude toward communicating may indeed influence the subsequent communication itself. Hart and coworkers extended Hart and Burks'

thinking, and identified three rhetorical postures.[22,23] At one end of the continuum is a *noble self* attitude, narrow in view and very self-oriented. At the other end is a *rhetorically reflective* attitude, which is strongly oriented to the other person and the situation. The *rhetorically sensitive* person approaches each situation as unique and weighs all the variables before speaking.

According to Hart and Burks, the rhetorically sensitive person is an "ideal" communicator, one who

1. Tries to accept role-taking as a part of human behavior
2. Seeks to distinguish between all information available and information acceptable for communication
3. Tries to understand an idea can be encoded in several different ways[22]

Perhaps rhetorical sensitivity can best be understood by examining the ends of the continuum—the noble self and the rhetorical reflector. Darnell and Brockreide label the noble self as one who

1. Sees any variation from their personal norms as hypocritical, as a denial of integrity and as a cardinal sin.
2. Views the self as the primary basis for making communicative choices. The needs of another person or pressures of a situation are considered to be of secondary importance if they are taken into account at all.
3. Tends to want control, rather than to share choices. Prefers to engage in monologue, rather than dialogue.[24]

The rhetorical reflector is characterized in the following manner:

1. Rhetorical reflectors have no "self" to call their own. The self developed for each communication act is inextricably bound up in the situation.
2. Communicative choices from reflectors arise from the perceived needs and wishes of the other person and the situation. They feel their way into the transaction and behave and become what they feel the other needs and wants.

3. Reflectors neither control nor share choices. Rather, from all the frames of reference, the self created plays the passive role and is acted upon as opposed to a proactive role. The only "choice" a reflector makes is to accommodate the choice of others.[24]

In contrast, the *rhetorically sensitive* person is one who recognizes that not all messages are suitable for all receivers. With skills, such as attending, active listening, and empathy, the rhetorically sensitive person takes into account the receiver's knowledge, background, experiences, emotions, and attitudes when encoding messages.

Rhetorical Sensitivity and Respiratory Care

Rhetorical sensitivity can help the respiratory therapist balance important professional responsibilities to the patient and to the respiratory care profession. Such a balance leads to professionally responsible respiratory care, as indicated in Figure 3–4. As depicted in the model, the vertical axis is a continuum of knowledge and skills for respiratory care professionals. These would include all the scientific, technical, and general professionalization issues addressed in respiratory care training programs, along with your ongoing learning on the job and through continuing education opportunities. The horizontal axis is a continuum of your communication and interpersonal skills and sensitivity with your patients and colleagues.

As discussed earlier in this chapter, having a high level of knowledge and skills *without* the communication and interpersonal skills to work well with your patients and colleagues will not foster professional effectiveness. In rhetorical sensitivity terms, you would be more likely to give "noble self" responses to patients, perhaps well grounded in technical knowledge but very insensitive to the patients themselves or the context of your work with them. On the other hand, high sensitivity to patients without the requisite professional knowledge and skills certainly would not qualify you to be a respiratory care professional and would be most like a "rhetorical reflector" posture. However sensitive a communicator you are, you would not belong in the field.

In between these two positions, however, as depicted by the shaded area in Figure 3–4, are those respiratory care professionals who have both the necessary professional skills and the communication–interpersonal skills to deliver them with a view to the patient and the context. In short, they have the skills to provide responsive, responsible respiratory care. Beyond baseline competency levels for entry into the field, our *responsible respiratory care* model accounts for increasing levels of knowledge, expertise, and growth in both areas, through your continuing education and commitment to renew and grow in the profession.

BASIC STRESS SKILLS

Although only brief mention can be made here, the extent to which you manage the inevitable stresses of working in respiratory care will enhance both the quality of your work and your personal sense of satisfaction in the profession. Several key concepts will follow, some of which you may wish to pursue in more detail through the sources cited.

Figure 3–4. A model illustrating the balance between technical knowledge and human skills to accomplish "responsible" patient care. When respiratory care practitioners operate outside the stippled area, knowledge and therapeutics are applied without interpersonal skills or communication occurs without technical substance.

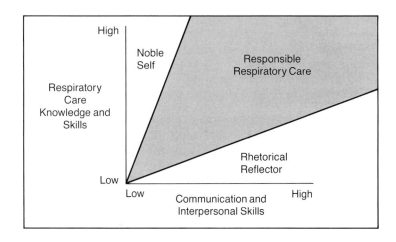

In general, does your being in respiratory care "fit" for you?

As cited in the model in Figure 3–4, your professional effectiveness depends both upon your responsibility to the profession and your responsibility to your patients. Although your very presence in a respiratory care training program may speak to your interest and commitment, it may be that the kinds of training, skills, and professional expectations of a respiratory therapist do not fit nearly as well for you as those of other important roles in health care or other professions. Can you imagine, for example, having an aversion to highly technical instruments and data, yet still expecting to enjoy work in respiratory care? Or can you imagine having a strong preference for working totally on your own and having absolute control over all decisions affecting a patient, yet knowing that you will be expected to work closely and cooperatively with many other health care professionals, some of whom often end up calling many of the shots (yes, we're aware of the pun!)?

Your careful self-assessment and career planning process need to be ongoing personal and professional issues for you, both for your own sense of career and life satisfaction as well as for the welfare of the innumerable patients whose lives are often quite literally in your hands. The literature abounds with excellent career-planning and decision-making texts; we refer you to two current sources as a point of departure.[25,26]

The way that you *think* about your work situation will strongly affect the amount of stress that you experience in it.

For example, to approach the day thinking, "This obviously is going to be a terrible day" will have a qualitatively different impact on you than to think "Today I have some important things to do, and I know they're going to matter to some people."

This is not a new notion—the ancient Greek philosophers wrote about the power of ideas on one's well-being, for example—but is worth considering as to its impact on your own self-care *and* your effectiveness in respiratory care. It is a core concept of Viktor Frankl's famous book *Man's Search for Meaning* about surviving imprisonment in a Nazi concentration camp,[27] and also is a cornerstone of one model of counseling called Rational Emotive Therapy (RET). This model encourages people to look at whether their beliefs are realistic.[28] Woolfolk and Richardson's excellent book *Stress, Sanity, and Survival* goes on to say

that our *perceptions* of situations can, all by themselves, trigger stress in our lives.[29]

The work of Suzanne Kobasa and her colleagues also points out that a person's commitment to a particular line of work and the felt sense of doing something that matters contributes to a hardier, more stress-resistant personality.[30] This also speaks to the importance of the way that you think about your work, whether in general or as you approach specific interpersonal situations. Assuming, for example, that your respiratory care responsibilities *do* matter, and that you carry them out in a professional manner to the best of your ability, may make it more likely for you to receive negative feedback and respond, "Thanks for the input," rather than to personalize the feedback and respond in a defensive way.

Having a clear view of the importance of your own respiratory care functions also will increase the likelihood that you will be able to adopt a positive, respectful perspective on the contributions of all members of the health care team (regardless of whether there is truly a team or the structure of the organization is hierarchical, with physicians on top).[12]

Being well yourself will help sustain you and prevent burnout in this high-intensity helping profession.

As a respiratory care professional, you will be delivering important services to others. You will be giving of yourself constantly. Your own self-care will have an important influence on your capacity to keep giving, day after day, in appropriate ways. Christina Maslach, the leading researcher on burnout, subtitled her book on the subject "*The Cost of Caring.*"[31] The very fact *that* you care about your patients and your profession makes you more vulnerable to burning out, and thereby speaks to the need for you to be actively involved in your own positive self-care.

Ardell, Travis and Ryan, and other authors have made important contributions to the burgeoning literature on wellness, which looks at the process of our being actively involved in the integration of our physical, intellectual, social, emotional, and spiritual well-being.[32,33] We would emphasize the *process* nature of wellness, because maintaining an ongoing balance among these dimensions of wellness is not achieved in a once-and-for-all way.

The key issue is remaining actively involved in our own self-care. By keeping ourselves "in tune," we can be there both personally and professionally.

The process of balancing may involve placing emphasis, at a given point, on physical fitness,[34-37] diet,[38,39] time management,[40] assertiveness skills,[41,42] difficult relationships,[43] or general stress management skills.[44,45]

Building and maintaining a support system is an important goal for respiratory care professionals.

From Harlow's early work with laboratory monkeys, to Spitz's parallel work with children in foundling homes, to more recent applications with a variety of populations, it is becoming increasingly clear that social support can play a crucial role in helping persons to cope.[46-52] Coping may involve the expected stresses of everyday life, as well as times of higher stress (e.g., examination period for respiratory care students). A sudden hospitalization is extremely stressful for most people.

▪ CASE STUDY: GOOD SELF-CARE FOR GOOD PATIENT CARE

DISCUSSION QUESTIONS

1. In the case study described earlier, on the assumption that you very likely will be walking into a stressful situation, what kinds of appropriate stress prevention skills or techniques will be important for you to utilize *before* you enter the room?

2. More generally, list 10 stress management or self-care skills that you utilize to take care of yourself in healthy ways. Consider the general issues mentioned in this chapter, but begin with the assumption that "all ideas are good ideas" for your list (i.e., feel free to include specific skills, behaviors, and so on, that have not been mentioned here). Of all the items on your list, which *two or three* are most essential for you to keep in your life so that you can remain a healthy, vital person and respiratory care professional?

3. What are the stress management and self-care issues in your own life that deserve more attention? Which one or two of them deserve your most concerted attention *now*?

Again, as a respiratory care professional who is expected to deliver high-quality, highly technical care to a wide array of patients, often in life-threatening situations, it seems essential that you know you have both professional and personal support to back you up. The support of other respiratory care professionals or of other members of the health care team can provide information, perspective, and encouragement in your work. The support of friends and loved ones *outside* the health care setting can provide needed perspective about your worth as a person as well as about your human limits on the job.

SUMMARY

This chapter has introduced information and skills to promote effective communication, positive working relationships, and coping skills for respiratory care professionals. We would emphasize, however, that these issues provide a framework or point of departure for your work, not a prescription for facing all of the inevitable complexities of this field, which is continuing to grow and evolve.

For example, in their chapter for the previous edition of this text, DeKornfeld and Scanlan addressed the gradual move away from a rigidly hierarchical health care delivery system toward one that operates on the team concept, in which *all* team members—physicians, nurses, technologists, aides, orderlies, and administrative support staff—are assumed to have important contributions to make toward patients' well-being.[53]

It is within this complex and still-evolving organizational structure that you as a respiratory care professional will provide service to patients. In some specific settings, the team concept will be alive and well, whereas in others a hierarchy—with physicians at the top and all other health care team members significantly down the pecking order—will be the case. Your understanding of the structure, roles, rules (explicit as well as unspoken), and expectations of the setting will help you to function effectively there, regardless of the norms. And your long-term commitment to refining and integrating your communication and interpersonal skills will continue to serve you as you deliver high-quality, responsive service in respiratory care.

REFERENCES

1. Verdeber RF: Communicate! Belmont, Calif, Wadsworth, 1987
2. Littlejohn SW: Theories of Human Communication. Belmont, Calif, Wadsworth, 1983

3. Ruben BD: Communication and Human Behavior, 2nd ed. New York, Macmillan, 1988

4. Berlo D: The Process of Communication: An Introduction to Theory and Practice. New York, Holt, Rinehart & Winston, 1960

5. McCroskey JC: An Introduction to Rhetorical Communication, 4th ed. Englewood Cliffs, NJ, Prentice Hall, 1982

6. DeVito JA: Human Communication. New York, Harper & Row, 1988

7. Malandro LA, Barker L: Nonverbal Communication. New York, Random House, 1983

8. Knapp ML: Nonverbal Communication in Human Interaction, 2nd ed. New York, Holt, Rinehart & Winston, 1978

9. DeVito JA: The Communication Handbook: A Dictionary. Philadelphia, Harper & Row, 1986

10. Ashforth O: Climate formation: Issues and extensions. Acad Manag Rev 10:837, 1985

11. Egan G: The Skilled Helper, 3rd ed. Monterey, Calif, Brooks/Cole, 1986

12. Larson G: Valley of the Far Side. Kansas City, Andrews, McMeel, & Parker, 1985

13. Ivey AE: Counseling and Psychotherapy: Skills, Theories, and Practice. Englewood Cliffs, NJ, Prentice Hall, 1980

14. Ivey AE: Intentional Interviewing and Counseling. Monterey, Calif, Brooks/Cole, 1983

15. Ivey AE, Authier J: Microcounseling, 2nd ed. Springfield, Ill, Charles C Thomas, 1978

16. Mehrabian A: Silent Messages. Belmont, Calif, Wadsworth, 1971

17. Rogers CR: Client-Centered Therapy. Boston, Houghton Mifflin, 1951

18. Rogers CR: On Becoming a Person. Boston, Houghton Mifflin, 1961

19. Rogers CR: A Way of Being. Boston, Houghton Mifflin, 1980

20. Burton GG (Speaker): The art of becoming a change agent. Pulmon Med Technol 1:58, 1984

21. Garber JJ: Improved doctor-patient communication: a means of reducing physician stress. Unpublished master's thesis, Winona State University, Minnesota, 1987

22. Hart RP, Burks DM: Rhetorical sensitivity and social interaction. Commun Monogr 39:75, 1972

23. Hart RP, Carlson RE, Eadie WF: Attitudes toward communication and the assessment of rhetorical sensitivity. Commun Monogr 17:1, 1980

24. Darnell D, Brockreide W: Persons Communicating. Englewood Cliffs, NJ, Prentice Hall, 1976

25. Bolles RN: What Color Is Your Parachute? Berkeley, Ten Speed Press, 1988

26. Hagberg J, Leider R: The Inventurers: Excursions in Life and Career Renewal, 3rd ed. Reading, Mass, Addison-Wesley, 1988

27. Frankl V: Man's Search for Meaning. New York, Washington Square Press, 1963

28. Ellis A, Harper RA: A New Guide to Rational Living. Englewood Cliffs, NJ, Prentice Hall, 1975

29. Woolfolk RI, Richardson FC: Stress, sanity, and survival. New York, Signet, 1979

30. Kobasa S: Stressful life events, personality, and health: An inquiry into hardiness. Person Soc Psychol 37:1, 1979

31. Maslach C: Burnout: The Cost of Caring. Englewood Cliffs, NJ, Prentice Hall, 1982

32. Ardell DB: High Level Wellness, 2nd ed. Berkeley, Ten Speed Press, 1986

33. Travis JW, Ryan RS: Wellness Workbook, 2nd ed. Berkeley, Ten Speed Press, 1988

34. Bailey C: Fit or Fat. Boston, Houghton Mifflin, 1978

35. Cooper KH: The New Aerobics. New York, Bantam, 1970

36. Fixx JF: The Complete Book of Running. New York, Random House, 1977

37. Sheehan GA: Dr. Sheehan on Running. New York, Bantam, 1978

38. Cumming C, Newman V: Eater's Guide: Nutrition Basics for Busy People. Englewood Cliffs, NJ, Prentice Hall, 1981

39. Orbach S. Fat Is a Feminist Issue. New York, Berkley, 1978

40. Lakein A: How to Get Control of Your Time and Your Life. New York, Peter Wyden, 1973

41. Kilkus SP: Adding assertiveness to the nursing profession. Nurs Success Today 3:17, 1986

42. Smith M: When I Say No, I Feel Guilty. New York, Bantam, 1975

43. Bramson RN: Coping with Difficult People. New York, Ballantine, 1982

44. Rice PL: Stress and Health: Principles and Practice for Coping and Wellness. Monterey, Calif, Brooks/Cole, 1987

45. Tubesing DA: Kicking Your Stress Habits. Duluth, Minn, Whole Person Associates, 1981

46. Albrecht TL, Adelman, MB: Social support and life stress. Hum Commun Res 11:3, 1984

47. Cobb S: Social support as a moderator of life stress. Psychosom Med 30:300, 1976

48. Harlow HF: Love in infant monkeys. Sci Am 200:68, 1959

49. Lynch JJ: The Broken Heart: The Medical Consequences of Loneliness. New York, Basic Books, 1977

50. Pearson JE: The definition and measurement of social support. J Counsel Dev 64:390, 1986

51. Spitz R: Life and dialogue. In Gaskill HS (ed): Counterpoint: Libidinal Object and Subject, p. 154. New York, International Universities Press, 1963

52. Veninga RC: A Gift of Hope. New York, Ballantine, 1985

53. DeKornfeld TJ: Ethical considerations and interpersonal relationships in respiratory care. In Burton G, Hodgkin J (eds): Respiratory Care: A Guide to Clinical Practice, 2nd ed, p. 58. Philadelphia, JB Lippincott, 1984

FOUR

The Physician and the Respiratory Care Team

Alan L. Plummer

The provision of respiratory care within the hospital has been in evolution since the early 1940s, when personnel dubbed "oxygen technicians" were utilized to deliver oxygen therapy.[1] Since that time there has been an expansion of services offered by the respiratory care department. As new information and technology continue to flow into the field, respiratory care will continue to grow and develop in the future. The practitioner providing respiratory care must be educated and trained in respiratory care, pulmonary and cardiac physiology, and the pathophysiology of diseases affecting the lungs, heart, and other organs. Respiratory care practitioners have had a close working relationship with physicians since respiratory care services were first organized.[1]

The respiratory care team usually includes the medical director, the patient's personal physician, respiratory therapists, nurses, and physical therapists (if chest physiotherapy is provided by the physical therapy department). In some circumstances nutritionists, pharmacokineticists, psychiatrists, and social workers may be added. The more complex the patient's problems, the greater the involvement necessary by members of the respiratory care team.

This chapter is written for the medical director of the respiratory care department, as well as other physicians who interrelate with the members of the respiratory care team.

DEFINITION OF RESPIRATORY CARE

The current definition of respiratory care is as follows:[2]

> Respiratory care is a life-supporting, life-enhancing health care profession practiced under qualified medical direction.* Respiratory care services provided to patients with disorders of the cardiopulmonary system include: diagnostic testing, therapeutics, monitoring, and rehabilitation. Patient, family, and public education are central to the mission of the profession. Respiratory care services are provided in all health care facilities and in the home.

---

* Medical direction means that the practice of respiratory care is provided under a medical director.

Other than the wide variety of functions and services available from the respiratory care department, the characteristic that distinguishes respiratory care from other allied health specialties is that respiratory care personnel must function under the aegis of a *qualified* physician medical director of respiratory care. This has been deemed necessary by the Joint Commission on Accreditation of Health Care Organizations (JCAHO, formerly JCAH) for hospital accreditation to occur,[3] and by Medicare, which requires a medical director of respiratory care as a condition to participate in Medicare.[4] This long-term association between physicians and respiratory care personnel has been present since the development of respiratory care (formerly oxygen or inhalation therapy) departments.[1] Over the years this cooperative venture has resulted in a strong bond between physicians and respiratory care personnel and has led to a common goal to provide optimal patient care to all patients with pulmonary and cardiac diseases. No other allied health department in the hospital, including nursing, physical therapy, and dietetics, has the physician input and leadership that the respiratory care department has. This should ensure that patient care delivered by respiratory care personnel is of the highest quality.

QUALIFICATIONS OF RESPIRATORY CARE PERSONNEL

Respiratory care services should be provided by well-trained personnel, preferably credentialed by the National Board for Respiratory Care (NBRC). Schools of respiratory care that offer 1 to 4 years of curriculum are widely available. Nontraditional educational courses, which provide home study courses supplemented by supervised clinical teaching in local hospitals, have been another avenue of education leading to credentialing by the NBRC. On-the-job training, which formerly was used to train respiratory care personnel before educational programs were designed, still may be necessary, but only nonskilled positions should be filled with these individuals. Some departments may employ nurses who are specifically trained in the care of patients with pulmonary and cardiac diseases and who also have training in respiratory care per se. Similarly, physical therapists trained in chest physiotherapy may be employed by the respiratory care department to provide that service.

THE MEDICAL DIRECTOR OF THE RESPIRATORY CARE DEPARTMENT

As mentioned previously, a medical director of the hospital respiratory care department is required for the hospital to meet JCAHO accreditation[3] and to participate in Medicare.[4] The Joint Commission on Accreditation of Hospitals (JCAH) initially developed the standards for accreditation in 1973 that mandated a medical director of respiratory care.[5] Although these standards have been revised over the years, the medical director of respiratory care has always been included as an essential element of JCAH standards. Similarly, the most recent revision of the Medicare conditions of participation elevated respiratory care services to condition status and dictated that these services be under the aegis of a medical director.[4]

It is essential that the medical director of a respiratory care department have the proper qualifications to carry out his or her functions and responsibilities. The National Association of Medical Directors of Respiratory Care (NAMDRC), the American College of Chest Physicians (ACCP), and the Board of Medical Advisors (BOMA) of the American Association of Respiratory Care (AARC) have jointly passed a statement defining a *qualified* medical director of respiratory care.[6]

> The Medical Director of any inpatient or outpatient respiratory care service, department, or home care agency shall be a licensed physician who has special interest and knowledge in the diagnosis and treatment of respiratory problems. Whenever possible, the medical director should be qualified by special training and/or experience in the management of acute and chronic respiratory disorders. This physician should be responsible for the quality, safety, and appropriateness of the respiratory services provided, and require that respiratory care be ordered by a physician who has medical responsibility for the patient. The medical director should be readily accessible to the respiratory care practitioners and should assure their competency.

The key points of this statement are that medical direction in respiratory care can occur both within and outside the hospital and that the medical director should be a physician who has received specific training in the care and treatment of patients with acute and chronic respiratory diseases. (Medical direction in home care and at alternative sites will be discussed later in this chapter.) The vast majority of medical directors of respiratory care are pulmonologists.[7,8] The next largest group is anesthesiologists, who once formed the largest group of medical directors of respiratory care until the large influx of specialists from pulmonary disease-training programs in the 1970s and 1980s. Medical direction in respiratory care departments can also be provided by thoracic surgeons, internists, and a few others who have an interest but no specific training in pulmonary diseases.[7,8] The latter situation tends to occur in small, rural hospitals.

RESPONSIBILITIES OF THE MEDICAL DIRECTOR

The diverse responsibilities of the medical director are outlined in Table 4–1.[9] It is important that the hospital imparts the authority to the medical director to carry out these responsibilities. Thus, the medical director must be able to make day-to-day decisions on selected departmental activities untethered by hospital administrators, chiefs of staff, or others to accomplish his or her objectives and fulfill his or her responsibilities.

The medical director is responsible for the overall function of the respiratory care department.[10] He or she should delegate much of the responsibilities for the day-to-day operation of the department to the nonphysician director of the department. However, it is the medical director's responsibility to ensure that this individual and his staff perform well, to assure a properly operating respiratory care department that delivers high-quality patient care. If this does not occur, the medical director should effect the proper changes to ensure a smooth-running, efficient operation.

The medical director is also responsible for the quality of care delivered to patients by respiratory care personnel. This responsibility is one of the principal reasons that a medical director of respiratory care has been mandated by JCAH and Medicare. Many of the functions carried out by the medical director (see following section) directly relate to this important responsibility.

The medical director must provide a liaison between the respiratory care department and the medical staff. New therapies that are instituted must be communicated to the medical staff so that they may utilize them. The medical staff may have therapies that they wish the respiratory care department to perform. Only by effective communication between the medical director and the medical staff can these be accomplished. Medical staff input is necessary to ascertain how well the respiratory care staff is performing patient care.

The respiratory care department is one department among many in the hospital. Activities of other departments may directly influence activities of the respiratory care department. Similarly, the respiratory care department's functions also impinge on the output from other hospital departments. It is very important that the medical director ensure that effective communication exists between the respiratory care department and other hospital departments so that activities of one do not compromise or negate the activities of another. If all activities are not coordinated, patient care may be adversely affected. It is the responsibility of the medical director to make certain that this does not happen.

Respiratory care technology continues to expand rapidly. It is an additional responsibility of the medical director to ensure that respiratory care personnel keep abreast of these technological advances, as well as the changes in the therapies offered through the respiratory care department. Departmental in-service education is essential to impart new knowledge to the staff. Education can occur through an ongoing, scheduled program of lectures and conferences, as well as through scheduled rounds with members of the department. The medical director should make sure that department personnel are given time to attend educational meetings outside the hospital that will upgrade the individual's knowledge in respiratory care. A knowledgeable staff is more likely to provide quality patient care.

It is important that the medical director practice medicine and be available for patient consultation by the medical staff. He or she should serve as a model for other physicians to follow in the care of patients with pulmonary diseases. It is very important that the hospital grant the medical director the privilege of practicing medicine within the hospital.

Finally, the medical director must keep abreast of regulatory efforts by federal and state agencies, as well as the JCAHO, to ascertain that the department is in compliance with these regulations.

Table 4–1 Responsibilities of the Medical Director of Respiratory Care[9,11,12]

---

1. Responsible for the overall function of the respiratory care department
2. Responsible for the quality of care delivered by respiratory care personnel
3. Responsible for providing a liaison between the respiratory care department and the medical staff
4. Responsible for providing a liaison among the respiratory care department, hospital administration, and other hospital departments
5. Responsible for the in-hospital education of the respiratory care personnel
6. Responsible for the quality of care provided to his or her patients and those patients seen in consultation
7. Responsible for the respiratory care department's compliance with federal, state, and JCAHO regulation

---

FUNCTIONS OF THE MEDICAL DIRECTOR

The functions of the medical director are many[9,11,12] and continue to expand as technological advances occur, as governmental laws and regulations change, and as third-party payers regulate reimbursement. These functions can be categorized into administrative, supervisory, educational, and clinical areas. The list in Table 4–2 shows general categories rather than the myriad of specific functions.

The ultimate effect of reviewing and updating all departmental policies and procedures is to assure a quality operation. A departmental *Policies and Procedures Manual* is an absolute necessity. It should be reviewed in toto at least every 3 years and modified each year as new procedures and policies are added.

The quality of care delivered by the department

Table 4–2   Functions of the Medical Director of Respiratory Care

I. Administrative
   A. Review and update of all departmental policies
   B. Review and update of all departmental procedures
   C. Review and institute effective new respiratory therapy procedures
   D. Participate in the selection of new employees and in the dismissal of old employees
   E. Participate in development of cost-effective departmental budgets
   F. Participate in the selection and purchase of equipment
   G. Participate in departmental quality assurance activities
   H. Participate in the day-to-day activities of the department to the degree necessary to ensure quality patient services
II. Supervisory
   A. Observe the activities of the respiratory care personnel
   B. Certify respiratory care personnel for invasive and other procedures
III. Educational
   A. Review all departmental educational programs
   B. Participate in all educational activities of the department
   C. Participate in educational activities of medical staff and other hospital departments
IV. Clinical
   A. Provide care for primary patients
   B. Be available for patient consultations
   C. Perform procedures commensurate with training and education

is directly dependent on the expertise and training of respiratory care personnel. The selection of quality personnel is essential; this must be a function of the medical director in concert with the technical director of the department. Selection of a new director or assistant directors must be done carefully to assure competence in the management of the day-to-day operations of the department.

The medical director must have input into the budgetary process to guarantee a cost-effective operation. This is particularly important in determining salaries and the purchase of equipment. The development of a quality assurance program will assist in developing cost-effective budgets.

Even though the medical director is responsible for the overall function of the department, he or she should delegate the oversight of the day-to-day departmental activities to the respiratory care department technical director and his or her staff. It is the medical director's responsibility to keep abreast of the departmental affairs and he or she can do this only by spending an adequate amount of time in the department on an almost *daily* basis. This is the best way to effect clear communication and cooperation between the medical director and the technical director of the respiratory care department.

The supervisory functions of the medical director (see Table 4–2) are important to make certain that the quality of care administered to patients is of high caliber. The more complex the care, the more observation is necessary. Those individuals performing invasive procedures, such as intubation, arterial puncture and cannulation, mechanical ventilation, and others, should be certified by the medical director; this certification should be in writing and placed in the employee's file. Certification should be completed only after the therapist has received proper training and has been directly observed performing the procedure or function by the medical director or his designee. This will ensure the competence of the respiratory care staff.

The medical director should participate in the development and delivery of all the educational functions of the department. Usually, an educational director or a therapist who functions in this capacity develops the department's educational programs. The medical director should deliver some of the conferences, participate in others, and develop rounds in which respiratory care personnel can participate. The in-service program should be mapped out well in advance. Consideration should be given to videotaping the conferences so that personnel on the evening or night shifts can see them. The medical director should participate in the conferences of the medical staff, to update the medical staff's knowledge in the field of respiratory care.

It is important that the medical director have the time to perform his or her patient care functions. Often these functions, if properly structured, will allow educational opportunities for the respiratory care personnel. The medical director should be available for consultations regarding other physicians' patients, particularly those receiving mechanical ventilation. He or she should have the ability to admit and care for his or her own patients, as well as to perform those procedures (bronchoscopy, thoracentesis, pleural biopsy, chest tube placement, intubation, arterial and venous line placement, and others) for which he or she is qualified by training.

The medical director must be available to the respiratory care department 24 hours a day.[9,11,12] In a large department, this function and other responsibilities and duties (see Tables 4–1 and 4–2) can be shared with assistant medical directors appointed to the department. In a small department, the medical director should designate a competent physician to handle these responsibilities whenever he or she is away or is otherwise unavailable.

The medical director should be compensated for the time and services he or she provides to the department. The amount of compensation should directly relate to the amount of time spent in the department and *not* be tied in any way to its productivity (e.g., percentage of gross or net revenues, number of patients, and such). The medical director should have a written contract with the hospital defining his or her authority, responsibilities, functions, and reimbursement.

HOSPITAL LIAISONS IMPORTANT TO THE MEDICAL DIRECTOR

One of the most important relationships is that between the medical director and the technical director of the respiratory care department. The medical director will spend most of his time with the technical director, discussing and solving problems concerning the operations of the department. Together they set up the goals and objectives of the department. This interaction can be a most mutually rewarding experience. A good working relationship is crucial to the proper functioning of the medical director and the ability to achieve the goals and objectives set. Over the years, several medical

directors have complained of difficulties in performing their role. Almost always the problem boils down to the fact that the medical and technical directors of the respiratory care department do *not* have a good working relationship, or that the medical director does not spend sufficient time in the respiratory care department, or a combination thereof. It is important for the medical director to meet with the technical director on an almost *daily* basis and with the assistant directors and the supervisory staff on a *regular* basis. Participation in departmental staff meetings or meetings among the departmental director, assistant director(s), and supervisory staff is a necessity and will give the medical director an excellent view of the overall function of the department. Regular discussions with individual members of the department are also very important. This will greatly enhance the medical director's familiarity with his or her staff. Often problems with patients are discussed, and these can be solved efficiently and effectively.

The medical director is responsible to the hospital administration for the overall function of the respiratory care department. Often he or she works with a specific hospital administrator. It is very important that the medical director develop a solid working relationship with the hospital administrator. They should meet, along with the technical director of the respiratory care department, on a scheduled basis throughout the year. At times, special projects or events will dictate that a special meeting be set up with the administrator either with or without the technical director being present. Communication is crucial to determine solutions for departmental problems and to achieve the goals set.

The medical director will interact with other departments within the hospital, especially nursing. The medical director will be viewed as representing the respiratory care department; hence, it is important that contacts with nursing administration be amiable and constructive. The same can be said about his or her relationship with other hospital departments. In some hospitals, chest physical therapy is under the aegis of the physical therapy department. Timing of respiratory therapy (e.g., bronchodilator aerosol delivery) with chest physiotherapy is important and will have to be arranged between these two departments if chest physiotherapy is not a function of the respiratory care department. Again, a healthy relationship at the top will ensure good cooperation among therapists from both departments.

In many departments, the pulmonary function laboratory is under the aegis of the respiratory care department.[7,8] If the pulmonary function laboratory is a separate department under the aegis of a separate medical director, it is particularly important that the medical director of the respiratory care department interact closely with his or her counterpart from the pulmonary function laboratory. The qualifications and function of a medical director of a pulmonary function laboratory and of the pulmonary function laboratory staff are well delineated[9,13,14] and will be discussed later in the chapter. The personnel and medical director of the pulmonary function laboratory can be valuable resources for the respiratory care department, particularly for in-service training and research.

In larger hospitals, an intensive care unit (ICU) or group of ICUs each may have a designated medical director. It is important that the medical director of the respiratory care department interact with his ICU counterpart because respiratory care personnel provide many important functions within the ICU. Input concerning the operation of ventilators and other respiratory care equipment within the ICU, as well as the efficient and effective use of respiratory care personnel within the ICU, are extremely important. A good working relationship will facilitate the accumulation of this valuable information.

Because of the ever-expanding knowledge and technology in the field of respiratory care, it is important that the medical director keep abreast of new developments in the field. This information is presented in specialty journals and during regional and national meetings of subspecialty societies (e.g., American Thoracic Society, American Society of Anesthesiologists, American College of Chest Physicians). The membership of the National Association of Medical Directors of Respiratory Care consists of only medical directors. The information disseminated from NAMDRC is directed solely to the medical directors of respiratory care. To enhance his function, the medical director should join NAMDRC.

THE MEDICAL DIRECTOR OF THE PULMONARY FUNCTION LABORATORY

The pulmonary function laboratory is an essential element in the diagnosis and evaluation of patients with pulmonary diseases. A medical director is required for the proper function of this laboratory so that the physiologic results reported are accurate and timely.[9,13,14] If the pulmonary function laboratory is under the aegis of the respiratory care department, the medical director of the respiratory care department may also function as the medical director of the pulmonary function laboratory. He or she may opt to allow another physician to be the medical director of the pulmonary function laboratory.

The medical director of the pulmonary function laboratory must be a physician, or the equivalent, who has been trained and has expertise in pulmonary physiology. He or she must have in-depth knowledge of the devices, the significance of the data obtained from these devices, and how the data apply to the patient. In addition, he or she should possess the qualifications listed previously for the medical director of the respiratory care department (see page 50).

The medical director of the pulmonary function laboratory is accountable to the hospital administration, the hospital staff, and the medical director of the respiratory care department if the laboratory is under the aegis of that department. He or she is responsible for the quality of the data generated by the laboratory. He or she must train the pulmonary function staff if they have not received training, ascertain that they meet the requirements necessary to be competent in pulmonary function testing,[14] and supervise their activities closely. The development of a policy and procedures manual for the laboratory is critical and should be done with staff input. The medical director is responsible for developing written protocols for each test. The tests chosen should have proper quality control programs to reduce errors and ensure accurate results. The medical director is also responsible for determining and minimizing the risks associated with arterial punctures, exercise testing, administration of medications, inhalation challenges, and the possible transmission of infection to patients and staff through the laboratory equipment.[9]

The medical director of the pulmonary function laboratory must read and interpret all pulmonary function tests leaving the laboratory.[9,13,14] The only exception to this is arterial blood gas (ABG) values, which should be interpreted and utilized at the bedside by the attending physician. If the attending physician has a question about the meaning of the ABG values, the medical director or his designee should be readily available to interpret the results on a 24-hour basis.[9]

The economic matters of the pulmonary function laboratory are also the responsibility of the medical director. It is also his or her responsibility to make sure that the laboratory complies with regulations set forth by federal, state, or volunteer organizations.

The medical director of the pulmonary function laboratory should have the freedom to perform all the clinical functions that the medical director of the respiratory care department is allowed (see Table 4–2). These are discussed on page 52.

THE ATTENDING PHYSICIAN AND THE RESPIRATORY CARE TEAM

The attending physician has the responsibility for the overall care of the patient. He or she must initially assess the patient's needs, utilizing his or her skill in history taking and physical diagnosis and integrating this information, plus other data from the x-rays, ECG, and the various laboratories, to reach a definitive diagnosis. Once a diagnosis has been made, an effective treatment program should be formulated and followed. The respiratory care team may aid in making the diagnosis by performing pulmonary function testing, including arterial blood gas analysis, and may play a large part in the treatment plan if the patient's primary problem resides in the airways or pulmonary parenchyma.

The level of expertise of the attending physician in managing patients with pulmonary diseases depends upon his or her previous training in caring for these patients. Those with training in medicine usually have a more extensive pertinent background than those trained in surgery or the surgical subspecialties, with the exception of thoracic surgery. In-depth training in the pathophysiology of the vast array of pulmonary diseases and their therapy occurs in pulmonary disease and critical care training programs. Depending upon his or her training, the attending physician's knowledge of the use of respiratory care modalities in the treatment of patients with lung diseases may be detailed or superficial.

Respiratory care orders, like any others, need to be complete and specific. A proper respiratory care order includes the mode of therapy, its duration and frequency, and the dose of medication given. For example, an acceptable order for aerosolized albuterol could be written: aerosolized albuterol 2.5 mg in 2 mL saline q 4 hours. Depending upon the disease being treated, the dose ordered and the frequency could be varied considerably. Specific prescriptions for the various modalities of respiratory care can be found in the chapters on oxygen therapy, intermittent positive-pressure breathing (IPPB), incentive spirometry, chest physiotherapy,

and mechanical ventilation. A computerized respiratory care ordering system greatly limits the number of options available and clearly defines the orders possible for respiratory care. It is the responsibility of the respiratory care team to develop a cost-effective menu of respiratory care orders that will aid the attending physician in ordering what his patient needs. All respiratory care modalities ordered, except for mechanical ventilation, should have an automatic cut-off at 72 hours so that unneeded therapies are not continued indefinitely and the utilization of necessary therapy is reduced appropriately. Orders for respiratory care modalities that are outside the menu offered by the respiratory care department should be evaluated by the medical director and a decision made after a discussion with the attending physician.

The respiratory care team can be very helpful to attending physicians. Because the patient is seen frequently during the day, sudden changes in the patient's condition can be observed by the respiratory care personnel and these changes should be communicated quickly to the attending physician. Therapeutic needs of the patient frequently diminish as he or she improves. The respiratory care personnel should suggest a reduction in the intensity of therapy to the attending physician when this occurs. The respiratory care team can monitor the patient's pulmonary function at the bedside by simple measurements of vital capacity, tidal volume, inspiratory and expiratory forces, arterial blood gas levels, and spirometry, including pulmonary flows, or peak flow. Not all patients require monitoring, but those who are most ill, particularly those in the ICU, should have appropriate monitoring at appropriate intervals. The respiratory therapist should suggest to the attending physician that respiratory monitoring be performed whenever the patient's respiratory condition deteriorates. If monitoring is already being performed, the respiratory therapist should inform the attending physician of any significant deterioration in pulmonary function. This is most likely to occur in patients receiving mechanical ventilation. Thus, by effective monitoring and delivery of therapy, the respiratory care team can be particularly helpful to the attending physician.

The medical director of respiratory care can be helpful to the attending physician in several other ways. The medical director can serve as a repository of knowledge for the attending physician to tap whenever he or she requires it. This may take the form of an informal "curbside consultation" when a specific question needs addressing, or the attending physician may request a formal consultation from the medical director when a complex patient management problem arises. Effective communication between the attending physician and the medical director should greatly facilitate patient care. The medical director should be involved in delivering conferences on timely topics in respiratory care to the hospital staff. In this milieu, information can be imparted quickly to many. Another effective mode of communication between the respiratory care personnel and the attending physician is a handbook describing all the respiratory care modalities delivered by the department, those pulmonary diseases that may benefit from each modality, and the proper manner in which to order each modality. Good communication, whatever form it takes, is essential between the respiratory care team and the attending physician. Each respiratory care department should work diligently to achieve and maintain this goal.

THE MEDICAL DIRECTOR IN SCHOOLS OF RESPIRATORY CARE

The rationale for the necessity of medical direction in respiratory care educational programs has been reviewed in detail in Chapter 2. The Joint Review Committee on Respiratory Therapy Education (JRCRTE) reviews all educational programs. The most common reason for failure of the educational program to be certified by the JRCRTE is inadequate input from the medical director of the program and from other physicians involved in the affiliated institutions.[15] The medical director of a school in respiratory care should have all the qualifications listed earlier for a qualified medical director of respiratory care[7] (see page 50), and have the ability to teach and assist the program director in program development. The medical director must be responsible for the quality and validity of the scientific and clinical content of the program taught by the faculty. It is important that he or she teach at least one course each term and be available for assistance to other faculty in the program.

The medical director of an educational program in respiratory care is responsible for obtaining input from physicians in the hospitals used for the clinical portion of the students' curriculum. Student contact with these physicians is important for the students' growth and development as respiratory care practitioners. Establishment of good rapport with physicians should be learned as a student

and perfected as a graduate respiratory care practitioner.

A more detailed description of the responsibilities and functions of the medical director in schools of respiratory therapy is given in the 1977 "Essentials" of respiratory therapy education, but not in the new Essentials recently adopted by the JRCRTE.[16]

MEDICAL DIRECTION OF RESPIRATORY CARE SERVICES IN THE HOME AND IN ALTERNATIVE SITES

Respiratory care services provided in the hospital must be under the direction of a medical director to receive hospital accreditation by the Joint Commission on Accreditation of Health Care Organizations (JCAHO)[3] and as a condition of participation in Medicare.[4] The medical director of respiratory care was mandated in the hospital to assure that the respiratory care services provided were appropriate for the patient population and were of high quality. Those who provide respiratory care services in the home and in alternative community sites have an obligation to provide quality respiratory care services similar to those provided in the hospital.

A medical director would seem a logical choice to assure that good quality respiratory care services are provided in sites outside the hospital.[17] The American College of Chest Physicians (ACCP), the National Association of Medical Directors of Respiratory Care (NAMDRC), The American Thoracic Society (ATS) and the Board of Medical Advisors (BOMA) of the American Association of Respiratory Care (AARC) feel strongly that a qualified medical director is needed to supervise respiratory care services outside the hospital.[11,18,19]

The qualifications, responsibilities, and duties of a medical director of a home care company or an alternative community site have recently been delineated.[18,19] The medical director should be a licensed physician who has had specialized training and clinical experience in caring for patients with acute and chronic respiratory diseases, particularly those requiring home mechanical ventilation.[18,19] He or she should be responsible for the quality and appropriateness of the medical services, which should be delivered in a safe and cost-effective manner.[19] The medical director should be accessible to the respiratory care staff wherever they practice outside the hospital, as well as to the patients' private physicians.[19] It is his or her responsibility to see that the respiratory care provided has been prescribed by the patient's personal physician.[11] The responsibility for the overall care of the patient resides with the attending physician.

The functions of the medical director should be mainly administrative and educational and are listed in Table 4–3. The medical director should be involved in activities that lead to the delivery of quality, cost-effective respiratory care. This care must be delivered by qualified practitioners; hence, adequate personnel job descriptions and policies must be in place. All aspects of patient care must be reviewed by the medical director, including all patient care policies, treatment protocols, and procedure manuals, to make certain that the care provided by the respiratory care staff is appropriate and of high quality. The equipment used should be safe and reliable. New therapies should be used whenever the staff has the expertise and training to institute their use. A quality assurance program

Table 4–3 Functions of the Medical Director for Respiratory Care Services Provided Outside the Hospital[7,17]

I. Administrative Functions
   A. Develop and review personnel policies and job description
   B. Develop and review standards of patient care, including treatment protocols and procedure manuals
   C. Review and update all medical services delivered to patients to ensure high quality and cost-effectiveness
   D. Assess existing and new equipment and its application for patient use
   E. Develop and review quality assurance measures
   F. Assist with budgeting and reimbursement from fiscal and regulatory agencies if requested
   G. Ensure that the respiratory care services provided are in compliance with safety regulations and other regulations dictated by local, state, and federal governments
   H. Ensure that accreditation standards are met for JCAHO
II. Educational Functions
   A. Develop and review all patient programs and educational materials
   B. Develop and maintain staff in-service and education programs
   C. Serve as a medical resource for inquiries from staff, patients, and attending physicians concerning patient care and disease processes
   D. Educate third-party payers and others regarding the cost effectiveness and importance of providing quality respiratory care outside the hospital

should be designed to assess the effectiveness of the care provided to patients; this is also necessary because technology continues to advance rapidly in the field of respiratory care. The medical director may be asked to assist in matters of budgeting and reimbursement, depending upon his or her interests and expertise. All respiratory care should be in compliance with current safety standards and other regulations dictated by federal, state, and local governments. The JCAHO has developed standards to be met by providers outside the hospital.[20] The purpose of these standards is to protect the patient, assure a high quality of care, and prevent system abuse. This is a voluntary process for any company or facility delivering medical care outside the hospital. If the entity for which the medical director functions decides to seek accreditation, the medical director should be of assistance in any way possible to ensure that the accreditation standards are met.

The educational functions of the medical director are very important. The patient programs offered and the patient educational materials utilized need to be reviewed and updated for accuracy and applicability to patient care. It is important that patients readily understand the materials. Only those programs that are medically correct and efficacious should be continued. Development of an ongoing in-service training program for the respiratory care staff is important to keep knowledge updated and to introduce new technology and therapy. The medical director should have a large input into this area. He or she must be available to serve as a resource for inquiries concerning pathophysiology of disease processes, treatment and prognosis, and other aspects of respiratory care from staff, patients, and attending physicians. The medical director may need to discuss the cost-effectiveness and appropriateness of the respiratory care programs offered with third-party payers (including Medicare) and others.

In a recent study, 27% of home health agencies (HHAs) and 28% of durable medical equipment companies (DMEs) were found to have a designated medical director.[21,22] The remainder of the medical input was provided by the attending physicians. In a survey of skilled nursing facilities (SNFs), only 58% provided respiratory care services, and another 14% planned to provide these services in the future.[23] Of those SNFs providing respiratory care services, medical supervision was provided by a department medical director in only 17% of the facilities. The facility medical director provided the service in 34%, the attending physicians in 33%, and the remainder (16%) apparently had no medical supervision.[23] It has been suggested that all entities providing respiratory care services outside the hospital have input from a *qualified* medical director.[18,19] If a home care company or alternate site facility is part of a national corporation that has a medical director, input from the medical director may not meet the needs of the local company or facility, in which case a qualified, local medical director should be available.

The compensation for medical director services outside the hospital should be reasonable and commensurate with the time and effort expended. Reimbursement should *not* be based on the number of patients treated or on a percentage of the revenues from the hospital, home care company, or alternative community site facility.

FUTURE DIRECTIONS IN MEDICAL DIRECTION OF RESPIRATORY CARE SERVICES

In response to the institution of the Prospective Payment System (PPS), the AARC appointed a Task Force on Professional Direction composed of respiratory therapists and physicians in 1985. Its purpose was to determine the scope of practice of respiratory care, at that time, and to develop a "blueprint for action" for the future.[24] The task force developed its data base from six national surveys of respiratory care department managers (including a second survey), hospital administrators, medical directors of respiratory care departments, and program directors of respiratory therapist- and respiratory therapy technician-training programs. In addition to the "traditional" services administered,[25] it was found that nearly 80% of all hospital respiratory care departments also delivered nontraditional services in many areas, but most frequently in health promotion, cardiac or pulmonary rehabilitation, noninvasive cardiac diagnostics, home care or durable medical equipment, and electroencephalography.[24] The addition of nontraditional services was seen as a move by the hospitals to improve efficiency of operations and reduce costs. Traditional and nontraditional services were being provided by the same number or fewer staff in 76% of the hospitals.[24] These findings bring up some interesting points for the medical director of respiratory care. It appears that hospitals are attempting to control costs (which is good) but are attempting to provide more services with the same or fewer staff. The latter could lead to a decrease in the quality of respiratory care delivered (which is not good). The medical director will need to work diligently with his or her department technical director to avoid a reduction in the quality of services delivered by the respiratory care department, under any circumstances. If new services are added to the department, it is necessary that qualified, trained personnel deliver these services. This may mean hiring personnel who do not have respiratory care training or credentialing. The medical director will need to sharpen his or her skills and knowledge in the nontraditional areas while keeping abreast of the programs made in the technology and scientific basis of respiratory care. It may even be necessary to add one or more other medical directors with expertise in other fields (e.g., cardiology) if these services expand and the medical director of respiratory care does not feel comfortable advising in these nontraditional areas. The addition of a medical director (or directors) outside the area of respiratory care should be viewed as a positive step in the growth of the respiratory care department, affording all involved the opportunity to expand their knowledge base and provide improved patient care.

CONCLUSIONS

The future appears bright for the medical director and the respiratory care department. It is exciting to belong to a field that continues to grow in knowledge and scope of activities. One of the reasons respiratory care will continue to advance, in spite of forces present that could stifle progress, is the close relationship between physicians and respiratory care personnel fostered over the years. It is clear that working together to accomplish goals and objectives has worked in the past and will be successful in the future.

Finally, on a personal note, it has been, and will continue to be, a definite pleasure serving as a medical director of a respiratory care department. One of the highlights of the day is to go into the department to meet with the technical director and other members of the department. Being a medical director is fun and rewarding, both personally and professionally!

REFERENCES

1. Young JA, Singletary WS: History of the inhalation therapy–respiratory care profession. In Burton GG,

Hodgkin JE (eds): Respiratory Care: A Guide to Clinical Practice, pp 3–16. Philadelphia, JB Lippincott, 1977

2. American Association of Respiratory Care: Definition of respiratory care. Dallas. AARC, 1987

3. Joint Commission on Accreditation of Health Care Organizations: 1988 Accreditation Manual for Hospitals. Chicago, JCAHCO, 1988

4. Medicare conditions of participation. Fed Reg 51:116, 1986

5. Joint Commission on Accreditation of Hospitals: 1976 Accreditation Manual for Hospitals, pp 161–164. Chicago: JCAH, 1976

6. National Association of Medical Directors of Respiratory Care: NAMDRC definition of a qualified medical director of respiratory care. Washington, DC, NAMDRC, 1986

7. American Association of Respiratory Care: 1983 Human resources survey. Dallas, AARC, 1983

8. National Association of Medical Directors of Respiratory Care: Membership survey. Washington, DC, NAMDRC, 1987

9. National Association of Medical Directors of Respiratory Care: Position statement: Duties and responsibilities of medical directors of respiratory care services and pulmonary function laboratories. Washington, DC, NAMDRC, 1987

10. Yanda, RI: The Management of Respiratory Care Services. New York, Projects in Health, 1976

11. American Thoracic Society: Position paper: Medical director of respiratory care. Am Rev Respir Dis 138:1082, 1987

12. Miller WF, Plummer AL et al: Guidelines for organization and function of hospital respiratory care services. Chest 78:79–83, 1980

13. ATS Respiratory Care Committee Position: The director of pulmonary function laboratory. ATS News 4:6, 1978

14. American Thoracic Society: Position paper: Pulmonary function laboratory personnel qualifications. Am Rev Respir Dis 134:623–624, 1986

15. Burton GG: The physician and the respiratory care team. In Burton GG, Hodgkin JE (eds): Respiratory Care: A Guide to Clinical Practice, 2nd ed., pp 82–90. Philadelphia, JB Lippincott, 1984

16. American Medical Association: Essentials of an approved program for the respiratory therapy technician and the respiratory therapist. Chicago, Council on Allied Health Education, 1977

17. Plummer AL: Medical direction of home care. Respir Manag 17:9, 1987

18. American Association of Respiratory Care: Medical direction for respiratory care services provided outside of the hospital. Dallas, AARC, 1989

19. National Association of Medical Directors of Respiratory Care: NAMDRC position statement on medical direction of home health care. Washington, DC, NAMDRC, 1988

20. Joint Commission on Accreditation of Health Care Organizations: Standards for the accreditation of home care. Chicago, JCAHCO, 1988

21. American Association of Respiratory Care: 1987 Human resources survey. Home health agencies. Dallas, AARC, 1987

22. American Association of Respiratory Care: 1987 Human resources survey. Durable medical equipment companies. Dallas, AARC, 1987

23. American Association of Respiratory Care: 1987 Human resources survey. Skilled nursing facilities respondents. Dallas, AARC, 1987

24. American Association of Respiratory Care: The impact of prospective payment on the respiratory care profession. Report of the Task Force on Professional Direction. Dallas, AARC, 1986

25. American Association of Respiratory Care: The role of the respiratory care practitioner in the provision of respiratory care services in hospitals and alternative sites. Dallas, AARC, 1987

FIVE

Legal and Ethical Concerns in Respiratory Care

Thomas J. DeKornfeld

The problems of health care delivery are not limited to the prevention, diagnosis, and treatment of disease. They also include, in an ever-increasing degree, the legal and ethical concerns that are characteristic of our complex and rapidly changing civilization. No practitioner in any phase of the health care delivery system can afford to ignore the legal implications of health care or the ethical principles that impinge so profoundly on the provider–consumer relationships. To cover both the legal and ethical concerns in one brief chapter is not easy and, obviously, the material must be presented in a highly condensed fashion. Many areas can be touched upon only briefly, and some areas of importance will not be addressed at all.

There is merit in discussing legal and ethical issues as a single unit, since there is considerable overlap between the two. The primary distinction is that the law is a public matter, set down in writing, and not subject to individual interpretation. Ethics, on the other hand, is largely an emotional issue, an area of deeply felt personal beliefs, rarely codified and subject to wide individual interpretation. The two areas overlap: many areas in the realm of ethics have been given a statutory underpinning, and many areas of law are the result of fundamentally ethical concerns, namely, the distinction between right and wrong.

The basic principles of both areas will be discussed separately. The second half of the chapter will attempt to meld the two areas into an issue-oriented whole.

In much of the following discussion, the role of the physician is emphasized because, under our present system of health care delivery, the physician is still the primary contractor and most of the health care providers function as assistants or legal "servants" of the physician or as employees of the hospital. There are exceptions to this, of course, and nurse practitioners, other health practitioners, and some respiratory therapists function as independent contractors and are thus subject to the same legal and ethical constraints and liabilities as the physician.

LEGAL RELATIONSHIPS

PHYSICIAN–PATIENT RELATIONSHIP

The physician–patient relationship is the basis of all medical practice. Whenever an individual contacts a physician and the physician agrees to provide a service to that person, a legal relationship is established that cannot be unilaterally dissolved (by the physician) without certain clearly defined conditions. This does not mean that the physician must "accept" every patient. In fact, the physician is quite at liberty not to accept any patient, and no reason need be given for such a refusal. Even under emergency conditions, no legal requirement forces a physician to render a service if the physician chooses not to do so. There are some exceptions to this rule; for example, a physician employed by a hospital to provide medical services in the emergency room or a "walk-in clinic" must render appropriate services to *all* patients. Similar principles apply to all employed physicians whose conditions of employment imply or, indeed, specify that they must render services to certain groups of patients or employees. Physicians working in public institutions may not refuse any patient in violation of constitutional or statutory mandate.

Ethical considerations make it improper for a physician to refuse his services to a patient in need, but no legal constraints force him to do so. However, as soon as the physician indicates a willingness to see a patient or listen to a complaint, a legal relationship has been established. The physician now has the duty to act with due care, to provide this patient with the proper information or services appropriate to the situation.

In general, the physician–patient relationship can exist under one of two legal theories. Under the *contract theory*, a direct or implied contract exists between the two parties. The physician agrees to provide a service for a fee. This theory is not a particularly good one, for it applies poorly to emergency situations, when the service is rendered without the expectations of a direct fee. The second theory holds that accepting a patient creates a *professional relationship* in which the physician accepts the responsibility for rendering due care. This professional relationship, legally, falls under the law of tort and, indeed, courts generally view the physician–patient relationship in this light. Personal contact is not necessary for establishing a professional relationship. For example, a radiologist viewing x-ray films or a pathologist examining a surgical specimen has a professional relationship with the patient and owes the patient due care as a professional obligation.

The professional relationship will remain in effect until either the patient chooses to select a different physician or the physician withdraws from the case. If the physician unilaterally decides to discontinue medical care of the patient without adequate warning and without appropriate provision for replacement, this results in injury to the patient, *abandonment* is said to occur. This can serve as the basis for legal action on the part of the patient. The fact that a patient does not follow the physician's instructions may constitute adequate reason for a physician to withdraw from the care of the patient,

but only if reasonable notice is given, if there is an equally competent replacement available, and if the patient understands and agrees.

Thus, the first component of the physician–patient relationship is that a *duty* exists. Second, the physician must use reasonable skill and care in providing his or her services. This is the fundamental consideration of health care and, probably, the most difficult one to define or quantify. No physician or other health care provider is expected to function perfectly or even consistently above the average. The general standard, however, to which all health care providers must conform has been nicely stated by the court in *Blair v Eblen*:[1] "A physician is under a duty to use that degree of skill which is expected of a reasonably competent practitioner in the same class to which he belongs, acting in the same or similar circumstances."

This definition does not exclude the honest differences of opinion that are quite common in health care. If there are two or more options by which a condition can be diagnosed or treated, any one of these options can be chosen, provided that at least a "respectable minority" of the profession support that choice. Even if, in retrospect, another option may have been better, the standard has not been violated if the choice was "reasonable."

The profession generally has no written disease- or condition-specific standards, and it has been reluctant to establish such. Consequently, deviations from the standard have to be determined by a judge or jury. Because the jury probably has inadequate knowledge to make such decisions, expert testimony is required to educate the jury by explaining the medical facts and by giving testimony on the standards of care. In the past, these standards of care had to conform to the standards of the community and to the level of care appropriate to the training and experience of the physician who provided the care. Presently, the "locality rule" has been rejected and, for medical specialists, standards of care reflect national, rather than regional or local, standards. Presumably the same would apply to credentialled respiratory therapists.

The standard of care for a specialist should be that of a reasonable specialist practicing medicine in the light of present-day scientific knowledge. Therefore, geographic conditions or circumstances control neither the standard of specialist's care nor the competence of an expert's testimony.

The third component of a tort is that there have to be damages. If there are no damages, the patient is not entitled to compensation, even though the health care provider may have been negligent. Obviously, the patient is at liberty to, and probably should, switch doctors, but there is no legal foundation for seeking compensatory payments since there was no injury.

The forth and final component of a tort is that there has to be a proximate causal relationship between the negligence and the damages. In other words, the injury must be the direct result of a breach of the standard of care. The case of *Fayson v Saginaw General Hospital*[2] illustrates this important point. Because of the unquestioned negligence of an anesthesiologist, Fayson aspirated gastric contents and developed acute respiratory distress syndrome (ARDS). In the intensive care unit (ICU) he was entrusted one evening to a licensed practical nurse (LPN) with no experience and no instruction. The respirator became disconnected, the alarm was turned off, and the LPN failed to recognize the problem. When it was pointed out to **her** by the patient's wife, the LPN ran out of the room in search of the registered nurse (RN). Fayson suffered severe brain damage. A jury found the anesthesiologist not liable and held the hospital liable for the incompetence of its employee.

Negligence, although by far the most common cause for a malpractice suit, is by no means the only reason why a patient may start litigation against a health care provider. Other reasons for a consumer–provider suit include assault and battery, breach of confidentiality, invasion of privacy, fraud, and several others.

Assault and battery, in common parlance, is considered to be the application of a baseball bat to somebody's head. In legalese, assault and battery means the unauthorized touching of another person's body, for whatever reason. In other words, every person has the absolute right to decide what will be done to him or her, and every diagnostic or therapeutic manipulation that is done without the patient's permission technically constitutes assault and battery. Consequently the patient must *consent* to whatever the health care provider recommends or wishes to do. The necessary components of consent are that it must be free, that it must be informed, and that the patient must be legally able to grant consent.

The *freedom of consent* principle applies primarily, although not exclusively, to experimental work and was first formulated in the Nuremberg Declaration,[3] following World War II, as a consequence of the experimentation performed on prisoners in German concentration camps.

The problem of *informed consent* is considerably more complicated. The patient is entitled to the opportunity to make an intelligent choice between treatment and no treatment or between two different types of treatment, but this is not accomplished easily. It is impossible to detail all the possible complications that might ensue from the administration of a drug or from a surgical or medical procedure, and the law does not require this. Nevertheless, all health care providers must make a reasonable effort to explain (in lay language) the major hazards of any proposed drug or treatment. In addition, a patient must be given the opportunity to ask questions or seek advice from an outside source. No patient should ever be misled, and serious hazards, if known, should always be explained in as much detail as needed, to enable the patient to make a choice or at least to understand the hazards to which he or she will be subjected. When possible, such explanations should be given even for such relatively innocuous procedures as oxygen administration, humidity therapy, or intermittent positive-pressure breathing.

Before any "treatment" is given, it is important that the patient understands what the treatment is, its purpose, its risks, the availability of reasonable alternatives, and the benefits that should be derived from it. Questions must be answered and, if the patient refuses the treatment, under no circumstances should it be administered. It is the patient's absolute and unquestionable privilege to refuse a diagnostic or therapeutic procedure. Even if consent is obtained, the patient has the right to withdraw such consent at any time and without having to state any reason for so doing. If a patient refuses consent, the possible hazards of this decision must also be explained. The court in *Truman v Thomas*[4] concluded that "If a patient indicates that he or she is going to refuse a risk-free test or treatment, then the doctor has the additional duty of advising of all material risks of which a reasonable person would want to be informed before deciding not to undergo this procedure."

The last, but by no means least, component of consent is that it must be valid (i.e., it must be granted by a person who is legally entitled to do so). In general, only a competent adult can give consent for himself or herself. Adulthood is a matter of age and is determined in all states by statute. If may be as young as 18 or as old as 21 years. All health care providers must be aware of local laws. Competence is more difficult to determine, and every adult is considered to be competent unless declared to be incompetent by a court of law. A patient may behave in the most bizarre fashion and even claim to be Napoleon, but he still may be legally competent. This places the provider, at times, in a very difficult dilemma. The usual solution is to seek consent from the family. This may be comforting to the provider, but has no legal significance whatsoever. A spouse or another family member has no legal right to consent for a "conscious and competent" family member.

If the patient is unconscious or patently incompetent, in cases of life-threatening emergencies, and when consent cannot be obtained, physicians may proceed with life-saving measures. Courts have decided that this is entirely proper in those situations for which it can be reasonably assumed that the patient would have given consent had he or she been able to do so.

For minors, the parent or legal guardian must give consent. There are, however, some situations in which a minor can legally consent. A minor is considered legally "emancipated" if he or she is married, a member of the armed forces, living away from the family home and providing for himself or herself, or if he or she is declared "adult" by a court. In most states, there are also statutory exceptions. These usually are in the realm of reproductive problems or sexually acquired diseases.

Consent need not be in writing, although most institutions have policies to this effect. The consent form should be signed by the patient, by the person obtaining the consent and, if possible, by a witness not involved directly in that patient's care. The simple, all-inclusive consent form that patients formerly signed on admission, which gave "permission" to a physician to do anything and everything, is no longer considered sufficient. The consent form should specify the diagnostic or therapeutic manipulation to which the patient consents and should have a space for the likely complications, particularly if these complications are serious, disfiguring, disabling, or likely to interfere with the patient's quality of life.

The next legal aspect of the physician–patient relationship is the *confidentiality* of the information that the physician obtains. Everything a patient confides to his or her physician, everything that forms part of the patient's record must remain absolutely confidential and cannot be revealed without the patient's permission. This includes not only the physician's notes, but also the nurses' notes, respiratory care notes, laboratory data, and all personal, technical, or other information that may be contained in the patient's chart. The observations made by the nurse or by the respiratory therapy technologist are a part of the confidential legal document and must be handled with the same concern for confidentiality as the admission diagnosis, history, or physical findings.

From a practical viewpoint, all persons who may need information about the patient's care must have access to the record, including nurses, respiratory therapists, and others who participate in the patient's care. The rule of confidentiality, therefore, is extended to this group as well, and it must be respected strictly and without exception. It is an inexcusable breach of this rule to discuss a patient's problems in public, and even discussion among professionals should be limited to the nature of the problem, without identification of the patient. Although it is common practice to discuss "an interesting case" with colleagues, unless this is done for the purposes of consultation or teaching and unless the patient's anonymity is preserved or his consent for disclosure is obtained, this is a breach of confidence that is actionable.

Breach of promise is a rare, but not unheard of, cause for litigation. If a health care provider is stupid enough to guarantee results, the patient may very well sue under the legal theory of breach of promise if the results are not as expected. Technically, every time we tell a patient: "Don't worry, everything will be all right," we make a promise. Fortunately, courts have ruled that for a breach of promise to be actionable, the promise has to be made in writing or has to be made under circumstances from which its contractual nature is evident.

A less rare and very disturbing suit is one brought on the basis of *fraud.* This usually means that a patient has been told that a test or procedure had been performed when, in fact, the test or procedure was not performed, but the patient was charged for the service. Fraud is a criminal charge that will lead not only to a heavy fine and possibly a prison sentence, but almost certainly to loss of license.

PATIENT–HOSPITAL RELATIONSHIP

Until recently, the relationship of the patient to the hospital was quite similar to that of a guest to a hotel. The hospital was obligated to provide a safe, salubrious environment, room and board, and the facilities and personnel necessary for a physician to practice his trade. The hospital was further obligated to provide safe and usable equipment and personnel who either participated with the physician in the care of the patient or who were responsible for the proper functioning of the building as a hotel and restaurant. The hospital did not have any responsibility for the quality of medical care being practiced in the facility, although, traditionally, it participated with the medical staff in administrative decisions pertaining to practice privileges and to other similar items. Although the hospital employed and compensated the nurses and other health practitioners and was responsible for their actions, they were frequently held to be under the control of the physicians. It was the physician who was responsible for the employee's error under the doctrine of the borrowed servant.

Before Darling (see below), the hospital was liable only for harm to the patient caused by personnel, equipment, or circumstances under its control. This situation has now changed dramatically. The celebrated case of *Darling v Charleston Community Hospital*[5] has established the principle, at least in Illinois, that the hospital, through its lay governing board, is responsible for the standards of medical care practiced in the hospital. This means that the hospital, as a corporate entity, may be held responsible if it permits the physicians on its staff to practice below acceptable standards and the hospital had the ability to prevent harm. In other words, the hospital board of trustees must make sure that there is a suitable medical staff organization, that there are bylaws governing the activities of the medical staff, that the standards set by the Joint Commission on Accreditation of Healthcare Organizations (JCAHO) are met, and that the medical staff properly polices itself according to stated specific procedures.

The most important case since Darling on this matter has been *Gonzales v Nork*,[6] which was decided by the California Supreme Court in 1978. This is a case in which the issue of the hospital's corporate responsibility was carefully investigated and in which Mr. Justice Goldberg, in a most convincing and literate opinion, concluded that

> . . . the hospital by virtue of its custody of the patient, owes him a duty of care; this duty includes the obligation to protect him from acts of malpractice by his independently retained physician who is a member of the hospital staff, if the hospital knows, or has reason to know, or should have known that such acts were likely to occur.

A much more frightening decision was rendered in *Corleto v Shore Memorial Hospital*.[7] In this New Jersey case, a court held the medical staff, collectively, and the medical staff members, individually, liable for the negligence of a staff member.

In the United States, with few exceptions, all practicing physicians have some form of hospital affiliation that can take one of two basic forms: The physician may be employed by the hospital, or the physician may be granted practice privileges in the hospital without being in any way compensated by the hospital or in the hospital's employ. The number of hospital-based and hospital-paid physicians is increasing steadily. In this system, physicians function legally as employees of the hospital, receive all or most of their compensation from the hospital, and perform specific tasks for the hospital that may be administrative, educational, patient care, or a combination of these. In this situation, the source of professional incomes is either a salary from the hospital or a salary from an agency or organization that operates the hospital and employs the physician. An example of this latter situation is the federal or state government that employs physicians in the armed forces, Public Health Service, Veterans Administration, or other federal or state organizations. Certain nongovernmental organizations may also employ physicians, who then perform all or most of their work in a hospital with which they have no financial relationship. Examples of this type of practice are the hospitals maintained by industrial or labor organizations and major prepaid hospital plans such as the Kaiser-Permanente group in California and the proliferating health maintenance organizations (HMOs). Another type of hospital-based practice is that of the full-time medical director of the respiratory care department, the emergency room physicians, and the medical director of intensive care units, among others.

The most common form of practice in the United States is still the private "fee-for-service" practice, in which the physician bills the patient for services rendered and payment is made by the patient or by a third-party payer (i.e., an insurance company).

The legal situation differs depending on which of the foregoing relationships exists between the physician and the hospital. If the physician is a full-time employee of the hospital, the relationship is simple and clear, and the hospital is responsible for the action of the physician as long as he is performing his duties within the context of his employment. If the physician, however, is granted only "hospital privileges" (i.e., he is admitted to the hospital staff and has the prerogative of admitting patients to the hospital and directing their care while in the hospital), the legal situation is much more complex.

Every hospital staff, comprising all the physicians with privileges in the hospital, traditionally establishes its own bylaws, which are then approved by the hospital's governing body. These bylaws specify the categories of staff privileges and the conditions under which physicians are eligible for staff positions. In addition, the bylaws also establish the staff organization and deal with such matters as continuing education requirements, quality assurance, meetings, elections, and the steps for due process to be followed for admission to the dismissal from the staff.

The medical staff bylaws may also limit certain physicians, on the basis of training, to the performance of certain patient services. For instance, in a number of hospitals only trained obstetricians are permitted to perform forceps deliveries or cesarean sections, whereas family practitioners may perform uncomplicated manual deliveries. In others, the care of patients who require ventilatory support may be limited only to those physicians trained and experienced in such activity (ventilator privileges). The bylaws may also specify the requirements for mandatory consultation. In one hospital, for example, no patient may be given continuous respirator care without the approval of a chest physician or an anesthesiologist.

Until the Darling decision, the hospital had no control over the physicians who enjoyed staff privileges in the hospital. As long as the physicians were willing to abide by the bylaws of the medical staff and maintained their license to practice medicine, the only controls over the quality of their practice were the elasticity of their conscience and the very mild peer pressures exerted by their colleagues. The fear of a suit for negligence also may have contributed to the quality of care. It has certainly forced most practitioners to practice a more defensive type of medicine, which may have benefited the patient's health, but, most certainly, has affected his or her pocketbook.

Changing attitudes toward the hospital's legal liability have made it imperative that the hospital's bylaws and medical staff regulations be carefully reviewed and conform with current practices. The steps for admission to the medical staff and, particularly, the disciplinary mechanisms whereby physicians can be corrected by their peers or dismissed from the staff must be specific and in accordance with due process. Highly desirable disciplinary measures have been frustrated when the physician or employee to be disciplined could show that due process had not been followed.

The Darling, Gonzales, and Corleto decisions raise some particularly awkward problems, not only for the formally constituted medical staff organizations of the hospital, but also for all hospital employees, particularly nurses and respiratory therapists. The operative phrase in all the foregoing cases was the ". . . the hospital knew or should have known . . ." that a physician was incompetent. The only way the hospital can know this is when somebody tells them. The implication is obvious: The hospital administration must establish quality assurance, credentials, and tissue committees and must make sure that these committees report regularly on any staff member who appears to violate the standards set for the institution; also, any employee who has information suggesting professional incompetence has the obligation to bring this matter to the attention of the hospital administration in a formal way—by an appropriate reporting mechanism. This may take various forms but is usually an "incident report" addressed to the hospital administration that outlines the alleged incident, identifies the persons involved and, most important, identifies the person filing the report.

Thus, the employees' duty is clear: They must report the negligent or incompetent colleague, even though this duty leaves them with a painful and potentially dangerous dilemma. Very few people enjoy "blowing the whistle" on a colleague, and the traditional relationship between physicians and nonphysicians makes it very difficult for the latter to "rat" on the former. Furthermore, the suggestion of professional incompetence will have to be substantiated before the medical staff organization, and failure to do so may leave the complainant liable to disciplinary action, possible dismissal, and even legal action for damages. Therefore, the decision to report or not to report observed deviations from the standard of care must remain an individual one. To report is an ethical and legal requirement, but one not without individual hazard; not to report is a "cop-out" that may also have legal implications, because the withholding of such information may very well implicate the person as sharing the responsibility for future damages. Yet, as Mr. Justice Goldberg has stated in the *Gonzales v Nork* case:

> As for the doctors on the Mercy Staff, two thoughts keep going through my mind. The one is from Dr. Jones [physician on the Mercy Staff]: "No one told anyone anything." The other is from Edmund Burke [an 18th century English politician]: "The only thing necessary for the triumph of evil is for good men to do nothing."

Of particular interest in this context is Public Law 99660, also known as the Health Care Improvement Act of 1986. This places a heavy reporting responsibility on the hospitals and state licensing boards and grants immunity to those who report on a physician or dentist's malpractice or other disciplinary action. Public Law 99660 will undoubtedly profoundly affect the practice of medicine once the Federal Disciplinary Data Bank is in operation.

PHYSICIAN–TECHNOLOGIST RELATIONSHIP

Under the bylaws of the American Association for Respiratory Care and the National Board of Respiratory Care, and under the standards published by the JCAHO, respiratory therapy technologists must work under competent medical supervision. Although there have been many unfortunate exceptions, this relationship has generally been mutually beneficial, and the medical director concept has worked well whenever there was a concerned, competent physician to serve in this capacity. The relationship between the technologist and the medical director or any other physician comprises personal, professional, and legal elements.

The legal relationship between a physician and a technologist depends largely on whether the technologist is employed by the physician. If an employer–employee relationship exists, then the legal liability that the physician has for the actions of the technologist is clear and well established in law. The doctrine of *respondeat superior* states that the "master" is responsible for all damages caused by the "servant." The terms master and servant, although not current in their social connotation, are still very much a feature of current legal practice. Nevertheless, to be liable for the actions of an employee, certain legal requirements must be met. It must be shown that the employee acted within the scope of his or her employment; that he or she was, in fact, negligent; and that this negligence was the proximate cause for the alleged injuries. Of these, the first one needs some additional comment.

A physician employer of a respiratory therapy technologist would not be responsible if the technologist drove a car under the influence of alcohol while on vacation and caused damage to person or property. This situation is clear, but in other instances, a jury would have to decide the limits of liability. If, for example, a respiratory therapy technologist in the hospital administers IPPB therapy to a patient, and at the end of treatment decides to adjust a surgical dressing or an orthopedic appliance, thereby causing some injury to the patient, this act is clearly outside the professional competence of the respiratory therapy technologist. That task does not form part of his or her usual and customary activities, and it would thus be a matter for a jury to decide whether the employer was responsible for this action of the employee.

Another delicate area in the physician–technologist relationship is the legal situation that arises when a technologist executes an order that is clearly improper and for which the technologist, by virtue of his training, could or should have known that the order, if followed, was likely to lead to an injury to the patient. The classic example is the misplaced decimal point. Let us assume that 0.5 mL of isoproterenol (Isuprel) is intended for a bronchodilator aerosal treatment, but, because of haste or carelessness, the order reads 5.0 mL. What is the responsibility of the technologist charged with delivering the treatment? Should he or she go ahead? Should he or she refuse to administer the potentially harmful dose, or should he or she arbitrarily change the dose to what is considered safe and appropriate? Few, if any, legal precedents give a clear answer to this dilemma in respiratory care.

If the technologist knowingly administers a dose that is clearly in excess of the usual and customary dose, he or she may be held responsible as the direct tort feasor, even though the primary responsibility is still the physician's who issued the incorrect order. I believe that, under the circumstances, the technologist has the duty to contact the responsible physician or, in his or her absence, the medical director of respiratory therapy and seek clarification or correction of the unusual order. The technologist should neither carry out nor willfully ignore or modify a physician's order without taking all necessary steps to have the situation clarified. I feel that carrying out an obviously dangerous and probably erroneous order places the technologist in legal jeopardy. Willfully ignoring or modifying an order, without seeking competent advice, may place the technologist in jeopardy as far as his or her employment is concerned. A technologist can certainly refuse to carry out any order, but by so doing, may leave himself open to severe and justifiable criticism if it should turn out that the order was indeed appropriate for that particular patient, who suffered injury in consequence of the technologist's refusal to carry out the order. Generally, it seems a wise policy to have technologists question all orders that they do not fully understand. With few exceptions, physicians will appreciate the opportunity to rectify an error or to explain the reason for orders that may appear unusual or excessive.

If the technologist is employed by the hospital, the physician may still be liable under the doctrine of the *borrowed servant*. This doctrine states that a "superior" who has the power and the right to control the activities of the employee of another person or organization is responsible for the negligence of that employee.

TECHNOLOGIST–HOSPITAL RELATIONSHIP

There are two levels of relationship between respiratory therapy technologists and the hospital in which they work and by which they are employed. One level relates to the professional activities of the technologist; the other relates simply and exclusively to the nonprofessional employer–employee interaction that is no different from the relationship of any employee to any employer.

Under current legal practice, the hospital, as a corporate entity, will be responsible for the technologist's negligence under *respondant superior*, a responsibility that may or may not not be shared by the nonemployer physician, as discussed earlier. It therefore behooves the hospital to insure, and to insure adequately, against claims for damages because of the negligence of its employees.

Legal Implications of Employment

Employment is a contract that establishes a legal relationship between employer and employee. The offer of a job to an applicant, and its acceptance by the applicant, establish a contractual relationship between the two parties that entails clear and binding conditions, which, if broken by either party, open the door to legal remedies.

Under federal and state regulations, all offers for employment must be made in good faith and the job must be available to all qualified applicants regardless of age, sex, race, religion, physical handicap, or national origin. There are a few exceptions to this rule, for example, when the nature of the job demands certain physical characteristics that can be met only by males or females. In addition, child labor laws clearly specify the conditions under which minors can be permitted to work.

Under the present regulations of the *Fair Employment Practice Act*, each job vacancy in any public institution must be advertised in suitable and appropriate media, giving a description of the job, qualifications for employment, approximate salary range, and any other pertinent data that would enable potential candidates to determine their interest in or suitability for the job.

Applicants must then complete a formal job application outlining their vital statistics, previous training, work record, and references for past performance. For many positions a personal interview is required, and for certain types of technical jobs a specialized examination may be administered. From this information, the employer makes a decision and selects the most suitable candidate for the job, preparing a written justification both for selecting that particular candidate and also for turning down the other candidates whose basic qualifications conformed with the advertised job specifications. Once the candidate is selected and an appropriate salary has been agreed on, the employee is processed through various initial stages of employment including the completion of paper documentation that serves to establish the new employee as a full-fledged member of the organization.

New employees, with some exceptions, are usually placed on probation for 3 to 6 months, during which orientation and in-service training take place. During this time, the employer is at liberty to discharge the probationary employee if it becomes evident that the job and the employee are not well suited. After the probationary period, the employee becomes a "regular," who is entitled to the elaborate and often cumbersome mechanisms designed to protect him or her against any capricious and arbitrary actions on the part of the employer.

When a respiratory technologist accepts a position offered in good faith, a contract is established that is binding on both him or her and the employer. Breaking the contract and walking away from the job, particularly in a supervisory position, is a breach of contract under the law and a reprehensible act by any civilized standard of behavior. It places a significant burden on the hospital and on the remaining members of the department. It also adversely affects patient care and, thereby, infringes quite clearly on the principles of ethics that must guide all health professionals.

In fact, one of the most common complaints of hospital administrators and medical directors has been the extreme mobility of respiratory therapists. Even the maintenance of an accurate state respiratory care chapter mailing list has become a herculean task, further demonstrating the problems. It is a fundamental human endeavor to improve one's economic and occupational status, and every serious attempt to grow in one's chosen field is both laudable and in the best interests of the profession as a whole. Nevertheless, "job-hopping" places an extreme hardship on individual departments and hospitals, particularly those whose salary structure is relatively inflexible because of the funding mechanisms under which they operate.

Salary

Every employee is entitled to financial compensation commensurate with the type of employment that he or she is expected to assume and with the training and experience of the employee. Salaries should be negotiable within certain ranges established by the employer's salary and wage officers. The salary may be calculated on an hourly, monthly, or annual basis, and payments may be made weekly, biweekly, or monthly.

Fringe Benefits

In almost all employment situations, except for part-time or temporary employees, the salary package includes a variety of fringe benefits, including Social Security benefits, retirement programs, health and accident insurance, life insurance, vacation and sick time, and occasional financial support for continuing education.

Working Conditions

The employer is obliged to provide adequate working areas that meet the requirements of fire and occupational safety. Increasing concern over exposure to low-level toxic substances and the traditional lack of protection against dust and other pulmonary irritants have led to significant improvements in environmental controls. Much still needs to be done in this area, and the rapidly increasing number of identified carcinogens and teratogens makes the environmental protection process of employees an expensive and complex matter.

Grievance Mechanism

Most employers establish written policies for handling complaints, even if collective-bargaining agreements do not extend to all employees. The due process of law, discussed earlier, clearly applies to all grievance procedures, and most employees are entitled to have their complaints heard and adjudicated by an orderly and well-established mechanism.

The legal obligations of the employee are much more difficult to categorize with any degree of pre-

cision. Basically, employees commit themselves to perform their legitimately assigned duties satisfactorily, to keep their employer's interests at heart, and to perform "an honest day's work." Employees must also protect the employer's property as far as possible, maintain a clear distinction between "mine and thine," and give the employer adequate notice, such that a replacement can be obtained without a major disruption of work schedules or patient services.

LAWS AFFECTING HEALTH CARE DELIVERY

Licensing

The right to practice medicine has been interpreted to be a guarantee made to all citizens by the United States Constitution. Interpretation of the Constitution over the years, however, has also clearly established the principle that the states have the right to protect the public and to enact laws to promote the public welfare. This prerogative of the states has been upheld by the United States Supreme Court in several decisions. States may, through appropriate and legally constituted boards, regulate the practice of medicine and other modalities of health care. All states have enacted laws to establish legal bodies and boards to determine the minimum requirements that health professionals must meet before they are admitted to the particular practice of their choice. The prototype of these bodies is the State Board of Medical Examiners, which comprises physicians and consumers who are charged with establishing the criteria for practice in the state. These criteria usually include graduation from an approved school, a certain period of practical experience after graduation, and the satisfactory completion of a number of written or oral examinations or both. Other requirements include such variables as good moral character and not having been guilty of a felony involving moral turpitude.

The problem of licensure in respiratory care is complex, consisting of emotional, political, economic, and administrative components. The AARC has thrown its considerable political and financial resources on the side of licensure and has provided strong support to the chartered affiliates in their efforts to gain formal recognition from the state. To date, this endeavor has been successful in 26 states, although it is likely that over the next few years an increasing number of jurisdictions will grant respiratory care practitioners recognition in the form of licensure or registration.

The arguments in favor of a licensure are

largely emotional. It does appear strange that this health profession, which has a very real potential to do serious and permanent damage to patients, should not be regulated, whereas occupational therapists, marriage counselors, and watchmakers are. The argument that licensure will improve the quality of care and will eliminate the substandard practitioner is, at best, questionable. First, new licensing laws almost invariably "grandfather" the current practitioners so that it will take many years before all licensed practitioners will have met the minimal licensing requirements. Second, all licensing regulations set the entry requirements at a very low level and rely heavily on the educational system and one or two examinations to determine competence. It does not require much thought to realize that similar regulations for other currently licensed health care providers have fallen far short of assuring uniformly competent care. A good exam-taker is not necessarily a good practitioner, and even the best practitioner makes mistakes.

If the license will not truly assure uniformly competent care, what will it do? In my opinion, (1) it will increase health costs. This is inevitable because the licensing and regulatory process is an expensive one and also, because of licensure, the practitioners will expect to be compensated at a higher level. (2) It will decrease the mobility of the practitioners from one jurisdiction to another. (3) It will narrow the gap between the therapists and the technicians, as the state will recognize providers at one level only. In view of these questions, one might ask: Is licensure really justified for respiratory care practitioners?

Regulation

State medical boards are also charged with regulating the professionals whom they admit to practice. This regulatory or disciplinary function of the boards is also an extension of the police powers of the state. Any licensed health professional who violates a section of the practice act and is brought to the attention of the board will be investigated and sanctioned, if the allegations prove to be true. Sanctions may vary from a reprimand to probation, fine, limitation of practice, suspension, or revocation of the license. The major areas wherein practitioners may violate the public health code include practice below minimal standards, sexual abuse of patients, physical or emotional impairment, criminal behavior affecting the ability to practice, and misuse or diversion of controlled substances.

To regulate, supervise, and fully enforce licens-

ing and regulation in medicine and in other health fields, the state boards must be strengthened. They must be properly financed and staffed, and given every fiscal, legal, and political support needed to perform their difficult mandate. Although peer reviews, societal forces, and the federal government all contribute to quality control in health care and toward the improvement of health services, the true power remains with the state licensing boards. Only these boards can effectively stop bad practitioners by revoking their license to practice. It seems most appropriate that the boards exert this power fairly but vigorously, and that they be given the means to do so.

The medical practice acts were the first ones to be established, but the last few decades have seen significant proliferation of licensing bodies for other health professions. Nurse practice acts, pharmacy practice acts, dental practice acts, and a number of other practice acts are now established in all 50 states. Several states have also established licensing regulations for some of the so-called technical specialties. These acts are similar in general form and intent to the medical practice acts and serve to establish the criteria that have to be met before a license is issued to an applicant in that particular phase of health care.

There is considerable pressure to lower the barriers that make the move of a licensed health professional from one state to another cumbersome and, occasionally, all but impossible. The United States Congress has made attempts to enact legislation making licensure by endorsement easier and more uniform. The Federation of State Boards of Medicine has worked for the same goal. The problems of moving from one state to another have been somewhat simplified, but as long as the constitution is not amended and the states have the right to regulate their internal affairs, it is unlikely that national licensure will become a reality in the forseeable future.

FEDERAL HEALTH LEGISLATION: PAST, PRESENT, AND FUTURE

The right of the states to license certain purveyors of services has been a well-established legal principle, and we have discussed some of the problems of licensing in the health delivery field. This section will comment on recent federal laws and some projected health legislation that will profoundly modify the practice of medicine and the entire system of health care delivery.

Under the Harris–Kefauver Amendment to the

Food and Drug Act of 1962, the methods whereby new drugs could be put on the market were defined, and the manufacturers of drugs were forced to prove both effectiveness and safety of literally thousands of different pills, lotions, and other concoctions with which the public was "treated." The benefits of the act were significant indeed. It controlled the frequently unscientific and shoddy methods whereby new drugs were put on the market and also tended to decrease the appearance of useless or harmful substances under the guise of "medication."

More recently, amendments to the Social Security Act of 1935 have profoundly affected the practice of medicine. These amendments have established not only the principle that health care is a *right* (at least, for large parts of the population), but also that the *quality* of care is a legitimate concern of the government, which finances a very significant portion of its cost. Particular reference is made to Public Law 92-603, the so-called Professional Standards Review or PSRO law that stipulates very clearly the right of government to supervise and, where necessary, to regulate the standard of medical care, at least in those areas where the cost of this medical care is borne by the public through Social Security funds.

Other laws that affect the health and well-being of the population include Public Law 91-596, enacted in 1970, known as the Occupational Safety and Health Act (OSHA). This act, not for the first time (but more effectively), attempts to regulate the working conditions of the millions of men and women whose health is seriously jeopardized by the disinclination of industry to expend the necessary funds for the creation of a salubrious working environment.

A companion piece to this law is Public Law 92-573, known as the Consumer Product Safety Act, which states, among its purposes, to protect the public against unreasonable risks of injury associated with consumer products and to assist consumers in evaluating the comparative safety of consumer products.

These four acts have made giant strides in assuring the American public of a high standard of medical care, better drugs, safer products, and decent working conditions. More recently the Tax Equity and Fiscal Responsibility Act of 1983 (TEFRA) and the already cited Health Care Quality Improvement Act of 1986 have already and will continue to affect health care in the United States.

Unfortunately, the laws must be enforced by imperfect human beings; consequently, the lag is usually significant between the enactment of a useful piece of legislation and its satisfactory implementation for the common good. Frequently, Congress fails to provide adequate funds for enforcement of the legislation, and occasionally the best-intentioned laws fail because special-interest groups have enough power to block the enactment of laws that may decrease the profits of their industries or the earning powers of certain persons.

The only prediction that can be made with a reasonable degree of certainty is that governmental regulatory activities will continue and are likely to increase. Consumers will continue to demand ready access to quality health care, and the health care industry will be expected to provide this. Judging from past experiences, this is unlikely to happen, unless the education and control of the health care professionals and the regulation of the health care industry become truly societal responsibilities.

THE AVOIDANCE OF LEGAL ENTANGLEMENTS

This discussion of the legal considerations of health care delivery should properly conclude with comments on how to avoid getting sued and how to optimize the chances of winning a suit that cannot be avoided. A suit for malpractice is, at best, a nuisance and, at worst, a professional and financial disaster. Whether innocent or not, the defendant's reputation suffers by the mere fact of being sued, and even complete legal vindication is insufficient to wash away the stigma entirely. Although I feel strongly that patients have not only the right to sue if they are injured by professional negligence, but the obligation to do so, it is the responsibility of the health professional to avoid such suits whenever possible and proper.

Improved Consumer–Provider Relationships

By far the most important single factor in the establishment of good consumer–provider relationship is the scrupulous attendance to the ethics and practice of the profession. Performance as a careful, conscientious, concerned practitioner may not grant immunity from litigation, but it will most certainly be the strongest bulwark against it. It would be presumptuous to attempt a discussion of the details of "good health care" in the framework of this short chapter, but it is certainly appropriate to point out that the major elements of good care are concern and competence. *Concern* incorporates such intangibles as caring for the patient as a human being, approaching all problems with humility and respect, wanting to do the "right thing," and striving to live up to the best traditions of a noble profession.

Competence is defined as being duly qualified, answering all requirements, and having sufficient ability. Thus competence incorporates far more than the minimum legal standards under which a professional is permitted to practice. It includes an ongoing educational process, a "keeping up" with the field, a recognition of one's limitations, and the courage of one's convictions, provided these are based on erudition and not on stubbornness and pride. Continued competence is a quality that the consumer has the right to expect. Although it is impossible to know all new developments in a rapidly expanding field of knowledge, we must continue the educational process from the first day in school to the last day of practice. The moment this continuum stops, the professional begins to deteriorate. Even the medical giants of the previous generation would be charlatans if judged by contemporary standards. Continued education is, and has been, an ethical requirement for all health professionals; it has now become a legal one in most states.

Improved Communication

The second important factor is good communication between provider and consumer. "Communication" is a much abused word, and "lack of communication" has been blamed for everything from the decline and fall of the Roman Empire to the unseasonable weather that appears to afflict all regions most of the time. Certainly, lack of adequate communication is indeed responsible for much misunderstanding in the field of health care delivery and consumer–provider relationships. *Communication*, in this context, means an exchange of ideas between the provider and consumer leading to a thorough understanding of the problem, of the proposed plan of diagnosis and treatment, and of the probabilities of cure or complications. With few exceptions, patients are reasonable and do not expect miracles, provided they understand the issues involved in their disease and realize that the health professional is sincerely concerned and committed to do his or her best. No patient will tolerate being misled, few patients will tolerate being ignored, and most patients wish to be informed about their health care management. Unfortunately, this participatory management is foreign to the training of most health professionals. In addition, it also takes considerable time that many health professionals neither have nor wish to give.

Regardless of the reasons for it, poor communications between provider and consumer are responsible for a significant percentage of all actions under the law of negligence. The most likely patient to sue is an angry patient, and patients usually feel anger not because of a bad result but because of a real or perceived lack of understanding of the issues involved. These patients are "mad" at their doctor or other health care provider because of lack of courtesy, lack of adequate time spent with the patient, the appearance of always being in a hurry, the feeling that the doctor "doesn't care," or that the patient is only "a case." This is also the reason why the doctor with the impeccable bedside or office manners gets away with terrible things, whereas the highly competent, but rude and overbearing physician, is a common target for litigation. Health care providers have obligations to their patients beyond competence and skill. They must be able to communicate with the patient at the patient's level of understanding and must make the time available to satisfy the reasonable patient. Ten minutes spent with a patient may save 10 days spent in a court room.

Improved Records

The third most important feature in the avoidance of legal troubles is the maintenance of good records. Most people, including health care practitioners, feel a general contempt for records and record-keeping. They settle for the minimum acceptable and begrudge every moment they spend or should spend in recording their observations, actions, conclusions, and results. Most physicians consider it beneath their dignity to keep detailed, meticulous records, and many of them consider it contrary to their freedom of action if the hospital or a peer group insists that records be kept fully, accurately, and informatively. Yet many negligence suits won by plaintiffs are won because of poor records, and most of the suits won by defendants are won because there was documented evidence of everything that happened in the case of the plaintiff patient.

Review of many hospital or office records reveals an appalling lack of pertinent information, and it is a rare record, indeed, that permits an outsider to reconstruct precisely the patient's problems, the events in the hospital, the justification for these events, and the results of diagnostic and therapeutic manipulations.

Worse even than the incomplete record is the record that a physician or other health worker considers as the suitable medium for witticisms or, worse, unfounded or unjustified comments on the actions of other health professionals. There is no excuse for any professional to use a legal document, such as a medical record, for the ventilation of personal criticism or petty jealousies. The medical record is not the suitable medium to try to correct errors in management.

There is even less excuse for making incorrect entries on a medical record. This constitutes not only a complete breach of professional ethics, but is also fraud, and thereby, subject to legal action. I have found, in reviewing many records, repeated evidence of treatments recorded but not given and of laboratory tests being entered without their ever having been performed. This despicable practice not only reflects the dishonesty of the so-called health professional but may also have catastrophic results for the patient. It is impossible to find words strong enough to condemn this totally unacceptable practice.

The requirement for keeping good records is not only a legal and professional one, but has become a financial one as well. Third-party payers require that the record show evidence of the care provided so that compensation can be made. Certain procedures, for example, the "routine" preoperative chest x-ray, are no longer reimbursed unless there is a documented medical rationale for them. It is likely that this list will grow in view of the increasing concern about escalating hospital and medical costs.

Risk Management

A relatively new concept in legal protection is known as risk management. Hospitals and other health care facilities establish an office in which specially trained personnel assume the responsibility of dealing with "incidents" that may lead to litigation. The risk managers must be informed immediately when anything happens that was unforeseen or potentially dangerous. The risk manager then contacts all appropriate persons involved in the incident, makes sure that the records are in good order, acts as the spokesperson for the institution and staff and, simultaneously, acts as the ombudsman for the patient and the family. Speaking

from personal experience at the University of Michigan, I can assure you that a good risk management team can save an immense amount of grief and millions of dollars.

Malpractice Insurance

All health care professionals who provide health care as independent contractors should carry malpractice insurance so that patients may be adequately compensated for injury without financial ruin for the health professional. For many years, the malpractice insurance business was stable, and many insurance companies issued policies to cover professional negligence. In recent years, partly in consequence of increasingly large judgments and settlements, but mainly because of general economic problems in the insurance business, the insurance premiums have increased enormously. In fact, this problem has become a recurring national crisis. A number of insurance companies have discontinued writing this type of policy, and even those that continue to do so have increased the premiums to exorbitant levels.

In several states tort reform legislation has been enacted in the past few years, mostly under enormous pressure from the health and insurance industries. These laws have been helpful in some areas, but they do not resolve the basic conflict, and it seems extremely unlikely that the solution to the "malpractice crisis" lies in statutory reforms of the fundamental laws governing personal or professional liability.

If indeed the solution to "malpractice" comes from legislation, it is very probable that the solution is going to be worse than the problem and will lie in the area of a totally controlled health care delivery system.

ETHICAL CONSIDERATIONS

Ethics may be defined as a branch of philosophy that deals with the fundamental values in life. Good and bad, right and wrong are the central concepts of the ethicist and, through the ages, ethicists have struggled to define and to apply these concepts. Every society, from the most primitive to the most sophisticated; every religion, from the most austere to the most permissive; and, indeed, every learned profession has evolved some set of rules, some moral precepts, or some "ethical" standards to regulate individual and interpersonal behavior.

Medical ethics has only recently come to be viewed as a subset of general ethics that governs the nontechnical interphase between the health professional and the patient, both individually and as a society. The ethics literature of the 19th and early 20th centuries accepted that physicians were governed only by a "professional ethic" that allowed them to do what others, following ordinary ethics, could not. The revelations of the Nuremberg trials, the exponential growth of scientific knowledge, and the increasingly sophisticated technical and pharmacologic armamentarium led to the realization that general ethical principles had to apply to all, regardless of profession.

MAJOR TRENDS IN ETHICAL THOUGHT

The history of Western ethical thought starts in Greece in the 4th century B.C. with the efforts of Socrates, Plato, and Aristotle. Their attempts to distinguish right from wrong objectively and to find a rational explanation for human motivations and human behavior have influenced ethical thought to this day.

Roman Catholicism held almost universal sway during the first 16 centuries of the Christian era, and impressed its own ethical views on Europe. The Church equated right and wrong, good or bad with whatever was pleasing or displeasing to a remote Deity as recorded in writings directly or indirectly attributed to Him. Catholic philosophers from Ambrose to Aquinas tried to harmonize natural law and divine will and put a rational base under the "Golden Rule." Interestingly, Catholic ethicists and philosophers have been preeminent in contemporary medical ethics, with the same respect for logic and reason that characterized the great early thinkers of the Church.

The questioning spirit of the 18th century crystallized the two major directions of modern ethical thought, which had been present in a more diffuse fashion in the writing of pagan and Christian ethicists. These two major strands of ethical thought may be termed utilitarianism and formalism or deontologism.

Utilitarianism, most clearly defined in the writings of Jeremy Bentham[8] and John Stuart Mill,[9] holds that an act is good if its results are good and is bad if its results are bad. Thus, an act, in itself neutral or even harmful to an individual is *good* if its long-term results benefit a larger group or humanity itself. Even though it carries overtones of the allegedly Jesuitical "the end justifies the means," a modified utilitarianism is one of the basic principles of medical ethics.

Formalism or deontologism largely disregards the result of an act and looks at the act itself as being either good or bad. According to formalistic thinking, wrongful acts, such as telling lies, are never permissible, even though the results may be most beneficial. The foremost proponent of this ethical theory was the German philosopher Immanuel Kant.[10]

Despite the best intentions, adherence to theoretical concepts of ethics may lead to legal entanglements and to awkward interpersonal confrontations. It is, I believe, one of the major emotional problems in modern health care delivery that so many of the situations we encounter in our daily activities do not lend themselves to simple theoretical solutions. No rule can be applied universally, and the more closely a health professional attempts to be strictly "ethical" according to one of the major ethical philosophies, the more likely he or she will wind up in a morass of dilemmas. In fact, most of the so-called ethical issues in health care delivery can be resolved by remembering some basic principles and applying them, with suitable modifications, to the specific issue or to the individual situation. The ancient precept *primum non nocere* (first of all do no harm), expanded by the Golden Rule, "do unto others. . . ," will resolve most problems.

One point fundamental to all interpersonal relationships must be emphasized: Good manners, courtesy, and respect for others' feelings and rights are the keystones that keep the edifice of society from collapsing.

ETHICAL DYNAMICS OF INTERPROFESSIONAL RELATIONSHIPS: THE TEAM CONCEPT

Traditional interprofessional relationships in health care delivery were predicated on a rigid caste system, with the physician on top followed, in descending order, by nurses, technologists, aides, and orderlies. These relationships were paternalistic and authoritarian. Personal relationships were held to a minimum, except among persons on the same level in the professional, administrative, or corporate structure. This system was not designed for personal contentment, and it is a tribute to human resilience that it was not only quite efficient, but also that its different components functioned competently and appeared reasonably satisfied with their role. In these relationships there was little reciprocal respect; what held the system together was discipline and an unquestioning acceptance of traditional authority.

During the past 30 years these emotional and behavioral relationships have undergone a gradual but accelerating change. Many factors have contributed to this change, including a decline in the perceived stature of the medical profession, a dramatic improvement in the educational sophistication of the nonphysician health care providers, a realization that nonphysicians could make major contributions to the health care system, and a universal democratization of society as a whole. One significant result of these different movements has been the slow evolution of the team concept in health care delivery.

The fundamental tenet underlying the team concept is that its members have specific contributions to make that are of comparable value and that all must function harmoniously for the end result to be optimal. There has been a definite blurring of the lines of responsibility. A number of activities traditionally considered nursing functions have been assumed by technical specialists, and there has even been some exchange among the technical specialist groups.

A brief inspection of the system as it exists at present reveals that, indeed, the tightly structured caste system in health care delivery has largely disappeared; each group within the system has now assumed a quasi-collegial relationship vis-à-vis the other groups. These changes have also had a profound effect on the emotional relationships within and between the health professions. The caste system required a great deal of respect from the lower orders in return for authoritarian paternalism, quite similar to the structure of the Victorian family. There the father (physician) made all decisions and bestowed praise or punishment as he saw fit. The mother (nurse) backed the father's authority and contributed a certain humanizing influence. The children (technologists, aides, orderlies) were to be seen but not heard. They were to "behave" at all times, "do as they were told," and be grateful for every small kindness shown to them by the Jovian parent.

Changes came slowly but inexorably. Industrial relationships were the first to change under the leadership of the great founders of the labor movements. Two world wars made their contribution, and since about 1950 there has been an accelerating trend toward the "democratization" of all forms of

social organizations, from the family to the armed forces. Health care could not remain immune, and the aforementioned changes finally reached this almost unique survivor of the paternalistic, quasi-feudal model of interpersonal relationships.

These changes, spurred by both external and internal forces, have led to the gradual evolution of the health care team. The concept is certainly not new. Small teams have functioned in some areas for many years. Psychiatric hospitals have led in this area, and even 30 years ago teams of physicians, nurses, social workers, occupational therapists, and, rarely, some nonhealth professionals met to plan the management of individual patients. Similar teams became active in the management of emergency situations, cardiopulmonary resuscitation, and in the care of critically ill patients. These teams were still under the nominal leadership of the physician, although individual team members were frequently placed into decision-making roles, depending on the requirements of specific problems.

Unfortunately, the team concept, while receiving much verbal support, failed to achieve general acceptance for two major reasons. First was turf protection and the unwillingness of most people to recognize their own limitations or the abilities of others. The second and perhaps equally important cause for the failure of the team concept must be attributed to our educational institutions. For a group to function well as a team, the individual members must have a thorough understanding of each other's roles, duties, and abilities. This is impossible *unless* the team members receive much of their training jointly and are exposed to both basic educational experiences and clinical learning situations as a group. To date, attempts to provide such joint learning opportunities and experiences have been few and largely unsuccessful.

I believe that no substantial, rational advance in education or formal team development will take place until there is a strong societal mandate enforced by economic sanctions for failure to comply. This is likely to take years. What posture, then, should the individual health care provider assume *now* vis-à-vis colleagues in the other health professions? More precisely, what should the attitude of respiratory therapists be in relationship to physicians, nurses, physical therapists, and others who may have direct input into the management of patients served by respiratory care?

Foremost, the roles that each plays in the care of the patient must be understood. The respiratory therapist who aims to be more than a mechanic must have a good working knowledge of the medical problems of pulmonary patients and a thorough understanding of the diagnostic and therapeutic considerations that the physician brings to bear on the problem. The respiratory therapist must understand the contribution nurses have to make, both in the narrow sense as providers of bedside care, and in the broader sense as consumer educators and coordinators of the health care team. The same principles apply to working with physical therapists, occupational therapists, and others.

The keys to this complex relationship are respect, good manners, equanimity, humor, humility, and, most important, a single-minded, inflexible devotion to the well-being of the patient.

MAJOR CONTEMPORARY PROBLEMS IN HEALTH ETHICS

Problems of Life and Death

Subsumed under the somewhat pretentious title of "problems of life and death" are such ethical problems as abortion, the management of the defective newborn, the problems of death and dying, and the problem of euthanasia.

Few, if any, of the ethical issues are as replete with emotional content, personal and religious prejudices, and attempts to resolve the insoluble as the issue of abortion. The 1973 Supreme Court decisions (*Roe v Wade*[11] and *Doe v Bolton*[12]) have settled some of the legal aspects of the dispute, without having resolved any of the ethical or moral issues involved.

The two sides of the argument can be stated briefly. The extreme antiabortionists believe that human life begins at the moment of conception. It necessarily ensues then that interferences with this "human," with intent to destroy, must be considered murder and is thus forbidden by divine and human law. The only exception most of the proponents of this view are willing to allow falls under the heading of self-defense; the fetus may be "destroyed" if its continued existence seriously jeopardizes the mother's survival. Tubal pregnancy or removal of the cancerous pregnant uterus would be examples of such exceptions. Conservative antiabortionists may still consider this "homicide" but are willing to concede that it is "justifiable homicide," or that it is but a "side-effect" of a primarily ethical "lifesaving" action. This latter idea is known as the *Doctrine of Double Effect*. At the other end of the spectrum, the most liberal proabortionists claim that the fetus in utero is not a person but an integral part of the mother's body, and as such the mother has the right to dispose of it until the moment of delivery. The arguments raised by this group include both ethical and legal ones and include references to the constitution and to the moral right of a person to the pursuit of happiness and to complete control over her own body.

Both of these extremes are difficult to defend rationally; indeed, such extreme views are held by only a relative few of the opposing groups. The more enlightened antiabortionists concede that the mother's survival is not the only justification for abortion, but that pregnancy ensuing from forcible rape or incest may also be terminated. A further concession, although usually the last one made by the most liberal of the antiabortionists, is the recognition that medically proven serious physical or emotional disturbances occasioned by pregnancy may, under certain circumstances, be acceptable as a reason for terminating the pregnancy.

Proabortionists commonly base their views on the principle that there is a point in the intrauterine development of the fetus when it changes from a "nonperson" to a "person," and, consequently, may be aborted before this point at the mother's discretion. Abortion after this critical turning point must be governed by compelling medical reasons only. Cultural, historic, and even scientific arguments are marshalled to determine when this change takes place and when a crude assembly of cells suddenly becomes a human being entitled to all the rights and protections that society has traditionally granted to human beings.

Societal arguments on abortion are even more difficult to defend. Some opponents of abortion argue that once this type of "murder" is sanctioned, we are all embarked on a "slippery slope" that leads inevitably to a total disintegration of social mores and to a chaos of unimaginable brutality. Some proponents of abortion cite overpopulation, the mental health of the unhappy mother and the unwanted child, and numerous other irrelevant considerations in their attempts to justify abortions entirely at the discretion of the mother and her attending physician. A recent decision by the Supreme Court and several laws enacted by state legislatures have further complicated this issue. How it will ultimately be resolved remains an open question.

Respiratory therapy personnel have little, if any role in decisions on abortion, other than in reference to their own personal and family life. In the next ethical dilemma, the problem of the severely handicapped neonate, they do become involved professionally.

Despite the availability of intrauterine diagnostic techniques and legally available abortion services, many infants are born with severe congenital deformities that would prove fatal unless corrected surgically or that would make impossible a decent quality of life, with or without therapy. The second group presents a relatively minor ethical problem. Any newborn, regardless of how grotesque or how severely damaged, who would survive with standard care cannot be willfully and intentionally put to death without incurring the appropriate prosecution for willful homicide. The problem becomes much more complex when sophisticated life-support machinery is required to maintain this infant or if surgical intervention becomes necessary to prevent the infant's inevitable death.

As with most ethical problems, this one cannot be discussed intelligently without a reasonable understanding of the legal issues involved. Two fairly recent cases illustrate this problem. In the "Johns Hopkins case,"[13] which was not submitted to a court for decision, an infant was born with intestinal atresia and with what appeared to be severe Downs' syndrome. The intestinal atresia was surgically correctible, and it was thought likely, with modern medicine, that this mentally deficient infant could be physically rehabilitated. The parents, after much discussion and agonizing, refused permission to operate, and the infant was allowed to die of starvation in about 2 weeks. During this time it was given minimal supportive care and was the center of considerable emotional turmoil among the nurses and other health professionals who were forced to stand by and watch it die. Much has been written about this case by writers representing a wide spectrum of philosophical and political orientations. Surprisingly, the condemnation of the parents and the Hopkins' physicians was practically unanimous.

The second case did involve a court decision in Maine[14] concerning a neonate who suffered from many grossly deforming congenital defects and who also had a tracheoesophageal fistula (TEF). This was the most immediately life-threatening deformity, although other defects were such that it was impossible to suppose a satisfying quality of life for the infant. The parents refused to consent to the TEF repair. The physicians at the Maine Medical Center petitioned the court to assume guardianship over the child and to authorize the surgery. The court ruled that surgery should be performed because ". . . the most basic right enjoyed by

every human being is the right to life itself." The court also found that this right started with the moment of birth. Pursuant to this decision, the operation was performed.

Such decisions surrounding the crib or incubator on whether to save a profoundly damaged "life" or whether to let it die are among the most difficult ethical and moral issues. Currently there are no clear guidelines, and responsible thinkers have doubted whether such guidelines are possible. The argument again ranges from the doctrinaire "we always must do everything to maintain life" to the nihilistic "we must save only those who are likely to be fulfilled and fulfilling human beings."

I believe that there is a minimal quality of life below which existence is, at best, humanoid. No newborn should be willfully and arbitrarily sentenced to live its life in pain, misery, and discomfort while placing an enormous emotional and economic burden on its family and on society as a whole. The parents have the right both legally and ethically to refuse extraordinary means to salvage what, in their opinion, would be an unacceptable quality of life. The obvious and, unfortunately, unanswerable question is that of the level below which the quality of life is not acceptable. There is no generalization that can be universally applied to this situation; this is the most excruciating dilemma with which parents can be confronted. All thinking and feeling parents must resolve this question for themselves and would be well-advised to seek assistance in this decision from physicians involved in the care of the infant and from whoever is serving as a spiritual advisor to the family. If a conflict arises between the family and the physicians, the only resource is to refer the matter to a court.

This judicial action may have the virtue of appearing dispassionate, and it tends to disregard the burden it may place on the family or on society for many years to come. Seemingly, there should be a minimum standard below which no extraordinary means of support should be used. At the least, the newborn must show some evidence that it is likely to have the cardinal human characteristics of cognition and emotion. Without these, whatever the newborn is, it is not a human being, and neither law nor morality would be served by maintaining it in a vegetative state.

During the eight years from 1980 to 1988 a new development was seen. The federal government, under the leadership of President Reagan and Attorney General Meese, chose to insert their heavy foot into this sensitive ethical web. The federal government first mandated that an emergency "hotline'' number be displayed prominently in all obstetrical centers inviting family or bystanders to call the emergency number if there was any suggestion that a neonate was not provided with all possible ordinary or extraordinary means of maintaining life. The lawsuit that ensued was decided against the government.

Next the government got involved in a celebrated case known widely as the Baby Jane Doe case.[15] This case, involving a newborn with spina bifida and paraplegia, was first dealt with by the New York court system. The parents and the physicians at Stonybrook Medical Center agreed not to subject this child to extensive and most probably unsuccessful surgery. They were dragged into court by an out-of-state lawyer and, indeed, the lower court instructed the physician to proceed with the surgical procedure. In appeal the New York Court of Appeals, in a very sharply worded opinion, reversed the lower court. At this point the federal government reeopened the suit under the discriminatory statute, claiming that the baby was discriminated against as a handicapped person. The federal judge ruled against the Attorney General with the finding that the drafters of the antidiscrimination (civil rights) statutes clearly had no such situation in mind when they enacted this law.

One result of all this meddling by the federal government was the mandatory establishment of ethics committees in all health care facilities where babies were born or cared for. These ethics committees have only an advisory role, but they must be consulted in all cases of an impaired newborn.

A similar and yet distinct ethical and legal problem arises at the opposite end of human existence. The normal process of aging inevitably leads to physical, mental, and emotional deterioration, which is usually gradual but may, on occasion, be sudden and dramatic. When it occurs, its manifestations may be primarily physical, as in many terminal illnesses, or mental, as when brain damage occurs because of trauma, hypoxia, or various external or internal causes such as senility or chronic brain syndrome.

The problem is similar to that of the severely damaged newborn, but there are some significant differences. These differences flow from the fact that adults may be in a position to make decisions for themselves or may have left instructions about their desires for a certain course of action to be taken should such a catastrophe occur. Furthermore, there are significant economic and emotional differences between letting a baby die or letting an old person die. Babies rarely have substantial estates, and inheritance is rarely a consideration. Babies, at least ideally, have the possibility of a long and happy life before them. Old people can look forward only to death as a relief from the burden of life.

In the conscious adult the situation is simple. Under constitutional guarantees, a person has the unquestioned right to determine whether diagnostic and therapeutic manipulation shall be performed, and every adult has the right to refuse health care even though such refusal will inevitably lead to death. Both court decisions and the overwhelming weight of ethical writing clearly distinguish between such a refusal to be treated for a terminal illness and suicide. Catholic theologians have taught and are teaching that, although suicide is a deadly sin, refusal to engage in any extraordinary activity to prevent death cannot be considered suicide and consequently is not banned by the Catholic Church. The emphasis is on the word "extraordinary." Theologians and ethicists generally contend, although for different reasons, that the person has a duty to maintain the body in good health and to do everything reasonable and proper to avoid illness or to regain health. Where "reasonable and proper" ends and "extraordinary" begins has never been accurately defined, is subject to individual interpretation, and is likely to change with the development of new technology.

Freedom of choice, however, is not absolute. The state has the right, through legislation and judicial decisions, to set some limits to constitutional guarantees. Just as it was held that yelling "fire" in a crowded theater could not be excused under the guarantee of "free speech," the state also has the right to quarantine and to treat patients with infectious diseases, to insist on the immunization of school children, to demand premarital blood tests, and to allow other "invasions of privacy," if these steps are in the evident interest of society as a whole.

If the adult patient is unconscious or otherwise incompetent to make a decision, the situation becomes more complicated, particularly if there are no real indications of the wishes of the person involved. Some states have enacted (or are now considering) "right to die" legislation.[15] According to these states, a person of sound mind may formally request that no extraordinary means be used to prolong life should that person be unable to make the decision. To die with dignity is just as much an inalienable right as living in dignity. Yet thoughtful and kind physicians, other health practitioners, and family members regularly and commonly deny this right to their patients or relatives. These are deep, dark waters that must be navigated with the utmost care, since the choices range from euthanasia to the indefinite maintenance of the living dead.

To kill another human being willfully is homicide. Euthanasia or "mercy killing" is homicide, even though performed with the purest and most humane motives. Whether there are circumstances in which an outright positive act, designed solely to produce death, may ever be justified is difficult to answer. The proponents of euthanasia feel strongly that the answer to this question is, yes! There are situations, they believe, in which a conscious adult may reasonably request to be "put to sleep" or even for which parents are entitled to make this decision for a badly damaged infant. The opponents of euthanasia claim that the answer is a categorical and unalterable, no! Opponents admit that some people may be better off dead and that an unqualified denial of euthanasia condemns some patients or infants to a degrading, quasi-human, or subhuman existence for an indefinite period. The arguments against euthanasia usually fall into one of two broad categories. It is claimed that both divine and human law demand that life not be taken except in war, self-defense, or (perhaps) as the punishment for certain heinous crimes. It is also claimed by those who do not necessarily insist on the total sanctity of life that permitting euthanasia is wrong, primarily because it is the thin edge of the wedge that leads inevitably to the elimination of increasing numbers and groups of undesirables. Ultimately it could lead to political or racial mass murder.

I find it very difficult to accept such reasoning. Those who truly believe in the Divine mandate "Thou shall not kill" should oppose killing absolutely in every form, including self-defense, judicial execution, and war. Once one is willing to accept one form of homicide, it appears illogical to deny categorically the potential appropriateness of another form of equally justifiable homicide. The second argument about the thin edge is even more specious. Making the leap from cheerfully circumscribed voluntary euthanasia to political genocide is an absurd conclusion or inference.

Whatever the arguments may be, it is quite evident that American society is not prepared to accept euthanasia as an option at this time. Let us therefore examine the next level of activity designed for terminally ill and for those who are suffering gravely and irreversibly. Is there anything short of active euthanasia that is acceptable legally and ethically, that will benefit hopeless sufferers, and that has the support of the health care community?

Several suggestions have been made. Most common are those related to "making the patient comfortable" and to "not doing anything" that may prolong the patient's life. Liberal use of morphine and other narcotic analgesics are indicated in patients with preterminal and terminal pain. How much is given and how often is a medical decision. In an adult patient with severe pain, 15 mg of morphine would not be considered excessive. Given to elderly patients regularly, morphine is likely to keep the patient quite comfortable and, indeed, may ease and speed the transition from "this world to the next."

Is this euthanasia? Most ethicists will argue that it is not, whereas some maintain that, in some respects, it is just that. Most thoughtful health care providers will agree, however, that this method of managing the desperately, terminally, and painfully ill is not only ethically permissible but often mandated. Legally it is very unlikely to be questioned unless the narcotic is administered in a single dose, large enough to be incompatible with survival.

Withholding medication or other therapeutic modalities is a related but more difficult issue. Pneumonia was once referred to as "the old person's friend" because it was one of the most frequent and gentle causes of death in elderly patients in the preantibiotic era. Now old patients who wish for death and who do get pneumonia can be "treated" and given weeks, months, or even years of existence that they do not really want. The question once again arises, "Is it permissible, ethically and legally, to withhold antibiotics from these patients, thus allowing them to die, without interfering artificially in a natural process?"

Recently the most hotly debated issue in this area concerns the ethical–legal considerations of withholding parenteral hydration or nutrition. Some years ago in California two physicians were charged with homicide for stopping intravenous fluids on a vegetative patient.[17] More recently, in Florida[18] and New Jersey[19] decisions fell on the opposite side and found there was no difference ethically or legally between discontinuing a ventilator and discontinuing artificial hydration and nutrition. In this area the Opinion of the AMA Council on Ethical and Judicial Affairs, issued on March 15, 1988 summarized the position of organized medicine very well, and clearly stated that the continuation of artificial feeding and hydration, whether through tubes or IVs was a medical measure that could be terminated just as artificial ventilation could be terminated.

A related issue concerns the problem of cardiopulmonary resuscitation. To resuscitate or not to resuscitate is a medical decision. Writing "no code" orders is legally permissible and ethically sound and has been upheld by one of the most conservative jurisdictions.[20] Health care providers must remember that it is easier not to start resuscitation and not to connect a patient to a ventilator than to stop. Resuscitation should be started only if the victim can be reestablished as a functional human being, and should be discontinued when obvious evidence of significant central nervous system damage appears. It is very easy to be righteous in this area, but those of us who have resuscitated decerebrate patients and then were involved in their care are inclined to be pragmatic, even to the point of therapeutic nihilism.

Problems of Behavior Modification and Genetic Engineering

Few areas of medical intervention are fraught with more promise and more potential danger than behavior control and its prospective application: genetic screening and genetic engineering.

Behavior modification by psychosurgery was quite popular some years ago but has been largely terminated under societal pressure and at least one major lawsuit.[21] Behavior modification by psychotherapy, with or without psychopharmacology, is the currently accepted technique for the management of certain mentally ill patients.

There are few violent or potentially dangerous mental patients who are not subjected to some form of psychotherapy and to the administration of various psychoactive drugs during voluntary or involuntary commitments to a mental institution. Both psychotherapy and psychopharmacology are not without hazard, and their long-range effectiveness has been greatly exaggerated, as evidenced by the frequent reports in the daily press relating the violent crimes committed by treated and released former mental patients. It is difficult to understand a system that protects the mentally ill but is unable to protect their innocent victims. Legalists and civil libertarians are rarely around when the victims of their protégés are brought to the emergency room raped, beaten, stabbed, shot, mutilated, or dead. Constitutional freedoms are important and governmental or individual excesses must be controlled, but there must be a balance at which individual rights and societal rights are placed into proper perspective.

This same balance should be achieved in genetic counseling and genetic engineering. It is well known that a considerable number of serious diseases are transmitted from parent to child: sickle cell anemia, hemophilia, thalassemia, Down syndrome, Klinefelter syndrome, cystic fibrosis, Morton syndrome, retinoblastoma, some forms of muscular dystrophy, phenylketonuria, and others. These genetically linked illnesses present two major problem areas: the identification and counseling of the carriers; and the statutory enforcement of preventive sterilization, amniocentesis, and abortion.

Both areas are fraught with the greatest dangers to individual liberties, whereas at the same time, the societal cost of total nonfeasance in this area is enormous. As usual, a compromise will have to be found. Few people will object to voluntary screening for the carrier state in adults who may be heterozygotes, and only those who object to all abortions will find fault with the decision to terminate a pregnancy when amniocentesis reveals a homozygote fetus. It is the duty of the family practitioner and the obstetrician to be fully aware of the family history of their patients and to counsel them on the principles of mendelian genetics and the statistical likelihood of affected offspring. Then, the patients can make a rational decision on marriage and procreation. The use of voluntary genetic counseling seems appropriate. Prospective mothers and fathers should be concerned with the odds of having "normal" children and should take chances in this area only after careful and reasoned deliberation. Amniocentesis should be performed if there is a high index of probability for a genetically malformed fetus. Abortion should be discussed with the prospective parents and should be made available in a timely and medically proper fashion. Not to do so is to deprive the parents of their right to make decisions and may indeed leave them and the medical advisors open to the dangers of "wrongful life" litigation.

Finally, a new area of controversy has emerged concerning the new methodologies of genetic engineering. It has become possible in recent years to make changes in the genetic patterns of certain bacteria, and even certain higher-order animals, that allow scientists to create hitherto unknown forms of life. A case in point is the so-called recombinant DNA research. New technology has made it possible to split the DNA helix carrying the genetic messages, splice in DNA fragments from other organisms, and reintroduce the "new" DNA into a host. In this way it may become possible to develop new strains of microorganisms that could for example, make insulin, decrease the incidence of cancer, and make vast amounts of nutrient protein. It may, of course, also be possible to create a Frankenstein's monster and let loose on an unsuspecting world new life forms of unimaginable tenacity and ferocity.

Therefore, thoughtful scientists and philosophers have argued vigorously against pursuing studies in this field. The arguments have been both objective and emotional. It was believed that the possible dangers of this work were so great and so unpredictable that they outweighed the possible benefits. Others argued that there were areas of possible knowledge that were best left unknown. Yet others condemned any research in this area as being contrary to the desires of the Creator.

None of these arguments appears to be convincing. The benefits of creating new life forms may be substantial and, indeed, may herald a new and better life for humanity. The dangers may be real but can be minimized, and should not be allowed to influence the new technologies. The theological arguments are unanswerable and need no answer. If the Creator does not wish humans to work in this area, it is safe to assume that the Creator will make his will known in no uncertain terms.

Problems of Allocation of Scarce Health Resources: Triage

It is a generally accepted principle that all residents of the United States are entitled to health care; it is an unfortunate, but inevitable, corollary of this principle that not all citizens can be furnished optimal health care at all times. There are manifold reasons for both the principle and the corollary. In its simplest terms, it has become a political necessity, and indeed an electioneering slogan, that all health care is a right and that every man, woman, and child is "entitled" to health care. Whether it is considered a constitutional guarantee or whether simply something on which all decent people agree is immaterial. The fact remains that for the past half century, at least, there has been an increasing tendency to provide optimal health care to all who need it, at all times and in all geographic locations.

Desires once again outran performance and, in fact, there were major discrepancies both in the availability and in the quality of health care. These differences were geographic and economic. Rural areas and inner cities were underserved, as were the poor, regardless of geographic distribution. All efforts to the contrary, both the quantity and quality of health care services were superior in medium-sized towns, in the more affluent suburbs, and in those areas where health care delivery was associated with academic health centers. Thus, even in this wealthiest of all countries, it has been impossible to assume optimal health care to all. There are insufficient facilities, insufficient personnel at all levels, and insufficient money to provide everything to everybody.

The solutions to this problem are almost entirely economic, and only to a limited extent personal and professional. Governmental priorities must be adjusted so that not only a larger share of the budget is devoted to health, but that within the health budget a larger share is devoted to health care delivery where it is most urgently needed. The full weight of the federal and state governments must be applied to this issue.

Other concerns that confront health planners on the national level are the problems of allocating limited resources. Health care is an enormous arena composed of numerous related and yet quasi-independent segments. Once the fact is accepted that resources are limited and that the first priority must be the provision of minimally acceptable health care to all, how should the remainder of the resources be allocated? Numerous options are available.

Most of the funds could be devoted to research in the hope that the major contemporary scourges—cancer, heart disease, and chronic respiratory ailments—can be eliminated or at least significantly reduced. The funds could also be used to continue to provide the most sophisticated scientific technologies to the relatively few who would benefit the most from them. Such items as open-heart surgery, organ transplant, chronic renal dialysis, magnetic resonance imaging, and other similar "luxuries" come to mind immediately. Another solution would be to devote most of the remaining funds to preventive medicine and health maintenance. Health education is yet another option, as is the establishment of geriatric facilities, hospitals, drug treatment centers, chronic care facilities, and the like.

None of the foregoing can possibly be singled out as uniquely deserving support, and societal funds will have to be divided among all of them. The relative importance of the various areas and the sums allocated to them should, however, be decided immediately. How these decisions are made and what the ultimate outcome of this decision-making process will be concerns us all. They are not, ethical or moral decisions, strictly speaking, and yet they clearly have a major ethical component. To direct funds away from open-heart surgery and toward rehabilitation centers for drug addicts, to take money from diabetes research and spend it on chronic care facilities for retarded children, to stop funding health education and establishing hospitals or hospices for the terminally ill, all are ethical concerns. Society in general, and the health care provider community in particular, cannot delay making such choices.

The second major allocation of resources issue involves individuals and decisions made at the local level. *Triage* is a term well known in military medicine. It means that when a large number of injured must be cared for, preference is given to those with minor injuries who can be treated rapidly and in whom the chances for full recovery are great. The heavily injured who would consume a disproportionate share of the available resources are left to the last, even if this means that some of them may die before care can be provided. In civilian practice, triage usually takes a very different form. The issue is rarely one of emergency management of large groups but is usually one of selecting small groups from a large pool for treatment modalities or drugs that are available in limited quantity. When penicillin first became available in very limited amounts, physicians had to make choices in their allocation of the "miracle drug." Should they treat the mayor of the town who had gonorrhea or the principal of the high school who had pneumonia? Should the youngster with otitis media be given preference over the waitress with an infected hand?

The first renal dialysis unit established in Seattle was a similar sphere for decision-making.[22] The number of patients with terminal renal failure was much larger than the number that could be accommodated in the limited facilities of the dialysis unit. Choices had to be made, and these choices were matters of life and death. The questions are obvious: "Who should make this choice, and on what basis?"

The basic ethical dilemma can be stated simply: "If not all can be saved, who shall be saved?" To answer this dilemma, a fundamental value judgment must be made. If we assume that all human beings have the same value and that there is no difference between a child with Down's syndrome

and a Nobel Laureate in medicine from the point of view of intrinsic "humanness," the selection process must be made by chance. Random selection by some form of lottery or selection on a "first come, first served" basis may well be the most appropriate. This method has advocates among the major ethicists of our time.

A highly respected contemporary ethicist has taken a diametrically opposite position. In a somewhat different context, Edmund Cahn held that, if not all could be saved, none should be saved. Cahn finds a recourse to chance unacceptable because it abrogates responsibility and rationality.[23] The less radical opponents of the random selection approach advocate a selection system based on "merit" or "value," in combination with the highest probability of success. Selection would first be made on the basis of life expectancy and likelihood of cure. A second consideration would be given to such factors as the number of family members who depend on the patient. Finally, past societal services rendered or potential future societal contributions would be weighed in making choices between individuals.

The medical choices and the family choice are relatively clear. Given the limited nature of the resources, preference may well be given to those in whom the treatment is likely to be successful and who, by virtue of age, would benefit for the longest time. In the family criterion, the provider for a group of small children may well be awarded preference over the lonely bachelor or spinster. The societal value choices are much more complex. Past services rendered have generally been recognized as meritorius, and indeed both a logical and ethical case can be made for rewarding those who have already made contributions to society. More difficult to assess is a person's potential future value. Is a promising artist, athlete, or politician worth more than a skilled mechanic, promising physician, or brilliant engineer? Should there be a premium on "scarcity," or should "utility" be a primary determinant? If we accept the proposition that value judgments of this type are acceptable on ethical grounds, who is to make the selection and how can the selection process be freed from subjective factors?

Because of their proximity to the problem, physicians have traditionally been in a position to make the selections, and indeed have done so in many instances. Yet nothing in the training or education of physicians qualifies them to make such choices in any area except the strictly medical one. Physicians, as a group, are no more qualified to make societal value judgments than are lawyers, merchants, or housewives as groups. Who, then should make the selection, and how should the selection be made? In the absence of any agreement between providers and consumers, a scheme that has considerable appeal has been suggested by Rescher.[24] Selection for life-saving therapy would be performed as a three-tiered process. The first level of selection would be made by health care personnel on medical grounds. The likelihood of success and the life expectancy of the candidate would be evaluated according to the best available estimate; those who fall below a minimally acceptable level would be eliminated from further consideration. The next level of selection would be done from the reduced group by a lay panel using the criteria of familial and social value. From these two selection processes, a more or less homogeneous group would remain in whom the medical indications and the social indications are both favorable. The final selection from this group would then be made by chance, by lottery, and not on a first-come, first-serve basis. This scheme does not pretend to be "optimal," but it may well be "acceptable" and does attempt to let health providers make medical decisions, society make societal decisions, and chance make the final decision.

The Acquired Immunodeficiency Syndrome Problem

The appearance and identification of the human immunodeficiency virus (HIV) and the rapid spread of an almost invariably fatal infectious disease has created massive ethical problems. Acquired immunodeficiency syndrome (AIDS) patients were considered to be a major menace to the community, and there was an almost hysterical fear of even being in the same room with a patient suffering from this disease. There are numerous cases on record in which AIDS patients were refused admission to hospitals or in which hospital personnel refused to care for patients, if admitted. From an ethical point of view there is no excuse for such a medieval attitude. Refusing to care for an AIDS patient is strongly reminiscent of the handling of lepers in allegedly less enlightened periods of world history.

The mode of transmission of the HIV virus is well known. It can be transmitted only by body fluids, and the survival time of the virus outside the body is apparently quite limited. The chances of becoming infected by casual contact are minimal, if any. Nevertheless, health care providers should protect themselves by using strict isolation techniques with gown, cap, gloves, mask, and goggles, whenever they are engaged in the active care of an AIDS patient.

The second major ethical–legal problem with AIDS is the question of mandatory testing. This is an extremely sensitive area, and there are widely divergent opinions concerning the propriety of testing for AIDS on a compulsory basis or unbeknownst to the the person. To some extent, this issue is analogous to the involuntary or compulsory testing for narcotics or other central nervous system–active substances in certain population groups.

It is my strong feeling that testing for AIDS without the patient's consent constitutes assault and is thus actionable. Under no circumstances should this test be performed without consent. Only the legislature can mandate compulsory testing, and if the legislature wishes to exempt AIDS testing from the protection of the constitution, legislation to this effect would have to survive a constitutional challenge in the US Supreme Court. I doubt very much if this is possible.

The Ethics of Experimentation

Because respiratory care personnel are increasingly engaged in research and because some of this research frequently involves patients, some thoughts on the ethical and legal requirements of human experimentation may be appropriate.[25]

The findings of the international tribunal that tried the major Nazi war criminals sent a wave of shivers around a world already numb with the horrors discovered in the German concentration camps. Not only were millions of racially or politically "undesirables" put to death, but there was irrefutable evidence that brutal and frequently fatal experiments had been conducted by medical practitioners on hundreds of prisoners. To prevent a repetition of such barbaric acts, the tribunal announced a code of ethics for human experimentation known as the Nuremberg Code (1946–1949). The code states that no person shall ever be used as an experimental subject unless he or she consents voluntarily; that there be no other way to gain the same information; that risks never outweigh the benefits; that the experiments be conducted only by experienced and careful scientists fully aware of their responsibilities to the subject; and that the subject be free to withdraw from the experiment at any time and for whatever reason.

Considerable amplification of this code was

provided by the Declaration of Helsinki, a statement by the World Medical Association. This declaration, issued in 1964 and revised in 1965, lays down the basic principles of ethical medical research and distinguishes between clinical research and nontherapeutic biomedical research on human subjects.[26]

Following the discovery of some scandalous experimentation in allegedly reputable hospitals, the Surgeon General of the United States in 1981 issued a set of guidelines[27] governing human experimentation in the United States. These guidelines, since expanded, now regulate all research done under federal grants or in federal institutions. Indeed, most health care facilities have voluntarily expanded the scope of these guidelines and now insist that all investigations involving human subjects conform, regardless of funding source. The core of these guidelines (now regulations) is the establishment of an institutional review board (IRB) that is charged with reviewing and monitoring all projects that involve human subjects.

These IRBs are composed of senior members of the medical staff representing various disciplines and varied research backgrounds. Other nonmedical members also must participate. Careful minutes are kept and reviewed periodically by federal inspectors. The committees have considerable authority to request modifications in the proposed investigations and may even refuse permission to engage in certain types of "research."

Generally, human experimentation takes two major forms: therapeutic or physiologic. Therapeutic experimentation, in turn, may have two major subsets: the testing of drugs or techniques on patients who may benefit from the new drug or technique, or the testing on healthy volunteers before introduction into the clinical area. The Food and Drug Administration (FDA) requires that all new drugs have initial testing performed in healthy adults to ascertain the safety of the new agent. These are usually small-scale studies that involve a few volunteers in whom very elaborate laboratory and other studies are performed and to whom the new drug is administered in increasing doses, usually to the limits of tolerance. Traditionally, many of these so-called Phase I studies were performed on prisoners in state penitentiaries. This was, in many ways, an ideal arrangement because there were usually numerous volunteers, the experimental conditions could be rigidly controlled, and costs of the studies were relatively low. More recently, the freedom of consent of a prison population was questioned and today this very useful form of study has been largely abandoned.

The second step in therapeutic testing involves the use of the new drug or technique in small and carefully selected groups of patients. Initially these studies are controlled with extensive laboratory tests. In the case of drug evaluation studies, they serve to establish an approximate effective dosage range while checking for changes in laboratory variables.

The third phase is larger in scale, involves more patients, uses less laboratory control, and introduces a standard drug for the sake of comparative effectiveness. If the experimental drug still looks promising and has an acceptable incidence of side effects, it enters the final phase of testing. In this phase, large, multicenter studies are conducted to reaffirm the effectiveness of the new agent and to look for the rare complication that may appear only after widespread use.

Fundamental to all these studies is valid, free, and informed consent. Assuming that such consent is obtained, few will argue that such therapeutic trials are immoral or unethical.

Generally the same principles apply to therapeutic experiments conducted on minors or others who cannot give valid consent. If the new agent or technique clearly shows potential benefit for the patient in the study, the parent or guardian need not have ethical scruples in consenting for the child or ward. For an older child it is desirable, although not legally required, that permission for the study be obtained from the youngster.

Even though the well-controlled therapeutic study is less controversial than other forms of human experimentation, some serious ethical questions can be raised. Let us assume that a new antimicrobial agent is to be tested that is allegedly effective against a certain type of serious infection. Second, assume that agents effective against this particular microorganism already exist. Is it justifiable to subject patients in life-threatening situations to a drug of unproven value, when the patient could be treated effectively with a known agent? The answer I believe, is a highly qualified yes. This type of study is permissible only if the new drug shows unusual promise. It must be safer—that is, have fewer side effects—be more effective, or be cheaper. Lacking these potential benefits, a strictly "me too" study is ethically highly suspect.

Another area of real doubt regards therapeutic studies for which the nature of the agent requires the introduction of a placebo control. The ground rules should be the same. If consent can be obtained and if the participant's life is not threatened by being randomly assigned to the placebo group, the study may go forward. If the patient may be seriously jeopardized, even the best consent is insufficient, and such studies should not be performed.

The problem is entirely different if the proposed study is not therapeutic, but the purpose of the investigation is to obtain better understanding of physiologic or pathophysiologic principles. Occasionally these studies may benefit successive generations of patients, but in most other instances they serve only to increase the fund of human knowledge, without any foreseeable benefits to anyone except the investigator. Some ethicists believe that such studies are never permissible. This extreme position, like all extreme positions, is indefensible. Experiments that increase our understanding of physiology and pathophysiology are not only permissible but even desirable, provided certain very rigid conditions are met in the experimental design. These conditions can be stated as follows:

1. The risk of the study to the participants must be minimal and may at no time include the possibility of permanent harm of any kind.
2. The design of the study must be such that results, positive or negative, have statistical validity. Badly designed, predictably inconclusive studies are never justified.
3. Physiologic studies should not be performed on patients and should be performed only on healthy volunteers. Pathophysiologic studies must be performed on patients, but are legitimate only if there is minimal or no risk and if the patients understand very clearly that no benefit will accrue to them.
4. Such studies are probably never justified on minors or incompetents.
5. Inducement to participate should never be of a nature to make a rational decision difficult.
6. Studies may produce psychological damage as well as physical damage. Emotional trauma is more difficult to predict and much more difficult to correct. If there is any doubt, the experiment should not be performed.

Experimentation in medicine is as old as medicine itself. Any "first" in therapy—from the first incantation of the neolithic shaman to the first transplantation of a human heart—is an experiment, for there is not previous experience to serve as a predictor of result. The entire field of contemporary health care is based on experiments that were performed on patients by healers who tried new methods to treat illness. All of us are the beneficiaries of previous human experimentation; indeed, many of us would not be alive if we had not been treated with a drug or a surgical procedure that was "experimental" at one time. It is therefore absurd to maintain that human experimentation is wrong; that it is always an invasion of the sanctity of the human body; and that it should not be permitted under any circumstances.

The current fashion of protesting against most things regrettably includes protesting against experimentation both human and animal. Human experimentation and its ethical parameters have been discussed in the foregoing. Animal experimentation is an entirely different matter. Animals have no "rights," but humans have a duty to treat animals humanely. It is just as absurd to advocate that no animal should ever be used for experimentation as it is to say that there should be no parameters beyond which animal experimentation is not ethically permissible. This entire matter is discussed in depth by Professor Cohen.[28] I most strongly urge all readers interested in this subject to read his paper.

OTHER ETHICAL CONCERNS

The Impaired Health Professional

The problem of the impaired health professional is becoming a major issue, and all health care providers must learn to cope with it. Many of us have colleagues or associates who are becoming or have become incompetent because of senescence, alcoholism, drug abuse, emotional instability, or chronic illness. What is our ethical and (perhaps) legal obligation when we recognize that a physician, nurse, respiratory therapist, or other hospital worker no longer functions as well as he or she did in the past? He or she behaves erratically, shows wide mood swings, is forgetful, may become slovenly in appearance, or may show other evidence of emotional or physical deterioration. The surgeon whose tremor is no longer controllable, the respiratory therapist who "forgets" what treatments have to be given, the nurse who makes repeated mistakes in scheduling patients or who makes errors in medication—all are people who need help and who constitute a real or potential menace to the patient. Yet many of these people are our friends, our superiors, our colleagues. What is our duty; what do we have to do?

It is very easy to be categorically righteous and say that the impaired colleague must be reported to the proper hospital authority and removed from any patient care situation. Actually it is very difficult to do this. Few of us relish the thought of "reporting" or "squealing" on a fellow health worker. There is the fear of reprisals, there is the possibility of error, there is the very real possibility that our motives will be misunderstood. At the very least, we are almost certain to lose the friendship of the person whose failings we bring to the attention of the administration. The other side of the coin is equally awkward. If we do or say nothing and if because of this a patient is hurt, we have a heavy burden of responsibility to carry and may even be legally liable. To me, the latter is the greater of two evils; I believe that we must not, and cannot, stand by in splendid inactivity and hope that all will come out well. We must take active steps to assure the safety of the patients and must do this in a way that will cause the least pain or stress to the health professional involved.

If it is an employee, the first step is a private session to make friendly inquiries, to offer assistance, and to make the individual aware that his or her problem has become known and that there is every intent to be supportive and helpful. Suggestions can be made for early retirement, professional assistance, or referral to appropriate local agencies. In some instances this type of informal action may suffice, and the employee will voluntarily seek assistance or, if necessary, ask for leave of absence or reassignment to a less sensitive position. Some employees will not have been aware of their problem and will honestly be grateful for help and advice. If the employee denies any problem or becomes defensive or even abusive, the good supervisor will pursue the matter through the proper established channels, making certain that all allegations are fully documented and that the employee is given every possible assistance.

The problem is more complex if the impaired person is in a different health profession and, particularly, if that person is higher in the organizational structure of the institution, either by seniority or by the nature of his or her profession. The obligation is still clear. If a respiratory therapist be-

lieves that a nurse or a physician is impaired and may be dangerous to patients, the respiratory therapist must not console himself that this is "not his or her business." In this situation, the medical director of the respiratory therapy department is the appropriate recipient of a documented report. It is then the medical director's task to bring this matter to the attention of the hospital administration and the appropriate person in the medical staff organization.

What if it is the medical director who becomes impaired? Here, much depends on the interpersonal relationship that exists between the technical director and the medical director. If this relationship is a good one, the technical director may be able to have a frank and friendly discussion with the medical director and indicate the concerns that have been raised by members of the department. If the relationship is such that a conversation of this type is impossible, the technical director has no choice but to report to the hospital administrator. This is a tough step to take, and it is possible that the technical director who chooses this route may encounter serious criticism and even threats. It takes a good, strong person to have the courage of his convictions and to do the right things, even at the price of personal inconvenience and risk.

Professional organizations and the regulatory agencies are trying very hard to come to grips with this problem. To date, they have not been very successful. Several states have enacted legislation dealing with this matter. Although only beginnings, these are encouraging actions.

The Dishonest Employee

Somewhat akin, and yet sufficiently different, is the problem of the dishonest employee and the ethical and legal burden this places on us all. There must be few of us who, on occasion and usually in a very minor way, have not failed to distinguish between the property of the employer and the perquisites of the employee. The list of such minor peccadilloes is long and includes such items as using hospital stationery for personal correspondence, making personal calls and even long-distance calls from hospital telephones, snitching food in the cafeteria, swiping a few aspirin tablets at a nursing station, taking a bottle of hand lotion home, and so forth. More significant thefts include books from the library, surgical instruments for home workshops, scrub suits to be used as pajamas, and so on. Finally, there are the more serious thefts that include money and other valuables, major equipment, and indeed almost anything that is not a structural component of the building.

Everyone will agree that stealing a patient's pocketbook or a hospital television set is reprehensible, and yet most people will see little if anything wrong with the "minor thefts." From a purely ethical point of view there is no difference between a sheet of stationery and a television set, even though the law does distinguish on the basis of monetary value, and even the strictest employer is likely to ignore the pettiest of petty pilfering.

As employees, we do have a clear and binding duty to protect our employer's property, both from others and from ourselves. The excuses that "it does not matter" or "they'll never miss it" or "it's just a few cents' worth" are, at best, shabby. Whether we should take any action for the sake of a roll of tissue paper is another question. It is ethically wrong, but it may be practical if we look the other way and do not antagonize everybody for trivia. It would almost certainly accomplish nothing, make a lot of enemies, and place us into the invidious position of intolerable righteousness. The situation is quite different if the thefts involve more costly items. Here, I believe, our duty is clear. We must report it with the awareness that apprehension of the thieving coworker will lead to loss of his or her employment, probably criminal prosecution, and possible incarceration.

The Wrong Order

In respiratory care it is quite common to find orders that are incomplete, incorrect, or even potentially harmful. Most departments have policies that address this issue, but in many departments this situation is left to the discretion of the individual practitioner. The temptation is great to ignore the wrong order and to do what is deemed appropriate. This I believe to be ethically unsound and legally tenuous. No order should be willfully ignored or capriciously modified. The proper way to deal with this situation is to contact the physician who wrote the order and request a clarification or correction. If the physician is not available, the medical director of respiratory care should be contacted and asked to assume responsibility for the evaluation of the situation and to endorse, cancel, or modify the order. If the medical director also is unavailable and no other physician is willing or able to assume responsibility, the respiratory therapist faces a dilemma. Should he or she follow the order, or should the order be modified or ignored? I believe that in this situation the therapist should use his or her best judgment and do what, by training and experience, appears to be the right course of action. It is absolutely essential, however, that this action is carefully documented in the record and that a written justification is given for the decision. If the therapist decides to follow an order that appears to be in error, it is critical that the patient be observed continuously and that treatment be discontinued at the first sign of side reactions. Again, full documentation of the action is necessary.

These problems test the system and quickly point out weaknesses. The unavailable medical director and the careless ordering physician are not uncommon. Written policies, for handling improper orders should be included in respiratory care department policy and procedure manuals. Nonetheless, the good training and mature judgment of the therapist may be tested and found wanting. The reaction of the physician whose order was changed may be indicative of his or her education or personality. An incorrect order may occur anywhere and at any time. Handling it properly, and with no bad feelings on any side, indicates mature professional relationships and is a good measure of the professional ethics of the health care providers.

Sexual Harassment

An ethical problem as old as humanity is the relationship of the sexes. In recent years this problem has become accentuated by the increasing entry of women into the job market and the appearance of women in occupations and careers that were previously considered exclusively male domains. Women entering these fields have to overcome prejudice, hostility, and humiliation. They are the target of abuse and discrimination, are considered easy prey for the predatory man, and are frequently the subject of covert or overt sexual harassment. This may take many forms, from the smutty joke and "accidental" body contact, to frank sexual advances, including crass sexual blackmail. From an ethical and legal point of view the issues are relatively simply. No woman should ever be made to suffer discrimination or humiliation because she is a woman. Employees or coworkers must be treated with the same courtesy, consideration, and respect regardless of whether they are male or female.

Unfortunately, matters that may be ethically obvious and simple are very complex and perhaps even unresolvable in real life. Sexual impulses are among the strongest known urges, and to expect that all intersexual problems can be eliminated by regulations is absurd. Once again, the issue is one of degree. Sexual favors should never be demanded in exchange for retention in a job or promotion. All women should be able to follow effective grievance procedures and receive the full protection of the administrative system in case of sexual harassment or abuse. Predominantly female occupations, such as nursing, physical therapy, occupational therapy, and clerical and secretarial work, must have the same formal recognition, job description, salary potential, and general consideration as the still primarily male occupations. Once we proceed beyond these areas, however, we rapidly reach an area in which ongoing contact between young or not so young men and women will inevitably lead to behavior that some will consider offensive, some flattering, some amusing, and some will view with righteous indignation.

There is no ready answer to this problem, and it is the function of the department managers to keep interpersonal behavior consistent with professional decorum. As in so many other situations, good manners and good taste will accomplish more than rigid rules or the loftiest ethical principles. Although sexual harassment has a peculiarly and distressingly male connotation, much trouble can be avoided if the women's behavior is also kept within the same decorous bounds. Unnecessarily provocative behavior or dress is an invitation to trouble, and the woman who flaunts her femininity or who tries to use it for advantage is just as guilty of sexual harassment as the man who is weak enough or stupid enough to fall for it.

Another area of ethical concern is the relationship between therapists and patients. Although sexual misbehavior between health professionals is regrettable, sexual misbehavior between health professionals and patients is intolerable and is almost certain to lead to a loss of license, if it is brought to the attention of the appropriate regulatory agency.

A different, but still related, issue is the way health professionals address patients of the same or opposite sex. Customs change, and it has become quite common that coworkers, even of widely differing age and opposite sex, address each other by their first name. This is alleged to foster camaraderie and promote cheerfulness and cooperation. Perhaps so, and perhaps it is quite acceptable between members of the health team. I do not believe it is

acceptable between health professionals and patients. To address an adult patient, particularly a middle-aged or elderly patient, as Mary or Jane is not only rude but condescending and suggests a feeling of superiority. Even more objectionable are terms of endearment—"honey," "cutie," or "dearie" have no place at the bedside. Patients appreciate being treated with courtesy, and a proper form of address is certainly part of elementary courtesy.

SUMMARY

This chapter has presented, in a very condensed form, some of the legal and ethical concerns that have become major societal issues in the second half of the 20th century. The presentation stresses the practical aspects of very complex issues, and it is hoped that it will assist the respiratory care worker in avoiding legal entanglements. Every individual must come to grips with the ethical issues presented and somehow has to decide for himself or herself, on which side of the issue to take a stand. Like religion or politics, discussions on ethics can clarify the issues, but only very rarely can they change deeply felt convictions or overcome legitimate conscientious scruples. It is my hope that this chapter has helped the reader to make up his or her mind. I do not delude myself that I was able to convince anybody of anything, let alone everything!

REFERENCES

1. Blair v Eblen 461 SW 2d 370 (Ky 1970)
2. Fayson v Saginaw General Hospital Saginaw C. Circuit Ct. Mich. 1978
3. The Nuremberg Code—trial of war criminals before the Nuremberg Military Tribunals under Control Council Law No 10. Vol. II, Nuremberg, 1946–1949
4. Truman v Thomas 611 P 2d 902 (Cal. 1979)
5. Darling v Charleston Community Hospital 33 Ill 2d 3213 and 211 NE 2d 252, (Ill. 1965)
6. Gonzales v Nork 131 Cal Reptr 717 (Cal. 1976)
7. Corleto v Shore Memorial Hospital 350 ATL 2d 534 (N.J. 1975) and 138 N.J. Supreme Court (1975)
8. Bentham J: In LeFleur J (ed): An Introduction to the Principles of Morals and Legislation. New York, Hafner Press, 1948
9. Mill JS: Utilitarianism and Other Writings. Cleveland, Meridian, 1962
10. Kant I: Groundwork of the Metaphysics and Morals. New York, Harper & Row, 1964
11. Roe v Wade 410 U.S. 113, 1973

12. Doe v Bolton 410 U.S. 179, 1973
13. Gustafson JM: Mongolism, parental desires and the right to life. Perspect Biol Med 16:229, 1973
14. In re Houle. 74–145 Supreme Ct. Cumberland Co., Maine (Feb. 14, 1974)
15. Weber v Stonybrook Hospital 469 NYS 2d 63 (1983) and U.S. v University Hospital 729 F 2d 144 (2nd Circuit 1984)
16. Veatch RM: Death, Dying and the Biological Revolution. New Haven, Yale University Press, 1976
17. Barber v Superior Court 147 Cal. App. 3d 1006 (Ct. of Appeals 1983)
18. Corbett v D'Alessandro # 85-1052 Fla Distr. Ct. of Appeals (April 18, 1986)
19. In re Jobes # 4971-85E N.J. Superior Ct-Chancery Division, Morris Co. (April 23, 1986)
20. In re Dinnerstein 380 NE 2d 134, Mass 1978
21. Kaimowitz v Department of Mental Health N.E. 73-19434, A.W. Circuit Ct. Wayne Co. Mich. 1973
22. Anonymous: Scarce medical resources. Columbia Law Rev 69:620, 1969
23. Cahn E: The Moral Decision. Bloomington, Indiana University Press, 1955
24. Resher N: The allocation of exotic medical life saving therapy. Ethics 79(3):173, 1969
25. Chatburn RL, Hess D: The role of educators in clinical research [editorial]. Respir Care 32:321, 1987.
26. Declaration of Helsinki. Tokyo, World Medical Association, rev ed. 1965
27. Federal Register 46(Jan):8366, 1981
28. Cohen C: The case for the use of animals in biomedical research. N Engl J Med 315:865, 1986

■ SIX

The Modern Respiratory Care Department

Ray H. Ritz

Managers of respiratory care departments of today must deal with a "business" environment significantly different than that of the past 20 years. The responsibility of leadership requires an ability to cope with a variety of dynamic and interrelated factors. Diagnostic Related Groupings (DRGs), the Prospective Payment Systems (PPS), and Joint Commission on Accreditation of Health Care Organizations (JCAHO) regulations are now facts of life. Institutions place a high priority on reducing the patient's length of stay in the hospital, whereas society expects high-quality health care for all. Rapidly evolving technology requires a high level of sophistication among respiratory care practitioners. Studies of population demographics suggest probable staffing shortages throughout the next decade. A more culturally varied work force will require more open-minded and creative leaders. Service, as well as product quality considerations, will become increasingly important. These and other challenges will shape the modern respiratory care department well into the next century.

This chapter will provide an overview of the administrative organization of a respiratory care department, the management of personnel and budget, the assurance of quality, and the effect of current and future trends on respiratory care delivery. Techniques in handling specific situations may vary, but the importance of leadership will always remain constant. Good managers must find the balance between the art of inspiring people and the science of organizing them.

ORGANIZATION OF A RESPIRATORY CARE DEPARTMENT

Without a functional organizational matrix, communication is difficult and responsibility is unclear. The organizational chart in Figure 6–1 displays a chain of command for a moderate to large respiratory care department.[1] Although there are variations in this basic approach, most departments will find it offers logical flow. The size of the department and the personal style of the manager will control the level of complexity. Let us examine the relationship that some of the different components of the organization maintain with one another.

The hospital board of directors helps define the mission of the institution, including what portion of the community the hospital is to serve and the general philosophy of operation. The role of the hospital administration is to develop a global plan, or strategy, to complete this mission. These operational goals are passed on to the various departments, which then draft a set of action plans. The process works best when each level ensures feedback and advice during the development of these service and quality objectives.

The role of the medical director of a respiratory

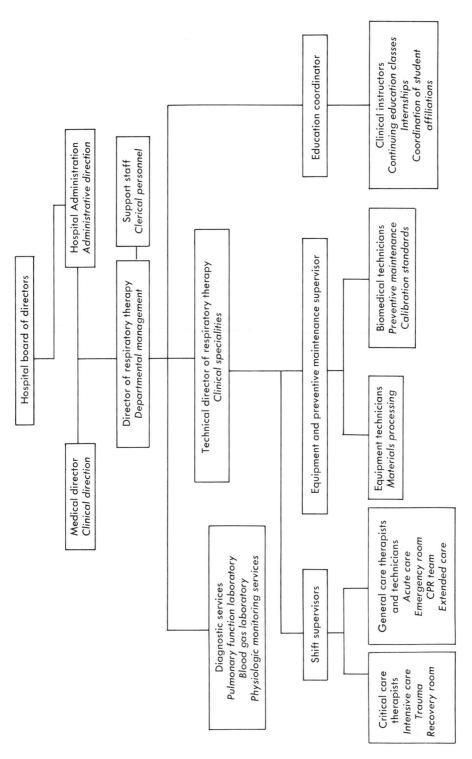

Figure 6–1. The traditionally organized, centrally managed and controlled respiratory care department. (McDonald PM: The organization and service of a respiratory therapy department. In Spearman CB, Sheldon RL, Egan DF: Egan's Fundamentals of Respiratory Therapy, 4th ed. St. Louis, CV Mosby, 1986)

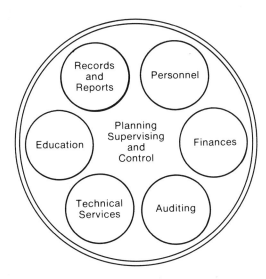

Figure 6–2. Centralized management. In a department operated in this fashion (a rearrangement of Fig. 6–1 into a Venn diagram), one person plans, supervises, and controls, essentially carrying out all management functions himself. The external circle represents the total sphere of his influence.

care department is to assure that the department provides appropriate and safe patient care. One could oversimplify the relationship between the departmental medical director and the hospital administration by portraying the medical director as the advocate of quality at any price, and hospital

Figure 6–3. The metamorphic state of management. As the department expands and the centralized administrative structure (*see* Fig. 6–2) becomes inadequate to handle increasing job pressures, additional staff will be given authority by the director to supervise those functions that have evolved to a point requiring semiautonomy.

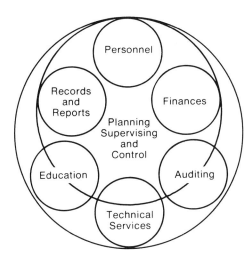

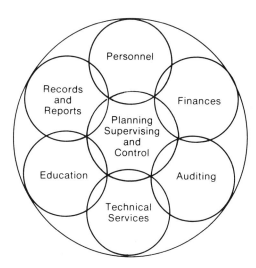

Figure 6–4. Decentralized management. As the department continues to expand to its fullest potential and adds additional management staff, the director will continue to maintain his or her role of delegating authority to those functions, although the interrelationships become more complex.

administration as focused only on a program's economic impact to the institution. Conflicts may arise and the *department manager* can, and must, act as the bridge between the two. When working optimally, this portion of the organizational structure should function in a symbiotic fashion and benefit all.

A pyramid-shaped organizational chart (see Fig. 6–1) is traditional and, at least on the surface, appears logical and clear. On the one hand, it is an accepted part of the science of management. How things work within the pyramid are a function of the art of management. How successfully managers communicate objectives and implement systems depends on how well they understand and motivate the staff. A small department will not have the complexity and layering of a large department, but the general function will be similar. In a small department, the responsibility for supervising staff and maintaining an educational program may reside directly with the manager. Equipment processing and repair may be done by staff therapists. A larger department may require more compartmentalization, with area supervisors controlling their section's day-to-day operations and reporting to the manager.

Descriptions in previous editions of this text demonstrate the concept of centralized (Fig. 6–2), metamorphic (Fig. 6–3), and decentralized management (Fig. 6–4) quite elegantly. In smaller departments, a centralized form of management may be ideal. The manager in this environment tends to be a "jack-of-all-trades." The larger and more complex the department, the greater the need for decentralization. In reality, a manager will find that he or she must monitor the department closely and allow some portions to become autonomous, while personally providing close supervision to other areas.

Knowing when to "back off" and when to "step in" is a trait of a skilled manager. Different personnel, changes in attitudes, or increasing or decreasing complexity in a segment of a department can make a unit more, or less, effective. Employees with admirable attitudes but limited experience may need only minimum direction, as the manager increases his responsibilities and grooms them into excellent supervisors. On the other hand, a historically effective supervisor may become "burned out" or distracted and need more motivation or assistance than in the past. Failure of a manager to adequately monitor or understand area operations will seriously affect departmental performance. One must not forget that while moment-to-moment control of a portion of the department may be delegated to a subordinate, the responsibility for its performance may never be lifted from the departmental manager.

DEVELOPING LEADERS

When decentralizing a portion of a department, the process of choosing the correct person to lead that area is crucial. A poor choice seriously compromises the ability to achieve departmental objectives. Leadership positions should be filled by individuals who consistently show good judgment, creativity, and organizational skills. They should provide good role models for those working with them, be fair, and be effective communicators. The manager must spend an adequate amount of time with these leaders to develop and refine the necessary skills in them and to ensure that they fully understand the desired objectives.

A manager must be willing to relinquish some control and accept some failures as part of the process of growing. Delegation of increased responsibility to subordinates has the effect of promoting their sense of ownership in a system.[2]

Managers who do not delegate responsibilities may find themselves overwhelmed with detail work and with no one available to assist them. It is wise to groom every employee to his or her highest level of potential. Not all will become leaders, but a manager can often be pleasantly surprised.[3]

Communication between the manager and the staff must occur in both directions. A manager's ability to listen to the staff can encourage new ideas and prevent "groupthink." Groupthink is the condition in which members of a group maintain a narrow set of concepts and reject anything outside the consensus.[4] This inbreeding limits creativity and independence.

Education plays a key role in developing staff into resourceful problem-solvers. Learning to be a leader is quite different from learning the technical aspects of patient care. Many institutions and continuing education services offer courses on a variety of supervisory and nonsupervisory topics. They can stimulate people and allow them to develop their own style of leadership. All levels of staff should be offered this training. Those who participate in the training may have a clearer understanding of the role of their supervisors.

Managers should challenge staff in a stimulating, positive fashion. Most individuals will strive to meet the expectations of peers and supervisors. A manager's role is to guide those expectations to match the departmental objectives and standards. It is the manager's obligation to support those who will accept the increased responsibility. Making someone responsible for something without giving him or her the authority and support to control the outcome is unfair, and it can be a source of frustration.

PERSONNEL

The most valuable resource of a respiratory care department is its people. Nothing happens without them. A manager has no more important task than to recruit, orient, and maintain an adequate number of employees. The skill with which this is done will have great impact on the department's ability to be successful. The pool of candidates coming into the profession in the 1980s and 1990s will be predictably small and competition for them understandably fierce. The Joint Review Committee for Respiratory Therapy Education (JRCRTE) reported a steady decline in the number of graduate technicians and therapists entering the profession from 1984 to 1987. During the same time, the 1986 Human Resources Survey of the American Association of Respiratory Care (AARC) estimated almost 3000 vacant positions in the United States. This was an average of 0.6 full-time equivalents, (FTEs) per department, and they occurred when most departments were stabilizing or reducing their personnel budgets.

RECRUITMENT

In most departments, recruitment is a process that must be kept active 12 months a year. The first hurdle a manager must cross is to cause a prospective employee to apply for a position. Advertising locally in newspapers, professional newsletters, and at local professional meetings is relatively quick and easy. These efforts reach practitioners who are more immediately available for employment. Maintenance of a close relationship with local respiratory care schools and assisting with their recruitment are also important. The response to recruitment efforts can be somewhat erratic, much like fishing: sometimes they're biting and sometimes not! Perhaps the best local advertisement is a staff that is technically competent and that displays high morale and professionalism to others.

When the local pool of recruits is not adequate, advertising in other metropolitan areas may be productive. Advertising in national professional journals is not a quick way to resolve an immediate staffing problem but is part of a long-range recruiting plan. It may take as long as 3 months before an advertisement is actually run.[5] One then has to go through the interview and reference-checking process and wait for the employee to relocate. There are times when this is perfectly acceptable, as when recruiting for an upper-level position, but staffing shortages usually occur suddenly and replacement staffing is needed quickly. If staffing shortages are frequent albeit unpredictable, regular national advertising can help keep a steady flow of inquiries coming.

Budget and acuteness of need will dictate the effort and expense of advertising. Even when professionally done, large layouts are no guarantee of attracting responses. The more positive and professional description is usually better. A quick follow-up to inquiries, which may include a mailing or a brief telephone call, is necessary. There is truth to the adage, "Advertising can be expensive but staffing shortages can cost more."

INTERVIEWING

The process of interviewing a candidate should include a series of general questions designed to begin the dialogue. Each interviewer has his or her own style to cover the following general areas:

- Previous employment history
- Educational background
- Job expectations
- Areas of strength and limitations

When questioning a candidate about technical issues, one should be careful not to play "Guess what I'm thinking." The candidate most likely knows little about your institutional policies or style, so questions should be general and pertain to accepted community standards. Questions on race, color, religion, creed, marital status, children, or sexual preference may violate state and federal law and should not be asked. Interviewers should limit themselves to those lines of inquiry that give job-related information. All persons who participate in the interview are part of the employment process and must follow these guidelines.

Inquiry about an applicant's strengths and limitations helps the manager get a feel for how a person perceives himself (although it is rare for someone to describe himself as lazy, inept, or hostile). Perhaps the most illuminating part of assessing a potential employee is the checking of his references. Previous employers and program instructors can provide valuable insights. Some applicants look apparently reliable on paper, only to have reference checks uncover a trail of disappointed past employers. One poor reference may not be conclusive, but several should raise a red flag. References should be questioned about the applicant's work ethic, attention to detail, ability to get along with others, absenteeism, and eligibility for rehire.

STAFFING SHORTAGES

Another avenue available to provide adequate staffing is the use of per diem and agency personnel. Per diem employees work on an "as-needed" basis and generally do not receive benefits such as medical coverage and vacation time. Agency staffing is contracted through an outside company and may often cost as much or more than the use of permanent staff at overtime wages. Each of these approaches has its own advantages and drawbacks. However, when permanent staff is unavailable, these may be the only options.

Judicious use of overtime and temporary staff can reduce the impact of a staffing crisis and also ease the stress inflicted on permanent employees. The ideal scenario involves use of these staffing options during periods of abnormally high volume or during a temporary staffing shortage. In reality, many departments must use these options continuously to maintain adequate staffing during normal times. This is not necessarily bad, because it allows the department to cancel staffing if volume decreases quickly. Adjusting the mix of full-time/part-time, per diem/agency personnel is part of the art of management. Each manager must look for the best solution for his or her department in balancing what is most economical and yet maintains adequate quality.

The performance of agency and per diem employees should be monitored at least as closely as that of permanent staff. Often their orientation to individual institutions (provided by a staffing agency) covers only very basic information. One may not be able to expect the same problem-solving or technical skills in an agency employee as from one's own staff. Agency and per diem staff may need additional information tools that permanent staff do not. It is helpful to develop succinct policy statements or procedural summaries that clarify confusing but commonly encountered issues.

ORIENTATION

Once employees are recruited, an effective orientation will prepare them for their job responsibilities. Orientation may consist of anything from a 1-day tour and description of expectations to a thorough exposure to departmental and institutional policies and procedures. The more demanding the job, the more detailed the orientation. There are several components of the orientation process that help ensure success. An organized outline of the expected skills and access to written departmental policies and procedures help a new employee acclimate to the department. Exposure to tasks should progress from basic to advanced.[6] Records must be kept that document an individual's ability to perform specific procedures and his or her knowledge of institutional policies. These records must be maintained in the employee's personnel file to meet various credentialing agencies' requirements.

Orientation personnel should be trained to ensure that new employees receive all necessary support. Also, a consistent method of evaluating performance during orientation is important. If more than one person participates in a new employee's orientation, it is necessary to ensure effective communication among them.

MAINTAINING AND GROOMING EMPLOYEES

A manager's expectations define the professional standards of the department. The staff's performance is based on the manager's ability to communicate those expectations. If one hires people with acceptable skills and work ethic, the job is simply to "focus" them on specific "targets." Unreasonable expectations create frustration for both the manager and the employees. For example, reason-

able expectation may be for staff to perform 6 hours of direct care per 8-hour shift. It may be unfair to expect them to provide an additional 2 hours of direct care per shift because another staff member is absent and has not been replaced.

A manager must provide employees with the necessary tools needed to perform their jobs. These tools are information, clear policies or procedures, reliable equipment, adequate supplies, and administrative support. Breakdowns in the system are often related to the lack of one of these tools. Looking at problems and complaints from a viewpoint of "What missing resource or information would fix this?" provides a more positive framework for managing a group and is far superior to simply blaming individuals or performance.

Managers and supervisors should be trained in the techniques of handling a difficult employee. Seminars that develop a process for effective coaching and counseling help avoid mistakes or resolve problems in the work place. Training provided by the institution's staff-development program or by educational services can be helpful. In the past, many managers and supervisors have been promoted on the basis of their clinical skills. This is no longer entirely sufficient. The art and science of management is complicated and may not always parallel clinical abilities. Periodic reexposure to the concepts of effective management is helpful to all leaders, just as continuing education is to clinical staff.

POLICY AND PROCEDURE MANUALS

One of the most important and fundamental tools required by respiratory care practitioners is a clear and comprehensive *policy and procedure manual*. This document will define the standards of care and expectations of the staff. Careful organization will enhance its usefulness and make revisions less difficult. A policy and procedure manual will require constant updating and revision as changes occur.

When constructing a policy and procedure manual, all clinical procedures should be included. Pertinent personnel issues, such as sick time use or how to request vacation, should also be addressed. Policies on employee safety, infection control, and how to respond to a physician's order that is unclear must be available.

The first step in this organizational process is to determine how the document will be used. Unfortunately, most written policy or procedure manuals are infrequently referred to by the staff. Only when a specific question needs to be clarified will the document be consulted, and the reader will probably spend as little time reading it as possible. The following are features of a well-constructed manual:

1. The manual should contain information on frequently asked questions or complex issues.
2. Individual policies or procedures should be clear and brief.
3. Topics should be easy to find.
4. The manual should be updated or revised at regular intervals.

The distinction should be made between policies and procedures. *Policies* state departmental standards but do not describe how to perform the actual task. They should not be lost in the body of text of the task description but should stand alone. Written *procedures*, on the other hand, should outline the steps necessary to complete a task. With extubation as an example, a policy statement would be as follows:

Policy: Removal of an artificial airway is to be done only after a physician's written order is entered into the patient's medical record.

The written procedure would then list the equipment needed and actions taken by the practitioner. When constructing a written procedure, one should include all basic components. Making the description too detailed or wordy has several negative effects. The reader will have difficulty finding specific important information quickly. Also, there are likely to be many minor yet acceptable variations that a clinician may employ, given the circumstances at the time.

Some shortcuts can be taken. Manufacturers' operation manuals for various devices (ventilators, monitors, and such) can be made available and referred to instead of rewriting this information. Only unusual operations or modifications of these devices that are specific to one's particular institution need to be constructed.

Brief comments can highlight items that pertain to patient safety or that are frequently confusing. Again, the manual writer should keep the procedure description succinct and clear. One rule of thumb to use is: If it takes longer than 60 seconds to read a policy or procedure, one should review it for unnecessary content.

The key to making information quickly retrievable is a well-organized table of contents and an index. The table of contents should list policies and procedures in a logical order and group similar topics together. An alphabetical index is helpful for large manuals in which information on one topic is referred to in several different areas. A numbering system that facilitates clear organization of categories must also accommodate periodic additions.

ONGOING EDUCATION

Ongoing education helps employees improve their knowledge base and skill levels, which results in improved quality. It also serves to maintain their interest in and passion for their job. By providing new and challenging issues for the staff, one avoids the stagnation that occurs from lack of stimulation. Ongoing education provides employees with the tools they need to deal with the challenges of tomorrow's problems. The AARC recommends 25 hours each year of continuing education for respiratory care practitioners;[7] the continuing education can be linked to enhanced job performance.[8]

Education should be offered to all levels in a department, from the manager to the equipment technicians. It should include programs that not only improve job performance but also promote job satisfaction and safety. Because most respiratory care departments operate 24 hours a day, accommodations should be made to reach those employees who work evenings, nights, and weekends. Videotaping programs can be an effective way to accomplish this if an institution has the necessary equipment.

Records must be maintained of participation in educational programs. An easy way to document participation and comprehension is to administer a post-test, which should be simple and quick to take. The answers should be heavily emphasized in the presentation. The goal is to ensure that all participants are able to achieve an adequate number of correct responses. If this does not happen, the quality of the educational program or the clarity of the post-test should be reassessed.

EVALUATIONS

Regular performance reviews can be one of the most-effective methods of communicating with an employee. An evaluation should never be used as a disciplinary action but as an opportunity to improve an employee's overall job performance or behavior.

The evaluation interview should be held in a comfortable location and without interruptions. Keep the evaluation objective. Avoid being too lenient or strict: one is too wishy-washy, the other too demanding and critical. Be careful not to rate an employee's overall performance on one good or bad characteristic. Avoid the tendency to rate all employees as average. Let them know about their successes and their limitations.

Be specific when discussing concerns and accomplishments. It is a good idea to maintain a regular diary that notes significant comments about each staff member. Vague or generalized statements can be antagonistic and appear unfair. The reviewer should avoid being defensive and concentrate on facts. Responses should be made to objections and problems, without being judgmental. The interview should end on a positive note. Emphasis is best placed on how to improve performance and on follow-up plans that promote employee growth.[9] Whenever possible, employee compensation should be linked to performance, with performance objectives clearly understood by both the employee and the employer.

SCHEDULING

The provision of creative, yet adequate, staffing patterns will have a significant effect on the quality of a department. Recruitment and retention can be enhanced by offering patterns that meet the differing needs of staff members. At the same time, the manager must assure adequate productivity and quality of care. With more single parents in the work force and an increasing priority on leisure time activities, managers must consider more nontraditional methods of staffing.

Today's work force commonly works 8-, 10-, and 12-hour shifts. Part-time work is often a necessity for one or both members of a working couple. However, respiratory care departments typically remain predominantly 24-hours-a-day, 7-days-a-week operations, and this often results in scheduling conflicts. Regardless of the scheduling pattern a department uses, it is often a topic of great debate among the staff.

Rotating shifts may have the advantage of reducing shift rivalry, but studies show that worker efficiency and satisfaction can decline in this environment.[10] Straight-shift patterns may satisfy those who are allowed to work their preferred shift, but conflict between one shift's staff and another may be accentuated. Also, requiring new employees to begin their work careers on night shift may impair recruitment.

The length of time for shifts can affect a department as well. Although 8-hour shifts may promote consistency and follow-through, employees have fewer days off. A person working 12-hour shifts may enjoy the long stretches off,[11] but a manager may find it difficult to assign that person a project that requires daily attention. Ten-hour shifts can help provide a staffing overlap to complete scheduled treatments or procedures. However, if procedures are not grouped into set time slots, 10-hour shifts may not be economical.

To determine the number of staff assigned to a given work shift requires an assessment of the volume of work that must be done during different periods of the day. (This topic is addressed in detail in the section on monitoring departmental productivity later in this chapter.) It is important to note that one shift, staffed 7 days a week, needs approximately 1.4 to 1.6 full time equivalents (FTEs) for each position filled. An FTE is defined as 40 hours a work per week × 52 weeks = 2080 hours per year, including vacations, education time, and sick leave.

PROSPECTIVE PAYMENT AND SCOPE OF PRACTICE

Respiratory care departments tend to provide a wide variety of patient care services that are based on each institution's need. Those services can be separated into two types: traditional and nontraditional. *Traditional* services are those that are common and well accepted in most departments. *Nontraditional* services include those that may not be directly related to respiratory care but share similar levels of technology. The spectrum of services a department offers defines its scope of practice. All services and equipment must be paid for, and changes in how hospitals costs are reimbursed have significantly affected the services offered of practice by many departments.

In 1983, in the face of escalating health care costs, Medicare implemented the Prospective Payment System (PPS), which limits reimbursement to hospitals on the basis of a patient's Diagnostic Related Grouping (DRG). If a hospital spends more money caring for a patient than the DRG allows, the hospital loses money. This method of reimbursement has had the profound effect of changing departments from revenue centers into cost centers. The elimination or control of unnecessary or inappropriate services and procedures became essential cost-cutting measures in every respiratory care department. Theoretically, the most efficient method

TYPES OF RESPIRATORY CARE SERVICES

Traditional

Airway management
Bronchial hygiene
Oxygen–aerosol therapy
Mechanical ventilation
Consultation–educational
Pulmonary diagnositics
Assessement/Monitoring

Nontraditional

Invasive cardiac diagnostics
Extracorporeal circulation
Health promotion
EEG laboratories
Cardiopulmonary rehabilitation
Homecare
Noninvasive cardiac diagnostics
Bronchoscopy services
Hyperbaric oxygen therapy
Smoking intervention programs
Sleep disorders laboratories

for a hospital to deal with this new limitation on reimbursement is to increase the total number of admissions while simultaneously reducing the length of stay for each patient. Practically, the "sicker in, quicker out" patient flow through was born.

A survey by the AARC in 1986 attempted to determine the range of services offered in typical respiratory care departments and quantify the effect of the PPS.[12] The survey solicited responses from department managers, medical directors, and hospital administrators. The findings demonstrated that respiratory-related admissions had increased or remained stable in most hospitals and that the overall length of stay had decreased. Additionally, between 1984 and 1986, the demand for respiratory care services had increased or remained stable in most departments, although those same departments experienced a reduction or no change in their staff budget. This would require that an overall improvement in operational efficiency occur for these departments to handle the increase in patient acuity levels.

Although not indicated in the survey, departments may have improved the utilization of their employees by several methods. The respiratory care practitioner is generally well trained for various technical procedures and can operate a variety of sophisticated instruments. Procedures such as incentive spirometry, aerosol medications, and the setup of simple forms of supplemental oxygen therapy might be easily assumed by the nursing staff, thereby enabling the respiratory care staff to act as a consulting service and to provide more technically demanding respiratory care procedures. If these options are chosen, the respiratory care department must continue to be a consulting resource to the nursing staff for these procedures

and monitor for acceptable quality and appropriateness of therapy. Nursing services feel themselves as much constrained by PPS as respiratory care services; therefore, this transference of duties often is not practical.

Another effect of the PPS was to increase the range of services delivered by respiratory care departments. According to the AARC study, most respiratory care departments (94% to 100%) provide traditional services, defined as (1) diagnostic pulmonary tests, (2) respiratory therapy procedures, (3) therapeutic gas administration, (4) chest physiotherapy, and (5) ventilatory support. The acquisition of additional, nontraditional services is now common, and departments often provide one or more nontraditional services. These services include (1) invasive cardiac diagnostics, 11%; (2) noninvasive cardiac diagnostics, 54%; (3) extracorporeal circulation, 4%; (4) health promotion, 64%; (5) electroencephalography (EEG), 37%; (6) cardiopulmonary rehabilitation, 43%; (7) home care and/or durable medical equipment (DME), 34%; and (8) other services, 40%. The technology used in these nontraditional services is similar to that which is common in much of the traditional services provided by respiratory care departments; therefore, the staff is usually well prepared to acquire the necessary skills. Additionally, the 24-hour-a-day operation of respiratory care departments allows adequate access to those services.[12]

The consolidation or clustering of various smaller services under one management umbrella also serves to reduce operational cost to the hospital. Determining a department's scope of service depends on, among other things, the staffing considerations of both respiratory care and nursing departments. An understaffed respiratory care department may be forced to relinquish certain procedures. Shortages of nurses may require the assumption of new responsibilities. Although some departments relinquish to the nursing staff much of the basic floor care (incentive spirometery, basic O_2 therapy, or administration of aerosol drugs), others may assume responsibility for services that nursing cannot provide. Generally, smaller hospitals have required respiratory care departments to provide a wider range of nontraditional services, but this trend continues to grow in departments of all sizes.

Given the need to reduce the average length of hospital stay, it is predictable that *home care* and *health promotion* are some of the more common inclusions in today's respiratory care department. Hospital administrators who responded to the AARC survey gave these nontraditional services a high priority. These same administrators gave a strong vote of confidence to the ability of respiratory care departments to successfully manage the acquisition of new services. Interestingly, the consensus was that respiratory care managers should aggressively seek out these new areas and expand their role in such important activities.

The process of using respiratory care staff for nontraditional services is enhanced by adequate preparation of respiratory care students. Educators who responded to the survey indicated that, generally, students were well trained in noninvasive cardiac diagnostics, health promotion, cardiac or pulmonary rehabilitation, home care, and various other services.

QUALITY ASSURANCE

A quality assurance (QA) program should monitor a department's activities to assure appropriate responses for a specific need. Quality assurance must cite examples of adequate quality and the achievement of a successful outcome. Institutional and departmental accreditation is based on meeting standards set by the Joint Commission on Accreditation of Healthcare Organizations (JCAHO), and reimbursement for services is contingent on achieving this accreditation. A poor QA program can limit adequate reimbursement, in addition to depriving patients of quality health care.

In 1986, the JCAHO launched its "Agenda for Change." As the commission stated, "The goal of this program is to develop an outcome oriented monitoring and evaluation process that will assist health care organizations in improving the quality of care they provide."[13]

Hospitals must move away from audits that look retrospectively at records. These are simply quality control monitors and do not directly address outcome. Today's approach requires daily monitoring of frequently performed activities (called *volume indicators*) for both appropriateness and effectiveness. Evidence must be provided showing that activities create a beneficial outcome for the patients. This includes daily documentation that correct therapy is provided, costs are kept to a minimum, and the patient's response to therapy is evaluated at appropriate intervals. Put in slightly different terms, today's QA is documentation that supervisors are performing their jobs effectively.

Quality assurance must be applied to all significant facets of a department, including payroll, equipment processing, continuing education, and preventive maintenance.[14] It can be an effective tool in pinpointing and resolving problems. The key to meeting current standards and making QA a powerful problem-solving tool is to construct a system that meets the following criteria:

1. QA should document daily supervisory activities.
2. Documentation should be easy to do and clear.
3. All staff should have some responsibility in QA.
4. QA should maintain or improve operations.

HOW TO CONSTRUCT A MONITOR

An effective monitor should be easy for staff to understand, simple to perform, and provide a complete data base. These criteria may seem to be incompatible, but the goal is achievable. The following steps allow the construction of a QA monitor and evaluation device:[15]

1. Determine the primary components of an activity.
2. Determine the factors that indicate the appropriateness or maintenance of a quality environment.
3. Establish criteria that define acceptable levels of performance.
4. Designate responsibility for the monitor.
5. Collect and analyze data.
6. Report findings and recommendations to the hospital QA committee and effected personnel.
7. Initiate corrective actions that resolve identified problems.

8. Remonitor the activity to determine conformity with institutional standards after corrective measures are implemented.

There are two classifications of QA monitors. *Periodic monitors* are those that are applied to various aspects of the departmental operation for a designated period. At the end of the collection period, if the activities are within conformity of institutional standards, the monitor is terminated. If standards are not met, corrective actions are implemented and the activity is remonitored at an appropriate interval. Virtually every type of departmental activity should be the focus of a monitor at some time.

The other type of monitor, *continuous*, is reserved for those activities for which nonconformity with institutional standards carries significant risk to patients or departmental operations. Such ongoing monitors are sometimes called *rolling audits*. The monitoring of equipment disinfection and use of oxygen and bronchodilator aerosols are examples of the types of procedures that might be continuously monitored.

Another type of activity that may merit a continuous monitor is one for which acceptable consistent conformity is difficult to obtain. An adequate documentation in the patient's chart of services rendered by respiratory care staff is a common problem in many departments. A review of the last 24 hours of charting is a common supervisory task, and documentation of this supervisory activity is an important QA monitor.

The application of monitors should be predicated on their benefit. Although it is appropriate to demonstrate that quality is provided, data for data's sake serve no purpose. Overmonitoring an activity that clearly functions well is not an effective use of departmental resources. The goal should be to strive for appropriate, effective, and efficient operations.

A sample monitor might evolve as follows: A supervisor has received numerous comments from the clinical therapists indicating that chest physical therapy is being ordered for patients who may be able to manage their own pulmonary hygiene with a less labor-intensive form of therapy. The fact that increased supervisor's time was being spent addressing this issue is evidence a monitor is needed.

The first step is to develop a list of indications for chest physical therapy. These may include radiographic findings, ability to clear secretions, and the acuity of illness. The quality of the patient's cough and level of cooperation and various laboratory findings are also considered. If physicians of various services order the therapy, each service should have an opportunity to review the criteria developed. Because the monitor will be conducted by respiratory therapists, the data gathered should be easily acquired from the patient's chart or physical examination.

A systematic method of rating the positive or negative effect of these items is then developed. This prevents distortion of the assessment from personal bias. Adequate peer review of the rating system by various physicians and therapists will help improve its accuracy. In the sample monitor shown in Figure 6–5, the area of the lung in which a lesion occurs is entered. The quality of the patient's cough, sputum characteristics, and cooperation can be noted with a check mark. This allows the form to be quickly and consistently filled out. Subjective comments can be noted and reviewed as monitor data are returned. If the same comments occur frequently, the monitor may require adjustment. A list of alternative therapies is available for the evaluator to choose from. A monitor such as the example in Figure 6–5 might take about 15 to 30 minutes to fill out for each patient and is done only when therapy is initially ordered.

Instructions must be developed so that the individuals who will apply the monitor can use it in a consistent fashion. This also must be constructed with adequate peer review at both therapist and physician levels. One method of ensuring consistent use of a monitor is to have several staff members assess the same patient and compare their recommendations. After consistency is achieved, the monitor is again applied. To avoid skewed results, study all patients or a random selection. It is just as important to determine when chest physical therapy is properly ordered as it is to find when it is not. Those physicians who use it correctly can be your best allies in educating their colleagues.

When the monitor has been applied to a designated number of patients, the preliminary data are reviewed to determine if the monitor answered the question, "Is chest physical therapy ordered according to accepted criteria?" Commonly, one finds that adjustments in the monitor or additional education of those applying it are required. After the monitor is "debugged," it is again applied.

After adequate data have been obtained, they are analyzed and reported. The process of adequately reporting QA data is extremely important, as it provides additional support for promoting

Instructions

Upon receiving any initial chest physiotherapy order, assess the patient, review the medical record, and consult with other care givers (nurses, therapists, & physicians). Complete form and make any additional comments regarding information not gathered by monitor. Return completed form to departmental QA coordinator.

Patient: _____ ID #: _____
Unit/Bed: _____ Managing Service: _____
Ordering Physician: _____
Current Order/Date: _____
Diagnosis: _____

Clinical Findings
CXR-Date: _____

	Location	Score
Atelectasis	_____	+30
Diffuse Infiltrates	_____	+30
Lung Abscess	_____	+30
Focal Infiltrates	_____	+30
Foreign Body	_____	+30
Pleural Effusion	_____	0

Examination

Breath Sounds	Location	Score
Clear/Equal	_____	−30
Decreased	_____	+10
Absent	_____	+20
Gurgles	_____	+15
Crackles	_____	+5
Wheezes	_____	0

Cough		Score
None	_____	+20
Poor	_____	+20
Fair	_____	0
Good	_____	−30

Cooperation		Score
Excellent	_____	−20
Needs Encouragement	_____	0
Unconscious	_____	+10
Uncooperative	_____	−10
Ambulatory	_____	−10

(continued)

Figure 6—5. Respiratory care pulmonary hygiene evaluation monitor.

change. Reports should be submitted to the institutional QA board, the department medical director and staff, and other affected parties.

In the foregoing example, the monitor found that chest physical therapy was utilized inappropriately or at an unacceptable frequency: a logical response is to require a review of future therapy to ensure that it fits accepted criteria. The design of this QA monitor makes possible its easy conversion into a Respiratory Care Pulmonary Hygiene Consultation Form. When countersigned by the medical director, it can serve as an effective tool for educating other physicians in choosing the most appropriate and cost-effective therapy.[16,17]

Types of Monitors

Because the activities and services of a respiratory care department are varied, so are the methods of monitoring those activities.

Examination

Complications of Therapy   Score
    Extreme Pain   _____   −15
    Shortness of Breath   _____   −10
    SaO2 < 90% c Therapy _____   −30
    Refuses Therapy   _____   −30

Sputum
Color: Yellow/Green _____ +15 Clear _____ −10
Quantity: Lg _____ +20 Med _____ +10 Sm _____ 0 None _____ −20
Consistency: Thick _____ +10 Thin _____ 0
Hemoptysis (frank) _____ −100 (direct contraindication)

    Labs
       Temp (TMAX)   _____
       pH   _____
       PaO2   _____
       PaCO2   _____
       SaO2   _____
       FiO2   _____
TOTAL SCORE: _____
Comments: _____
_____
_____

Recommendations

_____ Continue Current Therapy
_____ Discontinue Current Therapy or:

Change To:
                 (Frequency)   (Frequency)
    DB & Cough   _____   ETT Suction Only   _____
    NT Suction Only   _____   IPPB Trial   _____
    CPT to _____   _____   Hyperinflation   _____
            lobe

Respiratory Therapist: _____ Date: _____

Figure 6—5 (continued)

Charting Monitors

Most (if not all) activities carried on at the bedside must be charted. Reviews of these records can help ensure that procedures are performed according to the ordered frequency or institutional standards. This is also an important area for monitoring, because reimbursement may depend on adequate documentation of billable procedures. There is an increasing trend to perform these monitoring activities with computerized devices.

For this type of monitor to conform to today's standards, data must be reviewed and gathered on a regular basis. Timely feedback can be provided to the authors of the charting. It is a simple matter to then maintain records on historical conformity and current trends.

Some methods to improve QA are

- To provide the staff with a uniform set of responses that document specific procedures and therapies
- To compartmentalize the charting forms so that procedures that require little description can be simply checked off
- To place items that require description in designated areas of the form for quick location by the reviewer

Bedside Observations. Observation of direct patient care activities can be useful in determining a practitioner's conformity with institutional policy. The drawback to this method of monitoring is that performance during observation may be different from that when unobserved. Observation by an unknown data collector may avoid this complication. Observing compliance with handwashing policy is an example of a monitor that can be done in this fashion.

Satisfaction Questionnaires. Although the responses may often be subjective, surveys obtained from patients, nurses, and physicians can reveal areas in which service is lacking or quality is good. They provide an insight to departmental performance that may be distinctly different from that held by those inside the work group.

How To Report a Monitor

There are two components to reporting a monitor: what to report and whom to report it to. The report should describe what the focus of the monitor was and the criteria defining acceptable quality or appropriateness (or both). Data collected are summarized to show the results in a clear and concise fashion. A target level of conformity must be designated and the incidence of nonconformity reported. The report should also describe any proposed corrective actions that are recommended. If the monitor's purpose was to observe the effect of a change in practice, the previous conformity or outcome should be compared with the current level. The next scheduled period of monitoring should also be noted.

Reports are submitted to the institutional QA board and to any other affected personnel. Because quality assurance is such an integral aspect of today's health care, the use of the influence of the institutional QA board may be one of the most effective means of instituting a multidisciplinary change.

BUDGET

Much of a respiratory care department manager's responsibility includes measuring and counting activities and calculating the cost to provide service. Each institution will require departments to budget and monitor performance, with various degrees of complexity; as costs increase and reimbursement becomes more limited, the need for tight budgetary control becomes even more important.

A hospital administrator must ask if the cost of operating a respiratory care department is justified by the service it provides. The department manager must respond by demonstrating that appropriate standards are maintained in three areas: (1) staff productivity, (2) operating costs, and (3) quality of care.

MONITORING DEPARTMENTAL PRODUCTIVITY

In light of the ever-increasing costs of health care, adequate monitoring of staff productivity serves several useful purposes. The ability to justify staffing budgets to administration depends on a manager's ability to provide data that demonstrate departmental staff is not underutilized. Conversely, assuring that staff are assigned appropriate workloads helps ensure that patients receive safe and high-quality care. Before DRGs and the transformation of respiratory care departments from revenue centers into cost centers, many departments maintained this balance by depending on a "gut feeling."

The evolution of productivity monitoring systems has gone from departmentally developed systems designed for institutional use to systems with a much grander purpose. These second-generation systems were developed by professional associations and were intended both to be used for departmental management and to allow a creation of data bases from information supplied by numerous subscribers. These data bases were then used to assist in the development of appropriate professional and operational standards. An example of one such system is that mandated by the Washington State Hospital Commission for use by all respiratory care departments in that state.[18] This Uniform Reporting System (URS) assigns a designated time value to each procedure, derived by analyzing data supplied by numerous departments. In the Washington URS, some procedures lack a preassigned time value. These tend to be procedures that can vary substantially from patient to patient in the same institution (e.g., CPR, patient transports, or discharge planning).

Measuring Productivity

The determination of an appropriate level of productivity for a department is one of the most important questions a manager must consider. It can justify virtually every aspect of the departmental budget. Appropriate personnel and supply budgets cannot be constructed without knowing the level of resources required to perform a given number and mix of procedures. The essential tool needed for the manager to monitor productivity is a system that accurately reports the amount of time spent with patients and the types of procedures performed.

A substantial amount of departmental productivity is generated by support staff productivity and is difficult to quantify. However, this direct patient care activity justifies a department's existence. Consequently, a department must produce an adequate number of appropriate direct care hours (DCH) or it risks FTE reductions and budget cuts. A reliable method of relating the type and volume of procedures to the number of staff needed to perform those procedures is an essential tool for managers.

The first step in determining an appropriate productivity level for a department is to assign time values to each direct patient care procedure. All specific components of a procedure must be clearly defined, in advance, and each activity monitored several times to determine the average time needed to complete it. Complete procedures generally include the following:

COMPONENTS OF DIRECT CARE HOURS

- Order verification and chart review
- Handwashing, gloving, and so on
- Bedside equipment preparation
- Dialogue with patient
- Pretherapy assessment
- Administration of therapeutic modality
- Post-therapy assessment
- Charting

Staff members can spend a substantial amount of time involved in activities not included in the foregoing list. The following components and activities do not contribute to DCH and, therefore, can be considered "indirect activities" or nonproductive hours:

INDIRECT ACTIVITIES

- Travel to and from patient area
- Phone interruptions
- Complications (e.g., chart not available)
- Supervision and QA monitoring
- Staff education
- Personal fatigue, other

Once each procedure has an assigned time value, the manager simply multiplies the number of times each is performed by its relative time value to get total DCH. This is compared with the total number of hours worked in the department in the same period to calculate the overall percentage productivity for the department.

The AARC and other producers of management tools have developed various URSs. There are three reasons to consider such a system instead of developing one's own. First, one of the major components of the JCAHO's Agenda for Change is a data-reporting and analysis system that provides institutions feedback about their performance. Data of this nature will be essential for JCAHO to monitor institutions, and all institutions will be required to submit reports in the same format. No single URS has been designated as "the" system of choice, but a national system may be developed in the future. Second, constructing a system from scratch requires a great investment of time and resources. Even installing an "off the rack" system can be a formidable task, but it may be cheaper and more comprehensive than one developed internally. Finally, by using time values that represent a professional standard, a manager can pinpoint areas of departmental efficiency and inefficiency.

A URS is not intended to be a billing system, but it can be incorporated into one. By combining personnel time with the cost of supplies and other resources used, a weighted value can be assigned to each procedure. This is commonly called a *relative value unit* (RVU). Two procedures that require the same time to complete may have different RVUs, based on the comparative total cost of each. An RVU system can be a valuable tool to monitor total direct expenses as related to the number of procedures performed, but it may be less well-suited to monitoring productivity.

Setting a Productivity Standard

Once productivity can be measured, a standard must be set for the department.[19] Determination of this value is not a simple matter. The DCHs can only be performed by staff that do patient care. Support staff, such as supervisors, secretaries, equipment technicians, and such, generally will not contribute to this statistic. To determine the maximum amount of DCHs a department can produce, a manager must calculate how many hours an FTE works per year, less the nonproductive, paid hours such as vacation, sick, and holidays. The following is an example of this calculation:

Total paid hours/FTE = 2080 hr/yr	Non-	
Sick leave (8 hr/mo) = −96 hr/yr	productive	
Vacation (8 hr/mo) = −96 hr/yr	hours	
Paid Holiday (11/yr) = −88 hr/yr		
Total Working hr/yr/FTE = 1800 hr/yr	Productive hours	

Next the manager must determine how many direct care hours an FTE can produce per shift. Assuming that in an 8.5-hour shift each employee gets 30 unpaid minutes for meals, there is still a substantial amount of nondirect care time required. These activities include report (1.0 hour) and breaks (0.5 hour), which leave 6.5 hours available for direct care per FTE.

$$
\begin{array}{rl}
\text{Total hr/shift} = & 8.5 \text{ hr/shift} \\
\text{Unpaid meal period} = & -0.5 \text{ hr/shift} \\
\text{Two 15-min breaks} = & -0.5 \text{ hr/shift} \\
\text{Two 30-min reports} = & -1.0 \text{ hr/shift} \\
\hline
\text{Maximum possible} & \\
\text{DCH/FTE/Shift} = & 6.5 \text{ hr/shift}
\end{array}
$$

This means that one direct patient care FTE could produce a maximum of 1462.5 DCH per year for a productivity of 81.25%. This leaves no time for travel, interruptions, complications, and so on. If indirect activities such as those listed previously equal 1.0 to 1.5 hours per shift (and they most likely do), then productivity for direct care providers can fall to 69% to 62% or lower. The percentage of productivity will vary from department to department, based on structure and institutional nuances. The physical layout, variety of patient problems, and type of hospital can have great effect on productivity.

Once a productivity level is designated for a department, the following formula will supply an approximation of the maximum possible DCHs for a given number of staff who provide direct patient care:

(No. clinical FTEs × Pd hr) × % Productivity = Projected DCHs

DIRECT OPERATING EXPENSES

The direct operating expenses of a department can be divided into two distinct types of costs: the fixed costs that are fairly constant, regardless of patient volume, and variable costs that rise and fall in response to the number of admissions and the severity of illness of the patients. An example of some of the components of these categories follows:

SALARY EXPENSES

Fixed Costs	Variable Costs
Administration	Therapists
Supervision	Technicians
Clerical	Diagnostic staff
Equipment technicians	

NON-SALARY EXPENSES

Fixed Costs	Variable Costs
Depreciation	Medical supplies
Facility overhead	Non-medical supplies
Durable equipment	Drugs
Office supplies	Equipment rentals

The ratio of fixed to variable costs will fluctuate according to the departmental organization and structure. The more personnel a department utilizes for nonpatient care activities, the greater the fixed costs in relation to the variable. For example, a department that cleans and processes its own equipment will have a higher fixed/variable ratio than a department that has central service provide that function. Once the proper balance is achieved between these two types of costs, the manager must then monitor variable expenses to ensure that the department responds appropriately to its fluctuating environment.

Variable Expenses

Variable expenses are directly related to cost of labor and supplies required for each type of procedure. The number of times each procedure is performed is multiplied by the labor and supply costs to obtain the total cost. It is relatively simple to determine the supply cost of a procedure. For each procedure, a list of required supplies is defined and the cost of the items totaled. The labor costs are calculated in a similar fashion. If staff efficiency is high, the overall labor costs are low, relative to the number of procedures performed.

Fixed Expenses

The number of clerical staff, equipment processing and maintenance personnel, supervisors, educators, and so on will depend on the organization and structure of both the department and the hospital. The manager must carefully assess the productivity and function of these support areas to assess their costs versus services provided. Once this level is determined, it becomes part of the "fixed costs" of the department. Perhaps the easiest method of determining the fixed costs is to subtract the patient care–related variable costs from the total operating costs. The remainder will include some variable expenses, such as office supplies, replacement of minor equipment, and other miscellaneous items, but most will be fixed costs.

Constructing a Target Operating Budget

Once the fixed-to-variable-expense ratio has been set for a department and an appropriate productivity level is designated, construction of a target operating budget becomes a logical process. A target budget should estimate the operational funds required, based on a prediction of departmental activity for a given period.[20] A historical review of departmental spending and productivity will help the manager determine those items. With the labor and supply costs of the direct patient care defined and a historical trend of spending on fixed expenses and other related costs, a manager must now examine factors that may affect future trends. Typically, those factors may include

- Changes in regional population
- New or deleted services or programs
- Inflation
- New technology
- Changes in reimbursement or funding sources

Any of these items can precipitate an increase or decrease in the proposed budget. Once approved, the target budget becomes nothing more than a yardstick. As the demand for services changes, the appropriate adjustments should be made in staffing and spending. This method of variable budgeting requires close monitoring, but offers the manager the ability to best utilize institutional resources while delivering safe and appropriate care.[21]

The Capital Budget

Capital purchases are those that institutions define as major purchases, commonly exceeding a fixed dollar amount (e.g., $500). These purchases are generally made from funds separate from a department's operating budget. Justification of capital purchases generally includes patient safety, improved efficiency, improved quality, maintenance of operations, and new program support. It is helpful to show that new equipment can offer improved performance at reduced operating costs. Competition for funds is usually stiff, and the justification may require detailed estimates on operational costs, usage, and ability to generate revenue.

COMPUTERS IN RESPIRATORY CARE

The widespread application of computers in respiratory care poses an exciting challenge. Today's modern department can use computers for most clerical and record-keeping duties. The application in the clinical portion is also important. The computerization of a department need not happen all at once, although careful selection of microprocessor-controlled devices can save future dollars. When considering the purchase of a computer system, a careful investigation of all costs must be undertaken. A reasonably powerful complete computer system can be obtained for a modest investment. Once the system is installed, a manager may find that the cost of training and software far outstrips the initial purchase.

Substantial improvement in office efficiency and productivity can be gained with the use of word processors and electronic spreadsheets. Production and storage of any type of communication, policy, or report is easily done with any word processor, and updating can be accomplished quickly.

Detailed record keeping is extremely time consuming if done by hand. The use of an electronic spreadsheet or data base software can make the recording and monitoring of equipment maintenance simple. Monitoring departmental productivity, patient billing, quality assurance monitors, budgeting projections, and many more functions are readily processed by computers.

Before computerizing an office several questions should be considered:

1. What "hardware" is needed? One should accept the fact that whatever computer you buy today will be slower and less powerful than next year's version. The same is true of software. The limitations of a system are usually related to the user and not the computer. Some software has specific hardware requirements, such as minimum memory levels, hard memory disk drives, color display, or other unique options. This is a constantly evolving technology, and planning for expansion and increased functionality is appropriate. The option of upgrading memory and storage capacity should always be available.

2. What "software" is needed? Each department must define its own needs, but virtually all can make use of word processor and electronic spreadsheet. Both of these can be

easily mastered and can improve productivity and recordkeeping. For more sophisticated tasks, such as billing and inventory control, a data base program may be helpful. Any number of utility programs are available to maintain and repair both hardware and software. They are used to repair and retrieve lost data, diagnose system problems, and perform a host of complicated services. The type of software available is limited only by one's imagination.

3. What data will the computer manage? Information that is compiled over time and used for budgeting and tracking of spending patterns is tailor-made for electronic storage. This includes payroll, inventory control, billing, accounts payable, and much more. The more the complexity of these operations grows, the more a computer system can improve efficiency.

4. How much training will be needed? A sound fundamental knowledge of how computers and programs operate is extremely helpful, but not absolutely essential, for all users. Introduction to microcomputers is commonly offered at colleges, universities, and staff development programs and is well worth the time. Top of the line software generally comes with both written instructions and tutorial programs that teach the user by hands-on application. This is often enough, but again, classes are frequently available from numerous sources, including the vendor.

There are also pitfalls involved with computers. During the learning phase, productivity is often compromised. Each new piece of software purchased must be learned by someone. This means that if you collect software like baseball cards, either you will spend all your time learning it or it will sit around unused. Buying software that is too sophisticated may keep you from using your system. The more powerful a piece of software, the more difficult it is to operate.

Departmental operation can become very dependent upon a computer system. Therefore, a backup system, access to technical programming, and repair skills are all-important if a system goes "down."

Unless programming is a hobby for the respiratory care manager, it is generally not of great value. Commercially available software can save you time

and money, and the department members can become skillful in operating it. One can get bogged down in months of programming and can soon incur more costs than the use of a consultant who could install a system and train the staff in less time.

If a department is going to fully utilize computers, it must also have the resource to maintain them. Hard drives and memories must be organized and periodically cleaned out. Repairs must be made to damaged data. Data must be manipulated and analyzed. Once a department computerizes its functions, there is always more to learn about computer applications and utilization.

The computerization of patient care records is a completely different process, which can be separated into several layers. The first layer is the use of microprocessor-controlled equipment (Box). Today, this includes almost every device that operates electrically. Computer-controlled ventilators, physiologic monitors, diagnostic devices, and others all become more complex each year. One must decide what level of sophistication is appropriate for their institution. Devices should operate in an intuitive fashion and provide accurate and useful data.

The next step is to have all the data-generating devices deliver their information to a central-processing unit. There, many magical feats might be accomplished. The patient's complete medical record might be maintained for quick review. Data from numerous sources could be displayed on the same screen to see the effect and interdependency of various actions. The "paperless chart" may not yet have arrived, but prototypes are now being used, and this may be common in the respiratory care practice of the future.

As progress on developing the paperless chart is made, work is also being done on "closing the

---

COMPUTER-CONTROLLED DEVICES

Ventilators
Pulse oximeters
Capnographs
Apnea monitors
Transcutaneous pH, O_2, and CO_2 monitors
Humidifiers
ECG/blood pressure monitors
Hemodynamic monitors
Metabolic monitoring systems
Pulmonary function systems
Blood gas analyzers

loop." This is the phrase used to describe the process of feeding data acquired by physiologic monitors to devices such as ventilators, and the adjustments being made automatically. This evolution does not threaten our profession, but, instead, demands that respiratory care practitioners and managers keep pace with new changes and challenges.

The ability of a respiratory care department to provide appropriate, effective patient care and operate in a responsible and adaptive fashion is directly related to the quality of its leadership. Communication and accountability must be clear. Personnel should be treated with respect and fairness. They require support and guidance when dealing with difficult problems. The financial operation of a department needs the same type of frequent assessment that a patient needs. A consistent and effective method of assuring quality is required. The promotion of professionalism and personal growth at all layers of a department is paramount. The role of a manager is to organize a department in a fashion that results in the achievement of these goals. This process is the marriage between the art and the science of managing people.

REFERENCES

1. McDonald PM: The organization and service of a respiratory therapy department. In Spearman CB, Sheldon RL, Egan DF (eds): Egan's Fundamentals of Respiratory Therapy, 4th ed. St. Louis, CV Mosby, 1968
2. Hertzberg F: One more time: how do you motivate employees? Harvard Bus Rev Sept/Oct:109–210, 1988
3. Hersey P, Blanchard K: Management of Organizational Behavior: Utilizing Human Resources. Englewood Cliffs, NJ, Prentice Hall, 1987
4. Janis I: Victims of Groupthink: A Psychological Study of Foreign Policy Decisions and Fiascos. Boston, Houghton Mifflin, 1983
5. Fink J, Fink A: The Respiratory Therapist as Manager. Chicago, Year Book Medical Publishers, 1986
6. Pomerleau K: Organizing an effective orientation program. AARTimes 12:29–32, 1988
7. Continuing education: AARC position statement. AARTimes 10(5):1–64, 1986
8. Continuing education: does it affect job performance? AARTimes 8(5):25–30, 1984
9. Neal JA: Effective Phrases for Performance Appraisals: A Guide to Successful Evaluations. Perrysburg, OH, Neal Publishing Inc., 1987
10. Czeisler CA, Martian MC, Coleman RM: Rotating shift work schedules that disrupt sleep are improved by applying circadian principles. Science 217:460–462, 1982
11. Bunch D: Twelve hour day. AARTimes 5:38–39, 1981
12. American Association for Respiratory Care: The impact of prospective payment on the respiratory care profession. AARC, 1986
13. Joint Commission on Accreditation of Healthcare Organizations. Agenda for change update: Vol. 1, No. 1, JCAHO, 1986
14. Bader BS: Quality assurance: shaping up your board. Healthcare Executive (May/June):26–29, 1987
15. Joint Commission on Accreditation of Healthcare Organizations: HAP scoring guidelines, 1987
16. Shapiro B, Cane R, Peterson J, Weber D: Authoritative medical direction can assure cost–beneficial bronchial hygiene therapy. Chest 93:1038–1042, 1988
17. Walton JR, Shapiro BA, Harriston CH: Review of a bronchial hygiene evaluation program. Respir Care 28:174–178, 1983
18. The Uniform Reporting System Board of the Washington State Society for Respiratory Care: The uniform reporting system manual for hospital based respiratory therapy departments in Washington State. Seattle, Washington State Society for Respiratory Care, 1988
19. Herkimer AG: Understanding Hospital Personnel Management. Rockville, Md, Aspen Publishers, 1986
20. Herkimer AG. Understanding Health Care Budgeting. Rockville, Md, Aspen Publishers, 1988
21. Herkimer AG. Variable budget: A management tool for laboratory financial planning and control. Am J Med Technol 49:421–427, 1983

SEVEN

Evaluation, Maintenance, and Quality Control of Respiratory Care Equipment

Dean Hess
Garry Kauffman

Respiratory care, perhaps more than any other health care profession, involves the use of equipment. This equipment is therapeutic and diagnostic in nature. Malfunction of respiratory care equipment can be life threatening or can result in misdiagnosis. Respiratory care practitioners must be able to troubleshoot equipment malfunctions, conduct necessary preventive maintenance, and assure the quality of diagnostic test results. In this chapter, we will discuss topics related to equipment evaluation, maintenance, and quality control. Our intent is to provide practical information in a generic manner that will be useful to respiratory care practitioners.

STANDARDS ORGANIZATIONS

A number of organizations have published standards related to respiratory care equipment (Table 7–1).[1,2] These standards have been developed by organizations of individuals who are considered authorities in the content of a specific standard. Standards are usually consensus statements developed through the cooperation of manufacturers, consumers, government, and academia. Compliance with these standards is usually voluntary, but there may be considerable professional pressure to adhere to recognized standards. Standards may become law. For example, building codes in some municipalities may include standards developed by one or more standards organizations.

The National Bureau of Standards (NBS) develops measurement methods, instrumentation, and measurement standards. Although the NBS was established by Congress in 1901, it does not establish or enforce mandatory standards. The NBS ensures that the American system of measurement is internationally compatible.

The International Standards Organization (ISO) was established in 1946 to facilitate international coordination in the unification of international standards. In 1988, the ISO represented 73 countries. The ISO develops standards in virtually every area of technology, except electrotechnical matters. The International Electrotechnical Commission (IEC) is the world standards authority for electrical and electronic engineering.

The American National Standards Institute (ANSI) serves as the national standards coordinating organization in the United States. ANSI is not a governmental agency; unlike many countries, there is no standards organization that is part of the United States government. ANSI is the American representative to the ISO and the Pan American Standards Commission.

The American Society for Testing and Materials (ASTM) is a technical and scientific organization that was formed for the development of standards on characteristics and performance of

Table 7—1 Standards Organizations and Specific Standards Related to Respiratory Care Equipment

ORGANIZATION	EXAMPLES OF STANDARDS
American National Standards Institute (ANSI) 1430 Broadway New York, NY 10018	ANSI Z79.2 Tracheal tube connectors and adapters ANSI Z79.3 Oropharyngeal and nasopharyngeal airways ANSI Z79.6 Breathing tubes ANSI Z79.7 Breathing machines for medical use ANSI Z79.9 Humidifiers and nebulizers for medical use ANSI Z79.10 Requirements for oxygen analyzers for monitoring patient breathing mixtures ANSI Z79.13 Oxygen concentrators for medical use ANSI Z79.14 Tracheal tubes ANSI Z79.16 Cuffed orotracheal and nasotracheal tubes
American Society for Testing and Materials (ASTM) 1916 Race Street Philadelphia, PA 19103	F 920 Specification for minimum performance and safety requirements for resuscitators F 965 Specification for rigid laryngoscopes F 927 Specification for pediatric tracheostomy tubes F 984 Specification for cutaneous gas monitoring devices F29.02.01 Cuffed tracheostomy tubes F29.03.01 Standard specification for ventilators intended for critical care F29.03.05 Standard specification for blood gas analyzers F29.03.07 Standard specification for humidifiers F29.03.08 Standard specification for oxygen analyzers for monitoring patient breathing mixtures F29.03.09 Standard specification for electrically powered homecare ventilators F29.03.10 Standard for pulse oximeters
American Association for the Advancement of Medical Instrumentation (AAMI) 1901 North Fort Myer Drive Suite 602 Arlington, VA 22209	AAMI SS-D Spirometers AAMI MIM Guideline for establishing and administering medical instrumentation maintenance programs AAMI SCL safe current levels for electromedical apparatus
Compressed Gas Association (CGA) 1235 Jefferson Davis Highway Arlington, VA 22202	C-9 Standard color marking of compressed gas cylinders E-7 Standard for flowmeters, pressure reducing regulators G-4 Oxygen G-7 Compressed air for human respiration P-2 Characteristics and safe handling of medical gases V-5 Diameter index safety system
National Committee for Clinical Laboratory Standards 771 E. Lancaster Avenue Villanova, PA 19085	C12 Tentative standard for definitions of quantities and conventions related to blood pH and gas analysis C21 Devices measuring PO_2 and Pco_2 in blood samples C27 Blood gas pre-analytical considerations: specimen collection, calibration, and controls H11 Percutaneous collection of arterial blood for laboratory analysis
National Fire Protection Association (NFPA) Batterymarch Park Quincy, MA 02269	50 Bulk oxygen systems 53 M Fire hazards in oxygen enriched atmospheres 56 B Respiratory therapy 56 H Home use of respiratory therapy 76 B Safe use of electricity in patient care areas 99-1987 Standard for health care facilities
Underwriters Laboratories (UL) 1285 Walt Whitman Road Melville, NY 11747	252 Compressed gas regulators 407 Manifolds for compressed gas

Form Approved; OMB No. 0910-0143

Medical Device & Laboratory Product Problem Reporting Program	DATE RECEIVED
	ACCESS NO

1. PRODUCT IDENTIFICATION:

Name of Product and Type of Device
(Include sizes or other identifying characteristics and attach labeling, if available)

_____

_____

Manufacturer's Name _____

Manufacturer's City, State, Zip Code _____

_____

Is this a disposable item?   YES ☐   NO ☐

Lot Number(s) and Expiration Date(s) (if applicable)

Serial Number(s)

Manufacturer's Product Number and/or Model Number

2. REPORTER INFORMATION:

Your Name _____   Today's Date _____

Title and Department _____

Facility's Name _____

Street Address _____

City _____ State _____ Zip _____ Phone ( ) _____ Ext: _____

3. PROBLEM INFORMATION:

Date event occurred _____

This event has been reported to: Manufacturer ☐ FDA ☐

Please indicate how you want your identity publicly disclosed:

Other _____

No public disclosure ☐

To the manufacturer/distributor ☐

To the manufacturer/distributor and to anyone who requests a copy of the report from the FDA ☐

If requested, will the actual product involved in the event be available for evaluation by the manufacturer or FDA?   YES ☐   NO ☐

Problem noted or suspected (Describe the event in as much detail as necessary. Attach additional pages if required. Include how and where the product was used. Include other equipment or products that were involved. Sketches may be helpful in describing problem areas.)

RETURN TO	OR	CALL TOLL FREE ANYTIME
United States Pharmacopeia 12601 Twinbrook Parkway Rockville, Maryland 20852 Attention: Dr. Joseph G. Valentino		**800-638-6725*** IN THE CONTINENTAL UNITED STATES *In Maryland, call collect (301) 881-0256 between 9:00 AM and 4:30 PM

FORM FDA 2519f (3/85)

Figure 7—1. Medical device problem reporting form used by USP.

materials, products, systems, and services. ASTM is the world's largest source of voluntary consensus standards.[1]

The Occupational Safety and Health Administration (OSHA) sets standards for protection of employees in the workplace. Thus, OSHA sets standards related to the safety of hospital employees, rather than the safety of patients. The Centers for Disease Control (CDC) sets standards related to infection control within the hospital to protect both the hospital employee and patients.

Professional organizations have also developed standards related to the practice of respiratory care. The American Association for Respiratory Care (AARC) has adopted a number of "Position Statements,"[3] the American Heart Association has established standards for the performance of cardiopulmonary resuscitation,[4] the American Thoracic Society has established standards for spirometry,[5–7] and standards for quality control of blood gas analysis have been established by the College of American Pathologists and the American Thoracic Society. Through its voluntary accreditation procedures, the Joint Commission on Accreditation of Healthcare Organizations (JCAHO) also establishes standards.

The Emergency Care Research Institute (ECRI) is a nonprofit biomedical testing laboratory dedicated to medical equipment evaluation and technology assessment. The Health Devices Program of ECRI is recognized as an important source of information on medical devices. ECRI publishes a monthly *Health Devices* journal, twice-monthly *Health Device Alerts,* and *Hazard Bulletins* whenever a problem is deemed serious enough to require an immediate warning. Many detailed objective evaluations of medical devices are published in *Health Devices.*

The National Committee for Clinical Laboratory Standards (NCCLS) represents a cross section of professions, industry, and government. The NCCLS promotes the development and the voluntary use of national and international standards and guidelines that are needed for improved operation of clinical laboratories. The NCCLS has developed several consensus standards related to blood gas analysis.

The United States Pharmacopeial Convention (USPC), publishers of the *United States Pharmacopeia (USP),* also serves as the governmental agency for reporting medical equipment problems. This Product Problem Reporting Program is a practitioner-oriented system to communicate health hazards and product problems to government and industry. Equipment problems are reported to the USPC using a standard format (Fig. 7–1). A copy of the report is forwarded by the USPC to the Food and Drug Administration (FDA) and the manufacturer of the device identified in the report, which should initiate corrective action.

ROLE OF THE FOOD AND DRUG ADMINISTRATION

In 1976, Congress enacted the comprehensive Medical Device Amendments to the federal Food, Drug, and Cosmetic Act. Before 1976, medical devices could be marketed without review by the United States Food and Drug Administration (FDA). The principal purpose of the Medical Device Amendments was to ensure that new devices are safe and effective before they are marketed.[8–12] From a statutory standpoint, a *medical device* is defined as any item promoted for some medical purpose that does not rely on chemical action for its desired effect. It has been estimated that there are more than 1700 different types of medical devices affected by this legislation. This includes 50,000 separate products from 7000 manufacturers.

The 1976 legislation divided medical devices into three classes (Table 7–2) and seven categories

Table 7–2 FDA Classification of Devices

Class I: General Controls—These are the least-controlled devices, and include devices such as nasal cannulae and suction catheters. Devices in this class are required to comply with regulations regarding registration, premarketing notification, record keeping, labeling, reporting of adverse experiences, and good manufacturing practices.

Class II: Performance Standards—Devices assigned to this class must meet federally defined performance standards. These standards specify the minimal acceptable performance for these devices. Devices such as mechanical ventilators are assigned to this class. Although equipment assigned to this class must meet performance standards, for bureaucratic reasons very few performance standards have yet been written.

Class III: Premarket Approval—These are the most-controlled devices. Devices assigned to this class cannot be marketed until the manufacturer demonstrates their safety and effectiveness to the FDA's satisfaction.

Table 7–3 FDA Categorization of Medical Devices

Preamendment devices: Devices on the market before May 28, 1976 (when the Medical Device Amendments were enacted).
Postamendment devices: Devices put on the market after May 28, 1976.
Substantially equivalent devices: Postamendment devices that are substantially equivalent to preamendment devices.
Implanted devices: Devices inserted into a body cavity (either a surgically formed or naturally occurring cavity) and intended to remain in place for at least 30 days.
Custom devices: Devices specifically designed for a particular patient; these devices are not available for general commercial distribution.
Investigational devices: Devices undergoing clinical investigation under the authority of the FDA.
Transitional devices: Devices that were regulated as drugs before May 28, 1976, but are now defined as medical devices.

(Table 7–3). The regulatory authority granted to the FDA depends upon this complex classification and categorization scheme. The regulation of new medical devices is based primarily on an evaluation of risk. This differs from the regulation of new drugs, in which standards of safety and effectiveness are uniformly applied.

Because the FDA has not developed performance standards for Class II devices, there are two principal routes to the market for a new device. Premarketing notification is all that is required if the manufacturer can establish substantial equivalence (this is commonly referred to as "510(k) notification," because it is covered by section 510(k) of the Medical Device Amendments). Otherwise, premarketing testing and approval are required. In most cases, manufacturers are able to establish substantial equivalence. About 55 substantial equivalent premarketing notifications are filed for each premarketing approval.

EVALUATION OF AGREEMENT BETWEEN DEVICES

When a new medical device is introduced, its performance is usually compared with that of a commonly accepted standard device. If there is good agreement between the new device and the standard device, then the new device is considered acceptable for use. Such comparisons are frequently published in the respiratory care literature, but the methodology of these studies is poorly understood by many respiratory care practitioners. These studies may not be properly conducted, the data may not be analyzed correctly, and the conclusions may not be supported by the data.

An appropriate comparison device must be chosen to evaluate a new device. This will usually be a commonly accepted standard device. For example, a new electronic spirometer might be compared with a water-sealed spirometer.[13–15] To evaluate a new pulse oximeter, it would be appropriate to compare its saturation with a CO-oximeter saturation measured on simultaneously obtained arterial blood.[16,17] It would not be correct, however, to compare the pulse oximeter saturation with a saturation calculated from Pa_{O_2}. Before the devices are compared, it is also important to assure that the standard device is performing optimally.

The new device should be evaluated with clinically appropriate conditions. A spirometer should be evaluated using test signals that include the variety of physiologic signals obtained during health and disease. A ventilator should be evaluated using the variety of conditions in which ventilators are used. Devices should also be evaluated using the range of conditions encountered clinically. For example, evaluation of a pulse oximeter at saturations of 75% to 100% is more useful than an evaluation at saturations of 90% to 100%.

Depending upon the device, evaluations may be performed using models, animals, normal volunteers, or patients. Lung models might be used to evaluate spirometers or ventilators. Normal volunteers can be exposed to hypoxic gas mixtures to evaluate the saturation response of pulse oximeters. However, evaluations based solely on data obtained with lung models, animals, or normal volunteers should be interpreted cautiously, because these results do not always extrapolate well to sick patients.[18]

A repeated measures design is often used for equipment evaluation. This means that each test signal is repeated several times, which allows the evaluation of precision (repeatability or reliability) as well as agreement (validity). A repeated measures design also allows statistical analysis of the results.

The conclusions of many published equipment

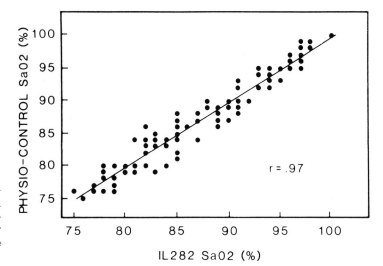

Figure 7—2. Scattergram illustrating relationship between Sa_{O_2} measured by a pulse oximeter and a CO oximeter. (Hess D, et al: An evaluation of the accuracy of the Physio-Control Lifestat 1600 pulse oximeter in measuring arterial oxygen saturation. Respir Care 32:19–23, 1987, with permission)

evaluations are based upon either incorrect or incomplete statistical analysis. Statistical evaluation of agreement involves use of correlation and regression analysis, t-test analysis (or analysis of variance), calculation of bias and precision, and calculation of the intraclass correlation coefficient.

A scattergram can be drawn to illustrate the relationship between the two devices (Fig. 7–2). On a scattergram, the value of the new device is plotted on the y-axis and the value of the comparison device is plotted on the x-axis. If agreement is good, the scatter of the data points will approximate a straight line with a slope of 1.0.

Statistically, the relationship between the devices being evaluated is determined by calculation of the correlation coefficient (r). A perfect direct relationship produces $r = 1$, a perfect inverse relationship produces $r = -1$, and no relationship produces $r = 0$. It should not be surprising if the correlation between two devices that are designed to measure the same thing is good. However, it is important to recognize that the correlation between two devices can be perfect ($r = 1$ or $r = -1$), but agreement between the two devices might be poor (Fig. 7–3).[19] For example, if the new device consistently produces a value that is half of that produced by the reference device, then correlation will be good, but with poor agreement.

Regression analysis defines the line that best fits the data. If the relationship is linear, the general form of the regression line is $y = mx + b$, where y is y-axis value, x is the x-axis value, m is the slope of

Figure 7—3. Correlation between conjunctival Po_2 and arterial Po_2, showing good correlation but poor agreement. The Pcj_{O_2} is significantly less than the Pa_{O_2}. (Hess D, et al: The relationship between conjunctival Po_2 and arterial Po_2 in 16 normal persons. Respir Care 31:191–198, 1986, with permission)

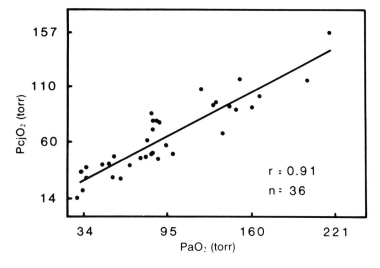

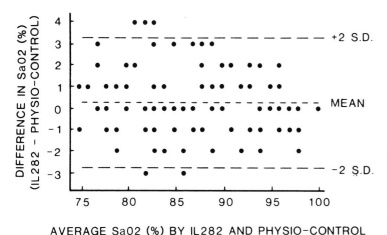

Figure 7—4. Plot of the difference in Sa_{O_2} measured by two devices (pulse oximeter and CO oximeter) against their mean, with mean difference (bias) and limits of agreement (± SD). (Hess D, et al: An evaluation of the accuracy of the Physio-Control Lifestat 1600 pulse oximeter in measuring arterial oxygen saturation. Respir Care 32:19–23, 1987, with permission)

the line, and b is the y-intercept of the regression line. The closeness of the points on the scattergram to the regression line is determined by the standard error of the estimate (SEE); about 95% of the data will lie within 2 SEE of the regression line for a normal distribution of data. If agreement is perfect, the slope of the regression line will be 1, the y-intercept will be 0, and the SEE will be 0.

Bland and Altman[20,21] have described a method to evaluate agreement that calculates bias and limits of agreement. *Bias* is defined as the mean difference between the two devices. The limits of agreement between the two devices are calculated as the mean ± 2 SD. If agreement is good, then the mean difference (bias) will be near zero, and the limits of agreement (precision) will be small. Bias and precision can be illustrated graphically by plotting the difference between the devices against the mean of the two devices (Fig. 7–4).

A more sophisticated technique for evaluation of agreement is calculation of the intraclass correlation coefficient (R_I), as described by Kramer and Feinstein.[22] The R_I can vary between −1 and +1, with higher scores reflecting better agreement. The calculation of R_I involves the use of repeated measures analysis of variance, which is beyond the scope of this discussion.

Data from the two instruments can also be compared by t-test analysis or analysis of variance. Such analysis determines whether there is a statistically significant difference between the instruments. However, this analysis is of limited usefulness because it does not determine the magnitude of the difference between the instruments.

After the data are statistically evaluated, they may still be difficult to interpret. Acceptable agreement is a value judgment that can be supported by the sophisticated evaluation of data. When reports of equipment evaluations are published, it is important that sufficient data are provided for the readers to enable them to make independent interpretations of the data.

Evaluation of agreement between instruments is meticulous and time consuming. Such thorough evaluations may exceed the budgetary constraints and resources of many respiratory care departments. However, results of equipment evaluations are commonly reported in the medical literature. Respiratory care practitioners should appreciate the methodology of these evaluations, so that published studies of equipment evaluations can be critically evaluated.

EVALUATION EQUIPMENT

The previous section discussed the evaluation of new devices introduced to the market. In this section, instruments to evaluate respiratory care equipment will be discussed. The evaluation instruments described here might be found in respiratory care departments and be used for day-to-day evaluations of equipment performance. These instruments include signal generators, measurement equipment, and test lungs. Equipment is needed to evaluate pressure, flow, volume, time, temperature, and humidity (Table 7–4).

Signal generators are used to produce a standard signal to evaluate instruments. For example, a supersyringe (or calibration syringe) (Fig. 7–5) is used to produce a reproducible known volume to

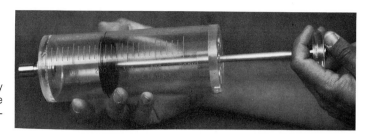

Figure 7–5. Calibrated "super syringe." Generally available from 500-mL to 5-L sizes, these syringes provide a very accurate source for volume standardization, particularly in devices that are flow independent.

Table 7–4 Devices Available for Everyday Evaluation of Respiratory Care Equipment

MEASUREMENT	EVALUATION DEVICE
Pressure	Water or mercury column
Volume	Supersyringe
	Calibrated spirometry system
Flow	Precision Thorpe tube
	Calibrated spirometry system
Time	Stopwatch
Temperature	Mercury thermometer
Humidity	Hygrometer

evaluate volume-measuring equipment (such as spirometers).

Pressure manometers are commonly used on respiratory care equipment. Because of their convenience and low cost, aneroid gauges are often used for this purpose. Pressure might also be measured with an electronic pressure transducer. The accuracy of manometers (such as aneroid gauges or electronic transducers) can be checked with a water or mercury column (Fig. 7–6). When evaluating the accuracy of pressure gauges, it is important that they are evaluated over the entire range of pres-

Figure 7–6. (A) Water column to evaluate accuracy of pressure manometers. (B) Mercury column to evaluate accuracy of pressure manometers.

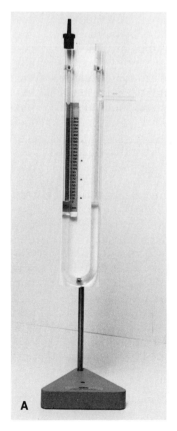

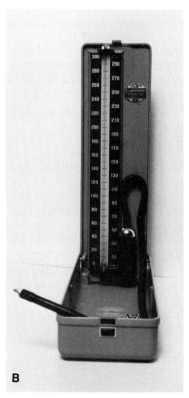

A

B

sures for which the gauge is clinically used. A wide range of pressure gauges is used in respiratory care equipment (from a few cmH$_2$O to over 2000 psi). The accuracy required of these gauges depends upon their application.

The accuracy of flow gauges (flowmeters) can be evaluated with a precision Thorpe tube (Fig. 7–7). These precision devices are factory calibrated for specific gas composition and barometric pressure. They are not backpressure-compensated; thus, any restriction to their outflow will cause them to be inaccurate.

Because of its accuracy, availability, and ease of use, the water-sealed spirometer (Fig. 7–8) is commonly used as a volume reference device. The water-sealed spirometer can also provide a hard-copy permanent record. If the water-sealed spirometer is used with a kymograph, flow can also be evaluated. To assure validity of results with a wa-

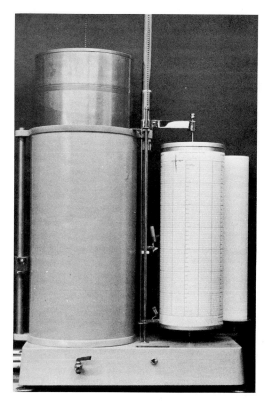

Figure 7–8. A Collins 13.5-L water-seal spirometer. This device is one of the most commonly used "volume standards" in respiratory care.

ter-sealed spirometer, the spirometer should be checked for leaks, the bell factor should be confirmed against a supersyringe, and the kymograph speed should be checked against a stopwatch. To evaluate large volumes, a 120-L Tissot spirometer can be used (Fig. 7–9). In place of a water-sealed spirometer, any other calibrated spirometry system can be used to evaluate volume and flow.

The standard temperature monitor is a mercury thermometer. Electronic thermometers (Fig. 7–10) may be more convenient to monitor temperature in some applications, but the accuracy of these must be confirmed by evaluating them against a mercury thermometer. The standard device to monitor relative humidity is the dry bulb—wet bulb hygrometer (Fig. 7–11) or the sling psychrometer (Fig. 7–12). Electronic devices are also available to monitor humidity (Fig. 7–13).

Much respiratory care equipment is electronically powered. The electrical safety of this equipment must be assured before the equipment is put

Figure 7–7. Thorpe tube-type flowmeter standardization devices. *A, B,* and *D* are custom-built units calibrated for 735-mmHg atmospheric pressure and for air measurement. Flows of more than 600 L/min can be measured accurately by the larger unit. *C* is a set of three flowmeters calibrated at 760-mmHg (sea level) atmospheric pressure, for use with oxygen.

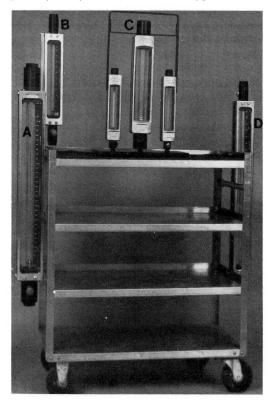

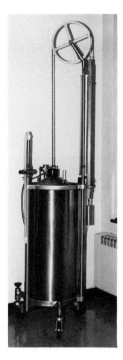

Figure 7—9. Tissot spirometer.

Table 7—5 Suggestions for Safe Use of Electrical Equipment

- Do not use cheater adapters to convert three-prong devices to two prongs
- Use only grounded outlets
- Use only hospital-grade outlets and plugs
- Do not pull electrical plugs out by the cord
- Do not touch electrical equipment with wet hands
- Use electrical plugs with transparent covers
- Do not store liquids on electrical devices
- Do not allow patients to use home equipment in the hospital unless that equipment meets hospital leakage current standards
- Promptly repair defective electrical devices
- Have equipment and outlets checked regularly for leakage current
- Do not touch two pieces of grounded electrical equipment simultaneously
- Do not assume that properly operating equipment is safe
- Be skeptical about the safety of electrical devices

into use, and periodically thereafter. It is particularly important that equipment be evaluated for leakage current (Fig. 7–14). Leakage current is electricity that is accidentally applied to the external chassis of the equipment, and, thus, poses a potential electrical shock hazard. Electrical safety standards have been established by the AAMI, NFPA, and ANSI. Electrical leakage current should be as low as possible and generally should not exceed 100 μamp. Because the purpose of the ground plug is to minimize the shock hazard associated with leakage current, it is also important that the integrity of the ground plug is assured. Assuring the electrical safety of equipment is usually the responsibility of the biomedical department of the hospital, but it is the responsibility of all respiratory care practitioners to be vigilant regarding electrical safety (Table 7–5).

The Timeter RT-200 Calibration Analyzer (Fig. 7–15) is a commercially available device for evaluation of respiratory care equipment. The RT-200 can be used to evaluate a wide range of pressures, flows, and volumes. This versatile device can be used to evaluate many respiratory care devices, is simple to use, and is very accurate. The RT-200 is factory-calibrated with high-precision instruments, many of which are traceable to the National Bureau of Standards.

A variety of test lungs are available to simulate a realistic patient load when testing ventilators and resuscitators. Ventilator performance should be evaluated with such a simulated patient load, and

Figure 7—10. Electrical and mercury thermometers.

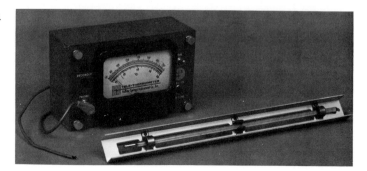

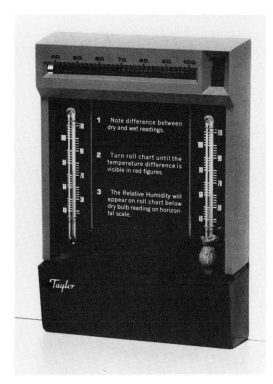

Figure 7–11. Dry bulb–wet bulb hygrometer.

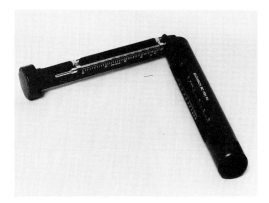

Figure 7–12. Sling psychrometer.

ANSI has recommended specific resistances and compliances for such testing (Table 7–6). A simple inexpensive rubber test lung can be used (Fig. 7–16), but this does not allow resistance and compliance to be quantitatively varied. More sophisticated test lungs allow the resistance and compliance to be varied quantitatively. Examples of these include the Vent-Aid Training Test Lung (Fig. 7–17) and the Bio-Tek Adult Ventilator Tester VT-1 (Fig. 7–18).[23]

Many ventilators feature spontaneous breathing modes such as intermittent mandatory ventilation (IMV), continuous positive airway pressure (CPAP), and pressure support. Evaluation of spontaneous breathing modes requires the ability to simulate spontaneous breathing. Several systems have been described to evaluate spontaneous breathing modes. One of these uses a modification of an Emerson 3-PV Ventilator (Fig. 7–19),[24] and the other uses a modification of the Vent-Aid Training Test Lung in combination with an Emerson 3-PV Ventilator (Fig. 7–20).[25–27]

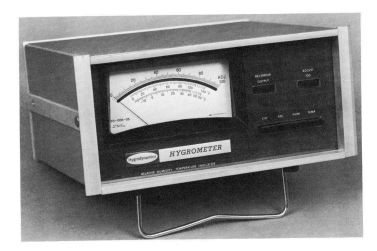

Figure 7–13. Electrical hygrometer for measuring relative humidity and accurate temperatures on an analog meter or a recording device.

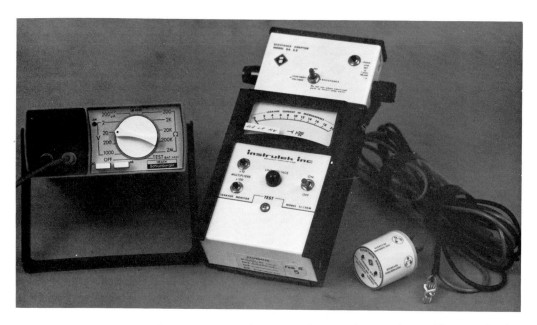

Figure 7—14. Electrical leakage detectors and receptacle ground tester. The ground tester tests the correctness of wiring of the electrical receptacle.

EQUIPMENT ACQUISITION

Dramatic increases in the costs of health care and health care equipment have occurred in recent years. As a result, the decision process used to acquire respiratory care equipment has become one of the most important functions of the respiratory care department. Historically, third-party payers have fi-

Table 7—6 Compliances and Resistances Suggested by ANSI for Testing Ventilator Performance

CATEGORY	CONDITION	COMPLIANCE (mL · cm H$_2$O^{-1})	RESISTANCE (cm H$_2$O · L^{-1} · sec^{-1})
Adult	1	50	5
	2	50	20
	3	20	5
	4	20	20
Pediatric	1	20	20
	2	20	50
	3	10	20
	4	10	50
	5	3	20
	6	3	50
	7	3	200
Neonatal	1	3	50
	2	3	200
	3	1	50
	4	1	200
	5	1	500
	6	1	1000

Figure 7—15. Timeter RT-200 Calibration Analyzer.

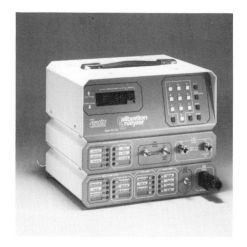

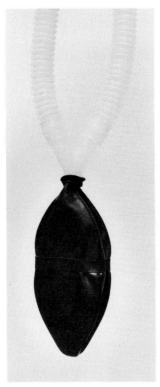

Figure 7—16. Inexpensive rubber test lung.

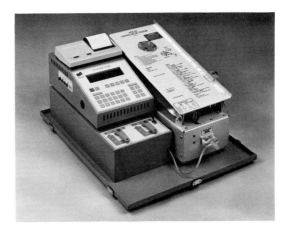

Figure 7—18. Bio-Tek VT-1.

nanced capital equipment acquisitions, as well as other materials and equipment needs of hospitals. However, with the introduction of prospective payment, monies are no longer as readily available for the purchase of health care equipment.

A major goal of the respiratory care department thus becomes one of objectively and critically eval-

Figure 7—17. Vent-Aid Training Test Lung.

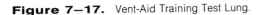

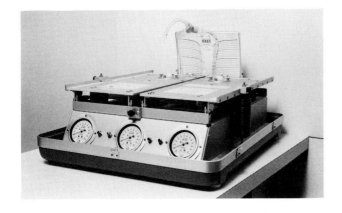

uating all equipment and supplies to ensure that the equipment will meet the current and anticipated needs of the hospital, will function in a reliable and dependable manner, will perform adequately over its service life, and is as inexpensive as possible to perform the required function. In other words, the cost-effectiveness of the equipment must be established.

Respiratory care equipment and supplies can be divided into two categories: capital and noncapital. Although the definition of *capital equipment* varies from hospital to hospital, it generally refers to equipment that is more expensive (e.g., more than 500 dollars) and has an expected service life of more than a few years (e.g., more than 5 to 7 years). *Noncapital equipment* usually refers to less expensive equipment with a shorter service life. A mechanical ventilator is an example of a capital equipment item, whereas a flowmeter is an example of a noncapital equipment item.

There are three primary acquisition options available for capital equipment: outright purchase, short-term rental, and long-term lease (which may include a purchase option). Historically, most respiratory care equipment has been purchased as a direct one-time payment to an equipment vendor. This remains the primary method by which respiratory care equipment is acquired. Owing to budgetary constraints, however, other innovative methods of acquiring capital equipment have evolved.

Short-term rental of equipment has become more popular in recent years. A common example is the rental of ventilators during seasonal busy periods to supplement existing inventory. The rationale for short-term rental is that it provides equip-

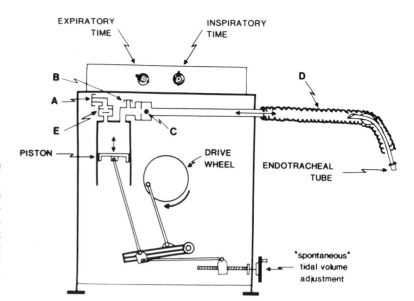

Figure 7–19. A mechanical model of spontaneous ventilation using an Emerson 3-PV. *A,* Inlet of the piston is occluded; *B,* exhalation valve orifice is occluded; *C,* one-way valve at piston outlet is removed; *D,* wide-bore tubing is attached to outlet of ventilator; *E,* one-way valve at piston inlet has no practical use. (Banner MJ, Hurd TE, Boysen PG: A mechanical model of spontaneous ventilation. Crit Care Med 12:986–987, 1984. © by Williams & Wilkins, 1984, with permission)

ment during high-demand periods and does so within the fiscal constraints of the hospital because a large single payment is not required. For example, if the history of a respiratory care department demonstrates that four ventilators a day are required for 8 months of the year, but seven ventilators a day are required for the remaining 4 months of the year, then it might be more cost-effective to purchase four ventilators and rent additional ventilators only when they are needed.

Evaluation for use of short-term rental equipment must compare the trade-off of rental equipment versus on-site availability of the equipment. On-site availability of the equipment offers the advantages of immediate access to the equipment and a high level of familiarity with the equipment by the respiratory care staff. Advantages of short-term rental include less lump-sum capital budget expen-

ditures, less time and expense in performance testing and maintenance of the equipment, and less expense in cleaning and sterilization of the equipment. Disadvantages of short-term rental equipment include lack of immediate availability of the equipment, the time and expense required to arrange for the use of rental equipment, and less familiarity with the equipment by the respiratory care staff.

The newest capital equipment acquisition method is the long-term lease arrangement, which may include an option to purchase. Recognizing the increased difficulty that hospitals are experiencing in the lump-sum method of capital equipment acquisition, manufacturers and equipment vendors have introduced a variety of lease options. These range from simple-structured plans that permit the hospital to pay a monthly fee throughout

Figure 7–20. A mechanical model to evaluate spontaneous breathing. (Op't Holt TM et al: Comparison of changes in airway pressure during continuous positive airway pressure (CPAP) between demand valve and continuous flow devices. Respir Care 27:1200, 1982, with permission)

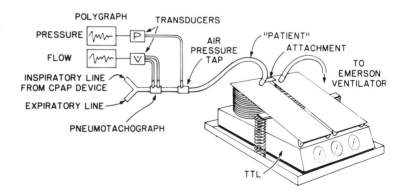

the length of the contract, to sophisticated contracts with variable time payments leading either to a termination point or a buy-out option.

Long-term lease options permit improved cash flow because the equipment is not purchased outright, and allow the respiratory care staff to become familiar with the equipment (unlike short-term rental). Although long-term lease contracts vary among manufacturers and vendors, they often include a provision for preventive maintenance to be performed by the manufacturer or vendor. Although a long-term lease may improve cash flow, the hospital ultimately pays more for the equipment than the original purchase price. If the long-term lease includes a buy-out at the end of the lease, the hospital in essence purchases a used piece of equipment.

Decisions concerning capital equipment acquisition are not simple. The successful respiratory care department will match the clinical needs of the department to the financial status of the hospital. Before capital equipment is acquired, it should be thoroughly evaluated by bench testing and clinical application. The equipment should be subjected to the variety of circumstances that might be encountered clinically. For the most thorough evaluation, acquisition decisions should be made by a group of persons including respiratory care clinical staff, respiratory care supervisory staff, nursing personnel, biomedical personnel, and physicians (e.g., respiratory care medical director).

Noncapital respiratory care equipment includes low-cost reusable supplies (e.g., oxygen flowmeters, hoses, adapters), and disposable supplies (cannulae, masks, ventilator circuits). The procurement of routine respiratory care equipment (such as flowmeters) is simple in that these devices are usually purchased as needed according to usage levels. Issues of controversy regarding noncapital devices include (1) disposables versus nondisposables and (2) reuse of single-patient-use (disposable) supplies.

Until the early 1970s, the use of reusables versus disposables was not a major issue because inexpensive plastics were not readily available. However, since that time, the low cost of disposable plastics has convinced many respiratory care departments to utilize at least a portion of their daily supply needs as disposables. When considering the issue of disposables versus nondisposables, at least four issues must be addressed: (1) construction quality, (2) safety in handling, (3) infection control, and (4) total costs.[28]

Although the quality of disposables was a serious limitation of early plastic products, the importance of this issue has decreased significantly. The quality of most disposable equipment today is similar to that of their nondisposable counterparts.

The safety in handling issue remains significant. The handling safety and infection control of disposables pose fewer problems than those for reusable products. Conversely, the multistage process of processing reusables poses some degree of risk of operator injury in that the person handling soiled patient care equipment has an increased risk on contracting a disease secondary to the handling of infectious materials.

The cost of disposables versus reusables is an important consideration. Reusable devices require a greater amount of personnel time and material expense to disassemble, clean, sterilize, and package the equipment. The cost of disposable equipment includes both direct costs (e.g., purchase price and the mechanics of ordering) and indirect costs (e.g., disposal, handling, and storage). A comparison of the components of total cost of disposable versus reusable equipment is provided in Table 7–7. As a general rule, disposable equipment is less expensive at low usage volume because of the lower fixed costs. At high usage volume, reusables are less expensive (Fig. 7–21).[28]

Another issue related to the use of disposable equipment deals with the reuse of this equipment. There has been a tendency in some respiratory care

Table 7–7 Comparison of Components of Total Cost of Disposed Disposables and Reusables

COST	DISPOSABLE DEVICE	REUSABLE DEVICE
Purchase	Low	High
Ordering	High	Low
Storage	High	Low
Cleaning	None	High
Disassembly/ reassembly	None	High
Repair	None	High
Repackaging	None	High
Sterilization	None	High
Wastage	High	Low
Disposal	High	Low
Transporting	High	High

(Adapted from Walton JR: A new controversy in respiratory equipment management: reusables versus disposables versus reused disposables. Respir Care 31:213–217, 1986)

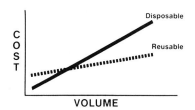

Figure 7–21. Relationship between total cost and usage volume of disposed disposables and reusables. (Walton JR: A new controversy in respiratory equipment management: reusables versus disposed disposables versus reused disposables. Respir Care 31:213, 1986, with permission)

departments to clean and sterilize disposable respiratory care equipment for reuse. It must be recognized that a considerable portion of the product liability of disposable equipment may shift from the manufacturer to the hospital if such equipment is reused. The decision to reuse equipment marked "single-patient-use" or "disposable" should be made only after the advice of legal counsel has been obtained. Because of differences in law among states, it is unwise to base this decision upon the practice of other institutions without legal advice.

Equipment purchase decisions must be individualized to the specific needs of the hospital and the respiratory care department. These decisions will be based upon the financial status of the hospital, the clinical requirements of the department, and the skills of the respiratory care, nursing, and physician staff.

EQUIPMENT MAINTENANCE AND QUALITY CONTROL

Like decisions on the acquisition of equipment, decisions on the institution of a comprehensive equipment maintenance program are complex. In today's world of complex electronics and litigation-conscious consumers, the roles of the manufacturer, biomedical personnel, and clinical personnel are not always clear. The following sections provide general guidelines for the roles of various participants in a comprehensive equipment maintenance program. This information provides general guidelines to be used in concert with each specific piece of equipment's prescribed maintenance program, as recommended by the manufacturer. These general guidelines are applicable to a wide range of equipment.

ROLE OF THE MANUFACTURER

Historically, the most common method for equipment repair and maintenance was to return the device to the manufacturer or manufacturer-authorized dealer. However, this method does not apply to all pieces of equipment in a modern respiratory care department. One of the more important considerations in choosing to return a device to the manufacturer is the amount of time that the device will be out of service. With some of the more complex pieces of equipment (e.g., ventilators), many manufacturers specify the amount of time that a particular repair or overhaul will require. However, many nonroutine repairs may take variable amounts of time. The astute respiratory care manager will define this downtime as precisely as possible to acquire the appropriate amount of equipment to balance finances with efficiency.

The location of the repair service can be a major factor in the determination of the appropriate quantity of equipment. In most cases, a local repair center will provide a quicker turnaround time than one in another part of the country. The respiratory care department should require a written quote from the repair center of the amount of repair time to expect. Some manufacturers confine their sale of certain units to defined geographic areas so that they can provide the necessary level of service on a consistent basis.

Size and initial cost of the equipment will also be deciding factors in determining which devices to return to the manufacturer. Devices such as flowmeters and oxygen analyzers typically require only simple, inexpensive maintenance and usually do not require the expense and downtime of returning the equipment to the manufacturer. On the other hand, large and expensive equipment (e.g., pulmonary function equipment and critical-care monitoring equipment) cannot be easily shipped without risk of damage because of their size and delicate construction. For such equipment, it is common to have the factory representative provide service within the respiratory care department. Most manufacturers of such equipment have established mobile service units for such repairs.

Warranties and guarantees influence equipment maintenance and repair. These vary widely in scope and are modified by changes in laws from state to state. The reader is encouraged to utilize existing legal and administrative support personnel within his or her institution to discern the implication of specific warranties and guarantees before the acquisition of any medical equipment.

In 1984, the American Association for the Advancement of Medical Instrumentation (AAMI) published a *Guideline for Establishing and Administering Medical Instrumentation Maintenance Programs*, which details the roles and responsibilities of the medical equipment manufacturer:

> In addition to providing medical instrumentation of high quality, fabricated in accordance with good manufacturing practices and other legal and ethical requirements, the manufacturer has the responsibility to help assure the proper care and safe and effective use of the medical equipment. There is a special need for the manufacturer to provide documentation and support thorough enough to enable trained personnel to readily identify and repair equipment malfunctions, and to offer realistic preventative maintenance guidelines that will assure that equipment safety and performance can be maintained cost-effectively.

This suggests that the manufacturer should provide appropriate documentation (e.g., specifications, operating manuals and instructions, warranty and certification information, quality control specifications), provide user support (e.g., in-service training, technical training, and applications information), provide maintenance support, and provide timely and detailed updates.

ROLE OF THE HOSPITAL BIOMEDICAL DEPARTMENT

The hospital biomedical department plays an important role in the maintenance of medical equipment. This department has the advantages of being within the hospital, having personnel with the specific skill needed to maintain equipment, and having channels of communication with the respiratory care department as well as with manufacturers. The biomedical department is also well informed of the various safety standards and regulations concerning respiratory care equipment.

To institute a comprehensive maintenance program, personnel from both the respiratory care department and the biomedical department should meet to discuss the use of each piece of equipment that is to be regularly serviced within the hospital. Both departments together must establish how the equipment will be used, how repair and maintenance procedures will be conducted, what standards of performance are required by various accrediting agencies and the manufacturer, what special training will be required for the biomedical

personnel to retain competence with maintenance of the equipment, and what record-keeping systems will be used. The equipment inventory and maintenance history records should be available to both the respiratory care and biomedical departments for concurrent review and for review by outside inspection agencies such as the JCAHO.

Although the biomedical department will be responsible for maintaining specified devices for respiratory care, this does not eliminate the respiratory care department's overall responsibility for the safe and effective use of each device. In many cases, the biomedical department staff have been primarily established to service electronic equipment and may be unfamiliar with the pneumatic devices that respiratory care practitioners utilize. Therefore, the biomedical staff may require reeducation, some of which manufacturers may provide. Additionally, it is appropriate, in some instances, for the respiratory care department to supply qualified personnel to the biomedical department for the design or implementation of maintenance procedures and protocols.

The AAMI has addressed the desired roles and responsibilities of the biomedical department. These duties include provision of technical support in evaluating the equipment before acquisition, the performance and inspection of newly acquired equipment, the maintenance of service and repair records to detail the specific corrective and preventive maintenance procedures applied to each piece of equipment, the establishment of a comprehensive preventive maintenance program, and an ongoing training program for all biomedical personnel to ensure their continuing competency.

ROLE OF THE RESPIRATORY CARE DEPARTMENT

The respiratory care department is the principal department responsible for the maintenance program relating to respiratory care equipment. The amount and scope of maintenance procedures accomplished by the respiratory care department depend upon the scope of the hospital, types of equipment used, sophistication of the equipment, space available to house personnel and testing equipment, and the sophistication of the respiratory staff in equipment testing and maintenance.

The personnel involved in the actual repair and maintenance of the equipment must be qualified to provide the desired services. Their initial training and continuing education must be documented for medicolegal–accreditation reasons. Respiratory

Table 7—8   Responsibilities of Respiratory Care Department and
Biomedical/Manufacturer/Authorized Repair Center

EQUIPMENT	CHECKS BY RESPIRATORY CARE PERSONNEL	ADDITIONAL CHECKS BY BIOMEDICAL/MANUFACTURER/ AUTHORIZED REPAIR CENTER
Flowmeters	Leaks Flow valve Structural defects Accuracy	Clean internally Replace faulty parts Calibration
Regulators	Inlet and outlet threads Leaks Check outlet pressure	Clean internally Calibration Check safety valves
Manometers	Zero adjust Replace lens	Calibration
Compressors	Excess noise Water discharge Outlet pressure External filters Outlet flow Electrical cord	Electrical components Electrical leaks Shock mounts Internal filters Internal leaks
Air–oxygen blenders	FiO_2 accuracy Outlet pressure Inlet filters Alarms and bypass	Calibration Replace faulty internal parts
Oxygen analyzers	Zero meter Calibration Battery check Drying agents Electrode change Electrolyte change Membrane change Alarms	Internal calibration Replace internal parts
Gas-powered resuscitators	Leaks Valve operation Pressure pop-off Pneumatic hose Structural defects Outlet flow Outlet pressure FiO_2	Inlet filters Replace internal parts
Manual resuscitators	Leaks Valve action Pressure pop-off Structural damage	Pressure testing for valve integrity Replace faulty part
Respirometers	Structural damage Accuracy Battery check Water accumulation Zeroing of meter	Clean and adjust Electrical service Replace internal parts
Pneumatic nebulizers	Leaks Structural damage Aerosol generation FiO_2	Aerosol volume output Aerosol particle size Heater function
Ultrasonic nebulizers	Aerosol generation Fan noise Water leakage Structural damage Electrical cord	Electrical leakage Aerosol volume output Aerosol particle size

(continued)

Table 7–8   (continued)

Equipment	Checks By Respiratory Care Personnel	Additional Checks By Biomedical/Manufacturer/ Authorized Repair Center
Humidifiers	Leaks	Water output
	Heater function	Electrical leak test of heater
	Integrity of internal parts	Heater calibration
	Gas temperature	Relative humidity output
Ventilators	Pressure	Electrical leak testing
	Flow	Precision dynamic testing of all ventilator functions
	Leaks	
	PEEP	Routine preventive maintenance according to manufacturer specifications
	Inspiratory hold	
	Sensitivity	Replacement of internal parts
	Volume delivered	
	Alarms	
	Pneumatic tubing	
	Structural damage	
	Rate	
	Sigh rate and volume	
	Pop-off and pressure limits	
	Filters	
	Compressor noise	
	Circuit competence	
	FiO_2	
	High pressure lines	
	Electrical cord	
Alarms	Visual indicators	Electrical leakage
	Audio indicators	Precision calibration
	Delay timer	Replace internal parts
Pulse oximeter	Accuracy check	Internal calibration
	Cable and probe	Electrical leakage
	Battery check	Replace internal parts
Blood gas analyzer	Quality control program	Preparation of calibration gases
	Electrode cleaning and replacement	Electrical leakage
	Electrode membrane change	Replace internal parts
	Calibration	Electronic testing
	Temperature check	Preparation of quality control materials
	Replace gas lines	
Transcutaneous monitor	Calibration	Electrical leakage
	Electrode membrane change	Preparation of calibration Gases
		Replace internal parts
Capnograph	Calibration	Electrical leakage
	Filter changes	Preparation of calibration gases
		Replace internal parts
Pulmonary function equipment	Accuracy testing	Electrical leakage
	Calibration	Dynamic testing
	Filter changes	Replace internal parts
	Hoses and filters	Preparation of calibration gases

care practitioners must understand the proper use and performance of the equipment they use and should be able to perform many of the simple repair and maintenance tasks. It is the responsibility of the hospital to assure that all respiratory care practitioners can recognize equipment malfunctions and take corrective actions. Those persons with training in both respiratory care and mechanical or electrical engineering possess the greatest skills for more complex equipment maintenance. Many respiratory care departments select an individual from the clinical staff with "mechanical" abilities to be trained on-the-job and through specialized training provided by manufacturers, local colleges or universities, or in-house by a biomedical engineer. Regardless of the individual selected to perform equipment maintenance, it is critical that continuing education programs are structured to maintain the individual's competence.

As is shown in Table 7–8, much respiratory care equipment can be serviced either totally or in part by in-house respiratory care practitioners. However, some equipment may not be serviced within the respiratory care department without violating the warranty or guarantee. If warranty service is mandated and the equipment is shipped to the manufacturer or authorized repair center, the respiratory care department must document this action. Subsequently, the documentation detailing the maintenance performed should accompany the device upon return to the hospital.

The responsibility of the respiratory care department does not cease with the return of the serviced equipment from the manufacturer or vendor. The department should provide feedback to the manufacturer concerning repair records, availability of parts, downtime, outcome of service and repair procedures, and performance specifications. This dialogue provides an added measure of quality control for the department and gives valuable feedback to the manufacturer to assist in future equipment development.

Regardless of whether the respiratory care department, in-house biomedical department, manufacturer, or authorized repair center performs the service, the hospital is always legally responsible for the proper function of all medical devices. Legal problems can be avoided by documentation of the maintenance procedures for each piece of equipment, departmental policies and procedures related to equipment maintenance, and the training and continuing education for those persons performing equipment maintenance.

ROLE OF CONTRACT SERVICES

A more recent option in the maintenance of respiratory care equipment is the emergence of specialized contract services. Contracts vary greatly, but the most common involves payment for specific service on specified devices. The respiratory care department, in concert with the biomedical department, must ensure that all of the details are specified (e.g., number of service visits/per device per year, whether parts are included, and so on) before entering into a contract with such companies. For many "high-tech" medical devices, excluding the cost of parts may significantly increase the total maintenance costs of the device.

Although the development of such contracts requires much time to ensure the appropriateness of the cost for services provided, they do offer several advantages. The contract company provides the necessary space, testing equipment, parts inventory, and skilled personnel to free the hospital from these costs. A specified minimal cost for maintenance can be predetermined, and the hospital may negotiate repair and maintenance warranties beyond that expressed by the manufacturer. Downtime and repair costs can often be more precisely determined by the hospital than is possible with geographically distant manufacturers. Although the hospital continues to carry the largest share of legal responsibility for the ultimate safety and effectiveness of the medical devices, such contracts provide some sharing of this legal burden by the contract services. Many contract companies also rent equipment, which can serve both to reduce downtime (i.e., negotiating the delivery of replacement equipment when the hospital's is being serviced) and to provide additional equipment during periods of high utilization.

MAINTENANCE REPAIR RECORDS

Regardless of who performs the maintenance, it is important that the respiratory care department maintains proper documentation of all equipment. All such documentation must provide sufficient detail to meet legal and accreditation standards; this is particularly important for JCAHCO accreditation. Appropriate record-keeping of equipment maintenance should document the following:

- Routine preventive maintenance
- Equipment malfunctions, reasons for the malfunctions, and actions taken to correct the malfunctions

- The frequency and dates of major equipment overhauls
- Parts and labor costs
- Interactions with the biomedical department, maintenance contractors, and manufacturers

QUALITY CONTROL

An important part of a preventive maintenance program is a quality control program. Such a program ensures that equipment is performing optimally. For diagnostic equipment, the quality control program assures the validity of test results. For therapeutic equipment, the quality control program assures that the equipment is properly functioning. Components of a quality control program for a spirometer,[29–31] blood gas analyzer,[32] and ventilator are listed in Table 7–9. To assure optimal performance of all equipment, the respiratory care department must document appropriate quality control procedures for all equipment. An important component of quality control is a well-educated staff. An astute respiratory care practitioner will recognize equipment malfunction and take the necessary corrective actions. Another important component of all quality control programs is the performance of all manufacturer-suggested preventive maintenance.

MAINTENANCE OF RESPIRATORY HOME CARE EQUIPMENT

In recent years, the use of respiratory home care equipment has increased. As a result, there is an increased need to assure the proper function of that equipment.

Proper maintenance of respiratory home care equipment should begin before the patient leaves the hospital. A thorough in-hospital training program by hospital staff should be conducted with the patient and his or her family (or others assisting with the patient's care at home). It is important that the hospital staff use the exact equipment that the patient will use at home for this training. This training program should include a detailed explanation of the role of the patient and the durable medical equipment (DME) supplier in the maintenance of the equipment. The program should also include a discussion of the disassembly and reassembly of the equipment (as appropriate), evaluation of its proper performance, its correct use, and care and maintenance.

It is very important that the patient learns how to clean and disinfect the equipment. The patient, or another person who is assisting with the patient's home care, should be taught the procedure for disassembly, cleaning, disinfection, reassembly, and storage.

The patient should be provided with a written description that explains, in simple terms, the correct use of the equipment and how to evaluate its performance. He or she should learn not only how the equipment functions normally but also how to detect some of the common equipment malfunctions.

On a predetermined maintenance schedule, each piece of home care equipment should be replaced by a duplicate piece. In this way, appropriate preventive maintenance of the equipment can be performed. The responsibility for this is usually that of the DME supplier. A reliable supplier will also visit the patient's home periodically to evaluate and reinforce the proper use and performance of the equipment; this responsibility is shared by the patient and the supplier.

Table 7–9 Components of a Quality Control Program for a Spirometer, Blood Gas Analyzer, and Ventilator

SPIROMETER

- Qualified staff
- Manufacturer-suggested preventive maintenance
- Leak testing
- Calibration checks with 3-L syringe
- Recorder speed with stopwatch

BLOOD GAS ANALYZER

- Qualified staff
- Manufacturer-suggested preventive maintenance
- Commercial or tonometered quality control materials
- Plots of quality control results using Levy-Jennings plots
- Duplicate testing on independently calibrated instruments
- External proficiency testing

VENTILATOR

- Qualified staff
- Manufacturer-suggested preventive maintenance
- Comprehensive between-patient bench testing of performance
- Frequent (every 2–4 hours) performance checks of in-use equipment

REFERENCES

1. Identifying standards. How to find if a standard exists. ASTM Stand News (Apr):44–47, 1989
2. Hiegel ME, Pacela AF: The Guide to Biomedical Standards. Brea, Calif, Quest Publishing, 1985
3. American Association for Respiratory Care: Position Statements. Dallas, AARC
4. American Heart Association: Standards and guidelines for cardiopulmonary resuscitation and emergency cardiac care. JAMA 255:2841–3044, 1986
5. Gardner RM, Clemmer TP: Selection and standardization of respiratory monitoring equipment. Respir Care 30:560–569, 1985
6. Gardner RM, Hankinson JL, West BJ: Evaluating commercially available spirometers. Am Rev Respir Dis 121:73–82, 1980
7. Standardization of spiromentry—1987 update. Respir Care 32:1039–1060, 1987
8. Bancroft ML, Steen JA: Health device legislation: An overview of the law and its impact on respiratory care. Respir Care 23:1179–1184, 1978
9. Gardner RM: The Medical Devices Act and mandatory standard promulgation: What are the implications for respiratory care? [editorial]. Respir Care 31:881–882, 1986
10. Gardner RM: Federal medical device regulations: What are the implications for respiratory care? Respir Care 33:258–263, 1988
11. Goodwin G: Governmental regulation of medical devices. Respir Care 33:251–257, 1988
12. Kessler DA, Pape SM, Sundwall DN: The federal regulation of medical devices. N Engl J Med 317:357–366, 1987
13. Hess D, Lehman E, Troup J, Smoker J: An evaluation of the P.K. Morgan Pocket Spirometer. Respir Care 31:786–791, 1986
14. Hess D, Chieppor P, Johnson K: An evaluation of the Respiradyne II spirometer. Respir Care 32:1123–1130, 1987
15. Hess D, Kacer K, Beener C: An evaluation of the accuracy of the Ohmeda 5410 spirometer. Respir Care 33:21–26, 1988
16. Hess D, Kochansky M, Hassett L, Frick R, Rexrode WO: An evaluation of the Nellcor N-10 portable pulse oximeter. Respir Care 31:796–802, 1986
17. Hess D, Mohlman A, Kochansky M, Kriss T: An evaluation of the accuracy of the Physio-Control Lifestat 1600 pulse oximeter in measuring arterial oxygen saturation. Respir Care 32:19–23, 1987
18. Harris KW: The role of the respiratory care practitioner in the evaluation of medical devices. Respir Care 33:264–273, 1988
19. Hess D, Evans C, Thomas K, Eitel D, Kochansky M: The relationship between conjunctival P_{O_2} and arterial P_{O_2} in 16 normal persons. Respir Care 31:191–198, 1986
20. Altman DG, Bland JM: Measurement in medicine: The analysis of method comparison studies. Statistician 32:307–317, 1983
21. Bland JM, Altman DG: Statistical methods for assessing agreement between two methods of clinical measurement. Lancet 1:307–310, 1986
22. Kramer MS, Feinstein AR: Clinical biostatistics LIV. The biostatistics of concordance. Clin Pharmacol Ther 29:111–123, 1981
23. Torzala T: Ventilatory performance testing. Med Electronics (June):70–79, 1987
24. Banner MJ, Hurd TE, Boysen PG: A mechanical model of spontaneous ventilation. Crit Care Med 12:986–987, 1984
25. Katz JA, Kraemer RW, Gjerde GE: Inspiratory work and airway pressure with continuous positive airway pressure delivery devices. Chest 88:519–523, 1985
26. Lampotang S, Gravenstein N, Banner MJ, Jaeger MJ, Schultetus RR: A lung model of carbon dioxide concentrations with mechanical or spontaneous ventilation. Crit Care Med 14:1055–1057, 1986
27. Op't Holt TB, Hall MW, Bass JB, Allison RC: Comparison of changes in airway pressure during continuous positive airway pressure (CPAP) between demand valve and continuous flow devices. Respir Care 27:1200–1209, 1982
28. Walton JR: A new controversy in respiratory equipment management: Reusables versus disposables versus reused disposables. Respir Care 31:213–217, 1986
29. Gardner RM: Calibration and quality control in the pulmonary laboratory—why? Respir Care 28:745–746, 1983
30. Quality assurance in pulmonary function laboratories. Am Rev Respir Dis 134:625–627, 1986
31. Shigeoka JW: Calibration and quality control of spirometer systems. Respir Care 28:747–753, 1983
32. Elser RC: Quality control of blood gas analysis: A review. Respir Care 31:807–816, 1986

The Rational, Scientific Basis of Respiratory Therapy Techniques

EIGHT

Respiratory Gas Exchange Mechanisms

J. Robert Kinker, Jr.
F. Herbert Douce

The primary function of the lung is gas exchange. In the process of gas exchange, the lung delivers atmospheric air from our external environment into our internal blood gas-transport system. Gas exchange occurs by exposing approximately equal volumes of air and blood, interfacing over a large surface area, so that efficient exchange of oxygen and carbon dioxide may occur. The lung also has secondary functions, such as the storage of a small amount of blood, filtration, metabolic capabilities, and the biosynthesis of certain compounds. Abnormalities of gas exchange are the most obvious manifestations of pulmonary disease, but disturbances of the secondary functions of the lung may also occur.

In addition to the pulmonary system, several other body systems play vital roles in gas exchange. The nervous system controls ventilation; the musculoskeletal system overcomes the mechanical work of breathing; the circulatory system delivers carbon dioxide to the lungs and oxygen to body tissues; and the renal system helps control the stimulus to breathe. Each of these body systems plays a role in the gas exchange process and has several complex interdependent physiologic mechanisms that can support or impair the gas exchange process. When gas exchange is impaired, the result is a lack of oxygen and an excessive accumulation of carbon dioxide in the blood, which can hinder energy production and utilization, impair mental capability, cause cardiac arrhythmias, and result ultimately in tissue death.

The respiratory care team is primarily concerned with the distribution and magnitude of pulmonary ventilation, although respiratory care techniques may also influence other physiologic processes of gas exchange, such as the flow and distribution of pulmonary blood. It is a constant challenge to the respiratory care clinician to assess the efficacy of each mechanism of the gas exchange process. Especially in a life-threatening situation, a rapid, accurate, and well-considered assessment to determine the impaired mechanism, followed by the proper support of that failing mechanism, makes the difference in quality patient care and may save a life.

A GAS EXCHANGE ANALOGY

Oxygen and carbon dioxide move between the external air and the metabolizing cells of the body by the processes of bulk flow and simple diffusion from areas of high to low partial pressures. The delivery of gases from the external atmosphere through the tracheobronchial pathways to the parenchyma of the lungs is similar to the water cycle (although the role of fluid and gas are reversed).

In the water cycle, water from heavy rains flows down hills through a series of channels and over waterfalls and pools to a general area, such as a pond, much like the air in the alveoli, where gas and fluid interface. The water in the pond evaporates at a rate dependent on the capacity of the air to hold water and the surface area of the pond. Although the water cycle occurs without a barrier between the water surface and the air, it is similar to the exchange of gases through the alveolar-capillary membrane into the blood transport system. The success of the water cycle depends on adequately matched amounts of air and water, or, in the respiratory system, air and blood, as well as membrane diffusion processes. Success of the water cycle is gauged by the partial pressure of H_2O in the air. In the human physiologic gas exchange system, measurement of the partial pressures of oxygen and carbon dioxide (P_{O_2} and P_{CO_2}) of arterial blood is reflective of the exchange of these gases from the external environment to the blood transport system.

The internal gas exchanger distributes oxygenated blood to the tissues and removes carbon dioxide and other metabolic end products from them. It comprises the left ventricle and systemic arteries, capillaries, and veins containing hemoglobin. The internal gas exchanger is in series with the external, cellular, and subcellular gas exchangers. In the last-named compartment, molecular oxygen enters into substrate oxidation by acting as a terminal electron acceptor. For instance, in the metabolism of glucose, the reaction, $C_6H_{12}O_6 + 6O_2 \rightarrow 6CO_2 + 6H_2O$ + ATP (energy), requires an intracellular P_{O_2} of less than 5 torr and is responsible for about 70% of the total oxygen consumption.

Figure 8–1 is a model of the total respiratory gas exchange mechanism as an engineer might envision it. The external gas exchanger comprises two parallel pumps, one for air and one for blood, in series with two sets of parallel conducting tubes (the tracheobronchial tree and the pulmonary arterial circulation) and an interface at which air and blood come into close contact (the alveolar-capillary membrane).

Implied in Figure 8–2 is the concept that all

Figure 8–1. A model of the respiratory gas exchange mechanisms. T-B tree, tracheobronchial tree (airways); P-V tree, pulmonary vascular tree (pulmonary arterial system). (Modified from Gee JBL, Robin ED: Disorders of respiratory gas transport and metabolism. In Scientific Clinician, Vol 1, Unit 2. New York, McGraw-Hill, 1966.)

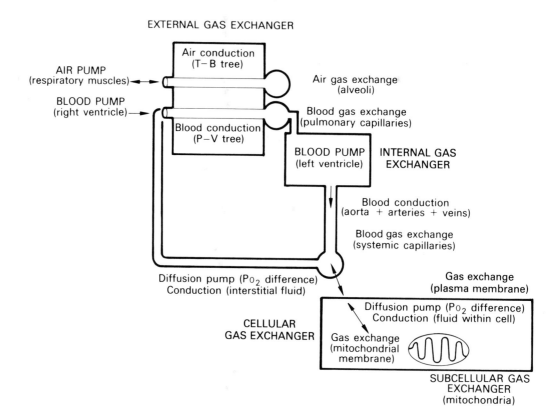

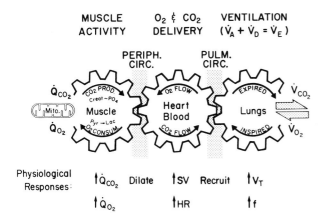

Figure 8–2. A model of the key components of gas exchange. This model emphasizes the interdependence of these gas-exchange mechanisms. (Wasserman K, Hansen JE, Sue DY, Whipp BJ: Principles of Exercise Testing and Interpretation. Philadelphia, Lea & Febiger, 1987, with permission)

pumps and tubes must be functioning simultaneously and continuously and, in the blood circulation, hemoglobin must be contained as the biochemical transport vehicle for oxygen. Of most importance is the understanding that, in engineering terms, the gas exchange mechanism is a "go–no–go" system; that is, if one part of the system fails, even though the others are temporarily functioning adequately, the overall function of the system will be impaired.

To understand the gas exchange process, it is first important to understand the anatomy and physiology of the lung and the gas transport system. The respiratory care clinician should be familiar with these components of gas exchange from birth to the adult, from the upper airways to the lower airways, from the control of ventilation to the pumping mechanism of air movement. It is not only important to understand these components of gas exchange and the gas exchange process, but the respiratory care clinician should be able to integrate this knowledge in daily patient care.

PULMONARY ANATOMY AND PHYSIOLOGY

The components of the pulmonary system consist of the upper airways, the central airways, the peripheral airways, the terminal respiratory unit, and the alveolar-capillary units. Effective gas exchange is dependent upon the structure and integrity of each of these components.

SUBDIVISIONS OF THE LUNG

Anatomically, the right lung has three lobes: upper, middle, and lower. The left lung has two lobes: upper and lower. Analogous to the right middle lobe the left lung has an anterior, lower portion of the upper lobe called the lingula. These lobes are further divided into segments, as depicted in Figure 8–3. Another useful illustration of the bronchopulmonary segments is found in Chapter 23. Each segment has its own airway and arterial and venous circulation, which allows any diseased segment to be surgically removed, if necessary. Knowledge of the location of each segment is of further importance to the respiratory care practitioner when applying appropriate bronchopulmonary hygiene techniques, particularly during percussion–vibration and postural drainage procedures (see Chap. 23), when localizing and interpreting abnormalities in the chest x-ray (see Chap. 12), and when accurately localizing physical findings in the chest.

Physiologically, the lungs can be divided into four lung volumes and four capacities; a *capacity* is the sum of two or more lung volumes. The lung volumes and capacities that are most important for gas exchange are the functional residual capacity, tidal volume, and inspiratory reserve volume. The *functional residual capacity* is the volume of gas in the lungs following a normal exhalation; it serves as a reservoir and maintains alveoli in their partially expanded state. With each inspiration the *tidal volume* delivers new atmospheric gas to the lungs, and with each expiration removes carbon dioxide from the lungs. The *inspiratory reserve volume* allows us to sigh and reinflate partially collapsed alveoli. The names, abbreviations, normal adult values, and interrelationships of lung volumes and capacities are shown in Figure 8–4.

UPPER AIRWAYS

Air is delivered to the lungs through the nose to the nasopharynx and then through the branching airways, where about 23 to 25 divisional generations later it reaches the alveoli, where gas exchange takes place. The nose, pharynx, hypopharynx, and the larynx are the great "air conditioners" of the upper airway. Air is warmed and humidified; soluble noxious gases are absorbed into the fluid lining the walls; and particles larger than 50 μm in diameter are removed in these intricate passages. Nearly one-third of patients with chronic obstructive pulmonary disease have associated upper airway disease (Table 8–1).

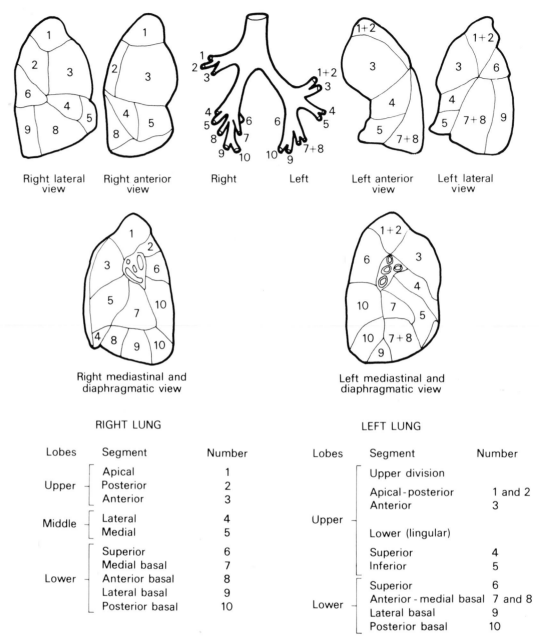

	RIGHT LUNG			LEFT LUNG	
Lobes	Segment	Number	Lobes	Segment	Number
Upper	Apical	1	Upper	Upper division	
	Posterior	2		Apical-posterior	1 and 2
	Anterior	3		Anterior	3
Middle	Lateral	4		Lower (lingular)	
	Medial	5		Superior	4
Lower	Superior	6		Inferior	5
	Medial basal	7	Lower	Superior	6
	Anterior basal	8		Anterior-medial basal	7 and 8
	Lateral basal	9		Lateral basal	9
	Posterior basal	10		Posterior basal	10

Figure 8–3. Pulmonary lobes and segments. The diagram views the lungs in the lateral, anterior, and mediastinal diaphragmatic projections. The numbered airways correspond to the bronchopulmonary segments.

CENTRAL AIRWAYS

The central airways consist of the trachea, the main stem bronchi, the lobar, segmental, and 18 generations of subsegmental bronchi (Table 8–2). The sole function of the central airways is to conduct gas by bulk flow from the larynx to the distal airways; the central airways are also known as the conducting airways, the cartilaginous or large airways. The trachea is supported by the hyoid bone, and its caliber is maintained by anterior U-shaped cartilaginous rings; a membranous portion is located posteriorly.

Total lung capacity (TLC) 6000 mL	Vital capacity (VC)	Inspiratory reserve volume (IRV) 3600 mL	Inspiratory capacity (IC) 3600 mL
		Tidal volume (V_t) 500 mL	
		Expiratory reserve volume (ERV) 1200 mL	Functional residual capacity (FRC) 2400 mL
	Residual volume (RV) 1200 mL	Residual volume (RV) 1200 mL	

Figure 8—4. The names, abbreviations, normal adult values, and interrelationships of the lung volumes and capacities.

At the bifurcation of the trachea, a complete cartilaginous ring called the *carina* joins the trachea with the main stem bronchi that serve each lung. In the bronchi, the cartilaginous rings are replaced by a circumferential structure of cartilaginous plates, which irregularly encircle the airway. These plates are interconnected by a strong fibrous layer intermeshed with circularly arranged smooth muscle.

The bronchial smooth muscle is innervated by the vagus nerve. When bronchial smooth muscle is stimulated, the muscle contracts and the airway lumen becomes smaller and constricted, causing an increase in airway resistance. The role of the autonomic nervous system in maintaining normal airway caliber is discussed elsewhere (see Chap. 19).

The surface of the cartilaginous central airways is lined with pseudostratified, columnar, ciliated epithelium (Fig. 8–5A) interspersed with clear goblet cells that secrete thick viscid mucus. Beneath the epithelium, cartilaginous rings, and plates there are nests of mucous glands that connect with the airway lumen by ducts (Fig. 8–6). These glands secrete a mixture of thick and thin mucus, and they secrete their products with vagal stimulation. Both the submucous glands and cartilage gradually disappear distally as the airways become smaller with each bifurcation.

The surface of the epithelial cells is coated by a thin, complex layer of mucus secreted by the glands just described. This mucous blanket is propelled toward the pharynx by hairlike structures called *cilia* at a rate of about 1000 strokes per minute. Adverse conditions, such as cigarette smoking, drying of the airways, alcoholism, and hypoxia, interfere with ciliary action and may suppress it altogether. Ciliary function may be overwhelmed by an excessive thickness of the overlying mucous coat in cystic fibrosis or during exacerbations of asthma or chronic bronchitis. The ability of ciliated epithelium to regenerate after damage is not known. At biopsy or autopsy in patients with chronic bronchitis, one often sees replacement of the ciliated epithelium with squamous metaplasia, as shown in Figure 8–5B. The only way secretions can pass such damaged areas is by coughing or suctioning, which produces blasts of air shearing off the secretions; postural drainage may also enhance mobilization of secretions in damaged airways.

The cartilaginous airways comprise a large part of the *anatomic dead space,* which is the portion of the airways containing no alveoli and thus taking no direct part in gas exchange. The volume of this

Table 8–1 Associations Between Upper Airway Diseases and Chronic Obstructive Lung Diseases

LUNG DISEASE	COMMONLY ASSOCIATED UPPER AIRWAY CONDITIONS
Bronchial asthma	Allergic rhinitis, nasal polyposis, sinusitis
Chronic bronchitis	Sinusitis (recurrent tonsillitis)
Bronchiectasis	Sinusitis (Kartagener syndrome with situs inversus)
Emphysema	Elevated nasal airway resistance (mechanism unknown)

Table 8–2 Description of the Human Airways*

STRUCTURE	NO. UNITS	GENERATION	MEAN DIAMETER (mm)	AREA SUPPLIED	CARTILAGE	SMOOTH MUSCLE	EPITHELIUM	NUTRIENT CIRCULATION
CONDUCTIVE ZONE								
Mouth nasopharynx, oropharynx	1	0		Both lungs				
Trachea	1	I	18	Both lungs	U-shaped	Closes open end of cartilage	Columnar ciliated	Bronchial circulation
Bronchus	2	II	13	One lung				
Lobar bronchi	4→5	II→III	7→5	Lobes	Irregular helical-shaped	Helical bands		
Segmental bronchi	18	III	4	Segments				
Smaller bronchi	32 → 2,000	III	3→1	Secondary lobules				
TRANSITIONAL AND RESPIRATORY ZONE								
Bronchioles Terminal bronchioles	4,000 → 65,000	IV→XIV	1→0.5	Primary lobules	Absent	Muscle bands between alveoli	Cuboidal	
Respiratory bronchioles	130,000 → 500,000	XV→XX	0.5				Cuboidal to flattened cuboidal	Pulmonary circulation
Alveolar ducts	1,000,000 → 4,000,000	XXI→XXII	0.3	Alveoli		Thin bands in alveolar septa	Alveolar epithelium	
Alveolar sacs	8,000,000	XXIII	0.3					

(Data modified from Weibel ER: Morphometry of the human lung. New York, Springer-Verlag, 1963)
*The first 16 generations make up the conductive zone, the sole purpose of which is to transport gases to and from the distal transitional and respiratory zone. Distal to the alveolar sacs are the alveoli themselves (see text).

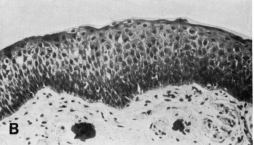
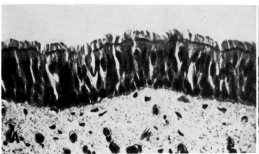

Figure 8—5. Normal pseudostratified columnar ciliated epithelium (*A*) is contrasted with that seen in chronic bronchitis (*B*). Note the replacement of the normal ciliated epithelium by metaplastic squamous cells (*B*).

space is about 150 mL in an average adult, approximately 1 mL/lb (~2 mL/kg) of ideal body weight. The blood supply of the central airways is from the *bronchial circulation*, which arises from the aorta. A large portion of the venous drainage from this circulation returns to the left atrium of the heart, thereby contributing to the normal anatomic shunt. A shunt is blood that bypasses its normal route through the lungs where gases are usually exchanged.

With a cross-sectional area of approximately 5 cm², the trachea is the largest single central airway, but with each airway bifurcation the resulting total cross-sectional area of the next airway generation increases. According to Poiseuille's law, resistance to air flow is inversely related to the fourth power of the radius and, because the cross-sectional area of an airway is directly proportional to the square of the radius, resistance decreases with the increasing cross-sectional area in the branching airways. At each bifurcation of the airways the radius decreases, but the *sum* of the diameters of all the passageways increases; therefore, resistance to airflow decreases from the trachea to the terminal respiratory bronchioles, the cross-sectional area of which is approximately 1000 cm². The pressure required to move air through the large central airways is normally 1.6 cmH₂O/L/sec, approximately 80% of the total airways resistance of 2.0 cmH₂O/L/sec.

In the large airways, particles from 2 to 10 μm in diameter impact at the bifurcations or settle onto their surfaces by sedimentation. Such particles are usually transported by the mucociliary escalator out of the airways to the pharynx, where they are swallowed or expectorated. Particles smaller than 2 μm and relatively insoluble gases are not efficiently removed by solution, impaction, or sedimentation; these penetrate deeper into the lung.

Figure 8—6. Cross-sectional view of cartilaginous central airway. *L*, lumen; *E*, epithelial surface; *M*, smooth muscle; *G*, submucous gland; *C*, cartilage.

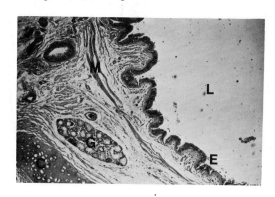

PERIPHERAL AIRWAYS

The cartilaginous plates of the bronchi gradually disappear, and noncartilaginous airways begin to appear at approximately the 12th airway generation. The noncartilaginous airways are collectively called the *peripheral airways*, the distal airways, or the small airways with diameters smaller than 2.0 mm. These airways can also be classified as membranous airways or bronchioles; the final generation of bronchioles is known as *terminal bronchioles*. The airway epithelium also gradually changes from pseudostratified, ciliated, and columnar, interspersed with goblet cells, to more cuboidal ciliated cells in the bronchioles. *Clearance* of inhaled material from the airways occurs by ciliated cells bathed in a fluid composed of both a watery protein layer from the Clara cells and secretions from the goblet cells. In bronchitis the number of goblet cells and inflammatory cells in the large bronchioles may markedly increase.

The terminal bronchioles are the smallest conducting airways and have a diameter of about 0.6 mm, but the sum of all the diameters, or the cross-sectional area of the terminal bronchioles, is much larger than the central airways. As a result of the relatively large cross-sectional area, the resistance to airflow is relatively small and approximately 20% of the total airway resistance. In comparison with the central airways, the bronchioles have proportionally more smooth muscle and connective tissue that contains more elastic fibers. With the lack of supporting cartilage, these airways are more susceptible to severe bronchospasm and significant increases in airway resistance.

The bronchial arterial system anastomoses with the pulmonary artery through a network of capillary plexus at the junction of the conducting airways and the terminal respiratory units.[2]

TERMINAL RESPIRATORY UNIT

The structures distal to the terminal bronchioles have been called the terminal respiratory unit (TRU), the respiratory zone, acinus, or secondary lobule. These structures consist of the respiratory bronchioles, their subdivisions, alveolar ducts, alveolar sacs, and individual alveoli. Five to ten acini constitute the primary pulmonary lobule.

The respiratory bronchioles have occasional alveoli budding from their walls, and they are supplied by the pulmonary circulation rather than the systemic bronchial circulation; this is the start of the respiratory zone of the lung where trans-membrane gas exchange becomes possible. There are about 100,000 TRUs in adults and, within each TRU, there are approximately 3000 alveoli; all together there are approximately 300,000,000 alveoli.

Within the acinus, or secondary lobule, the respiratory bronchioles are continuous with the terminal bronchioles. They are smaller than 0.5 mm in diameter and are supported solely by the connective tissue framework of the lung. The smooth muscle, so prominent in the bronchioles, becomes less clearly defined in the respiratory bronchioles, and the epithelial mucosa becomes entirely monolayered. Only occasional cilia are seen, but no goblet cells. Clara cells, which are believed to secrete a

serous fluid, are interspersed with a cuboidal epithelium.

The distance from the terminal bronchiole, at which point bulk gas flow ceases, to the alveolar-capillary membrane is at most 5 mm. The movement of gases in this area occurs by simple diffusion and kinetic motion. The respiratory zone makes up most of the resting lung volume, approximately 2400 mL in an average adult.

ALVEOLAR-CAPILLARY UNIT

The alveolar-capillary unit (Fig. 8–7) is the fundamental unit of gas exchange. It is composed of a polygonal-shaped alveolus, about 150 μm in diameter, surrounded with pulmonary capillaries. About 300 million such units are in the adult human lung.[3] The membrane separating capillary blood from the alveolar air space is between 0.01 and 0.5 μm in width. The alveolar-capillary membrane has a total surface area of 50 to 100 m^2 (about the size of a tennis court), depending on body size, and is extremely well suited to its function of gas exchange.

In the healthy lung, the alveolar-capillary membrane is highly permeable to gases and relatively impermeable to the liquid constituents of blood, although small amounts of blood constituents flow to and from the pulmonary lymphatics at all times. Approximately equal volumes of air and blood must interface in the alveolar-capillary units for effective gas exchange to occur. Optimally, there is a good, but variable, "matching" of air and blood flows to the lung. Neither a ventilated, nonperfused alveolus ("deadspace ventilation") nor a perfused, nonventilated alveolus ("physiologic right-to-left shunt") function as gas exchange participants.

Several factors are involved in the transport of gases across the alveolar-capillary membrane. These include the solubility of the gas consistent with Henry's law, the molecular weight of the gases consistent with Graham's law, the thickness of the membrane, the membrane surface area exposed to the gas, the available pulmonary capillary blood volume to exchange the gas, the pressure gradient of the gas across the membrane, the reaction rate of the gas with hemoglobin, and the affinity of the gas with that respiratory pigment. Many diseases can affect each factor of the exchange of the gases across the membrane. For example, thickening of the alveolar-capillary membrane, as in interstitial pulmo-

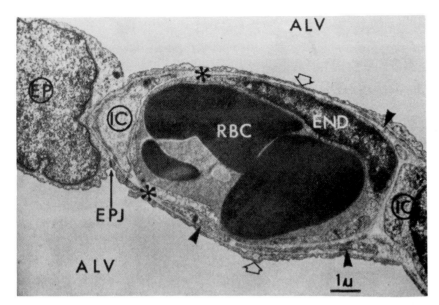

Figure 8—7. Portion of an interalveolar septum lined by thin cytoplasmic processes (*open arrows*) of type I pneumonocytes (EP) (original magnification (×10,000). A junction (EPJ) between two epithelial cells is shown on the left side. A capillary, lined by endothelium (END) and containing three red cells (RBC), occupies the central portion of the septum. The interstitium contains interstitial cells (IC) and processes of fibroblasts (*solid arrows*). Between the endothelium and epithelium, the interstitial space is very narrow. In some areas (*) the interstitium is represented only by fused epithelial and endothelial membranes, thereby reducing the space between air and blood to a layer 10 nm thick. (Fishman AP, Pietra GG: Handling of bioactive materials by the lung. N Engl J Med 291:884, 1974, with permission)

nary fibrosis, can be severe enough to cause a shunt effect that inhibits the exchange of oxygen into the capillary blood, resulting in hypoxemia.

ALVEOLAR CYTOARCHITECTURE

As seen in Figure 8–7, the alveolar-capillary unit comprises several types of cells. Knowledge of the metabolism and function of these cells is increasing (Table 8–3). The thin, type I epithelial cells are known to have a relatively rapid turnover, to be oxygen-sensitive, and to be involved early in oxygen toxicity. Type I cells have extensive cytoplasmic extensions that facilitate gas exchange. The fatter granular pneumocytes, or type II "corner" cells, are fewer, have fewer organelles in the cytoplasm, and are involved in the production of *surfactant*. The importance of this material will be discussed later.

Large cells with wrinkled cytoplasmic surfaces are also scattered around the alveoli. These cells

Table 8—3 Alveolar Cell Types, Their Function, and Known Metabolic Profile

CELL TYPE	FUNCTION	ENERGY REQUIREMENT	SUBSTRATES
I	Structural support; gas transfer	Low	Glucose
II	Surfactant production	Probably high	Glucose, fatty acids, lipids, amino acids
Macrophages	Scavenger/phagocyte	High	Glucose
Endothelial cells	Gas transfer	High	Biogenic amines, adenine, nucleotides, prostaglandins(?), polypeptide hormones, lipids

are the *alveolar macrophages*, the scavengers of the alveoli. They are thought to originate in bone marrow and to function in the removal of the dead cells, which regularly scale off into the alveoli, and are then swept up and out of the lung by the mucociliary escalator. Because of their accessibility by bronchoalveolar lavage, alveolar cell metabolites have been widely studied.

Under inflammatory conditions, migratory white blood cells (polymorphonuclear neutrophils; PMNs) and lymphocytes aggregate at the junction of the respiratory bronchioles and the alveolar ducts. These lymphocytes and PMNs provide an important immediate local defense against microorganisms and allergens.

INTERAIRWAY AND INTRA-ALVEOLAR COMMUNICATIONS

Various types of airway intercommunications are important in the pathophysiology of emphysema and in the spread of alveolar disease. The interlobular septa are not clearly defined in the central portions of the lung, and extension of disease through these communications may explain the more rapid spread of alveolar lesions, such as bronchopneumonia. These junctions can pass particles with a molecular weight of up to 60,000 daltons (e.g., albumin) in acute pulmonary edema or nearly 500,000 daltons in the adult respiratory distress syndrome (ARDS). The alveolar pores of Kohn and the bronchiolar communication channels of Lambert are largely responsible for the collateral movement of air throughout the lung. When obstruction occurs proximal to these pores and channels, a shunt occurs because of lack of ventilation into this unit, whereas perfusion to the unit continues.

The alveolar pores of Kohn are smoothly rounded and occasionally reinforced by a ring of elastic tissue (Fig. 8–8). There is an increase in the size and number of pores with increasing age, corresponding to the enlargement of the air spaces. With the aging process, the pores of Kohn show a propensity for the lung borders, especially in the apices of the upper and lower lobes. They are frequently identified in patches near the hila and also near the larger bronchi and blood vessels.[4]

The bronchiolar channels, described by Lambert in 1955, are connections between the bronchioles and adjacent alveoli. As many as five of these connections have been observed in a single terminal bronchiole. These channels are lined with cuboidal epithelium and are one of the prime sites for carbon deposits from smoke or coal dust, a condition called anthracosis.

EMBRYOLOGY AND GROWTH OF THE LUNG

The fetal lung is not used as an organ of gas exchange; fetal gas exchange is accomplished by the placenta. Knowledge of fetal lung development, specifically development near the end of the sec-

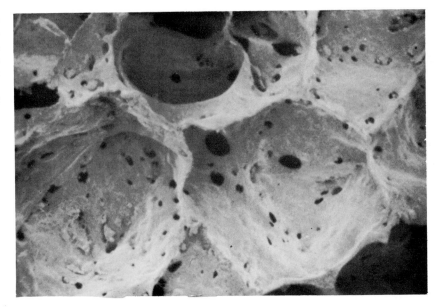

Figure 8–8. Scanning electron micrograph showing an alveolar duct surrounded by alveoli. Note the holes in the alveolar walls (pores of Kohn) and the rough cells lining some of the alveoli (alveolar macrophages). (Courtesy of C. E. Cross, MD, University of California at Davis)

ond trimester and during the third trimester of pregnancy, is vitally important for respiratory care practitioners because premature babies are often born in these stages of development with life-threatening gas exchange problems.

In general, the three stages of fetal lung development are consistent with the trimesters of pregnancy. During the first trimester, organogenesis of the lung occurs as the pseudoglandular phase of fetal lung development; during the second trimester, organ differentiation occurs as the canalicular phase of fetal lung development; and during the third trimester, organ maturation occurs as the alveolar phase. The alveolar phase includes anatomic and biochemical maturation processes that continue up to 8 years of age.

In the embryo, the first accumulation of cells that will ultimately develop into pulmonary tissue arises from the primitive pharynx. By about the fourth week of gestation it forms primitive right and left lung buds. By the end of the pseudoglandular phase, at 16 weeks of gestation, the lobes of the lungs are formed and the cartilaginous trachea and bronchi are virtually complete, including their epithelia.

By the end of the canalicular phase, at 24 weeks of gestation, the bronchial tree has developed 20 generations of branches, up to and including the terminal bronchioles; pulmonary arterioles have developed; the diaphragm is functional; and fetal breathing movements occur. During gestation, the lung serves as one of the main sources of amniotic fluid, and fetal breathing mixes pulmonary fluid containing surfactant with amniotic fluid, which can be sampled by amniocentesis and analyzed to determine fetal lung biochemical maturation.

The alveolar phase of development begins when alveoli develop in the respiratory bronchioles at about 24 weeks of gestation; alveolar ducts and sacs develop subsequently. Also at about 24 weeks lamellar bodies first appear in the granular pneumocytes, which will begin to produce limited amounts of pulmonary surfactant at about 26 weeks. Coincident with alveolar development is pulmonary capillary development.

By the beginning of the third trimester, approximately 28 weeks, the alveolar type I cells are mostly cuboidal, and the pulmonary capillaries have medial hypertrophy, making gas exchange possible but highly inefficient. The alveolar type I cells and pulmonary capillaries become thin and adjoined at 30 weeks and continue to proliferate until almost 8 years of age.

The pulmonary system is the final life-sustaining organ system to mature in the fetus and, at some point during fetal lung development, there is a point of viability outside the uterus. Fetal lung development, specifically the ability of the lung to perform gas exchange, may be accelerated by several factors, including maternal hypertension, cardiovascular disease, hemoglobinopathies, and uteroplacental insufficiency; pharmacologic acceleration may also occur with maternal administration of corticosteroids. Maternal diabetes mellitus and hyperglycemia may decelerate fetal lung development. New mechanical ventilatory techniques, as well as other advances in respiratory care, nutrition, and infection control, have slowly moved the theoretical point of viability into the final weeks of the second trimester of pregnancy. Many babies with gestational ages as young as 24 weeks survive and do well, even though the ability of the lungs to perform gas exchange has not been fully developed.

At birth, the airless alveoli quickly expand during the first few breaths of life, and the functional residual capacity is established by trapping some of each inspired volume (Fig. 8–9). Gas exchange in infants is less efficient than in adults because of smaller and fewer alveoli, resulting in relatively less gas exchange surface area and a greater tendency to collapse. The full-term infant has the nor-

Figure 8–9. Schematic representation of volume–pressure relationships in the lungs of newborn infants during the first (——), second (– – –), and third (XXX) breaths. (Avery ME: In pursuit of understanding the first breath. Am Rev Respir Dis 100:295, 1969, with permission)

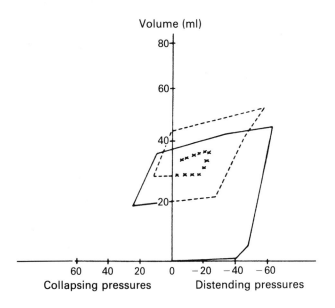

mal complement of airways down to the terminal bronchioles, which will continue to lengthen and enlarge. The respiratory bronchioles, alveolar ducts, and alveoli will increase in number until about age 8 and in size throughout adulthood. The average alveolar diameter is around 50 μm between ages 1 and 2 and about 200 μm at aged 70. By way of comparison, in emphysema the alveoli are enlarged to more than 225 μm in diameter.

Gas exchange in infants is also influenced by perinatal circulation. In the normal newborn, the mean pulmonary artery pressure is slightly less than the aortic pressure, and within the first 12 hours of life a left-to-right shunt through a patient ductus arteriosus is common. After 24 hours of life, the pulmonary artery pressure begins to decrease; by the third day of life, it normally has decreased by 50%. During this early newborn period, pulmonary vascular resistance may increase significantly with acidosis and hypoxemia, and the newborn's normal left-to-right shunt may reverse to a right-to-left shunt, further compromising gas exchange. Persistent pulmonary hypertension of the newborn may develop and last up to 4 days from the onset of acidosis and hypoxemia.

SURFACTANT AND THE ROLE OF SURFACE-ACTIVE FORCES IN THE LUNG

Were it not for the presence of surfactant, alveoli and the bronchioles would tend to collapse, especially during expiration when their size normally becomes smaller. Surfactant is produced by the type II alveolar cell. It is a phospholipid composed mainly of dipalmitoyl lecithin; its production depends on an adequate blood supply to the lung parenchyma, and its ability to reduce surface tension may be related to blood pH. The effect of this material is to reduce surface tension, especially as the radii of the alveoli and the small airways decrease.

The importance of this material will be appreciated by a consideration of the Laplace's law $P = 2T/r$, wherein the pressure P, inside a spherical structure with radius r is related to surface tension T. For a given surface tension, the pressure required to keep a sphere from collapsing will be greater as the radius decreases. At end-expiration the alveolar radius decreases, and the alveolar pressure is essentially atmospheric. With the reduction in alveolar radius, surface tension would rise to critical levels causing collapse. Surfactant reduces the amount of surface tension and becomes more concentrated and effective as the alveolus becomes smaller.

Surfactant allows the alveoli and small airways to remain open at low transpulmonary pressures. A reduction in surfactant promotes alveolar instability and atelectasis and may seriously affect gas exchange. Depletion of surfactant may occur after repeated bronchial lavage, in near-drowning victims, after open-heart surgery in which extracorporeal membrane oxygenation is used, after exposure to high concentrations of oxygen, in oxidant airpollution–induced toxicity, and in the neonatal and adult respiratory distress syndromes. An excess of surfactant is thought to be present in the relatively rare condition known as pulmonary alveolar proteinosis. The exact nature of the removal and fate of surfactant is unclear at present. Problems of neonatal surfactant deficiency are now treated routinely with artificial or bovine surfactant or surfactant removed from human placentas.

THE THORAX AS AN AIR PUMP

The bony thorax and respiratory muscles function as a pump with variable frequency and variable volume displacement to deliver atmospheric air to the alveolar-capillary surface. The components of the bony thorax consist of the thoracic spine, ribs, scapulae, clavicles, and sternum. The respiratory muscles consist of the internal and external intercostals, scaleni, sternocleidomastoids, trapezi, and rhomboids. The primary respiratory muscle of inspiration during tidal breathing is the diaphragm. During inspiration the diaphragm flattens in the process of contracting and enlarges the thoracic cavity in a longitudinal dimension. The ribs articulate on the thoracic spine in such a way as to elevate and widen the thorax during inspiration; this movement increases the transverse dimension of the thorax and is called the "bucket-handle" motion. The sternum moves outward from the spine, and this movement increases the anterior to posterior dimension and is called the "pump-handle" motion. Although the ribs are raised during inspiration by contraction of the internal intercostals, contraction of both sets of intercostal muscles provides rigidity to the intercostal spaces. With exercise and in disease states associated with increased work of breathing, the accessory muscles of breathing, including the intercostals, scaleni, sternocleidomastoids, trapezi, and rhomboids, become involved in inspiration.

The *diaphragm* is a dome-shaped fibromuscular separation between the chest and the abdomen. The central portion of the diaphragm is made up of tendinous tissue and at the periphery consists of skeletal muscle, which attaches to the chest wall. The muscle fiber composition of the diaphragm is 75% high-oxidative fibers, which are highly resistant to endurance fatigue. When high-resistance workloads requiring strength are placed on the diaphragm, these muscle fibers quickly fatigue. In addition, like other skeletal muscles the diaphragm adapts to chronic resistance loads. The diaphragm may function voluntarily when one takes a deep inspiration, or it may function involuntarily during normal breathing at rest or during sleep. The diaphragm is innervated by the phrenic nerve arising from cervical spinal cord roots (C-3, C-4, and C-5). At the time of diaphragmatic contraction, the transabdominal pressure gradient is increased. During normal breathing, a synchronous interaction occurs between the rib cage, the diaphragm, and, to a lesser extent, the abdominal musculature. Current data suggest that the diaphragm is the "prime mover" of normal resting ventilation and that other muscular movements may be secondary.[5]

The *pleural space* is essentially a closed, potential space delineated by the visceral and parietal pleural. With enlargement of the thorax during inspiration, the intrapleural pressure falls, becoming more subatmospheric, and a pressure gradient develops between the mouth, which is at atmospheric pressure, and the alveoli, which is at subatmospheric pressure. This pressure gradient during tidal breathing is between −3 and −5 cm H_2O and is enough to ensure tidal volumes of between 300 and 750 mL of air per breath, provided that airflow resistance is not abnormally high.

Expiration during quiet breathing is a passive process that requires no muscular contraction, unless airway resistance is abnormally high or pulmonary compliance is abnormally low. Expiration is normally achieved by recoil of the lung parenchyma and chest wall. The abdominal muscles are the major muscle group active during expiration. During forced expiration or with deep, rapid breathing, such as occurs during exercise, the contracting abdominal muscles depress and lower the thoracic cage, causing positive intra-abdominal and intrapleural pressure. Such events also occur during coughing, sneezing, and the performance of the Valsalva maneuver.

The muscular work of the respiratory air pump is so small that it consumes less than 5% of the total oxygen consumption of the body at rest when the minute ventilation is 6.0 L/min; during severe exercise, when the minute volume is in excess of 100 L/min, 30% of the total oxygen consumption is consumed by the respiratory muscles. The oxygen cost of breathing increases markedly when the airway resistance is high or the compliance of lung is low. In addition, if the ventilation is "wasted" on underperfused areas of the lung, the normally efficient breathing and gas exchange processes become very inefficient.

When the oxygen cost of breathing or energy demand exceeds the oxygen supply, the gas exchange system must be supported. For example, when the oxygen cost of breathing exceeds approximately 40% of resting oxygen consumption, a mechanical ventilator may be necessary to support the ventilatory muscles.[6]

CONTROL OF RESPIRATION

The arterial pH and Po_2 respond to changing metabolic demands with a fidelity that is relatively unparalleled in nature.[7] From a resting ventilation of 6.0 L/min to maximal exercise of 100 L/min, the normal healthy adult does not demonstrate a significant change in PaO_2. The $Paco_2$ does not change until the onset of metabolic acidosis, when carbon dioxide is excreted in an attempt to compensate for the lactic acidosis. The complex neural and humoral mechanisms whereby alveolar ventilation is regulated are only now beginning to be understood. The literature on respiratory control is exceedingly complex, and the interested reader should refer to the bibliography and to Chapter 35 for additional information.

NEURAL CONTROL OF RESPIRATION

Attempts to understand respiratory rate and periodicity have caused us to reinterpret studies wherein various portions of the brain or brain stem were transected or electrically stimulated. When the upper cervical spinal cord is severed, voluntary and rhythmic contraction of the main respiratory muscles is not possible. Breathing is the only automatic function subserved entirely by skeletal muscle. In contrast, the heart continues to pump blood when completely denervated.

The respiratory system is under both voluntary and involuntary control. The behavioral or voluntary centers are located in the motor cortex of the forebrain and the limbic cerebral area. Efferent output fibers descend through the corticospinal and rubrospinal tracts in the dorsal and lateral spinal cord. Certain conscious acts, such as speaking, response to anxiety or fear, voluntary hyperventilation, and breath-holding, interfere with the rhythmic respiratory pattern and are mediated by means of these pathways. The automatic system has its origins, which are not completely localized, in areas of the lower pons and medulla. The afferents (inputs) for this system come from peripheral chemoreceptors, the glossopharyngeal and vagus nerves, and various proprioceptors. The efferents involve the phrenic nerve, which innervates the diaphragm, and cells in the ventral and lateral columns of the upper thoracic spinal cord, which innervate the intercostal muscles. Mitchell and Berger admit that despite more than a century of study, the nature of the cellular organization of those parts of the brain stem (pons and medulla) responsible for respiratory rhythmicity "still remains one of the mysteries of neuro and respiratory physiology."[8]

To complicate matters further, the way in which the voluntary and involuntary pathways are integrated in the spinal cord is still debatable, although the location of the tracts themselves is well known. The effect of lesions in the cerebral cortex, midbrain, brain stem, and spinal cord on respiratory rate, depth, and periodicity is discussed in Chapter 35.

HUMORAL CONTROL OF RESPIRATION

Chemoreceptors are located in the carotid and aortic bodies and in the medulla. These structures provide the afferent signals for the chemical control of respiration. The respiratory controller responds to these signals by adjusting the level of ventilation to maintain the arterial P_{CO_2} as constant as possible, combating the effects of increased $[H^+]$ or decreased P_{O_2}.

Carotid and Aortic Bodies (Peripheral Chemoreceptors)

The peripheral chemoreceptors are stimulated by an elevation of arterial P_{CO_2} or elevation of $[H^+]$ (metabolic acidosis), but most importantly by a fall in the oxygen tension of arterial blood. The *carotid bodies* are found at the bifurcation of the common carotid arteries, and their afferents to the medulla pass through the glossopharyngeal nerve (IX). The *aortic bodies* are located near the arch of the aorta, with afferents conveyed by the vagus nerve (X).

When these structures are denervated in animals, the ventilatory response to hypoxemia is severely blunted. In humans, the aortic bodies respond readily to hypoxemia, with the carotid bodies having less of a role, except in rare instances. The hyperpnea seen with carbon dioxide inhalation is depressed only slightly by denervation of the aortic and carotid bodies. When increased P_{CO_2} or $[H^+]$ is combined with hypoxemia, however, a considerable increase in ventilation occurs when these centers are intact.

The effects of hyperoxia result in only a mild reduction in ventilation and a clinically insignificant increase in Pa_{CO_2} in the normal healthy individual. In the chronically hypoxemic patient, however, hyperoxia may cause a significant rise in Pa_{CO_2}, resulting in respiratory acidosis and serious side effects (so-called carbon dioxide narcosis.)

Medullary Chemoreceptors

Chemosensitive areas responsive to changes in P_{CO_2} and $[H^+]$ exist in the medulla. These *medullary respiratory centers* are influenced primarily by the $[H^+]$ of cerebrospinal fluid (CSF), which, unlike blood, has a less effective buffer system, so that changes in P_{CO_2} produce maximal changes in $[H^+]$. For example, the CSF protein level is low, compared with that of blood proteins, which are an important buffer. Furthermore, the concentration of CSF HCO_3^- is lower than plasma and does not respond rapidly to changes in arterial P_{CO_2}. The medullary centers respond more slowly to abrupt changes in P_{CO_2} than do the peripheral chemoreceptors, which respond in seconds.

Figure 8–10 summarizes current thinking on the interaction of peripheral and central chemoreceptors in the cortical control of ventilation.

OTHER (NONCHEMICAL) INFLUENCES

Nonchemical influences include the voluntary or behavioral system just discussed, joint proprioceptors, and stretch receptors, which inhibit inspiration, located in the smooth muscle of the airways. In association with this last-mentioned group, deflation receptors exist that stimulate inflation; collectively, these form the *Hering-Breuer reflexes*.

In summary, the sites or mechanisms by which respiratory rhythmicity occurs have still not been completely identified or illustrated, but the search continues.

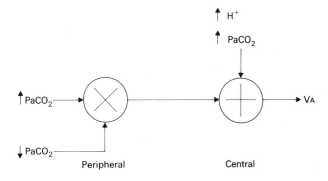

Figure 8–10. Peripheral and central chemoreceptor and ventilatory control: Note that the effects of hypoxemia and hypercapnia on peripheral chemoreceptors are multiplicative. Carbon dioxide and [H+] stimulate central chemoreceptors in a fashion additive to the peripheral afferent input. (Modified from Cunningham DJC: Integrated aspects of the regulation of breathing: a personal view. MTP International Review of Science, Physiology Series 1, Vol 2. Baltimore, University Park Press, 1974)

BRONCHIAL AND PULMONARY CIRCULATIONS

BRONCHIAL CIRCULATION

The bronchial circulation arises from tributaries from the aorta and nourishes the entire tracheobronchial tree down to the terminal bronchioles. The respiratory bronchioles, alveolar ducts, and the alveoli normally receive oxygenation and metabolic substrates from the pulmonary arterial circulation. At the junction of the terminal bronchi and respiratory bronchioles there is a rich anastomosis between capillaries supplied by both bronchial and pulmonary arteries. Most bronchial venous drainage is into the left atrium, contributing to the normal anatomic shunt.

The bronchial circulation is hypertrophied in chronic bronchitis, and even more so in brochiectasis. In these conditions, rupture of these vessels can occur, producing hemoptysis.

PULMONARY ARTERIAL CIRCULATION

The pulmonary circulation has an intricate role in the exchange of oxygen and carbon dioxide. Several factors will determine the effectiveness of the pulmonary circulation in the exchange of respiratory gases. These factors include the total blood volume in the lungs, the regional differences in the capillary blood volume, and the hematocrit of blood in the pulmonary capillaries. In addition, other factors that affect the binding of oxygen to the hemoglobin are important in the exchange and transport of oxygen. A few of the most important factors include the transit time of the erythrocyte in the capillary, the partial pressure of oxygen in the domain of the capillary, and the hemoglobin dissociation curves of oxygen and carbon dioxide. All of these influences of pulmonary circulation form an interweaving network for effective gas exchange.

The lung must also participate in acid–base homeostasis, as well as provide respiratory gas exchange; thus, the respiratory processes are clearly interlocked with circulatory processes, in addition to electrolyte and water balance, temperature control, and metabolism. The lungs, through alveolar ventilation, excrete the major portion of the acid load of the body by eliminating carbon dioxide, which is excreted as a gas through pulmonary ventilation, although it exists transiently as a potent and highly dissociable acid (H_2CO_3) in the body.

The right ventricle delivers the entire cardiac output to the pulmonary arterial circulation. The right ventricle may be described as a variable-displacement, variable-frequency blood pump that produces a pulsatile flow. By special techniques this pulsatile flow may be theoretically observed in the smallest of pulmonary capillaries, although not all pulmonary capillaries are perfused at resting cardiac output. The output of the right ventricle varies from about 5 L/min at rest to more than 20 L/min during severe exercise.

The lung can be thought of as a network of interlacing capillaries and alveoli separated only by the fine and delicate alveolar-capillary membrane (Fig. 8–11). At any time, the volume of blood in the pulmonary capillaries (Vc) is between 75 and 150 mL; this increases by about 100 mL during peak exercise, presumably by vascular "recruitment" (opening of normally closed capillaries, or distention of underperfused capillaries).

The average time in which blood resides in alveolar capillaries and is exposed to alveolar air is about 0.75 seconds a rest. During exercise this residence time is shortened considerably. When gas exchange between alveolar and incoming fresh air is incomplete or alveolar-capillary thickening prolongs transmembrane diffusion time, ventilation–perfusion mismatch occurs, and saturation of capillary blood with oxygen is incomplete. These relationships worsen further during exercise and may result in hypoxemia or hypercapnia, or both, limiting exercise performance and increasing dyspnea.

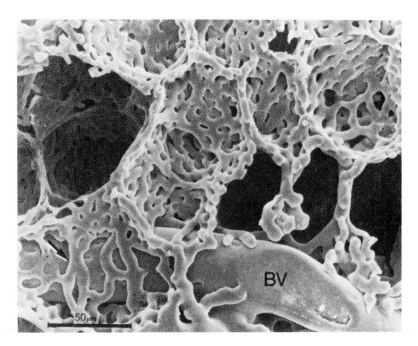

Figure 8—11. A three-dimensional view of the pulmonary capillaries surrounding the alveoli. This demonstrates the intermeshing of the pulmonary capillaries. A blood vessel is also visible. (Guntheroth WG, Luchtel DL, Kawabori I: J Appl Physiol 53:510, 1982, with permission)

The main pulmonary artery divides at the hilum into a left and right pulmonary artery. These further subdivide, generally paralleling the divisions of the airways, down to about the level of the terminal bronchiole (Fig. 8—12). Unlike the diminishing stiffness of the walls of the branching airway, the pulmonary circulation tends to gain stiffness as it branches, although the pulmonary capillaries are believed to be distensible with increasing blood volumes. The proximal pulmonary arteries make up what is known as the *capacitance* portion of the pulmonary circulation. Here, the ves-

Figure 8—12. The pulmonary arterial circulation closely follows the arborizing, branching airway. This photomicrograph demonstrates this relationship. A, airway; a, pulmonary arterial segment.

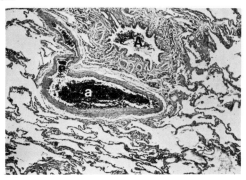

sel walls largely consist of elastic tissue and resemble the aorta and larger systemic blood vessels.

In the normal adult human lung, pulmonary blood vessels 0.1 to 1.0 mm in diameter have media consisting of smooth muscle fibers bounded by internal and external elastic laminae. These vessels and the pulmonary capillary network compose the *resistance* portion of the pulmonary circulation. The walls of the muscular pulmonary arteries lie close to the bronchioles, respiratory bronchioles and alveolar ducts. When the blood vessels become smaller than 0.1 mm (at the level of the terminal bronchioles), the walls of the pulmonary arterioles have a large proportion of smooth muscle, which may contract under various stimuli, most notably hypoxemia and acidosis.

Finally, at the level of the pulmonary arterioles (<0.1 mm in diameter), the muscular layer gradually disappears until the vessel wall contains only the endothelium and an elastic lamina. These vessels directly supply the alveolar ducts and alveoli, ending in the pulmonary capillaries.

Studies have shown that the pulmonary arterioles arborize into a system of pulmonary capillaries that encase the interdigitating alveoli, much as a lace napkin might lie over the top of an open umbrella. The diameter of the pulmonary capillaries is about 10 μm, just enough for red blood cells to pass through end-to-end. This meshwork of pulmonary capillaries rejoins to form the pulmonary venules,

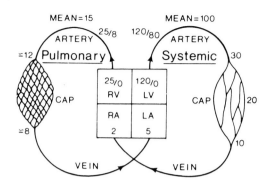

Figure 8–13. Heart chamber and vascular pressures in the greater (systemic) and lesser (pulmonary) circulations. To a certain extent, particularly in the lung, these pressures are modified by hydrostatic differences. Numbers are mmHg. (West JB: Respiratory Physiology: The Essentials. Baltimore, Williams & Wilkins, 1974, with permission)

which subsequently drain into the pulmonary veins and the left atrium.

Generally, the pulmonary arterial circulation should be thought of as one with high compliance, for which vascular resistance is less than one-fifth that of the systemic circulation. A mean pulmonary arterial pressure of less than 12 mmHg at rest and 15 mmHg during exercise propels the entire cardiac output through the pulmonary circulation. The function of this circulation is to distribute the right ventricular stroke volume over the nearly 100-m² surface area of the alveolar-capillary membrane.

A knowledge of normal cardiac chamber and vascular pressures is essential in understanding many of the pathologic conditions that will be discussed in later chapters. Figure 8–13 illustrates these relationships. The resting right ventricular pressure is 25/0 mmHg. Cardiac output from this circulation drains into the left atrium, which has a mean pressure of about 5 mmHg. The etiology of acute respiratory failure can be separated into pulmonary, cardiac, or combined cardiopulmonary causes by measurement of these chamber and vascular pressures, using the Swan–Ganz catheter.[9]

PULMONARY VENOUS SYSTEM

Like the arteries, the pulmonary veins initially are in proximity to the bronchi. At the very periphery of the lung the veins move away from the bronchi and pass between the lobules, whereas the arteries and bronchi travel together down into the center of the lobules. The pulmonary veins possess thinner walls than do the arteries, having a less-developed muscular layer at all stages of life.

GAS EXCHANGE

MATCHING OF AIRFLOW AND BLOOD FLOW

Gas exchange occurs optimally if ventilation ($\dot{V}$) and perfusion ($\dot{Q}$) are adequately matched. As mentioned earlier, blood flow per unit of lung volume is greatest in the gravity-dependent portions of the lung, largely because of the generally passive nature of the pulmonary arterial circulation, such that the blood flows unopposed primarily to the gravity-dependent areas of the lung. Ventilation is also greatest in dependent lung areas, largely because of the geometry of the lung and the greater distending forces (negative intrathoracic pressure) generated in the bases of the lung by the contraction of the diaphragm. The ratio of ventilation to perfusion ($\dot{V}/\dot{Q}$,) is highest in the nondependent (upper) parts of the lung, about unity in midlung (i.e., the level of the third and fourth ribs in the upright position), and lowest in the dependent portions of the lung. The average of these $\dot{V}/\dot{Q}$ ratios is normally 0.8 in the standing adult and varies with body position.

Ventilation–perfusion inequality is the most common cause of hypoxemia, which can be the result of a relative or absolute shunt, dead space ventilation, hypoventilation, or a combination of these conditions. When hypoventilation of some alveoli occurs, the carbon dioxide content can be normally maintained by overventilating other alveoli to compensate for the underventilated alveoli. However, it is not possible to compensate for the oxygen deficit caused by underventilated alveoli, because of the difference in the solubility and hemoglobin dissociation curves of the two gases and other considerations.

Underventilated alveoli are continually perfused with blood that passes by poorly oxygenated, thereby causing a shunt. An example of an absolute shunt occurs in the congenital heart disease, tetralogy of Fallot. In this disease blood bypasses the lungs, going directly from the right ventricle to the left ventricle through a ventricular septal defect, resulting in venous admixture. No matter how high the Pao₂ is in the lungs, there is little improvement in the Pao₂. Some diseases create a relative shunt that is responsive to hyperoxia; an example of such a disease is one involving diffusion impairment across the alveolar-capillary membrane.

Dead-space ventilation occurs when alveoli are

ventilated but the interfacing capillaries around the alveoli are underperfused or not perfused at all (wasted ventilation or alveolar dead space). Figure 8–14 shows three schematized units in which abnormal V/Q relationships are compared with normal. Since abnormalities of ventilation/perfusion ratios cause most of the gas exchange abnormalities found in various pulmonary disease states, it is important to consider each disease in terms of the question, "What is the ventilation–perfusion abnormality?" Only when this is understood will the respiratory care practitioner be able to determine the appropriate therapy and the limitations of this therapy for improving the disease state. A classic treatise on this important topic has been prepared by West.[10]

SYMPTOM–PATHOLOGY RELATIONSHIPS OF GAS EXCHANGE

All pulmonary pathologic processes can result in impairment of the gas exchange process. Diseased lungs may become a significant impediment to oxygen exchange in all the disease states described in Section Three of this volume, although the early stages of lung disease may go unnoticed until the disease progresses. In the later stages of lung disease, the delivery of oxygen and removal of carbon dioxide may be impaired to the extent that work production is limited and severe disability may result. In conjunction with impaired gas exchange, the sedentary life-style of lung-disease patients results in a greater than normal demand on the gas exchange process because of atrophied and inefficient muscles.

Figure 8–15 illustrates a hypothetical, yet practical, relationship between increasing pulmonary abnormalities and symptoms. Few symptoms of lung disease are expressed in the early stages of the disease process. When first injured or otherwise affected, the lung remains adequately efficient in performing its task of gas exchange. The effects of cigarette smoking, industrial exposure, or air pollution may continue for years without any significant abnormality in gas exchange or disability on the part of the patient. Furthermore, the most common symptoms of pulmonary disease, shortness of breath and cough, are often considered by the victims of pulmonary disease as the expected effects of air pollution, cigarette smoking, obesity, or age. This is a real tragedy when it occurs in early pulmonary disease that could be diagnosed and stabilized or reversed.

The right side of Figure 8–15 shows the effects of the progression of pulmonary disease to the point that symptoms become apparent. Any one of the interdependent gas exchange mechanisms in Figure 8–1 can be affected by the disease in Table 8–4, resulting in failure of the gas exchange system. For example, with early obstructive lung disease the patient can be medically managed, the disease process can be stabilized, and some symptoms may be reversed. With the insult of secondary complications, such as airways edema, small pneumothoraces, pleural effusions, or segmental pneumonia, the gas exchange impairment may become more severe and may only be reversed if the patient is still within the zone of potential stability. The reversal of this acute secondary disease is limited to the severity of disability caused by the patient's

Figure 8–14. Ventilation–perfusion relationships in normal and diseased lungs. Areas resembling *C* occur at the apices of normal lung, which are underperfused relative to ventilation, and resemble *B* at the bases, where the converse occurs.

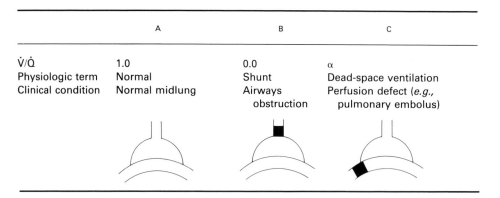

	A	B	C
V̇/Q̇	1.0	0.0	α
Physiologic term	Normal	Shunt	Dead-space ventilation
Clinical condition	Normal midlung	Airways obstruction	Perfusion defect (*e.g.*, pulmonary embolus)

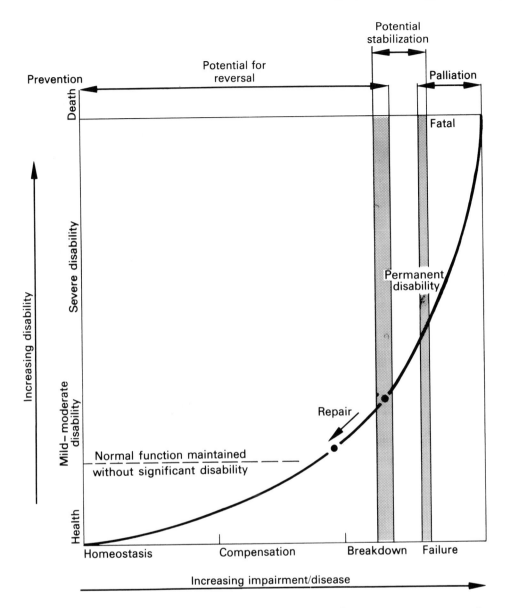

Figure 8—15. Early in the course of progressive pulmonary disease, symptoms are scarcely noted by the patient because of the enormous physiologic functional reserve of the lung (see text). With more advanced disease, small exacerbations or complications cause successively more disability. (Adapted from Hatch TF: Changing objectives in occupational health. Am Ind Hyg Assoc J 23:1, 1962)

permanent chronic pulmonary disease, which may be further advanced by the secondary disease.

With more advanced disease, severe disability will occur because of the severely impaired pulmonary system limiting the gas exchange process. At this stage in the progression of the disease process, even minor complications will result in exacerbations and failure of the pulmonary system that frequently cannot be reversed, and only supportive or palliative care may be all the clinician has to offer the patient. Respiratory care practitioners may be involved in the complete disability–impairment spectrum of pulmonary disease, from smoking cessation education and epidemiologic pulmonary function testing to care of critically ill patients and the rehabilitation process.

Table 8—4   Clinical Application of Gas Exchanger Model*

EXCHANGER COMPONENT	SITE OF ABNORMALITY	EXAMPLES OF DISEASES AFFECTING	BEDSIDE FINDINGS
EXTERNAL			
Air pump	Control of ventilation	Respiratory-depressant drugs, CO_2 narcosis, carotid body excision, sleep apnea	Hypopnea or apnea
	Neuromuscular	Cervical spine injury, poliomyelitis, myasthenia gravis	Hypopnea or apnea; may observe diaphragmatic or chest wall weakness
	Chest wall	Trauma, pleurisy, pleural effusion, kyphoscoliosis, obesity	Restricted chest wall expansion
	Parenchymal	Pulmonary fibrosis, congestive heart failure, respiratory distress syndrome	Shallow rapid breathing, rales
Blood pump	Right ventricle	Infarction (rare) Failure of, secondary to pulmonary hypertension	Elevated CVP RV gallop, $P_2 > A_2$
Tracheobronchial tree	Airways	Foreign bodies, sputum, bronchospasm, external compression, tumor	Wheezes, rales, sputum production
Terminal respiratory unit	Respiratory bronchioles and alveoli	Emphysema	Decreased breath sounds, expiratory prolongation
		Pulmonary (alveolar) edema	Moist rales, LV gallop
Pulmonary vascular tree	Pulmonary arteries and capillaries	Pulmonary emboli, hypoxia-induced pulmonary vasoconstriction, essential pulmonary hypertension	Signs of cor pulmonale
	Pulmonary venous system	Pulmonary venous hypertension	Signs of left ventricular failure
Air–blood interface	Alveolocapillary membrane	Pulmonary edema, hyaline membrane disease, pulmonary fibrosis, adult respiratory distress syndrome	Tachypnea, rales (x-ray and D_LCO much more sensitive)
INTERNAL			
Blood conduction	Arteries and capillary lumen	Atherosclerosis (*e.g.,* coronary artery disease, emboli, extravascular pressure producing ischemia—plaster casts)	Asymmetrical or absent pulses, arrhythmias, etc.
	Hemoglobin	Anemia, hemoglobinopathies, carbon monoxide poisoning	Pallor in anemia, rubor in carbon monoxide poisoning

* See Figure 8–1.

LIMITATIONS OF THE GAS EXCHANGE SYSTEM

Several years ago a young athlete, who previously had one entire lung removed for cavitary pulmonary tuberculosis, went on to win an international tennis meet in Mexico City, more than 7500 feet above sea level. This is an extreme example of just how much loss of respiratory functional reserve can occur before gas exchange impairment and disability become apparent. As mentioned previously, the exchange of oxygen and carbon dioxide is directly or indirectly essential for energy production. The consumption of oxygen is an indicator of the aerobic production of energy. Because energy provides the capacity to perform work, human work performance is highly correlated with the maximal amount of oxygen that can be consumed ($\dot{V}o_2$ max). In the aerobically trained elite athlete, the maximal $\dot{V}o_2$ may be higher than 70 mL/kg/min (5–6 L/min). This is an energy expenditure of over 20 times the resting level of 3.5 mL/kg/min.

Maximal work performance is not only limited by the aerobic energy system but also by metabolic acidosis. The less efficient the aerobic system is, the more the reliance on anaerobic energy sources. When the anaerobic system is accelerated to the point that lactic acid is elevated above resting levels (the anaerobic threshold), lactic acidosis ensues, with a blood pH as low as 7.00 and a muscle pH as low as 6.40 at maximal exercise, resulting in fatigue. The quantity of work that can be performed at the anaerobic threshold is closely related to the work rate that can be tolerated for long periods; work above the anaerobic threshold rapidly results in fatigue.

Many healthy individuals become dyspneic during stressful work or exercise requirements; their dyspnea is not due to limited pulmonary gas exchange. Dempsey has recently theorized that the upper limit of gas exchange or maximum oxygen consumption is limited by the diffusion of oxygen across the alveolar-capillary membrane only in ultraelite endurance athletes.[11] In these athletes, at maximum exercise, some oxyhemoglobin desaturation is present. The reason for inadequate gas exchange at maximal exercise in these elite athletes is believed to be the tremendous cardiac output, which pushes the blood through the pulmonary capillaries so fast the oxygen does not have time to completely saturate the hemoglobin. This oxyhemoglobin desaturation may be aggravated by alveolar hypoventilation or $\dot{V}/\dot{Q}$ mismatching. This is similar to the pulmonary-disease patient, who de-

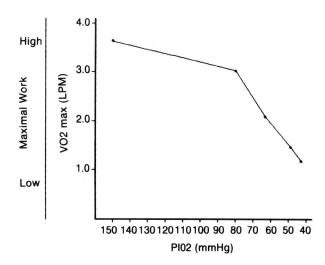

Figure 8—16. This figure demonstrates the effect of hypoxia on maximal oxygen consumption ($\dot{V}o_2max$) and the ability to perform work in young athletes with excellent health. Notice that there is a markedly rapid decline in $\dot{V}o_2max$ below a P_iO_2 of 80 mmHg. The clinical implications of the effects of hypoxia are important to consider when solving the problems of deficient gas exchange in hypoxemic patients. However, hypoxemia may limit exercise performance because of dyspnea before gas exchange limitations are reached. (Adapted from data in Sutton JR, Reeves JT, Wagner PD et al: Operation Everest II: oxygen transport during exercise at extreme simulation altitude. J Appl Physiol 64(4):1309, 1988)

saturates during exercise or activities of daily living because of hypoventilation, $\dot{V}/\dot{Q}$ mismatching or alveolar-capillary diffusion defects. The effect of hypoxemia on maximal work performance is illustrated in Figure 8–16.

In normal persons, another extreme stress on gas exchange that is relevant to pulmonary disease occurs at *high altitude.* As the result of lower inspired and alveolar partial pressures of oxygen, gas exchange at high altitude limits maximal work capacity. At high altitudes the low partial pressure of oxygen results in a lower pressure gradient for oxygen diffusion across the alveolocapillary membrane and, therefore, a lower PaO_2.

REFERENCES

1. Macklem PT, Mead J: Resistance of central and peripheral airways measured by a retrograde catheter. J Appl Physiol 22:395, 1967
2. Murray JF: The Normal Lung: The Basis for Diagnosis and Treatment of Pulmonary Diseases. Philadelphia, WB Saunders, 1976
3. Angus EE, Thurlbeck WM: Number of alveoli in the human lung. J Appl Physiol 32:483, 1972

4. Cordingley JL: The pores of Kohn. Thorax 27:433, 1972
5. Goldman MD, Mead J: Mechanical interaction between the diaphragm and rib cage. J Appl Physiol 35:197, 1973
6. McDonald NJ, Lavelle P, Gallacher MN, Harpin RP: Use of oxygen cost of breathing as an index of weaning ability from mechanical ventilation. Intensive Care Med 14:50–54, 1988
7. Wasserman K, Burton GG, Van Kessel AL: Interactions of physiologic mechanisms during exercise. J Appl Physiol 22:71, 1967
8. Mitchell RA, Berger AJ: Neural regulation of respiration. Am Rev Respir Dis 3:206, 1975
9. Stevens PM: Assessment of acute respiratory failure: Cardiac versus pulmonary causes. Chest 67:1, 1975
10. West JB: Ventilation/Bloodflow and Gas Exchange, 2nd ed. Oxford, Blackwell Scientific, 1970
11. Dempsey JA: Is the lung built for exercise? Med Sci Sports Exerc 18:143–155, 1985

BIBLIOGRAPHY

The Gas Exchange Process

Johnson RL: The lung as an organ of oxygen transport. Basics RD 2(1), 1973 (published by the American Thoracic Society). An excellent description of the circumstances by which the lungs, whose function at sea level is usually not rate-limiting in exercise, may be so when derangements in alveolar ventilation or pulmonary diffusion occur.

Wasserman K, Whipp BJ: Exercise physiology in health and disease. Am Rev Respir Dis 112:219, 1975. This classic "state-of-the-art" discussion, although tedious reading in spots, will be particularly helpful to the reader who has access to an exercise physiology laboratory, which can be used to advantage in localization of defects in the respiratory–cardiovascular gas transport chain.

Embryology and Growth of the Lung and Surfactant

England M: Color Atlas of Life Before Birth: Normal Fetal Development. Chicago, Year Book Medical Publishers, 1983. Remarkable color photos of gross fetal cardiopulmonary development.

Thibeault DW, Gregory GA: Neonatal Pulmonary Care, 2nd ed. Norwalk, Conn, Appleton–Century–Crofts, 1986. A literature review with 2213 references, not for the novice.

Avery ME: The Lung and Its Disorders in the Newborn Infant, 3rd ed. Philadelphia, WB Saunders, 1975. Chapters 1 through 4 are pertinent to this section.

Scarpelli EM (ed): Pulmonary Physiology of the Fetus, Newborn, and Child. Philadelphia, Lea & Febinger, 1975. A classic.

Hills BA: The Biology of Surfactant. New York, Cambridge University Press, 1988.

The Thorax as an Air Pump

Peters RM: The Mechanical Basis of Respiration: An Approach to Respiratory Pathophysiology. Boston, Little, Brown & Co, 1975. Chapters 1, 4, and 9 are concise treatments of complex topics.

Functional Anatomy

Negaishi C: Functional Anatomy and Histology of the Lung. Baltimore, University Park Press, 1972. A definitive, beautifully illustrated treatise, well worth including in any departmental library.

NINE

Pulmonary Function Tests

Paul L. Enright
John E. Hodgkin

Respiratory therapists are often asked to perform pulmonary function (PF) testing at the bedside or in the emergency room, and they are frequently responsible for operating the hospital's pulmonary function laboratory. Pulmonary function testing offers many opportunities for a respiratory therapist because the indications for testing are many, the economics are positive, and the tests are currently underutilized by most physicians.

Evaluation of pulmonary function benefits many types of patients. Pulmonary disease may frequently be detected by PF tests years before the onset of signs or symptoms. Early detection of pulmonary disease helps the physician convince patients to stop smoking, reducing the risk of both cardiovascular and pulmonary disease. Test comparison helps the physician to determine whether a specific therapeutic regimen is beneficial. Shortness of breath is a common complaint for which PF tests can help differentiate between a cardiac and a pulmonary cause. The PF tests performed before planned surgery help to reduce the incidence of postoperative pulmonary complications by identifying patients at increased risk. Finally, patients who feel that their ability to work is limited by shortness of breath can be objectively evaluated by PF tests. The results often carry considerable legal and economic consequences. This chapter will first introduce the reader to the most important and most frequently performed PF tests. Those at the end of this chapter are not usually available in smaller laboratories. For each test you will learn why physicians order the test (indications), what equipment is necessary to perform the test (you will often be asked to specify and purchase instruments), how to perform the test, how to calibrate the instruments and obtain accurate results (quality control [QC]), how to calculate the results and normal values, and finally, what the results mean clinically (interpretation).

SPIROMETRY

Several types of tests can be performed with a spirometer. We will first consider the most frequently performed test—the *forced vital capacity (FVC) maneuver*.

INDICATIONS

Spirometry is the most commonly performed PF test because it is quick, safe, and inexpensive. It is a screening test for pulmonary disease, just as blood pressure measurement is a screening test for hypertension. All current and former cigarette smokers over the age of 40 should be tested; 15% to 33% of them will have abnormal spirometry results, and their abnormal rate of decline of lung function will probably return to normal if they stop smoking.[1]

Table 9–1   Indications for Pulmonary Function Tests

Identify the high risk smoker
Early detection of lung disease
Follow the course of lung disease
Measure therapy effectiveness
Determine the cause of dyspnea
Evaluate the risk of postoperative complications
Evaluate effects of occupational exposures
Determine degree of impairment (medicolegal)

Table 9–1 lists the indications for spirometry, which is usually performed before any of the other PF tests.

EQUIPMENT

Several types of spirometers are available—from traditional 1000-dollar manual volume spirometers to 5000-dollar computerized flow spirometers (Table 9–2). Manual spirometers should be avoided for frequent testing because manual calculations are time-consuming and error-prone. Independent evaluations of commercial spirometers[2] show that only half of the volume-sensing and half of the flow-sensing spirometers meet the American Thoracic Society's (ATS) spirometry standards [3] (Table 9–3).

Table 9–2   Types of Spirometers and Examples

TYPE	EXAMPLES
VOLUME SENSING	
Water-sealed	Collins Survey
Bellows	Med Science Wedge
Dry rolling seal	Spirotech, Spirometrics
FLOW SENSING	
Fleisch pneumotach	Welch Allyn PCheck
Metal screen	Vitalograph Alpha
Disposable screen	Puritan Bennett PB900
Vortex shedding	Riko Spiromate

The primary advantage of volume-sensing spirometers is better long-term accuracy if calibration is not done regularly. Flow-sensing spirometers are smaller, less expensive, and easier to clean, but must be calibrated every day to maintain accuracy. Both types may be automated with a microprocessor or a personal computer. Hand-held spirometers are flow-sensing. Nonautomated, manually operated spirometers are volume-sensing.

Table 9–3   ATS 1987 Spirometry Standards

1. Minimum graph	RANGE	SIZE
Volume	7 L	7 cm
Flow	12 L/sec	6 cm
Time	15 sec	40 cm

2. Daily calibration check with a 3.00-L syringe to better than 3% accuracy for FVC
3. Daily leak check for volume spirometers with no volume change after 1 minute with a 3-cm H_2O internal pressure applied
4. Quarterly speed check for volume spirometers with 1% accuracy using a stopwatch
5. Less than 1.5 cm H_2O/L/sec backpressure at 0–12 L/sec airflow
6. Temperature measured in the spirometer within 1°C for each subject (test only between 17–40°C).

PROCEDURE

The FVC maneuver requires considerable cooperation from the patient. You must first explain the test and then demonstrate the maneuver. The patient must then perform at least three acceptable and two reproducible maneuvers while you provide enthusiastic coaching. Traditionally, a volume–time tracing called a spirogram was produced (Fig. 9–1), but submaximal efforts are more easily detected by viewing the flow–volume curves produced by an automated spirometer (Fig. 9–2). If three acceptable maneuvers are not produced after eight attempts, testing should be rescheduled.

QUALITY CONTROL

Submaximal FVC efforts mimic disease patterns, potentially resulting in "false-positive" interpretations. Vigorous coaching and close observation of the patient's "body language" during his or her efforts is essential. You must also learn to recognize the patterns of unacceptable maneuvers (Fig. 9–3).[4] After three acceptable maneuvers are obtained, you must then check them for reproducibility. The two highest FEV_1s should match within 5% or 0.1 L, and the two highest FVCs should match within 5% or 0.1 L (whichever is greater). If a flow–volume display is available, the peak expiratory flow rates (PEFR) give an excellent index of effort and should match within 10%.

The accuracy of all types of spirometers should

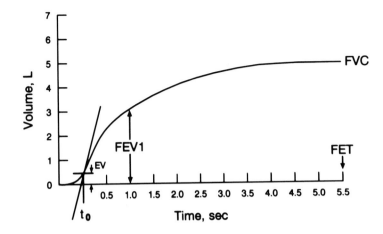

Figure 9–1. Traditional volume–time spirogram. The FVC maneuver starts at the lower left corner at full inhalation. The FVC is the total exhaled volume at the end of the maneuver's plateau (FVC = 5.0 L in this example). The start of the maneuver is determined by "back extrapolation": a tangent is drawn through the steepest portion of the maneuver, intersecting the baseline at time zero (t_0). The FEV_1 occurs 1 second after time zero (FEV_1 = 3.0 L here). The extrapolated volume (EV = 0.5 L here) and the forced expiratory time (FET = 5.5 sec here) are measured as quality control checks. (© Mayo Foundation)

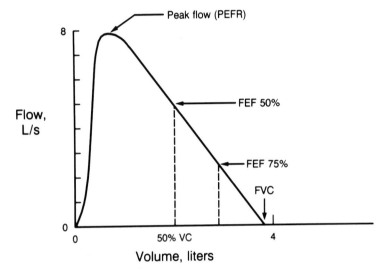

Figure 9–2. Flow–volume curve from a normal subject. The maneuver starts at the lower left corner. Flow increases rapidly to a peak (PEFR) and then decreases evenly until all of the forced vital capacity (FVC) is exhaled. Instantaneous flows at 50% and 75% of the FVC are sometimes measured. The FEV_1 and the forced expiratory time (FET) cannot be measured directly from a flow–volume curve. (© Mayo Foundation)

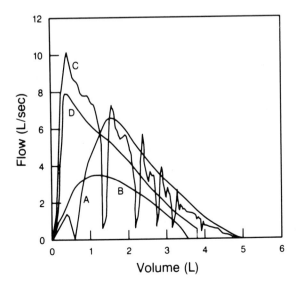

Figure 9–3. Unacceptable FVC maneuvers. Maneuver *A* shows a hesitating start. Maneuver *B* shows poor peak flow effort; the patient did not blast out the air quickly. The jagged lines of maneuver *C* are due to coughing throughout the maneuver. Coughing is unacceptable during the first second of the maneuver because it lowers the measured FEV_1. The vertical drop at the end of maneuver *D* occurred when the patient quit too soon (premature termination of effort). (© Mayo Foundation)

be checked using a 3.00-L syringe at least daily. The resulting volumes should be within 3% of 3.00 L. Volume spirometers should also be checked daily for leaks by placing a weight on the bell or piston and watching for at least 1 minute to be sure that it does not change position. At least quarterly, further QC checks should include a linearity check over the entire range of flows (0–12 L/sec) and volumes (0–7 L or more); a stopwatch should be used to ensure that the chart speed is accurate to within 1%.

To reduce the risk of cross-contamination from spirometers, always use a new mouthpiece and a clean breathing tube for each patient, avoid inhalation from the spirometer, and dry the inside of the spirometer at the end of each day. Consider the use of disposable flow sensors or a separate spirometer for infectious patients, such as those with tuberculosis, hepatitis, or acquired immunodeficiency syndrome (AIDS). After testing such patients, wipe all surfaces exposed to exhaled air with a detergent solution while wearing rubber gloves, soak all hoses and the spirometer interior in an activated glutaraldehyde solution for at least 20 minutes, then dry all surfaces before using the spirometer to test another patient.

CALCULATIONS

The FVC maneuver measures both flow and volume. Flow is best represented by the FEV_1, which is the average flow during the first second. Its name, *forced expiratory volume in 1 second*, comes from the old method of measuring it directly from a spirogram (see Fig. 9–1). A method called back-extrapolation is used to determine the onset (zero time) of the maneuver. The many other indices of flow that can be measured from FVC maneuvers are generally unnecessary or misleading.

The *forced vital capacity* (FVC) is the volume of air exhaled during the FVC maneuver. It is measured from the point of maximal inhalation to the point at which the patient cannot exhale any more air. This may take only 3 seconds in normal children, but more than 30 seconds in adults with emphysema.

The FEV_1 is often divided by the FVC to obtain the FEV_1/FVC ratio. This ratio is a sensitive index of borderline-to-mild airways obstruction and is also helpful in differentiating obstructive from restrictive pulmonary disease. It is decreased in obstruction and is normal or increased in restriction. Normal adults are able to exhale more than 70% of the FVC in the first second (this ratio decreases

with age). The maximal midexpiratory flow rate or forced expiratory flow between 25% and 75% of the FVC ($FEF_{25\%-75\%}$) is also used by some physicians as a sensitive (but highly variable) index of borderline-to-mild obstruction.

The maximum flow that can be achieved during the FVC is known as the *peak expiratory flow rate* (PEFR). The PEFR is a good index of the amount of effort (blast) during the first part of the FVC maneuver, but is not a good measure of obstruction because of this "effort dependence." The PEFR is not easily measured by volume spirometers and must be determined either by flow–volume curves or by using a peak flowmeter.

Normal values for spirometry results are determined from large studies of supposedly "normal" subjects. Older studies were flawed by including smokers, using obsolete equipment or techniques, or not including enough subjects from wide ranges of age or height. The studies of Miller,[5] Crapo,[6] and Knudson,[7] done since 1980, provide accurate predicted equations and normal ranges for white adults. The lower limit of the normal range for FEV_1 and FVC is about 80% of the mean predicted value. It is more accurate, however, to define the normal range as excluding the bottom 5% of the "normal" population. Use of this "95% confidence interval" is necessary to define the normal range of the FEV_1/FVC ratio, the $FEF_{25\%-75\%}$, and most other pulmonary function variables.

The predicted values for nonwhites are not well established, but are estimated by multiplying the white adult predicted values by 0.85 for blacks, Asians, and East Indians. Predicted values depend largely on height, which must be measured accurately in stocking feet.

INTERPRETATION

Submaximal efforts must always be excluded by inspection of the spirometry tracings before attempting to interpret the results. The most common spirometry abnormality is airways obstruction, demonstrated by reduced flow rates, a reduced FEV_1/FVC ratio, and a reduced FEV_1 (Fig. 9–4). The degree of impairment (abnormality) is best determined by the percentage predicted FEV_1, since the FEV_1 decreases linearly with worsening obstructive lung disease (Fig. 9–5). Most adults with an FEV_1 below 1 L are short of breath with only mild exertion and meet the American Thoracic Society (ATS)[8] and Social Security department's criteria for total disability from chronic obstructive pulmonary disease (COPD).[9]

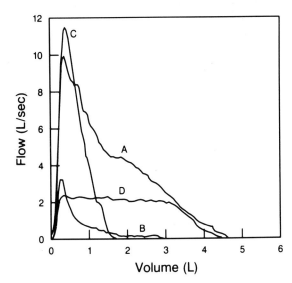

Figure 9—4. Flow–volume patterns of spirometric abnormality. Patient A is normal. Patient B has severe obstruction (COPD) resulting in small flows. Patient C demonstrates moderate restriction caused by interstitial fibrosis, resulting in high flows but a low volume. Patient D has a fixed upper airways obstruction (UAO) from tracheal stenosis; his expiratory flow is limited to a maximum of about 2 L/sec, causing a plateau pattern. (© Mayo Foundation)

Table 9—4 Types of Pulmonary Disease

I. *Obstructive Pulmonary Disease*
 1. Emphysema
 2. Chronic bronchitis
 3. Bronchial asthma
 4. Bronchiectasis
 5. Cystic fibrosis
 6. Tracheobronchomalacia
II. *Restrictive Pulmonary Disease*
 A. Intrapulmonic
  1. Interstitial fibrosis
  2. Pulmonary edema
  3. Pneumonia
  4. Vascular congestion
  5. Adult respiratory distress syndrome
  6. Pneumoconioses
  7. Sarcoidosis
 B. Extrapulmonic
  1. Thoracic
   a. Kyphoscoliosis
   b. Multiple rib fractures
   c. Rheumatoid spondylitis
   d. Thoracic surgery
   e. Pleural effusion
   f. Pneumothorax or hemothorax
  2. Abdominal
   a. Abdominal surgery
   b. Ascites
   c. Peritonitis
   d. Severe obesity
  3. Neuromuscular defects
   a. Poliomyelitis
   b. Guillain-Barré syndrome
   c. Myasthenia gravis
   d. Tetanus
   e. Drugs (e.g., curare, kanamycin)
  4. Respiratory center depression
   a. Narcotics
   b. Barbiturates
   c. Anesthesia

A reduction of the FVC below 80% predicted with a normal FEV_1/FVC ratio is probably due to one of many kinds of restrictive lung disorders (Table 9–4). When obstruction is present (a reduced FEV_1/FVC ratio) *and* the FVC is also reduced, the tendency to interpret a "mixed pattern" of obstruction and restriction should be avoided without measurement of absolute lung volumes, since the low FVC is frequently due to air-trapping secondary to the obstructive disease rather than to a concomitant restrictive disorder. (See Figure 9–5 for a flow diagram for interpretation of spirometry results.)

COMPARISON STUDIES

INDICATIONS

Because the normal range for spirometry values is so wide (80%–120% predicted), it is often useful to compare a patient's current results with his or her own previous results (Table 9–5).

Isoproterenol given by metered-dose inhaler (MDI) is the bronchodilator (BD) most commonly used for testing because its onset of action is rapid and its effects short-lived. If a patient is known to have heart disease, it is prudent to substitute a β_2-adrenergic bronchodilator such as albuterol.

Methacholine is a bronchoconstricting agent that should normally be given only to patients with normal baseline spirometry (or borderline obstruction) in whom asthma is suspected but not confirmed.[10] These patients often have chronic cough, chest tightness, or wheezing only during upper respiratory infections or after exercise in cold weather. Exercise testing for exercise-induced bronchospasm (EIB) is probably unnecessary if a methacholine challenge test is negative.

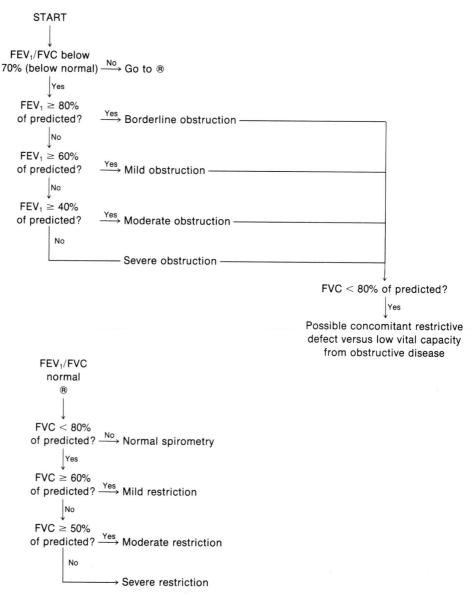

Figure 9–5. Spirometry interpretation. Always start by using the FEV$_1$/FVC ratio to determine if obstruction exists. Grade the degree of obstruction using the percentage of predicted FEV$_1$. If the FEV$_1$/FVC ratio is normal, check for restriction using the FVC. If both the FEV$_1$/FVC ratio and the FVC are above the lower limit of normal range (LLN), spirometry is normal. (© Mayo Foundation)

EQUIPMENT

Several nebulizers and a compressor and dosimeter are useful for methacholine challenges. Drugs and oxygen for treating an acute asthma attack should be readily available. A treadmill or bicycle ergometer and electrocardiogram (ECG) monitor are used for exercise testing. Metered-dose inhalers alone are needed for post-BD testing.

PROCEDURE

The FEV$_1$ is the most reproducible PF parameter; hence, when the patient has airways obstruction, the FEV$_1$ should be followed. When following patients with restrictive disorders, the FVC is compared. The FEF$_{25\%-75\%}$ and other ratios such as the FEV$_1$/FVC should not be used for comparisons because both their numerator and denominator often change.

Table 9—5   Spirometry Comparison Studies

STUDY	INDICATION	AGENT	TIME INTERVAL
Pre- and post-BD	Baseline obstruction, broncho-dilator response	Isoproterenol Albuterol Ipratropium	5 min 15 min 45 min
Methacholine challenge	Suspect asthma but normal baseline spiro	0.1–25 mg/mL methacholine	1 min after each dose
Exercise	Suspect exercise-induced bronchospasm	6–10 min of exercise	6 and 20 min after exercise
Therapeutic intervention	Evaluate effectiveness of chronic therapy	Steroids and bronchodilators	6–8 wk
Work shift	Suspect occupationally in-duced asthma	Dusts, chemicals	8 hr work shift
Trend analysis	Evaluate effects of chronic exposures	Time	1 yr

The technique for administering drugs from a metered-dose inhaler is important. You should first explain and demonstrate the correct maneuver. It is better for you (not the patient) to actuate the MDI. Consider using a spacer if the patient cannot inhale slowly. Be sure to wait for maximal bronchodilation before repeating the FVC maneuvers: 5 minutes after isoproterenol, 15 minutes after albuterol, and 45 minutes after ipratropium.

Methacholine is mixed from a commercially available powder and serial dilutions added to nebulizers.[10] Starting with the smallest concentration, five deep inhalations are administered, followed by two reproducible FVC maneuvers. Exhalation need continue only 3 to 4 seconds because only the FEV_1 is measured. If the FEV_1 decreases less than 20%, the next higher concentration is administered, and so on, up to a maximum concentration of 25 mg/mL.

Isoproterenol is given if FEV_1 decreases more than 20% following methacholine. You should also make a note of any symptoms of coughing, wheezing, dyspnea, or chest tightness provoked by the methacholine; however, disturbing asthma attacks almost never occur.

The goal of exercise testing for EIB is to raise the patient's heart rate to greater than 85% predicted for at least 6 minutes using a treadmill, bicycle, or free running. Noseclips are recommended to bypass the "air-conditioning" of the nose.

QUALITY CONTROL

Optimal accuracy is needed for comparison studies because 10% or 0.2-L changes in the FEV_1 are often considered significant. Repeat tests should be performed by the same technician with the same spirometer, and calibration must be done daily. Maximal efforts should be confirmed by watching for maximal inhalations and by obtaining reproducibly high PEFRs, otherwise apparent changes in the FEV_1 could be due to only a difference in effort.

CALCULATIONS

The percentage change in FEV_1 should be calculated compared with the baseline value. Because measurement errors of up to 0.2 L are common, the absolute change in liters should be calculated when severe obstruction was present at baseline. For instance, an increase from 1.00 L to 1.15 L is a +15% change, but the 0.15 Liter improvement could have been due to measurement errors. Normal subjects improve their FEV_1 by up to 9% following a bronchodilator. Normal subjects can be given five breaths of 25 mg/mL methacholine with less than a 20% decrease in their FEV_1.

The normal annual change in FEV_1 caused by aging alone is about −30 mL/yr after age 30, whereas cigarette smokers developing COPD have an accelerated decline of −60 to −120 mL/yr.[1] At least five annual measurements of the FEV_1 are usually necessary before an individual's rate of decline can be accurately estimated. Trend analysis involves calculating the slope of the regression line of these annual FEV_1 measurements over time (Fig. 9–6).

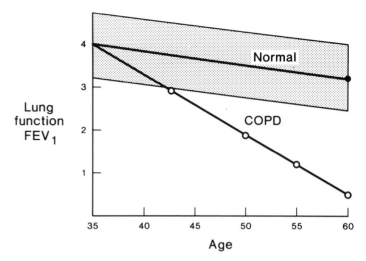

Figure 9—6. Trend analysis of annual changes in pulmonary function. The normal rate of FEV₁ decline for adults is 30 mL/yr. Smokers developing COPD have declines greater than 60 mL/yr. Smoking cessation will stop this abnormal rate of decline. (© Mayo Foundation)

INTERPRETATION

An acute increase in FEV_1 of 15% and 0.2 L after a bronchodilator is considered a significant response, indicating "reversible" airways obstruction.[12] An acute response to a bronchodilator suggests the presence of asthma, although a response may sometimes also be seen in patients with chronic bronchitis. Lack of an acute response, however, does not rule out benefit from long-term therapy with bronchodilators or steroids.

For methacholine challenge tests, a positive response is a 20% or greater reduction in the FEV_1 following five breaths of 25 mg/mL or less of methacholine (Fig. 9–7). A positive response is evidence of "airways hyper-reactivity." Almost all asthmatics will have a positive response if their medications are withheld; however, a few persons without any asthma-like symptoms will also have a positive response.

A 20% or greater fall in the FEV_1 at 6 and 20 minutes after exercise is considered positive for exercise-induced bronchospasm (EIB), seen in most patients with asthma. However, a negative response does not rule out asthma.

A reproducible 15% reduction in the FEV_1 after an 8-hour workshift indicates work-induced bronchospasm, according to cotton dust standards. For long-term trend analysis in adults, a greater than 60 mL/yr decrease in the FEV_1 is considered an abnormal rate of decline (significantly greater than the 30 mL/yr expected from aging alone).

FORCED INSPIRATORY FLOWS

INDICATIONS

The *forced inspiratory vital capacity* (FIVC) test is indicated whenever an upper airway obstruction is suspected, especially in patients with inspiratory stridor (Table 9–6). The FIVC test is not useful for routine outpatient screening.

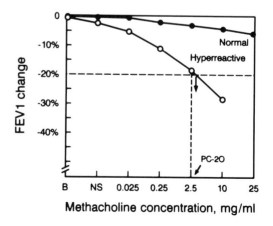

Figure 9—7. Methacholine challenge results. The patient inhales increasing concentrations of nebulized methacholine with the FEV₁ measured after each dose. The FEV₁ of normal subjects will not drop 20% even after the highest concentration. The FEV₁ of patients with airways hyperreactivity (and all asthmatics) will drop by 20% or more indicating a "positive response." The test may be summarized by the Pc₂₀, the concentration that causes a 20% fall in the FEV₁ (about 2.5 mg/mL in this example). (© Mayo Foundation)

Table 9—6 Indications for FIVC Test

Suspected upper airways obstruction
Stridor (noise on forced inspiration)
Hoarseness
Recent general anesthesia, then dyspnea
Neck surgery
Neck masses
Normal spirometry but low MVV

EQUIPMENT

The FIVC can be performed on spirometers that allow forced inhalation maneuvers to be graphed on a flow–volume curve. Volume spirometers that return to zero volume automatically (using gravity or a spring) cannot be used. A volume–time spirogram is not adequate for judging the degree of effort or for interpreting the results.

PROCEDURE

Forced inspiratory maneuvers are started by a slow complete exhalation followed by a maximally rapid deep inhalation. The common practice of performing FIVC maneuvers immediately after FVC maneuvers should be avoided, as the subject may not exhale completely because of air-trapping, and the best FIVC maneuver often does not follow the best FVC maneuver. The FIVC results are very depen-

dent on effort, much more so than FVC results. It is useful to almost scare the patient into inhaling quickly by coaching loudly. At least three reproducible maximal maneuvers should be obtained.

QUALITY CONTROL

The FIVC maneuver graphs should be displayed superimposed at the onset of inhalation and checked for reproducibility. The inspiratory volumes should match within 5%, and the peak inspiratory flows should match within 10%. The spirometer's inspiratory flow calibration should be checked by simulating inhalation with a 3.00-L syringe at different speeds. The FIVCs obtained should all be within 3% of 3.00 L.

CALCULATION

The shape of the FIVC curves is most important. Although some instruments measure parameters from the FIVC, there are no good predicted values available. The inhaled volume and peak inspiratory flows should be used primarily for quality control to check for maximal and reproducible efforts.

INTERPRETATION

A reproducible plateau of forced inspiratory flow may indicate an upper airway obstruction (UAO) (Fig. 9–8).[13] If a similar plateau exists during ex-

Figure 9—8. Flow–volume loop patterns caused by three types of upper airways obstruction (UAO). (*A*) A variable, extrathoracic UAO is commonly due to vocal cord paralysis. The vocal cords are forced wider during forced exhalation but narrow during forced inhalation (because of negative pressure in the airway), creating an inspiratory plateau. (*B*) A fixed UAO, such as tracheal stenosis, is unaffected by pressure differences across the airway, resulting in limited flow (a plateau) both during forced exhalation and inhalation. (*C*) Less commonly, a variable, intrathoracic UAO, such as a tumor near the carina, opens during forced inhalation but narrows during forced exhalation, limiting expiratory flow. (© Mayo Foundation)

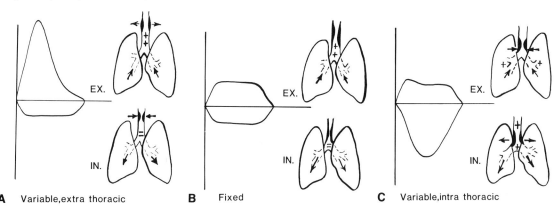

A Variable, extra thoracic   **B** Fixed   **C** Variable, intra thoracic

halation, the obstruction is "fixed" (as in tracheal stenosis), but if there is a sharp peak flow during exhalation, the obstruction is "variable" and extrathoracic (as in vocal cord paralysis). False-positive results occur frequently because of submaximal efforts. A plateau during forced exhalation with maintenance of peak flow during forced inhalation is indicative of a "variable" intrathoracic obstruction. Confirmation of a UAO is necessary, with tracheal x-rays, computed tomography scans, or direct visualization.

RESPIRATORY PRESSURES

INDICATIONS

Measurement of *maximal inspiratory and expiratory pressures* (MIP and MEP) is indicated when respiratory muscle weakness is suspected clinically or to follow patients with neuromuscular diseases that may involve the diaphragm. These pressures may be markedly decreased in the presence of normal lung volumes and blood gas levels. Maximal respiratory pressures are also useful as an index of a patient's ability to be weaned from mechanical ventilation.

EQUIPMENT

Maximal respiratory pressures are measured using simple mechanical pressure gauges (0 to -100 cmH_2O for MIP and 0 to $+300$ cmH_2O for MEP). Electronic pressure gauges for this purpose have also recently become available. A large rubber mouthpiece must be pressed *against* the lips for MEP maneuvers. A 1-mm diameter leak is introduced intentionally to reduce the effect of the patient generating pressure with his or her cheeks. A tracheostomy tube fitting with the breathing hole plugged during measurements is used for intubated patients.

PROCEDURE

The maximal inspiratory pressure maneuver starts by complete exhalation, then a maximal attempt to inhale from the pressure gauge, sustained for 2 seconds (like trying to suck up a thick milkshake through a narrow straw). At least two reproducible maneuvers should be obtained and the best reported. Maximal expiratory pressure starts with complete inhalation, followed by a maximal attempt at exhalation (like trying to blow up a small balloon). Always make a note of the patient's apparent degree of effort.

QUALITY CONTROL

Maximal respiratory pressures are very effort-dependent. False-positive results often occur because of poor coaching or malingering. The pressure gauges should be calibrated regularly with a mercury manometer (blood pressure type) before use. Five percent accuracy at 100 cm H_2O is acceptable. A large, firm rubber mouthpiece is necessary for MEP measurements to allow a firm seal against the lips, otherwise MEP will be underestimated. The pressures should be sustained for 1 second because short "peaks" may be due to only cheek muscles being used.

CALCULATIONS

The average normal MEP for adults is about 200 cm H_2O for men and 140 cm H_2O for women. The normal MIP is about 100 cm H_2O for men and 70 cm H_2O for women. The lower limit of the normal range is about 65% of the predicted value.[14]

INTERPRETATION

Reduction of MIP indicates diaphragm (inspiratory muscle) weakness, whereas a reduced MEP indicates expiratory muscle weakness. Respiratory pressures may be reduced by generalized weakness, malnutrition, unilateral diaphragm paralysis, myasthenia gravis, amyotrophic lateral sclerosis (ALS), muscular dystrophy, hypothyroidism, and steroid myopathy.

MAXIMAL VOLUNTARY VENTILATION

INDICATIONS

The *maximal voluntary ventilation* (MVV) maneuver has traditionally been used for preoperative testing and disability determinations, but is losing favor because of its lack of specificity. Patients who are debilitated or who have heart disease should probably not have MVV tested. The MVV is not a screening test, for it is insensitive to both obstructive and restrictive pulmonary diseases; however, the MVV is useful when performed before exercise testing so that it may be compared with the exercise ventilation. Avoid performing MVV maneuvers on patients known to have asthma since it may provoke bronchoconstriction.

EQUIPMENT

The MVV tests can be performed on many but not all spirometers. A 15-second volume–time graph is necessary. Volume spirometers are preferred because their large dead-space volume tends to prevent hypocarbia during the rebreathing maneuver.

PROCEDURE

The MVV maneuver simulates breathing during strenuous exercise, but only lasts for 15 seconds. Rapid, deep breaths usually give the best results (Fig. 9–9). Vigorous coaching is necessary throughout the maneuver. Several minutes of rest are necessary to avoid fatigue and hyperventilation before the maneuver is repeated.

QUALITY CONTROL

The MVV is very effort-dependent. The MVV maneuvers must last for at least 10 seconds to avoid overestimation of the MVV. The breathing pattern should be relatively regular.

Figure 9—9. Maximal voluntary ventilation (MVV) maneuver tracings. The patient breathes rapidly in and out of a spirometer for 15 seconds. Note the lower tidal volumes produced by the patient with a restrictive disorder and the slower breathing rate, with increasing lung volume, produced by the patient with airways obstruction. The MVV is an estimate of the maximal ventilation that could be achieved in 1 minute. The normal MVV for an adult male is about 150 L/min.

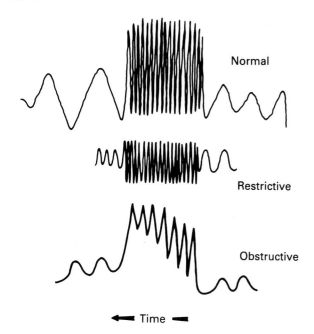

CALCULATIONS

The MVV is calculated by multiplying the accumulated exhalation volume during 12 seconds by 5. The respiratory rate should also be reported. The predicted MVV can be quickly estimated by multiplying the predicted FEV_1 by 40. Because of its wide variability, the lower limit of the normal range is about 65% of the predicted value.

INTERPRETATION

A reduction of the MVV is nonspecific—it may be due to upper or lower airways obstruction, restriction, muscle weakness, or poor effort.

LUNG VOLUMES

INDICATIONS

Traditionally, four lung volumes have been recognized. Combining these volumes results in four "capacities" (Fig. 9–10). Those that cannot be measured with only a spirometer are the *total lung capacity* (TLC), *residual volume* (RV), and *functional residual capacity* (FRC). Measurement of these "absolute lung volumes" is useful whenever the vital capacity is reduced. Because the FVC maneuver often causes airways to collapse in patients with obstruction, when reduction of the FVC is noted, the *slow vital capacity* (SVC) should also be measured. If the SVC is normal, a coexisting restrictive pattern is ruled out; if the SVC is also reduced, absolute lung volumes should be measured to evaluate for a coexisting restriction of lung volumes (Fig. 9–11).

EQUIPMENT

Four methods are available for determining absolute lung volumes (Table 9–7). Equipment costs range from 300 dollars for a simple planimeter to 30,000 dollars for an automated body plethysmograph (body box) system. (See Ref. 15 for a good description of methods of measuring lung volumes.)

Body boxes are of three types: variable-pressure, variable-volume, and flow. Variable-pressure boxes are used more commonly because they are easier to keep accurately calibrated. The body box method is not only more rapidly performed than the other methods, it also gives accurate measurements in the presence of obstructive airway disease. A minor drawback is that some patients are claustrophobic in a box.

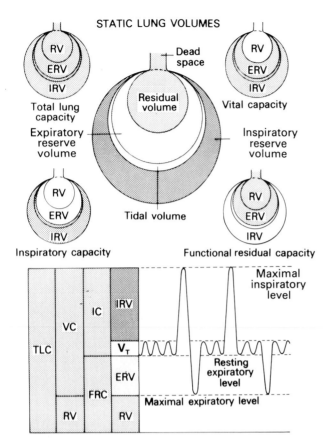

Figure 9–10. Division of total lung capacity into lung volumes and lung capacities. In the small diagrams surrounding the large central one, the shaded areas outline the volumes that constitute the various lung capacities. (Adapted from Comroe JH Jr et al: The Lung: Clinical Physiology and Pulmonary Function Tests, 2nd ed. Chicago, Year Book Medical Publishers, 1962)

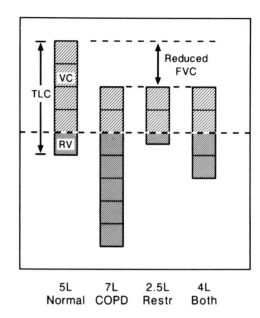

Figure 9–11. Spirometry measures only the vital capacity (VC, above the dashed line). The residual volume (RV) and, therefore, the total lung capacity (TLC) are "absolute" lung volumes, usually measured with a body box or inert gas technique. For comparison, the first patient in this example has normal lung volumes, but the latter three patients all have a VC of only half normal. Knowledge of their absolute lung volumes allows a diagnosis of COPD when the TLC is increased (hyperinflation), restriction when the TLC and RV are reduced, and a mixed pattern when the TLC is reduced but the RV is enlarged. (© Mayo Foundation)

PROCEDURES AND CALCULATIONS

Body Box Procedure

The patient sits quietly breathing through a pneumotach inside the box (Fig. 9–12). At the end-tidal position (FRC), a shutter is occluded in the breathing tube. The patient continues momentarily to try to breathe against this obstruction, and the changes in mouth pressure and box pressure are measured. The shutter is then opened and the patient is asked to inhale completely (to TLC) through the pneumotach, as inspiratory capacity (IC) is measured by integrating the pneumotach flow.

Body Box Calculations

The principle of measurement of thoracic gas volume in the body plethysomograph is based on Boyle's law:

Table 9–7 Methods of Measuring Absolute Lung Volumes

METHOD	ACCURACY	COST ($)	TIME (MIN)	SENSORS
Body box	++++	30,000	5	Pressure transducers
Helium dilution	++	20,000	20	Helium analyzer
Nitrogen washout	++	20,000	20	Nitrogen analyzer
CXR planimetry	+++	300	10	Planimeter

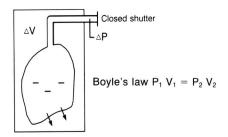

Figure 9–12. Body plethysmography. The patient sits in a box and attempts to inhale when the shutter closes. The change in pressure at the mouth (ΔP) and change in the box volume (ΔV) are measured with electronic transducers. The air in the thorax when the shutter was closed is calculated from Boyle's law. (© Mayo Foundation)

$$P_1V_1 = P_2V_2$$

The starting alveolar pressure, P_1, new alveolar pressure, P_2, and change in alveolar volume, V_2, are measured when the shutter is closed. From these data, the starting volume, V_1, is calculated. The volume measured when the shutter closed is the FRC (but is often called the thoracic gas volume, TGV, or V_{tg}) and is added to the IC measured when the shutter opens to obtain the TLC.

Helium Dilution Procedure

The study starts with about 10% helium in a bag-spirometer system (Fig. 9–13). Helium is used because it is relatively inert and does not leave the alveoli to dissolve in lung tissue or blood. The starting concentration of helium in the lungs is zero. The patient is switched from breathing room air

Figure 9–13. Helium dilution method. The patient begins to breathe air from a spirometer containing 10% helium. The helium is diluted by the air in the patient's lungs but is not absorbed by the body. The helium concentration of the system is monitored until it stops changing (equilibration). (© Mayo Foundation)

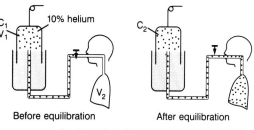

Before equilibration   After equilibration

$$C_1 \times V_1 = C_2 \times (V_1 + V_2)$$

C = concentration of helium

Solved for V_2 = volume of gas in the lungs

into the bag-spirometer system at the end-tidal position (FRC). He or she then rebreathes the helium mixture from the bag-spirometer system until equilibration between the lungs and bag-spirometer system is reached.

Helium Dilution Calculation

By knowing the new concentration of helium in the system, F_E, along with the starting volume of gas, V_S, and helium fraction in the equilibrated bag-spirometer system, F_S, the starting lung volume, FRC, can be readily calculated:

$$VFRC = V_S\,(F_S - F_E)\,/F_E.$$

Nitrogen Washout Procedure

The subject begins to breathe 100% oxygen at the end-tidal position (FRC). The concentration of nitrogen is measured at the mouth (Fig. 9–14). The gas in the lungs at the start of the test contains about 80% nitrogen. As the patient breathes 100% oxygen, the nitrogen is "washed out" of the lungs.

Nitrogen Washout Calculation

By measuring the volume of gas exhaled during the study and the fraction of nitrogen in this gas, the volume of nitrogen in the lungs at the start of the test can easily be calculated. Because this represents approximately 80% of the gas, FRC can be calculated. A minor correction is made for the small amount of nitrogen present in "100%" oxygen that passes from the blood and lung tissue into the alveoli during the washout study.

CXR Planimetry

A good estimate of the TLC can be easily obtained from a standard posteroanterior and lateral chest x-ray (CXR) taken at full inhalation. One technique involves making 28 measurements with a ruler, and the other utilizes a drafting instrument called a planimeter. The separate outlines of the right and left lungs are traced on the posteroanterior view, and then the area of both lungs is traced on the lateral view with the planimeter which measures the enclosed areas (Fig. 9–15). The three areas are then used in a simple empirically determined equation to estimate the TLC. The results are usually within 5% of the body box technique in both children and adults.

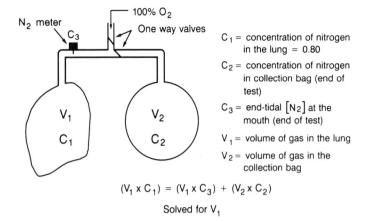

C$_1$ = concentration of nitrogen in the lung = 0.80

C$_2$ = concentration of nitrogen in collection bag (end of test)

C$_3$ = end-tidal $[N_2]$ at the mouth (end of test)

V$_1$ = volume of gas in the lung

V$_2$ = volume of gas in the collection bag

$$(V_1 \times C_1) = (V_1 \times C_3) + (V_2 \times C_2)$$

Solved for V$_1$

Figure 9—14. Nitrogen washout. The patient begins to inhale 100% oxygen with each breath, thereby washing out all of the nitrogen in the lungs. All of the exhaled nitrogen is collected and measured. (© Mayo Foundation)

QUALITY CONTROL

The major disadvantage of the gas analysis methods for determining lung volumes is that some alveolar gas is usually trapped in the lungs of patients with moderate to severe obstructive airway diseases; therefore, all of the nitrogen will not wash out during the short time that the test is performed, or the alveolar gas will not reach true equilibration for helium. The standard length of time for the nitrogen washout test is 7 minutes; however, in patients with COPD, complete washout may take 20 to 30 minutes. Therefore, lung volumes determined using these gas analysis methods may be gross underestimates.

Leaks can also cause large measurement errors in the gas analysis methods. Leaks commonly occur around the mouthpiece, through cracks in the tubing, and because of punctured eardrums. The vacuum pumps used by nitrogen analyzers can lose their efficiency, the needle valves clog, and the sensors get dirty. These problems can be detected by

Figure 9—15. Determination of total lung capacity (TLC) by chest x-ray planimetry. The areas outlined in the PA and lateral chest films are measured with an inexpensive planimeter, and simple calculations are made to determine the TLC. (Harris TR, Pratt PC, Kilburn KH: Total lung capacity measured by roentgenograms. Am J Med 50:756, 1971)

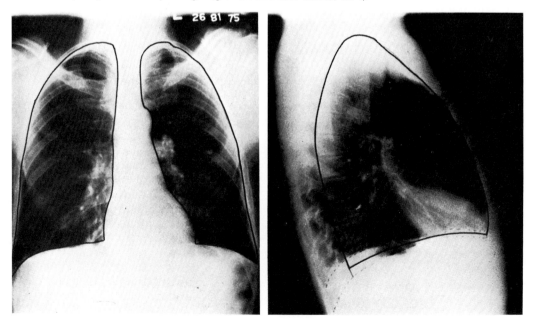

daily calibrations using at least two known concentrations of test gas.

The body box pressure transducers are very sensitive to temperature changes and overpressure. A small 30-mL sinewave pump should be used at least daily to calibrate the box pressure and a water manometer used to calibrate the mouth pressure to within 5% accuracy. A 1.00- or 3.00-L syringe emptied at several rates should calibrate the pneumotach to within 3% accuracy.

INTERPRETATION

Normal adults' TLC should not decline as they grow older, but their RV will slowly increase, resulting in a gradual decline in their vital capacity. The lower limit of the normal range for the TLC is about 80% of the mean predicted value—a decrease in TLC below this indicates a restrictive process. A restrictive process will usually reduce all lung volumes proportionately. (Refer back to Table 9–4 for a list of causes of restriction.)

Even mild degrees of airways obstruction often cause the RV to increase. As obstruction worsens, the TLC will increase, eventually causing "hyperinflation" to be seen on the chest x-ray and a barrel chest noted on physical examination. Hyperinflation may be defined as a TLC above 140% predicted or an RV/TLC ratio above 140% predicted. Hyperinflation occurs both with asthma (decreasing rapidly with treatment) and emphysema.

DIFFUSING CAPACITY

INDICATIONS

Diffusing capacity measured with carbon monoxide ($D_{L_{CO}}$), also called transfer factor in Europe, determines the ability of gases to cross the alveolar-capillary membrane. Carbon monoxide (CO) is used because of its great affinity for hemoglobin and its normally low concentration in the blood before testing.

When airways obstruction is present on spirometry, measurement of the $D_{L_{CO}}$ helps to distinguish among the various causes of obstruction. The $D_{L_{CO}}$ is reduced in emphysema, normal in simple chronic bronchitis, and normal or increased in asthma.

When spirometry and lung volumes show restriction, $D_{L_{CO}}$ measurement helps to distinguish between chest wall and interstitial disease. The diffusing capacity test is probably the most sensitive indicator of early interstitial lung disease (such as the *Pneumocystis* pneumonia seen in patients with AIDS) and vasculitis and is also used to determine response to specific therapy. In patients with cancer, the $D_{L_{CO}}$ is sensitive for detecting lymphangitic spread of cancer to the lungs and lung fibrosis caused by radiation therapy and chemotherapy.

EQUIPMENT

The $D_{L_{CO}}$ measurement requires one of three types of carbon monoxide analyzers: infrared, fuel cell, or gas chromatograph. All three require that water vapor and carbon dioxide be removed first (Fig. 9–16). A thermal conductivity helium analyzer is usually used to simultaneously measure alveolar volume. Most laboratories have finally replaced "homemade, Rube Goldberg"–appearing apparatus with an automated system that costs between 15,000 and 30,000 dollars and also measures spirometry and lung volumes.

PROCEDURE

The technique most widely used is the single-breath method ($D_{L_{CO}}$-SB). The exact procedure has recently been standardized by the American Thoracic Society.[16] The patient should be asked to refrain from smoking for 24 hours before the test and should not eat or exercise for 1 hour before the test.

Explain the test and demonstrate the breathing maneuver. The patient must be seated wearing noseclips. Starting at RV, the patient rapidly inhales to TLC a gas mixture containing 0.3% carbon monoxide (CO) and 10% helium, then holds his or her breath for 10 seconds before exhaling rapidly. After 1 L of dead space is cleared, 1 L of exhaled alveolar gas is sampled. Wait at least 4 minutes (to eliminate the test gas from the lungs), then repeat the test. Obtain at least two acceptable tests with $D_{L_{CO}}$ values that match within 3 mL/min/mmHg. Report the mean $D_{L_{CO}}$ and V_A of all acceptable tests.

Rebreathing and steady-state exercise methods of $D_{L_{CO}}$ measurement are less frequently used because standards for them are not widely accepted.

QUALITY CONTROL

Many factors affect the $D_{L_{CO}}$, often causing differences in the reported $D_{L_{CO}}$ between laboratories testing the same individual. A fully automated system with recently updated computer software, as well as careful technique, is necessary to obtain

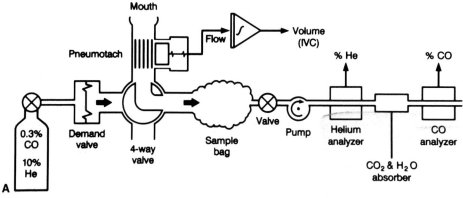

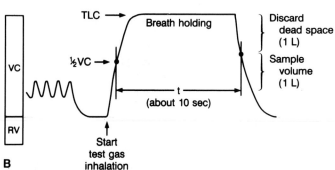

Figure 9—16. *(A)* Measurement of diffusing capacity. The patient inhales a full breath of a test gas containing 0.3% carbon monoxide (CO) and 10% helium. He holds the test gas in his lungs for 10 seconds. Some of the CO is taken up by his red blood cells and the helium is diluted. As he exhales, deadspace gas is discarded and the next liter of air (exhaled into the sample bag) is analyzed for CO and helium. *(B)* The single-breath D_{LCO} maneuver. After complete exhalation (to RV), the patient quickly inhales a full vital capacity of test gas, holds his breath for 10 seconds, then quickly exhales.

results reproducible within 3 mL/min/mmHg. Daily leak tests and volume calibration checks must be done. The CO analyzer is usually at fault when inaccurate measurements are obtained. A 2% error in the CO analyzer will result in more than a 10% error in the reported D_{LCO}; therefore, the accuracy and linearity of the CO analyzer must be checked at least quarterly and found to be within 1%. The chemical absorbers frequently used to prevent carbon dioxide and water from entering the CO analyzer must also be checked daily.

A "biologic control" is also necessary to check D_{LCO} instruments. Test yourself or another non-smoker without lung disease every week. After at least five measurements, determine the mean and standard deviation (SD) of the results. Thereafter, plot the results; if the current D_{LCO} is greater than 2 SD from the mean of the previous results, recheck the D_{LCO} system thoroughly, fix the problem, and repeat the test to validate the repair.

Individual D_{LCO} maneuvers are unacceptable (and should be discarded) if any of the following occurs:

- The volume of test gas inhaled is less than 90% of a previously measured slow vital capacity

- Inspiratory time is more than 2.5 seconds
- Breath-hold time is less than 9 seconds or more than 11 seconds
- Washout volume is less than 500 mL
- Sample size is less than 500 mL
- Sample collection time is more than 3 seconds

CALCULATIONS

Think of D_{LCO} as the uptake of carbon monoxide. It is reported in milliliters of CO that diffuse per minute across the alveolar-capillary membrane per millimeter of mercury pressure (D_{LCO} = mL/min/mmHg). The pressure is the difference in the partial pressure of CO between alveoli (the driving pressure) and the blood in pulmonary capillaries (the back pressure).

Some laboratories also report the ratio of D_{LCO}/V_A, where V_A is the alveolar volume at which D_{LCO} was measured. The D_{LCO}/V_A tends to remain normal in restriction caused by chest wall disorders. (This ratio is called Krogh's constant in Europe.) The V_A is equivalent to the TLC; since it is measured by the single-breath helium dilution method, however, the V_A measured in severely obstructed patients will be somewhat lower than the TLC measured by other methods.

Because the uptake of CO also depends on the number of red cells in the blood, $D_{L_{CO}}$ will decrease in anemia with no lung disease. For example, an anemic patient with a hemoglobin value of 7 gm/dL and a measured $D_{L_{CO}}$ value of 20 mL/min/mmHg would have a $D_{L_{CO}}$ value of 30 if he were transfused to reach a normal hemoglobin (Hb) of 15 gm/dL. Consequently, if the patient's hemoglobin value is available, both the uncorrected $D_{L_{CO}}$ and Hb-corrected $D_{L_{CO}}$ values are reported. The formula for adjusting the $D_{L_{CO}}$ for anemia is

$D_{L_{CO}}$ (Hb-corrected)
$$= (10.22 + Hb) \, D_{L_{CO}} \text{ measured}/1.7 \, Hb$$

The $D_{L_{CO}}$ normally declines with aging in adults. The lower limit of the normal range is about 80% of the mean predicted value, but is more accurately defined by the 95% confidence interval.

INTERPRETATION

The $D_{L_{CO}}$ is diminished in patients with interstitial lung diseases, emphysema, pulmonary vascular diseases, and anemia. The reduced $D_{L_{CO}}$ of emphysema is due to loss of alveolar-capillary membrane area (permanent destruction of lung tissue). A declining $D_{L_{CO}}$ in a patient with sarcoidosis or interstitial pneumonitis–fibrosis suggests a poor response to the therapy initiated (usually corticosteroids). The $D_{L_{CO}}$ is a very sensitive test for early interstitial lung disease. It is often reduced in pulmonary sarcoidosis, vasculitis, scleroderma, and *Pneumocystis* pneumonia, when the chest x-ray, lung volumes, and resting arterial blood gas values are still within normal limits.

An increase in the $D_{L_{CO}}$ above 120% predicted may occur in asthma (for unknown reasons), polycythemia (because of the increased number of red cells in the lungs), during or immediately following exercise, and in patients with left-to-right cardiovascular shunts.

EXERCISE TESTING

INDICATIONS

Cardiopulmonary exercise testing was previously confined to research laboratories, but is now clinically useful for the following:

- To measure a person's ability to perform work (disability evaluation)
- To measure cardiovascular fitness for vigorous sports (maximal oxygen uptake)
- To help differentiate between cardiac and pulmonary causes of dyspnea
- To determine the need for and dose of ambulatory oxygen
- To assist in developing a safe exercise prescription for patients with cardiovascular or pulmonary disease
- For predicting the morbidity of lung resection

Contraindications include recent heart attack, severe hypertension, aortic stenosis, or worsening angina.

EQUIPMENT

The minimum equipment necessary includes a treadmill with 0–5 mph and 0–20% grade adjustments (or a calibrated bicycle ergometer), ECG monitor, and pulse oximeter. For noninvasive oxygen uptake measurement add a low-resistance breathing valve, mixing chamber, pneumotach, and oxygen analyzer (Fig. 9–17). Complete breath-by-breath computerized systems add fast-responding O_2 and CO_2 gas analyzers and cost more than 50,000 dollars. Cardiac output may be estimated using a CO_2 rebreathing or acetylene method. Invasive studies may add radial artery cannulation for blood gas and lactate measurements or right heart catheterization with monitoring of PA and wedge pressures.

The technician should have CPR certification and a resuscitation cart with a defibrillator; oxygen must be in the room, and a physician should normally be present to monitor the ECG for signs of ischemia (ST segment depression) or malignant arrhythmias (which are more likely to occur during the recovery period). A 12-lead ECG system is best for detecting ischemia.

PROCEDURE

Attach the ECG electrodes securely, calculate the predicted maximal heart rate (HR) for the patient (220 minus age), adjust the cycle seat height (for a cycle ergometer), then instruct him or her that maximum effort is required for a valid test. Monitor the HR, blood pressure (BP), oxygen saturation (Sp_{O_2}), and ventilation ($\dot{V}e$) during an initial 3- to 5-minute resting period. Start the workload at a level judged to be easy for the patient (1.7 mph at 0 grade or 50

Figure 9—17. Exercise-testing equipment. The speed and grade of the treadmill control the workload. The ECG is monitored for arrhythmias and heart rate (HR). Oxygen saturation may be monitored noninvasively with a pulse oximeter. The patient inhales room air through a low-resistance breathing valve. Exhaled air is mixed and then sampled for oxygen and carbon dioxide concentrations. A pneumotach measures exhaled airflow and the signal is integrated to give minute ventilation ($\dot{V}e$). Alternately, a bicycle ergometer may replace the treadmill, a radial artery cannula may be placed to measure arterial blood gas and lactate levels, and a mass spectrometer may replace the individual gas analyzers.

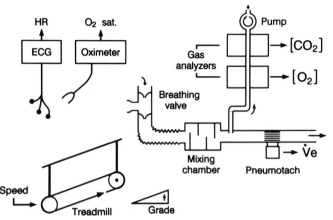

watts) and then increase it at 1- to 3-minute intervals, measuring HR, BP, Sp_{O_2}, and $\dot{V}e$ at the end of each interval. Return the workload back to the lightest level for a "cooldown" period only when the patient is exhausted, has chest pain suggesting angina, or develops serious arrhythmias. Record the symptoms that limited further exercise and continue monitoring for 5 minutes.

QUALITY CONTROL

Before each test, check the pneumotach for 3% accuracy at high- and low-flow rates using a 3.00-L syringe. Gas analyzers must also be calibrated to within 0.1% accuracy before each test, using at least two calibrated reference gases. The delay times of gas analyzer outputs in breath-by-breath computerized systems can be a major source of error and should be remeasured periodically and whenever tubing changes are made.

Perform a biologic control by testing a laboratory technician each week or month, depending on test volume. Collect exhaled gas in large Douglas bags during 1-minute intervals at high and low workloads. The volume and gas concentrations in the bags must then be checked with a large-volume spirometer (Tissot) and mass spectrometer or gas chromatograph, respectively, and compared with results from the pneumotach and gas analyzers. Keep a log of the results at each workload—the intraindividual variability of $\dot{V}e$ and $\dot{V}o_2$max measurements should be less than 10%.

Every 2 months check the indicated treadmill speed for 1% accuracy by measuring the length of the belt and counting the number of cycles per minute, using a stopwatch at two different speeds. Also check the indicated grade for 1% accuracy. Ask hospital safety engineers to check the electrical leakage current of the instruments at least yearly.

CALCULATIONS

The best overall indicator of cardiopulmonary health and physical fitness is the maximum oxygen uptake ($\dot{V}o_2$max), which is usually normalized for body weight in kilograms (mL/kg/min). Predicted $\dot{V}o_2$max and other exercise variables should be calculated from data from a large study.[18] The $\dot{V}o_2$max is about 30–45 mL/kg/min in sedentary persons, whereas athletes may achieve an oxygen consumption of over 80 mL/kg/min. The $\dot{V}o_2$max from a bicycle ergometer is about 90% of that achieved by the same person on a treadmill. In some patients with cardiac disease, it may be risky to perform "maximal" exercise; thus, various submaximal exercise test regimens, including measurement of the anaerobic threshold (the $\dot{V}o_2$ at which blood lactate increases) have been developed.

The O_2 pulse ($\dot{V}o_2$/HR) at maximum exercise should be greater than 8 mL O_2/beat in women and 12 in men. Maximum ventilation ($\dot{V}e$) achieved should be about 60% of the previously measured MVV. (If the MVV is less than 40 times the FEV_1, poor MVV effort should be suspected.) The ratio of dead space to tidal volume (V_D/V_T) should be less than 0.25 during exercise (this calculation requires arterial blood gas measurements). The anaerobic threshold should normally be reached at or above a $\dot{V}o_2$ of 40% of the predicted $\dot{V}o_2$max.

INTERPRETATION

Maximal effort probably has been obtained if any of the following occurs at the end of exercise:

$\dot{H}R > 90\%$ predicted max
$\dot{V}e_{max} \geq 80\%$ of MVV
$\dot{V}o_2max \geq 85\%$ predicted
Blood lactate > 8 mM

The test result is considered normal if the patient achieves an oxygen consumption ($\dot{V}o_2max$) of 85% or more of predicted[18] (Table 9–8). The most common cause of low oxygen consumption is deconditioning, indicated by normal ventilation, normal oxygen saturation, and a normal to low O_2 pulse response to exercise. Cardiovascular diseases generally cause a high heart rate for a given workload, a low O_2 pulse, and sometimes angina or abnormal ECG findings. A cardiovascular limitation to exercise should also be suspected if the anaerobic threshold is reached at a lower oxygen consumption than expected.

Exercise limitation caused by moderate COPD or restriction is accompanied by a high minute ventilation relative to workload, which quickly approaches the resting MVV, and oxygen desaturation, while the ECG and HR respond normally. Pulmonary vascular diseases (such as primary pulmonary hypertension) are noted for an increased V_D/V_T at rest that does not fall with exercise, and considerable oxygen desaturation.

LUNG COMPLIANCE

INDICATIONS

Lung compliance testing measures the elastic recoil or stiffness of the lungs. It is more invasive than other PF tests because the patient must swallow an esophageal balloon. Lung compliance is usually measured only when other PF tests give equivocal results or require confirmation by additional data.

EQUIPMENT

Lung compliance studies are often performed in a body box because the necessary mouth shutter, pneumotach, and 60-cmH_2O range pressure transducer are already available; only an esophageal balloon needs to be added. However, lung compliance can be measured without a body box.

PROCEDURE

Lung compliance is normally measured under static conditions (no airflow) as the change in volume produced by a unit change in pressure: $C = \Delta V/\Delta P$. Prepare the esophageal balloon, mark the position 50 cm from the tip and fill it with 0.5 mL of air. Give the patient a glass of water. Dip the balloon in 4% lidocaine jelly and gently guide it straight backward through the more patent nostril. When it reaches the back of the throat, tell the patient to quickly drink the water as you advance the catheter. The balloon will usually be swallowed down the esophagus. Advance it to the 50-cm mark and have the patient breathe to and from the spirometer or pneumotach as you watch the volume and pressure changes. Withdraw the balloon 10 cm if the pressure is positive during inspiration, indicating that it is in the stomach. Tape the catheter to the nose when it is correctly positioned.

Ask the patient to inhale to TLC and then close the shutter for 3 seconds several times as he slowly exhales. He or she should relax each time you close the shutter. Repeat this procedure two or three more times.

To measure *static lung compliance* in mechanically ventilated patients, apply an inspiratory hold after the tidal volume has been delivered, either by using a prolonged inspiratory plateau or by occluding the exhalation port. Note the mouth pressure obtained and the tidal volume. Repeat the procedure twice and report the average values.

Table 9–8 Exercise Response Interpretation

	DECONDITIONING	CARDIAC	COPD	FIBROSIS	PULMONARY–VASCULAR
$\dot{V}o_2max$	Low	Low	Low	Low	Low
HR/workload	High	High			High
MVV–$\dot{V}e_{max}$	High	High	Low	Low	
O_2sat			Low	Low	++Low
O_2 pulse	Low				Low
V_D/V_T			High	High	++High

QUALITY CONTROL

Before each test, calibrate the spirometer with a 3.00-L syringe for 3% accuracy and the pressure transducer with a U-tube manometer at 50 cm H_2O for 5% accuracy. Check the balloon for patency and leaks. Check the mouthpiece and shutter assembly to be sure it does not leak when the shutter is closed. Ignore any occlusions when the volume changed or the pressure did not remain constant.

CALCULATIONS

Two components contribute to overall compliance of the respiratory system (C_{RS}): the lung itself (C_L) and the chest wall (C_W). Pressure–volume (PV) curves can be made by measuring the pressure developed at many lung volumes. The driving pressure (Prs) equals alveolar pressure (Palv) minus atmospheric pressure or pressure at the body surface (Pbs): Prs = Palv − Pbs. The pressure used to develop the PV curve of the lung itself is the transpulmonary pressure (i.e., alveolar pressure minus pleural pressure): P_L = Palv − Ppl. In developing the chest wall PV curve, the pressure across the chest wall is used (i.e., atmospheric pressure minus pleural pressure): Pw = Pbs − Ppl. Alveolar pressure is equivalent to pressure at the mouth when there is no airflow (Palv = Pm).

Compliance is often reported as a single value from that portion of the PV curve 1 L above end-tidal volume, but you should plot all of the pressure and volume pairs from each valid occlusion and draw a line between them. The normal static compliance for the lung and the chest wall systems is the same (i.e., 0.2 L/cm H_2O). The compliances of the total respiratory system, lung, and chest wall are related in a reciprocal fashion: $1/C_{RS} = 1/C_L + 1/C_W$. Normal C_{RS} = 0.1 L/cm H_2O.

Compliance is related directly to lung volume and, thus, is meaningless unless related to the patient's lung volume. For example, the compliance of a newborn lung is almost the same as the compliance of an adult lung when expressed as liters per cm H_2O per liter of lung volume. When the difference in lung volume is not taken into account, the neonate's lung compliance is about 0.006 L/cm H_2O, whereas the adult's lung compliance is about 0.2 L/cm H_2O. Therefore, it is helpful to divide lung compliance (C_L) by the lung volume at which the measurement is made (V_L), to give a parameter known as *specific compliance*.

Compliances of the chest wall and total respiratory system are not routinely measured because they are affected by skeletal muscle contraction. Therefore, unless the muscles are totally relaxed, the measurements are invalid. Lung compliance, on the other hand, can be determined readily, even if the subject is not relaxed.

For patients requiring mechanical ventilation in an intensive care unit, it is often valuable to follow an estimate of lung stiffness known as *effective compliance*. The usual way of determining this measurement is to divide the tidal volume delivered by the peak inspiratory pressure required to deliver the volume. It is often mistakenly assumed that "compliance," when determined this way, is a reliable indicator of lung stiffness. However, the peak pressure required to deliver the tidal volume is influenced by factors in addition to lung compliance: airway resistance and chest wall compliance. Also the peak pressure increases, without any change in airway diameter or respiratory system stiffness, if the tidal volume or the inspiratory flow rate is increased. Therefore, since this parameter is not solely an estimate of lung compliance, it is more accurately known as *effective compliance, dynamic*.

If one applies an inspiratory hold after the tidal volume has been delivered to mechanically ventilated patients, either by using a prolonged inspiratory plateau or by occluding the exhalation line, one can obtain a measurement of the "static" pressure required to hold the lung at this inspired tidal volume point. By dividing the tidal volume by this new static pressure, you obtain a value known as *effective compliance, static*. This allows accurate determination of respiratory system compliance changes, because airway resistance is now eliminated as a factor.

INTERPRETATION

An abnormally high lung compliance in a patient with obstructive pulmonary disease indicates the presence of anatomic emphysema, which destroys lung tissue, making the lungs easy to distend. Lung compliance is normal in chronic bronchitis and bronchial asthma. Reduced lung compliance suggests the presence of interstitial or alveolar filling lung disease, which makes the lungs stiffer (Fig. 9–18).

Chest wall compliance (C_W) may be decreased in patients who have kyphoscoliosis, ankylosing spondylitis, prominent obesity, severe pectus excavatum, and neuromuscular disorders associated with spasticity of the muscles. A reduced compliance of the lung or chest wall results in increased

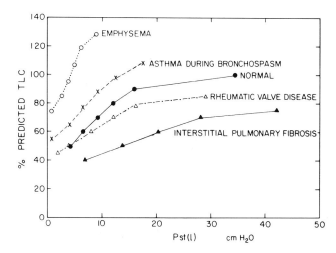

Figure 9—18. Pressure–volume curves for the lungs. The pressure is measured by an esophageal balloon when a shutter is closed at different lung volumes. The change in lung volume on the vertical axis is measured by a spirometer. Examples include a normal curve, a curve demonstrating the increased compliance of emphysema, and curves showing reduced compliance as seen with interstitial and alveolar lung disease. (Bates DV, Macklem PT, Christie RV: Respiratory Function in Disease, 2nd ed. Philadelphia, WB Saunders, 1971)

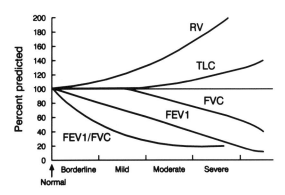

Figure 9—19. Changes in pulmonary function parameters as the degree of airways obstruction worsens from borderline to very severe. The FEV_1/FVC ratio becomes abnormal first (is most sensitive). Note the linear decline in FEV_1. As the patient becomes short of breath with moderate obstruction, the FVC decreases and the TLC increases (with emphysema) as progressive air trapping occurs. (© Mayo Foundation)

work of breathing because the pressure required to produce a volume change is increased.

In mechanically ventilated patients, changes in respiratory system stiffness are usually the result of pulmonary edema or pneumonitis but may also be due to factors other than lung compliance, such as changes in chest wall compliance secondary to muscle spasm or abdominal distention.

CONTROL OF BREATHING

Factors that stimulate the ventilatory drive and, thereby, control breathing include hypoxemia, hypercapnia, and acidosis. Some patients partially or completely lose the ability to respond to these ventilatory stimuli. The response to these factors can be measured in a few laboratories.[5,15]

PATTERNS OF IMPAIRMENT

OBSTRUCTIVE PATTERN

Refer to Figure 9–19 for a diagram of how pulmonary function parameters change as an obstructive airways disease progresses over time, from mild to severe. During the asymptomatic early stages, the

FEV_1/FVC ratio becomes abnormal first, followed by a linear decline in the FEV_1. As the patient becomes symptomatic with moderate obstruction, air-trapping causes an increase in the RV and a decrease in the FVC. In the late stages of emphysema, the TLC increases (hyperinflation) because of further air-trapping. If the obstruction is due to emphysema, the $D_{L_{CO}}$ will decrease. Refer to Table 9–9 for patterns of pulmonary function abnormality.

RESTRICTIVE PATTERN

All lung volumes are reduced in restrictive disorders. Expiratory flow rates that are more reduced than the reduction in VC suggest the presence of concomitant obstructive airway disease. Although the FEV_1 and FVC are reduced, the FEV_1/FVC ratio is normal or increased in pure restrictive disease. This helps to differentiate the reduced FEV_1 of obstructive disease from that of restrictive disease. The RV/TLC ratio is usually normal in pure restrictive disease.

COMBINED OBSTRUCTIVE AND RESTRICTIVE PATTERN

Patients occasionally have more than one disorder, which may result in a combined obstructive and restrictive pulmonary function abnormality. Examples include emphysema (obstructive) with mild congestive heart failure (restrictive), or tracheal stenosis (obstructive) with obesity (restrictive). The

Table 9–9 Patterns of Pulmonary Function Abnormality

	NORMAL	OBSTRUCTION	RESTRICTION	MIXED
FEV_1/FVC	≥90% predicted	Low	Normal to high	Low
FEV_1	≥80% predicted	Low	Low	Low
FVC	≥80% predicted	Normal to low	Low	Low
TLC	80%–120% predicted	Normal to high	Low	Normal to low
RV/TLC	25%–40%	High	Normal	High

VC is reduced in combined obstructive and restrictive disease. The flow rates are reduced disproportionately to the reduction in VC, reducing the FEV_1/FVC ratio.

A common error is to assume that a reduced FVC indicates the presence of restrictive pulmonary disease. The FVC (and slow VC) may be reduced solely because of air-trapping from obstructive airway disease. To be certain that restrictive disease is present, in association with a reduced VC and reduced FEV_1/FVC ratio, one should demonstrate that a reduced TLC is present. Serial changes in the TLC might be helpful. For instance, the TLC in a patient with emphysema may change from above normal to normal as a concomitant restrictive process is developing. The RV/TLC ratio will be increased in the presence of combined obstructive and restrictive disease.

Refer to Figure 9–20 for an efficient method of evaluating pulmonary function. This method starts with simple screening spirometry; other, more expensive tests are added depending on the spirometry results.

REFERENCES

1. Camilli AE, Burrows B, Knudson RJ, Lyle SK, Lebowitz MD: Longitudinal changes in FEV_1 in adults. Effects of smoking and smoking cessation. Am Rev Respir Dis 135:794–799, 1987
2. Nelson SB, Gardner RM, Crapo RO, Jensen RL: Performance evaluation of contemporary spirometers. Chest 97:288–297, 1990
3. American Thoracic Society Statement: Standardization of spirometry—1987 update. Am Rev Respir Dis 136:1285, 1987
4. Enright PL, Hyatt RE: Office Spirometry. A Practical Guide to the Selection and Use of Spirometers. Philadelphia, Lea & Febiger, 1987
5. Miller A: Pulmonary Function Tests in Clinical and Occupational Lung Disease. Orlando, Grune & Stratton, 1986
6. Crapo RO, Morris AH, Gardner RM: Reference spirometric values using techniques and equipment that meet ATS recommendations. Am Rev Respir Dis 123:659, 1981
7. Knudson RJ, Lebowitz MD, Holberg CJ, Burrows B: Changes in the normal expiratory flow–volume curve with growth and aging. Am Rev Respir Dis 127:725, 1983
8. American Thoracic Society Statement: Evaluation of

Figure 9–20. Flow chart for efficient evaluation of pulmonary function. Start with spirometry. Obstruction is probably due to asthma if the FEV_1 increases to near normal (following bronchodilator inhalation), and is probably due to emphysema if the diffusing capacity (D_{LCO}) is low. If spirometry is normal in a patient with symptoms suggesting asthma, a positive methacholine challenge supports a diagnosis of asthma. Restriction is probably due to an interstitial lung disease if the D_{LCO} is low. (© Mayo Foundation)

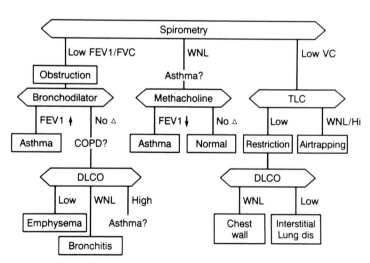

impairment/disability secondary to respiratory disorders. Am Rev Respir Dis 133: 1205, 1986

9. Disability Evaluation under Social Security, a Handbook for Physicians. Washington, DC, HEW Publication No SSA 79-10089, 1979

10. Chatham M, Bleecker ER, Norman P, Smith PL, Mason P: A screening test for airways reactivity. Chest 82:15, 1982

11. Dockery DW, Speizer FE, Ferris BG et al: Cumulative and reversible effects of lifetime smoking on simple tests of lung function in adults. Am Rev Respir Dis 137:286–292, 1988

12. Lorber DB, Kaltenborn W, Burrows B: Responses to isoproterenol in a general population sample. Am Rev Respir Dis 118:855–856, 1978

13. Acres JC, Kryger MH: Clinical significance of pulmonary function tests: Upper airway obstruction. Chest 80:207–211, 1981

14. Black LF, Hyatt RE: Maximal respiratory pressures: Normal values and relationship to age and sex. Am Rev Respir Dis 99:696–702, 1969

15. Clausen JL: Pulmonary Function Testing Guidelines and Controversies. New York, Academic Press, 1982

16. American Thoracic Society Statement: Single breath carbon monoxide diffusing capacity (transfer factor), recommendations for a standard technique. Am Rev Respir Dis 136:1299, 1987

17. Hansen JE, Sue DY, Wasserman K: Predicted values for clinical exercise testing. Am Rev Respir Dis 129:S49–S58, 1984

18. Wasserman K, Hansen JE, Sue DY, Whipp BJ: Principles of Exercise Testing and Interpretation. Philadelphia, Lea & Febiger, 1987

BIBLIOGRAPHY

Two recent journals have devoted entire issues to the field of pulmonary function testing. They are highly recommended as representative of state-of-the-art thinking on the topics considered in this chapter.

Journal Conference, St Petersburg, Florida: Pulmonary function testing. Respir Care 34:647 pp, 1989

Mabler DA (ed): Pulmonary function testing. Clin Chest Med 10(2):129, 1989

TEN

Blood Gas Analysis and Acid–Base Physiology

James A. Peters
John E. Hodgkin
Clarence R. Collier

The evaluation of oxygenation and acid–base status in critically ill patients is crucial to proper management. An arterial blood gas (ABG) is used to measure or assess (1) oxygenation, (2) ventilation, and (3) acid–base status. Normally, the body regulates these different parameters automatically, but when patients are severely ill with respiratory or kidney disorders, acid–base regulation becomes compromised. This necessitates greater intervention by the medical team. However, with more intervention comes the need for accurate feedback, so that one can know if the therapeutic maneuvers were sufficient to correct for ventilation, oxygenation, or acid–base abnormalities. An ABG provides this physiologic feedback. In some cases, noninvasive transcutaneous oxygen ($PtcO_2$) monitoring may be all that is needed; however, at present, this monitoring does not provide all the needed information for most clinical situations.

Arterial blood is most frequently used for analysis because it comes directly from the lung and heart organs and, therefore, is representative of how well the lungs exchanged respiratory gases. Analysis of oxygen (O_2) and carbon dioxide (CO_2) levels in peripheral *venous* blood can be quite misleading, reflecting as it does the metabolic activity of the limb from which the blood was obtained. Peripheral venous blood analysis will not reflect the acid–base status of the rest of the body. Additionally, one would have to guess how well the lungs were blowing off CO_2 because one would not

know if a high CO_2 level was generated by the tissues from which the blood was drawn, or if it was already high when it arrived there in the arterial blood. In short, it is impossible to properly manage critically ill patients without using ABG data.

The proper technique for performing arterial punctures can be easily learned by respiratory therapists and nurses; hence, physicians need not be available to obtain samples. Proper maintenance of blood gas equipment, with accurate calibration and performance of quality control, is essential to assure valid results. The newer blood gas machines have improved the accuracy and reliability of measurements with their automated calibration and internal controls.

ARTERIAL PUNCTURE

Arterial blood samples may be drawn from multiple sites. Samples are most commonly obtained from the radial artery, brachial artery, or femoral artery. It is important to consider the availability of collateral circulation when selecting a site for arterial puncture. Both the radial and brachial arteries normally have excellent collateral blood flow; however, there is a marked lack of collateral flow if the femoral artery becomes obstructed in the area just below the inguinal ligament. Because radial artery puncture is relatively safe, and the site easily accessible as well as convenient for checking collateral circulation, this site is preferable.

A modified Allen test is used to assess for adequacy of collateral circulation.[1,2] After the patient has made a fist to force blood from the hand, pressure is applied to compress both the ulnar and radial arteries. When the hand is relaxed, the palm and fingers are blanched. Obstructing pressure is then removed from the ulnar artery while the radial artery remains compressed. If the ulnar artery is patent, the hand should quickly become flushed within 10 to 15 seconds. If this does not occur, radial artery puncture should be avoided in that wrist. Once adequate collateral circulation has been demonstrated, the patient is prepared for puncture of the radial artery.

It is recommended that the person performing the arterial puncture sit in a chair at the patient's bedside. At times, what appears to be an "easy stick" turns out to be more challenging than anticipated. If one is standing and bending over while "chasing" an elusive artery, fatigue sets in quickly and is soon followed by slips in proper technique. The patient's arm should be positioned comfortably, using a rolled or folded towel to hyperextend the radial or brachial site. The anticipated puncture site should be carefully palpated to determine the position and course of the artery. The skin surface should then be cleansed thoroughly with 70% isopropyl alcohol before the arterial puncture.

The use of a local anesthetic is usually recommended because it can help relieve apprehension (of both patient and therapist), minimize hyperventilation, improve compliance with subsequent punctures, and is believed to be helpful in reducing the likelihood of arterial vasospasm. With a disposable 3-mL syringe or a 1-mL insulin syringe and a 25-gauge, ⅝-in needle, 0.25 mL to 1.0 mL of 2% lidocaine (Xylocaine) (*without* epinephrine) can be injected subcutaneously above the artery and then into deeper tissues around the artery to achieve anesthesia, provided the patient gives no history of allergy to local anesthesia. One should wait for 2 or 3 minutes after injecting the lidocaine before beginning the arterial puncture to allow for the full anesthetic effect to take place. The effect begins to wear off in about 15 or 20 minutes.

The ABG syringe can be of a plastic material or glass. Previously, the plastic syringes were more permeable to gas diffusion and therefore were avoided. Now, prepackaged ABG puncture kits use preheparinized (1000 unit/mL) plastic syringes, which have proved to be very satisfactory[3] and have the added benefit of being disposable. Although the older glass syringes were easy to use, they required more care for cleaning, reassembling, and lubricating with heparin and had the possibility of breakage. A 21-gauge, 1-inch short-bevel needle is most commonly used. The heparin in the syringe is swirled around and the excess expelled. Excess heparin in the syringe can raise the PO_2 of the blood drawn into the syringe, as heparin has a PO_2 of about 150 mmHg (at sea level) which will mix with the sampled blood. To further minimize this error, an adequate amount of blood should be obtained, such that the heparin/blood ratio is negligible. Some ABG syringe manufacturers have tried to minimize this even more by using dried heparin to coat the inside of the syringe.

When palpating the position of the artery, use the fingers of the opposite hand (e.g., the left hand to palpate the right radial artery). The syringe, with the needle bevel facing cephalad and being held like a pencil, is directed through the skin toward the artery at approximately a 45° angle. Advancement should be slow. if the needle is advanced too rapidly, it may pass through the artery without blood being obtained. On occasion, it is only while slowly *withdrawing* the needle that blood begins to enter the syringe. Repositioning of the needle may be necessary because the artery often rolls to one side or the other during the procedure. Gently palpating for the artery with the opposite hand while the needle is inserted into the tissue helps one determine where the needle might need to be positioned next. Sometimes, palpating too firmly (although you may not think you are) occludes the artery enough that blood does not flow into the syringe, even though the artery has been penetrated. *Never* reposition the needle until after bringing the tip back up to the subcutaneous tissue, to avoid severing vessels or tendons with the sharp needle.

When the needle enters the artery, blood will readily fill the syringe without aspirating because arterial blood is normally under high pressure. With the needle in the artery, a pulsation should be visualized. If no pulsation is present, one should suspect that the needle is in a vein rather than in an artery. It is recommended that during the ABG procedure, the hand holding the syringe should be rested against the patient's wrist (if drawing a radial sample). This makes the practitioner's hand steadier and also will prevent the patient from jerking his or her hand back if a sensitive area is hit.

About 3 mL of blood should be obtained. This allows for expelling bubbles from the sample, for repeating the analysis to double-check a reading, and provides an adequate heparin/blood ratio.

When the needle is withdrawn, a folded 4 × 4-in gauze should be placed over the site and *firm* pressure applied for a minimum of 5 minutes—longer if the patient is anticoagulated or has a bleeding disorder. This is a most important part of the procedure. If any bleeding occurs at the end of this time, pressure should be maintained until no further bleeding occurs. A protective gauze strip can be placed over the folded 4×4 pad and around the wrist, and an elastic bandage then placed *partly* around the wrist to continue pressure on the puncture site. Placing the elastic bandage all the way around the wrist would cause it to act like a tourniquet, which of course is undesirable. It is customary to leave this pressure dressing on for 2 hours. It is convenient to write on the dressing the time it can be removed so other hospital personnel will not remove it prematurely.

Arterial blood gas samples should be obtained anaerobically. Any air bubbles in the syringe should be expelled immediately from the sample. The sample should then be placed in a cup of crushed ice and delivered immediately to the blood gas laboratory for proper analysis. Because blood cells continue to live (and be metabolically active) after being drawn up into the syringe, warming of the specimen and a delay in analysis results in a lower PaO_2 and a higher $PaCO_2$ than at the time of sampling. Although it is preferable to analyze the sample immediately, it is acceptable to delay analysis up to 2 hours if the sample is iced immediately after drawing.

It is strongly recommended that practitioners drawing blood wear latex gloves to minimize the risk of exposure to blood. Needles should never be recapped or covered with two hands because the risk of puncturing oneself is high. Using only one hand or specially designed needle-recapping devices should be standard practice.

MEASUREMENTS OF OXYGENATION

Numerous factors can be evaluated to determine whether tissue oxygenation is adequate. Each of these measurements yields information helpful in managing the patient properly. A thorough understanding of the significance of each of these factors, as well as a knowledge of their limitations, is critical.

OXYGEN TENSION

The partial pressure of oxygen, created by the random collision of molecules of the gas, may be read-ily measured. This tension may be measured in inspired gas (PiO_2), arterial blood (PaO_2), venous blood (PvO_2), and capillary blood (PcO_2). Formulas for calculating PiO_2 are as follows:

1. Dry gas formula:

$$PiO_2 = PB \times FiO_2$$

where PB = barometric pressure and FiO_2 = the fractional concentration of inspired oxygen. At sea level, with an FiO_2 of 0.2093 (approximately 21% oxygen) the PiO_2 for room air would be

$$PiO_2 = 760 \text{ mmHg} \times 0.21 = 159 \text{ mmHg}.$$

2. Humidified gas formula:

$$PiO_2 = (PB - \text{water vapor pressure}) \times FiO_2$$

For room air at sea level:

$$PiO_2 = (760 \text{ mmHg} - 47 \text{ mmHg}) \\ \times 0.21 = 149 \text{ mmHg}$$

in humidified room air with a normal water vapor pressure.

The PaO_2 is a measure of the partial pressure of oxygen dissolved in the plasma of arterial blood and is usually reported in millimeters mercury (mmHg).* Torr is equivalent to millimeters of mercury (mmHg) and has been used by some in honor of Torricelli, the inventor of the barometer. The amount of gas (O_2) dissolved in the blood is directly proportional to the partial pressure of the gas above the fluid (Henry's law) and the gas's solubility. The solubility coefficient of O_2 in plasma is quite low (0.00003 mL O_2/mL plasma/mmHg); therefore, the actual amount of O_2 dissolved or carried in the plasma is very small and is not sufficient to support life without the presence of hemoglobin. However, the PaO_2 is the most important determinant of the amount of oxygen that binds to hemoglobin.

The *alveolar oxygen tension* (PAO_2) may be calculated from the alveolar air equation as follows:

$$PAO_2 = PiO_2 - \frac{PACO_2}{R} \\ + \left[PACO_2 \times FiO_2 \times \frac{1 - R}{R} \right]$$

This is valid if there is no carbon dioxide in the inspired gas. R is the respiratory exchange ratio and

* To convert pressure from mmHg to kilopascals (kPa), use the following formula: $PkPa = P \text{ mmHg} \times 0.1333$.

represents the ratio of CO_2 production to O_2 uptake. (This is equivalent to the respiratory quotient, RQ, when in a steady-state.) Since the term in square brackets is a small correction factor (2 mmHg, when $FIO_2 = 0.2093$, $PACO_2 = 40$ mmHg, and $R = 0.8$) and $PACO_2$ is assumed to be equivalent to $PaCO_2$, many reduce the formula to the following:

$$PAO_2 = PIO_2 - \frac{PaCO_2}{R}$$

If $R = 0.8$, then this becomes

$$PAO_2 = PIO_2 - PaCO_2 \times 1.25$$

The factor 1.25 (1/0.8) changes slightly with changes in FIO_2. Some present the alveolar air equation as follows (assuming $PACO_2$ is equal to $PaCO_2$):

$$PAO_2 = PIO_2 - PaCO_2 \times \left[\frac{1}{R} - FIO_2 + \frac{1-R}{R}\right]$$

This can be rewritten as

$$PAO_2 = PIO_2 - PaCO_2 \times \left[FIO_2 + \frac{1-FIO_2}{R}\right]$$

Assuming an R of 0.8, while the patient breathes room air, this equation simplifies to

$$PAO_2 = PIO_2 - PaCO_2 \times 1.20$$

The respiratory exchange ratio R, if not measured, is assumed to be 0.8 (assuming that carbon dioxide production $[\dot{V}CO_2]$ is 200 mL/min and O_2 uptake $[\dot{V}O_2]$ is 250 mL/min at rest, so $\dot{V}CO_2/\dot{V}O_2 = 200/250 = 0.8$). The R can range from about 0.7 with fat metabolism to 1.0 with carbohydrate metabolism and even higher in states of excess $\dot{V}CO_2$. However, when plugging different values into the alveolar air equation, it changes the actual PAO_2 very little. Therefore, under most clinical situations the simplified equation, which assumes an R of 0.8, will suffice. PIO_2 may be calculated from the foregoing gas formulas, and the $PaCO_2$ is a directly measured value.

Calculation of alveolar PO_2 allows one to determine the alveolar–arterial oxygen difference $[P(A-a)O_2]$. The PaO_2 "normally" decreases with age as a result of a worsening ventilation–perfusion mismatch.

The normal PaO_2 for a person breathing room air may be predicted with the following formulas:
Predicted PaO_2 (ages 14–84, supine)[4]

$$= 103.5 - (0.42 \times age) \pm 4.$$

This was the formula from Sorbini's data at 500-m

Table 10–1 Normal, Supine PaO_2, and $P(A-a)O_2$ Values (Sea Level)

AGE (yr)	PaO_2 (mmHg)	$P(A-a)O_2$ (mmHg)
20	96–104	< 5
30	92–100	< 9
40	88–96	< 13
50	84–92	< 17
60	79–87	< 22
70	76–83	< 26
80	71–79	< 30
90	66–74	< 35

elevation.[4] When the data are corrected for a barometric pressure of 760 mmHg, the formula for predicting the normal supine PaO_2 at sea level becomes:

$$= 109 - (0.43 \times age) \pm 4.$$

The predicted PaO_2, according to Mellemgaard[5] (ages 15–75, seated),

$$= 104.2 - (0.27 \times age) \pm 6$$

Table 10–1 gives examples of age-predicted PaO_2. Because the PaO_2 *decreases* with age, then the alveolar–arterial oxygen difference increases with age. It is invalid to assume that the standard normal PaO_2 is 80 to 100 mmHg and the normal $P(A-a)O_2$ is 10 to 15 mmHg, since these "normal" values do not take age into account. From the foregoing formulas, it should also be recognized that the PaO_2 is usually lower when the patient is supine than when upright.

It is sometimes useful to determine the a/A O_2 *ratio* (PaO_2/PAO_2).[6] Whereas the $P(A-a)O_2$ varies as the FIO_2 is changed, the a/A O_2 ratio remains relatively stable. One can, therefore, use the a/A O_2 ratio as an index to the status of lung function when the oxygen concentration being delivered to the patient is altered. The a/A O_2 ratio can also be used to predict what a new PaO_2 will be when the FIO_2 is changed or to help choose the FIO_2 needed to obtain a desired PaO_2. To determine new FIO_2:

New $FIO_2 =$
$$\frac{[\text{Desired } PaO_2/(PaO_2/PAO_2)] + (PaCO_2/R)}{(P_B - 47)}$$

OXYGEN SATURATION

Oxygen saturation is a measurement of the amount of oxygen bound to hemoglobin compared with hemoglobin's maximum capability for binding oxygen.

$$\% \ O_2 \ \text{saturation} =$$

$$\frac{mL \ O_2 \ \text{bound to hemoglobin} \times 100}{\text{maximum mL of } O_2 \ \text{hemoglobin is capable of binding}}$$

The O_2 saturation is expressed as a percentage, with normal commonly being listed as equal to or greater than 96%; however, normal oxygen saturation is decreased with aging because the normal PaO_2 decreases with age (see Table 10–1).

The characteristic relation between PO_2 and O_2 saturation is known as the *oxygen dissociation curve* (Fig. 10–1). This relationship is described by an **S**-shaped curve. At higher oxygen tensions the curve is relatively flat; at lower oxygen tensions the curve becomes quite steep (more vertical). This relationship is one of the most fundamental concepts of respiratory physiology. A clear understanding of these relationships enables one to make better use of transcutaneous oximetry. Table 10–2 provides a useful way of expressing the oxygen dissociation curve. From a review of Table 10–2, it can be seen that for a given pH range one can approximate the PaO_2 if the O_2 saturation is known, especially in the steep portion of the curve.

The flat part of the oxyhemoglobin dissociation curve is an advantage in the lung where, despite significant drops in alveolar oxygen tension, the hemoglobin in the pulmonary capillaries will still bind O_2, almost to full capacity. For example, the PAO_2, and thus the PaO_2, may drop significantly because of obstructive airway disease; however, unless the PaO_2 is below about 60 mmHg, the O_2 saturation in the blood that leaves the pulmonary capillary will be almost normal.

The steep portion of the curve is an advantage at the tissue level, where small decrements in PO_2 result in a rapid release of O_2 by hemoglobin, characterized by a rapidly decreasing O_2 saturation. In other words, as O_2 tension drops at the tissue site, the hemoglobin molecule readily releases it to make it available for tissue use. Thus, PaO_2 is a more sensitive indicator of mild hypoxemia than is O_2 saturation because the upper portion of the curve is relatively flat and the O_2 saturation will change only slightly at first while the PO_2 is decreasing.

It should be noted that O_2 saturation is *not* dependent upon how much hemoglobin is present. It depends only on how much O_2 is actually bound to hemoglobin compared with how much it could carry. Thus a patient who is very anemic can have a normal O_2 saturation but be experiencing tissue hypoxia. It is important, therefore, to include O_2 in the evaluation of body oxygenation (see discussion under O_2 Content).

P_{50} Measurement

Multiple factors may alter the position of the oxygen dissociation curve. As a general rule those factors that shift the curve to the *right* are an advantage to the patient, since a rightward shift reflects a *reduced* affinity of hemoglobin for oxygen, resulting in an increased release of oxygen to the tissues. A shift to the *left* indicates that hemoglobin's affinity for oxygen is *increased*, so that hemoglobin will less readily release oxygen to the tissues.

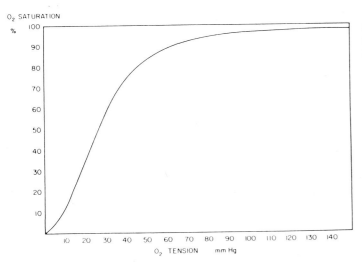

Figure 10–1. Oxyhemoglobin dissociation curve, showing relationships between PO_2 and O_2 saturation. (Bates DV, Macklem PT, Christie RV: Respiratory Function in Disease, 2nd ed. Philadelphia, WB Saunders, 1971)

Table 10—2   Tabular Form of Oxygen Dissociation Curve

pH	7.20	7.30	7.35	7.40	7.45	7.50
PO_2			O_2 Saturation			
10	10.2	11.7	12.4	13.3	14.3	15.4
20	26.9	31.1	33.2	35.5	38.1	40.9
30	46.4	52.4	55.1	58.0	61.0	64.1
40	63.1	68.9	71.4	73.9	76.3	78.8
44	68.5	73.9	76.1	78.4	80.6	82.7
48	73.0	78.0	80.0	82.0	83.9	85.8
52	76.9	81.4	83.2	84.9	86.6	88.2
56	80.2	84.2	85.8	87.3	88.8	90.2
60	82.9	86.5	87.9	89.3	90.6	91.8
64	85.2	88.4	89.7	90.9	82.0	93.0
68	87.2	90.0	91.1	92.2	93.1	94.0
72	88.8	91.4	92.3	93.2	94.1	94.9
76	90.2	92.5	93.3	94.1	94.9	95.6
80	91.4	93.4	94.2	94.9	95.5	96.1
90	93.7	95.2	95.7	96.3	96.8	97.2
100	95.2	96.4	96.8	97.2	97.6	97.9

The P_{50} measurement is a way of expressing the position of the oxygen dissociation curve and is defined as the PO_2 at 50% O_2 saturation, at a pH of 7.40, PCO_2 of 40 mmHg, and temperature of 37°C. Normally, the P_{50} is about 26.5 mmHg. An increased P_{50} (e.g., P_{50} of 30 mmHg) would indicate that the oxygen dissociation curve is shifted to the right (Fig. 10–2).

Factors known to shift the curve to the right include chronic hypoxemia, acidosis, hypercapnia, and fever. Alkalemia, hypocapnia, and hypothermia shift the curve to the left. Changes in pH, PCO_2, and temperature affect hemoglobin's affinity for oxygen but will not affect the P_{50} measurement if, as is standard practice, the P_{50} is determined with the blood at a normal pH, PCO_2, and temperature. Some do calculate the P_{50} at the patient's temperature, PCO_2, and pH that exist in the blood sample (in vivo P_{50}).

The importance of 2,3-diphosphoglycerate (2,3-DPG), a red-cell phosphate-containing molecule that is synthesized from the glycolytic pathway and affects hemoglobin's affinity for oxygen, is well recognized. If the level of 2,3-DPG increases in the red blood cell, hemoglobin's affinity for oxygen is decreased, thereby making more oxygen available to the tissue. This is a compensatory mechanism by which tissue oxygenation can be aided in the face of hypoxemia. Hypoxia results in an increased 2,3-DPG level in the red blood cell, thus increasing oxygen release from hemoglobin. This is one of the methods by which humans adapt to the hypoxia of high altitude or chronic disease. The 2,3-DPG molecule binds to the globin portion of the hemoglobin molecule, which results in a structural

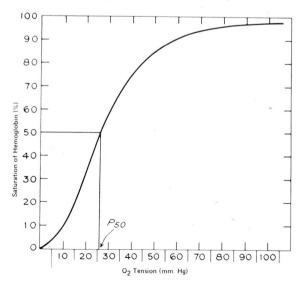

Figure 10—2. Oxyhemoglobin dissociation curve depicting the P_{50} (PO_2 at 50% O_2 saturation). The P_{50} is normally approximately 26.5 mmHg. (Comroe JH Jr: Physiology of Respiration. Chicago, Year Book Medical Publishers, 1974. Data of Severinghaus JW: J Appl Physiol 21:1108, 1966)

repositioning of the tertiary arrangement of the amino acids. This alters the ease with which oxygen can bind or be released from the iron-containing heme portion.[7]

Pyruvic kinase deficiency and thyrotoxicosis also result in an increased 2,3-DPG level. A decrease in 2,3-DPG levels, such as occurs in hexokinase deficiency and myxedema, results in a shift of the oxygen dissociation curve to the left (i.e., decreased P_{50}).

Blood preserved in acid citrate dextrose (ACD) loses most of its red cell 2,3-DPG within several days, whereas blood preserved in citrate phosphate dextrose (CPD) maintains its 2,3-DPG levels for weeks.[8] Thus, ACD-preserved blood more than several days old when transfused raises the hemoglobin level and oxygen-carrying capability; however, the hemoglobin in these red cells does not normally release oxygen to the tissues for the first 18 to 24 hours after infusion. Blood banks now generally use CPD rather than ACD for preserving blood.

Certain congenital hemoglobinopathies also result in a shift of the oxygen dissociation curve. For example, hemoglobin Kansas shifts the curve to the right, resulting in improved oxygen release to the tissues. On the other hand, hemoglobin Rainier shifts the curve to the left, resulting in impaired oxygen release. Patients with hemoglobins that shift the curve to the right may present with anemia, whereas patients with hemoglobins resulting in a decreased P_{50} may present with polycythemia. When carbon monoxide binds to hemoglobin (carboxyhemoglobin), the curve is also shifted to the left.

Fetal hemoglobin (hemoglobin F) results in a curve that is markedly shifted to the left. It helps the fetus to obtain more oxygen from the mother during intrauterine life. Normally, fetal hemoglobin rapidly disappears after birth; otherwise, oxygen release from hemoglobin to the tissues would be grossly impaired. Table 10–3 provides a list of factors that shift the oxygen dissociation curve.

The P_{50} can be calculated from blood gases from a single sample of blood, without tonometry, with results within 2 mmHg of standard P_{50} measurements when the O_2 saturation in the sample is between 20% and 90%.[9,10]

OXYGEN CONTENT

The oxygen content, although often not reported by the laboratory, is actually more important than the PaO_2 or oxygen saturation since it is a quantitative measure of the amount of oxygen present in the blood. It is reported as "mL of oxygen per 100 mL of whole blood" or as "volumes percent." There are two components to the oxygen content.

1. The amount of oxygen dissolved in plasma:

$$PO_2 \times 0.003 = \text{mL } O_2 \text{ dissolved}$$
$$\text{per 100 mL whole blood}$$

2. The amount of oxygen bound to hemoglobin:

$$\text{Hemoglobin g\% } \times 1.39^* \times O_2 \text{ saturation} =$$
$$\text{mL } O_2 \text{ bound to hemoglobin}$$

Calculation of the normal O_2 content for arterial blood with a PaO_2 of 100 mmHg, a hemoglobin of

---

* The factor 1.34 has been used for many years; however, studies using hemolyzed blood have suggested that 1.39 may be more valid.[11]

Table 10–3 Factors That Shift the Oxygen Dissociation Curve

TO THE LEFT	TO THE RIGHT
Alkalosis	Acidosis
Hypocapnia	Hypercapnia
↓ 2,3-DPG	Fever
Hexokinase deficiency	↑ 2,3-DPG
Myxedema	Pyruvic kinase deficiency
ACD-preserved bank blood	Thyrotoxicosis
Certain congenital	Hypoxia
hemoglobinopathies (e.g.,	Anemia
hemoglobin Rainier)	Certain congenital
Fetal hemoglobin	hemoglobinopathies (e.g.,
Carboxyhemoglobin	hemoglobin Kansas)

15 g% and an O_2 saturation of 98% would be as follows:

1. The amount of oxygen dissolved in the plasma:

$$100 \text{ mmHg } PO_2 \times 0.003 =$$
$$0.3 \text{ mL } O_2 \text{ per } 100 \text{ mL blood}$$

2. $15 \text{ g\%} \times 1.39 \times 0.98 = 20.4 \text{ mL } O_2$ bound to hemoglobin per 100 mL blood:

$$O_2 \text{ content} = 0.3 + 20.4 =$$
$$20.7 \text{ mL } O_2 \text{ per } 100 \text{ mL whole blood}$$

Normally the tissues, as a whole, extract only about 25% of the oxygen carried in the arterial blood. The normal venous oxygen content is about 15 mL of oxygen per 100 mL blood. One of the mechanisms by which tissues cope with hypoxemia or with increased oxygen demand is to increase the amount of oxygen extracted from the blood. However, some tissues have less capability for increasing extraction than others. The heart normally extracts 60% to 70% of the oxygen in the coronary arterial blood; therefore, it is more perfusion-dependent. The skeletal muscles extract about 40% of the oxygen available to them at rest, the brain 30%, and the kidneys 6%. During maximal exercise only about 25% of the oxygen content of arterial blood returns to the heart (i.e., mixed venous oxygen content is about 5 mL oxygen per 100 mL blood).

Figure 10–3 is a diagrammatic representation of the effect of shifts of the oxygen dissociation curve on oxygen content and the amount of oxygen available to the tissues. A reduced P_{50} results in an increased oxygen content in the venous blood, indicating that less oxygen has been released to the tissue.

Measurements of oxygen content are particularly important in the following conditions:

Anemia. An anemic patient may have a normal PaO_2 and O_2 saturation and be suffering from tissue hypoxia because of the reduced oxygen-carrying capacity resulting from severe anemia.

Carbon Monoxide Poisoning. Carbon monoxide binds to hemoglobin with an affinity 210 times greater than that of oxygen. In this situation the PaO_2 may be relatively normal, yet the patient suffers from tissue hypoxia because of the reduced O_2 saturation and O_2 content. If the O_2 saturation is calculated (with a "normal" oxygen dissociation curve) from a measured PaO_2, both the reported O_2 saturation and O_2 content values will be incorrect in a patient with carbon monoxide poisoning. As mentioned earlier, carboxyhemoglobin also results in a leftward shift of the oxygen dissociation curve, which further contributes to tissue hypoxia.

Methemoglobinemia and Sulfhemoglobinemia. Abnormal types of hemoglobin result in an inability of hemoglobin to bind oxygen. Again the PaO_2 may be relatively normal, and yet the patient will have substantial tissue hypoxia because of the reduced O_2 saturation and O_2 content. Here also, unless the O_2 saturation is measured directly, one will calculate a falsely high O_2 content.

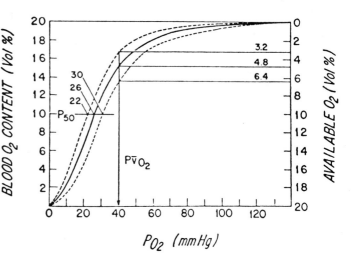

Figure 10–3. Effect of shifts of the O_2 dissociation curve on O_2 content and the amount of oxygen available to the tissues (assuming a $P\bar{v}O_2$ of 40 mmHg). The isopleths represent different P_{50} values, ranging from 22 to 30 mmHg. A reduced P_{50} is associated with an increased O_2 content in the venous blood, indicating that less oxygen has been released to the tissue (low A–V O_2 difference). (Snider GL: Clinical Interpretations of Blood Gases. Audiographic series, Vol 1. American College of Chest Physicians)

MIXED VENOUS PO_2 ($P\bar{v}O_2$)

Of equal importance to the O_2 content in terms of oxygen delivery to the tissues is the cardiac output.

O_2 delivery = arterial O_2 content × cardiac output

An arterial blood sample can provide data about the PaO_2, O_2 saturation, P_{50}, and O_2 content. It does not, however, provide information on cardiac output, effectiveness of tissue perfusion, and quantity of oxygen being extracted by the tissues.

The measurement of PO_2 in a blood sample taken from a central venous catheter or the pulmonary artery ($P\bar{v}O_2$) provides an indication of the adequacy of tissue oxygenation. At rest, the normal $P\bar{v}O_2$ is 35 to 40 mmHg. A value less then 35 mmHg in a critically ill patient suggests that oxygen extraction is increased and tissue oxygen delivery may be inadequate. One must then look at the multiple factors involved in oxygenation to determine the cause for the tissue hypoxia. An arterial–venous O_2 content difference greater than 5 vol% would similarly suggest that delivery of oxygen to the tissues may be inadequate. Unfortunately, the $P\bar{v}O_2$ may occasionally be normal in spite of serious tissue hypoxia (e.g., with septicemia). In septic patients, arteriovenous shunting occurs, so that blood bypasses tissues and less oxygen is extracted from the blood. If tissue metabolism is markedly reduced, as occurs in cyanide poisoning (which inhibits cytochrome oxidase of the respiratory transport chain), the difference between arterial and venous O_2 content and PO_2 narrows, even though severe cellular hypoxia is present. Measurement of the PO_2 from a peripheral venous sample may be misleading because it provides information relating only to the adequacy of oxygenation in the tissue being drained by that particular venous system. One must also be careful in interpreting the $P\bar{v}O_2$ because it mostly represents the blood returning from tissue with higher perfusion and does not adequately represent the oxygen extraction in tissues with low perfusion.

In patients with the adult respiratory distress syndrome (see Chap. 32), the implementation of positive end-expiratory pressure (PEEP) along with mechanical ventilation can be lifesaving; however, PEEP can occasionally reduce cardiac output. In such patients, the introduction of PEEP might result in actual worsening of tissue oxygen delivery. If the PaO_2 improves with the introduction of PEEP but the $P\bar{v}O_2$ decreases, worsening of tissue oxygenation has occurred, most likely as a result of reduced cardiac output. One of the techniques for determining the optimal level of PEEP is to select the amount of PEEP that results in the highest $P\bar{v}O_2$.[12] The $P\bar{v}O_2$ can also be very helpful in determining the amount of supplemental oxygen needed (i.e., the FiO_2 needed to provide satisfactory oxygenation of the tissues). One should remember that the $P\bar{v}O_2$ represents a sample of blood from all perfused organs of the body. Some organs may be hypoxic despite a normal $P\bar{v}O_2$.

CAUSES OF HYPOXEMIA

The measurement of PaO_2 is commonly used to determine whether hypoxia is present. However, hypoxemia properly refers to low O_2 concentration in the blood. Arterial O_2 content may be normal, despite a reduced PaO_2, if the hemoglobin is increased. On the other hand, the O_2 content may be significantly reduced from anemia despite a normal PaO_2. Hypoxemia and tissue hypoxia are not the same thing: tissue hypoxia may be present despite a normal arterial O_2 content.

Altitude

An obvious cause for reduced arterial oxygen tension is a decreased PiO_2. This most commonly results from living at high altitude. When patients with pulmonary disease are discharged from a hospital located at a low altitude (e.g., sea level) and return to their homes at a higher altitude (e.g., 5000-ft elevation), their arterial PO_2 may drop significantly. This must be kept in mind when determining whether supplemental oxygen will be needed for the patient at discharge. Furthermore, the PiO_2 in pressurized aircraft is equivalent to that found at approximately 5000- to 8000-ft elevation, and this must be taken into account should the patient plan to travel in airplanes. Table 10–4 is a brief reference table showing the relationship between altitude, barometric pressure, and PO_2. If one eliminates altitude there are basically four causes for hypoxemia: (1) overall hypoventilation, (2) ventilation–perfusion mismatch, (3) diffusion defect, and (4) shunt.

Overall Hypoventilation

The minute ventilation may be decreased as a result of a reduction in tidal volume, slowing of respiratory rate, or both. Alveolar ventilation drops as a result of the decreased minute ventilation, resulting in hypoxemia and, as will be explained later, hypercapnia (an elevated PCO_2). The differ-

Table 10—4 The Relationship Between Altitude and PO_2

ALTITUDE (ft)	BAROMETRIC PRESSURE (mmHg)	AMBIENT AIR PO_2 (mmHg)	ALVEOLAR PO_2 (mmHg)
Sea Level (0)	760	159	102
5,000	630	132	75
8,000	564	118	63
10,000	523	110	57
12,000	483	101	54
15,000	412	90	52
20,000	349	73	35
30,000	226	47	9

ential diagnosis of factors that produce hypoventilation includes respiratory center depression owing to drug overdose, effects of anesthesia during the early postoperative period, excessive postoperative analgesia, the pickwickian syndrome, thoracic deformities such as kyphoscoliosis and rheumatoid spondylitis, and neuromuscular disturbances.

Ventilation–Perfusion Mismatch

Ventilation–perfusion ($\dot{V}/\dot{Q}$) mismatch is the most common cause of hypoxemia. When units of lung are underventilated relative to their perfusion (low $\dot{V}/\dot{Q}$), the pulmonary capillary blood that leaves these units is underoxygenated, and hypoxemia results. Examples include bronchospasm, mucoid obstruction of the airway with resultant atelectasis, obstruction of airways associated with chronic bronchitis, emphysema, pneumonia, and pulmonary edema. High $\dot{V}/\dot{Q}$ units do not directly cause hypoxemia because the blood perfusing these units becomes well oxygenated.

Diffusion Defect

The alveolocapillary membrane may occasionally be thickened to the extent that diffusion is reduced enough to result in hypoxemia. This is unusual, however, because normally at rest the hemoglobin in the pulmonary capillary is fully saturated by the time the blood is one-third of the way past the alveolus. The alveolocapillary membrane can be widened substantially without resting hypoxemia occurring. In most interstitial lung diseases (e.g., sarcoidosis, pulmonary fibrosis, and interstitial pneumonitis), hypoxemia is due to $\dot{V}/\dot{Q}$ mismatch rather than to diffusion defect. Therefore, it is a misnomer to refer to these diseases as "alveolocapillary block syndrome."

Shunt

Anatomic (or congenital) right-to-left shunts, such as the tetralogy of Fallot and pulmonary ateriovenous fistulas, result in hypoxemia. Shunts that are correctable with proper respiratory care (commonly referred to as "physiologic shunts") also cause hypoxemia; for example, in lobar atelectasis resulting from a mucous plug obstruction, if the collapsed area of lung continues to be perfused, this functions as a shunt (i.e., the blood does not come in contact with normally ventilated alveoli).

With proper evaluation the cause of a patient's hypoxemia may be determined. The $P(A-a)O_2$ is normal in the presence of overall hypoventilation and high altitude and is increased in the other three causes of hypoxemia ($\dot{V}/\dot{Q}$ mismatch, diffusion defect, and shunt). A "rule of thumb" that works reasonably well for determining the cause of hypoxemia in adult patients is to note the sum of the PaO_2 and $PaCO_2$. If, when inhaling room air, the sum is between 110 and 130 mmHg, the cause of the hypoxemia is overall hypoventilation. If the sum is less than 110 mmHg with room air or when receiving supplemental oxygen, the cause is $\dot{V}/\dot{Q}$ mismatch, diffusion defect, or shunt. If the sum is more than 130 mmHg in adults and the laboratory report states that the patient was inhaling room air, one should suspect an error; either the patient was receiving supplemental oxygen or an error was made in the PaO_2 or $PaCO_2$ measurements. In children or teenagers, the sum of the PaO_2 and $PaCO_2$ may normally be above 130 mmHg. These general observations apply to most adults and can be helpful if one has difficulty in clinically evaluating the cause of an abnormal $P(A-a)O_2$.

With the use of the $P(A-a)O_2$ or the sum of the PaO_2 and $PaCO_2$, one can differentiate hypoxemia owing to overall hypoventilation from other causes of hypoxemia. One must then look at other tests to differentiate $\dot{V}/\dot{Q}$ disturbance, diffusion defect, and shunt. Such measurements as the nitrogen washout and helium dilution tests give evidence for the presence of $\dot{V}/\dot{Q}$ mismatch and nonuniform ventilation. Comparison of pulmonary ventilation and perfusion lung scans can give a semiquantitative analysis of $\dot{V}/\dot{Q}$ matching over the lung fields.

The carbon monoxide diffusing capacity test can evaluate the patient for the presence of a diffusion defect. The diffusing capacity is a fairly sensitive indicator of the presence of interstitial lung disease. In the presence of obstructive airway disease, a reduced diffusing capacity is indicative of emphysema.

The presence of a shunt can be detected by giving the patient 100% oxygen. The patient breathes 100% oxygen for about 20 minutes, and then an arterial sample is obtained. For a patient at sea level, there is about a 5% shunt for every 100 mmHg the PaO_2 is below 550 to 600 mmHg. This rule of thumb works reasonably well down to a PaO_2 of 100 mmHg. One should remember that everyone normally has about a 2% to 4% shunt. Unfortunately, the administration of 100% oxygen to detect a shunt in patients with diseased lungs has a major drawback: when alveoli that are supplied by partially obstructed airways are filled with a high percentage of oxygen, they are prone to collapse. Alveoli that normally contain a large amount of nitrogen resist collapse because nitrogen is not significantly absorbed by the blood perfusing the alveo-

lus; however, when this nitrogen is replaced by oxygen, which is readily absorbed by the blood that comes in contact with the alveolus, the alveolus can rapidly collapse (absorption atelectasis), resulting in a shunt. Therefore, administration of 100% oxygen in diseased patients may indeed produce a significant shunt. In patients with hypoxemia resulting from overall hypoventilation, $\dot{V}/\dot{Q}$ mismatch and diffusion defect, inhalation of 100% oxygen will correct the hypoxemia—that is, the PaO_2 should reach the level expected for normal subjects inhaling 100% oxygen.

Table 10–5 summarizes the laboratory clues to the various causes of hypoxemia.

EVALUATION OF ACID–BASE STATUS

GENERAL CONCEPTS

The body always strives to maintain the extracellular fluid (ECF) hydrogen ion concentration [H$^+$] within a narrow range—35 to 45 nmol/L (pH 7.35 to 7.45). This is vital for proper functioning of body enzyme systems. If the blood becomes too alkaline or acidic, life-threatening changes can occur. The body has three lines of defense against changes in [H$^+$]: (1) *buffers*, which are immediate but temporary; (2) *lungs*, which work fast and excrete up to 20,000 mmol/day of acid in active adults; and (3) *kidneys*, which act slowly and are responsible for disposing of about 60–80 mmol of acid per day.

Buffers are substances that minimize the change in the concentration of hydrogen ion (or pH) in a solution when hydrogen or hydroxyl ions are added or removed. A *buffer system* is a mixture of a weak acid and its conjugate base. Most of the hydrogen ions added to this mixture combine with the base, and most of the hydrogen ions removed from the mixture by adding base are replaced from the acid of the acid–base pair.

Important in the immediate defense against changes in the hydrogen ion concentration are the following buffer systems: (1) bicarbonate (HCO_3^-), (2) hemoglobin, (3) proteins, and (4) phosphate. Hemoglobin, quantitatively, plays one of the most important roles in buffering in the process of carbon dioxide metabolism. Since all ECF buffers are in equilibrium, changes in one of the buffer systems reflect changes in all of them. In studying and evaluating acid–base physiology, the CO_2/HCO_3^- system is used because of convenience and because it is easy to measure. The pH and $PaCO_2$ are measured, but bicarbonate is calculated from these two

Table 10–5 Determination of the Causes of Hypoxemia

	$P(A-a)O_2$	$PO_2 + PCO_2$ (mmHg)
Overall hypoventilation	Normal	110–130 on room air
$\dot{V}/\dot{Q}$ mismatch*	Increased	<110 on
Diffusion defect†	(in all	room air or
Shunt‡	three)	on oxygen

*V/Q lung scans are useful in demonstrating mismatching.
†Use diffusing capacity test (DLco).
‡Detect by placing patient on 100% O$_2$.

values. From these values, the acid–base status of the body is determined. Measurements of these parameters are usually obtained from arterial blood.

To properly evaluate a patient's acid–base status requires careful review of a patient's history, ABG, and serum electrolyte values. One cannot look at any one acid–base measurement; rather, one must look at a combination of factors to arrive at a proper interpretation before appropriate treatment is initiated. Assessing serial ABGs values is also helpful in making a correct assessment. An understanding of the individual factors of the CO_2/HCO_3^- system is necessary for proper interpretation of acid–base physiology.

Carbon Dioxide Tension

Carbon dioxide is produced by every cell of the body and can be thought of as the "metabolic smoke." There is a minimum of about 200 mL CO_2 ($\dot{V}_{CO_2}$) produced each minute. The "smoke," of course, must be ventilated off, and this requires proper functioning of the lungs. The respiratory center in the brain is normally very sensitive to small changes in CO_2 levels and strives to maintain the partial pressure of the arterial CO_2 ($PaCO_2$) in the range of 35 to 45 mmHg. By definition, alveolar hypoventilation is present if the $PaCO_2$ is greater than 45 mmHg (*hypercapnia*). Alveolar hyperventilation is indicated by a $PaCO_2$ less than 35 mmHg (*hypocapnia*). A high minute volume is not synonymous with alveolar hyperventilation; for example, in severe pneumonia or obstructive airway diseases an elevated $PaCO_2$ may be present despite the presence of an increased minute ventilation when most of the increased ventilation is dead-space ventilation owing to a high dead space/tidal volume ratio. Many also confuse *tachypnea* (rapid breathing) with hyperventilation; however, by definition, *alveolar hyperventilation* is present only when the $PaCO_2$ is lower than normal (<35 mmHg).

The $PaCO_2$ represents the respiratory component of an acid–base disturbance. It is the product of the following relationship:

$$PaCO_2 = \frac{\dot{V}_{CO_2} \times 0.863}{\dot{V}_A}$$

The factor 0.863 corrects for the fact that $\dot{V}_A$ (alveolar minute ventilation) is reported in liters per minute (L/min) (BTPS), whereas $\dot{V}_{CO_2}$ (CO_2 production) is reported in milliliters per minute (mL/min) (STPD). The $PaCO_2$ is affected by both the ventilation and the metabolic rate (production), but it is *regulated* by ventilation. Carbon dioxide behaves as an acid

in the body, as can be seen from the hydration reaction of CO_2 and H_2O:

$$CO_2 + H_2O \xrightleftharpoons{CA} H_2CO_3 \leftrightharpoons HCO_3^- + \boxed{H^+} \; \text{acid}$$

The reaction is facilitated in the red blood cells (RBC) and the kidney cells by the enzyme carbonic anhydrase (CA), which speeds up the reaction some 13,000 times. As can be seen here, the more CO_2 that is produced, the more the chemical equation is shifted to the right, producing more acid. At the tissue sites, the buffer systems are crucial in maintaining a normal pH. In the lungs, the reaction moves to the left and CO_2 is blown off, thereby eliminating the acid.

Figure 10–4 summarizes the major reactions in the transport of CO_2 in the body. Carbon dioxide can be transported to the lungs from the tissues in six forms (see Fig. 10–4). When CO_2 enters the plasma, it may (1) remain dissolved in plasma, (2) become bound to plasma proteins to form carbamino compounds, or (3) join with water to form carbonic acid and then hydrogen ion and bicarbonate. However, most CO_2 enters the RBC where it again may (1) be present as dissolved CO_2, (2) become bound to the globin portion of hemoglobin, forming *carbaminohemoglobin*, or (3) join with water to form carbonic acid and then hydrogen ion and bicarbonate. Since there is no carbonic anhydrase in the plasma, the amount and speed of plasma formation of H_2CO_3 is slow. The bulk of the CO_2 readily moves into the RBC (CO_2 is freely permeable to all body compartments) because there is a pressure gradient favoring its diffusion in that direction. Inside the RBC, the carbonic anhydrase (CA) rapidly helps convert CO_2 to H^+ and HCO_3^-. The HCO_3^- then rapidly diffuses out of the RBC into the plasma because there is now a greater concentration of bicarbonate inside the RBC than outside in the plasma, and the RBC membrane is permeable to this anion. About 60% to 90% of the CO_2 is transported from the tissues to the lung in the form of HCO_3^-, with most of this having been formed in RBC, but transferred out to the plasma for transport. Some 10% to 20% of the CO_2 is transported as carbamino compounds, with less than 10% being transported as dissolved CO_2.

Meanwhile, hydrogen ion that is formed in the process is immediately buffered by the hemoglobin molecule, minimizing the change in pH. The increase in hemoglobin acidity favors release of oxygen to the tissues. The concentration of anions (HCO_3^- and Cl^-) inside the red cells relative to that in the plasma is increased, bringing water into the

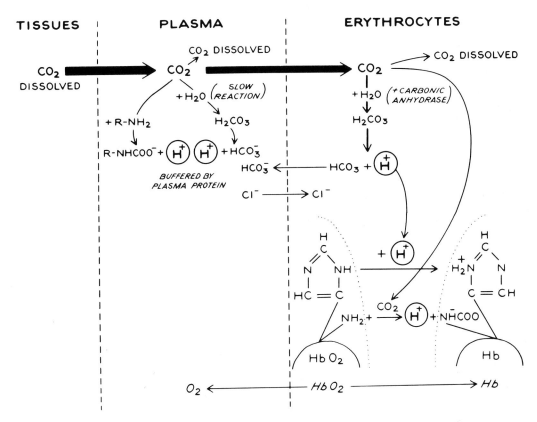

Figure 10—4. Carbon dioxide transport in blood. About 70% to 80% of CO_2 is transported as HCO_3^- in the plasma, 10% is carried as carbamino compounds both inside and outside the cell, and about 7% as dissolved CO_2. The reverse of these reactions occurs when the blood reaches the lungs, allowing rapid elimination of CO_2. (Comroe JH Jr: Physiology of Respiration. Chicago, Year Book Medical Publishers, 1974. Redrawn from Davenport H: The ABC of Acid-Base Chemistry, 5th ed. Chicago, University of Chicago Press, 1969)

cells. Thus, the venous hematocrit is slightly larger than that of arterial blood. This has erroneously been called the "chloride shift," probably because Hamburger did not have a ready method of measuring bicarbonate when he described the phenomenon. When the RBC reaches the lungs, these chemical reactions are reversed and CO_2 is unloaded while O_2 is taken up.

Plasma Bicarbonate

Bicarbonate (HCO_3^-) is normally in equilibrium in plasma, in RBCs, and in other body cells, as depicted previously in the hydration reaction of CO_2 and H_2O ($CO_2 + H_2O \overset{CA}{\underset{CA}{\rightleftarrows}} H_2CO_3 \rightleftarrows H^+ + HCO_3^-$). Plasma bicarbonate is usually referred to as the metabolic component of an acid–base disturbance.

Normally, the arterial plasma bicarbonate is in the range of 22 to 26 mEq/L (or mmol/L). Although influenced by pulmonary ventilation, to a small extent, by the foregoing reaction, HCO_3^- is mainly regulated by the kidneys. If one acutely hypoventilates, resulting in an increased CO_2 tension, the equilibrium reaction shifts to the right, resulting in a slight, instantaneous increase in plasma bicarbonate. Therefore, the plasma bicarbonate not only represents the renal-regulated or metabolic component but also is slightly affected by acute changes in alveolar ventilation.

The production of bicarbonate is also dependent upon other nonbicarbonate buffers.

$$Metabolism \rightarrow CO_2 + H_2O \rightarrow$$
$$H_2CO_3 \rightarrow H^+ + HCO_3^-$$
$$\downarrow$$
$$\boxed{H^+ + Fixed\ Buffers}$$

When $[H^+]$ is formed in the foregoing reactions, HCO_3^- is also produced. It is the capacity of the fixed buffers in the body that limit the amount of H^+ that can combine with buffers and the amount of HCO_3^- formed. Bicarbonate can also be readily formed when acid leaves the body, such as through emesis or nasogastric suctioning.

Bicarbonate is also influenced by electrolytes. Potassium (K^+) and HCO_3^- are inversely related. In acidosis or excesses of hydrogen ion, serum K^+ levels increase and serum HCO_3^- levels decrease. Chloride, being an anion, will *inversely* affect HCO_3^- levels because the body strives to maintain electroneutrality. Thus, as chloride levels increase, the HCO_3^- levels decrease. Administration of HCl, ammonium chloride, or potassium chloride (when hypokalemia is present) is effective in treating metabolic alkalemia.

The regulation of plasma bicarbonate is predominantly carried out by the kidney. Although the lungs can vary the CO_2 level in the blood within minutes, it takes hours to days for the kidney to change the bicarbonate level in the plasma. The reabsorption of sodium from the urine by the kid-

ney cell and its return to the blood is accompanied by the regeneration of bicarbonate (Fig. 10–5). Normally, about 99% of the bicarbonate filtered through the glomerulus is returned from the renal tubule to the blood by the reabsorption (reclamation) mechanism depicted in Figure 10–5 (mechanism A). Normally, about two-thirds of the acid excreted in the urine is in the form of ammonium chloride (e.g., through the glutamine mechanism), and one-third is in the form of titratable acid (e.g., NaH_2PO_4).

If respiratory acidosis caused by hypercapnia (elevated $PaCO_2$) occurs, the kidney attempts to compensate for this by regenerating extra bicarbonate. On the other hand, when respiratory alkalosis caused by hypocapnia (a decreased $PaCO_2$) occurs, the kidney reduces the amount of bicarbonate regenerated, resulting in increased hydrogen ion in the plasma, in an attempt to compensate for the alkalosis. Carbonic anhydrase is present in the kidney cell, resulting in acceleration of the reaction,

$$CO_2 + H_2O \xrightarrow{CA} H_2CO_3.$$

The bicarbonate–carbonic acid system is the

Figure 10–5. Mechanisms for reabsorption of sodium from the urine into the blood (take place in the distal convoluted tubule and collecting duct system). Mechanism *A* depicts the usual mechanism for reabsorption of bicarbonate from the glomerular filtrate. In mechanism *B*, H^+ is excreted in the form of "titratable acid." In mechanism *C*, the glutamine mechanism, H^+ is excreted in the form of NH_4Cl. C.A., carbonic anhydrase.

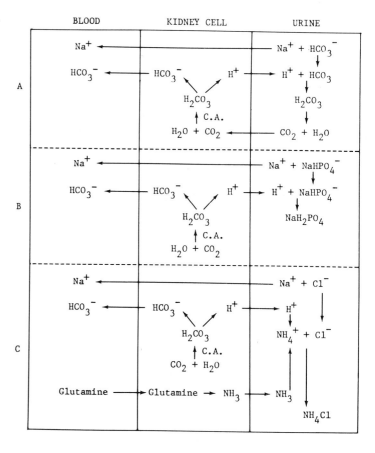

most important pH-maintaining system of the body. It removes the acid H_2CO_3 and functions equally well at all ranges of pH. This unique property is due to the volatility of CO_2. So, in addition to the simple chemical buffering (around pH 6.1), the levels of CO_2 can be increased or decreased as needed by the lungs, and the kidneys adjust the balance of cation concentration (primarily Na^+ and K^+) with "non-buffer" anions (primarily Cl^-).

pH MEASUREMENT

The measurement most commonly used to reflect the hydrogen ion concentration of the blood is the pH (puissant hydrogen). The Brønsted-Lowry concept defines an acid as a proton donor and a base as a proton acceptor. The proton is H^+. The proton acceptors are the various conjugate bases. *pH* is defined as the negative logarithm of the hydrogen ion concentration, $[H^+]$. For instance:

$$[H^+] = 40 \times 10^{-9}$$
$$\begin{aligned} pH &= -\log (40 \times 10^{-9}) \\ &= -\log 40 - \log 10^{-9} \\ &= -1.6 - (-9) \\ &= 7.4 \end{aligned}$$

Normally, the arterial blood pH is in the range of 7.35 to 7.45. The relationship between pH and $[H^+]$ is illustrated in Table 10–6.

Table 10–6 The Relationship Between pH and Hydrogen Ion Concentration

pH	$[H^+]$ (nmol/L)
7.0	100
7.1	80
7.2	60
7.3	50
7.4	40
7.5	30
7.6	25
7.7	20
7.8	15
7.9	12.5
8.0	10

From a pH of 7.2 to 7.5 there is a relatively linear relationship between pH and $[H^+]$. For each 0.01 pH change there is a 1 nm/L $[H^+]$ change.

An estimate of hydrogen ion concentration can be made from the following formula:

$$[H^+] = 24 \times \frac{PCO_2 \text{ mmHg}}{HCO_3^- \text{ mEq/L}}$$

Acidemia is present if the pH is lower than 7.35, and *alkalemia* is present if the pH is higher than 7.45.* The presence of a normal pH, however, does not rule out an acid–base disturbance.

The relationship of pH to the HCO_3^-/H_2CO_3 system is shown below:

1. K = the dissociation constant of a buffer solution (the number of molecules that separated into H^+ and HCO_3^-). There is a different K constant for each type of buffer. For the bicarbonate system:

    $$K \text{ of } H_2CO_3 = 7.85 \times 10^{-7}$$

2. pK = the pH at which the associated and dissociated molecules are present in equal amounts (50 : 50). This is the pH at which maximum buffering occurs.

    $$\begin{aligned} pK &= -\log K \\ &= -\log (7.85 \times 10^{-7}) \\ &= 6.1 \end{aligned}$$

3. pH is defined by the classic Henderson–Hasselbalch equation:

    $$\begin{aligned} pH &= 6.1 + \log \frac{[HCO_3^-]}{[H_2CO_3]} \\ &= 6.1 + \log \frac{[HCO_3^-]}{0.03 \times PaCO_2} \end{aligned}$$

Since the PCO_2 is easier to measure than the H_2CO_3, $PaCO_2$ is used in the equation instead. As an example (assuming HCO_3^- = 24 mEq/L and $PaCO_2$ = 40, then H_2CO_3 = 40 × 0.03 = 1.2 mEq/L):

$$pH = 6.1 + \log (24/1.2) = 7.40$$

As described previously, the kidneys regulate the HCO_3^- and the lungs regulate the $PaCO_2$, the acid–base balance of the body could be conceptually viewed as follows:

$$pH \sim \frac{\text{kidneys}}{\text{lungs}} \text{ or } \frac{\text{metabolic}}{\text{respiratory}}$$

---

* Commonly, the terms acidosis and alkalosis are used; however, because arterial blood analysis measures only the blood pH, acidemia and alkalemia are theoretically preferable.

OTHER BUFFER SYSTEMS

Several buffer systems, in addition to the bicarbonate–carbonic acid system, operate in the blood to minimize the wide fluctuations of pH that might occur if respiratory or metabolic aberrations are present.

Protein Buffers

Quantitatively, hemoglobin is the most important "chemical buffer" in *whole blood* because of its important role of buffering [H$^+$] created during carbon dioxide metabolism. Plasma proteins are the most important "chemical buffers" (Pr$^-$/HPr) in plasma, but, quantitatively, plasma proteins are less important than hemoglobin.

Phosphate Buffer System

The phosphate buffer system is relatively unimportant quantitatively as a blood buffer system. Phosphate is an important intracellular buffer.

There is an interrelationship between the bicarbonate–carbonic acid buffer system and the other body buffers.

$$CO_2 + H_2O \underset{CA}{\rightleftharpoons} H_2CO_3 \rightleftharpoons H^+ + HCO_3^-$$
$$+$$
$$BUF^-$$
$$\Updownarrow$$
$$HBUF$$

Each of the three buffer systems of blood acts to minimize the effect of excess hydrogen or hydroxyl ions, but only the nonbicarbonate buffers (hemoglobin, plasma proteins, and phosphate) buffer the effect of a rising or falling PCO$_2$. This effect is expected because the PCO$_2$ is part of the bicarbonate–carbonic acid system.

In Vitro and In Vivo Buffer Systems

The effectiveness of a buffer system is proportional to its concentration. Most of the nonbicarbonate buffers of the extracellular fluid (ECF) are concentrated in the blood compartment, but the PCO$_2$ and bicarbonate are rather evenly distributed to the interstitial fluid as well as to the blood plasma. Because in an adult the ECF volume is about three times the blood volume, the effective concentration and, hence, buffering power of nonbicarbonate buffers in the entire ECF is only about one-third of that in the blood. It is these considerations that cause the arterial blood in a living subject to react differently than the same blood in a test tube when subjected to changes of PCO$_2$.

MEASUREMENTS TO EVALUATE THE METABOLIC COMPONENT

The respiratory component of acid–base balance is evaluated by measurement of the PCO$_2$. No excess or deficit of fixed acid or base will influence this evaluation. Measures of the metabolic component will be discussed next.

Plasma Bicarbonate

Plasma bicarbonate should always be calculated from the measured PCO$_2$ and pH. This can be done quickly using the nomogram of Figure 10–6, or the formula: [HCO$_3^-$] = antilog (pH − 6.1) 0.03 PCO$_2$. A line connecting the PCO$_2$ and pH is extended to the HCO$_3^-$ line. As noted earlier, the plasma bicarbonate, to a small degree, is quickly affected by respiratory changes. Many experienced physicians simply make a qualitative mental correction of the bicarbonate for the respiratory effect. The effect is never greater than about 4 mEq/L of HCO$_3^-$. There are several indirect calculations to quantitate the respiratory correction. They can all be calculated by using a nomogram, but the best one can be calculated in one's head at the bedside if the laboratory has not calculated it (see discussion on Extracellular Fluid Base Excess).

In Vitro Corrections

These calculations are all based on the buffering power of whole blood in the test tube. Whole blood has a nonbicarbonate buffer value of 30 mEq/L [H$^+$] per pH unit or slykes (sl),[13] which means that it would take 30 mEq/L of H$^+$ added in the form of carbonic acid to change the pH 1 unit.

Standard Bicarbonate. The *standard bicarbonate* has been defined as the plasma bicarbonate concentration when the blood has been equilibrated at a PCO$_2$ of 40 mmHg, a temperature of 37°C, and the hemoglobin is 100% saturated with oxygen. This measurement theoretically allows one to look at the "metabolic component" of a plasma bicarbonate, eliminating the "respiratory component." For example, in acute respiratory failure, with a PaCO$_2$ of 85 mmHg, the plasma bicarbonate may be slightly increased; however, the standard bicarbonate would still be normal. The acute elevation in plasma bicarbonate as a result of the hypercapnia is

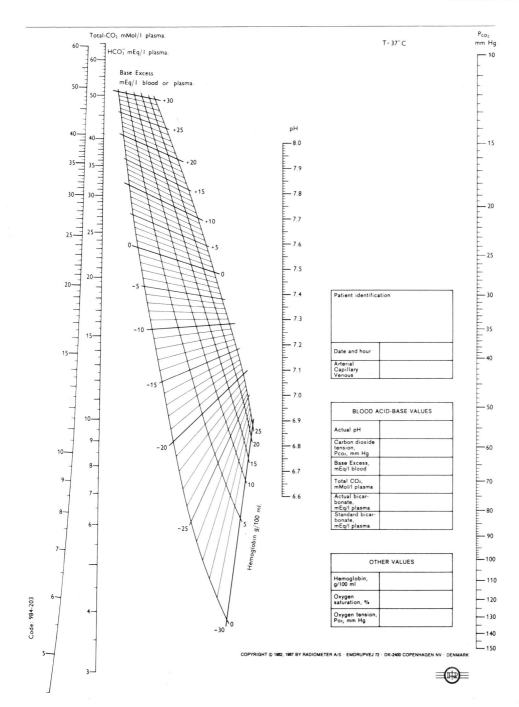

Total-CO₂ mMol/l plasma.

HCO₃⁻ mEq/l plasma.

Base Excess
mEq/l blood or plasma.

T-37°C

P_CO₂
mm Hg

pH

Patient identification

Date and hour

Arterial
Capillary
Venous

BLOOD ACID-BASE VALUES

Actual pH

Carbon dioxide
tension,
Pco₂, mm Hg

Base Excess,
mEq/l blood

Total CO₂,
mMol/l plasma

Actual bicar-
bonate,
mEq/l plasma

Standard bicar-
bonate,
mEq/l plasma

OTHER VALUES

Hemoglobin,
g/100 ml

Oxygen
saturation, %

Oxygen tension,
Po₂, mm Hg

Hemoglobin g/100 ml.

Code: 984-203

Figure 10—6. Siggaard–Andersen alignment nomogram for determination of base excess, total CO₂, actual bicarbonate, standard bicarbonate, T_{40} bicarbonate, and BE_{ECF}. *See* Appendix A for methods of calculation. (Reproduced by permission of O. Siggaard-Andersen and Radiometer A/S, Copenhagen, 1963)

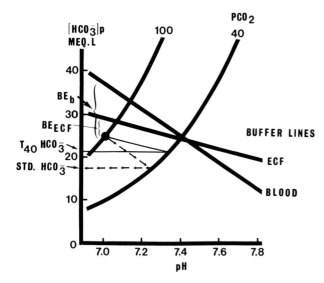

Figure 10–7.   In this graph, the $[HCO_3^-]$ of the plasma is plotted against the pH. The CO_2 isopleths are curved lines. The buffer lines represent the nonbicarbonate buffer value of ECF and blood, respectively. The buffer lines represent the average pathway for pure respiratory (PCO_2 changes in the respective compartments. The slope of the lines is the buffer value of about 10 for ECF and about 30 for blood. The slope $\Delta HCO_3^-/\Delta pH$, whereas buffer value was defined in the text as ΔH^+ added/ΔpH. The ΔHCO_3^- is stoichometrically identical with the ΔH^+ added for CO_2 as shown by the equation

$$CO_2 + H_2O \rightleftharpoons H_2CO_3 \rightleftharpoons H^+ + HCO_3^-.$$

Most of the H^+ is buffered by the nonbicarbonate buffers, but the $[HCO_3^-]$ remains as a quantitative marker of the $[H^+]$ added. The solid point (●) represents a patient with acute respiratory failure and a mild metabolic acidosis caused by lactic acidemia owing to hypoxia.

Measured values are

$$PCO_2 = 100 \text{ pH} = 7.01.$$

Calculated values are

$$(HCO_3^-)p = 24;$$
$$BE_{ECF} = -5; \ BEb = -12;$$
$$T_{40} = 21; \ STD \ HCO_3^- = 17.$$

The BE_{ECF} or BEb can be determined graphically from the deviation of the patient point from the ECF or blood buffer lines, respectively. Because of inhomogeneities within the compartments, the values obtained in this way are larger than the true values obtained from Figure 10–6. The BEb correction factor = 1 − 0.0143 Hb (g/dL). The BE_{ECF} correction is very small and can be ignored.

The $T_{40} HCO_3^-$ and standard HCO_3^- may be determined by extending a line from the patient point parallel to the ECF or blood buffer lines, respectively. The HCO_3^- level at the point of intersection with the $PCO_2 = 40$ line is the desired value.

due to an increased respiratory component rather than to a metabolic increase in bicarbonate. The normal standard bicarbonate is 22 to 26 mEq/L. A graphic solution for standard bicarbonate is shown in the example in Figure 10–7. The standard bicarbonate works fairly satisfactorily to correct for the respiratory component of bicarbonate when hypocapnia is present. In the presence of hypercapnia, however, it is unreliable, as is explained in the discussion of In Vivo Corrections.

Buffer Base.   The buffer base includes the total concentration of anions in the blood available to buffer the hydrogen ion chemically or by elimination of carbon dioxide. The buffer base thus includes bicarbonate, hemoglobin, plasma proteins, and phosphates. The normal buffer base with a hemoglobin value of 15 g% is 48 mEq/L.

In pure respiratory acid–base disturbances, the buffer base theoretically should remain normal. For example, in acute hypercapnia

$$\uparrow CO_2 + H_2O \rightarrow H_2CO_3 \rightarrow H^+ + HCO_3^-$$
$$+$$
$$BUF^-$$
$$\downarrow$$
$$HBUF$$

The BUF^- includes hemoglobin, plasma proteins, and phosphate buffers. An increased $PaCO_2$ results not only in an increased hydrogen ion level, but also in an increased plasma bicarbonate level as well. The interaction with the other buffer systems, however, results in an equal reduction in the nonbicarbonate buffers (BUF^-). Because the buffer base comprises bicarbonate and the other buffers (BUF^-), the total buffer base should remain normal in the presence of a pure respiratory acid–base disorder. However, in vitro and in vivo changes in buffer base in response to changes in $PaCO_2$ are different, as will be described. In vitro determinations are fairly satisfactory in the presence of hypocapnia but are unreliable with hypercapnia, as is explained under In Vivo Corrections. Changes in buffer base are commonly described in terms of base excess.

Base Excess of Blood.   Base excess of blood (BEb) is another way of reflecting an increase or decrease in the buffer base. Normally, the BEb is − 2 to +2 mEq/L. A BEb greater than +2 means that acid has been removed or base has been added, and a BEb less than −2 means that acid has been added or base removed. The BEb represents the amount of fixed acid needed to titrate the blood pH to 7.40

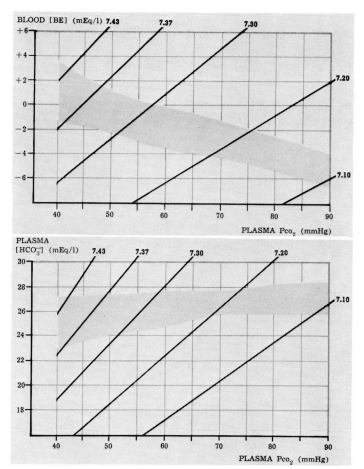

Figure 10—8. Ninety-five percent confidence-limit bands for acute CO_2 retention. Note that the blood base excess does drop below −2 with acute CO_2 retention even though there has been no change in "metabolic component." (Winters RW et al: Acid–Base Physiology in Medicine, 2nd ed. Cleveland, London Co, 1969)

after the blood has been equilibrated to a PCO_2 of 40 mmHg. A negative BEb would require titration with a base. The BEb is represented graphically in Figure 10–7 and can be calculated accurately from Figure 10–6.

This is an elegant way to quantitate the metabolic component of the blood, but unfortunately it is an in vitro measure. The BEb will not change if CO_2 is added to blood in vitro, but if it is added to blood in a living patient the BEb will decrease, as shown in Figure 10–8. Therefore, this test is of limited usefulness in the presence of hypercapnia. When hypocapnia is present, BEb is a fairly reliable indicator of the metabolic component of the plasma bicarbonate.

In Vivo Corrections

In vivo corrections are better than the in vitro calculations because they represent the state of the entire extracellular fluid, not just the blood. The T_{40}

bicarbonate and the base excess of the ECF (BEecf) are available in vivo measurements and are calculated essentially the same way as the standard bicarbonate and BEb, but the buffer value of the ECF is used instead of that of blood. An acute elevation of $PaCO_2$ owing to alveolar hypoventilation does result in an increase in plasma bicarbonate and a decrease in the other buffers; however, because the capillary wall is permeable to bicarbonate but not to the principal nonbicarbonate buffers (i.e., proteins), some of the bicarbonate formed in response to acute hypercapnia diffuses through the capillary wall into the interstitial fluid. The bicarbonate formed as a direct result of the buffer response to acute hypercapnia is distributed throughout the extracellular fluid space; thus, the increase in blood bicarbonate is only about one-third that which would be seen in an in vitro system with a single volume of distribution. Therefore, the increase in plasma bicarbonate in vivo in response to acute CO_2 retention is less than would occur in a setting in vitro, making standard bicarbonate, BBb, and BEb unreliable indicators of the metabolic component of the plasma bicarbonate in acute hypercapnia. Because the reduction in nonbicarbonate buffers is the same but the increase in plasma bicarbonate is less than would occur in vitro, the total blood buffer base or blood base excess may, in fact, decrease in association with acute hypercapnia. In this situation, the decrease in blood buffer base or blood base excess would not then represent a superimposed metabolic disturbance (e.g., metabolic acidosis), but would be related only to the in vivo response to acute CO_2 retention.

Superficially, it appears that the pathway of acute hypocapnia is the same for in vitro blood as for a living subject. The effect of acute hypocapnia on in vitro blood is exactly what would be predicted by extrapolation from hypercapnia experiments. In the living subject, however, very frequently a true superimposed metabolic acidosis occurs that is due to a lactic acidosis. The lactic acidosis may be produced by a reduced blood flow to some tissues caused by hypocapnia and alkalemia or by reduced excretion or reduced metabolism of lactate owing to the same causes. The T_{40} bicarbonate and BE_{ECF} measures reveal the presence of this metabolic acidosis, but the in vitro measures do not show it. With hypocapnia, in vitro and in vivo changes in standard bicarbonate, buffer base and base excess, are similar.

T_{40} Bicarbonate.

Because it was recognized that, with acute hypercapnia, the increase in plasma bicarbonate that occurs in vivo is less than that which occurs in vitro and, therefore, that in vitro nomograms used to calculate standard bicarbonate might be invalid, a new calculation known as the T_{40} bicarbonate was developed.[14] A method of calculating it graphically is shown in Figure 10–7. It can also be calculated accurately from Figure 10–6. A bedside estimation can be done by assuming that an acute increase in $PaCO_2$ of about 15 mmHg will increase the plasma bicarbonate by about 1 mEq/L. The change in plasma bicarbonate expected to occur with acute carbon dioxide retention would be

$$\Delta HCO_3^- = \frac{\text{observed } PaCO_2 - 40}{15}.$$

The T_{40} bicarbonate is equal to the observed plasma bicarbonate minus the bicarbonate expected to occur secondary to the acute CO_2 elevation. For example, if the $PaCO_2$ equals 85 mmHg, then

$$\Delta HCO_3^- = \frac{85 - 40}{15} = 3 \text{ mEq/L}.$$

If the observed plasma $HCO_3^- = 28$ mEq/L, then

$$T_{40} \text{ bicarbonate} = 28 - 3 = 25 \text{ mEq/L}.$$

Therefore, in this example, the slightly elevated bicarbonate was due to acute CO_2 retention and did not indicate increased metabolic bicarbonate.

Because changes in plasma bicarbonate with acute CO_2 retention are different in vivo than in vitro, T_{40} bicarbonate is a more reliable measure than is standard bicarbonate in patients with acute hypercapnia. In acute hypocapnia, T_{40} bicarbonate may also be more reliable than standard bicarbonate because it can detect the concomitant lactic acidosis better than the standard bicarbonate does.

Use a ratio of 5:1 (PCO_2/plasma bicarbonate) for estimating the decrease in T_{40} bicarbonate in the presence of acute CO_2 reduction ($PaCO_2$ less than 35 mmHg).[15] The T_{40} bicarbonate becomes more inaccurate when a large metabolic component is also present.

Base Excess of Extracellular Fluid.

The base excess of ECF (BE_{ECF}) is easy to calculate accurately, even at the bedside, and is a measure of the metabolic component of the entire ECF, provided the patient has been in a quasi-steady state for about 10 minutes. It can be defined as the *titratable basicity* of the ECF. In other words, it represents the amount of fixed base or acid that would have to be added to the ECF to bring the pH to 7.4 after the PCO_2 has been brought to 40 mmHg.[16,17]

The calculation is shown graphically in Figure 10–6. The BE_{ECF} is the deviation from the ECF buffer line. The BE_{ECF} can also be calculated from Figure 10–5, but a quite accurate bedside calculation is

$$BE_{ECF} = \Delta HCO_3^- + 10 \Delta pH,$$

where

$$\Delta HCO_3^- = \text{actual } HCO_3^- - 24$$

and

$$\Delta pH = \text{actual pH} - 7.4.$$

The approximate slope of the ECF buffer line is 10 mEq bicarbonate per liter per pH unit. (The slope depends on the hemoglobin concentration of the blood and on the ratio of blood volume to ECF volume.) A slope of 11.6 was obtained in a group of normal subjects. The value of 10 makes the calculation easier.

COMPARISON OF IN VITRO AND IN VIVO MEASURES

By using the following set of numbers from an arterial blood analysis, compare the in vitro and in vivo measures:

	MEASURED	NORMAL
pH	7.14	7.35–7.45
PaCO$_2$	85 mmHg	35–45 mmHg
Plasma HCO$_3^-$	28 mEq/L	22–26 mEq/L
Standard HCO$_3^-$	21 mEq/L	22–26 mEq/L
T$_{40}$ HCO$_3^-$	25 mEq/L	22–26 mEq/L
BBb	44 mEq/L	46–50 mEq/L
BEb	−4 mEq/L	−2 to +2 mEq/L
BEecf	1.4 mEq/L	−2 to +2 mEq/L

BEecf in this example, is derived as follows:

$$\begin{aligned} BE_{ECF} &= (\Delta\ HCO_3^-) + 10\ (\Delta pH) \\ &= (28 - 24) + 10\ (7.14 - 7.40) \\ &= (4) + 10\ (-0.26) \\ &= 4 - 2.6 \\ &= 1.4\ mEq/L \end{aligned}$$

The plasma HCO$_3^-$ is slightly elevated; however, the T$_{40}$ HCO$_3^-$ and the BEecf are normal, which indicates that the increased plasma HCO$_3^-$ is of respiratory origin, from the hypercapnia, rather than of metabolic origin. The reduced stan-

dard bicarbonate, BEb and BBb are inaccurate because they are derived from in vitro observations that are different from in vivo observations in acute hypercapnia. The reduced blood buffer base and BEb result from the leakage of HCO$_3^-$ from the blood into the perivascular tissues, which occurs in vivo with acute hypercapnia. The normal BEecf accurately indicates that this is a pure respiratory acidosis, with a normal metabolic component.

A study of Figure 10–7, reveals the following relationships between BEb and BEecf and standard bicarbonate and T$_{40}$ bicarbonate:

Below pH 7.4, BEb < BEecf
Above pH 7.4, BEb > BEecf
Above PCO$_2$ 40 mmHg, standard HCO$_3^-$ < T$_{40}$ HCO$_3^-$
Below PCO$_2$ 40 mmHg, standard HCO$_3^-$ > T$_{40}$ HCO$_3^-$

The BEecf is the only test of the four that is indicative of the metabolic component under all circumstances. The reasons for the superiority of the BEecf are twofold: First, the BEecf uses in vivo buffer values to compute the metabolic component. Hence, the value of BEecf is realistic and can be directly applied to living subjects. Second, the BEecf is a measure of the amount of strong base that needs to be added or removed to make the pH 7.4 *after* the PCO$_2$ has been made 40 mmHg. The T$_{40}$ bicarbonate is an in vivo measure but suffers from the fact that with a marked metabolic component, especially a severe metabolic acidosis, the intersection of the in vivo buffer line with the PCO$_2$ 40-mmHg line will

Table 10–7   Comparison of In Vitro and In Vivo Measures of Metabolic Component

	pH	PaCO$_2$	PLASMA HCO$_3^-$	BEecf	T$_{40}$ HCO$_3^-$	BEb	STANDARD HCO$_3^-$
Acute hypercapnia	↓ ↓	↑	↑	N	N	↓	↓
Chronic hypercapnia	↓	↑	↑ ↑	↑ ↑	↑ ↑	↑	↑
Metabolic acidosis	↓ ↓	↓	↓ ↓	↓ ↓	↓	↓ ↓ ↓	↓ ↓ ↓
Metabolic alkalosis	↑	↑	↑	↑	↑	↑ ↑	↑ ↑
Acute hypocapnia	↑ ↑	↓	↓ ↓	↓	↓	N	N
Chronic hypocapnia	↑	↓	↓ ↓ ↓	↓ ↓ ↓	↓ ↓ ↓	↓ ↓ ↓	↓ ↓ ↓
Mixed respiratory and metabolic acidosis	↓	↑	N or ↓	↓	↓	↓ ↓	↓ ↓
Mixed respiratory and metabolic alkalosis	↑	↓	N or ↑	↑	↑	↑ ↑	↑ ↑

occur at an abnormal pH. This will produce values for T_{40} bicarbonate that are qualitatively but not quantitatively correct.

The one drawback of the BEecf calculation is that it assumes a blood/ECF volume ratio of 1 : 3. In conditions of severe overhydration or underhydration and with a newborn or very young child, this assumption is incorrect. In pediatric disease, it is probably better to look at the plasma bicarbonate and not to correct it for a respiratory component. This has the effect of assuming that the effective nonbicarbonate buffer value of the fluid compartments is zero. This undoubtedly is not true, but it probably is very low.

Table 10–7, shows a comparison of plasma HCO_3^-, T_{40} HCO_3^-, BEecf, standard HCO_3^-, and BEb in typical clinical disorders. The plasma HCO_3^- gives values that might be misinterpreted in respiratory abnormalities, with or without a primary metabolic component. The T_{40} HCO_3^- may be misleading in severe acidosis. The standard HCO_3^- and BEb have the greatest potential of misinterpretation qualitatively and quantitatively. The BEecf may be misleading in small children or marked fluid imbalance, but otherwise is based on the most sound physiologic grounds. All tests will give qualitatively correct results in very severe acid–base imbalances of any kind, but in the less severe cases the in vitro tests and, to a lesser extent, the plasma HCO_3^- and the T_{40} HCO_3^- may be misinterpreted.

NORMAL ARTERIAL AND VENOUS ACID–BASE VALUES

Normal arterial values include pH 7.40; $PaCO_2$, 40 mmHg; bicarbonate, 24 mmol/L; compared with venous values of pH 7.37, PCO_2, 46 mmHg; and bicarbonate, 26 mmol/L. Thus, it can be seen that venous values for acid–base data normally are quite similar to arterial values, whereas oxygenation values are normally significantly different between arterial and venous blood. An example of normal arterial values would be a PO_2 of 80 mmHg, O_2 saturation of 94%, and O_2 content of 20 vol%, compared with normal venous values of PO_2, 40 mmHg, O_2 saturation, 75%; and O_2 content, 15 vol%. Then, as stressed earlier, venous blood analysis gives no reliable estimate of arterial oxygenation data.

Furthermore, it has recently become apparent that arterial acid–base data may not reflect venous values in patients with hypotension, heart failure, and during cardiopulmonary resuscitation.[18,19] In these conditions, the arterial pH and PCO_2 may be normal in the presence of severe acidosis and hypercapnia in the peripheral venous blood. Recent studies[19,20] suggest that central venous and pulmonary arterial blood have virtually identical pH and bicarbonate values; hence, one does not need to go through the more risky, technically demanding, and expensive placement of a pulmonary artery catheter to assess venous acid–base data.

Whereas arterial measurements provide an assessment of ventilatory function, venous data provide an assessment of tissue acidity and adequacy of oxygenation. To correct venous hypercapnia and acidosis when the arterial PCO_2 and pH are normal, it is necessary to improve circulation. An increase in alveolar ventilation is unlikely to help with venous acidosis and hypercapnia when arterial PCO_2 and pH values are already normal. In the presence of severe respiratory failure, arterial hypercapnia and venous hypercapnia develop simultaneously; consequently, there is no significant increase in the arteriovenous difference for pH and PCO_2. The precise role for venous blood gas measurements is still to be determined. It has been noted, for example, that during mild exercise the $PaCO_2$ remains near 40 mmHg, whereas the $P\bar{v}CO_2$ may rise to 60 mmHg or more.[21] During anaerobic exercise, hyperventilation results in hypocapnia, whereas the venous PCO_2 may rise to 70 mmHg or higher.[21] Whether venous hypercapnia in the presence of a normal $PaCO_2$ will be a guide to impending or existing circulatory impairment needs additional evaluation. Venous assessment of oxygenation data can provide better clues to the adequacy of tissue oxygenation than arterial measurements in many patients.

Usually the plasma bicarbonate measured on a chemistry panel is slightly higher than that calculated from the pH and PCO_2 measured in the blood gas laboratory. Whereas arterial blood samples are usually kept anaerobic and cool and are analyzed soon after withdrawal, clinical laboratory samples are usually venous, may not be anaerobic, and often are analyzed hours after the sample has been obtained. In autoanalyzers used in most clinical chemistry laboratories, the CO_2 is measured after the plasma is acidified, resulting in more CO_2 being released from the blood. There may also be some loss of CO_2 while the plasma is in the sample cups. Clinical laboratory bicarbonate (total CO_2) values are often higher than those of arterial HCO_3^-. In essence, the clinical laboratory total CO_2 (commonly reported as HCO_3^-) reports both dissolved CO_2 and HCO_3^- as one value. If one converts arterial $PaCO_2$ to milliequivalents per liter by multiplying the $PaCO_2$ by 0.0301 and then adds this value to the calculated arterial HCO_3^-, the two values will often be quite close. Venous CO_2 content is also slightly higher than arterial CO_2 content because of CO_2 liberated from the tissues. If the PCO_2 and pH measurements in the blood gas laboratory are accurate, then the calculated plasma bicarbonate from the blood gas laboratory should be accepted as valid if there is a significant discrepancy between that value and the one reported by the clinical laboratory.

CAUSES OF ACID–BASE IMBALANCE AND ACID–BASE DISORDERS

Respiratory acidosis is caused by hydrogen ion accumulation as a result of hypercapnia.

$$\uparrow CO_2 + H_2O \rightarrow H_2CO_3 \rightarrow H^+ + HCO_3^-$$
$$+$$
$$BUF^-$$
$$\downarrow$$
$$HBUF$$

The increased PCO_2 results in increased hydrogen ion concentration and acidosis. The plasma HCO_3^- level is increased slightly as a result of hypercapnia.

Respiratory acidosis may be due to overall hypoventilation associated with respiratory center depression and neuromuscular disturbances in the presence of normal lungs, or it may indicate respiratory failure associated with COPD (e.g., emphysema and chronic bronchitis). Other disorders, such as severe pulmonary edema caused by left ventricular failure and significant pulmonary embolism, may also result in respiratory acidosis.

Respiratory Alkalosis

Hypocapnia (decreased $PaCO_2$ caused by hyperventilation) results in a loss of hydrogen ion.

$$\downarrow CO_2 + H_2O \leftarrow H_2CO_3 \leftarrow H^+ + HCO_3^-$$
$$+$$
$$BUF^-$$
$$\uparrow$$
$$HBUF$$

Plasma bicarbonate decreases slightly in this reaction. Respiratory alkalosis is commonly associated with neurogenic hyperventilation, interstitial lung diseases, pulmonary embolism, asthma, hyperventilation syndrome, and severe hypoxemia.

Metabolic Acidosis

Metabolic acidosis may occur because of the increased metabolic formation of acids by the body (e.g., diabetic ketoacidosis and lactic acidosis), reduction in excretion of acids by the kidney (e.g., acidosis associated with renal failure), or the exogenous addition of acids to the bloodstream (e.g., ammonium chloride or hydrochloric acid).

$$CO_2 + H_2O \leftarrow H_2CO_3 \leftarrow \uparrow H^+ + HCO_3^-$$
$$+$$
$$BUF^-$$
$$\downarrow$$
$$HBUF$$

This primary increase in hydrogen ion results in both a reduction in plasma HCO_3^- and BUF^- levels, resulting in a reduction in buffer base and base excess of blood and of the ECF.

Metabolic acidosis may also result from a loss of plasma bicarbonate (e.g., diarrhea, excessive loss associated with an ileostomy, and excess renal loss [renal tubular acidosis]) or from the exogenous administration of acetazoamide (Diamox), a carbonic anhydrase inhibitor that blocks the regeneration of bicarbonate in the kidney.

$$CO_2 + H_2O \rightarrow H_2CO_3 \rightarrow H^+ + \downarrow HCO_3^-$$
$$+$$
$$BUF^-$$
$$\downarrow$$
$$HBUF$$

A loss of plasma bicarbonate results in increased hydrogen ion formation. Both HCO_3^- and BUF^- levels are reduced, resulting in a reduction in buffer base and base excess of both blood and ECF. The BEb will show a greater deficit than the true deficit of the ECF as shown by the BEECF.

In patients with metabolic acidosis, evaluating the "anion gap" can be a clue to the presence and cause of the acid–base disturbance. Normally, the difference between the major plasma cation (sodium) and the sum of the major plasma anions (chloride and bicarbonate) is about 10–15 mEq/L. For example:

Cation	Anion
Na^+ = 140 mEq/L	Cl^- = 100 mEq/L
	HCO_3^- = 25 mEq/L
Total = 140 mEq/L	Total = 125 mEq/L

If the difference is greater than 15, the anion gap is increased. This suggests the presence of other circulating anions, as would be seen with diabetic ketoacidosis, lactic acidosis, uremic acidosis, and the

Table 10–8 Causes of Increased and Decreased Anion Gap

CAUSES OF INCREASED ANION GAP

Increased unmeasured anion:
Organic anions: lactate, ketone acids
Inorganic anions: phosphate, sulfate
Proteins: increased albumin
Exogenous anions: salicylate, formate, nitrate, penicillin
Others: paraldehyde, uremia, ethylene glycol, methanol, salicylate poisoning, hyperosmolar hyperglycemic nonketotic coma
Decreased unmeasured cation:
Altered minerals: decreased K, Ca, Mg
Laboratory error

CAUSES OF DECREASED ANION GAP

Increased unmeasured cation:
Altered minerals: Increased K, Ca, Mg
Retention of abnormal cations: IgG, lithium, tromethamine
Protein: decreased albumin
Laboratory error

---

ingestion of methanol, paraldehyde, ethylene glycol, and salicylates. If metabolic acidosis is due to the simple addition of hydrogen ion (e.g., from HCl or NH_4Cl) or the loss of HCO_3^- (e.g., from diarrhea or acetazolamide administration), the anion gap is normal. In assessing a metabolic acidosis condition, looking at the anion gap as well as the serum potassium level, is helpful in identifying the cause of the metabolic acidemia. Table 10–8 identifies those things that can alter the anion gap. Table 10–9 lists various causes of metabolic acidemia, including those that elevate the anion gap and those conditions that are associated with a normal anion gap. Normal anion gap metabolic acidosis can be further classified into conditions commonly associated with hyperkalemic and hypokalemic states.

The anion gap can be increased by (1) decreased unmeasured cations, (2) increased unmeasured anions, or (3) laboratory error. Anion gap caused by unmeasured cations rarely is seen, for only minor changes in these cations become incompatible with life. The most common cause of an increased anion gap is the presence of increased unmeasured anions, such as lactic acid, ketoacids, and acids that accumulate in renal failure.

Bicarbonate therapy should be considered for severe metabolic acidosis. If bicarbonate therapy is desirable, arterial blood gas results can be used as a guideline to therapy. Because venous hypercapnia may worsen with intravenous bicarbonate adminis-

tration (e.g., during CPR), assessing venous values may become more common.

The total deficit in buffer base of the ECF compartment is easily calculated by multiplying BE_{ECF} by the ECF volume. If we assume that the ECF volume is 24% of the body weight in kilograms, the equation is:

$$\text{Deficit in } BE_{ECF} = 0.24 \times \text{wt (kg)} \times BE_{ECF}.$$

For instance, if the weight is 70 kg and $BE_{ECF} = -10$ mEq/L, then

$$\text{deficit in } BE_{ECF} = 0.24 \times 70 \times (-10) = -168 \text{ mEq}.$$

If the acidosis affected only the ECF compartment in the foregoing example, 168 mEq of bicarbonate would completely correct the metabolic deficit of the ECF, and if the $PaCO_2$ were 40 mmHg, the pH would be 7.40. Of course, the acidosis will not involve only the ECF compartment, but will also include the intracellular fluid (ICF) compartment. Ex-

Table 10–9 Causes of Metabolic Acidosis

NORMAL ANION GAP METABOLIC ACIDOSIS

Hyperkalemic Causes
  Acidifying Agents
    Ammonium chloride
    Calcium chloride
    Arginine
    HCl
  Adrenal Deficiency
    Mineralocorticoid deficiency
  Renal Pathology
    Amyloidosis
    Hydronephrosis
    Sickle cell nephropathy
    SLE interstitial nephritis
    Early nonspecific renal failure
Hypokalemic Causes
  Diarrhea
  Ureterosigmoidostomy and malfunctioning ileostomy
  Renal tubular acidosis
  Acetazolamide therapy

ELEVATED ANION GAP METABOLIC ACIDOSIS

Lactic acidosis
Renal failure
Ketoacidosis
Toxins
  Salicylates (overdose)
  Ethylene glycol
  Methanol
  Paraldehyde

---

perience has shown that the total body deficit may be two to four times the ECF deficit, and it has been observed to be as high as eight times the ECF deficit. If there are continuing losses of bicarbonate, these must also be replaced.

If one wanted to return the pH to 7.40 (assuming the PCO_2 remained the same), then about one-half of the calculated deficit in BE_{ECF} would be infused intravenously, a blood gas sample would be drawn in about 20 minutes, the new BE_{ECF} would be calculated, and about one-half of the new deficit would again be given intravenously. This approach could be continued until the desired pH is achieved.

In diabetic ketoacidosis with a pH below 7.1, it may be desirable to give enough bicarbonate to raise the pH to at least 7.1. This objective will require only comparatively small amounts of bicarbonate. In the treatment of severe diabetic ketoacidosis, large fluid volumes are administered. These large volumes will produce dilutional acidosis (diluting the bicarbonate concentration, whereas the PCO_2 remains constant or may even rise). Overtreatment with bicarbonate in diabetic ketoacidosis is undesirable.

Principles of bicarbonate therapy in lactic acidosis are similar to those in ketoacidosis. There is evidence that vigorous bicarbonate therapy may make lactic acidosis worse (as well as worsening venous hypercapnia).

Metabolic Alkalosis

The loss of hydrogen ion by nasogastric suction or excessive diuretic and steroid therapy results in metabolic alkalosis.

$$CO_2 + H_2O \rightarrow H_2CO_3 \rightarrow \downarrow H^+ + HCO_3^-$$
$$+$$
$$BUF^-$$
$$\uparrow$$
$$HBUF$$

Both plasma bicarbonate and BUF^- are increased, resulting in an increase in buffer base and base excess of both blood and ECF.

Hypokalemia can cause and perpetuate metabolic alkalosis. Because sodium reabsorption in the distal convoluted tubule and collecting duct system can be accomplished by excretion of either hydrogen or potassium ions into the urine in exchange for sodium ions, a deficit of potassium means that the hydrogen ions are used mainly for this sodium reclamation, resulting in continuous bicarbonate regeneration (see Fig. 10–5).

An increased plasma bicarbonate associated with injudicious use of exogenous intravenous or oral bicarbonate may also result in metabolic alkalosis.

$$CO_2 + H_2O \leftarrow H_2CO_3 \leftarrow H^+ + \uparrow HCO_3^-$$
$$+$$
$$BUF^-$$
$$\uparrow$$
$$HBUF$$

The increased HCO_3^- is associated with an increased BUF^-, resulting in an increase in the buffer

Table 10–10 Common Causes of Acid–Base Disturbances

RESPIRATORY ACIDOSIS

Overall hypoventilation
  Pickwickian syndrome
  Drug overdose
  Head injury
  Neuromuscular disturbance
    (*e.g.*, myasthenia gravis)
  Kyphoscoliosis
Chronic obstructive lung disease
Pulmonary edema, severe

RESPIRATORY ALKALOSIS

Neurogenic hyperventilation
Interstitial lung diseases
Pulmonary embolism
Acute asthma
Hyperventilation syndrome

METABOLIC ACIDOSIS

Increased metabolic formation of acids
  Diabetic ketoacidosis
  Uremic acidosis
  Lactic acidosis
Exogenous addition of acids
  Ammonium chloride
  Hydrochloric acid
Loss of bicarbonate
  Diarrhea
  Ileostomy loss
  Renal tubular acidosis
Exogenous administration of acetazolamide (Diamox)

METABOLIC ALKALOSIS

Loss of hydrogen ion
  Nasogastric suction
  Persistent vomiting
  Diuretic therapy
  Steroid therapy
Exogenous bicarbonate

---

base and base excess of both blood and ECF. The BEb will show a greater excess than the true excess of the ECF, as shown by the BEECF. Table 10–10 provides a list of acid–base disturbances.

INTERPRETATION OF ACID–BASE DISORDERS

In attempting to properly interpret acid–base disorders, one must remember the basic relationship implied in the Henderson–Hasselbalch equation:

$$pH \sim \frac{HCO_3^-}{PCO_2} \sim \frac{\text{Metabolic component}}{\text{Respiratory component}}$$

Two of the three factors in this relationship must be known to evaluate accurately the acid–base disturbance.

When interpreting acid–base data, one should look at the pH to determine whether acidemia or alkalemia is present, remembering that a normal pH does not rule out an acid–base disorder. If the pH is in the normal range (7.35 to 7.45), *and the* $PaCO_2$ and HCO_3^- are in their normal ranges, then the acid–base status is normal. If the pH is below 7.35, then an acidemia exists. If the pH is above 7.45, an alkalemia exists.

When the pH is outside of the normal range, the cause must be determined. One must then look at the $PaCO_2$ value to see if it is above or below its normal range (35 to 45 mmHg). The same must then be done with the HCO_3^- value to see if it is above or below its normal range (22 to 26 mEq). A look to see which parameter is out of the normal range will reveal the system responsible. For example, if the pH is on the acid side (below 7.35) and the $PaCO_2$ is greater than 45 mmHg, a respiratory acidemia exists. If the kidneys are functioning normally, they will start retaining bicarbonate to offset the respiratory acid (CO_2). If the bicarbonate was still in the normal range when the ABG was obtained, the respiratory condition would be identified as an *acute* respiratory acidemia. However, if the pH was in the normal range with the $PaCO_2$ above 45 mmHg, most likely the body has *compensated* for the hypercapnia. Because the kidney takes a while to respond to changes in CO_2, this second condition would be termed *chronic* or compensated respiratory acidemia. When the pH is in the normal range, but the carbon dioxide and bicarbonate are not, the primary problem can usually be determined by noting the direction the pH has moved from 7.4. Any value above 7.4 is *toward* the alkaline side. Any value below a pH of 7.4 is *toward* the acid side. Because the body will not overcompensate, finding the pH on the acid side (below 7.4) will suggest that the

primary problem is "acid." Since in our chronic respiratory acidosis example the CO_2 is also on the "acid side" (greater than 45 mmHg), the respiratory system is likely responsible for the primary problem. Remember that large changes of pH (from normal) suggest an *acute* process. Small changes of pH, with large deviations in HCO_3^- or PCO_2 suggest a *chronic* process.

Not all acid–base disturbances are as straightforward as the foregoing example of the simple disorder. The use of an acid–base nomogram or acid–base rules of thumb (Table 10–11) can help one decide whether a given change in CO_2 or HCO_3^- alone can account for the change in pH.

When evaluating the metabolic component, the plasma bicarbonate is what one should look at first. However, because there is a small respiratory component to the plasma bicarbonate, the T_{40} bicarbonate and BEECF more accurately reflect the metabolic component of the plasma bicarbonate, (especially in the presence of hypercapnia), with the BEECF being the more accurate of the two.

One should decide whether "compensation" is present. If a primary respiratory acidosis has occurred, for example, within hours the intracellular buffers will contribute to an increase of plasma bicarbonate and BEECF. Also within hours, the kidney will begin to alter the plasma bicarbonate in an attempt to compensate for the respiratory disturbance. The kidney response is slow, requiring 72 hours or more for maximal effect. If a primary meta-

Table 10–11   Rules of Thumb to Determine If Simple or Mixed Acid–Base Disorder Exists

CONDITION	PaCO₂ (mmHg)	HCO₃⁻ (mEq)
Acute hypercapnia	↑ 10	↑ 1
Chronic hypercapnia	↑ 10	↑ 3.5
Acute hypocapnia	↓ 10	↓ 2
Chronic hypocapnia	↓ 10	↓ 4.5
Metabolic acidosis	↓ 12	↓ 10
$PaCO_2 = (1.54 \times HCO_3^-) + 8.36*$		
Metabolic alkalosis	↑ 6	↑ 10

The changes (increase or decrease as indicated by the arrows) are from normal values, PaCO₂ of 40 mmHg and HCO₃⁻ of 24 mEq/L. For a "simple" disorder to exist, a given change in PaCO₂ will result in the predicted change in HCO₃⁻. If the suggested change is not present, then a mixed acid–base disorder is very likely.
*This formula can be used for determining the expected PaCO₂ for a "simple" metabolic acidosis.

bolic disorder occurs, within minutes the lungs will begin to compensate for the metabolic disorder by altering alveolar ventilation to change the $PaCO_2$. It may take up to 12 hours for the lungs to compensate maximally. In the past, the presence or absence of compensation has been categorized as follows:

1. *Uncompensated.* The presence of an abnormal pH owing to deviation of one component, with the other component still within normal limits (e.g., presence of metabolic acidosis with a $PaCO_2$ still within the normal range).
2. *Partially compensated.* Deviation of one component with the other component changing appropriately to compensate for the acid–base disorder. However, the pH is still abnormal.
3. *Completely compensated.* Deviation of one component with an appropriate change of the other component so that pH has been restored to normal (i.e., between 7.35 and 7.45).

It is now well recognized that with a *major* deviation from normal of one component, it is not possible for the other component to restore the pH to normal; for example, with severe diabetic ketoacidosis, it is impossible for the lungs to increase alveolar ventilation sufficiently to reduce the $PaCO_2$ to the extent by which pH would be restored to normal. Also, in the presence of severe chronic respiratory failure, the normal kidney will not regenerate enough bicarbonate to return the pH to the normal range.

Because physiologic compensatory mechanisms are unable to compensate fully (i.e., return the pH to normal) for *major* deviations in acid–base status, it has become apparent that determining the extent to which one could maximally return the pH toward normal would be more appropriate. Studies in animals and humans have helped determine the degree of compensation that can be expected for any given disturbance.

One way of evaluating the compensation is to consider the acid–base data from such studies. In a group of 100 subjects, the results are distributed in a bell-shaped curve. It has become accepted to compare a patient's acid–base data with the middle 95% of the curve, recognizing that 2.5% of the subjects' data will be above and 2.5% below the mid-95% of subjects. These data have been developed

into 95% *confidence-limit bands* that aid in the proper interpretation of various acid–base disturbances. These bands have been developed for both acute and chronic acid–base disturbances. In the presence of acute hypercapnia, for example, one can determine the appropriate pH, plasma bicarbonate, and BEb (see Fig. 10–8) or BEECF (Fig. 10–9) for any given $PaCO_2$. In the presence of chronic hypercapnia, one can determine the expected pH to be achieved for a certain level of $PaCO_2$ (see Fig. 10–9); for example, a $PaCO_2$ of 85 mmHg and a pH of 7.38, under the old acid–base terminology, would be interpreted as a completely compensated respiratory acidosis. Examination of this point on Figure 10–9 reveals, however, that it lies considerably to the right of the 95% confidence band for chronic hypercapnia, indicating that the level of plasma bicarbonate and BEECF is inappropriately high for this $PaCO_2$ and that the patient has a chronic respiratory acidosis with a *superimposed* metabolic alkalosis.

The proper terminology for compensation using 95% confidence-limit bands would express the compensation as "maximal" or "less than maximal" (see Fig. 10–9 for further examples of 95% confidence-limit bands). It is impossible to interpret acid–base disorders accurately and completely without a knowledge of (1) the duration of the acid–base disturbance (observation of serial arterial blood gas values are often helpful for this); (2) the patient's clinical condition (i.e., whether disorders are present that could lead to respiratory or metabolic acid–base disturbances), and (3) the electrolytes (i.e., anion gap).

Occasionally one will have a "combined" or "mixed" acid–base disturbance; for example, if changes in both the PCO_2 and plasma bicarbonate would result in acidosis, the patient would have a combined respiratory and metabolic acidosis. Mixed respiratory and metabolic alkalosis may also occur. (See Table 10–10 for some of the causes of acid–base disturbances.) Familiarity with the vari-

Table 10–12 Summary of Arterial Blood Gas Interpretation Guidelines

---

1. Evaluate oxygenation status
2. Check pH, then $PaCO_2$ and HCO_3^-
3. Check if ABG data is consistent with a simple disorder (rules of thumb or nomogram)
4. Check anion gap, if a metabolic acidemia is present
5. Compare interpretation with clinical history

Siggaard-Andersen Acid-Base Chart

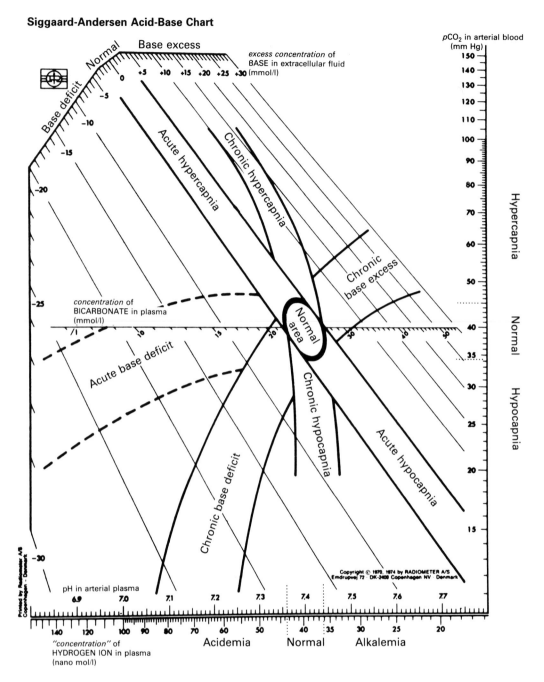

Figure 10—9. Depiction of 95% confidence-limit bands by Siggaard-Andersen. (Reproduced by permission of O. Siggaard-Andersen and Radiometer A/S, Copenhagen, 1971.) Note that extracellular fluid base excess is depicted on this "in vivo" nomogram.[17] The BEecf remains normal with acute hypercapnia, whereas the blood base excess, depicted in Figure 10–8 decreases.

ous causes of altered acid–base balance will facilitate proper treatment. To facilitate rapid bedside interpretation of acid–base disturbance when an acid–base nomogram is not available, Table 10–11 lists the rules of thumb for determining if a simple acid–base disorder or mixed disorder exists. If the PCO_2 or the bicarbonate values follow the rules listed in Table 10–11, then a simple (unmixed) disorder exists. If the carbon dioxide or bicarbonate values do not follow the rules, then there is a mixed acid–base disturbance present.

Table 10–12 summarizes the steps necessary for ABG interpretation. It is important to develop the habit of analyzing each blood gas in a systematic way so as not to miss important diagnostic information.

For a discussion of the methodology of arterial blood gas analysis, see Appendix A. For useful guidelines relating to oxygenation and acid–base disorders, see Appendix B. For examples of the proper interpretation of arterial blood gas data, see Appendix D.

REFERENCES

1. Allen EV: Thromboangiitis obliterans: Methods of diagnosis of chronic occlusive arterial lesions distal to the wrist with illustrative cases. Am J Med Sci 178:237, 1929
2. Greenhow DE: Incorrect performance of Allen's test—ulnar artery flow erroneously presumed inadequate. Anesthesiology 37:356, 1974
3. Winkler JB, Huntington CG, Wells DE, Befeler B: Influence of syringe material on arterial blood gas determinations. Chest 66:518, 1974
4. Sorbini CA, Grassi V, Solinas E: Arterial oxygen tension in relation to age in healthy sujects. Respiration 25:3, 1968
5. Mellemgaard K: The alveolar–arterial oxygen difference: Its size and components in normal man. Acta Physiol Scand 67:10, 1966
6. Gilbert F, Keighley JF: The arterial/alveolar oxygen tension ratio: An index of gas exchange applicable to varying inspired oxygen concentrations. Am Rev Respir Dis 109:142, 1974
7. Perutz MF: Hemoglobin structure and respiratory transport. Sci Am 239(6):92–120, 1978
8. Shafer AW, Tague LL, Welch MH et al: 2,3-Diphosphoglycerate in red cells stored in acid–citrate–dextrose and citrate–phosphate–dextrose: Implications regarding delivery of oxygen. J Lab Clin Med 77:430, 1971
9. Aberman A, Cavanilles JM, Weil MH et al: Blood P_{50} calculated from a single measurement of pH , PO_2, and SO_2. J Appl Physiol 38:171, 1975
10. Collier CR, Hackney JD, Mohler JG: Use of extracellular base excess in diagnosis of acid–base disorders: A conceptual approach. Chest 61:6S 1972
11. Kelman GR: Computer program for the production of O_2–CO_2 diagrams. Respir Physiol 4:260, 1968
12. Suter PM, Fairley HB, Isenberg MD: Optimum end-expiratory airway pressure in patients in acute pulmonary failure. N Engl J Med 292:284, 1975
13. Woodbury CW: Body acid–base state and its regulation. In Ruch TC, Patton HD (eds): Physiology and Biophysics, Circulation, Respiration and Fluid Balance, 20th ed. Philadelphia, WB Saunders, 1974, pp 480–524
14. Armstrong BW, Mohler JG, Jung RC et al: The in vivo carbon dioxide titration curve. Lancet 1:759, 1966
15. Armstrong BW: Rapid changes in $PaCO_2$ and HCO_3. Respir Care 21:808, 1976
16. Collier CR: Oxygen affinity of human blood in presence of carbon monoxide. J Appl Physiol 40:487, 1976
17. Siggaard-Andersen O: An acid–base chart for arterial blood with normal and pathophysiological reference areas. Scand J Clin Lab Invest 27:239, 1971
18. Weil MW, Rackow EC, Trevino R, Grundler W, Falk JL, Griffel MI: Difference in acid–base state between venous and arterial blood during cardiopulmonary resuscitation. N Engl J Med 315:153, 1986
19. Adrogue HJ, Rashad MN, Gorin AB, Yacoub J, Madias NE: Assessing acid–base status in circulatory failure: Differences between arterial and central venous blood. N Engl J Med 320:1312, 1989
20. Adrogue HJ, Rashad MN, Gorin AB, Yacoub J, Madias NE: Spurious assessment of systemic acid–base status by arterial sampling in circulatory failure: The case for central venous blood gases. Proc Am Soc Nephrol 21:66A, 1988
21. Astrand PO, Rodahl K: Textbook of Work Physiology. New York, McGraw-Hill, 1970, p 216

ELEVEN

History and Physical Examination of the Respiratory Patient

Robert L. Wilkins
John E. Hodgkin

This chapter will serve as a foundation on which clinicians can build effective bedside patient assessment skills. The careful observation and documentation of changes in a patient's signs and symptoms often provide the initial diagnostic clues. Good bedside examination techniques also can promote the development of rapport between patients and clinicians and offer an inexpensive and noninvasive way for clinicians to collect reliable data that will help guide them in determining the appropriate course for the remaining assessment process and establishing an effective treatment plan.

Good assessment techniques apply not only to the care of patients in acute care facilities, but also to those in nursing homes and in home care settings in which laboratory and x-ray data are not readily available. Such skills are valuable both to physicians making the initial diagnosis of the patient and to respiratory care practitioners formulating and evaluating patient care plans.

Some clinicians rely almost entirely on arterial blood gas measurements, chest x-rays, and pulmonary function data to evaluate a patient's respiratory function status. Over-reliance on these assessment parameters, however, can cause the clinician to overlook important findings that would be revealed by questioning and examining patients carefully.

INTERVIEWING AND THE MEDICAL HISTORY

With the onset of respiratory disease, patients typically have one or more characteristic symptoms. The initial patient interview should focus on identifying these symptoms and gathering pertinent details. Once treatment has begun, clinicians should interview patients periodically to determine how the respiratory care plan is affecting the patient's symptoms.

GUIDELINES FOR INTERVIEWING

With experience, clinicians develop their own interviewing styles. Beginners, however, are best advised to begin with a traditional approach.

Provide Privacy and Quiet

The examiner always should conduct the interview in a quiet environment in which the patient feels comfortable. All noisy distractions, such as radios or televisions, should be turned off. Many people are uneasy about discussing their symptoms in front of others; any guests, therefore, should courteously be asked to step out of the room. In a semiprivate room or ward, drawing the curtain around the patient's bed can help put the patient more at ease.

211

Introduction and Explanation of Purpose

Examiners should begin all patient interviews by introducing themselves briefly and explaining the reason for the interview and examination. A friendly, natural introduction is both polite and professional, and can reduce a patient's anxiety considerably and help establish rapport.

Having concrete goals for the interview helps clinicians get directly to the point and avoid wasting time with vague questions. Interviewers without a specific purpose may not be sure what to ask and, therefore, often miss important facts about changes in the patient's symptoms.

Adjust the Length of the Interview to the Patient's Condition

Patients who are short of breath or in pain are not prepared to answer numerous or lengthy questions. In such situations interviews should be brief, tactful, and direct. Later, when the patient is more stable and comfortable, examiners can probe for the details surrounding the onset of symptoms.

Listen and Observe Carefully

The ability to listen carefully is a true art and a vital clinical skill. Like all arts, however, listening requires effort, concentration, and practice. Nevertheless, clinicians who make the effort to focus all their attention on their patients' words will find that good listening skills often make the difference between whether a crucial detail is documented or overlooked.

Letting patients talk and encouraging them by nodding and saying, "yes," "go on," and the like can help draw out important details. When necessary, the examiner should check for understanding by paraphrasing and summarizing: "So what you're saying is. . ."

An important part of listening is expressing genuine concern for patients. One way concern can be conveyed is by establishing eye contact. This can give patients the impression that their words and feelings are important. Interviewers focusing on equipment or other activities in the room usually make only brief eye contact with patients who, as a result, may feel their comments are inconsequential.

Careful observation of patients' facial expressions and body language during the interview can help examiners identify their mood, mental state, and ability to understand and respond to questions. For instance, if patients are disturbed or confused by a question, their gestures and expressions will convey this immediately. Inspection of the patient will be discussed in more detail under physical examination.

Word Questions Carefully

Questions worded in a way that leads the patient to feel a certain answer is expected are termed "leading" or "biased" questions. Inexperienced examiners often use leading questions and, thereby, severely limit the value of the information obtained. For example, "Is your shortness of breath better now?" may give the patient the impression that a "yes" answer is expected and a "no" answer would disappoint the interviewer. Because many patients want to cooperate, they may answer "yes" even if they are unsure. A better way to ask the question is "How is your breathing?" This conveys no expectations to the patient and, therefore, should provide more reliable data.

Open-ended questions or statements are worded in such a way that the patient must provide more than a simple yes or no answer. This kind of question encourages patients to talk more freely and, therefore, is appropriate for the initial interview when the examiner is attempting to identify all the patient's symptoms and record pertinent details surrounding each one. Open-ended questions require organized narrative answers and, consequently, are especially valuable when assessing a patient's level of intelligence and mental alertness. An example of an open-ended question is: "Tell me how your breathing has been lately."

A disadvantage to open-ended questions is that they require more time to answer. They also may cause patients to digress. Accordingly, open-ended questions should not be used heavily during brief interviews when evaluating the patient's response to therapy.

Closed-end or direct questions require a plain one- or two-word answer. For example, "Is your cough productive?" can elicit only a "yes" or a "no." Direct questions are good for brief interviews such as those before and after a treatment, because they help prevent patients from rambling. Direct questions should not be used in a rapid-fire manner because they can overwhelm the patient and may give the impression that the interviewer is in a hurry.

Use a Common Language

Interviewers should speak clearly, simply, and confidently, using familiar words and expressions. During the interview, terms and phrases such as "COPD" or "dyspnea" that are likely to be alien to patients should be avoided. Many patients are insecure about asking for definitions of terms they do not understand because they feel this makes them look ignorant. As a result, they may misunderstand the question and, therefore, give inaccurate answers. A skilled examiner will assess the patients' level of education and familiarity with their disease and choose appropriate terminology.

SYMPTOMS OF RESPIRATORY DISEASE

Patients with respiratory disease may complain of a variety of symptoms, including shortness of breath, cough, sputum, and chest pain. Clinicians are responsible for knowing the potential causes and characteristics of these symptoms. This knowledge will help them choose the appropriate questions to ask and, thereby, lead to a more accurate assessment.

Shortness of Breath

When patients are short of breath or complain of difficult breathing, this is known as *dyspnea*. Dyspnea is a normal condition following exercise, but a sudden increase in breathlessness or a sudden decrease in tolerance for exercise is an important finding that is common in patients with respiratory disease.

Dyspnea is frequently caused by the patient's sensing that the work of breathing is excessive for the level of exertion. Diseases that cause an increase in the work of breathing frequently cause dyspnea. Elevation of airway resistance, such as occurs with bronchospasm, and decreases in lung or chest wall compliance, such as occurs with pneumonia, will cause an increase in the work of breathing. In addition, conditions that increase the drive to breathe, such as hypoxemia or acidosis, may cause or add to the patient's sensation of breathlessness. Table 11–1 lists the potential causes for dyspnea.

An increase in the awareness of normal breathing also may cause the patient to feel breathless. This is usually the result of anxiety. In such cases, the patient's breathing is often irregular with frequent sighs, or it may be associated with hyperventilation.

Table 11–1 Potential Causes of Dyspnea

PULMONARY DISORDER

Airway
  Laryngospasm
  Bronchospasm
  Excessive secretions
  Tumor
  Foreign body
Parenchyma
  Pneumonia
  Pulmonary edema
  Tumor
  Fibrosis
Vasculature
  Thromboemboli
  Fat emboli
  Foreign body
  Tumor
Pleura
  Effusion (fluid, blood, chyle)
  Air (pneumothorax)
  Fibrosis
  Tumor
Respiratory musculature
  Phrenic nerve dysfunction
  Systemic neuromuscular disease
  Nutritional depletion
Thoracic cage
  Kyphosis
  Scoliosis
  Kyphoscoliosis
  Flail chest
Miscellaneous
  Anemia
  Increased metabolic rate
  Breathing carbon monoxide
  Breathing at high altitude
  Psychogenic

The details surrounding the dyspnea are important to identify. Dyspnea occurring after lying supine or prone is termed *orthopnea*. This is common in patients with congestive heart failure (CHF). Dyspnea that occurs upon sitting or standing is called *platypnea*; it is commonly seen in patients with chronic obstructive pulmonary disease (COPD) and in post-pneumonectomy patients. It is believed to be the result of sudden alterations in $\dot{V}/\dot{Q}$ occurring with positional changes.[1,2]

Paroxysmal nocturnal dyspnea (PND) is the sudden onset of dyspnea occurring while a patient is sleeping. This complaint is common in patients with CHF and often is relieved when the patient sits up. A similar pattern of dyspnea is seen in patients with COPD. As pulmonary secretions collect in the airways during sleep, the patient's breathing becomes more difficult. With COPD, the shortness of breath may improve quickly following expectoration of the secretions or inhalation of bronchodilator, whereas with CHF the patient usually has to sit up for 30 to 60 minutes before the dyspnea improves.

Changes in the patient's dyspnea will vary from case to case. In asthmatics, dyspnea will often resolve quickly with the inhalation of bronchodilators that reduce airways resistance. In patients with permanent changes in lung pathology, such as occur with emphysema or pulmonary fibrosis, dyspnea may respond poorly or only partially to treatment.

Cough

Cough is one of the most frequent complaints of patients with respiratory disease. The sudden, forceful expulsion of air from the lungs is helpful in clearing airway secretions and other material from the tracheobronchial tree. Coughing also protects the lungs against aspiration. Coughing may be induced by inflammatory, mechanical, thermal (breathing hot or cold air), or chemical stimulation of the cough receptors lining the airways.

Whenever possible, the effectiveness of the patient's cough should be evaluated. A weak or ineffective cough may result from a poor inspiratory effort, weak accessory respiratory muscles, elevated airways resistance, or reduced elastic recoil of the lung, as in emphysema. Strategies such as improving the patient's inspiratory effort with coaching and administering appropriate pain medication to patients after surgery can enhance the cough's effectiveness.

The most frequent cause of cough is a viral respiratory infection. In such cases the cough initially is usually dry, acute, and nonproductive. Chronic cough is common with chronic bronchitis. Patients with chronic coughing may cough so habitually that they become unaware of the frequency. Questioning the patient's family members, therefore, may reveal useful information. With chronic bronchitis, the cough often is productive, especially in the morning upon rising. Asthmatics often complain of cough, either in conjunction with dyspnea or as the sole complaint.[3,4]

Sputum Production

Secretions from the tracheobronchial tree are known as *phlegm*. When phlegm passes through the oral cavity during expectoration, it may be altered by secretions from the mouth, nose, sinuses, or pharynx and then is called *sputum*. When pa-

Table 11—2 Disease States Associated with Abnormal Gross Appearance of the Sputum*

TYPE OF SPUTUM	LUNG ABSCESS	ACUTE BRONCHITIS	CHRONIC BRONCHITIS	PNEUMONIA	PULMONARY EDEMA	BRONCHIECTASIS	TUBERCULOSIS	LUNG CANCER	PULMONARY INFARCTION	BRONCHIAL ASTHMA	CYSTIC FIBROSIS	ASPIRATION PNEUMONIA
Mucoid (white or clear)			X							X		
Mucopurulent		X	X								X	
Purulent (yellow or green)	X	X		X		X						X
Fetid	X					X					X	X
Bloody		X		X	X	X	X	X	X			
Frothy, sometimes pink					X							

* The most characteristic sputum appearance, consistency, and odor are listed.

tients complain of a productive cough, the duration of sputum production, character of the sputum, and the presence or absence of blood should be determined.

A variety of terms may be used to describe sputum. *Mucoid* sputum is clear, thin, and elastic in consistency and is common in diseases that inflame or irritate the airways. *Purulent* sputum is yellow-green in color and usually more viscous, containing numerous pus cells, generally signaling the presence of bacterial infection. Staining yellow-green sputum can help in determining the source of the problem; with bacterial infection neutrophils are prevalent, whereas with allergy eosinophils predominate. Patients with chronic sputum production of mucoid or, occasionally, purulent sputum often have chronic bronchitis. *Fetid* sputum is foul-smelling and often occurs in large quantities as a result of airway infections. The chronic production of large amounts of purulent, occasionally blood-streaked, and fetid sputum suggests bronchiectasis (Table 11–2).

The expectoration of blood-tinged or bloody sputum is termed *hemoptysis.* It is common not only in bronchiectasis but also in pneumonia, pulmonary emboli, and bronchial carcinoma. Bronchitis also can cause blood-streaked sputum; the production of frankly bloody sputum is more often seen in pulmonary infarction, bronchial carcinoma, and tuberculosis (see Table 11–2).

Chest Pain

Chest pain is another common complaint of patients with respiratory disease. Respiratory disease may cause chest pain that arises from the chest wall or originates in the viscera and is conducted through the afferent fibers of the autonomic nervous system.

Chest wall pain is usually sharp and well localized in the lateral or posterior chest. When such pain increases with deep inspiration or coughing, it is called *pleuritic* pain. Pleuritic pain is caused by irritation, inflammation, or trauma of the parietal pleura: it is common with pneumonia, chest trauma, spontaneous pneumothorax, pulmonary embolism, and pulmonary malignancies.

Visceral pain is poorly localized but often described as substernal or central, and may radiate to the arm, back, or jaw. This type of pain occurs with diseases of the heart (myocardial ischemia) and aorta and the esophagus, as well as with neoplasms of the major bronchi and tumors of the mediastinum.

EXAMINATION

Patients are examined to identify the physical signs of disease. Once a patient enters treatment, examination is done to evaluate how the signs change in response to therapy. Before examining patients, examiners should review the medical history to know what to look for.

ASSESSMENT OF THE VITAL SIGNS

Assessment of body temperature, respiratory rate, pulse rate, and blood pressure are the most commonly performed clinical measurements made by health care practitioners. Assessment of the vital signs represents a simple and noninvasive way to determine patients' general condition and evaluate their response to therapy.

Body Temperature

Normal body temperature varies somewhat among healthy persons but generally is approximately 98.6° F (37° C), with a daily variation of 1° to 2° F (0.5° C). This is the optimal range of temperature for the metabolic function of all cells. When body temperature varies markedly from the normal range, the metabolic rate and the demands on the cardiopulmonary system change commensurately. For example, as body temperature elevates the metabolic rate increases, resulting in more oxygen consumption and carbon dioxide production at the cellular level. A general rule-of-thumb is that for every 1° C elevation of body temperature, oxygen consumption increases about 10%. The cardiopulmonary system must work harder to meet the additional demand, generally causing a more rapid pulse and breathing rate. Patients with a diseased cardiopulmonary system may tolerate this additional demand poorly.

Body temperature can rise in response to strenuous exercise or disease. An elevated body temperature caused by disease is called *fever*, and the patient is said to be *febrile*. Febrile conditions are common in patients with viral or bacterial infections. The fever may be classified as continuous, intermittent, or remittent, according to its pattern over 24 hours. Intermittent fevers have noticeable peaks and drops, with the decreases reaching normal or below. This pattern is common in patients with pyrogenic infections. Remittent fevers show marked spikes, but do not return to normal levels between the peaks.

Hypothermia is present when the patient's body temperature is below the normal range. Although hypothermia is uncommon, it may occur in patients suffering from cold exposure and in patients with a damaged hypothalamus. Hypothermia reduces the metabolic demands of the body, lessening the need for gas exchange.

Body temperature is most often measured at one of three sites: mouth, axilla, or rectum. Compared with oral temperature, rectal temperature is normally about 1° F higher and axillary temperature is 1° F lower. The oral temperature registration is acceptable for the awake, adult patient and is a reliable site, even if patients are receiving oxygen by simple mask or nasal cannula.[5,6] In such situations, therefore, it is unnecessary to remove the oxygen mask or to take the temperature rectally. If heated or cool aerosol is being delivered to the patient by face mask, the oral temperature reading can be altered slightly.[7] The range of fluctuation, however, is probably too small to affect clinical decisions. The oral site should not be used in infants, comatose patients, or orally intubated patients.

Pulse Rate

The normal resting pulse rate ranges from 60 to 100 beats per minute in the adult (Table 11–3). Tachycardia is a common finding in patients with respiratory disease because an increase in the heart rate is an important compensatory mechanism for hypoxemia. Tachycardia is an attempt by the body to maintain adequate oxygen delivery to the tissues in the presence of hypoxemia. Tachycardia also may occur with anxiety, anemia, hypotension, fever, or as a side effect of certain medications, such as bronchodilators.

The pulse rate is most often assessed at the radial artery but may be more reliably measured at more central sites, such as the carotid, when cardiac output is reduced. The pulse should be assessed for strength and rhythm as well as rate. Weak peripheral pulses usually are a sign of diminished cardiac output. The presence of normal radial artery pulses with weak pulses in the ankles and feet is suggestive of atherosclerotic vascular disease in the lower extremities.

Respiratory Rate

The normal adult breathing rate at rest is 10 to 16 breaths per minute. An increase in the breathing rate, termed *tachypnea*, is common with exercise, fever, acidosis, hypoxemia, anxiety, or pain. *Bradypnea*, a reduced respiratory rate, is uncommon but may occur with hypothermia, head injuries, and drug overdose.

Patients should be unaware that the respiratory rate is being counted because their awareness may cause them to alter their breathing rate, thereby producing an invalid result. Counting the respiratory rate immediately after evaluating the pulse, while maintaining the fingers on the radial artery, can be a useful method because patients will think the pulse is still being counted.

Although it is useful to determine the respiratory rate, it should be remembered that the rate may be normal in the presence of respiratory disease. For example, the dead space–to–tidal volume ratio may be significantly increased in COPD patients, with a normal respiratory rate.

Blood Pressure

The force exerted by the blood against the wall of the artery as the heart contracts and relaxes is the arterial blood pressure. Systolic blood pressure is the peak force generated when the left ventricle contracts; diastolic arterial pressure is the force when the left ventricle is relaxed. The difference

Table 11–3   Normal Ranges for the Vital Signs

VITAL SIGN	NEWBORN	ADULT
Pulse rate	110–160/min	60–100/min
Respiratory rate	30–60/min	10–16/min
Body temperature	36.5–37.5° C	36.5–37.5° C
Blood pressure		
Systolic	50–70 mmHg	95–140 mmHg
Diastolic	30–50 mmHg	60–90 mmHg
Mean	38–52 mmHg	80–100 mmHg
Pulse pressure	15–25 mmHg	35–50 mmHg

between systolic and diastolic pressure is the pulse pressure.

Normal systolic arterial pressure ranges from 95 to 140 mmHg; normal diastolic pressure ranges from 60 to 90 mmHg (see Table 11–3). Normal pulse pressure is 35 to 50 mmHg. Mean arterial pressure is estimated by dividing the pulse pressure by 3 and adding this value to the diastolic pressure. The arterial blood pressure is determined by the force of the left ventricular contraction, the peripheral vascular resistance, and the blood volume.

Abnormally low blood pressure (hypotension) may be caused by poor left ventricular function, low vascular resistance, or an inadequate blood volume. Hypotension is said to be present when the blood pressure falls below 95/60 mmHg. Decreased regional blood flow is associated with dizziness, visual blurring, sweating, and occasionally syncope. Hypotension may indicate inadequate cardiac output, resulting in compromised tissue oxygenation. Further investigation is warranted when hypotension is present.

Hypertension is present when the blood pressure exceeds 140/90 mmHg. It occurs when elevated peripheral vascular resistance is present and causes a significant increase in the heart's work load. Hypertensive patients may complain of headache or blurred vision.

Because the arterial blood pressure provides a general indication of the patient's hemodynamic status, it is a popular parameter among clinicians. Blood pressure measurements, however, do not correlate closely with blood flow and, therefore, are not necessarily good indicators of cardiac output. In fact, normal blood pressure can occur simultaneously with poor cardiac output.

Arterial blood pressure is known to fluctuate physiologically with the respiratory cycle, falling during inspiration and rising during expiration. Normally, the fall in arterial pressure corresponds with inspiration ranges from 2 to 8 mmHg. One of the most common explanations for this phenomenon is that inspiration leads to a pooling of blood in the pulmonic vasculature and an increase in venous return.[8] The former effect predominates, causing a decrease in left ventricular output and, thereby, a decrease in arterial pressure. Further, it is proposed that the decrease in intrathoracic pressure occurring with inspiration is transmitted to the aorta, thus lowering systolic pressure temporarily. An exaggeration of this normal fall in systolic blood pressure occurring with inspiration is called *pulsus paradoxus*. This phenomenon frequently occurs when the breathing efforts increase as a result of, for example, severe airways obstruction associated with acute asthma.[9] In such cases the drop in systolic pressure with inspiration may exceed the upper limits of normal (8 to 10 mmHg), indicating that respiratory effects on hemodynamics are more intense than normal. When pulsus paradoxus is present, quantification of its degree should be documented, along with the patient's ventilatory status. Cardiac tamponade associated with pericardial effusion is another common cause of pulsus paradoxus.

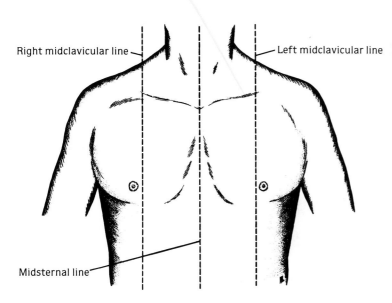

Right midclavicular line

Left midclavicular line

Midsternal line

Figure 11–1. Imaginary lines on anterior chest wall. (Reproduced by permission from Wilkins RL, Sheldon RL, Krider SJ: Clinical assessment in respiratory care. St Louis, CV Mosby, 1985)

LUNG TOPOGRAPHY

Clinicians can more accurately describe the location of abnormalities in the chest when they have a good working knowledge of chest topography (surface) landmarks and specific structures, such as lung borders and fissures.

Imaginary Lines

For reference, several vertical, imaginary lines are used. On the anterior chest, the midsternal line divides the anterior chest into two equal halves (Fig. 11–1). The left and right midclavicular lines parallel the midsternal line and run downward from the midpoints of the left and right clavicles, respectively.

The lateral chest is divided in half by the midaxillary line. The anterior axillary line parallels the midaxillary line and runs along the anteriolateral aspect of the chest. The posteroaxillary line runs vertically along the posterolateral chest (Fig. 11–2).

On the posterior chest wall three vertical lines are recognized: the midspinal and the left and right midscapular lines. The midspinal line runs down the spinal column, dividing the posterior chest into two equal halves. The midscapular lines parallel

Figure 11—2. Imaginary lines on lateral chest wall. (Reproduced by permission from Wilkins RL, Sheldon RL, Krider SJ: Clinical assessment in respiratory care. St. Louis, CV Mosby, 1985)

the midspinal line and run down through the middle of the scapulae (Fig. 11–3; note how the arms are positioned).

Thoracic Cage Landmarks

On the anterior chest, the manubriosternal junction often is visible and palpable. The manubriosternal junction is a ridge separating the body of the sternum from the manubrium. At this junction, the second rib articulates with the sternum (Fig. 11–4). With this as a reference point, examiners can count the anterior ribs and intercostal spaces. The intercostal spaces are numbered according to the number of the rib immediately above; for example, the first intercostal space is located between the first and second ribs. The manubriosternal junction is a useful reference point because it lies at the same level as the bifurcation of the trachea and the upper level of the atria of the heart.

On the posterior chest, the spinous processes of the vertebrae are useful landmarks. If patients are asked to extend the head forward and down, two prominent spinous processes usually will be visible at the base of the neck. The top one is the spinous process of the seventh cervicle vertebra (C-7); the bottom one is the spinous process of the first

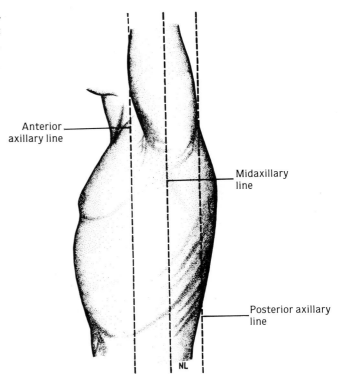

Anterior axillary line

Midaxillary line

Posterior axillary line

NL

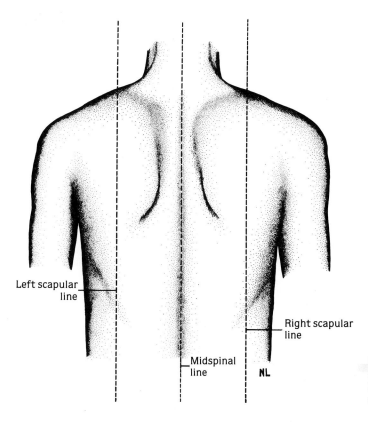

Left scapular line

Right scapular line

Midspinal line

NL

Figure 11–3. Imaginary lines on posterior chest. (Reproduced by permission from Wilkins RL, Sheldon RL, Krider SJ: Clinical assessment in respiratory care. St. Louis, CV Mosby, 1985)

thoracic vertebra. If only one spinous process is visible, it is usually C-7.

Lung Fissures

The right lung has two fissures: horizontal and oblique. The horizontal fissure runs from the fourth rib at the sternal border laterally to the fifth rib at the posteroaxillary line (Fig. 11–5). The horizontal fissure separates the right upper lobe from the middle lobe.

The oblique fissure is similarly located in both the left and right lungs. On the anterior chest it runs from the sixth rib at the midclavicular line upward and laterally through the fifth rib at the midaxillary line. It extends around on the posterior chest to approximately the third thoracic vertebra. On the posterior chest the oblique fissure divides the upper lobes from the lower lobes (see Fig. 11–5*B*).

INSPECTION AND PALPATION OF THE CHEST

Breathing Pattern

The patient's rate and pattern of breathing should be noted. Rapid and shallow breathing is consistent with a restrictive lung defect, whereas patients with COPD tend to breathe more slowly and deeply. The timing of the inspiratory and expiratory phases is also important to document. Prolonged inspiratory phases may be caused by upper airway obstruction; prolonged exhalation frequently is caused by intrathoracic airways obstruction.

The effort of breathing normally is minimal. When the work of breathing increases, as with airways obstruction or a reduction in lung compliance, the patient may begin to use the accessory muscles of breathing. This also occurs when the diaphragm becomes less functional, as with neuromuscular disorders or fatigue.

Tactile or Vocal Fremitus

The use of the palm or ulnar aspect of the hand to detect vibration of the chest wall can be helpful in detecting areas of consolidation. Vibration is increased over the consolidated area of lung; this is called increased tactile or vocal fremitus. Fremitus is diminished over areas of pleural effusion or pneumothorax.

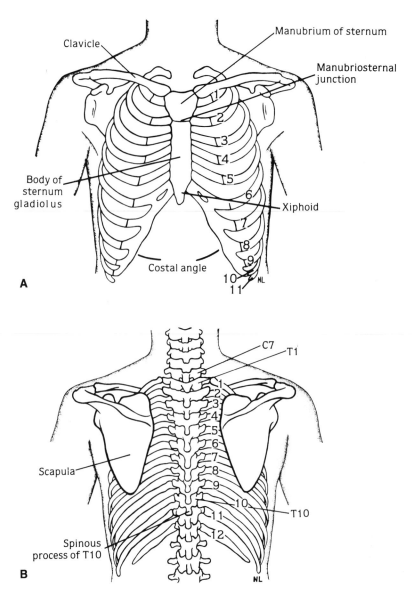

Figure 11—4. Bony structures of the thoracic cage; (A) anterior chest and (B) posterior chest. (Reproduced by permission from Wilkins RL, Sheldon RL, Krider SJ: Clinical assessment in respiratory care. St. Louis, CV Mosby, 1985)

Chest Expansion

The degree and symmetry of chest expansion should be observed. Normally, both sides expand equally during inhalation. With unilateral lung disorders such as pneumonia, pneumothorax, or pleural effusion, the affected side expands poorly, lagging behind the other. This can be confirmed by palpation for chest expansion. To palpate for chest expansion, examiners should place their hands over the anterolateral chest with the thumbs extended toward the xiphoid process. (This examination also can be done over the posterior chest.) The patient is instructed to exhale slowly and completely. After the patient has exhaled fully, the examiner secures the tips of his fingers gently against the sides of the patient's chest and extends the hands until just the thumbtips touch. The patient is instructed to take a full, deep breath. The examiner should note the distance each thumbtip moves from midline. Unilateral defects will cause one thumb to be pulled away from the midline to a

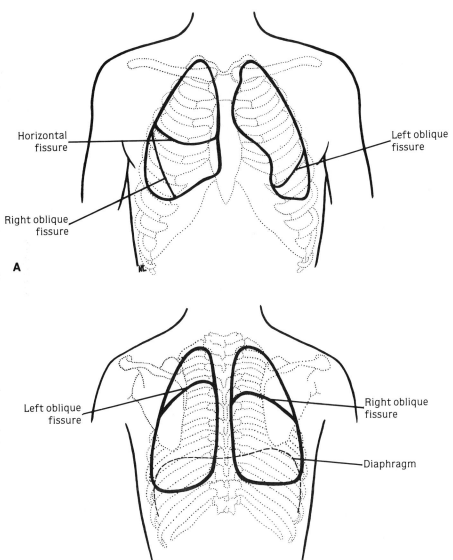

Horizontal fissure

Left oblique fissure

Right oblique fissure

A

Left oblique fissure

Right oblique fissure

Diaphragm

B

Figure 11–5. Topographical position of lung fissures on (*A*) anterior chest and (*B*) posterior chest. (Reproduced by permission from Wilkins RL, Sheldon RL, Krider SJ: Clinical assessment in respiratory care. St. Louis, CV Mosby, 1985)

lesser degree than the other. Bilateral disorders such as emphysema or neuromuscular disorders will cause both sides to expand poorly.

Chest Configuration

In the normal adult, the transverse diameter of the chest is greater than the anteroposterior (AP) diameter. With aging the AP diameter gradually increases; chronic obstructive lung disease, however, can cause premature increases. This condition is known as a barrelchest (Fig. 11–6). Barrel chest occurs when the lung loses its inward recoil.

The sternum may protrude abnormally inward (pectus excavatum) or abnormally outward (pectus carinatum). Severe cases of an inwardly depressed sternum may result in restrictive lung diseases.

Spinal column defects can be severe enough to alter the chest configuration. Abnormal anterior-to-posterior curvature of the spine is known as *kyphosis*, whereas lateral deviation is known as *scoliosis*. The presence of both anteroposterior and lateral

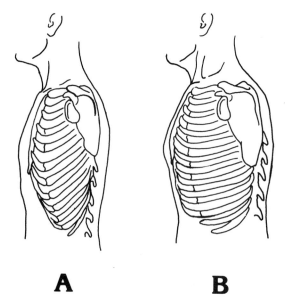

A   **B**

Figure 11—6. Normal (*A*) and barrell chest (*B*) configuration. Note horizontal position of ribs and hypertrophy of the scalene muscle in *B*. (Dexter JR, Wilkins RL: How to assess for COPD. Claremont, CA, Education Resource Consortium, 1987)

curvature defects is called *kyphoscoliosis.* This condition can be severe enough to result in a substantial restrictive lung defect.

Skin Color and Condition

If there is a history of recent trauma, the chest wall should be inspected for bruises and palpated for areas of tenderness and crepitus. When rib fracture occurs, the broken end of the rib may tear into the visceral pleura, causing air to leak into the subcutaneous tissues. This is known as *subcutaneous emphysema.* As the subcutaneous emphysema is palpated, a crackling sensation (crepitus) may be felt. The presence or absence of cyanosis should be noted. This condition is described in detail under Inspection and Palpation of the Extremities (later in this chapter).

Precordium

The chest wall overlying the heart is the precordium. The precordium is inspected and palpated for normal and abnormal pulsations. Normally, contraction of the left ventricle causes a pulsation to occur in the fifth intercostal space at the midclavicular line; this is referred to as the *apical impulse.* The apical impulse is usually visible and palpable in thin young men; obesity and hyperinflation of the lungs make it more difficult to detect.

The apical impulse may shift to one side with shifts of the mediastinum. A large pneumothorax or lobar collapse may produce such a shift. Left ventricular hypertrophy will cause it to shift laterally and become more prominent. Hypovolemia and hypotension cause a weak or absent apical impulse.

With right ventricular hypertrophy, a diffuse lifting impulse (heave) is often produced with each beat along the left sternal border. Patients with chronic lung disease that results in cor pulmonale are especially prone to this condition. If hyperinflation of the chest is present, the heave may be difficult to detect. In such cases, palpation of the epigastric area may allow identification of the heave associated with right ventricular hypertrophy.

CHEST AUSCULTATION

Chest auscultation is a simple and convenient way to evaluate the status of a patient's respiratory system. Although very popular among practitioners, its value is partially limited by the lack of standardized descriptive terminology and the lack of understanding among clinicians of the mechanisms responsible for production of normal and abnormal lung sounds.

For the purpose of this discussion, lung sounds can be divided into two types: breath sounds and adventitious lung sounds. Breath sound are the normal noises of breathing that can be heard over the airways and chest wall with the aid of a stethoscope. Adventitious lung sounds are abnormal noises superimposed on the breath sounds and usually are heard only with a stethoscope.

Breath Sounds

Normal breath sounds heard over the lung have been termed *vesicular,* and also are referred to as normal. Vesicular breath sounds are relatively soft, low-pitched sounds heard primarily on inspiration. The expiratory component is minimal and occurs only during the initial one-third of exhalation (Fig. 11–7).

Over the trachea a very different breath sound is heard. Tracheal breath sounds are loud, high-pitched sounds with approximately equal inspiratory and expiratory components. There also is a pause between the inspiratory and expiratory phases (see Fig. 11–7). This breath sound has been

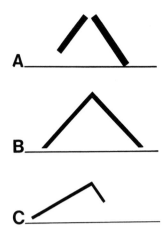

Figure 11—7. Breath sound diagrams: (*A*) normal tracheobronchial; (*B*) bronchovesicular; and (*C*) vesicular. Upstroke represents inspiration and downstroke expiration. The thickness of the line indicates intensity. (Reproduced by permission from Wilkins RL, Hodgkin JE, Lopez B: Lung sounds: a practical guide. St. Louis, CV Mosby, 1988)

referred to as *bronchial, tracheobronchial, tracheal,* or *tubular.*

Auscultation over the main stem bronchi should identify a softer version of the normal tracheal breath sound. This sound, called *bronchovesicular,* has equal inspiratory and expiratory components but no pause (see Fig. 11–7). Bronchovesicular breath sounds normally are heard on the anterior chest near the sternum at the first and second intercostal spaces. On the posterior chest, such sounds normally are heard only between the scapulae (Fig. 11–8).

The normal breath sounds just described are believed to be produced primarily by turbulent flow in the airways. The inspiratory component of the vesicular breath sound is believed to be produced more distally than the expiratory component. In fact, most evidence suggests that the inspiratory component is produced regionally within each lung and probably within each lobe.[10] The expiratory component of the vesicular breath sound is

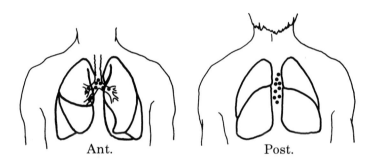

Bronchovesicular Breath Sounds

Figure 11—8. Position on anterior and posterior chest wall at which normal vesicular and bronchovesicular breath sounds are identified. (Reproduced by permission from Wilkins RL, Hodgkin JE, Lopez B: Lung sounds: a practical guide. St. Louis, CV Mosby, 1988)

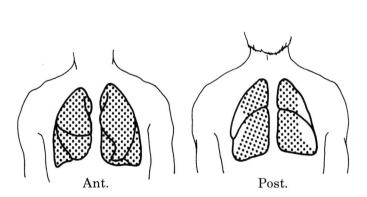

Vesicular Breath Sounds

believed to be produced in the larger airways where rapidly converging airstreams come together.[11,12] Because airflow is directed away from the chest wall during exhalation, the expiratory component fades away while the examiner is auscultating over the lung.

The differences in intensity (loudness) and pitch between the sounds heard directly over large airways (trachea) versus lung probably is caused primarily by the sound-filtering capabilities of normal lung. Normal lungs contain millions of air-filled alveoli that alter the high-pitched and loud tracheobronchial-type breath sounds to the softer, lower-pitched vesicular-type sound.[13]

Alterations in lung pathology can change the sound transmission characteristics of the lung. Increases in lung tissue density cause better sound transmission. As a result, louder or harsh breath sounds are heard over lung consolidation if a patent bronchus is present. If the consolidation is more significant, a tracheobronchial-type breath sound may be heard. This is common in patients with lobar pneumonia. Detection of this change in the breath sound requires the examiner to pay specific attention to the expiratory portion of the breath sound.

A decrease in lung tissue density, such as occurs with emphysema, provokes a reduction in the sound-transmitting ability of the lung, bringing about decreased breath sounds. Diminished or absent breath sounds also can be present when sound generation is limited by shallow or slow breathing and when sound transmission through the chest wall is reduced by obesity, pleural effusion, or other disorders.

Whispered pectoriloquy and *egophony* are encountered in lung consolidation. When an individual whispers "99" or "1,2,3," the sounds are transmitted poorly if auscultating over normal lung tissue. However, with consolidated lung, the sounds are transmitted more prominently, similar to what would be heard if the stethoscope were placed over the trachea. This phenomenon is called whispered pectoriloquy. Egophony refers to the phenomenon of a spoken /a/ sounding like /e/ when auscultating over consolidated lung. *Bronchophony* has been used to refer to the enhanced transmission of a spoken (not whispered) sound over an area of lung consolidation.

Adventitious Lung Sounds

Acoustical recordings of adventitious lung sounds have revealed two distinct categories: continuous and discontinuous.

Wheezes. Continuous adventitious lung sounds have a constant pitch but may be very short (0.25 sec), or long (several seconds) in duration. These sounds are more frequently heard during exhalation and are associated with airways obstruction (Table 11–4). A variety of terms have been used to

Table 11—4 Application of Adventitious Lung Sounds

LUNG SOUND	CLASSIFICATION	POSSIBLE MECHANISM	CHARACTERISTICS	CAUSES
Wheezes	Continuous	Rapid vibration of airway walls as airflow moves through obstructed airways; bronchospasm, mucosal edema	High-pitched or low-pitched; most often occur during exhalation	Asthma, bronchitis, congestive heart failure
Stridor	Continuous	Airways obstruction caused by inflammation	High-pitched; often inspiratory	Epiglottitis, croup, post-extubation
Crackles (late-inspiratory)	Discontinuous	Sudden expansion of atelectatic lung	Fine and diffuse	Atelectasis, pulmonary fibrosis, pulmonary edema, pneumonia
Crackles (early-inspiratory)	Discontinuous	Sudden opening of more proximal airways	Scanty and not affected by cough	COPD
Crackles (inspiratory and expiratory)	Discontinuous	Movement of airway secretions with breathing	Coarse and often clear with coughing	Bronchitis, respiratory infections

describe continuous adventitious sounds, but they are best described as *wheezes*. Although some clinicians still advocate using *rhonchus* to describe low-pitched, continuous, adventitious lung sounds, this term has been used in the past to describe a variety of sounds; it therefore lacks precision and should be abandoned.[14–16] Low-pitched continuous or snoring type sounds should be called low-pitched wheezes, and higher pitched or musical sounds should be called simply wheezes. The monophonic, continuous adventitious sound heard over the upper airways of a patient with upper airway obstruction is termed *stridor*.

Wheezes are believed to be produced by airway narrowing that initially causes rapid airflow through the site of obstruction. The rapid airflow decreases the lateral airway wall pressure and causes the opposite sides to be pulled into a partially obstructed or closed position.[17,18] Airflow is temporarily interrupted and airway pressure increases, partially opening the airway. Airflow speeds up again and the cycle rapidly repeats itself, causing vibration of the airway walls. This process continues until the airways obstruction is resolved or until the patient tires and cannot generate sufficient flow to cause vibration of the airway walls.

This condition is more likely to occur within intrathoracic airways during exhalation when they naturally become smaller.[18] During inhalation, chest expansion pulls the intrathoracic airways into a more open position; as a result, wheezing is not as likely to occur. With more severe or fixed airways obstruction, however, wheezing may be present during both inhalation and exhalation.

When wheezing is identified, three specific characteristics should be evaluated: pitch, intensity, and duration of the respiratory cycle occupied by wheezing. More severe airways obstruction is associated with louder, higher-pitched wheezing that is heard during inhalation and exhalation. As the airways obstruction is resolved by bronchodilators, the wheezing may change to a lower-pitched sound with reduced intensity. In addition, the wheezing often occupies a shorter portion of the patient's breathing cycle after therapy is initiated.[19] Clinicians should remember that severe airway obstruction can cause the patient to tire, producing reduced flow through the airways. As a result, wheezing may diminish in intensity and pitch. Evaluating multiple parameters, such as the vital signs, peak flow, and sensorium, will help the examiner distinguish between changes in wheezing caused by improvement and those resulting from fatigue. The presence of vesicular breath sounds in the absence of wheezing is a sign that airways obstruction is most likely minimal.[20,21]

Crackles. Discontinuous adventitious lung sounds are brief bursts of sound similar to the popping of bubbles. They are more frequently heard during inhalation and may be associated with restrictive or obstructive respiratory disorders. Discontinuous adventitious sounds frequently are called *rales*; however, this term, like *rhonchus*, has been used to describe an assortment of sounds.[16,22] Since the invention of the stethoscope of Laënnec,[23] "rales" has been used to denote all kinds of abnormal lung sounds. Because selective use of rales for discontinuous adventitious sounds may be misinterpreted, Forgacs and others have suggested use of the expression *crackles* for discontinuous adventitious sounds.[13,14] This use also has been endorsed by the ATS/ACCP Ad Hoc Subcommittee on Pulmonary Nomenclature;[24] however, the term rales remains popular.[25–27]

Crackles can be produced by several mechanisms. They may occur with the sudden opening of closed airways[13,28–30] or through the movement of excessive lung secretions with breathing.[31] Crackles produced by the sudden opening of small airways are inspiratory sounds generated by the rapid equalization of pressure between the patent and collapsed airways, causing the airways to snap open. When peripheral airways are collapsed as a result of atelectasis, pulmonary edema, or fibrosis, the crackles typically occur in the latter half of inspiration. In patients with fibrosis, the crackles are persistent in succeeding inspirations, even after a cough or deep breathing.[13,32] With atelectasis, the crackles often clear with several deep breaths, coughing, or changes in position. Crackles occurring early in inspiration can result from more proximal airways popping open.[13,33] More proximal airways may close during exhalation if bronchial wall compliance is increased or if the retractive pressure around them is low. Early-inspiratory crackles are common in patients with COPD. In such cases, the crackles tend to be fewer than in cases of interstitial fibrosis (see Table 11–4).

Crackles produced by the movement of fluid or excessive secretions in the lung tend to be low-pitched. They often are present during inhalation and exhalation and may clear somewhat with coughing or suctioning. When the airway narrows as a result of secretions, coarse crackles generated by excessive secretions often are accompanied by low-pitched wheezes.

Qualifying Adjectives. Examiners should listen for and document certain abnormal lung sound characteristics, most significantly the timing of the adventitious sounds within the patient's breathing cycle. Abnormal sounds should be described as inspiratory, expiratory, or both, and specific timing, such as "late-inspiratory," should be recorded.

Crackles should be described as "fine," "medium," or "coarse." Fine crackles are high-pitched, whereas coarse crackles are low-pitched, gurgling sounds. Medium crackles are somewhere in between. Wheezes should be described as "mild," "moderate," or "severe," according to their intensity.

Auscultation Technique

In preparation for auscultation, examiners should make the room as quiet as possible, and radios or televisions should be turned off. If possible, the patient should be sitting erect on the edge of the bed or chair with the chest exposed. Auscultation is best performed with the chest piece of the stethoscope directly against the patient's skin; hand-warming the chest piece before use is recommended.

Auscultation of the lungs is usually accomplished with the diaphragm of the stethoscope, while pressing the diaphragm firmly against the skin. The bell, generally used for listening for low-pitched cardiac sounds, may be helpful when listening between ribs in emaciated patients and over areas of the lungs in small children.

Conscious patients should be asked to breathe through an open mouth during the procedure, with inhalation a little deeper than normal and exhalation passive. Examiners must compare one side of the chest with the other by moving the chest piece back and forth from side to side in similar positions (Fig. 11–9). One full respiratory cycle should be

Figure 11–9. Auscultation sequence.

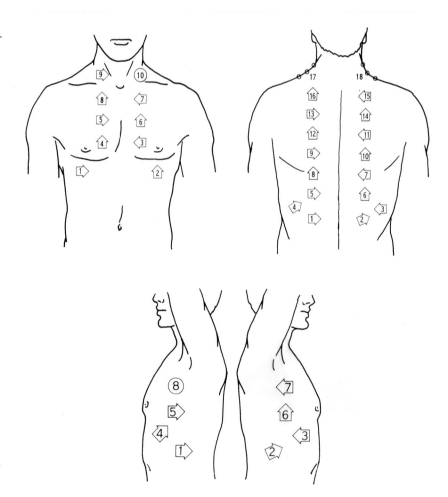

evaluated at each position, and the loudness, length, and adventitial components of inspiration and expiration should be documented. Changes in the breath sounds may be subtle at first. For example, in early lung congestion careful examiners will detect minor, but important changes, of the vesicular breath sound to a harsher sound with a more prominent expiratory component.

All areas of the anterior, lateral, and posterior chest must be evaluated. In the bedridden patient, hard-to-reach areas may reveal changes in lung sounds suggesting disease. To reach all areas in such cases, it may be necessary to roll the patient gently to one side.

Auscultating over chest hair may cause a crackling sound, similar to fine crackles, that could be misconstrued as a sign of lung disease. Wetting the chest hair may help reduce this problem. During the procedure, the tubing of the stethoscope should not rub against any object because artificial noise will be produced.

In bedridden patients suspected of having atelectasis, auscultating the dependent regions first may help the examiner detect the early signs of this disorder. Late-inspiratory crackles and harsh breath sounds occur first in the dependent regions because these regions are more prone to atelectasis. If nondependent regions are auscultated first, the initial deep inspiratory breaths may cause the atelectasis to clear temporarily. Subsequently, auscultation of the dependent regions may not disclose the early signs of atelectasis, causing appropriate treatment to be delayed.

CHEST PERCUSSION

Percussion is the tapping of an object in an effort to create a sound called a "percussion note." The percussion note helps the examiner evaluate the quality of the underlying tissues. Chest percussion is done to determine the relative amounts of air, liquid, or solid material in the underlying lung. In addition, it can be helpful in detecting the general position and relative range of motion for the diaphragm.

The technique most often used in percussion of the chest wall is the mediate or indirect method. The examiner places the middle finger on the left hand (if right-handed) firmly against the patient's chest. The tip of the middle finger of the right hand is used to strike the distal joint of the left middle finger with a quick, sharp blow (Fig. 11–10). Movement of the hand striking the chest should be generated at the wrist, not at the elbow.

Percussion over the lung fields should be done systematically, testing comparable areas on both sides of the chest consecutively. Comparing one side with the other is especially valuable in detecting subtle unilateral defects. Percussing over bony structures such as the scapulae or sternum is not of value and should be avoided. Asking patients to raise their arms above the shoulders will help move the scapulae laterally, minimizing their interference with percussion on the posterior chest.

Percussion over normal lung fields produces a sound that is easy to hear and is described as normal resonance. Increased resonance to percussion is present when hyperinflation of the lung occurs, as in acute asthma or emphysema. In such cases the increased resonance is bilateral, unless an underlying pneumonia also is present. Pneumothorax can cause a unilateral increase in resonance if it is of sufficient size (Table 11–5).

Increases in lung tissue density, such as occurs in pneumonia, atelectasis, or lung tumors, will cause a decrease in resonance to percussion. Pleural effusions also can cause a reduced resonance. The percussion note may be referred to as flat or dull when decreased resonance is pronounced.

Because the percussion vibrations only penetrate approximately 5 cm below the chest wall surface, abnormalities must lie within this range to be detected. Abnormalities that are deep and small will be undetected by chest percussion. In addition, the percussion note is difficult to assess in obese or highly muscular patients.

To measure diaphragmatic excursion, the examiner should instruct the patient to inhale deeply and hold his breath in. On the posterior chest wall at the left or right midscapular line, the examiner should percuss to identify the lowest margin of normal resonance and mark it. This point is assumed to be the position of the diaphragm at full inspiration. The patient should breathe normally for a few breaths, then exhale fully and hold this position. The examiner should then percuss up from the marked position to identify the diaphragmatic excursion of deep expiration, repeating the procedure on the opposite side.

Normally, diaphragmatic excursion is equal on both sides and approximately 4 to 8 cm, varying with the size of the patient. With severe pulmonary hyperinflation (emphysema) the diaphragm is low in position and has minimal excursion. Lobar collapse of one lung may pull the hemidiaphragm on the affected side up to a higher position. Neuromuscular diseases that affect the diaphragm will cause it to be elevated and immobile. Examiners

Table 11—5 Summary of Typical Physical Signs in the More Common Respiratory Diseases

PATHOLOGICAL PROCESS	MOVEMENT OF CHEST WALL	PERCUSSION NOTE	BREATH SOUNDS	ADVENTITIOUS SOUNDS AND ACCOMPANIMENTS
Consolidation: as in lobar pneumonia, extensive pulmonary infarction, or pneumonic tuberculosis	May be reduced on side affected	Dull	High-pitched, bronchial	Fine rales early; coarse rales later
Diffuse lobular pneumonia	Often symmetrically diminished	May be impaired	Usually harsh vesicular with prolonged expiration	Rhonchi and coarse rales
Pulmonary cavitation (typical signs present only when cavity is large and in communication with bronchus)	Normal or slightly reduced on side affected	Impaired	"Amphoric" or bronchial	Coarse rales
Atelectasis: from obstruction of major bronchus by secretions, carcinoma, foreign body, or tuberculous lymph nodes	Reduced on side affected	Dull	Diminished or absent if complete; high-pitched bronchial otherwise	Usually rales disappear after deep breath or cough
Bronchiectasis	Normal	Slightly impaired	Low-pitched bronchial	Coarse or sibilant rales
Pleural effusion or empyema	Reduced or absent (depending on size) on side affected	Dull to absent	Diminished or absent (occasionally high-pitched bronchial)	Pleural rub in some cases
Pneumothorax	Reduced or absent (depending on size) on side affected	Normal or hyper-resonant	Diminished or absent (occasionally faint high-pitched bronchial)	High-pitched rales when fluid present
Bronchitis (acute or chronic)	Normal	Normal	Vesicular with prolonged expiration	Usually with some coarse rales; occasionally wheezes
Bronchial asthma	Normal or symmetrically diminished	Normal or hyper-resonant	Vesicular with prolonged expiration	Mainly expiratory and high-pitched wheezes
Diffuse pulmonary emphysema	Symmetrically diminished en bloc motion	Usually hyper-resonant	Diminished vesicular with prolonged expiration	Wheezes coarse rales from associated asthma or bronchitis
Diffuse pulmonary fibrosis and other forms of interstitial lung disease	Symmetrically diminished	Normal	Harsh vesicular with prolonged expiration	Coarse rales (crackles) uninfluenced by coughing
Pulmonary edema	Normal or increased	Normal	Bronchial if interstitial: vesicular if alveolar-filling	Moist rales

should be aware that the exact position and range of motion of the diaphragm is difficult to detect by percussion.[34] This probably is due to its natural dome shape, with the center of the dome located 15 cm below the surface of the chest. Percussion, therefore, can only approximate diaphragm position and movement.

INSPECTION AND PALPATION OF THE NECK

The neck is inspected for jugular venous distention (JVD), which occurs when the right ventricle fails to pump blood forward through the pulmonary circulation at an adequate pace. This disorder is common in patients with chronic hypoxemic lung dis-

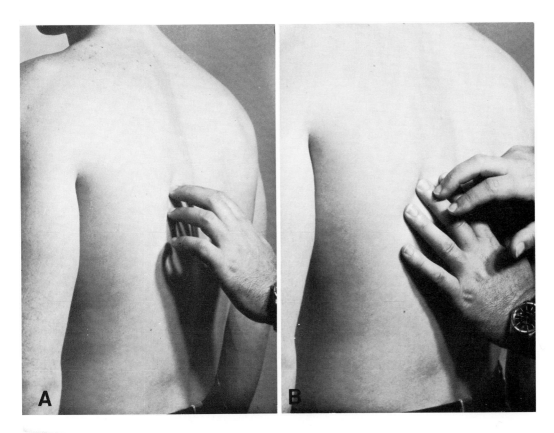

Figure 11—10. Technique for mediate or indirect percussion of the chest wall: (*A*) Placement of left (right) middle finger. (*B*) Strike distal joint with top of right (left) middle finger.

ease. The resulting pulmonary vasoconstriction increases the work load on the right ventricle, eventually causing right heart failure and JVD. Jugular venous distention also occurs with left heart failure (when it leads to right heart failure), constrictive pericarditis, cardiac tamponade caused by pericardial effusion, and massive pulmonary embolism.

To detect JVD the examiner should identify the level of the column of blood in the jugular veins with the head of the bed elevated 30° to 45° from horizontal. At this position, the level of the column of blood in the jugular veins normally is no higher than approximately 3 cm above the sternal angle. When JVD is present, the veins may be distended as high as the angle of the jaw (Fig. 11–11).

Use of the accessory muscles in the neck (scalene and sternocleidomastoid) indicates that the work of breathing (WOB) is increased. Elevated airways resistance or reduction in lung compliance is a common cause of an increase in the WOB. In patients with emphysema, flattening of the diaphragm occurs as a consequence of hyperinflation, leaving

it less effective. Consequently, the accessory muscles are utilized to enhance chest inflation.

The examiner palpates the patient's neck to identify the position of the trachea, which may shift toward one side with mediastinal tumors, tension pneumothorax, or collapse of one lung. The distance of the trachea from the head of each clavicle is determined to identify if it is midline. Palpation of supraclavicular lymphadenopathy or thyromegaly provides valuable information.

INSPECTION AND PALPATION OF THE EXTREMITIES

Cyanosis

Cyanosis is a bluish discoloration of the skin caused by excessive levels of desaturated hemoglobin. Cyanosis may be central or peripheral. Central cyanosis is generalized and often caused by severe respiratory disease that results in a significant drop in arterial saturation (<80%). It can also be caused

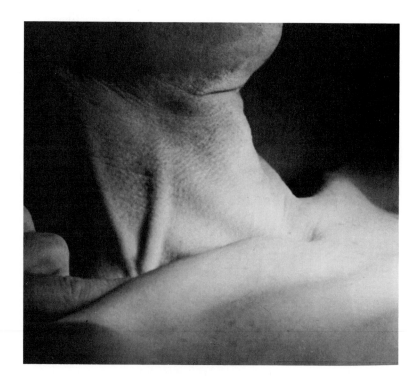

Figure 11–11. Photograph of jugular venous distention. (Reproduced by permission from Daily EK, Schroeder JP: Techniques in bedside hemodynamic monitoring, 2nd ed. St. Louis, CV Mosby, 1981)

by congenital heart diseases with right-to-left shunts. Peripheral cyanosis (acrocyanosis) is limited to the hands, feet, lips, and ear lobes, and results from reduced cardiac output that causes the circulating red blood cells to lose excessive amounts of oxygen because of prolonged transit time through peripheral capillaries. This decreases venous oxygen content, thereby causing peripheral cyanosis. Cool extremities typically are present when peripheral cyanosis is identified.

The ability to identify cyanosis is dependent on room lighting, the patient's skin color, and hemoglobin level. Cyanosis is not visible in anemic patients until the hypoxemia is severe. Conversely, polycythemic patients demonstrate cyanosis with mild to moderate hypoxemia. Measurement of the amount of oxygen in an arterial sample of blood is much more sensitive for detecting hypoxemia than waiting for the development of cyanosis.

Clubbing

Clubbing is defined as a painless uniform enlargement of the terminal segment of the fingers and toes. Although advanced clubbing is more obvious, early clubbing is difficult to identify. Changes in

the fingers and toes consistent with clubbing include a change in the angle between the nail and proximal skin to 180° or more, ratio of distal phalangeal depth to interphalangeal depth (DPD/IPD) greater than 1 (Fig. 11–12), sponginess of the nail bed, and increased nail curvature.

The exact mechanisms responsible for clubbing are unclear. Because clubbing is a common finding in patients with disorders, such as cyanotic heart disease, some clinicians believe that chronic tissue hypoxia is at least one cause.

Pedal Edema

Swelling of the ankles is a common finding in patients with chronic right heart failure. As the right side of the heart fails to pump blood adequately through the pulmonary circulation, the blood pressure in the venous system elevates. The increase in venous blood pressure promotes leakage of fluid from within the capillaries to the interstitial tissues. This occurs especially in the dependent areas such as the feet and ankles. Pedal edema may be described as pitting if firm pressure with the fingertip result in pits (indentations). When pitting edema is present, it should be evaluated for level of

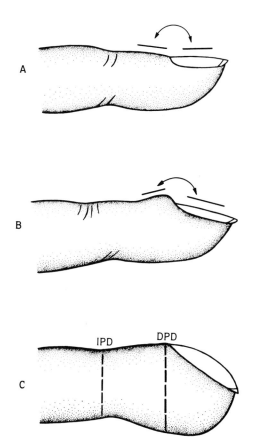

Figure 11–12. Normal digit configuration (*A*) and digital clubbing (*B*). Note how the angle between the nail and proximal skin exceeds 180°. Also (*C*) note how the distal phalangeal depth (DPD) is greater than the interphalangeal depth (IPD). (Reproduced by permission from Wilkins RL, Sheldon RL, Krider SJ: Clinical assessment in respiratory care. St. Louis, CV Mosby, 1985)

occurrence above the ankle in an effort to quantify its extent. Hepatomegaly (an enlarged liver) is also a common finding when pedal edema is due to right heart failure.

Capillary Refill

Capillary refill is assessed by pressing firmly for a brief period on the patient's fingernail and identifying the speed at which blood flow returns when the pressure is released. Normally, the capillary blood flow returns almost immediately. If cardiac output is below normal, capillary refill is slow, taking several seconds to appear. The extremities are usually cool to the touch when capillary refill is sluggish.

SUMMARY

A careful history and physical examination can provide valuable information that can lead to a correct assessment and appropriate therapy. Serial examinations provide useful information on the response to therapy. The clinician should avoid the temptation to rely mainly on radiographs, blood tests, and pulmonary function studies when evaluating a patient. Generally, a thorough history and physical examination should be the first step in patient assessment.

REFERENCES

1. Ault M, Robin ED: Platypnea (diffuse zone I phenomenon). N Engl J Med 281:1347, 1967
2. Begin R: Platypnea after pneumonectomy. N Engl J Med 293:342, 1975
3. Irwin RS, Rosen MJ, Braman SS: Cough, a comprehensive review. Arch Intern Med 137:1186, 1977
4. Carrao WM, Braman SS, Irwin RS: Chronic cough as a sole presenting manifestation of bronchial asthma. N Engl J Med 300:633, 1979
5. Hasler ME, Cohen JA: The effect of oxygen administration on oral temperature assessment. Nurs Res 31:265, 1982
6. Lim-Levy F: The effect of oxygen inhalation on oral temperature. Nurs Res 31:151, 1982
7. Yonkman CA: Cool and heated aerosol and the measurement of oral temperature. Nurs Res 31:354, 1982
8. Henkind SJ, Benis AM, Teichholz LE: The paradox of pulsus paradoxus. Am Heart J 114:198, 1987
9. Rebuck AS, Pengelly LD: Development of pulsus paradoxus in the presence of airway obstruction. N Engl J Med 288:66, 1973
10. Kraman SS: Vesicular (normal) lung sounds: How are they made, where do they come from, and what do they mean?
11. Kramin SS: Determination of the site of production of respiratory sounds by subtraction phonopneumography. Am Rev Respir Dis 122:303, 1980
12. Loudon R, Murphy RLH: Lung sounds. Am Rev Respir Dis 130:663, 1984
13. Forgacs P: The functional basis of pulmonary sounds. Chest 73:399, 1978
14. Robertson JA, Coope R: Rales, rhonchi and Laënnec. Lancet 2:417, 1957
15. Editorial: Say ninety-nine. Lancet 2:1258, 1986
16. Cugell DW: Lung sounds: Classification and controversies. Semin Respir Med 6:180, 1985
17. Murphy RLH, Holford SK: Lung sounds. Basics RD 8:1, 1980
18. Waring WW, Beckerman RC, Hopkins RL: Continuous adventitious lung sounds: Site and method of production and significance. Semin Respir Med 6:201, 1985
19. Baughman RP, Loudon RG: Quantification of wheezing in acute asthma. Chest 86:718, 1984
20. Marini JJ, Pierson DJ, Hudson LD, Lakshminarayan S: The significance of wheezing in chronic airflow obstruction. Am Rev Respir Dis 120:1069, 1979

21. Kraman SS: Lung sounds for the clinician. Arch Intern Med 146:1411, 1986
22. Hughes RL: When is a crackle not a rale? Chest 81:661, 1982
23. Andrews JL, Budger TL: Lung sounds through the ages. JAMA 241:2625, 1979
24. Report of the ATS–ACCP Ad Hoc Subcommittee on Pulmonary Nomenclature. Am Thorac Soc News 3:5, 1977
25. Wilkins RL, Dexter JR, Smith JR: Survey of adventitious lung sound terminology in case reports. Chest 85:523, 1984
26. Bunin NJ, Loudon RG: Lung sound terminology in case reports. Chest 76:690, 1979
27. Wilkins RL, Dexter JR, Smith MP, Marshak AB: Lung sound terminology used by respiratory care practitioners. Respir Care 34:36, 1989
28. Nath AR, Capel LH: Inspiratory crackles and the mechanical events of breathing. Thorax 29:695, 1974
29. Mitsuru M, Homma Y, Matsuzaki M: Production mechanism of crackles in excised normal canine lungs. J Appl Physiol 61:1120, 1986
30. Ploysongsang Y, Schonfeld S: Mechanism of production of crackles after atelectasis during low-volume breathing. Am Rev Respir Dis 126:413, 1982
31. Murphy RLH: Discontinuous adventitious lung sounds. Semin Respir Med 6:210, 1985
32. Forgacs P: Crackles and wheezes. Lancet 2:203, 1967
33. Nath AR, Capel LH: Inspiratory crackles—early and late. Thorax 29:223, 1974
34. Williams TJ, Ahmand D, Morgan WK: A clinical and roentgenographic correlation of diaphragmatic movement. Arch Intern Med 141:878, 1981

BIBLIOGRAPHY

Burton GG, Hodgkin JE: Respiratory Care: A Guide To Clinical Practice, 2nd ed. Philadelphia, JB Lippincott, 1984

Glauser FL: Signs and Symptoms in Pulmonary Medicine. Philadelphia, JB Lippincott, 1983

Hodgkin JE: Chronic Obstructive Pulmonary Disease: Current Concepts in Diagnosis and Comprehensive Care. Park Ridge, American College of Chest Physicians, 1979

Lehrer S: Understanding Lung Sounds. Philadelphia, WB Saunders, 1984

Prior JA, Silberstein JS, Stang JM: Physical Diagnosis: The History and Examination of the Patient, 6th ed. St Louis, CV Mosby, 1981

Seidel HM: Mosby's Guide to Physical Examination. St Louis, CV Mosby, 1987

Wilkins RL, Hodgkin JE, Lopez B, Lung Sounds: A Practical Guide. St Louis, CV Mosby, 1988

Wilkins RL, Sheldon RL, Krider SJ: Clinical Assessment in Respiratory Care. St Louis, CV Mosby 1985

TWELVE

Roentgenographic Diagnosis of Pulmonary Disease

Glen A. Lillington

A comprehensive review of chest roentgenography and the other modalities of chest imaging can scarcely be encompassed in a single chapter with a limited number of illustrations. This presentation, therefore, is introductory and will be directed toward three goals:

1. To acquaint paramedical readers with the terminology and some of the basic concepts pertaining to the imaging techniques employed in information gathering in patients with bronchopulmonary disease.
2. To demonstrate some of the "typical" radiologic patterns of abnormality, particularly those that occur in seriously ill patients and are associated with deterioration of pulmonary function.
3. To emphasize that radiologic analysis, although critically important in most instances, may be misleading in some situations. The stethoscope may at times be more sensitive and occasionally more precise than roentgenography.

SOME BASIC PRINCIPLES IN CHEST ROENTGENOGRAPHY

Roentgenographic visualization of body structures depends on the perception of contrast between tissues of differing radiodensities. As the roentgen beam passes through the tissues to register on the radiographic film, differential attenuation (absorption) of the beam by different tissues occurs. The greater the radiodensity of the tissue, the greater the absorption of the beam; as a result, the film image of the tissue or organ will be relatively white or *radiopaque*. Less dense tissues appear blacker on the film and are less radiopaque and more *radiolucent*.

Chest roentgenography is made possible by the widespread presence throughout the lung of relative radiolucency (blackness) owing to the air-filled alveoli. This provides contrast to the denser tissues such as bone, intrapulmonary vessels, and mediastinal structures, which are solid or fluid filled.

As *calcium* has the greatest radiopacity of any endogenous material, calcified structures are usually easily detected on the roentgenogram. Certain *exogenous substances* (tin, iodine, barium), which may occasionally appear in the thorax, have a "metallic density" similar to or greater than that of calcium. Body fluids and most tissues have a lesser degree of radiopacity, usually referred to as "water density" or "tissue density." The degree of radiopacity also depends on the *thickness* of tissue through which the beam has penetrated. For example, the heart, which is large, will appear more opaque than the much smaller right or left pulmonary artery.

In most lung diseases, the air density of the affected area of lung is replaced (or displaced) by the tissue or water density of the disease process, resulting in the appearance of *increased radiopacity*. Such abnormalities are commonly referred to as "shadows" or "infiltrates." The size, shape, distribution, location, and homogeneity of such shadows form *patterns* that provide clues to the radiologist in predicting the possible nature of the abnormality.

Certain thoracic diseases produce *increased radiolucency* owing to an increase in the air/tissue ratio in the affected area. This is most commonly due to a focal loss of lung tissue (emphysema, bullae, cavities), diffuse obstructive hyperinflation (asthma or a check-valve bronchial obstruction), or a collection of air in an abnormal location (pneumothorax or pneumomediastinum).

VALUE AND LIMITATIONS OF CHEST ROENTGENOGRAPHY

The chest roentgenogram is highly effective in the *detection* of abnormalities in the lungs. Routine chest roentgenography may reveal evidence of disease in asymptomatic patients with no abnormal signs on physical examination.

In addition to the detection of disease, the chest roentgenogram displays the *pattern* of abnormality. Pattern analysis provides valuable clues in determining the cause of the disorder. Only occasionally is the roentgenographic pattern specifically diagnostic. More commonly, the abnormal pattern suggests a limited number of diagnostic possibilities, which must then be further investigated by other techniques.

Serial chest roentgenograms obtained at appropriate intervals provide a dynamic portrait of the disease process. Information of this type has diagnostic value and prognostic implications and allows one to monitor the effectiveness of therapy.

In assessing the diagnostic implications of a normal chest roentgenogram, one must be constantly aware of the *limitations* of the technique. In patients with bronchial asthma or chronic bronchitis, for example, the chest roentgenogram may appear entirely normal even when the disease is severe. Emphysema may cause little change in the chest roentgenogram until an advanced stage has been reached. Primary lung cancer (bronchogenic carcinoma) usually cannot be detected by roentgenography until the tumor mass has reached a diameter of 1 cm or greater, by which time the tumor may have already been present for 10 years or longer. Relatively large lesions may be virtually undetectable on the chest roentgenogram if they are located in the "blind" areas where the lung tissue is obscured by overlapping opaque structures such as the heart, great vessels, or subdiaphragmatic solid organs.

Disorders of the ventilatory pump may occur in the absence of lung disease, and the chest roentgenogram may appear completely normal unless pulmonary complications, such as sputum retention, occur. Respiratory insufficiency may result from extrapulmonary abnormalities, including overdosage of sedative drugs, leading to respiratory center depression; trauma to the brain and spinal cord; and neuromuscular disorders, such as poliomyelitis and myasthenia gravis.

Conversely, moderate or even extensive abnormalities on the chest roentgenogram are not always accompanied by severe symptoms or marked abnormalities in pulmonary function. This discrepancy between radiologic appearance and pathophysiologic reality tends to occur most commonly in sarcoidosis, pneumoconiosis, and histiocytosis X.

NORMAL CHEST ROENTGENOGRAM

The standard (routine) chest roentgenographic study includes two views, each obtained with subject in the upright position: a film obtained in the posteroanterior projection (the PA film) and a lateral projection, either right or left (the lateral film). The exposures should be made with respiration suspended in the full-inspiratory position, with the subject properly positioned so that there is no rotation in either frontal or lateral projection, and with appropriate exposure techniques to enhance contrast without underpenetration or overpenetration.

When the patient is seriously ill, many or all of these ideal circumstances may be unattainable. The physician will often be required to examine and interpret a supine anteroposterior (AP) film that is badly overpenetrated or underpenetrated, obtained on a subject who was rotated and was in a state of submaximal inspiration and breathing at the time of exposure. A lateral film is rarely available under such circumstances. Such films can yield valuable diagnostic information provided one is fully aware of the many apparent but spurious abnormalities on such films, which are related solely to the suboptimal technique. Conversely, the radiologic appearance of actual disease that is present may be significantly modified by the suboptimal technique.

In situations in which the patient must have an

AP film while intubated, the respiratory care worker can assist the x-ray technician by inflating the patient's lungs before the film exposure, either with a resuscitation valve or bag or with the inspiratory hold or "sigh" control of the ventilator.

NORMAL RADIOLOGIC ANATOMY

A full description of the normal radiologic anatomy of the thorax is beyond the scope of this chapter, and the reader is referred to the classic descriptions in the standard texts (see Bibliography). Some pertinent data are included in the following description of the techniques of inspecting the radiographic film.

INSPECTION OF THE POSTEROANTERIOR CHEST FILM

It is a self-evident truth that an abnormality cannot be interpreted that has not first been detected. Many factors are operative in the unavoidable *observer error* that occurs in radiology,[5] but failures in perception can be reduced by following a standard search pattern in which the different areas and anatomic components of the chest roentgenogram are systematically inspected during the interpretative process (Fig. 12–1). The precise order in which one studies the various structures is less important than the consistency with which one applies the method.

The proper *positioning* of the patient is verified by comparing the relationship of the medial ends of the clavicles to the midline. Relatively minor degrees of rotation may create a spurious appearance of tracheal deviation, cardiac displacement, cardiomegaly, or widening of the vascular pedicle.

The *extrathoracic soft tissues* should be inspected briefly. If the patient is female, the breast shadows should be identified. Absence of one breast will result in relative hyperlucency over the lower lung on the affected side. Large breasts cause considerable haziness over the lower lung fields that may simulate pneumonia or pulmonary congestion. Nipple shadows may be mistaken for solitary nodules. The presence of subcutaneous emphysema may be apparent in the neck or lateral chest wall.

The *bony thorax* is inspected, including ribs, spine, manubrium, and scapulae. A cervical rib is present in 1% to 2% of normal persons. A search should be made for rib fractures and lytic lesions of bone. Rib fractures may be difficult to see in the

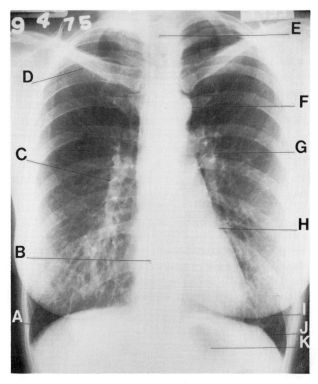

Figure 12–1. Posteroanterior (PA) chest roentgenogram of a young woman. (*A*) Right hemidiaphragm, convex upward with a clear costophrenic angle; (*B*) thoracic spine: (*C*) right hilum (the hilar opacity is mainly due to the pulmonary arteries); (*D*) right clavicle; (*E*) midline lucency caused by intratracheal air; (*F*) aortic knob (this becomes more prominent in older persons); (*G*) left hilum, usually higher than the right hilum; (*H*) left heart border; (*I*) interface representing the inferior margin of left breast; (*J*) left hemidiaphragm, usually a little lower than the right; (*K*) gas bubble within the stomach.

standard chest roentgenogram. Scapulae that overlie the lung may be confused with pleural or extrapleural lesions. The presence of kyphosis or scoliosis makes interpretation of the chest roentgenogram more difficult.

The *diaphragms* should have a normal rounded contour that is convex upward. The costophrenic angles should be clear. The right diaphragm is usually 2-cm higher than the left, and normally the dome is at the level of the anterior end of the sixth rib. Unilateral or bilateral elevation of the hemidiaphragms may have diagnostic significance.

The *mediastinal contour* should be inspected for shifting of the mediastinum from the midline position, cardiomegaly, abnormalities in position or size of the large vessel shadows, focal areas of mediastinal widening, and the presence of air or calcium within the mediastinum.

The *hilar areas* are inspected with particular attention to changes in size or position. The left hilum is usually about 2-cm higher than the right. Vertical displacement of the hilum, either cephalad or caudad, strongly suggests volume loss from a lobe of the lung on that side.

The *vascular pattern* in the lungs is assessed, tracing the vessels from the hilum to the periphery. The vascular shadows should progressively branch and diminish in size as one follows the vessels outward from the hilum to the periphery. Changes in the vascular pattern may be localized or generalized. Minor increases or decreases in vascularity are difficult to detect.

The *lung fields* are then searched for localized areas of increased or decreased translucency. The lung fields should be inspected in a systematic fashion from top to bottom, comparing one side

with the other. The *pattern* of the abnormality should be identified, when possible.

THE LATERAL CHEST ROENTGENOGRAM

The lateral chest roentgenogram (Fig. 12–2) is customarily obtained in conjunction with the standard PA film, although there is some evidence to suggest that the incremental diagnostic value is relatively low if the patient is asymptomatic. Nevertheless, the lateral view may yield important information about the mediastinum and hilar areas,[12] and it may detect pulmonary lesions not visible on the PA film.

By convention, the view obtained is a *left* lateral, with the film cassette against the left axilla. A right lateral roentgenogram is obtained only if there is reason to suspect that the right lung may harbor an abnormality.

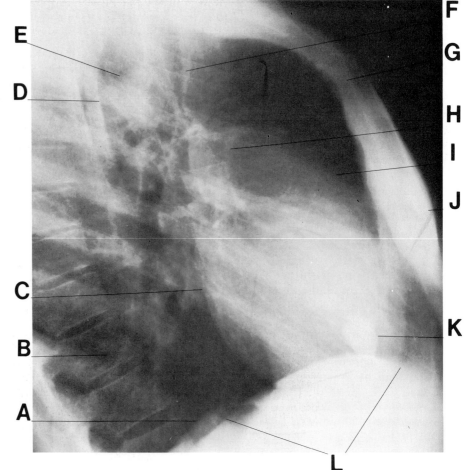

Figure 12—2. Chest roentgenogram in the right lateral projection. (*A*) left hemidiaphragm, the laterality of which can be determined in this particular case because the gastric air bubble can be seen; (*B*) thoracic spine (the intervertebral disk spaces are shown clearly; (*C*) posterior wall of the heart; (*D*) scapulae; (*E*) upper margin of the aortic arch; (*F*) anterior wall of the trachea (posterior to this is the tracheal air lucency); (*G*) sternum. The manubriosternal joint is visible; (*H*) right hilum, anterior to the left hilum in the lateral projection; (*I*) anterior border of the heart; (*J*) breast opacities; (*K*) rounded opacity caused by the presence of a small benign (fibrous) mesothelioma within the oblique fissure on the right (this is, of course, not a normal structure); (*L*) right hemidiaphragm.

ANTEROPOSTERIOR SUPINE CHEST FILM

The AP supine (or semierect) chest roentgenogram has inherent disadvantages that must be recognized if erroneous interpretations are to be minimized. The fact that the film was exposed with this technique is often indicated in some fashion. Radiologic clues that the projection is AP include high clavicles and transverse course of ribs (because the path of the roentgen beam often has a cephalad angulation) and the tendency of the scapulae to overlie the lung fields.

Assessment of heart size is difficult because the magnification effect on the heart and the elevation of the diaphragms often create an erroneous impression of mild cardiomegaly. The position-induced diaphragmatic elevation and the frequent failure of the patient to perform a maximal inspira- tion result in basilar haziness, suggesting pulmonary congestion or pleural effusion.

SPECIAL RADIOLOGIC TECHNIQUES

Special techniques are available to enhance the value of the radiologic examination. The most important techniques will be included here and discussed briefly.

CHANGES IN THE POSITION OF THE PATIENT

In addition to the standard PA and lateral projections, other views are sometimes helpful. *Oblique* projections aid in localizing lesions and, at times, detect evidence of disease that was not apparent on the standard films. The *apical lordotic* projection allows an improved view of the apical and subapical areas of the lungs (Fig. 12–3) and is particularly

Figure 12–3.   Value of the apical lordotic projection. (*A*) Posteroanterior chest film showing poorly defined consolidation (*arrow*) in the upper left lung deep to the clavicle and first rib. (*B*) Apical lordotic view clearly shows large ovoid mass in left upper lung field. Final diagnosis, established by biopsy, was bronchogenic carcinoma.

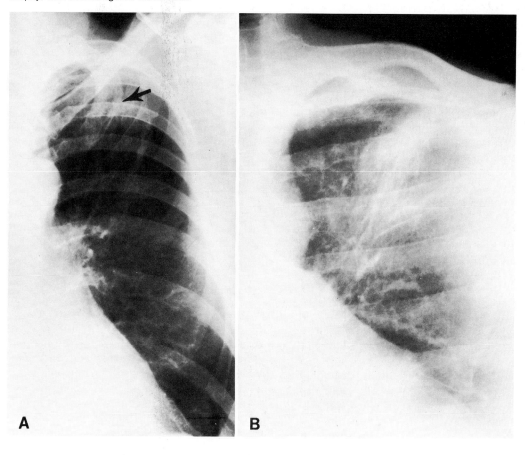

A   **B**

helpful in detection of chronic tuberculous disease. The *lateral decubitus* view is usually obtained with the affected side dependent and is particularly valuable in detecting the presence of small pleural effusions and in demonstrating that some large opacities seen on standard roentgenograms are caused by free pleural fluid and not by parenchymal consolidation. The shift in position will also shift fluid levels within pulmonary cavities, which at times is diagnostically helpful.

The *end-expiratory* PA chest roentgenogram is mentioned here for convenience. The end-expiratory film is compared with the standard end-inspiratory film. The comparison provides an objective measurement of diaphragmatic excursions and is valuable in detecting localized air-trapping within the lung. If a mediastinal shift is present, as in atelectasis or in obstructive hyperinflation, a change in the degree of shift may occur between inspiration and expiration, which is useful in determining which hemithorax is abnormal: the mediastinum appears to move toward the normal side on expiration. The end-expiratory film assists in the detection of small pneumothoraces.

CHANGES IN RADIOLOGIC CONTRAST

On occasion, it is useful to alter the technical factors affecting exposure and radiation density to produce an "overpenetrated" film that delineates certain abnormalities more clearly. This complements the standard chest roentgenogram but is never a substitute for it.

DIAGNOSTIC PNEUMOTHORAX AND PNEUMOPERITONEUM

The injection of gas into the peritoneal cavity (diagnostic pneumoperitoneum) has occasional usefulness in studying disease processes in or under the diaphragm. Air can be injected into a pleural cavity (diagnostic pneumothorax) to delineate certain pleural lesions more clearly, but this technique has been almost completely abandoned in favor of other modalities, such as computed tomography (CT) and sonography.

STANDARD TOMOGRAPHY

Body-section roentgenography (standard tomography, planigraphy, laminography, stratigraphy) facilitates the study of intrathoracic lesions obscured in standard chest roentgenograms by the superimposed opacities of overlying structures. Tomograms essentially consist of a series of roentgenographic sections that are "cut" (focused) at different depths. Each film shows a sharp image of the structures in that plane, with blurring of the images anterior and posterior to that plane. Tomograms are usually obtained in frontal (coronal) planes, but oblique or lateral (sagittal) plane projections may be useful in special circumstances.

Tomograms are particularly helpful in establishing the presence or absence of a disease process for patients in whom standard chest roentgenograms do not delineate the lesion clearly. The size and shape of the lesion, the sharpness of its margins, the presence of cavitation and calcification, and the surrounding vascular patterns are well demonstrated by tomography (Fig. 12–4). In addition, the patency of the tracheobronchial tree is well delineated by this technique.

BRONCHOGRAPHY

Bronchography requires the instillation of a radiopaque substance into the tracheobronchial tree. This adheres to the bronchial mucosa and allows radiologic visualization of the bronchi (Fig. 12–5). The standard bronchographic medium contains iodine, although barium has been used occasionally, and inhalation of tantalum dust has been employed in research studies. Bronchograms clearly show narrowing, dilatation, or obstruction of the bronchi. Bronchography causes some discomfort to the patient and increases hypoxemia and airway resistance, which involves an element of risk to the patient with diminished pulmonary function. The main contraindication to bronchography is allergy to the local anesthetic or to the bronchographic medium. The CT scan has largely replaced bronchography.

Bronchography of localized areas of lung can be accomplished by instillation of contrast through a fiberoptic bronchoscope that has been placed in the bronchus serving the region of interest.

ANGIOGRAPHY

Angiography is a contrast enhancement obtained by injection of a radiopaque medium into the vascular tree to determine the size, patency, and pattern of the blood vessels that are "downstream" from the point of injection. In the investigation of pulmonary diseases, injections of angiographic medium into appropriate areas may be used to opacify one or more of the following: the leg veins, the inferior vena cava, the superior vena cava and its tribu-

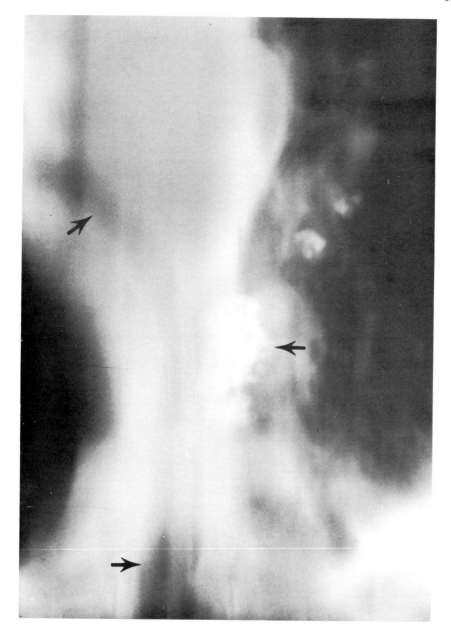

Figure 12—4. Standard tomographic cut in the coronal plane at 12 cm from the posterior thoracic wall. Tracheal air lucency is seen (*upper arrow*). A calcified mass of benign lymph nodes occupies the angle between the trachea and right main bronchus (*middle arrow*). Air in the left main bronchus is seen (*lower arrow*). (Lillington GA: A Diagnostic Approach to Chest Diseases, 3rd ed. Baltimore, Williams & Wilkins, 1987)

taries, the cardiac chambers, the pulmonary trunk and pulmonary arteries, the pulmonary veins, the aorta and its branches in the thorax or abdomen (including the bronchial arteries).

Pulmonary arteriography is probably the most commonly used of these procedures. It is employed primarily in diagnosing pulmonary embolism (see Chap. 36), but has other uses as well. *Bronchial arteriography* is sometimes utilized in the investigation and treatment of hemoptysis of unknown type; arteriography often localizes the site of bleed-

ing and provides guidance for therapeutic embolization of the bleeding vessel.

Contrast venography is primarily employed for the detection of obstruction in leg and thigh veins indicative of deep vein thrombosis.

FLUOROSCOPY

Fluoroscopy presents a continuous moving image of the area being examined. It provides a dynamic picture of the thorax and its contents during inspi-

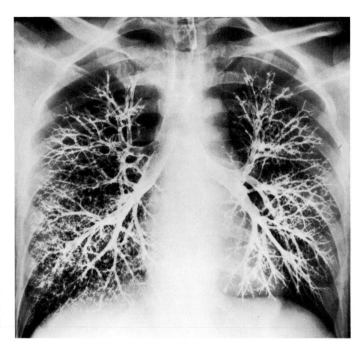

Figure 12—5. Normal bilateral bronchogram (posteroanterior view). Note the progressive diminution of airway caliber moving from the carina peripherally. The opaque medium coats the inner walls of the bronchial tree.

ration and expiration and throughout the cardiac cycle. Cinefluoroscopy will provide a permanent recording of the abnormalities visualized. Fluoroscopy is less sensitive than standard roentgenograms in detecting certain pulmonary lesions; therefore, it is an adjunct to standard chest roentgenograms, not a substitute for them. In addition, fluoroscopic examination entails a much greater radiation exposure than standard chest roentgenograms.

Fluoroscopy provides valuable information about the motion of the diaphragms and mediastinum and detects the presence of air-trapping. The relative expansion of the two lungs during inspiration is well shown. Mediastinal lesions can be better defined in terms of location and movement during breathing and swallowing. It is difficult, however, to differentiate the pulsatile expansion of a vascular mediastinal mass from the transmitted movement of a nonvascular mass adjacent to a large arterial vessel.

Fluoroscopic monitoring is employed during a barium swallow to detect abnormalities and displacements of the esophagus, and during needle aspiration biopsy of lung or mediastinum to guide needle placement. Fluoroscopy is sometimes used as a guide during bronchoscopic procedures, particularly biopsy of lesions beyond the visual field of the instrument.

RADIOLOGIC ESTIMATION OF PULMONARY FUNCTION

Numerous attempts have been made to use roentgenographic techniques for estimating the various functions measured by standard pulmonary function tests. The standard fluoroscopic methods obviously provide some information about the total expansibility of the lungs and the relative volume contributions of the two sides, but quantitation is extremely difficult. The specialized techniques of roentgen kymography and roentgen densitometry have shown a fairly good correlation with spirometric measurements of vital capacity and flow rates and have an advantage in that regional variations in these parameters are detectable. These methods have not found widespread application.

Total lung capacity can be measured fairly accurately from the standard end-inspiratory PA and lateral chest roentgenograms.[7] The method is tedious, however, and is not commonly used.

COMPUTED TOMOGRAPHIC SCANS

The widespread availability of computed tomographic (CT) scans of the thorax has had a major impact on the practice of pulmonary medicine. The method provides a series of cross-sectional (transverse) "tomographs" of the body structures at mul-

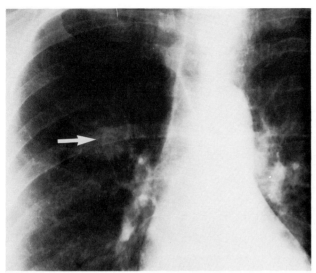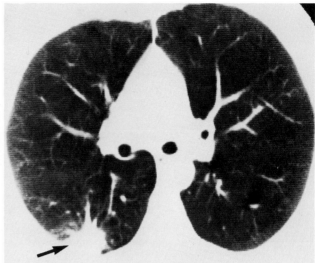

Figure 12—6.   Thoracic CT scan. (*Left*) The standard chest film shows a poorly demarcated mass (*arrow*) in the right lung. It was not clearly identified in the lateral projection film. (*Right*) CT scan shows the mass (*arrow*) in the right lung adjacent to the right posterior chest wall. This view is a transverse section just below the level of the carina, with the orientation as if the patient is lying supine and the observer is looking up toward the head.

tiple levels. Each image is generated by the computer and represents what a "slice" through the thorax at that particular level would look like (Fig. 12–6). Composite images in other planes can also be reconstructed.

The CT scan is a supplement to, not a replacement for, conventional chest radiography. It is particularly helpful in detecting or confirming the presence of a *mediastinal mass* and in determining its size, shape, location, and radiodensity. In the *lungs*, CT helps differentiate pleural from parenchymal masses, detects pulmonary nodules and subpleural lesions not visible on standard films or tomograms, and provides excellent demonstrations of the patterns of the abnormalities. Lesions in the bones and thoracic wall are seen very clearly.

Procedures such as needle biopsy can be carried out with CT guidance of needle emplacement. The full usefulness of the thoracic CT scan is still being determined.

With modern scanning devices, it is possible to perform the examination on critically ill patients receiving controlled ventilation (Fig. 12–7).

PULMONARY VENTILATION AND PERFUSION SCINTISCANS

Pulmonary scintiscanning is not, strictly speaking, a roentgenologic technique; the image is generated by the radiation emitted from radioisotopes introduced into the lungs.

Pulmonary scintiscans measure the volume and spatial distribution of ventilation and perfusion in the lungs. The standard *lung perfusion scintiscan* utilizes albumin particles that are tagged or labeled with a radioactive marker, such as iodine or technetium. This material is injected intravenously, and during its passage through the lungs some of the albumin particles impact in the small pulmonary capillaries. A scanning device is then passed over the thorax, and the pattern of γ-radiation is recorded as an index of the distribution and volume of perfusion in the lungs.

Similarly, the *ventilation scintiscan* assesses both the distribution pattern and the volume of ventilation within the lungs, measured by scanning the thorax while the patient takes one or several breaths of radioactive gas, usually xenon. Radioaerosols labeled with technetium also can be used; they have some technical advantages over xenon inhalation.

The diagnostic usefulness of ventilation and perfusion scintiscans lies in that a number of pulmonary diseases will give rise to abnormalities in either ventilation or perfusion, or both. Although the pattern that emerges is not entirely specific for any single process, it does delineate the physiologic abnormality that then can be correlated with

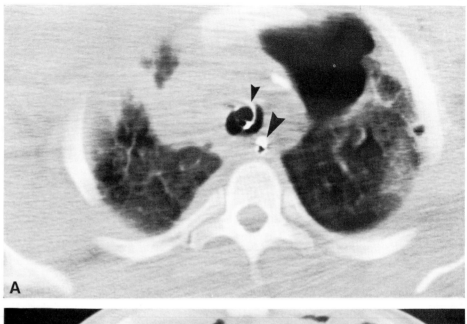

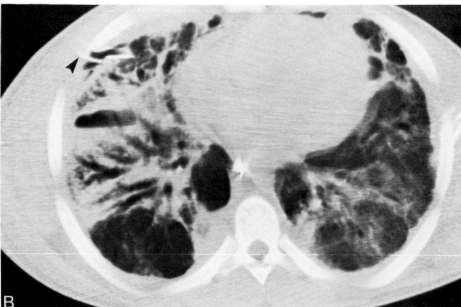

Figure 12—7.   Thoracic CT scans of a young man with chest and head trauma from a motorcycle accident. (*A*) This upper level "cut" shows an endotracheal tube (*upper arrowhead*) within the lumen of the trachea, and a small opaque gastric tube (*lower arrowhead*) within the esophagus. A bulla is present in the anterior portion of the left hemithorax. (*B*) The lower "cut," a few centimeters above the dome of the diaphragm shows a pleural drainage tube (*arrowhead*) entering the right pleural cavity anteriorly. There is extensive opacification throughout the right lung, with prominent air bronchograms. The gastric tube is still visible within the lower esophagus.

clinical and roentgenographic information to provide improved diagnostic precision.

Pulmonary scintiscanning is used most commonly in detecting and diagnosing *pulmonary embolism*. The lodgment of an embolus within a lobar or segmental pulmonary artery is followed by a marked decrease or complete absence of perfusion in the involved area. Ventilation to the area, however, is often fairly well maintained, at least for the first 24 to 48 hours. Ventilation–perfusion scans taken within the first 48 hours will often show a highly characteristic pattern of diminished or absent perfusion with normal ventilation (see Chap. 36). These are called "mismatching" defects. If the embolized area eventually undergoes infarction, ventilation will also decrease or disappear in the region of the perfusion defect. This type of combined or "matching" ventilation–perfusion defect is not specific for pulmonary infarction, however, but may also be seen with many other conditions, including pneumonia, asthma, emphysema, atelectasis, and bronchogenic carcinoma.[10]

Ventilation–perfusion scintiscans have some application in cases of *bullous emphysema*, particularly in selecting those patients who might benefit from surgical resection on the bullae. The technique has only limited usefulness in other pulmonary parenchymal and vascular conditions.

OTHER RADIOISOTOPIC TECHNIQUES

Radiolabeled gallium localizes in tissues that are inflamed or that have been invaded by malignant tumors. The gallium scan has been used to detect metastatic lung tumor in mediastinal lymph nodes, but CT is more sensitive and specific. Gallium is most commonly employed to determine if diffuse lung diseases such as fibrosing alveolitis or sarcoidosis are "active" and, therefore, potentially treatable. In the patient with *Pneumocystis carinii* pneumonia secondary to acquired immunodeficiency syndrome (AIDS), the gallium scan may show a diffuse increase in uptake of the isotope in the lungs before radiographic changes are clearly visible on the standard chest x-rays.

MAGNETIC RESONANCE IMAGING

Although the images generated by the magnetic resonance imaging (MRI) technique superficially resemble those produced by CT, the processes are quite different; MRI detects the radiosignals emitted when atomic nuclei are placed within a magnetic field and stimulated by radio waves. The images may be in any plane. In general, MRI is inferior to CT in imaging most intrapulmonary disorders, but the two processes are about equally effective in the study of lesions in the hilar areas or mediastinum. Magnetic resonance imaging is particularly valuable in the study of mediastinal vascular disorders such as aneurysms.

INTERVENTIONAL (INVASIVE) RADIOLOGY

Radiologic techniques can be employed to guide or monitor the performance of a number of invasive techniques.

Fluoroscopic guidance is sometimes employed during the course of *fiberoptic bronchoscopy*, primarily to monitor the positioning of biopsy forceps in distal areas of the lungs that cannot be visualized directly through the bronchoscope itself. *Transthoracic percutaneous needle aspiration biopsy* of lesions in the lung or mediastinum always requires radiographic guidance with fluoroscopy or CT.

Placement of a catheter in the bronchial artery for *bronchial arteriography* requires fluoroscopic guidance. As already noted, bronchial artery embolization can also be carried out for the treatment of severe hemoptysis.

DIAGNOSTIC ULTRASOUND

Ultrasonography is an important diagnostic tool in the investigation of certain cardiac abnormalities, but for technical reasons its applications in other forms of intrathoracic diseases are more limited.

Sonography is often helpful in the assessment of intrapleural fluid collections, both to detect free fluid and to localize pockets of loculated fluid within massive pleural densities. This may provide guidance for the emplacement of thoracentesis needles or intercostal drainage tubes. Subpulmonic and subphrenic collections of fluid may also be detected in this fashion. The position and degree of movement of the right hemidiaphragm can usually be determined. In some cases, sonography may provide guidance for needle aspiration biopsy of certain pulmonary and mediastinal lesions.

RADIOGRAPHIC PATTERNS OF LOCALIZED OPACIFICATION

Localized opacifications in the lungs may be single or multiple. The distribution of the opacities may be lobar, segmental, or nonsegmental.

Pulmonary consolidation is an opacification caused by displacement of alveolar air by fluid, tissue, or exudate. The distribution is lobar or segmental in some instances. There is usually no loss or gain of volume in the consolidated area.

Consolidation usually manifests a radiologic appearance called *alveolar filling*. An early radiologic sign is blurring of the normal vascular pattern in the consolidating area, with increasing loss of vessel outlines as the opacification increases. The opacification is due to the presence of multiple areas of alveolar filling, which are poorly circumscribed and confluent. Consolidation is usually nonhomogeneous, even when extensive, giving a patchy radiologic appearance (Fig. 12–8). Air bronchograms are usually detectable in nonobstructive consolidations.

Areas of consolidation may be single or multiple, unilateral or bilateral. Common causes include pneumonia (infectious or noninfectious), pulmonary edema, pulmonary contusion, chronic granulomatous diseases, localized alveolar cell carcinoma, and the early stage of pulmonary infarction.

Atelectasis is an opacification caused by loss of volume in a segment or lobe. When the collapse is due to complete obstruction of a bronchus, there is progressive resorption of air in the lung distal to the obstruction; the opacification will be homogeneous in appearance without air bronchograms (Fig. 12–9), and the entire lobe or segment will be involved. Pathologically, the alveoli are collapsed and airless rather than consolidated by alveolar filling. The vascular pattern is completely obliterated. Collapse of each lobe or segment has a specific and characteristic roentgenographic appearance.

Pleural effusion creates a homogeneous opacification that will usually have a characteristic localization and appearance. With the patient in the upright position, the opacity occupies the lower hemithorax, and its upper margin is poorly defined and concave upward. Atypical appearances may result if pleural obliteration impairs the free flow of fluid in response to gravitational forces. A large pleural effusion may mask the radiologic features of accompanying consolidation or atelectasis. If the pleural effusion is not too large and the underlying lung is normal, one may be able to discern a normal vascular pattern through the overlying pleural

Figure 12–8. Bacterial pneumonia, causing consolidation of the right upper lobe. This localized alveolar-filling process occupies most of the right upper lobe. Lucent air bronchograms can be seen within the consolidation, indicating that the opacity is alveolar, and that the upper lobe bronchus is patent. (*A*) PA projection with the consolidation sharply limited inferiorly by the horizontal fissure. Overlying the right hemithorax is a catheter taped to the anterior chest wall which then passes down the right subclavian vein and into the superior vena cava. The tip is obscured within the mediastinal opacity. Patchy, confluent, poorly circumscribed opacities can be seen in the lower left hemithorax. These are areas of bronchopneumonia. (*B*) Left lateral projection. The sternum is to the left; the spine to the right. The pneumonic consolidation is sharply demarcated inferiorly by the horizontal fissure (anteriorly) and by the oblique fissure (posteriorly). Foci of bronchopneumonia can be seen above the left hemidiaphragm posteriorly. The left diaphragm can be identified by its proximity to the gastric air bubble.

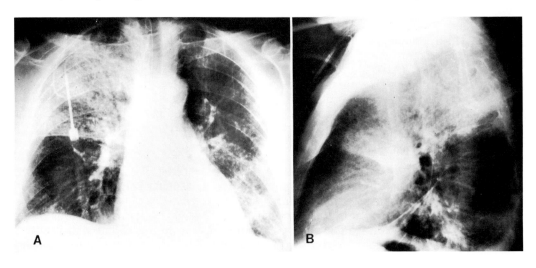

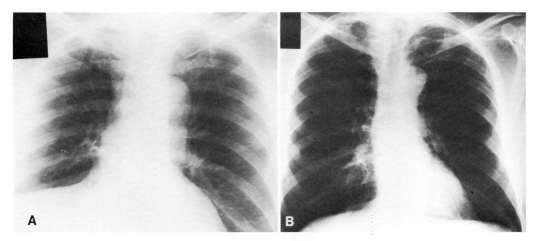

Figure 12—9. Atelectasis of the right lower lobe caused by sputum plug retention after intracranial surgery in an 18-year-old boy. (*A*) The PA view shows a collapsed and an airless right lower lobe which mimics an elevated right hemidiaphragm. The interface is at the level of the oblique (major) fissure, which is pulled downward by the collapse. (*B*) The same patient, 1 hour after bronchoscopic aspiration of the plug. The right lower lobe has reexpanded, and the diaphragm is now visible at its normal level.

opacity, particularly if the film is a little overpenetrated. This indicates the opacity is intrapleural and not intrapulmonary.

A *replacement opacity,* also called a "destructive" lesion, is one in which the normal lung tissue in the affected area has been replaced or displaced by a disease process. In some instances the normal tissue is pushed aside or compressed by a growing mass, whereas in other instances there has been actual tissue necrosis. Examples include intrapulmonary nodules and masses (many of which are malignant), tuberculous and fungal infections, necrotizing pneumonias, undrained lung abscesses, and complete infarcts. Such lesions, single or multiple, tend to be rather homogeneous in density and often sharply circumscribed, although the outline may be irregular.

PNEUMONIAS

Pneumonia is an inflammatory consolidation of the lung, usually caused by an infection with microorganisms. Other causes include inhalation or aspiration of toxic substances[3] or autoimmune processes. Most pneumonias are acute in onset, bacterial in etiology, and alveolar-filling in radiologic presentation. The opacification is usually nonhomogeneous provided that the bronchus to the area is not completely obstructed. Pneumonia sometimes shows lobar–segmental distributions (Figs. 12–8 and 12–10), but the involvement is incomplete in many instances.

BACTERIAL PNEUMONIAS

Bacterial pneumonias may be caused by a variety of pathogenic microorganisms that reach the lungs through inhalation or aspiration of infected secretions (commonly) or by hematogenous spread from an infection elsewhere (less commonly). Primary bacterial pneumonias caused by the pneumococcus (*Streptococcus pneumoniae*), Friedlander's bacillus (*Klebsiella pneumoniae*), or the staphylococcus (*Staphylococcus aureus*) are commonly *lobar* or *segmental* in distribution (see Fig. 12–8). Most commonly one lobe or segment is involved, although several areas of disease within different lobes are sometimes seen, particularly with staphylococcal pneumonia. These pneumonias are alveolar-filling in type, with confluent "fluffy" areas of opacity and air bronchograms contributing to the nonhomogeneity of the process.

Lobar bacterial pneumonias are often of the primary type but may be a complication of underlying lung disease, such as bronchiectasis or partial bronchial obstruction. Friedlander's pneumonia is particularly common in chronic alcoholics. Lobar pneumonias often have an acute onset with fever, cough, chest pain, dyspnea, and arterial hypoxemia. In occasional instances, lobar consolidations

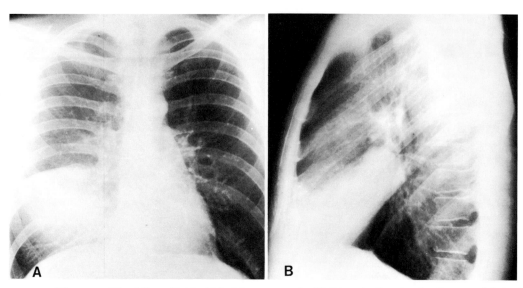

Figure 12–10. Right middle lobe pneumonia. (*A*) PA projection showing the consolidation with its characteristic triangular configuration. The upper border is limited by the horizontal (minor) fissure, and the lateral border by the oblique fissure. Note that the costophrenic angle is clear and the right heart border is blurred (the silhouette sign). (*B*) Lateral view showing the roughly triangular opacity overlying the cardiac opacity. The upper margin is often more sharply outlined than this.

may result from infection with tubercle bacilli or fungi.

Bacterial pneumonias caused by certain other microorganisms rarely show a lobar or segmental pattern and more commonly appear as multiple, poorly circumscribed areas of alveolar consolidation that may involve one or both lungs. This pattern is often referred to as *bronchopneumonia.* Organisms that commonly present in this fashion include *Streptococcus pyogenes, Haemophilus influenzae, Mycoplasma,* the coliform bacilli, *Pseudomonas, Proteus, Serratia,* and anaerobic bacteria. Staphylococcal pneumonias often show this pattern. Bronchopneumonias are often secondary to some other predisposing process, including the use of immunosuppressive drugs, general debility, aspiration, endotracheal intubation, prolonged antibiotic use, and contaminated inhalation therapy equipment.

Necrosis may occur with bacterial pneumonias, particularly those caused by *S. aureus,* aerobic gram-negative bacilli, and anaerobic organisms. Drainage of the necrotic material reuslts in the appearance of air-filled hyperlucent areas called *cavities* (Fig. 12–11). A cavity that changes rapidly in size (a pneumatocele) is a common complication in staphylococcal infections. A cavity secondary to necrotizing pneumonia is termed a *lung abscess.*

Bacterial aspiration pneumonia presents with single or multiple consolidation of dependent portions of the lungs caused by aspiration of infected pharyngeal secretions; it is most common in alcoholics and in patients with poor oral hygiene, particularly if obtunded. Nasogastric tubes, endotracheal tubes, and swallowing difficulties are frequent predisposing causes. The infecting organisms are usually anaerobes or gram-negative aerobic bacilli; necrosis and abscess formation are common.[2]

Bacterial pneumonias are commonly accompanied by *parapneumonic pleural effusions.* Occasionally frank empyema develops.

Certain bacterial pneumonias may initially appear to be nonbacterial because the organisms are rarely seen in sputum smears and are difficult to culture. These include *Mycoplasma pneumoniae* infection, one of the most common forms of pneumonia. Other examples are *psittacosis* (parrot fever) and *legionellosis* (Legionnaires' disease). Diagnosis is serologic or by lung biopsy. The radiologic pattern is usually bronchopneumonic.

VIRAL PNEUMONIAS

Viral pneumonias may present with a diffuse interstitial or alveolar-filling pattern. This is particularly

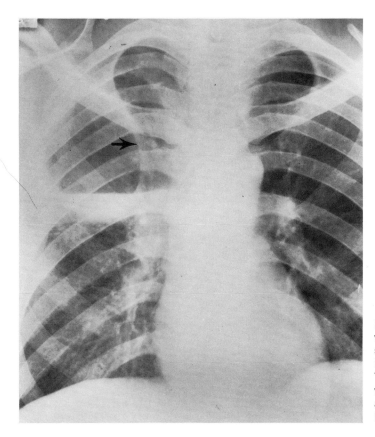

Figure 12–11. Lung abscess. A large thin-walled cavity is seen in the upper right lung, containing a small amount of opaque fluid. Note the horizontal air–fluid interface. The medial wall of the cavity is marked (*arrow*). The superior wall is hidden by the clavicle and the lateral wall is obscured by the ribs of the lateral chest wall. The antecedent necrotizing pneumonia that caused the cavity has largely cleared.

common with influenzal (Fig. 12–12) and cytomegalovirus infections, which may be accompanied by severe hypoxemia and increased lung stiffness sufficient to qualify these diseases as examples of adult respiratory distress syndrome (ARDS). Varicella (chickenpox) pneumonia in adults has a high mortality.

Many or most viral pneumonias, however, present as a patchy bronchopneumonia, which may be complicated by secondary bacterial infection. These illnesses may be only a temporary inconvenience to a previously healthy person but can produce a life-threatening respiratory insufficiency in the patient with chronic obstructive pulmonary disease (COPD).

Viral pneumonias caused by measles or varicella may appear on the roentgenogram as miliary lesions or multiple nodules, rather than as an alveolar-filling process.

TUBERCULOUS AND FUNGAL PNEUMONIAS

The tubercle bacillus and most fungi characteristically cause a chronic, slowly progressive, fairly well-localized destructive process that pathologically is often granulomatous. However, in the early primary stage of the infection, before the body develops resistance, single or multiple areas of pneumonia may occur with infection by the tubercle bacillus and certain fungi (*Coccidioides immitis* and *Histoplasma capsulatum*).

Other fungi may cause a pneumonic consolidation (sometimes rapidly spreading) if the host defenses have been compromised. Fungi that often behave in this fashion include *Cryptococcus neoformans*, the *Phycomycetes*, *Candida albicans*, and *Aspergillus fumigatus*. Infection with *Phycomycetes* (mucormycosis) is most commonly seen in diabetics. Candidiasis and aspergillosis may follow long-term antibiotic therapy and often occur in granulocytopenic patients and after the use of immunosuppressive drugs.

Chronic tuberculosis commonly presents as a somewhat indolent destructive granulomatous process in which consolidation, cavitation, fibrosis, and calcification are often present simultaneously. The apical and subapical areas of the lungs are most commonly involved (Fig. 12–13), and the dis-

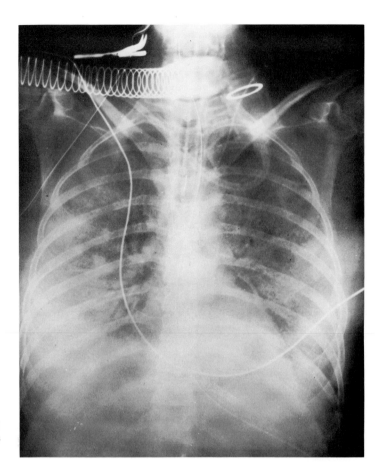

Figure 12—12. Diffuse alveolar consolidation caused by influenzal pneumonia. The diagnosis was proved by open lung biopsy and cultures.

ease is often bilateral. Quiescent "healed" tuberculosis may be converted to an active progressive disease by the use of adrenal corticosteroid drugs.

Certain fungal infections, particularly histoplasmosis and coccidioidomycosis, may demonstrate a similar clinical and radiographic pattern. Nocardiosis and actinomycosis may also behave similarly and are commonly included among the fungal diseases, even though the causative organisms are now classified as bacteria, rather than fungi.

PARASITIC PNEUMONIAS

Pneumonias caused by parasitic infections are rarely seen in nontropical climates, with two exceptions. Amebic infection in the liver may spread upward through the diaphragm to involve the right lower hemithorax, with roentgenographic changes indicative of pneumonic consolidation, pleural effusion, or pulmonary cavitation. Pneumonia caused by infection with *Pneumocystis carinii* presents as a diffuse alveolar-filling process and oc-

curs almost exclusively in immunosuppressed patients. It is particularly common in patients with AIDS.

NONINFECTIOUS PNEUMONIAS

On occasion, pneumonic consolidation may be due to physical or chemical irritation of the lung rather than to infection. Such pneumonias may be diffuse or localized in distribution.

The inhalation of *noxious fumes* (nitrogen dioxide, chlorine, sulfur dioxide, phosgene) may cause a diffuse pneumonic process that is acute, extensive, and often fatal. Silo-filler's disease is an acute hemorrhagic pneumonitis of farmers from inhalation of nitrogen dioxide formed during the ensilage process.

The aspiration of low pH gastric juice may cause a widespread pneumonic process called *peptic (acid) pneumonitis*. This syndrome is discussed in the section on diffuse alveolar diseases.

Lipoid pneumonia (oil granuloma) results from the habitual use of mineral oil or oily nose drops

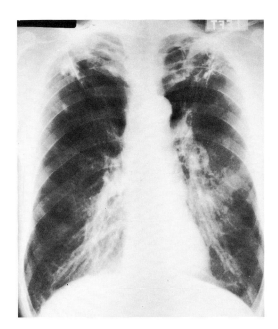

Figure 12–13. Bilateral apical and subapical tuberculosis. The lesions are fibrotic and calcified; however, active infection may be present in lesions that appear healed. This patient also has emphysema, which is indicated by the loss of lung markings in many areas of the lungs. Note the upward retraction of the left hilum, caused by fibrotic scarring and volume loss in the left upper lobe.

and presents radiologically as a localized chronic consolidation simulating carcinoma. Oily substances are easily aspirated because the material may pass through the vocal cords without exciting the protective cough reflex.

Localized noninfectious pneumonias, with solitary or multiple lesions, may occur in *systemic lupus erythematosus. Hypersensitivity pneumonitis (allergic alveolitis)* encompasses a group of diseases caused by inhalation of organic antigens. Examples include farmer's lung and bird-fancier's lung. The early stage of the reaction of the lung to *radiation* is pneumonic in type, although a rather dense interstitial fibrosis may eventually develop in the involved area.

ATYPICAL PNEUMONIA

The term *atypical pneumonia* dates back 50 years or more to the time when microbiologic sciences had developed sufficiently to permit the recognition that some cases of pneumonia were clinically different from the "typical" bacterial pneumonias,

and they were then classified as examples of "primary atypical pneumonia."

In current useage, the term denotes pneumonias that tend to have a gradual onset and are characterized by upper respiratory symptoms and systemic symptoms such as fever and malaise. The pneumonia, which is sometimes an unexpected chest x-ray finding, is usually nonsegmental. Sputum is scanty and nonpurulent, and examination of sputum by smears and standard bacterial cultures fails to identify a pathogenic bacterial cause.

Common forms of atypical pneumonia include mycoplasmal pneumonia, psittacosis, rickettsial pneumonia, legionellosis, and viral pneumonias. In some cases, primary tuberculous and fungal infections may present with this syndrome of atypical pneumonia.

SOLITARY AND MULTIPLE PULMONARY NODULES

A pulmonary *nodule* is a well-circumscribed, roughly spherical, solid intrapulmonary lesion usually larger than 1 cm in diameter. A circumscribed lesion larger than 4 cm in diameter is usually designated a *mass* lesion rather than a nodule. Some nodules develop cavitation, and many are calcified.

SOLITARY PULMONARY NODULES

The solitary nodule is most commonly a healed or healing infectious granuloma that may result from tuberculosis, coccidioidomycosis, or histoplasmosis. Less commonly the solitary nodule is a lung tumor, either benign or malignant. Primary malignant tumors are usually *bronchogenic carcinomas,* but occasionally the malignant lung nodule is a *solitary metastasis* from an extrapulmonary primary tumor. Other disease processes may occasionally present as a solitary nodule.

If serial chest roentgenograms show that the nodule has not increased in size over 2 years, or if it exhibits extensive calcification, it is safe to assume that the lesion is benign (Fig. 12–14). A nodule that fails to meet these criteria is potentially malignant and is usually subjected to needle biopsy or exploratory thoracotomy.[4]

MULTIPLE PULMONARY NODULES

Multiple nodules are usually due to intrapulmonary metastases from an extrapulmonary primary malignant lesion. Other causes include tuberculo-

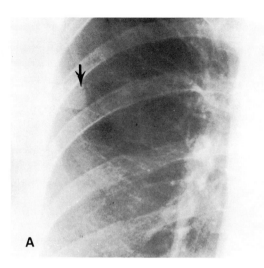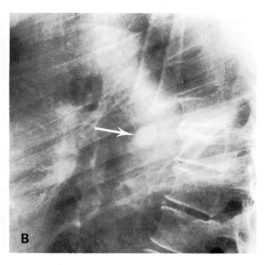

Figure 12–14. Solitary pulmonary nodule caused by coccidioidomycosis. (*A*) PA view of right hemithorax showing the 1.5-cm nodule situated far laterally (*arrow*) in the upper lung. (*B*) In the lateral view, the nodule is clearly seen overlying the shadow of the aortic arch, halfway between the hilar opacity and the thoracic spine. The nodule is calcified (*arrow*). (Lillington GA: A Diagnostic Approach to Chest Diseases, 3rd ed. Baltimore, Williams & Wilkins, 1987)

sis, fungal diseases, sarcoidosis, silicosis, and necrotizing granulomatous conditions such as Wegener's syndrome or lymphomatoid granulomatosis. The appearance of multiple pulmonary nodules in an immunosuppressed host strongly suggests opportunistic infection with fungi.

A solitary nodule has little, if any, deleterious effect on pulmonary function. Its importance is related to possible malignancy. Multiple nodules, depending partly on number, size, distribution, and etiology, may reduce lung volumes, but blood gas values are often little affected.

ATELECTASIS AND LOSS OF VOLUME

Atelectasis is a loss of volume of part (or all) of a lung. The airless atelectatic area is usually opaque. Although atelectasis may result from several difference mechanisms, the term is used most commonly in reference to those losses of volume caused by bronchial obstruction or cicatrization (scar formation).

OBSTRUCTIVE ATELECTASIS

Obstructive atelectasis may result from (1) extrabronchial compression from tumors or enlarged lymph nodes, (2) endobronchial diseases such as bronchial tumors (Fig. 12–15) or inflammatory strictures (Fig. 12–16), or (3) an intrabronchial

mass such as an exogenous foreign body or a large mucous plug (see Fig. 12–9). A movable intrabronchial mass may act as a "ball valve" that allows the air to be pumped out from the affected segment within minutes. More commonly, atelectasis results from the slow resorption of air in the bronchioles and alveoli distal to the completely obstructed bronchus.

CICATRIZATION ATELECTASIS

Cicatrization (scar) atelectasis may occur in the absence of significant bronchial obstruction. It is sometimes a complication of lobar or segmental pneumonia that fails to resorb and becomes "organized" and fibrotic. Contraction of the fibrosis decreases the lung volume. It may also develop as a complication of chronic fibrocaseous tuberculosis, usually involving an upper lobe.

SIGNS OF ATELECTASIS

The *indirect* signs of atelectasis are the secondary effects of collapse of a lobe or an entire lung. They are usually detectable on the chest roentgenogram and will suggest that volume loss has occurred, even if the opacification of the atelectic segment or lobe is not clearly seen. These signs include elevation of the hemidiaphragm on the affected side, shift of the mediastinum toward the affected side, a decrease in size of the rib interspaces over the af-

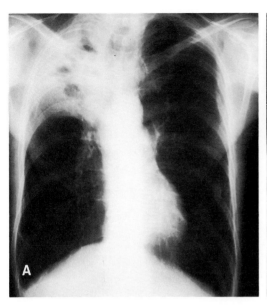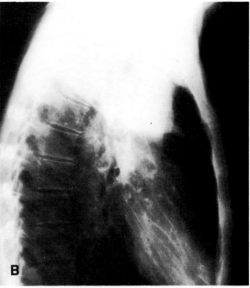

Figure 12—15. Obstructive pneumonitis of the right upper lobe secondary to bronchial occlusion by bronchogenic carcinoma. (A) In the PA view, the lobe has lost some volume, as shown by the elevation of the horizontal fissure, which demarcates the consolidation inferiorly, but the fissure has not rotated to the diagonal position that would be expected if marked loss of volume from complete atelectasis were present. Intralobar cavitation is secondary to necrotizing pneumonitis. (B) Lateral view shows fissures elevated, but retaining their normal angulation.

This man also has advanced pulmonary emphysema. In the PA view, the lungs are hyperlucent from hyperinflation and from widespread destruction of lung parenchyma and vessels. The diaphragms are low and flat, and the small heart appears to be "hanging" in the mediastinum above the left hemidiaphragm. In the lateral view, the diaphragms are flat and scalloped, and the sternodiaphragmatic angle is considerably greater than 90°. The retrosternal airspace is large and markedly hyperlucent.

fected hemithorax, and in many instances a compensatory hyperinflation of the adjacent lobes or of the opposite lung. A shift of the hilum, either upward or downward, is sometimes present.

The *direct* signs of atelectasis are the characteristic appearances on the standard chest roentgenograms of the collapsed opaque segment, lobe, or lung (see Figs. 12–9, 12–15, and 12–16).

DECREASED LUNG VOLUME OF OTHER TYPES

Decreased volume of the entire lung occurs when the stability of the chest wall is impaired, allowing the elastic recoil of the lung to effect a decrease in volume. Common examples include hemidiaphragmatic paralysis or eventration (Fig. 12–17) and multiple rib fractures with a flail chest.

The development of extensive pleural scarring (fibrothorax) renders the affected hemithorax smaller and less expansile. Finally, an expanding lesion within the lung, such as a rapidly growing tumor, a lung abscess, or an expanding tension cyst, may cause some compression of the adjacent normal lung. Although loss of lung volume is a feature of all these conditions, the term atelectasis is not used clinically under these circumstances.

The appearance in the pleural space of air (*pneumothorax*) or fluid (*hydrothorax, pleural effusion*) allows the lung to retract toward the hilum into a partially collapsed position. In these cases the loss of volume is generalized, not localized, is partial and not complete, and the radiologic picture is dominated by the primary intrapleural disturbance.

OTHER MANIFESTATIONS OF BRONCHIAL OBSTRUCTION

Bronchial obstruction will have differing effects on the distal lung, depending on the degree of obstruc-

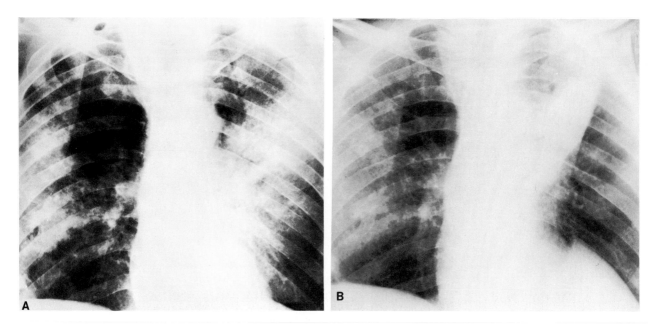

Figure 12–16. Consolidation of the left upper lobe, followed by atelectasis, in a case of active pulmonary tuberculosis. (*A*) PA view showing a fairly dense alveolar consolidation in the left upper lobe, with sparing of the apical segment, but involvement of the lingula. There is little loss of volume. In the right lung are several areas of tuberculous bronchopneumonia. (*B*) Two weeks later. The left upper lobe bronchus has become occluded, presumably by tuberculous endobronchitis, and the left upper lobe has become atelectatic, being smaller and denser. There is still some aeration within the apical segment. The left hemidiaphragm is now markedly elevated because of volume loss in the left lung.

tion and the rapidity with which it develops. Minor degrees of obstruction that have no major effect on airway dynamics will not result in roentgenologic changes. However, the presence of the localized obstruction may be apparent on auscultation over the affected area. A persistent localized wheeze or reduced breath sounds may be noted.

An obstruction large enough to impair the clearance of mucoid secretions from the distal lung predisposes toward *pneumonia* of the affected segment or lobe. This pneumonic consolidation will have the usual roentgenologic characteristics of a segmental or lobar alveolar-filling process and cannot be differentiated from nonobstructive pneumonias. If, however, the obstruction increases and becomes complete while the pneumonia is still present, the affected segment or lobe becomes completely airless but cannot shrink in volume because the alveoli are filled with inflammatory exudate. In such cases of *obstructive pneumonitis* ("drowned lung"), air bronchograms will be absent, allowing one to infer the presence of bronchial obstruction as the cause of the homogeneous opacification of the lobe (see Fig. 12–15). A complete bronchial obstruction that develops without secondary infec-

tion intervening will show the signs of *atelectasis* described previously.

An unusual but important manifestation of bronchial obstruction is *obstructive hyperinflation*, which occurs when the magnitude of the obstruction is such that it allows air to enter the lobe as the bronchus increases in size during inspiration, but prevents egress of air as the bronchus decreases in size during expiration. The hyperinflated lobe or segment is hyperlucent and virtually functionless. It may cause some compression atelectasis of the adjoining or contralateral nonobstructed lung segments or lobes. Bronchography is sometimes used to confirm the presence and site of obstruction. In clinical practice, bronchoscopic visualization with biopsy of the obstructing lesion is the most effective diagnostic tool.

PULMONARY CAVITIES AND CYSTS

A *cavity* is a hole within the lung parenchyma; it usually indicates that destruction of lung tissue has occurred, although sometimes it may result from the evacuation of a congenital fluid-filled cyst. The

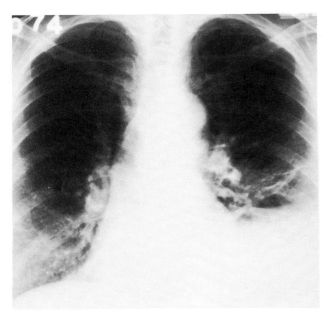

Figure 12—17. Eventration of the left hemidiaphragm: The elevated hemidiaphragm showed paradoxic movement on sniffing. Usually the upper margin of the eventrated hemidiaphragm maintains a sharp convex contour. Here, a previous pulmonary infection has resulted in pleural adhesions between the diaphragm and the lung. Horizontal streaks of "discoid" atelectasis can be seen. (Lillington GA: A Diagnostic Approach to Chest Diseases, 3rd ed. Baltimore, Williams & Wilkins, 1987)

terminology of cavitary lesions of the lung is confusing and somewhat inconsistent.

A *lung abscess* is a localized area of lung destruction caused by liquefaction necrosis, usually within an area of necrotizing pneumonitis caused by pyogenic bacteria. A lung abscess may present initially with the roentgenographic appearance of a solid mass; if the liquefied material then drains into a bronchus, the lung abscess will appear as a thick-walled, round cavity containing air and often an air—fluid level (see Fig. 12—11). Lung abscess is most commonly due to aspiration of anaerobic organisms, but may be a complication of other necrotizing pneumonias, particularly staphylococcal and aerobic gram-negative bacterial infections. Obstruction of a bronchus may cause a necrotizing process in the distal lung that eventually forms an abscess. Hematogenous spread of infection to the lungs may result in multiple abscesses.

Cavitation occurs commonly in pulmonary *tuberculosis* and in *fungal infections* of the lungs. These cavities may have thick or thin walls. Usually there are other lesions in neighboring portions of the lungs as well.

Bullae are thin-walled, focal areas of emphysema. They vary in size but sometimes may be several centimeters in diameter. The wall of the bulla may not be roentgenographically visible or may present as one or more "hairline" shadows that form part of the wall, but are not always continuous around the entire air-containing structure (Fig. 12—18). Bullae may occasionally occur in otherwise normal lungs, but they are usually a manifestation of diffuse obstructive emphysema. Secondary infection may occur, with the development of air—fluid levels, and the wall may then become thickened and more visible.

A *pneumatocele* is a bulla that results from a check-valve obstruction of a bronchus that causes the bulla to increase or decrease rapidly in size. It

Figure 12—18. Bullae in the upper right lung. Thin, hairline shadows of the walls of the bullae are shown (*arrow*). Within the bullae, there is little or no lung substance. This is a chest roentgenogram of a 76-year-old man with panacinar emphysema with bullous transformation.

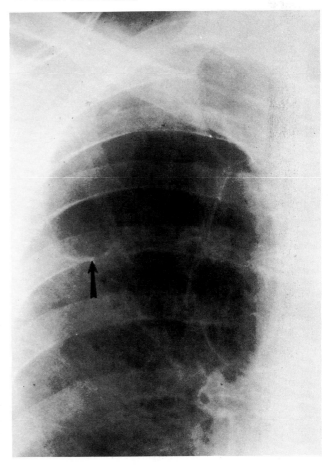

occurs most commonly as a complication of staphylococcal pneumonia.

Cavitation may occur within primary or secondary *neoplasms* of the lung, within *noninfectious granulomas* and, occasionally, within an *infarcted* area secondary to pulmonary embolism. Hemorrhage, often life-threatening, may occur within cavitary lesions. A lung abscess may be a source of dissemination of infection throughout the body, resulting in septicemia or, sometimes, brain abscesses.

A *cyst* is a thin-walled cavity that is usually congenital. Many cysts are originally fluid filled and contain air only if drainage of the contents has occurred. Bronchogenic cysts are oval, well-circumscribed, and opaque, and often hilar or mediastinal in location.

DIFFUSE AIRWAY OBSTRUCTION

The diffuse obstructive airway diseases are a group of conditions characterized by generalized airway narrowing, resulting in partial obstruction of most of the bronchi and bronchioles in the lungs. Examples include asthma, chronic bronchitis, emphysema, and pulmonary cystic fibrosis (mucoviscidosis).

Diffuse obstructive airway disease leads to increased airway resistance, manifested physiologically by decreases in airflow rates. The increased airway resistance may be present during both inspiration and expiration, or during expiration alone.

Roentgenologic changes in diffuse obstructive airway diseases may be very obvious or fairly subtle.[6] These changes, manifested in varying degrees by the different disease processes, include the following:

1. Hyperinflation: an increase in the total lung capacity as shown on standard end-inspiratory chest roentgenograms. The roentgenographic signs are depression and flattening of the diaphragms, a generalized increased translucency of the lung fields, and an increased size of the retrosternal airspace as seen on the lateral projection.
2. Air-trapping: a decreased ability to evacuate alveolar air during expiration. Detection of air-trapping requires an end-expiratory roentgenogram to compare with the standard end-inspiratory roentgenogram. Fluoroscopic examination will supply similar information.

3. Diminution or loss of interstitial tissue and pulmonary vessels: The loss of interstitial tissue is most apparent if bullae are present; demonstration of diminution in vasculature may require "full chest" tomograms or pulmonary angiography. It is now known that CT is the most sensitive and accurate modality for the identification and quantitation of lung destruction.
4. Increased lung markings: This occurs in some patients and is presumed to be caused by bronchial wall inflammation with thickening, and peribronchial fibrosis secondary to previous bronchopneumonic infections. This appearance is often referred to as the "dirty lung."

ASTHMA

Asthma is an intermittent or reversible form of diffuse airway obstruction that often begins in childhood and is characterized by bronchospasm, swelling of the bronchial mucosa, and plugging of the airways with tenacious mucus. In about 40% of cases the disease is associated with atopic allergy and is called *extrinsic* asthma; in the remainder of cases (*intrinsic* asthma) no definite allergic features can be identified, and the onset is often in middle age or later.

During symptom-free periods the chest roentgenogram usually appears entirely normal. During an acute asthmatic attack the airway obstruction is mainifested clinically by severe dyspnea and wheezing, and roentgenographically by reversible hyperinflation with some depression of the diaphragms and increased hypertranslucency. Destructive changes in the interstitial tissue do not occur, and the pulmonary vasculature is essentially normal. In short, an asthmatic attack may cause acute deterioration of pulmonary function, with relatively little radiographic change. In such cases the physical signs are diagnostic and more helpful than the roentgenographic features.[11]

Complications of asthma may give rise to roentgenographic abnormalities.[6] Recurrent infections result in thickened bronchial walls and a "tramline" appearance. Atelectasis may occur because of mucous plugs. Pneumomediastinum and pneumothorax may complicate asthma. Radiologic abnormalities in *allergic bronchopulmonary aspergillosis* (ABPA) include perihilar masses, consolidations, tramline shadows, nodules, and ring shadows.

CHRONIC BRONCHITIS

Chronic bronchitis is a chronic low-grade inflammation of the bronchi manifested by persistent cough and sputum production. Diffuse airway obstruction may be absent, mild, or severe. The chest roentgenogram often appears normal but may show the pattern of "increased lung markings." In some instances there is a superimposed reversible or asthmatic component (chronic asthmatic bronchitis), and, in these patients, hyperinflation and air-trapping are sometimes noticeable. Unless complicated by emphysema, chronic bronchitis is not associated with destruction of interstitial tissue or loss of pulmonary vasculature.

EMPHYSEMA

Emphysema is a destructive process in the pulmonary parenchyma, and the foregoing roentgenologic signs (including loss of interstitial tissue and pulmonary vessels, hyperinflation, and bullae) are most marked in this condition (see Figs. 12–13, 12–15, and 12–18). The diffuse airway obstruction is primarily expiratory, as the airways "collapse" during expiration. The presence of bullous disease ma be very striking. In advanced cases hyperinflation is usually quite apparent, both on physical examination and by roentgenographic studies. In many cases of emphysema, the chest roentgenogram appears normal.

PNEUMOTHORAX AND MEDIASTINAL EMPHYSEMA

Pneumothorax denotes the presence of air within the pleural cavity. Air may gain access to the pleural cavity through the chest wall, diaphragm, or mediastinum, or from the lung through the visceral pleura. Pneumothorax may be traumatic, iatrogenic, or spontaneous.

Roentgenographic recognition of a pneumothorax depends on the loss of volume of the affected lung. A hairline linear shadow representing the visceral pleura may be seen, separating the lung from the patternless hypertranslucency of the intrapleural air (Fig. 12–19). A small pneumothorax may be difficult to detect on the standard end-inspiratory roentgenogram. The pneumothorax is always more obvious if films are taken in the end-expiratory position, and this is a very useful diagnostic maneuver in questionable cases. The presence of underlying lung disease may be detected by the chest roentgenogram.

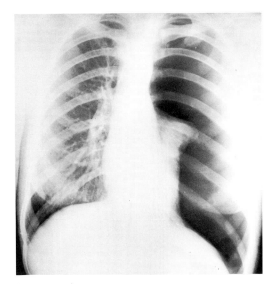

Figure 12—19. Massive left spontaneous pneumothorax in a young woman. The collapsed left lung forms a small opaque ball in the hilar area, whereas the rest of the hemithorax is filled with the patternless hypertranslucency of pleural air. Usually the lung does not collapse to this degree in spontaneous pneumothorax.

With a small pneumothorax, the air may be visible only in the apical and subapical areas. Pleural adhesions that prevent the retraction of portions of the lung may give rise to a loculated pneumothorax in which the intrapleural air is localized to one or more discrete areas, instead of involving the entire pleural space (Fig. 12–20). The concomitant presence of blood, pus, chyle, or serous effusion will result in an air–fluid level.

If a patient already has impaired pulmonary function, the development of a pneumothorax, even one that is small, may cause serious respiratory difficulty, which can, however, be quickly relieved once the correct diagnosis has been established and the air evacuated by closed intercostal drainage through a chest tube. Pneumothorax should be considered whenever there is an acute increase in dyspnea, particularly if unilateral chest pain is present.

TRAUMATIC PNEUMOTHORAX

Trauma may give rise to pneumothorax by several mechanisms, the most obvious being damage to the chest wall that allows atmospheric air to gain direct access to the pleural space. More commonly the underlying lung is lacerated, either from a penetrating foreign body or from injury to the lung by rib

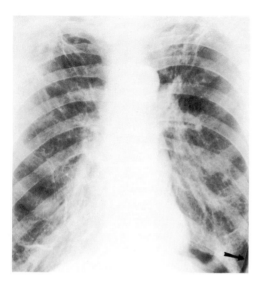

Figure 12—20. Small loculated pneumothorax at the left base. Compare with Fig. 12–13, which is an x-ray film of the same patient. Apparently, an emphysematous bleb has ruptured, allowing leakage of air into the pleural space, which is bound down by adhesions in most areas, except laterally and inferiorly at the left base.

fracture. Another mechanism is traumatic fracture of a bronchus with resulting air leakage.

IATROGENIC PNEUMOTHORAX

Iatrogenic pneumothorax is now the most common form of intrapleural air. Such pneumothoraces may be intentional (as in the induction of pneumothorax for diagnostic purposes), unavoidable (as in needle biopsy of the lung), or unintentional.

Iatrogenic pneumothorax usually results from inadvertent perforation of the lung during various diagnostic or therapeutic procedures, including thoracentesis, liver biopsy, pericardiocentesis, intercostal nerve block, stellate ganglion block, transbronchial or percutaneous lung biopsy, attempted cannulation of a subclavian vein, and surgical procedures (such as tracheostomy) at the base of the neck. Procedures such as transtracheal needle aspiration and endoscopic injury of the thoracic esophagus may result in mediastinal emphysema, which, subsequently, may rupture into the pleural space. Pneumothorax is, unfortunately, a rather common complication of mechanical ventilation.

SPONTANEOUS PNEUMOTHORAX

Spontaneous pneumothorax may occur as a complication of intrapulmonary or mediastinal disease processes. Most commonly, it is seen in young people and is caused by rupture of a bleb at the apex of a lung (See Fig. 12–19). It is essentially a benign disorder that may, however, be recurrent and eventually require surgical correction. Tuberculosis must be ruled out if the condition is recurrent. Pneumothorax resulting from intrapulmonary infectious diseases may be accompanied by empyema (*pyopneumothorax*).

MEDIASTINAL EMPHYSEMA

The term *mediastinal emphysema* (pneumomediastinum) denotes the presence of free air within the mediastinum. It may occur at any age. It may result from rupture of a major bronchus or the esophagus, or from the passage of air upward through the diaphragm or downward from the neck. Most commonly, it is secondary to an intrapulmonary rupture of alveoli with subsequent dissection of air centrally along the bronchovascular sheaths into the mediastinum. This may occur as the result of trauma or from spontaneous rupture of alveoli (seen most often in asthmatics, diabetics, and parturient women). It is a recognized complication of mechanical ventilation, particularly with positive end-expiratory pressure (PEEP) (*ventilator barotrauma*).

Roentgenographically, mediastinal emphysema is manifested by the presence within the mediastinum of one or more vertical linear hyperlucent streaks, most commonly appearing as an elevation of the mediastinal pleura from the underlying structures (Fig. 12–21). The roentgenographic changes are often subtle and frequently missed. The air may pass upward into the soft tissues of the neck and thoracic wall (subcutaneous emphysema), where it is easily visible on roentgenographic examination and equally easily detectable by palpation. Mediastinal emphysema often causes chest pain but usually has little deleterious effect on pulmonary function.

RADIOLOGIC PATTERNS OF DIFFUSE LUNG DISEASE

Patterns of multiple areas of increased opacification that are widely distributed throughout both lungs are seen relatively commonly.

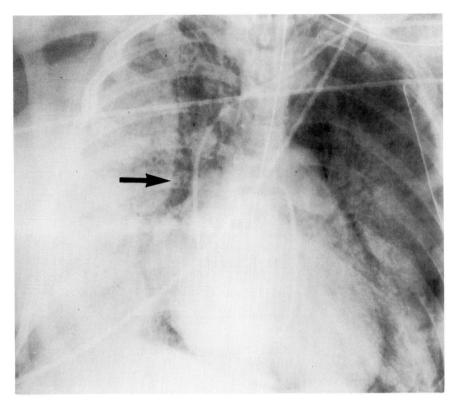

Figure 12—21. Mediastinal emphysema. PA view of a 16-year-old girl with ARDS and barotrauma. Note the tracheostomy tube, the Swan–Ganz catheter, and the chest tube draining air from the left pleural space. The mediastinal pleura (*arrow*) is lifted off by the air. Subcutaneous air can be seen in the pectoralis muscles and in the lateral chest wall.

Numerous diseases (well over 100) can cause diffuse pulmonary opacification. Differential diagnosis is somewhat simplified by the recognition that there are five basic radiologic patterns of diffuse lung disease: the alveolar-filling pattern, the interstitial pattern, the miliary pattern, the vascular pattern, and the bronchial pattern.

ALVEOLAR-FILLING PATTERN

The diffuse alveolar-filling pattern is characteristically comprised of "soft," fluffy, and poorly demarcated opacities, which are multifocal but widely distributed throughout the lungs. The individual opacities are 0.5 to 1 cm in diameter, but are usually sufficiently profuse that they are seen to overlap on the x-ray film and, thus, appear to coalesce to form larger, irregular, poorly demarcated opacities that may be several centimeters in diameter. The normal vascular pattern becomes blurred or even obliterated, as the alveolar opacification reduces the contrast between the air density of the lung and the water density of the vessels.

A bilateral perihilar (butterfly wing, bat-wing) distribution is sometimes seen when an alveolar-filling process diffusely involves the lungs (Fig. 12–22). Another diagnostically important manifestation of alveolar-filling disease is the air bronchogram. The consolidated alveoli around the bronchi and bronchioles provide contrast to the hyperlucent air within the bronchial tree, revealing a characteristic arborizing pattern (see Fig. 12–8). Occasionally, diffuse alveolar filling may also show a "ground-glass" appearance of diffuse granularity.

Functional Abnormalities with Alveolar-Filling Processes

Pulmonary function is usually markedly impaired with diffuse lung disease. Clinically, such patients are generally very dyspneic. Pulmonary function studies show the typical *restrictive pattern*: significant reductions in vital capacity (VC), residual volume (RV), and total lung capacity (TLC) without evidence of diffuse airway obstruction. The FEV_1/FVC ratio is normal or high. The lung is stiff and has a low compliance. The diffusing capacity is usually markedly reduced, and arterial blood gas values typically show severe hypoxemia associated with hypocapnia caused by secondary hyperventi-

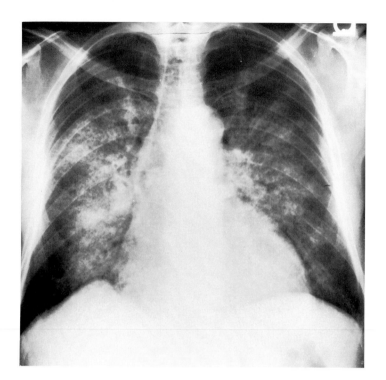

Figure 12—22. Bilateral perihilar distribution of pulmonary edema (the bat-wing or butterfly distribution). The soft, fluffy, poorly circumscribed and confluent alveolar-filling lesions are seen clearly. This appearance may occur with cardiogenic edema, but it is more characteristic of edemas caused by fluid overload or renal failure. Here, the patient had renal failure.

lation. On occasion, widespread involvement of alveoli may be associated with carbon dioxide retention. The arterial hypoxemia may be very profound, and even high-flow oxygen supplementation may fail to raise the arterial oxygen tensions to levels that will alleviate the tissue hypoxia. The hypoxemia is primarily caused by shunting of blood within the lungs.

The acute development of a diffuse alveolar-filling process frequently necessitates intubation and controlled mechanical ventilation, often with PEEP. Generally, the severity of the physiologic abnormality is paralleled by the extensiveness of the radiologic findings; progressive changes in the radiologic picture are useful indices to the success or failure of prevention or treatment.

The nature of the substance that is filling the alveoli can rarely be determined from the radiologic characteristics of the abnormality. Differential diagnosis, upon which successful treatment is based, depends on the associated clinical features and, at times, the results of bronchoalveolar lavage or lung biopsy.

Etiology of Diffuse Alveolar-Filling Patterns

Diffuse alveolar-filling diseases are relatively common. The most common forms are cardiogenic pul-

monary edema and ARDS. In AIDS patients, diffuse alveolar-filling is very likely to be due to *Pneumocystis carinii* pneumonia. The important causes of diffuse alveolar filling are shown in Tables 12–1 and 12–2. Some of these are discussed in the following.

Pulmonary Edema. Acute pulmonary edema is the most common cause of acute alveolar filling (see Fig. 12–22). *Hydrostatic* pulmonary edema is due to elevated pressures in the pulmonary capillaries or marked decreases in osmotic pressure. *Cardiogenic* pulmonary edema, the most common form of hydrostatic edema, usually results from left ventricular failure (which may have various etiologic factors) or from pulmonary venous hypertension, usually caused by mitral valve disease.

Roentgenologic characteristics of cardiogenic edema include cardiac enlargement, predominance of the pulmonary opacities in the lung bases bilaterally, Kerley B lines (thickened interlobular septa at the lung periphery), redistribution of pulmonary blood flow toward the upper lung fields, and pleural effusions in many cases.[8] Examination of the heart will usually reveal tachycardia and a gallop rhythm, and heart murmurs are often present. In the occasional patient in whom the diagnosis is in doubt, the demonstration of an elevated pulmonary

Table 12—1 Acute Diffuse Alveolar-Filling Diseases

PULMONARY EDEMA

1. Hydrostatic edema
   a. Cardiogenic
   b. Fluid overload, renal failure
2. Capillary leak edema

DIFFUSE INFLAMMATORY PROCESSES

1. Infectious diseases
   a. Viral pneumonias
   b. *Pneumocystis carinii* pneumonia (PCP)
   c. Other pneumonias (rarely)
2. Noninfectious
   a. "Shock lung" (ARDS)
   b. Aspiration (peptic) pneumonitis
   c. Toxic gas inhalation
   d. Fat embolism syndrome
   e. Drug-induced pneumonopathy
   f. Amniotic fluid embolism

INTRA-ALVEOLAR HEMORRHAGE

1. Bleeding diatheses
2. Anticoagulant overdosage
3. Idiopathic pulmonary hemosiderosis
4. Secondary hemosiderosis
5. Goodpasture's syndrome
6. Pulmonary vasculitis (Wegener's disease)

wedge pressure on right heart catheterization will strongly suggest the cardiogenic origin of the disorder.

Other types of hydrostatic pulmonary edema include *fluid overloads* caused by renal failure or excessive administration of intravenous fluids. In such patients the roentgenographic pattern is a little different in that the distribution of the intrapulmonary fluid is often central (paramediastinal), and significant widening of the "vascular pedicle" is almost invariably apparent.[8]

Capillary leak pulmonary edema may result from acute cerebral disorders (neurogenic edema), high altitude, uremia, intravenous overdosage of narcotic drugs such as heroin, aspirin overdose, transfusion reactions, near-drowning, allergic reactions to drugs, and ARDS.

Pulmonary edema may result from prolonged exposure to elevated inspiratory tensions of oxygen. Because diffuse alveolar-filling diseases are among the most common indications for the use of high-inspired oxygen concentration, the clinical

recognition of oxygen toxicity is obviously difficult.

The most common and most severe form by far is "shock lung," which is a major cause of ARDS (discussed in the next section Diffuse Alveolar Damage).

In these syndromes the heart is usually normal-sized and the alveolar opacities are scattered throughout all areas of the lung. The vascular pedicle is normal-sized and pleural effusions are rare.[8] The diagnosis can usually be established from a careful analysis of the history and surrounding clinical circumstances.

Unilateral pulmonary edema may occur if the patient has been lying for a prolonged time in a lateral decubitus position during the period when the edematous state developed. In rare instances, unilateral pulmonary edema may occur in the underlying lung after a rapid reexpansion of the lung by aspiration of a pneumothorax or pleural effusion.

Table 12—2 Conditions Associated with Adult Respiratory Distress Syndrome

SHOCK (ANY ETIOLOGY)

INFECTIONS

    Sepsis
    Pneumonias

ASPIRATION

    Peptic pneumonitis
    Near-drowning

INHALED IRRITANTS

    Chemical Fumes
    Smoke

DRUGS

    Paraquat
    Narcotics
    Oxygen (high concentrations)

MISCELLANEOUS

    Fat embolism
    Amniotic fluid embolism
    Head injury
    Acute pancreatitis
    Uremia
    Intravascular coagulation syndrome

Diffuse Alveolar Damage (Shock Lung). A diffuse hemorrhagic inflammatory intra-alveolar exudation may occur after stress, including shock, severe trauma, septicemia, and intra-abdominal catastrophies (see Table 12–2). The pulmonary abnormality usually begins 24 to 48 hours after the traumatic episode and is associated with severe dyspnea and profound hypoxemia. (This syndrome is discussed in detail in Chapter 32.) The profound physiologic disturbances that commonly occur in patients with diffuse alveolar disease are characterized by the term adult respiratory distress syndrome (ARDS). As alveolar edema is a major component of ARDS, these conditions are usually classified in the category of *noncardiogenic* pulmonary edema.

Although the exact pathogenesis is not well understood, capillary wall injury with excessive leakiness appears to be a major factor. The diagnosis is usually made from the roentgenographic appearance of severe widespread alveolar opacification occurring in the clinical circumstances mentioned. Clinically, the condition resembles acute pulmonary edema and, in many instances, the use of massive amounts of intravenous fluids in treating the preceding shock state may be a contributing factor to the development of ARDS. Once ARDS has developed, the pulmonary capillary wedge pressure is normal or low.

Infectious Pneumonias. Diffuse *viral pneumonitis* may result in a widespread alveolar-filling process and severe hypoxemia. Influenza virus, cytomegalovirus, and herpesvirus are the most common causes of diffuse viral pneumonias.

Pneumocystis carinii pneumonia (PCP) is typically diffuse and has both interstitial and alveolar-filling characteristics.

Noninfectious Pneumonias. Diffuse alveolar damage may result from massive aspiration of gastric juice with a low pH. *Peptic (acid) pneumonitis* usually causes enough damage to be classified as a form of ARDS. The opacification is usually widespread and bilateral (Fig. 12–23).

Diffuse alveolar damage may result from *inhalation of toxic gases* such as chlorine, SO_2, and NO_2 (silo-filler's disease). Ingestion of paraquat may result in a diffuse pneumonia that usually is rapidly fatal.

Fat embolism is a post-traumatic syndrome that is considered to be secondary to embolization of fat globules into the pulmonary capillaries, followed by enzymatic breakdown of the fats, with the release of fatty acids that irritate the lung. Presumably, the fat globules originate from traumatized tissues. The condition occurs almost exclusively in people with bone fractures. Although the radiologic abnormalities are similar to those in shock lung, fat embolism has some special clinical characteristics that usually allow its identification, and it usually responds more readily to therapy.

Figure 12–23. Peptic (acid) pneumonitis. A diffuse patchy alveolar opacification secondary to massive aspiration of gastric acid. Diagnosis often depends on the history of vomiting with aspiration, as radiologic differentiation from other causes of diffuse alveolar filling is usually impossible. This roentgenogram also shows artifacts peculiar to the intensive care unit: a midline tube passed down the esophagus for gastric decompression, two ECG leads, and a fine catheter, inserted in the right arm, that passes through the subclavian vein, superior vena cava, right atrium, right ventricle, the pulmonary trunk, and the right pulmonary artery.

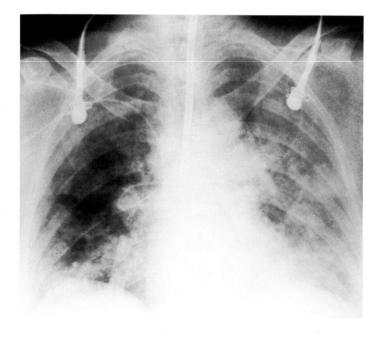

Intra-Alveolar Hemorrhage. Widespread intra-alveolar bleeding may result from spontaneous hemorrhagic states or from anticoagulant drug overdosage.

In many instances, hemorrhages are manifestations of *idiopathic pulmonary hemosiderosis*, which occurs primarily in children and adolescents, or *Goodpasture's syndrome*, which typically occurs in young male adults and is caused by an autoimmune disorder that damages the kidneys as well as the lungs. Clinical findings include the rapid development of a diffuse alveolar-filling process associated with a sudden fall in hemoglobin levels and, usually, hemoptysis. Recurrent attacks may lead eventually to diffuse interstitial fibrosis.

Diffuse alveolar hemorrhages may occur in cases of uremia and in patients with mitral stenosis. Diffuse bleeding can also be a manifestation of Wegener's granulomatosis and of systemic lupus erythematosus.

Aspiration Pneumonia. The aspiration of small or large amounts of liquid or semisolid material into the lungs may cause bronchial obstruction or a pneumonic consolidation.[2,3] Aspiration pneumonia actually occurs in three forms.

1. *Chemical* aspiration pneumonia (peptic pneumonitis, Mendelson's syndrome) is a diffuse alveolar-filling process that results from aspiration of gastric acid (see Fig. 12–23).
2. *Bacterial* aspiration pneumonia is a localized consolidation of dependent portions of the lungs caused by repeated aspirations of infected pharyngeal secretions. Lung abscess is a common outcome.
3. *Lipoid* pneumonia (oil granuloma) results from the habitual use of mineral oil or oily nose drops and presents radiologically as a localized chronic consolidation simulating carcinoma.

Chronic Alveolar-Filling Diseases. A number of diseases may occasionally be manifested with persistent diffuse alveolar opacification, including *sarcoidosis, infectious granulomas, alveolar cell carcinoma,* and *"alveolar" lymphoma.* An unusual cause of chronic alveolar disease is *pulmonary alveolar proteinosis.* Most of these conditions require a lung biopsy for diagnosis.

DIFFUSE INTERSTITIAL PATTERN

The interstitial tissue of the lung includes the alveolar walls, the intralobular vessels, the interlobular septa, and the connective tissue framework that surrounds the pulmonary arteries, veins, and bronchial tree. Opacifications resulting from diseases that primarily involve interstitial tissues have certain characteristics that often allow recognition of the roentgenographic pattern.

Diffuse interstitial diseases often show a pattern of *linear streaks* throughout the lungs. This phenomenon is primarily due to thickening of the interlobular septa and may be caused by fibrosis, granuloma, lymphangitic carcinoma, or interstitial edema. These linear streaks are called *Kerley lines,* which may be further differentiated into *A* lines (long linear streaks), *B* lines (short horizontal transverse streaks best seen at the periphery of the lower lung fields) (Fig. 12–24), and *C* lines (a diffuse reticular network caused by the overlapping of linear streaks running in different directions) (Fig. 12–25).

Perhaps the most characteristic feature of interstitial disease is *honeycombing,* which consists of multiple, rounded lucent areas up to 1 cm in diameter, outlined by the surrounding dense interstitial opacifications (Fig. 12–26). The air bronchogram effect is usually absent or not prominent in interstitial disease.

Many types of diffuse lung disease have both alveolar and interstitial components, with manifestations of both patterns radiologically. This is usually described as a "mixed" pattern. For example, cardiogenic pulmonary edema begins as septal thickening caused by edema and then evolves into diffuse alveolar-filling. In other cases, such as fibrosing alveolitis, ARDS, or desquamative interstitial pneumonitis, the initial manifestation is alveolar-filling that involves into an interstitial pattern owing to fibrosis.

Many diseases may give rise to a diffuse interstitial pattern (Table 12–3).

Diffuse Interstitial Pneumonitis

The most common condition in this category is *usual interstitial pneumonitis* (UIP), which is also known as *fibrosing alveolitis* or *diffuse pulmonary fibrosis.* Many cases are idiopathic, but some are secondary to (or associated with) underlying conditions, such as rheumatoid arthritis, scleroderma, inhalation of high oxygen concentrations (oxygen

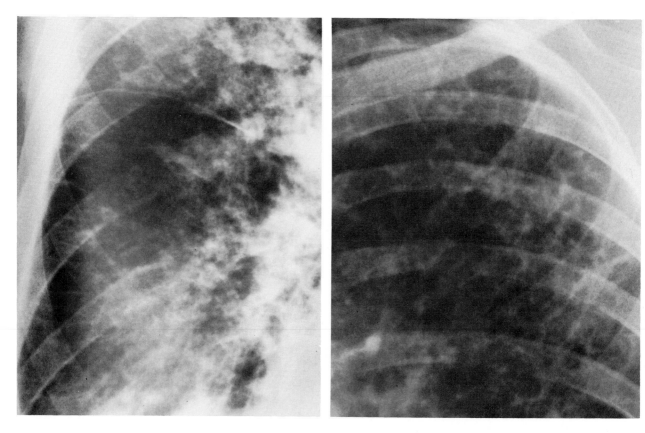

Figure 12—24.   (*Left*) Kerley B lines. These thin lines extend horizontally for 1–2 cm inward from the pleural surface and represent thickened interlobular septa. Here, they result from interstitial edema caused by pulmonary venous hypertension. Note scattered areas of alveolar-filling medially, which represent pulmonary edema of cardiogenic origin. (*Right*) PA view showing upper left lung in a 32-year-old woman with biopsy-proved eosinophilic granuloma (histiocytosis X). A reticular pattern is present, intermixed with blebs. This pattern may also occur with cystic fibrosis.

pneumonopathy), and the administration of drugs such as methotrexate, cyclophosphamide, busulfan, and others. In most cases, UIP is a slowly progressive disorder that results in a fibrotic "end-stage" lung.

Less common are *desquamative interstitial pneumonitis* (DIP) and *lymphocytic interstitial pneumonitis* (LIP). They may also progress to diffuse "end-stage" honeycomb lung in some instances.

Other Forms of Diffuse Interstitial Disease

Sarcoidosis is perhaps the most common diffuse interstitial process. Other conditions that commonly present with an interstitial pattern include *asbestosis, hypersensitivity pneumonitis, lymphangitic carcinomatosis,* and *eosinophilic granuloma* (histiocytosis X; see Fig. 12–24).

In most of these conditions, and particularly in the chronic ones, a lung biopsy is needed to establish the diagnosis. In some instances, the related clinical features will suggest the underlying etiology with considerable assurance.

Physiologically, the diffuse interstitial diseases are characterized by small stiff lungs with a reduced diffusing capacity and hypoxemia, usually without carbon dioxide retention. In fact, hypocapnia is common, caused by secondary hyperventilation. The hypoxemia can usually be relieved by a moderate enrichment of inspired air with oxygen. Generally, the severity of the physiologic abnormality is proportional to the extensiveness of the radiologic changes. However, there may be gross disparity between clinical status and radiologic abnormalities in sarcoidosis, the patient usually appearing much better than his chest x-ray film would indicate.

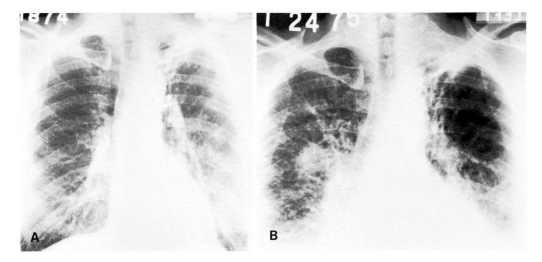

Figure 12—25.   Congestive heart failure. (*A*) PA chest film at a time when cardiac function was normal. In the left hemithorax, apical scarring and elevation of the left hilum have resulted from previous active tuberculosis, with loss of volume in the left upper lobe during the healing process. (*B*) Two months later, this man has suffered an acute myocardial infarction, and has developed left heart failure. The heart is enlarged. The hilar shadows are larger and have hazy margins. Pulmonary edema is present, manifested by a diffuse reticular pattern (Kerley C lines) and frank alveolar filling at the bases. The vascular shadows in the upper lung are accentuated because of redistribution of blood flow.

Figure 12—26.   Honeycomb lung in a patient with fibrosing alveolitis. The honeycomb cysts form dozens of rounded lucent areas, 5 to 10 mm in diameter, separated from each other by opaque fibrous tissue. These cysts are seen particularly well with CT.

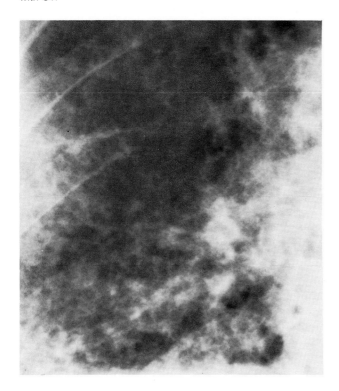

Table 12—3   Diseases with a Diffuse Interstitial Pattern

DIFFUSE INTERSTITIAL PNEUMONITIS/FIBROSIS

1. Fibrosing alveolitis (UIP)
   a. Cryptogenic (idiopathic pulmonary fibrosis)
   b. Secondary
      collagen–vascular diseases
      drug-induced pneumonopathy
2. Desquamative interstitial pneumonitis (DIP)
3. Lymphocytic interstitial pneumonitis (LIP)
4. ARDS (end-stage)

CONDITIONS INVOLVING LYMPHATICS

1. Sarcoidosis
2. Lymphoma
3. Lymphangitic carcinomatosis

INHALATIONAL DISORDERS

1. Asbestosis
2. Hypersensitivity pneumonitis

HISTIOCYTOSIS X (EOSINOPHILIC GRANULOMA)

LYMPHANGIOLEIOMYOMATOSIS

MILIARY PATTERN

The miliary pattern is a variant form of the interstitial pattern in which the chest roentgenogram shows a profusion of small nodules about 2 to 4 mm in diameter (Fig. 12–27). The prototype is miliary tuberculosis, but a diffuse fine nodularity of this type may also occur with fungal infections, sarcoidosis, certain pneumoconioses, metastatic tumors to lung, and varicella pneumonia (Table 12–4). The distinction between the interstitial and miliary patterns is often elusive, in which case the term *reticulonodular* disease may be used.

The severity of impairment of pulmonary function does not always correlate well with the severity of radiologic impairment in miliary disease. The critical task is to determine the etiology, particularly in infectious cases. Lung biopsy is often indicated.

Figure 12–27. Diffuse miliary nodules in a patient with disseminated coccidioidomycosis. The innumerable tiny nodules are well circumscribed and are 2 to 4 mm in diameter. A similar appearance occurs in miliary tuberculosis and, sometimes, is seen in certain fungal diseases, sarcoidosis, coal-worker's pneumoconiosis, and metastatic tumors.

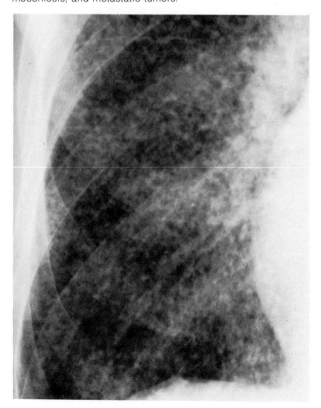

Table 12—4 Diffuse Miliary Processes

CONDITIONS CAUSED BY INHALATION

  Silicosis
  Coal worker's pneumoconiosis
  Berylliosis
  Hair-spray thesaurosis

CONDITIONS CAUSED BY HEMATOGENOUS/
LYMPHOGENOUS SPREAD

  Metastatic tumors
  Infections
    Tuberculosis,
    fungal, others
  Diffuse talc granulomatosis

SARCOIDOSIS

VASCULAR PATTERN

The pulmonary arteries and veins, as previously noted, form a somewhat indistinct branching pattern radiating peripherally from the hilum on the normal chest roentgenogram. Increases in the size of the pulmonary vessels cause an accentuation of this pattern. This accentuation superficially resembles interstitial disease and may be confused with it.

A *generalized increase in vascularity* may result from polycythemia, left heart failure, or congenital heart disease with left-to-right shunts. A striking feature of left heart failure is increased prominence and loss of marginal sharpness of the vessels in the upper lung fields (see Fig. 12–25). A spurious pattern of increased vascularity, particularly at the bases, may occur in normal lungs if the roentgenogram was obtained with the chest in the end-expiratory position.

Localized increases in vascularity are a common phenomenon in the redistribution of blood flow in patients with bullous emphysema.

Decreased vascularity may be focal, as in emphysema or pulmonary embolism, or diffuse, as in right-to-left shunts, pulmonic stenosis, and obstructive pulmonary hypertension. The central hilar vessels are often enlarged in obstructive pulmonary hypertension.

BRONCHIAL PATTERN

Diffuse involvement of the bronchial tree by inflammatory disease may result in roentgenographic abnormalities that somewhat resemble the diffuse interstitial pattern. This can result from thickened bronchial walls (as in chronic bronchitis, asthma, and bronchiectasis), from peribronchial scarring (as in mucoviscidosis or allergic bronchopulmonary aspergillosis), or from mucoid impactions within the bronchial tree. In patients with COPD, this appearance is often referred to as the "dirty lung"[6] and usually indicates that chronic bronchitis is a major component of the obstructive complex. The term "increased markings pattern" is also used.

The roentgen changes include focal linear streaks, fine ring shadows, irregular foci of opacification, and tramline shadows. If mucoid impactions are present, such picturesque terms as "toothpaste" shadows, "gloved-hand" shadows, and "frond-of-grapes" shadows are often employed.

PLEURAL EFFUSIONS

A *pleural effusion* is fluid within the pleural space. It may be blood (hemothorax), pus (empyema), chyle (chylothorax), or, most commonly, a relatively clear serous fluid, which is either a transudate or an exudate. The nature of the fluid cannot be determined from the roentgenographic appearance; its identification depends on aspiration of the fluid, followed by microscopic, bacteriologic, and chemical analysis.

The roentgenographic appearance of a pleural effusion depends upon the amount of fluid and whether loculations are present. A *small* effusion may show only haziness or obliteration of a costophrenic angle, sometimes seen better on the lateral view than on the PA projection. A *moderate-sized* effusion presents as a homogeneous opacity in the dependent portion of the thorax, with a poorly defined upper border that is generally concave and higher laterally along the chest wall (Fig. 12–28). The contour of the diaphragm is obliterated, both in the upright PA and lateral projections. A *very large* pleural effusion causes relatively complete opacification of the hemithorax, with relatively less opacity at the top than at the bottom and often with evidence of mediastinal shift toward the normal hemithorax.

The appearances just described are those with the subject in the upright position and with a pleural space not bound down to any major degree by adhesions. If the exposure is made with the subject in the *supine position*, the pleural fluid layers-out posteriorly, causing a diffuse haziness throughout the hemithorax.

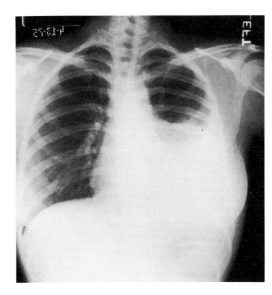

Figure 12—28. Moderately large pleural effusion caused by tuberculosis. There is a large homogeneous opacification in the lower half of the left hemithorax, with the upper border of the opacity being concave upward. There is some shift of the heart to the right.

A *subpulmonic* effusion forms between the lung and diaphragm with the patient in the upright position. It simulates elevation of the hemidiaphragm. An *interlobar* effusion collects within an interlobar fissure and resembles a mass lesion in the PA projection, but in the lateral view usually has a characteristic fusiform appearance. In all these cases, a film taken in the *lateral decubitus position* will usually show movement of fluid to the most dependent portions of the hemithorax, establishing the true nature of the opacity (Fig. 12–29).

TRANSUDATES

A transudative serous effusion results from changes in the hydrodynamic forces in the circulation. It may be regarded as a localized manifestation of a general tendency to form edema fluid. It most commonly is due to left heart failure. Other causes include cirrhosis and the nephrotic syndrome. In the cirrhotic patient the effusion is often right-sided, and associated with abdominal ascites; the intrapleural fluid, in such cases, may result from the passage of ascitic fluid through diaphragmatic pores or lymphatics into the thorax.

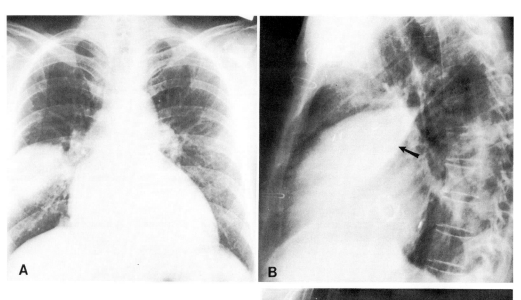

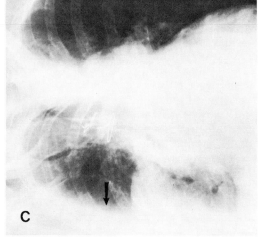

Figure 12—29. Loculated interlobar effusion. (*A*) PA chest film shows the fluid as a rounded opacity in the right hemithorax, resembling a tumor mass (pseudotumor). (*B*) Lateral film shows the characteristic fusiform appearance of an interlobar effusion (*arrow*), continuing upward as a thin diagonal line representing the upper portion of the oblique fissure. An artificial heart valve can be seen within the heart shadow, and surgical wires are seen encircling the sternum. (*C*) Right lateral decubitus film showing some passage of the pleural fluid out into the "lateral gutter," which is now the most dependent portion of the hemithorax.

EXUDATES

Exudative serous effusions result from irritation of the pleural membranes, secondary to inflammatory or malignant processes. Many inflammatory effusions are caused by an infection within the adjacent lung or mediastinum. An infection may also spread through the diaphragm to involve the pleural space; this occurs most commonly with subphrenic pyogenic abscess and with amebic infections of the liver.

Common causes of *inflammatory pleural* exudates include pneumonia, lung abscess, tuberculosis, fungal diseases, pulmonary infarction, acute pancreatitis, systemic lupus erythematosus, and the pleurisy of rheumatoid arthritis.

Malignant pleural effusions are most commonly caused by metastatic involvement of the pleura from bronchogenic carcinoma or an extrapulmonary primary malignancy. Malignant effusions may occur in patients with lymphoma. The most common primary malignant tumor of the pleural space is the diffuse pleural mesothelioma, usually secondary to asbestos exposure.

EMPYEMA

A purulent pleural effusion is usually secondary to pneumonia or lung abscess. Other causes of empyema include tuberculosis, fungal diseases, mediastinal abscess, and subphrenic abscess. In almost all instances the infecting organism can be easily cultured from the aspirated empyema fluid. Iatrogenic empyema may result from contamination of an uninfected pleural effusion by needles or drainage catheters passed into the pleural space.

The development of empyema is always a serious complication that requires prompt diagnosis and adequate mechanical drainage. Empyema should be considered whenever radiologic evidence of pleural effusion is present. Diagnosis depends on thoracentesis.

HEMOTHORAX

Blood in the pleural space usually results from chest trauma, either penetrating wounds or laceration of the lung by fractured ribs (Fig. 12–30). Some cases are secondary to leaking of an intrathoracic aneurysm; occasionally, it may occur with primary hemorrhagic disorders and anticoagulant drug use. Surgical intervention may be required for hemothorax, whether in the early stages to stop the hemorrhage, or in the later stage to remove the resultant

fibrin peel that may be encasing the lung and preventing adequate function on the affected side.

CHYLOTHORAX

Leakage of chyle from the thoracic duct is usually caused by chest trauma or by malignant obstruction of the thoracic duct. The fluid usually has a characteristic milky appearance, but in questionable cases the determination of the true nature of the fluid may require chemical studies. *Chyliform* and *pseudochylous* effusions, which resemble true chyle on gross inspection but can be differentiated chemically, are not due to leakage of chyle, but rather result from the endogenous formation of lipids within a chronic and highly cellular exudative effusion or empyema.

Pleural effusion of any type will reduce pulmonary function to the extent that the intrapleural fluid volume reduces lung volume. In addition, pleuritic pain, when present, impairs the patient's ability to take a deep breath and cough effectively, and the latter may lead to sputum retention.

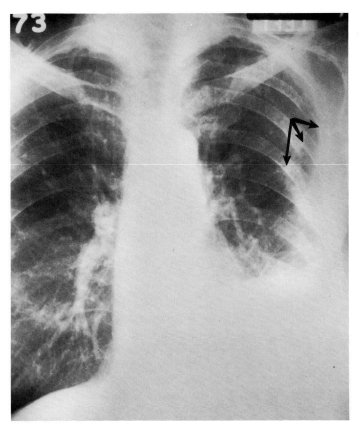

Figure 12—30. Left hemothorax secondary to rib fractures (*arrows*). The intrapleural opacity of the hemothorax cannot be distinguished from other types of fluid effusion.

DIAPHRAGMATIC ABNORMALITIES

The diaphragm is subject to relatively few primary disorders, but it is often affected by disease processes above or below it. *Bilateral depression* of the diaphragm is an important sign of hyperinflation and usually indicates emphysema or severe asthma. *Bilateral elevation* of the diaphragm may result from obesity, ascites, painful breathing, or inability of the patient to take a deep breath. It is a common finding in cases of bilateral pulmonary embolism (Fig. 12–31) and in roentgenograms obtained on obtunded patients lying in the supine position.

Unilateral elevation of the diaphragm may be an important sign of disease in or near the diaphragm and should never be ignored. Disorders *above* the diaphragm causing unilateral elevation include inflammatory or irritative processes in the adjacent lung and visceral pleura, for example, pulmonary embolism (with or without infarction), pneumonia, atelectasis, or pleurisy of any cause. *Diaphragmatic disorders* that cause unilateral elevation include paralysis, owing to phrenic nerve dysfunction, and eventration, which is a loss of diaphragmatic muscle with thinning of the organ, probably congenital in origin (see Fig. 12–17). Con-

Figure 12–31. Bilateral pulmonary emboli in a young woman. The degree of elevation of the left hemidiaphragm is indicated by the position of the gastric bubble (*arrow*). On the right, the hemidiaphragm is probably elevated as well, but it cannot be seen clearly because of overlying pleural fluid. The thick, horizontal, curved linear opacity in the right third anterior interspace is discoid atelectasis.

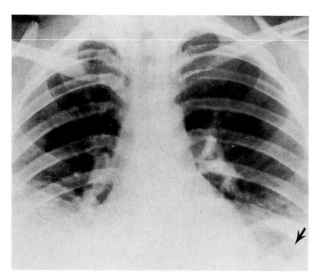

ditions *below* the diaphragm causing its elevation include subphrenic abscess (usually secondary to abdominal surgery or perforation of an abdominal viscus) and a large cyst or hematoma in the upper abdomen. On occasion, gross enlargement of the liver may cause diaphragmatic elevation. In most cases of an elevated hemidiaphragm, the respiratory excursions are reduced and will actually show paradoxic movement with phrenic nerve palsy.

A *diaphragmatic hernia* may simulate unilateral elevation of the diaphragm. In many instances, the hernia contains an air-filled viscus, the roentgenographic appearance of which aids identification.

PULMONARY EMBOLISM

The radiologic changes that accompany pulmonary embolism (see Chap. 36) are never distinctive, but they will often suggest the diagnosis and thereby indicate the need for more specific studies to identify positively the presence of the pulmonary embolus. In many instances, pulmonary scintiscans will establish the diagnosis with a high degree of assurance; in other cases pulmonary angiography is needed. It is critically important to recognize the clinical and radiographic findings that will suggest the possibility of pulmonary embolism.

Massive pulmonary embolism is caused by the impaction of one or more large thrombi in the pulmonary outflow tract or main pulmonary arteries. Clinical features include the sudden onset of dyspnea, tachypnea, tachycardia, retrosternal chest pain, and in many cases a precipitous fall in blood pressure because of low cardiac output. If the patient survives long enough for appropriate diagnostic studies to be performed, the standard frontal projection chest roentgenogram will show relatively clear or even oligemic lung fields, usually with unilateral or bilateral increased hilar size, secondary to enlargement of the capacitance portion of the pulmonary arterial circulation. Pulmonary angiography is indicated in such circumstances and is almost invariably diagnostic. The differential diagnosis includes acute myocardial infarction and leaking thoracic aortic aneurysms.

Pulmonary infarction is ischemic necrosis of an area of lung that occurs in a small percentage of cases of embolism. Infarcts are often multiple and appear on the chest roentgenogram as one or more areas of consolidation, large or small, always abutting on a visceral pleural surface (peripheral or interlobar) and often presenting a rounded contour on the margin facing the hilum (Fig. 12–32). Symptoms include dyspnea, tachypnea, pleuritic chest pain, and (often) hemoptysis. Pleural effusion is often present, and ipsilateral hilar enlargement with hemidiaphragmatic elevation is usually apparent. Infarcts occasionally undergo cavitation. Pulmonary scintiscanning is of limited value in such cases, since an infarct will show a matching ventilation–perfusion defect similar to that occurring with any type of pulmonary consolidation. However, because emboli are commonly multiple, the scans may show one or more mismatching defects in other nonconsolidated areas of lung that have been embolized but have not undergone infarction. Segmental pulmonary angiography is usually diagnostic. The differential diagnosis of pulmonary infarction includes pneumonia, atelectasis, and pleural effusion of other types.

Unexplained dyspnea is the presenting syndrome in patients who have single or multiple embolic occlusions in medium-sized branches of the pulmonary arteries, without the development of infarction. Pleuritic chest pain is unusual in these patients. The chest roentgenogram occasionally shows one or more oligemic, hyperlucent areas, but commonly is interpreted as normal. Careful review of such cases may show unilateral enlargement of the hilum or the lobar vessels, often associated with elevation of ipsilateral hemidiaphragm and the presence of discoid atelectasis, also called Fleischner's lines (see Fig. 12–31). Discoid atelectasis appears as one or more transverse linear shadows, 1 to 3 mm in diameter and extending 2 to 4 cm in length, usually horizontal, and mainly in the lower lung fields. The appearance of discoid atelectasis is not pathognomonic of pulmonary embolism, but it should always suggest the diagnosis. It may also result from any condition causing painful chest movement, including rib fractures, pleurisy, and upper abdominal surgery. The differential diagnosis of the "unexplained dyspnea" syndrome includes asthma, exacerbation of COPD, metabolic dyspnea, and psychogenic dyspnea.

Recurrent showers of small pulmonary emboli may result in clinical and radiologic evidence of *chronic pulmonary hypertension*, with right ventricular enlargement, bilateral hilar enlargement, and clear or oligemic lung fields. Exertional dyspnea and exertional chest pain are often present. Differentiation from primary pulmonary hypertension (plexogenic pulmonary hypertension; PPH) is often difficult, although recent work suggests that scintiscans and angiography are completely normal in PPH and mildly abnormal in cases of showers of small emboli. The "unresolved chronic embolism syndrome" caused by persistent embolic obstruction of lobar or central vessels[10] is usually accompanied by "high probability" scintiscans.

HILAR ENLARGEMENT

The hilum contains bronchi, lymph nodes, and blood vessels, but only the blood vessels are sufficiently large and radiopaque to contribute to the normal hilar opacity. The increased size of the hilum may be caused by vascular dilatation, enlargement of the hilar lymph nodes, or development of a mass lesion, such as a bronchogenic carcinoma, within the hilum. The differentiation between lymphadenopathy and vessel enlargement as the cause of hilar enlargement may require pulmonary angiography, CT, or MRI.

Figure 12–32. Small pulmonary infarct seen in this magnified view of the right costophrenic angle. The infarct is based on the pleural surface facing the adjacent costal chest wall and diaphragm, and the convex central border faces toward the hilum. Unfortunately, the diagnosis here was established by surgical removal of the lesion, which had been thought to be a tumor.

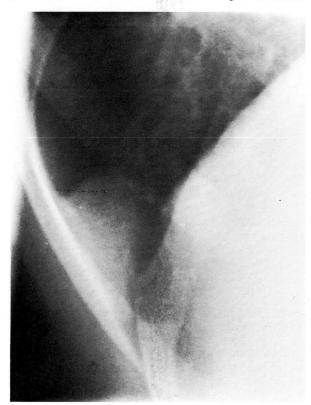

Unilateral nonvascular hilar enlargement may result from the development of an intrahilar mass lesion (tumor, bronchogenic cyst) or from the lymphadenopathy of tuberculosis, bronchogenic carcinoma, certain fungal diseases, and lymphoma. Unilateral enlargement is rare in sarcoidosis.

Unilateral vascular hilar enlargement is most commonly caused by pulmonary embolism, but there are several rare causes, including pulmonary artery aneurysms and poststenotic dilatation related to pulmonic stenosis.

Bilateral nonvascular hilar enlargement is most commonly caused by the lymphadenopathy of sarcoidosis (Fig. 12–33). Other causes of bilateral hilar adenopathy include lymphoma, leukemia, some fungal infections, and certain pneumoconioses.

Bilateral vascular hilar enlargement from dilated central pulmonary vascular shadows suggests pulmonary embolism, congestive heart failure (see Fig. 12–25), mitral stenosis, plexogenic pulmonary hypertension, cor pulmonale (pulmonary arterial hypertension owing to chronic lung disease), and congenital heart diseases associated with a left-to-right shunt. In most instances the peripheral intrapulmonary arteries are also distended and prominent, although in pulmonary embolism and in primary pulmonary hypertension the lungs are more commonly oligemic.

Figure 12–33. Bilateral hilar adenopathy in sarcoidosis. Such well-circumscribed, lobulated masses have been aptly described as having a "potato node" appearance. Compare with the poorly demarcated hilar enlargement seen in Figure 12–25.

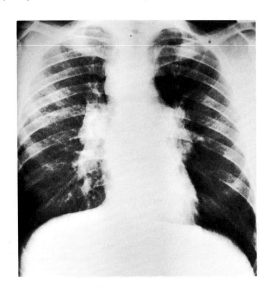

IATROGENIC DISEASES OF THE LUNG

An *iatrogenic* disease is one caused by some action (or occasionally lack of action) of the physician. The rising incidence of iatrogenic disease has now become a major medical problem. These "diseases" are related to the relentless increase in the number of invasive and potentially hazardous diagnostic procedures now available, and to the many toxic side effects of the powerful drugs and complicated therapeutic procedures in current use. Many iatrogenic diseases are unavoidable but predictable, and their prompt recognition depends on the physician's realization of their possible occurrence in certain clinical situations. The lungs are particularly susceptible to various iatrogenic diseases.

NOSOCOMIAL INFECTIONS

Pulmonary infections developing in hospitalized patients may result from invasion by the indigenous pathogenic microbiologic flora of the hospital or may be a manifestation of infection by "saprophytic" organisms that are normally present in the body, but that develop invasive potential because of reduced resistance in patients exposed to various diagnostic or therapeutic maneuvers. Predisposing factors include the use of broad-spectrum antibiotics or immunosuppressive drugs, invasive diagnostic or therapeutic procedures, swallowing difficulties allowing aspiration of food and infected pharyngeal secretions, tracheal intubation, and contaminated inhalation therapy equipment. Localization of the infection may be tracheobronchial, alveolar, or both.

Common infecting organisms include *Staphylococcus*, *Pseudomonas* and other aerobic gram-negative bacilli, anaerobic organisms, and bacteria and fungi normally of low pathogenicity, including *Aspergillus* and *Candida*. The roentgenographic features of nosocomial pneumonia are not characteristic, except that the lesions are less likely to be lobar or segmental in distribution and commonly are multiple, bilateral, and poorly circumscribed (bronchopneumonia). Common complications include cavitation and pleural effusion or empyema.

POSTOPERATIVE PULMONARY COMPLICATIONS

Pulmonary complications are a major cause of morbidity and mortality after surgical procedures, and their incidence is greatly increased if preexisting pulmonary disease is present (see Chap. 30).

Chronic obstructive airway diseases present the greatest hazard, because pulmonary function may already be borderline, and the inability of the patient to generate an effective cough postoperatively predisposes to sputum retention. Surgical procedures on the thorax itself or on the upper abdomen are more likely to be followed by postoperative pulmonary complications than procedures involving other areas of the body.

Atelectasis caused by obstruction of one or more bronchi by retained mucous plugs may occur during surgery or at any time in the postoperative period, but usually appears within the first few days. Roentgenographic signs include the changes indicating loss of volume and the opacity of the collapsed lobe or segment itself (see Fig. 12–9). The main contributing factor is the inability or unwillingness of the patient to cough effectively because of postoperative pain. In most instances postoperative atelectasis can be prevented by a vigorous program of pulmonary toilet, both before and after surgery. Treatment for atelectasis is simple and effective, provided the condition is recognized.

Postoperative *pulmonary embolism* may occur at any time in the postoperative period, but most commonly appears several days after the surgical procedure. The radiologic signs of pulmonary embolism have already been reviewed. Predisposing factors include obesity, polycythemia, heart disease, malignancy, and orthopedic procedures to the limbs, particularly the treatment of hip fractures. In most instances clear-cut evidence of underlying thrombophlebitis will not be detectable on physical examination.

Postoperative *respiratory insufficiency* has become increasingly common with the use of complicated surgical procedures on elderly or seriously ill patients. Chronic obstructive lung disease is the main predisposing factor. In many patients who develop respiratory insufficiency in the postoperative state, the chest roentgenogram shows no particular change from the preoperative film. The diagnosis depends primarily on arterial blood gas measurements. Prolonged, complicated surgical procedures associated with hypovolemic shock or sepsis may lead to the development of ARDS, in which case the chest roentgenogram reveals diffuse, patchy alveolar-filling process that develops 24 to 48 hours after the procedure.

DRUG-INDUCED DISEASES OF THE LUNGS

Certain drugs may have a direct toxic effect on the lungs. The prolonged use of high concentrations of *oxygen* in the inspired gas leads to hemorrhagic pulmonary edema, which is often not recognized because of the extensive radiographic abnormalities resulting from the underlying pulmonary disease that necessitated the oxygen therapy. *Allergic reactions* to drugs may cause pulmonary edema, asthmatic attacks, pulmonary vasculitis, or eosinophilic pneumonia.

Certain drugs (bleomycin, busulfan, methotrexate, and several others) may cause a *diffuse interstitial pneumonitis* and *fibrosis*. Methysergide may cause *mediastinal fibrosis*, with compression of the superior vena cava, the main bronchi, or the pulmonary veins. The prolonged use of adrenal corticosteroids often results in *mediastinal lipomatosis;* the fat deposits cause generalized mediastinal widening.

The intravenous use of narcotic drugs such as heroin may result in noncardiogenic *pulmonary edema.* β-Adrenergic drugs used in the therapy of premature labor may cause pulmonary edema, particularly in cases in which adrenal steroids are also employed.[9]

FLUID OVERLOAD

Hospitalized patients, particularly those in intensive care units, sometimes develop generalized fluid retention and pulmonary edema from vascular overload with intravenous fluids. This possibility must be considered in any patient receiving intravenous fluids who develops a diffuse alveolar-filling process. Congestive heart failure or renal failure are predisposing causes in some cases (see Fig. 12–22). The chest x-ray will usually show widening of the "vascular pedicle."[8] The diagnosis çan be confirmed, in most instances, by a careful study of intake/output data and serial body weights. In most patients, the central venous pressure and the pulmonary capillary wedge pressure are elevated.

COMPLICATIONS OF MECHANICAL VENTILATION

Mechanical ventilation, commonly used for maintaining life during episodes of respiratory insufficiency or respiratory failure, carries certain inherent hazards.[13]

Oxygen toxicity has already been mentioned. The inspired oxygen concentration must be maintained at the lowest level that will yield an arterial oxygen tension of 60 to 80 mmHg.

Endobronchial infections are common in intubated patients. Bacterial colonization of the upper tracheobronchial tree is unavoidable when an endotracheal tube is in place, but the incidence and severity of secondary infections can be minimized by strict adherence to appropriate technique. Endobronchial infections are manifested by purulent bronchial secretions, often without any radiologic abnormality indicative of parenchymal pneumonia. Inadequate sterilization of inhalation therapy equipment may result in a serious or even fatal pulmonary infection that is often bilateral and sometimes necrotizing (associated with cavity information).

Displacement of the endotracheal tube into the right main bronchus usually results in the rapid development of atelectasis of the left lung. Atelectasis is easily recognized by stethoscopic examination, and a chest roentgenogram is confirmatory. This disorder can be avoided by radiographic monitoring of the tube placement and by routine stethoscopic examination of the lungs of the intubated patient at appropriate intervals.

Pneumomediastinum and *subcutaneous emphysema* are infallible indices that air leakage is occurring (see Fig. 12–21). If a tracheostomy has been performed, the leakage of air may be occurring from the tracheal incision or from the surgical site. Air leakage may occur from transtracheal needle aspiration, even without barotrauma (Fig. 12–34).

In patients with barotrauma, alveolar rupture probably occurs first, with subsequent dissection of the air in a centripetal fashion along the bronchovascular bundles into the mediastinum and up into the subcutaneous tissues of the neck. This is commonly followed by development of a *pneumothorax*, and the appearance of subcutaneous air should indicate the need for immediate chest radiographic examination. Other clinical signs that indicate a pneumothorax include tachycardia, shock, and decline of arterial blood gas values. The intubated and sedated patient cannot always complain of chest pain or dyspnea. Roentgenographic recognition of a pneumothorax is simple if the collapse is massive, but the demonstration of a small amount of intrapleural air may require that the patient assume a somewhat upright position for the exposure of the film. The occurence of interstitial emphysema and pneumothorax is surprisingly uncommon with intermittent positive-pressure breathing but has a greatly increased incidence if PEEP is used.

RADIATION PNEUMONITIS AND FIBROSIS

Radiation therapy in or near the lungs may result in acute radiation pneumonitis or chronic radiation fibrosis. *Radiation pneumonitis* appears within 1 or 2 months after the start of therapy and is manifested roentgenographically as a soft, fluffy alveolar process, usually localized to the areas exposed to the radiation, although on occasion it may become generalized. *Radiation fibrosis* may be a sequela of radiation pneumonitis or may develop independently some months after radiation therapy has been completed. It is interstitial in its roentgenographic appearance and is characterized by its strict localization to the field of radiation exposure and its lack of segmental distribution. Secondary bronchiectasis within the involved area gives the infiltrate a nonhomogeneous character.

ENDOSCOPIC TRAUMA

Fiberoptic bronchoscopy is relatively atraumatic to the lung. Bronchoscopic biopsy of bronchial lesions may result in hemorrhage, more commonly with the larger-sized biopsies that are possible with the rigid bronchoscope. Bronchial bleeding may produce evidence of alveolar-filling consolidation in the affected lung area. Transbronchoscopic biopsies of peripheral lung may result in traumatic pneumothorax caused by penetration of the visceral pleura by the biopsy forceps (Fig. 12–35).

Figure 12–34. Subcutaneous emphysema in the neck secondary to transtracheal aspiration for diagnostic purposes. Multiple linear lucencies represent air within subcutaneous fat and cervical muscle bundles. The patient also has diffuse interstitial lung disease.

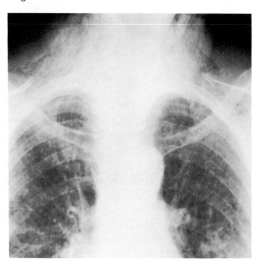

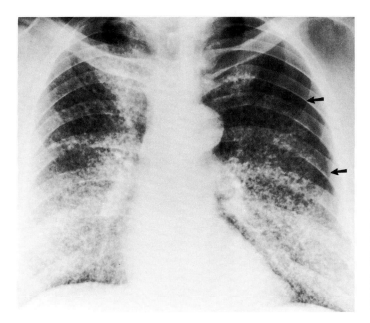

Figure 12–35. Left pneumothorax secondary to perforation of the visceral pleura during transbronchial lung biopsy with the fiberoptic bronchoscope. This complication occurs in approximately 5% of such biopsies. The diagnosis of miliary tuberculosis was established by the lung biopsy and the patient was treated successfully. Lung edge is marked (*arrows*). Note the absence of miliary lesions in the area of pneumothorax gas.

Esophageal endoscopic examination or bougienage may cause esophageal rupture, leading to acute mediastinitis. Roentgenographic findings include mediastinal widening, mediastinal emphysema, and often pneumothorax or hydropneumothorax. Esophageal perforation resulting from violent vomiting ("spontaneous" perforation of the esophagus) has identical radiologic characteristics.

OPPORTUNISTIC INFECTIONS

Opportunistic infections occur in patients with impaired host defenses. The "compromised host" may owe his or her vulnerability to the underlying disease (diabetes, impaired cellular or humoral immunity, granulocytopenia, splenectomy), to mechanical conduits (endotracheal tubes, intravenous catheters) that provide access for microorganisms, or to the effects of drugs (adrenal steroids, cytotoxic drugs).

The lungs are commonly the site of opportunistic infections. The organisms may have low pathogenicity under ordinary circumstances and, often, are normal body flora. The development of immune system compromise gives the organisms the opportunity to give rise to infection. A given opportunistic infection may be due to several organisms present simultaneously.

In the clinical and radiologic assessment of such patients, it must be remembered that the roentgenographic abnormality is not invariably caused by an infectious process. It may also be a manifestation of the primary underlying disease, an untoward reaction to treatment, or a nonspecific abnormality such as lymphocytic interstitial pneumonitis (Table 12–5).

The radiologic appearance of the lungs does provide some etiologic clues. *Lobar–segmental consolidation* suggests bacterial, fungal, or mycobacterial infections. *Multiple nodules* are often caused by fungal infections and, sometimes, by metastatic tumors. *Diffuse alveolar disease* suggests pneumocystis or cytomegalovirus infection, alveolar hemorrhage, oxygen toxicity, or drug reactions. *Diffuse interstitial disease* in a compromised host may result from viral infection, lymphoma, or the chronic stage of drug reactions, radiation fibrosis, and oxygen-damaged lung. *Miliary lesions* suggest mycobacterial and fungal infection.

PULMONARY MANIFESTATIONS OF AIDS

The acquired immunodeficiency syndrome (AIDS) resulting from infection with human immunodeficiency virus (HIV) eventually manifests pulmonary manifestations in almost all cases. The most common abnormality is *Pneumocystis carinii* pneumonia (PCP), but other infectious processes may be present, and noninfectious disorders may also develop in the lungs (Table 12–6). More than one disease process may be present in the lungs simultaneously.

Table 12—5 Pulmonary Disease in Compromised Hosts

OPPORTUNISTIC INFECTIONS

DRUG-INDUCED PULMONARY DISEASE

  Infections resulting from drug-induced immunosuppression
  Cytotoxic drug reactions
  Noncytotoxic drug reactions
  Radiation fibrosis
  Cardiogenic pulmonary edema [doxorubicin (Adriamycin)]
  Transfusion reactions
  Pulmonary oxygen toxicity

PULMONARY MANIFESTATIONS OF THE UNDERLYING DISEASE

  Metastatic tumor growth
  Lymphomas and leukemias
  Diffuse interstitial pneumonitis in the collagen–vascular diseases

COMPLICATIONS OF THE UNDERLYING DISEASE

  Infections
  Noninfectious processes
    Diffuse alveolar hemorrhages
    Cell lysis pneumonopathies
    Graph-vs.-host disease
    Pulmonary edema
    Kaposi's sarcoma

NONSPECIFIC INTERSTITIAL PNEUMONITIS

  LIP in AIDS
  Heart–lung transplants
  Bone marrow transplants

Table 12—6 Pulmonary Manifestations of AIDS

INFECTIOUS PROCESSES

  Pneumocystis carinii pneumonia
  Cytomegalovirus pneumonia
  Mycobacterium avium-intracellulare infection
  Tuberculosis
  Fungal pneumonias
  Bacterial pneumonias, including *Legionella*

TUMORS

  Kaposi's sarcoma
  Lymphomas

NONINFECTIOUS INTERSTITIAL PNEUMONITIS

  Nonspecific interstitial pneumonitis
  Lymphocytic interstitial pneumonitis

RADIOLOGY IN THE INTENSIVE CARE UNIT

Because patients in intensive care units tend to have life-threatening and rapidly changing pulmonary abnormalities, accurate interpretation is critically important, but the technical quality of the AP supine chest roentgenograms is often unavoidably suboptimal. Errors can arise from overinterpretation of "abnormalities" that may be spurious and caused by positional factors or differences in exposure on serial films. It has been wisely suggested that the interpreter of such roentgenograms attempt to provide answers to the following questions only:[1]

  • Is the film technically adequate?
  • Are there any rib fractures?
  • Are the endotracheal tube and intravenous lines correctly positioned?
  • Is there pulmonary consolidation? One should determine if there is consolidation and whether it has changed on serial films. Attempts to predict etiology may be seriously misleading.
  • Is pleural fluid present?
  • Is atelectasis present?
  • Is a pneumothorax present?

The interpreter must constantly remember that pneumothoraces and pleural effusions often have atypical appearances on AP supine films and that penetration and contrast vary from film to film.

THORACIC TRAUMA

Thoracic trauma may result in various physiologic and roentgenographic abnormalities in the thorax, the prompt recognition of which is imperative for successfully managing the patient. In most instances, the fact that trauma to the thoracic cage has occurred is apparent from the history or from superficial inspection of the thorax; however, if an unconscious patient is brought to the hospital emergency room and inspection of the thorax reveals no obvious evidence of injury, traumatic lung damage may go unrecognized. Thoracic trauma must be suspected in all such cases and appropriate roentgenographic studies carried out. The mechanisms of production of thoracic trauma and the nature of the resulting lesions are extremely varied. Some of the more common abnormalities will be mentioned.

RIB FRACTURES

Rib fractures may have a variety of possible consequences. One or two undisplaced rib fractures may have no deleterious effect other than pain, and they may be difficult to detect on standard roentgenograms. Special *rib films* may be needed to detect their presence. If the patient has COPD, the cough suppression induced by the pain of the fractures may result in atelectasis, pneumonia, or acute respiratory failure.

Multiple rib fractures will create an instability of the chest wall, known as *flail chest*, which may cause severe respiratory embarrassment. The modern treatment of flail chest with intubation and mechanical ventilation (internal pneumatic stabilization), often with pressure support, represents one of the more important advances in managing thoracic trauma. Flail chest is easily recognized on physical examination by the paradoxic movement of the traumatized unstable chest wall and can be confirmed radiographically by inspiration and expiration films.

Rib fractures may lacerate vessels and cause *hemothorax* (see Fig. 12–29) or may lacerate the lung and cause *pneumothorax*. The presence of air and fluid within the pleural space is manifested by the characteristic air–fluid interface, which cannot be seen, however, unless the roentgen beam is in the horizontal plane.

PENETRATING CHEST WOUNDS

Penetrating chest wounds cause pneumothorax by virtue of entry of air through the chest wall wound or by leakage of air from the lacerated lung. Intrapleural hemorrhage is common, and chylothorax appears if the thoracic duct is injured. Intrapulmonary hemorrhage occurs along the pathway of the penetrating foreign body within the lung.

NONPENETRATING TRAUMA

Nonpenetrating trauma may result in the formation of an intrapulmonary hematoma (*pulmonary contusion*), which appears roentgenographically as a poorly circumscribed opaque consolidation without localization to segmental boundaries. The opacity appears within hours after the injury and clears spontaneously within 1 or 2 weeks. Occasionally, closed-chest trauma may tear the lung internally to produce a pulmonary *laceration*—a cystlike hyperlucent space that may contain an air–fluid level because of intracavitary hemorrhage. *Tracheobronchial rupture* caused by nonpenetrating trauma results in pneumothorax, often accompanied by mediastinal and subcutaneous emphysema and frequently associated with fractures of the upper three ribs. Nonpenetrating trauma may cause hemothorax or chylothorax in some instances.

Mediastinal structures may be affected by nonpenetrating trauma. Traumatic pericarditis is often secondary to steering wheel injuries of the anterior chest. Traumatic rupture of the descending portion of the aortic arch may lead to formation of a false aneurysm, which presents on the chest roentgenogram as a left-sided mediastinal mass. Mediastinal hematoma resulting from traumatic injury of one or more small vessels causes generalized or diffuse mediastinal widening.

REFERENCES

1. Adams FG: A simplified approach to the reporting of intensive therapy unit chest radiographs. Clin Radiol 30:214, 1979
2. Bartlett JG: Anaerobic bacterial pneumonitis. Am Rev Respir Dis 119:19, 1979
3. Berkman YM: Aspiration and inhalation pneumonias. Semin Roentgenol 15:73, 1980
4. Cummings SR, Lillington GA, Richard RJ: Managing solitary pulmonary nodules: The choice of strategy is a "close call." Am Rev Respir Dis 134:453, 1986
5. Fraser RG, Paré JAP, Paré PE et al: Perception in chest roentgenology. In Diagnosis of Diseases of the Chest, Vol 1, 3rd ed, p 291. Philadelphia, WB Saunders, 1987
6. Heitzman ER: Chronic obstructive pulmonary disease. In The Lung: Radiographic–Pathologic Correlations. 2nd ed., p 422. St. Louis, CV Mosby, 1984
7. Miller RD, Offord KP: Roentgenologic determination of total lung capacity. Mayo Clin Proc 55:694, 1980
8. Milne ENC, Pistolesi M, Miniati M, Giuntini C: The radiologic distinction of cardiogenic and noncardiogenic edema. AJR 144:879, 1985
9. Milos M, Aberle DR, Parkinson BT et al: Maternal pulmonary edema complicating beta-adrenergic therapy of preterm labor. AJR 151:917, 1988
10. Moser KM, Daily PO, Peterson KL et al: Thromboendarterectomy for chronic, major vessel thromboembolic pulmonary hypertension in 42 patients: Immediate and long term results. Ann Intern Med 107:560, 1987
11. Palmer PES: Radiology of asthma. In Gershwin ME (ed): Bronchial Asthma, p 153. New York, Grune & Stratton, 1981

12. Proto AV, Speckman JM: The left lateral radiograph of the chest, Part I and Part II Med Radiogr Photogr 55:30, 1979; 56:38, 1980
13. Zwillich CW, Pierson DJ, Creagh CE et al: Complications of assisted ventilation. A prospective study of 354 consecutive episodes. Am J Med 57:161, 1974

BIBLIOGRAPHY

General Texts

Felson B: Chest Roentgenology. Philadelphia, WB Saunders, 1973

Felson B, Weinstein AS, Spitz HB: Principles of Chest Roentgenology: A Programmed Text. Philadelphia, WB Saunders, 1965

Forrest JV, Fiegin DS: Essentials of Chest Radiology. Philadelphia, WB Saunders, 1982

Lillington GA: A Diagnostic Approach to Chest Diseases: Differential Diagnoses Based on Roentgenographic Patterns, 3rd ed. Baltimore, Williams & Wilkins, 1987

Meschan I (ed): Roentgen Signs in Diagnostic Imaging, Vol 4 (The Chest), 2nd ed. Philadelphia, WB Saunders, 1987

Intensive Care and Interventional Chest Radiology

Lefcoe MS: Basic principles of chest x-ray interpretation in a critical care unit. In Sibbald WJ (ed): Synopsis of Critical Care, 3rd ed, p 77. Baltimore, Williams & Wilkins, 1988

Pinet F, Clermont A, Michel C, Celard P, Lagrange C: Embolization of the systemic arteries of the lung. J Thorac Imaging 2(2):11, 1987

Powner DJ: Pulmonary barotrauma in the intensive care unit. J Intensive Care Med 3:224, 1988

Wang KP (ed): Biopsy Techniques in Pulmonary Disorders. New York, Raven Press, 1989

Westcott JL: Transthoracic needle biopsy of the hilum and mediastinum. J Thorac Imaging 2(2):41, 1987

Pulmonary Scintiscans and Angiography

Markisz JA: Radiologic and nuclear medicine diagnosis. In Goldhaber SZ (ed): Pulmonary Embolism and Deep Venous Thrombosis, p 41. Philadelphia, WB Saunders, 1985

Thoracic CT Scans

Naidich D, Zerhouni E, Siegelman S: Computerized Tomography of the Thorax. New York, Raven Press, 1984

Magnetic Resonance Imaging

Carroll FE Jr: Lungs. In Partain CL, Price RR, Patton JA, Kulkarni MV, James AE Jr (eds): Magnetic Resonance Imaging, 2nd ed. Philadelphia, WB Saunders, 1988

Webb WR: Mediastinum and hila. In Partain CL, Price RR, Patton JA, Kulkarni MV, James AE Jr (eds): Magnetic Resonance Imaging, 2nd ed. Philadelphia, WB Saunders, 1988

Radiographic Patterns

Friedman PJ: Radiographic correlations. In Dail DH, Hammar SP (eds): Pulmonary Pathology, p 1095. New York, Springer-Verlag, 1988

Heitzman ER: Pattern recognition in pulmonary radiology. In The Lung: Radiologic–Pathologic Correlations, 2nd ed, p 70. St. Louis, CV Mosby, 1984

Atelectasis

Proto AV, Toscino I: Radiographic manifestations of lobar collapse. Semin Roentgenol 15:117, 1980

Infectious Processes

Genereux GP, Stilwell GA: The acute bacterial pneumonias. Semin Roentgenol 15:9, 1980

Janower ML, Weiss EB: Mycoplasmal, viral and rickettsial pneumonias. Semin Roentgenol 15:25, 1980

Palmer PES: Pulmonary tuberculosis—usual and unusual radiographic presentations. Semin Roentgenol 14:204, 1979

Pennington JE: Respiratory Infections: Diagnosis and Management, 2nd ed. New York, Raven Press, 1989

Diffuse Obstructive Airway Diseases

Bergin CJ, Muller NL, Miller RR: CT in the qualitative assessment of emphysema. J Thorac Imaging 1(2):94, 1986

Gaensler EA, Jederlinc PJ, Fitzgerald MX: Patient work-up for bullectomy. J Thorac Imaging 1(2):75, 1986

Pratt PC: Role of conventional chest radiography in diagnosis and exclusion of emphysema. Am J Med 82:998, 1987

Diffuse Lung Diseases

Bergin CJ, Muller NL: CT of interstitial lung disease: A new diagnostic approach. AJR 148:987, 1987

Genereux GP: Pattern recognition in diffuse lung disease: A review of theory and practice. Med Radiogr Photogr 61:2, 1985

Joffe N: The adult respiratory distress syndrome. AJR 122:719, 1974

Pulmonary Embolism

Alderson PO, Martin EC: Pulmonary embolism: Diagnosis with multiple imaging modalities. Radiology 164:297, 1987

Fleischner FG: Roentgenology of the pulmonary infarct. Semin Roentgenol 2:61, 1967

Lillington GA, Parsons GH: Acute pulmonary embolism. Hosp Med 16:11, 1980

Pulmonary Manifestations of AIDS

Stover DE, White DA, Romano PA, Gellene RA, Robeson WA: Spectrum of pulmonary diseases associated with acquired immunodeficiency syndrome. Am J Med 78:429, 1985

THIRTEEN

Diagnosis and Therapy of Sleep-Disordered Breathing

Joseph Kaplan

For centuries, physicians have recognized the importance of sleep as a restorative process, and a few have observed the alterations in breathing that sometimes occur during sleep. Although he was not aware of what is now called "sleep apnea," Broadbent[4] accurately described the phenomenon in 1877.

> When a person, especially advanced in years, is lying on his back in heavy sleep and snoring loudly, it very commonly happens that every now and then the inspiration fails to overcome the resistance in the pharynx, of which stertor or snoring is the audible sign, and there will be perfect silence through two, three, or four respiratory periods, in which there are ineffectual chest movements; finally, air enters with a loud snort, after which there are several compensatory deep inspirations...

In 1956, Burwell et al[6] first used the term *pickwickian syndrome* in a report on the association of obesity, hypersomnolence, and cor pulmonale. However, it was Gastaut et al[22] and Jung and Kuhlo,[31] in independent studies, who associated this syndrome with disordered breathing during sleep.

There have been several other major milestones in the search for understanding of sleep and breathing disorders. In the 1950s, the description of rapid eye movement (REM) sleep and its association with changes in autonomic function, including respiration, was published.[14] In 1969, a German team described the first successful treatment of sleep apnea by tracheostomy.[34] The use of technologic refinements such as oximetry[20,46,57] and inductance plethysmography[10] broadened our understanding. Finally, in 1981, Sullivan and his group[54] pioneered the development of nasal continuous positive airway pressure (CPAP), a new and effective nonsurgical treatment for sleep apnea.

These developments have led to a dramatic increase in the number of "sleep centers," and now sleep-disordered breathing has become a major interest of internists, pulmonologists, otolaryngologists, and respiratory therapists.

SLEEP PHYSIOLOGY

Sleep is an active and complex process that is characterized by a well-defined structure termed "sleep architecture." A person's 24-hour cycle has three distinct states: wakefulness, REM sleep, and non-REM (NREM) sleep (Fig. 13–1). Non-REM sleep has four stages: Stage 1 is the transitional phase between wakefulness and sleep and is characterized by a low threshold of arousal and a low-voltage electroencephalogram (EEG) that shows a mixed frequency of alpha and theta waves. As sleep deepens, bursts of high-frequency waves (sleep

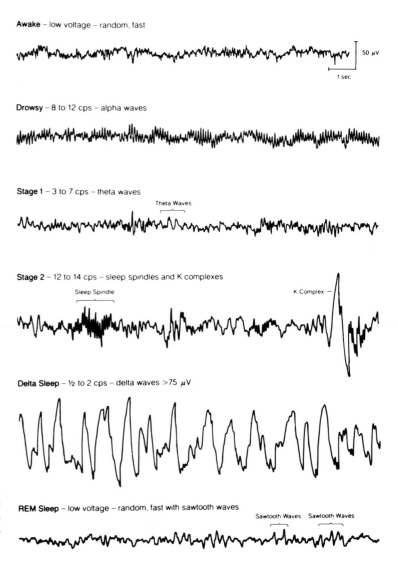

Awake – low voltage – random, fast

50 μV

1 sec

Drowsy – 8 to 12 cps – alpha waves

Stage 1 – 3 to 7 cps – theta waves

Theta Waves

Stage 2 – 12 to 14 cps – sleep spindles and K complexes

Sleep Spindle

K Complex –

Delta Sleep – ½ to 2 cps – delta waves >75 μV

REM Sleep – low voltage – random, fast with sawtooth waves

Sawtooth Waves Sawtooth Waves

Figure 13—1. Human sleep stages. (Hauri P: The Sleep Disorders [Current Concepts 8800-18], 2nd ed, pp 1–20. Kalamazoo, Michigan, The Upjohn Company, October 1982. By permission of the publisher)

spindles) along with K complexes and lower voltage are seen; this is stage 2 sleep. Stages 3 and 4 are also known as slow-wave or delta sleep. During slow-wave sleep, the arousal threshold increases and the EEG frequency slows and increases in amplitude. Non-REM sleep shifts from one stage to another up to 40 times during the night (Fig. 13–2).

The first REM period is preceded by a return to stage 2 sleep. The REM phase is identified by the rapid conjugate eye movements, detected by the electrooculograph (EOG), associated with a low-amplitude EEG and a decrease in muscle tone, as seen on the electromyogram (EMG) (Fig. 13–3). The REM sleep tends to occur three to five times per night, with progressive lengthening of each REM period so that the most REM sleep occurs early in the morning just before awakening (see Fig. 13–2).

CHANGES IN RESPIRATORY PHYSIOLOGY IN SLEEP

Small changes in breathing take place during NREM sleep.[40] The responses to hypoxia and hypercapnia are predictable, but the respiratory rate slows and peak instantaneous airflow rate and pressure developed against an occluded airway decrease, compared with wakefulness. Upper airway resistance increases owing to a decrease in upper airway muscle tone. Tidal volume increases as the result of increased duration during inspiration, but minute ventilation decreases.

In REM sleep, the changes in respiratory function are more significant than in NREM sleep.[40] The breathing pattern becomes rapid and irregular, and airflow is decreased. Tidal volume and inspiratory

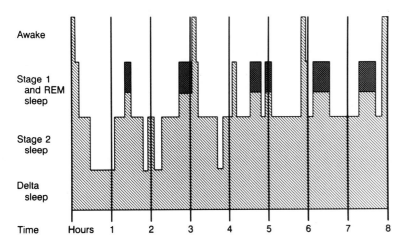

Figure 13—2. Typical sleep pattern of a young adult: Hatched area, stage 1 sleep; solid black area, REM sleep. (Hauri P: The Sleep Disorders [Current Concepts 8800-18], 2nd ed, pp 1–20. Kalamazoo, Michigan, The Upjohn Company, October 1982. By permission of the publisher)

times are decreased, and apnea and hyperpnea occur more frequently than in NREM sleep. Hypotonia of the intercostal muscles decreases or even eliminates costal breathing in REM sleep. Loss of muscle tone in the upper airway respiratory muscles leads to an increase in airway resistance. Finally, ventilatory responses to chemical stimuli and other respiratory reflexes are weakened. These changes make REM sleep a period of vulnerability for the person who has additional alterations in function as a result of a disease state.

DEFINITIONS

The term *sleep-disordered breathing* is applied to all types of abnormal respiratory patterns including apnea and hypopnea. *Sleep apnea* refers specifically to a pause in respiration with cessation of airflow occurring at the level of the nostrils and mouth and lasting for at least 10 seconds. Sleep apnea is classified into three types: (1) obstructive (Fig. 13–4A), occlusion of the upper airway and identified by the absence of airflow despite persistent respiratory effort; (2) central (see Fig. 13–4B), a failure of the respiratory center to initiate the impulses to activate the respiratory muscles and recognized as absence of airflow at the nose or mouth without any respiratory effort; and (3) mixed (see Fig. 13–4C), which has components of both obstructive apnea and central apnea.[24]

Sleep-related *hypopnea* is the situation of decreased airflow because of partial obstruction or central hypoventilation.[17] If the hypopnea is due to

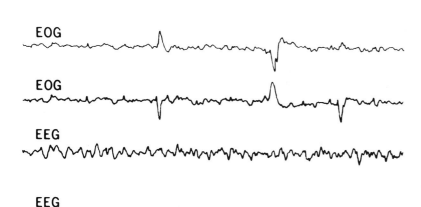

Figure 13—3. Polysomnographic tracing of the transition from NREM sleep to REM sleep: The EOG shows rapid conjugate eye movements associated with decrease in muscle tone (EMG) and a low-amplitude EEG. (Reproduced, with permission, from Orr WC, Altshuler KZ, Stahl ML [eds]: Managing Sleep Complaints, pp 11–28, Chicago, Year Book Medical Publishers, 1982)

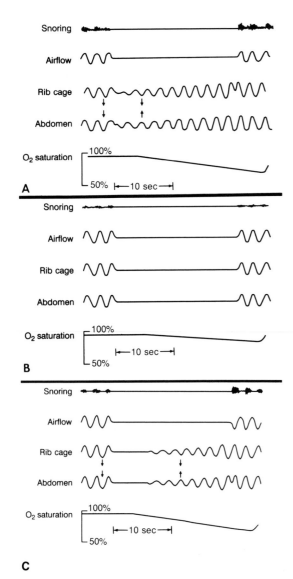

Figure 13—4. Types of sleep apnea. (A) Obstructive apnea: This is characterized by loud intermittent snoring, complete cessation of airflow, paradoxic movement of the chest and abdomen, and moderate to severe oxygen desaturation. (B) Central apnea: The features are absence of snoring, simultaneous cessation of airflow and respiratory effort, and, usually, only mild to moderate oxygen desaturation. (C) Mixed apnea: An initial central apnea is followed by an obstructive apnea that usually produces moderate to severe oxygen desaturation.

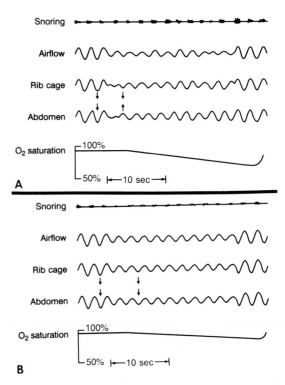

Figure 13—5. Hypopnea. (A) Obstructive type characterized by persistent snoring, decreased airflow, paradoxic movement of the rib cage and abdomen, and mild to moderate oxygen desaturation. (B) Nonobstructive type characterized by diminished snoring, persistent, but decreased, airflow, and rib cage and abdominal movements in phase; this usually is associated with mild oxygen desaturation.

ETIOLOGY AND PATHOPHYSIOLOGY

The *sleep apnea* syndrome is characterized by multiple obstructive or mixed apneas during sleep associated with repetitive episodes of inordinately loud snoring and daytime sleepiness. The key to the pathogenesis of this disorder lies in the function of the upper airway during sleep.

The oropharynx is the only collapsible segment of the upper airway, and its walls lack sufficient protection against forces that promote occlusion. Each inspiratory effort results in a decrease in intrapharyngeal pressure relative to atmospheric pressure and, therefore, a tendency for the pharynx to collapse. Normally, this tendency is resisted by the coordinated contraction of the oropharyngeal muscles during inspiration. This contraction results in both dilatation and increased tone (decreased compliance) of the airway. Factors that create a more negative intrapharyngeal pressure or decrease upper airway tone may shift the balance and result in occlusion of the airway.

partial obstruction, the movements of the chest and abdomen are out of phase and snoring is frequently heard (Fig. 13–5A). On the other hand, the nonobstructive hypopnea caused by central hypoventilation is characterized by decreased but in-phase chest and abdominal excursions with little or no associated snoring (see Fig. 13–5B).

In addition, any alteration in the anatomy of this critical segment of the airway favors collapse. A large tongue, redundant soft palate, shallow palatal arch, enlarged tonsils, narrow mandibular arch, and recessed mandible have all been implicated in the pathogenesis of obstructive sleep apnea.[18] Detailed measurements of the upper airway have revealed small but consistent anatomic abnormalities not only in the soft tissues of the pharynx, but also in the relationship of the hyoid bone (an anchor of the tongue) to the mandible.[44]

In view of the factors at work to keep the pharynx open, it is not difficult to understand the alterations that lead to occlusion. In sleep, especially REM sleep, muscle tone diminishes greatly, which favors collapse of the airway. Alcohol[29] or hypnotic drugs[16] may further diminish pharyngeal muscle tone. As muscle tone diminishes, airway resistance increases, and the diaphragm must contract more forcefully to overcome the increased resistance. This, in turn, decreases intrapharyngeal pressure and promotes closure. In addition, any process that increases upstream resistance (e.g., nasal obstruction) increases the risk for occlusive apnea.[28,61]

CLINICAL MANIFESTATIONS

Obstructive sleep apnea syndrome has a clear preponderance in middle-aged men and postmenopausal women,[33] although the disorder is seen in males and females of all ages.[2] Table 13–1 lists conditions that increase the risk of obstructive sleep apnea syndrome.

The two most common symptoms, seen in virtually all patients with significant disease, are snoring and excessive daytime sleepiness. The snoring typically is loud and intermittent. There are notable periods of silence when no audible breathing is detectable, despite persistent respiratory efforts. Daytime sleepiness may be severe, but the patient is usually a poor judge of the degree of the sleepi-

Table 13–1 Disorders Associated With Obstructive Sleep Apnea

Obesity
Nasal obstruction
Tonsillar hypertrophy
Macroglossia
Retrognathia, micrognathia
Acromegaly
Hypothyroidism

Table 13–2 Monitoring Options for Polysomnography

FEATURE	EQUIPMENT
EEG, EOG, EMG, ECG	Polygraph
	Standard electrodes
Airflow	Thermistor
	CO_2 analyzer
	Pneumotachograph
Respiratory effort	Inductance plethysmograph
	Intercostal EMG
	Esophageal balloon
	Strain gauge
Oxygenation	Oximeter, ear or finger

ness.[15] Relatives and friends frequently report that the patient falls asleep at inappropriate times, such as during meetings, movies, parties, or while driving. Patients have been referred to sleep disorder centers after motor vehicle or industrial accidents that apparently were caused by a low level of alertness.

The patient may experience other troublesome, although less common, symptoms such as increased body movements during sleep, morning headache, memory deficit, impotence, and personality change.[26]

Other findings reflect cardiovascular and respiratory responses to repeated apneas. Systemic hypertension is quite common,[19,32,35] and pulmonary hypertension is seen in advanced disease.[3,55] Cardiac rhythm disturbances have been reported,[25,37,56] but recent studies suggest that the incidence of life-threatening arrhythmias is low, especially if oxygen saturation is maintained above 60%.[47] Patients with sleep-disordered breathing and associated chronic lung disease or obesity may present with hypoxemia, hypercapnia, and cor pulmonale.[3]

DIAGNOSIS

Accurate diagnosis of sleep-disordered breathing requires all-night polysomnography. Table 13–2 lists the various types of equipment needed and the options available for recording each feature. Along with measurements of airflow at the nose and mouth, respiratory effort is monitored to differentiate central from obstructive apnea.

Measurements of oxygenation (oximetry) permit quantification of the severity of a disordered breathing event. Continuous ECG monitoring is helpful for identifying arrhythmias associated with disordered breathing events. The patient's body position is noted during polysomnography because many apneas are worse when the patient is in the supine position.[8]

In addition to the standard monitoring of cardiorespiratory function, sleep staging is crucial. An accurate description of the sleep architecture and the effect of disordered breathing on sleep continuity adds to the clinical interpretation. At least two EEG channels, an electrooculogram, and a chin electromyogram are required for this assessment. Because of the frequent association of abnormal movements of the extremities,[2] a leg electromyogram and video recordings are recommended.

The evaluation also should include a multiple sleep latency test (MSLT). This study provides objective evidence of the degree of daytime hypersomnolence[7] and also gives major clues regarding the presence of narcolepsy,[38,42,60] a condition that also causes daytime sleepiness and occasionally may coexist with sleep apnea.

The MSLT should begin 1.5 to 2 hours after the patient's usual nighttime sleep. Polysomnographic recordings are made during three to five naps spaced 2 hours apart throughout the day. Special attention is directed to the time it takes from "lights out" to the first clear evidence of sleep by EEG. This interval is termed *the sleep latency*. Table 13–3 shows the mean sleep latency in normals and in narcoleptic and non-narcoleptic patients with hypersomnia. If the patient demonstrates hypersomnolence and also a shortened REM latency, the diagnosis of narcolepsy is suggested.[38,42] The MSLT can be used along with nighttime polysomnography to monitor the response to therapy, because

treatment of nighttime apnea leads to improvement in daytime functioning.[60]

TREATMENT

As in other diseases, therapy is tailored to the individual. Patients with fewer than five apneas per hour of sleep usually require no therapy, but should be monitored over time for worsening of symptoms. Those with 5 to 30 apneas per hour have mild disease and will respond to simple measures such as avoidance of sedatives[16] and alcohol,[29] sleeping in the lateral position, and dieting to lose weight. Those with more than 30 apneas per hour or with mild disease but with cardiac arrhythmia or troubling daytime hypersomnolence are candidates for more aggressive treatment.

MEDICAL THERAPY

Nonpharmacologic approaches to obstructive sleep apnea remain the mainstay of therapy for patients with mild or moderate disease. Smith et al[49] found that moderate weight loss alone resulted in a significant decrease in obstructive sleep apnea and daytime hypersomnolence and an improvement in sleep architecture. However, most patients find weight reduction difficult to achieve and to maintain. In many instances, disordered breathing events are confined to the supine sleeping position, so training the patient to sleep in the lateral position frequently alleviates significant apnea.[8] Nasal[1] and oral[9] appliances have been developed to maintain airway patency during sleep, but they have not gained wide acceptance because of discomfort and

Table 13–3 MSLT Results for Various Groups

GROUP TESTED	n	*1000	1200	1400	1600	1800	Mean
		MEAN SCORES* BY TIME OF DAY NAP IS TAKEN					
Narcoleptics	49	3.05	2.74	2.42	2.26	4.07	2.91
Non-narcoleptics with hypersomnia	63	8.93	7.55	7.81	8.16	11.23	8.74
Controls	13	14.33	13.17	13.17	11.95	13.75	13.38

(Reproduced with permission, from Mitler MM: The multiple sleep latency test as an evaluation for excessive somnolence. In Guilleminault C (ed): Sleeping and Waking Disorders: Indications and Techniques, pp 145–153. Stoneham, Mass, Butterworths Publishers, 1982)
* Time to sleep onset, in minutes.

lack of effectiveness in moderate or severe disease.

The development of nasal CPAP by Sullivan et al[54] was a major advance in the nonpharmacologic treatment of obstructive sleep apnea. In many centers, nasal CPAP has replaced tracheostomy as the preferred mode of therapy in moderate or severe disease. This method uses a soft occlusive nasal mask held to the face by straps, an expiratory valve and tubing, and a blower system to produce continuous positive pressure ranging from 2.5 to 15 cmH_2O (Fig. 13–6). Nasal CPAP works by providing a pneumatic splint for the airway and thus prevents its collapse. In the laboratory, nasal CPAP virtually eliminates snoring and obstructive apnea when critical pressures are reached. Several studies have shown the high degree of efficacy of this form of therapy for obstructive sleep apnea, and a few reports claim effectiveness for central sleep apnea as well.[30]

There is little doubt that nasal CPAP is a highly successful treatment for obstructive sleep apnea in the laboratory, but approximately 20% of the patients fail to tolerate this therapy at home. Poor compliance results from the expense, the minor discomfort, and the pyschosocial problems associated with the nightly requirement for a nasal mask.

Several pharmacologic agents have been used for the obstructive sleep apnea syndrome, with mixed degrees of success. Protriptyline has been reported to decrease the frequency of obstructive apneas and to increase the oxygen saturation.[5,50] However, a recent controlled study failed to show any effect of protriptyline on symptoms or on polysomnographic criteria.[59] The use of protriptyline is limited by troublesome side effects, such as dry mouth, constipation, diaphoresis, urinary retention, and erectile impotence.

Progesterone has been tried for obstructive sleep apnea, but the experience is limited and the results are mixed.[41,52] Besides the lack of proven efficacy, the use of progesterone in men is limited by side effects such as hair loss and decreased libido.

Oxygen has been used with success in several types of sleep-disordered breathing. Oxygen therapy may produce a significant decrease in the total number of apneas as well as in the percentage of apnea time (duration of apneas divided by the total sleep time),[36] but individual apneas may become more prolonged. In NREM sleep, oxygen therapy decreases the apnea index and the peak decrease in oxygen saturation. In REM sleep, the disordered breathing improves but oxygen saturation does not. Oxygen therapy appears to have no effect on day-

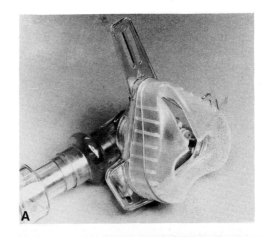

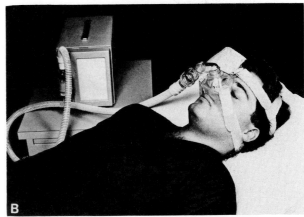

Figure 13—6. Continuous positive airway pressure (CPAP). (*A*) Standard adult nasal mask. (*B*) Nasal system in place on an adult (model is technician in Sleep Laboratory).

time sleepiness, as measured by the MSLT.[51] In patients with predominantly central and mixed apneas, oxygen administration results in a marked decrease in these apneas but a doubling in the number of obstructive apneas.[23] In view of the lack of a predictable response and the expense involved, polysomnography and MSLT are recommended before oxygen therapy is prescribed.

SURGICAL THERAPY

Several surgical approaches have been used to correct airway obstruction in patients with sleep apnea. Nasal septoplasty, in theory, should benefit the patient who has a collapsible pharynx, but the results have been inconsistent.[45] Because the risk of nasal surgery is low, an obvious defect in the nose should be corrected as the first step.

Tonsillectomy is an effective procedure in children, and a recent report[39] suggests that this procedure is of benefit in selected adults.

A more popular approach has been uvulopalatopharyngoplasty (UPPP), first developed by Fujita et al.[21] This procedure involves excision of redundant soft tissue, including the free margin of the palate, uvula, and posterior pharyngeal wall. Initial results were promising, but several studies have now found significant improvement in only 50% of the patients.[12] Studies are under way to determine which preoperative criteria will predict success. Despite the disappointing results with sleep apnea, the procedure has a higher success rate in treatment of snoring.[48] The UPPP may be complicated by worsening pharyngeal obstruction due to edema in the early postoperative period and, later, by nasal regurgitation.

Tracheostomy remains the most effective surgical therapy available and is essentially curative, regardless of the site or cause of obstruction.[27] The tracheostomy tube remains stoppered during the day and is opened by the patient at night to provide a "bypass" for the obstructed upper airway. Tracheostomy cannulas need not be cuffed and should be fenestrated to facilitate speech. This form of surgical therapy has been limited by the complications, which include bleeding, recurrent tracheitis and bronchitis, and granulation tissue formation.[13] Patients with a double chin may require lipectomy to avoid inadvertent blockage of the tracheostomy opening by excess adipose tissue. Tracheostomy should be reserved for the patient in whom conservative therapy has failed and who has disabling hypersomnolence, life-threatening cardiac arrhythmia, or cor pulmonale.

Gastric bypass and vertical banded gastroplasty have been used with some success in the obstructive sleep apnea syndrome.[11,53,58] In view of the other less invasive and more effective forms of therapy, this type of operation is rarely used.

Other experimental approaches that show promise in selected patients are mandibular osteotomy with hyoid bone advancement and combined maxillary, mandibular, and hyoid bone advancement.[43]

REFERENCES

1. Afzelius L-E, Elmqvist D, Hougaard K et al: Sleep apnea syndrome—an alternative treatment to tracheostomy. Laryngoscope 91:285–291, 1981
2. Ancoli-Israel S, Kripke DF, Mason W, Messin S: Sleep apnea and nocturnal myoclonus in a senior population. Sleep 4:349–358, 1981
3. Bradley TD, Rutherford R, Grossman RF et al: Role of daytime hypoxemia in the pathogenesis of right heart failure in the obstructive sleep apnea syndrome. Am Rev Respir Dis 131:835–839, 1985
4. Broadbent WH: Cheyne-Stokes' respiration in cerebral haemorrhage. Lancet 1:307–309, 1877
5. Brownell LG, West P, Sweatman P et al: Protriptyline in obstructive sleep apnea: A double-blind trial. N Engl J Med 307:1037–1042, 1982
6. Burwell CS, Robin ED, Whaley RD, Bickelmann AG: Extreme obesity associated with alveolar hypoventilation—a pickwickian syndrome. Am J Med 21:811–818, 1956
7. Carskadon M, Dement WC: Sleep tendency: An objective measure of sleep loss [Abstract]. Sleep Res 6:200, 1977
8. Cartwright RD: Effect of sleep position on sleep apnea severity. Sleep 7:110–114, 1984
9. Cartwright RD, Samelson CF: The effects of a nonsurgical treatment for obstructive sleep apnea: The tongue-retaining device. JAMA 248:705–709, 1982
10. Chadha TS, Watson H, Birch S et al: Validation of respiratory inductive plethysmography using different calibration procedures. Am Rev Respir Dis 125:644–649, 1982
11. Charuzi I, Ovnat A, Peiser J et al: The effect of surgical weight reduction on sleep quality in obesity-related sleep apnea syndrome. Surgery 97:535–538, 1985
12. Cohn MA: Surgical treatment in sleep apnea syndrome. In Fletcher EC (ed): Abnormalities of Respiration During Sleep: Diagnosis, Pathophysiology, and Treatment, pp 117–139. Orlando Fla, Grune & Stratton, 1986
13. Conway WA, Victor LD, Magilligan DJ Jr et al: Adverse effects of tracheostomy for sleep apnea. JAMA 246:347–350, 1981
14. Dement W, Kleitman N: Cyclic variations in EEG during sleep and their relation to eye movements, body motility, and dreaming. Electroencephalogr Clin Neurophysiol 9:673–690, 1957
15. Dement WC, Carskadon MA, Richardson G: Excessive daytime sleepiness in the sleep apnea syndrome. In Guilleminault C, Dement WC (eds): Sleep Apnea Syndromes, pp 23–46. New York, Alan R Liss, 1978
16. Dolly FR, Block AJ: Effect of flurazepam on sleep-disordered breathing and nocturnal oxygen desaturation in asymptomatic subjects. Am J Med 73:239–243, 1982
17. Edelman NH (ed): Contemp Issues Pulmonary Dis 5:1–264, 1986
18. Fletcher EC (ed): Abnormalities of Respiration During Sleep: Diagnosis, Pathophysiology, and Treatment. Orlando, Fla, Grune & Stratton, 1986
19. Fletcher EC, DeBehnke RD, Lovoi MS, Gorin AB: Undiagnosed sleep apnea in patients with essential hypertension. Ann Intern Med 103:190–195, 1985
20. Flick MR, Block AJ: Continuous in vivo monitoring of arterial oxygenation in chronic obstructive lung disease. Ann Intern Med 86:725–730, 1977
21. Fujita S, Conway W, Zorick F, Roth T: Surgical correction of anatomic abnormalities in obstructive sleep apnea syndrome: Uvulopalatopharyngoplasty. Otolaryngol Head Neck Surg 89:923–934, 1981
22. Gastaut H, Tassinari CA, Duron B: Étude polygraphique des manifestations épisodiques (hypniques et respiratoires), diurnes et nocturnes, du syndrome de Pickwick. Rev Neurol (Paris) 112:568–579, 1965

23. Gold AR, Bleecker ER, Smith PL: A shift from central and mixed sleep apnea to obstructive sleep apnea resulting from low-flow oxygen. Am Rev Respir Dis 132:220–223, 1985

24. Guilleminault C (ed): Sleeping and Waking Disorders: Indications and Techniques. Boston, Butterworths, 1982

25. Guilleminault C, Connolly SJ, Winkle RA: Cardiac arrhythmia and conduction disturbances during sleep in 400 patients with sleep apnea syndrome. Am J Cardiol 52:490–494, 1983

26. Guilleminault C, Eldridge FL, Tilkian A et al: Sleep apnea syndrome due to upper airway obstruction: A review of 25 cases. Arch Intern Med 137:296–300, 1977

27. Guilleminault C, Simmons FB, Motta J et al: Obstructive sleep apnea syndrome and tracheostomy: Long-term follow-up experience. Arch Intern Med 141:985–988, 1981

28. Heimer D, Scharf SM, Lieberman A, Lavie P: Sleep apnea syndrome treated by repair of deviated nasal septum. Chest 84:184–185, 1983

29. Issa FG, Sullivan CE: Alcohol, snoring and sleep apnoea. J Neurol Neurosurg Psychiatry 45:353–359, 1982

30. Issa FG, Sullivan CE: Reversal of central sleep apnea using nasal CPAP. Chest 90:165–171, 1986

31. Jung R, Kuhlo W: Neurophysiological studies of abnormal night sleep and the pickwickian syndrome. Prog Brain Res 18:140–159, 1965

32. Kales A, Bixler EO, Cadieux RJ et al: Sleep apnoea in a hypertensive population. Lancet 2:1005–1008, 1984

33. Katsumata K, Okada R, Ohta T et al: Incidence of sleep apnea syndromes in general patients at a hospital for internal medicine. Nagoya J Med Sci 48:47–53, 1986

34. Kuhlo W, Doll E, Franck MC: Erfolgreiche Behandlung eines Pickwick-syndroms durch eine Dauertracheakanüle. Dtsch Med Wochenschr 94:1286–1290, 1969

35. Lavie P, Ben-Yosef R, Rubin AE: Prevalence of sleep apnea syndrome among patients with essential hypertension. Am Heart J 108:373–376, 1984

36. Martin RJ, Sanders MH, Gray BA, Pennock BE: Acute and long-term effects of hyperoxia in the adult sleep apnea syndrome. Am Rev Respir Dis 125:175–180, 1982

37. Miller WP: Cardiac arrhythmias and conduction disturbances in the sleep apnea syndrome: Prevalence and significance. Am J Med 73:317–321, 1982

38. Mitler MM, van den Hoed J, Carskadon MA et al: REM sleep episodes during the multiple sleep latency test in narcoleptic patients. Electroencephalogr Clin Neurophysiol 46:478–481, 1979

39. Moser RJ III, Rajagopal KR: Obstructive sleep apnea in adults with tonsillary hypertrophy. Arch Intern Med 147:1265–1267, 1987

40. Orem J, Barnes CD (eds): Physiology in Sleep. New York, Academic Press, 1980

41. Orr WC, Imes NK, Martin RJ: Progesterone therapy in obese patients with sleep apnea. Arch Intern Med 139:109–111, 1979

42. Richardson GS, Carskadon MA, Flagg W et al: Excessive daytime sleepiness in man: Multiple sleep latency measurement in narcoleptic and control subjects. Electroencephalogr Clin Neurophysiol 45:621–627, 1978

43. Riley RW, Powell NB, Guilleminault C: Current surgical concepts for treating obstructive sleep apnea syndrome. J Oral Maxillofac Surg 45:149–157, 1987

44. Rivlin J, Hoffstein V, Kalbfleisch J et al: Upper airway morphology in patients with idiopathic obstructive sleep apnea. Am Rev Respir Dis 129:355–360, 1984

45. Rubin AHE, Eliaschar I, Joachim Z et al: Effects of nasal surgery and tonsillectomy on sleep apnea. Bull Eur Physiopathol Respir 16:612–615, 1983

46. Scoggin C, Nett L, Petty TL: Clinical evaluation of a new ear oximeter. Heart Lung 6:121–126, 1977

47. Shepard JW Jr, Garrison MW, Grither DA, Dolan GF: Relationship of ventricular ectopy to oxyhemoglobin desaturation in patients with obstructive sleep apnea. Chest 8:335–340, 1985

48. Simmons FB, Guilleminault C, Silvestri R: Snoring, and some obstructive sleep apnea, can be cured by oropharyngeal surgery: Palatopharyngoplasty. Arch Otolaryngol 109:503–507, 1983

49. Smith PL, Gold AR, Meyers DA et al: Weight loss in mildly to moderately obese patients with obstructive sleep apnea. Ann Intern Med 103:850–855, 1985

50. Smith PL, Haponik EF, Allen RP, Bleecker ER: The effects of protriptyline in sleep-disordered breathing. Am Rev Respir Dis 127:8–13, 1983

51. Smith PL, Haponik EF, Bleecker ER: The effects of oxygen in patients with sleep apnea. Am Rev Respir Dis 130:958–963, 1984

52. Strohl KP, Hensley MJ, Saunders NA et al: Progesterone administration and progressive sleep apneas. JAMA 245:1230–1232, 1981

53. Sugerman HJ, Fairman RP, Lindeman AK et al: Gastroplasty for respiratory insufficiency of obesity. Ann Surg 193:677–685, 1981

54. Sullivan CE, Issa FG, Berthon-Jones M, Eves L: Reversal of obstructive sleep apnea by continuous positive airway pressure applied through the nares. Lancet 1:862–865, 1981

55. Tilkian AG, Guilleminault C, Schroeder JS et al: Hemodynamics in sleep-induced apnea: Studies during wakefulness and sleep. Ann Intern Med 85:714–719, 1976

56. Tilkian AG, Guilleminault C, Schroeder JS et al: Sleep-induced apnea syndrome: Prevalence of cardiac arrhythmias and their reversal after tracheostomy. Am J Med 63:348–358, 1977

57. Trask CH, Cree EM: Oximeter studies on patients with chronic obstructive emphysema, awake and during sleep. N Engl J Med 266:639–642, 1962

58. Victor DW Jr, Sarmient CF, Yanta M, Halverson JD: Obstructive sleep apnea in the morbidly obese. Arch Surg 119:970–972, 1984

59. Whyte KF, Gould GA, Airlie MAA, et al: Role of protriptyline and acetazolamide in the sleep apnea/hypopnea syndrome. Sleep 11:463–472, 1988

60. Zorick F, Roehrs T, Conway W et al: Effects of uvulopalatopharyngoplasty on the daytime sleepiness associated with sleep apnea syndrome. Bull Eur Physiopathol Respir 19:600–603, 1983

61. Zwillich CW, Pickett C, Hanson FN, Weil JV: Disturbed sleep and prolonged apnea during nasal obstruction in normal men. Am Rev Respir Dis 124:158–160, 1981

Fourteen

Manufacture, Storage, and Transport of Medical Gases

James M. Webb
James Maguire
Thomas E. Sych

OXYGEN

ATMOSPHERIC CONTENT

Oxygen is the third most abundant atom in the universe, with hydrogen and helium first and second, respectively, and carbon and nitrogen fourth and fifth. Oxygen comprises only 0.09% of all the atoms in the universe. At the earth's crust, however, where oxygen is the most abundant atom, it comprises approximately 54% of all the atoms. There are approximately 37.7 examoles (Emol)* of oxygen in the atmosphere; 37.0 Emol are in the form of molecular oxygen and most of the rest is in the form of water vapor. In addition to molecular oxygen, the atmosphere contains several reactive gaseous species, including ozone. These other species are generally found at high altitude or in polluted environments.

The process of biologic photosynthesis is the main source and regulator of oxygen in the atmosphere. The greatest amount of oxygen is produced on land by terrestrial photosynthesis (0.0073 Emol/yr). Approximately 0.0037 Emol of oxygen per year are produced by oceanic photosynthesis, particularly close to land. The total production of oxygen for the earth is approximately 0.011 Emol/yr.

Photosynthesis is the process whereby light energy from the sun converts carbon dioxide and water into glucose and oxygen. The chemical agent necessary for this transformation is chlorophyll. Chlorophyll is a pigment that traps energy. Interestingly, the enzyme system that catalyzes the production of energy-rich compounds is the same as the enzyme system that allows energy release from these compounds, in the presence of oxygen, in the animal body.

$$6CO_2 + 6H_2O \xrightarrow[\text{Radiant energy}]{\text{Chlorophyll}} C_6H_{12}O_6 + 6O_2$$

The rate of photosynthesis is primarily influenced by two factors: an increase in oxygen and a decrease in carbon dioxide. Both factors decrease the rate of photosynthesis. Within the biosphere, the process of manufacturing oxygen is primarily the function of photosynthesis, and respiration is primarily the process by which oxygen is utilized. The end result of these two processes is a net production of oxygen that is practically zero. It takes approximately 3400 years for the oxygen in the air around the earth to be replaced.

The oxygen we breathe is necessary to support the metabolic process by which we convert carbohydrates, fats, and proteins into heat and energy. The amount of oxygen consumed by an average human being in a 24-hour period weighs about 2–5 lb (4.5–11.2 kg), which is roughly equal to the weight of the food that we consume in the same period of time. For our bodies to obtain this oxygen, we will

---

* One Emol represents 1×10^{18} mol, with 1 mol representing the gram molecular weight of the substance. For instance, 1 mol of free oxygen is 32 g, which corresponds to its molecular weight of 32.

1,000,000 CU. FT. OF DRY AIR CONTAINS	
781,400	CU. FT. NITROGEN
209,300	CU. FT. OXYGEN
9,300	CU. FT. ARGON
300	CU. FT. CARBON DIOXIDE
18	CU. FT. NEON
5	CU. FT. HELIUM
1	CU. FT. KRYPTON
1	CU. FT. HYDROCARBONS
.5	CU. FT. HYDROGEN
.08	CU. FT. XENON
.01	CU. FT. ACETYLENE

Figure 14—1. Specific identifiable gases contained in 1,000,000 cu ft of dry air. (Courtesy of Union Carbide Corp., Linde Division)

have to breathe approximately 500 ft³ (15,000 qt) of air (Fig. 14–1).

LABORATORY METHODS OF OXYGEN MANUFACTURE

Until the early 1900s the manufacture of oxygen was primarily a laboratory process. In 1774, Joseph Priestley liberated the first pure oxygen on record by concentrating the sun's rays through a magnifying glass on mercuric oxide.[1]

Several other methods may be used for preparing oxygen in the laboratory setting. Heating potassium chlorate in the presence of manganese dioxide, which serves as a catalyst, is one method. Another is the electrolysis of water. By volume, water contains two parts hydrogen to one part oxygen (by weight water contains one part hydrogen to eight parts oxygen). These elements can be split, leaving one part oxygen and two parts hydrogen. The difference between the volume and weight ratios can be explained by the fact that the atomic weight of oxygen is 16 times that of hydrogen.

The word *electrolysis* literally means "split by electricity". This is accomplished by passing an electric current through the water. Because water is a poor conductor of electricity, it is necessary to add a substance that will enable the electric current to pass through it. Generally, a trace of mineral or sulfuric acid is added to the water to facilitate the conduction of the current through the water. As the current passes through the water, bubbles of gas appear near the two electrodes. Oxygen collects in

the tube that contains the anode; the hydrogen collects in the tube containing the cathode (Fig. 14–2). As explained earlier, for every milliliter of oxygen produced there will be 2 mL of hydrogen.

Another method used for production of oxygen is the *LeBrin process,* by which oxygen is prepared from atmospheric air. This is an older process in which barium oxide (BaO) is heated to 500° C in air, producing barium peroxide. By raising the temperature of the barium peroxide to 800° C, oxygen and barium oxide will be liberated.

COMMERCIAL METHODS OF OXYGEN MANUFACTURE

Limited commercial production of oxygen began around the turn of the century with what was known as an "ozone generator." In this process, fused sodium peroxide interacts with water. This method was both expensive and cumbersome and, eventually, gave way to the common technique of

Figure 14—2. Apparatus used for the electrolysis of water.

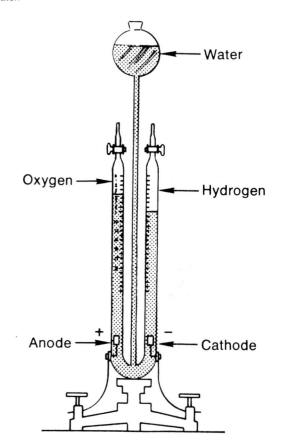

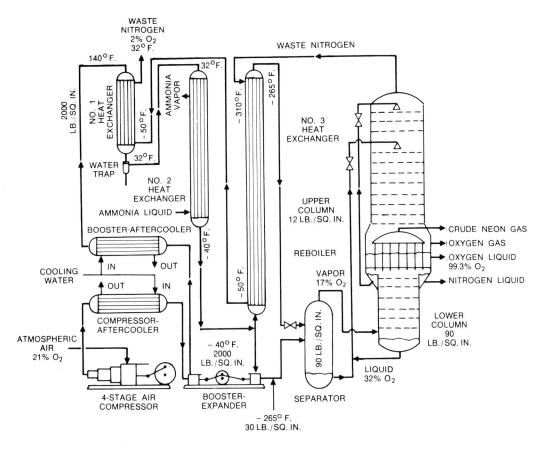

Figure 14—3. Air separation plant for the production of liquid oxygen. (Courtesy of Union Carbide Corp., Linde Division)

fractional distillation of liquefied air (sometimes referred to as the Joule–Kelvin method).[1]

According to the Joule–Kelvin principle, when gases, under pressure, are released into a vacuum, the molecules tend to lose kinetic energy. The molecules withdraw from each other and their cohesive attraction is lost in the vacuum. The loss in kinetic energy results in a decreased speed of the molecules, with a resultant lowering of the temperature, a necessary step for liquefaction of the air.

The complex process for the commercial preparation of oxygen can be divided into three stages: (1) purification of the air, (2) partial liquefaction of the air by refrigeration, and (3) separation of oxygen from nitrogen by fractional distillation of the partially liquefied air. To start the process, air is compressed to approximately 1500 lb/in.² gauge (psig) in a large compressor (Fig. 14–3). The initial increase in temperature caused by compression is reversed by a water-cooled heat exchanger. The air is then compressed further to approximately 2000

psig, after which it passes through an aftercooler and is delivered at room temperature to a countercurrent heat exchanger.

The purpose of the three-chamber countercurrent heat exchanger is to purify and liquefy the compressed air, partially through a refrigeration process. With waste nitrogen as a cooling agent, the first chamber cools the air below the freezing point of water, condensing most of the water out of the air. The compressed air enters this chamber and is cooled to approximately −50° F, and leaves the chamber at approximately 32° F (0° C).

In the second chamber of the heat exchanger, the compressed air first enters a forecooler and is cooled to approximately −40° F (−40° C) by the evaporation of liquid ammonia. At this point, any water remaining in the air is frozen out. The partially purified air is then transferred to the third chamber of the heat exchanger, where it is cooled to approximately −265° F. At this stage of the process, the extremely cold air is still compressed at 200 psig and will not liquefy, since the critical pressure of air is approximately 530 psig. At any pressure above 530 psig, the meniscus, or curved upper surface of the column of liquid under pressure, disappears and no separation between liquid and gas is evident; the air simply increases in density as it is cooled. Therefore, the extremely cold air–fluid

must be expanded to about 90 psig before it can be separated with a sizable fraction liquefied.

Still at −265° F, but expanded to a much lower pressure, the air leaves the heat exchanger and passes into a separator, where liquid and vapor are separated. These are pumped in separate streams into the distillation column. The pressure of the

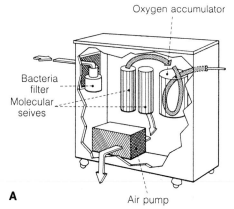

Figure 14–4. (*A*) Molecular sieve oxygen concentrator. (Courtesy of DeVilbis Company, Toledo, OH) (*B*) Membrane-type oxygen concentrator (enricher) flow diagram. (Courtesy of Oxygen Enrichment Company, Schenectady, NY)

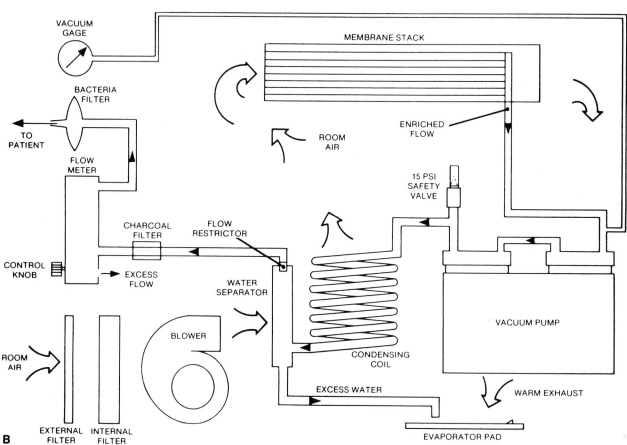

liquid air is expanded further to approximately 12 psig as it enters the distillation column, where it is separated into its component gases.

In the distillation column the liquid passes over cylindrical shells containing perforated metal trays that are spaced at regular intervals. The liquid passes over the trays, whereas the gas rises through the perforations and bubbles through the liquid. The gas that passes through the liquid becomes progressively richer in nitrogen, whereas the liquid becomes richer in oxygen.

The entire process actually takes place in two phases. Air, in the form of vapor, enters the very bottom of the column, and nitrogen gas leaves through the top of the column, leaving 99.9% pure liquid oxygen. The fractional distillation phenomenon can be explained through examination of the boiling points of various liquid gases. At 1 atmosphere (atm), oxygen has a boiling point of $-297°$ F, and nitrogen boils at $-320°$ F. The rare gases contained in the liquid oxygen in its first impure state also have lower boiling points than oxygen. Thus, by controlling the pressure and, therefore, the temperature within the two areas of the distillation column, the liquid nitrogen and other gases will evaporate faster, leaving pure liquid oxygen behind.

Two other methods of preparing oxygen for commercial use have been used on a limited basis. These are *solid oxygen systems,* in which a solid chemical is converted to medically pure oxygen, and a unit that removes a portion of the nitrogen from room air by drawing it through a *molecular sieve* (see Chap. 15 and Fig. 14–4).

COMPRESSED AIR

At atmospheric temperature and pressure, air exists as a colorless, odorless, tasteless gas mixture. In air for human respiration ("respirable air"), the primary constituents are oxygen and nitrogen. Although other trace gases may be present and are considered useful in industry and for scientific purposes, it has never been determined that these trace gases serve any physiologic role in respiration. Although nitrogen in the air does not serve any metabolic function, it aids in maintaining the inflation of the body cavities that are gas-filled, such as alveoli, sinus cavities, and the middle ear.

By increasing the forces acting upon it, air can be compressed. The percentage of oxygen in the air will remain the same; however, the partial pressure of the oxygen will increase. It is, therefore, critical to remember that even if the oxygen concentration is only 21%, in a chamber filled with air under pressure (e.g., in a multiplace hyperbaric oxygen chamber; see Chap. 16), most materials that are combustible will ignite more readily and burn much more rapidly than they would if the air were at normal atmospheric pressure.

Because atmospheric air contains a large variety of trace constituents, the Compressed Gas Association (CGA) has established a grading system for compressed air. This system limits the concentration of trace constituents for each specific grade. The oxygen concentration in all medically acceptable compressed air ranges from 19.5% to 23.5% oxygen, depending on the grade of air, with the balance being predominantly nitrogen. Grade J of the gas and grade B of the liquid are those most commonly used for medical purposes.

Compressed air, when handled properly and with the same caution as any other compressed gas, has many important uses. In many instances it can be liquefied and purified. Aside from its medical applications, compressed air is used in aerospace technology, undersea exploration, navigation, and atomic energy projects. It is necessary for tunnel construction and is used by industry and firemen in self-contained breathing devices.

The most common method of producing compressed air for human respiration is by the compression of normal atmospheric air at the point of use, although it can be transported to that point or synthetically produced by combining already purified components. The process involves various types of compressors that take in ambient air and compress it to the desired working pressure. The choice of compressor depends on the volume of air required and the pressure at which the air is to be used. Usually, a rotary or centrifugal compressor is used when less than 150 psig is required. The coaxial screw-type compressor is adequate for pressures ranging from 150 to 300 psig. The piston or diaphragm-type compressor is suitable for a wide range of pressures. For most hospital use, the piston, rotary, or centrifugal compressor would generally be considered adequate. In hospital systems, for which rate of consumption varies in the course of a day or week, an accumulator is recommended. It can be filled by the compressor and air withdrawn as needed.

There are two processes used in the manufacturing of liquid air. In the *Linde process,* air under pressure enters a tube and is then allowed to reexpand to atmospheric pressure. According to the Joule–Thompson effect, as the air reexpands, it produces a cooling effect. By the continual influx and reexpansion of the compressed air, the chamber eventually reaches a temperature at which the air will liquefy. This liquid air is accumulated at the bottom of the container. In this process a pressure of 200 atms is necessary for liquefaction.

The second process for producing liquid air is the *Claude process*. In this process air is compressed and passes through an orifice into a cylinder head. The expanding gas in the cylinder head causes a piston to compress additional fresh air. In this process, the cooling is obtained by the gas performing the external work of compressing a piston, and liquefaction is accomplished in a much shorter time and with a lower pressure (30 atm).

There are several important considerations in the manufacture of compressed air for human respiration. Proper lubrication and maintenance are essential to the efficient operation of the compressor. Compressors may be lubricated internally with water or with water to which a small amount of soap or natural mineral oil has been added. The bearings and working parts of most compressors are lubricated, but the cylinder and compressor chamber are not. The use of plastic or other low-friction seals on the piston has eliminated the need for lubrication in these areas. In the diaphragm-type compressor, the chamber is separated from the lubricated portions of the compressor by a diaphragm. Therefore, the chamber is considered to be unlubricated.

The compressor must be properly maintained. A compressor that is allowed to overheat may produce undesirable odors or even carbon monoxide caused by decomposition of lubricants. The compressor intake should be located away from the contaminating exhaust of automobiles, the gasoline or diesel engine used to drive the compressor, and other localized odors and contaminants. Activated charcoal may be used at the outlet of the compressor to remove odors and oil vapor. Desiccants or moisture-removal devices are necessary for the air to pass through before it reaches the charcoal, because the charcoal is most effective if kept dry. The type of filtering device used must be capable of functioning efficiently at the maximum anticipated degree of contamination that might exist in the incoming air.

If compressed air is to be used at temperatures below freezing, excess water vapor should be removed to reach a dew point below the minimum temperature anticipated to prevent the condensation of moisture from the air. It is also important to remember that as the compressed air passes through valves and regulators from a higher to a lower pressure, the temperature of the delivered air will be lower.

HELIUM

Helium is seven times lighter than air. Of all the elements, only hydrogen is lighter. It is noncombustible, nonexplosive, poorly soluble in liquid, and a good conductor of electricity, sound, and heat. As a gas, helium is odorless and tasteless, and is generally considered inert as it relates to the body.

One major source of helium is the natural gas fields around Amarillo, Texas, which contain approximately 2% helium. Other sources are found in Saskatchewan, Canada, and in areas near the Black Sea. The helium recovered from these natural fields is obtained by liquefaction and purification of the natural gas. Although helium can also be recovered from the atmosphere by fractional distillation, the amount recovered in this manner is so small that the process is commercially impractical.

One of the most important commercial uses of helium is as a cooling agent in nuclear reactors. Helium is used in cold-weather fluorescent lamps and in arc-welding as a gas shield. Because it is lighter than air, it is also used in some types of aircraft as a lifting gas. It provides protection in the production of metals, such as titanium and zirconium, and is useful for tracing leaks in refrigeration and other closed systems.

Because helium is a rare and limited natural resource, the cost of administering it for medical purposes is very high. The most common uses of helium in the medical setting are in the pulmonary function laboratory (e.g., in the helium dilution test for functional residual capacity and the volume isoflow test [see Chap. 9]). It is also used as the inflation gas in some intra-aortic balloon pump models.

Laboratory mixtures containing helium have found limited therapeutic usefulness in medicine (e.g., in ventilating patients with extremely high airway resistance and in the reduction of massive subcutaneous and mediastinal emphysema). The most economical means of administration is with a rebreathing system that uses a carbon dioxide absorption device to prevent carbon dioxide accumulation. Because helium is physiologically inert, it must be administered with oxygen. Mixtures containing helium and oxygen are supplied in several different compositions, of which the most common mixture is helium and 20% oxygen.

When administering the mixture, special flowmeters are required because the mixture is less dense than oxygen alone. If these special flowmeters are not available and regular oxygen flowmeters are used, it will be necessary to calculate the error in the flowmeter. The 80:20% mixture flows through restricted orifices 1.8 times more readily than 100% oxygen. To get the proper total flow of an 80:20% mixture, multiply the flow that is shown on the flowmeter by 1.8. To calculate a desired flow rate, divide the desired rate by 1.8 and adjust the flowmeter accordingly.

CARBON DIOXIDE

Carbon dioxide is a colorless, odorless gas about 1.53 times as heavy as air. It is abundant and constant in the atmosphere and is generated by the combustion of fuels, by respiration, by fermentation, and by the decay of animal and vegetable matter. The unrefined gas may be recovered from the gases found in some natural wells and springs. It is also a byproduct of the commercial production of ammonia.

Large-scale carbon dioxide production takes place primarily in lime kilns. The limestone is heated to a red glow in closed containers. Superheated steam is forced in at the bottom of the chambers; as it passes through the heated limestone, the steam carries with it the liberated carbon dioxide. The gas then passes out of the top of the chambers into coolers and compressors.

Carbon dioxide can be refined and purified to 99.9% or higher and is used medically in combination with oxygen. The gas itself is not toxic; in the absence of sufficient oxygen, however, it causes asphyxiation. The mixture of oxygen and carbon dioxide is sometimes called "carbogen."

The critical temperature of carbon dioxide is 83° F (28.3° C), and it is easily liquefied under pressure. When the pressure is released, part of the liquid vaporizes rapidly, but the rest solidifies into what is commonly called "dry ice." One of the most important commercial uses of carbon dioxide is as an expandable refrigerant. It is also used extensively to carbonate soft drinks and as a food preservative. Carbon dioxide is also used in metal welding and, in liquid form, is commonly used in fire extinguishers. Hospital usage of pure carbon dioxide is limited; however, it is frequently used in clinical laboratories for growing bacteriologic and tissue cultures. It is also used in a mixture of gases to calibrate blood gas measuring instruments.

TRANSPORTATION OF GASES

The federal Department of Transportation (DOT) was established by Congress in 1967 to coordinate the executive functions of all transportation agencies into a single governmental department. The rules for the transportation of compressed gases and cryogenic liquids and the requirements that are imposed on both the carriers and shippers fall under this department. The transportation agencies that are of greatest importance in the compressed gas and cryogenic liquid industry are

- The Federal Aviation Agency, which regulates shipment by air
- The Coast Guard, for transportation by water
- The Federal Railroad Administration, for shipment by railroad
- The Federal Highway Administration, for highway shipment

Further discussion of the roles and functions of these governmental agencies will be found later in this chapter.

Whenever compressed gases are transported in cylinders and caps are provided for valve protection, the caps should not be removed until the cylinder has reached its destination and is ready to be used. During the transport of cylinders of compressed gas or cryogenic liquids, protection against excessively high or low temperatures should be provided. *Provisions should be made to keep cylinders (compressed gas and liquid) upright at all times.*

STORAGE OF GASES

CYLINDERS

Nonflammable medical gases include oxygen, nitrous oxide, medical compressed air, carbon dioxide, helium, nitrogen, and various mixtures of these gases. Strict regulations for locating and maintaining bulk oxygen systems have been established by the National Fire Prevention Association (NFPA), subject to further control by local community fire and building codes.[3]

Storage rooms for cylinders should be dry, cool, well-ventilated, and fire-resistant. Subsurface locations should be avoided, and cylinders should never be stored in or near a hospital operating room. Care must be taken to assure that the temperature within the room does not exceed 125° F (51.7° C) and that any source of heat within the room is located well away from the cylinders. Full and empty cylinders should be stored separately. The storage layout should be carefully planned, such that older stock can be easily removed first, preventing unnecessary handling of the cylinders.

There must be separate storage areas for cylinders containing oxidizing gases that support combustion, such as oxygen and nitrous oxide, and for flammable gases. Such a precaution is critical. In the event of fire, the contents of the cylinders evacuate when the safety release valves open. In such cases, the oxidizing gases would then accelerate the combustion of any flammable gases in the area. As an added precaution, cylinders of carbon dioxide are, in themselves, good fire extinguishers.

Storage rooms for oxygen and nitrous oxide must be vented to the outside if the amount of gas to be stored is in excess of 200 ft³. The storage areas for these gases and flammable gases must have at least a 1-hour fire-resistance rating and may not be used for any purpose other than the storage of cyl-

Figure 14—5. Chained stands used to secure large gas cylinders. (Reproduced by permission from Eubanks DH, Bone RC: Comprehensive Respiratory Care, 2nd ed. St. Louis, CV Mosby, 1990)

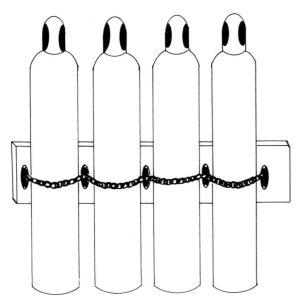

inders. Under no circumstances should flammable materials be stored in these areas.

The storage area should contain racks on fasteners to prevent the cylinders from falling over (Fig. 14–5), which could result in damage to cylinders or to persons who may be working in the area. Electric wall fixtures, receptacles, or switches must be installed no less than 5 ft above the floor as a precaution against damage to them from the cylinders.

Cylinders may be stored outside when necessary, but they should be protected from rusting caused by weather or contact with the ground. They should never be stored in areas where there is constant dampness, and they should be protected from continuous direct rays of the sun and excessive accumulations of ice or snow. Cylinders must never be stored where oil, grease, or other readily combustible materials may come in contact with them. They should also be protected against corrosive chemicals or fumes. It is good practice to store the cylinders in a locked area to prevent tampering by unauthorized persons.

BULK GAS SYSTEMS

The NFPA has also established regulations governing bulk oxygen systems for industrial or institutional use. A bulk oxygen system consists of an assembly of oxygen storage containers, pressure regulators, safety devices, vaporizers, manifolds, and interconnecting piping. By definition, the storage capacity of the system must be more than 20,000 ft³ of oxygen, including reserves on hand that are not connected to the system.

Oxygen containers in the bulk system may be stationary or moveable, and the oxygen may be either gas or liquid. The bulk system ends at the point where the oxygen first enters the supply line. It consists of the main equipment that actually supplies the system (primary supply), a secondary system that takes over when the primary supply is used up, and a reserve system that will function in an emergency when the primary–secondary operating supply fails.

The system must be located out-of-doors or in a building that is of noncombustible construction and adequately ventilated to the outside. If the system is located in a building, the building must be used for no purpose other than to house the system. The bulk system must be located above ground and in a place that is easily accessible for the mobile equipment used to supply it. Of special importance is that the system be located well away from expo-

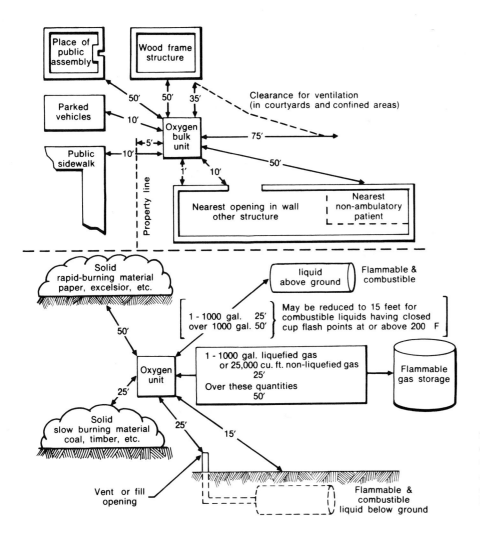

Figure 14—6. Distance between bulk oxygen systems and various nearby structures (not to scale). (Reproduced with permission from *Bulk Oxygen Systems at Consumer Sites* [NFPA 50] © 1974, National Fire Protection Assn., Boston, MA 02210)

sure to power lines, flammable or combustible liquid, or gas lines (Fig. 14–6).

There are three basic types of bulk systems for piping oxygen to a central supply area within a facility. In the manifold system, large cylinders are banked together and replaced when empty. Another system uses fixed cylinders that are refilled on location from a truck that contains liquid oxygen and converts the liquid to gas for pumping into the cylinders. In the third system, large cylinders are permanently attached to a trailer, and the entire trailer unit is replaced with the oxygen supply is used up. In all three of these methods, oxygen is supplied in gaseous form.

When large volumes of oxygen are used, the most practical and economical method for storage is the liquid bulk supply system (Fig. 14–7). Containers are constructed on the principle of a large thermos bottle, consisting of inner and outer steel shells separated by a vacuum, which effectively blocks the transfer of heat into the liquid. The containers are kept under a pressure not to exceed 250 psig and must be kept below −297° F, both in transportation and storage, to prevent the liquid from reverting to gas. Vaporizing units, consisting of finned tubing, are used to convert the liquid oxygen into gas. The size of the vaporizing unit is dependent on the rate of withdrawal from the vessel. Normally, water vapor from the air will condense and freeze on these units over a period of steady usage.

The location of the liquid storage system should be carefully planned. Again, the NFPA, along with local, state, and federal agencies, has created regulations, including safe limits for the

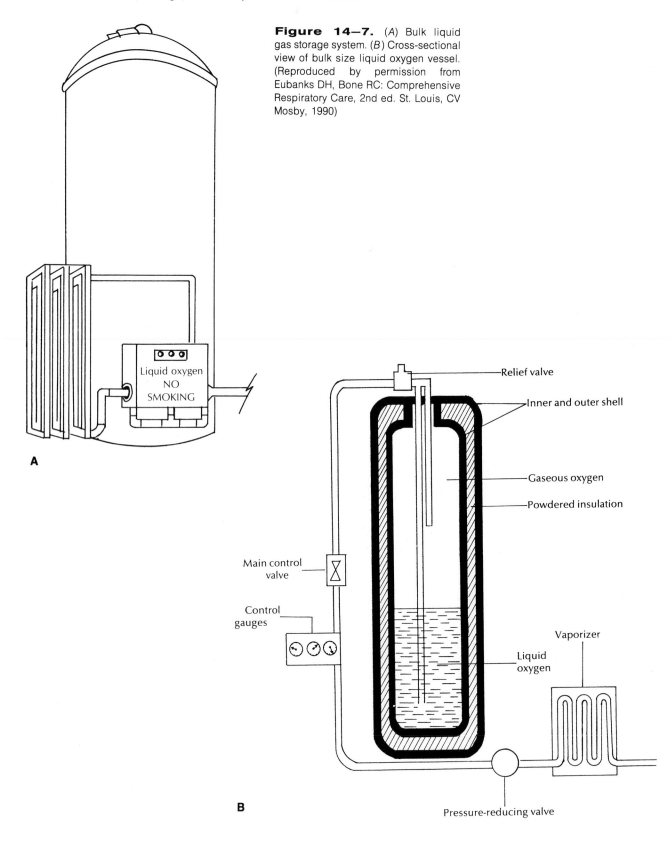

Figure 14—7. (*A*) Bulk liquid gas storage system. (*B*) Cross-sectional view of bulk size liquid oxygen vessel. (Reproduced by permission from Eubanks DH, Bone RC: Comprehensive Respiratory Care, 2nd ed. St. Louis, CV Mosby, 1990)

distances between the system and various points of exposure. At least 3 ft of a noncombustible surface should be extended in all directions from the storage tank. The area under the liquid delivery connections should be at least as wide as the mobile supply equipment and should extend at least 8 ft in both directions to prevent hazards from any leakage while the system is being filled. This surface must not be of asphalt paving because this type of paving may be considered to be combustible.

Under normal operating conditions, the liquid oxygen remains in the liquid state and is automatically transformed into gas as it passes through the vaporizing portion of the unit, upon demand by the user.

CRYOGENIC LIQUIDS

Many gases may be stored at low temperatures in the liquid form. Cryogenics is a science pertaining to materials at very low temperatures. Cryogenic liquids usually have temperatures of $-238°$ F $(-150°$ C) or below. Many medical and industrial gases are stored, transported, and handled in liquid form. The most common ones used for medical and industrial purposes are oxygen, nitrogen, argon, hydrogen, and helium. Neon, krypton, xenon, and rare atmospheric gases are used in industry. Natural gas (LNG) and carbon monoxide are also stored and handled as cryogenic liquids but are not usually considered industrial or medical gases. Liquefied ethylene, carbon dioxide, and nitrous oxide are not considered cryogenic because their normal temperature is above $-238°$ F $(-150°$ C).

The *boiling point* of a cryogenic liquid is the temperature at which the vapor pressure of the liquid equals the pressure exerted on the liquid by the atmosphere, or the temperature at which a liquid boils at 1 atm of pressure (Table 14–1). The highest temperature at which the substance can exist as a liquid is called the *critical temperature*. The pressure exerted by the vapor of the substance at the critical temperature is the *critical pressure*.

To change a gas to a liquid, it must be cooled below its critical temperature, then increasingly cooled to below its boiling point. The combination of compressing and cooling the gas is used, as previously described in the manufacturing process. Compression alone will not liquefy a gas if the gas remains at a temperature above its critical temperature. Warming allows the liquid to return to a gaseous state.

A *saturated liquid* is one that has stabilized at a given pressure and temperature. It does not vaporize into a gas, nor does the gas condense into a liquid. Water at a temperature of 212° F (100° C) at sea level is a saturated liquid. Applying more heat causes the water to vaporize or turn to steam yet the water itself does not become warmer.

If the pressure in a container of saturated liquid is decreased, the liquid becomes *"supersaturated"* or too warm to remain a liquid. The liquid begins to boil (removing heat from within itself) in an attempt to refrigerate or cool itself until an equilibrium is reached at the lower pressure. When boiling occurs, vaporization begins and continues until the liquid cools to the new saturation temperature or the vaporization restores the previous saturation pressure and temperature.

Boiling can occur when liquefied gases are transferred from one container to another. During the boiling period, the vaporized liquid is referred to as saturation loss. When pressure in a container of saturated liquid is increased, the liquid is capable of absorbing more heat (the boiling point is increased) without vaporization, but the liquid is not saturated until it reaches a state of equilibrium with pressure and its corresponding temperature.

Heat leak (loss rate/boil off) is the quantity of heat per unit of time that penetrates the cryogenic container through its insulation, piping, and supports, thereby causing vaporization of the cryogenic liquid. Factors affecting heat leak include ambient temperature, design and insulation of the cryogenic container, and perhaps damage to the vessel. Heat leak may be expressed in BTU per hour and loss rate in pounds per hour. The end result of heat leak is commonly referred to as normal evaporation rate (NER) and is expressed in pounds of liquid per day (24 hours).

Liquefied gases are stored and handled in double-walled, vacuum-insulated containers, sometimes referred to as Dewars. (James Dewar developed the first container of this type.) These containers must be made of suitable materials such as authentic steel, copper, or certain aluminum alloys. Other types of material become very brittle at cryogenic temperatures.

There are three major types of liquid storage cylinders—one for dispensing liquid or gas, one for gas withdrawal, and one for liquid withdrawal. Each type of cylinder has valves for filling, dispensing, pressure control, and pressure relief. Cryogenic liquids produce large volumes of gas when they vaporize. For example, the volume expansion ratio of oxygen is 860 : 1. Should there by a vacuum loss in the container, warming of the liquid begins and the liquid will vaporize. If the container were not

Table 14–1 Physical Properties of Cryogenic Liquids

	XENON (XE)	KRYPTON (KR)	METHANE (CH₄)	OXYGEN (O₂)	ARGON (AR)	MONOXIDE (CO)	NITROGEN (N₂)	NEON (NE)	HYDROGEN (H₂)	HELIUM (HE)
Boiling Point, 1 atm										
F	−163	−244	−259	−297	−303	−313	−320	−411	−423	−452
C	−108	−153	−161	−183	−186	−192	−196	−246	−253	−268
Melting Point, 1 atm										
F	−169	−251	−296	−362	−309	−341	−346	−416	−435	−*
C	−112	−157	−182	−219	−189	−207	−210	−249	−259	−
Density at B.P. and 1 atm. lb/cu ft	191	151	26	71	87	49	50	75	4.4	7.8
Heat of vaporization at B.P. Btu/lb	41	46	219	92	70	98	85	37	193	10
Volume expansion ratio, liquid at 1 atm and B.P. to gas at 70° F and 1 atm	559	693	625	860	842	680	696	1445	860	755
Flammable	No	No	Yes	No†	No	Yes	No	No	Yes	No

* Helium does not solidify at 1 atm pressure.
† Oxygen does not burn but supports and accelerates combustion. However, high oxygen atmospheres substantially increase combustion rates of other materials and may form explosive mixtures with other combustibles. Flammable temperatures in oxygen are higher than those in air.

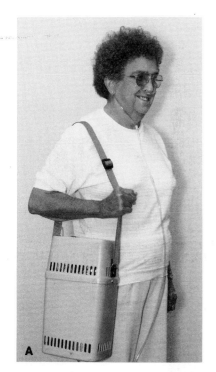

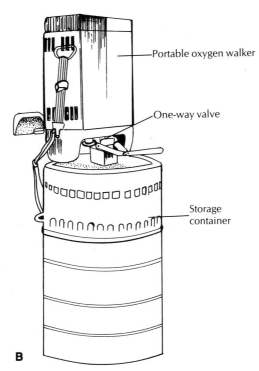

Portable oxygen walker

One-way valve

Storage container

Figure 14—8. (A) Patient carrying portable liquid oxygen reservoir, good for approximately 11 hours of average activity at 1 L/min flow. (B) Diagram of portable liquid oxygen container being refilled from a stationary liquid oxygen source. (Reproduced by permission from Eubanks DH, Bone RC: Comprehensive Respiratory Care, 2nd ed. St. Louis, CV Mosby, 1990)

fitted with overpressurization relief devices, the pressure within the vessel could become enormous.

Because of the smaller volume of cryogenic liquid compared with compressed gas, use of oxygen in the cryogenic liquid form has become economically popular and safe. The first tank-truck shipment of liquid oxygen occurred in 1932. These liquids are usually stored in containers requiring considerably less pressure than the pressure of compressed gas cylinders; thus, they are safer to transport and handle.

Cryogenic containers of liquid oxygen (referred to as stationaries or reservoirs) are an economical and safe means of providing oxygen in the home for those who require oxygen on a continuous basis (Fig. 14—8). The stationaries are filled (usually on a weekly basis) by home care distributors.

Smaller liquid oxygen containers (called portables) are used to provide mobility for the continuous oxygen user. The portables are filled as needed from the stationary source and provide approximately 4 to 8 hours of oxygen at 2 L/min. Portables weigh between 6 and 13 lb when full and may be carried by shoulder strap or a two-wheeled cart (Fig. 14—9).

Cryogenic liquid oxygen containers are usually more aesthetic than compressed gas cylinders, and are easier and safer to handle for the patient and the distributor. These units maintain pressures between 16 and 50 psig, much less than the pressure within a compressed gas cylinder.

Most safety precautions practiced when using compressed gases apply to the storage, handling, transportation, and use of cryogenic liquids. Some additional precautions are also necessary. Because cryogenic liquids are extremely cold, they can produce frostbite on exposed skin or eye tissue. If the liquid is spilled, it tends to completely cover the surface on which it is spilled. Vapors that originate from the spilled liquid are also extremely cold. Delicate tissue (such as the eye) can be injured by exposure to these cold gases. Skin contact with parts such as transfer lines or connections that have been exposed to cryogenic liquids can cause frostbite injury or cause flesh to stick to the cold object. Ob-

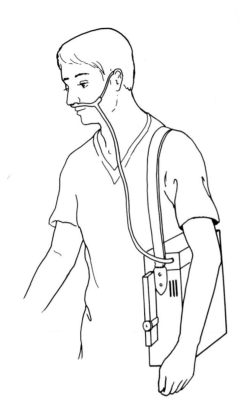

Figure 14—9. Person carrying portable, lightweight liquid oxygen container. (Reproduced with permission from Eubanks DG, Bone RC: Comprehensive Respiratory Care, 2nd ed. St. Louis, CV Mosby, 1990)

jects that are soft and pliable at room temperature are easily shattered or broken if they come into contact with a cryogenic liquid.

Liquid oxygen spills on surfaces contaminated with combustibles are conducive to fire on ignition for at least 30 minutes after the liquid, frost, or fog has dissipated. Use of liquid oxygen, the most commonly used gas in respiratory care, mandates following the standard safety practices required with the use of oxygen from any source.

As with compressed gases, labeling of cryogenic containers is regulated by the Food and Drug Administration (FDA), Department of Transportation (DOT), and Canadian Transport Commission (CTC). Generally, labeling requirements include the following: product name; hazardous components; a statement of hazards; signal work (i.e., danger, warning, or caution); precautionary measures; first aid instructions in case of fire, spill, or leak; and container storage and handling instructions. The gas supplier is responsible for ensuring that all

containers are properly labeled and that the label has all languages required by the regulatory agencies.

DISTRIBUTION OF GASES

OXYGEN PIPING

Because any bulk system ends at the point where the oxygen first enters the supply lines, a distribution system is necessary within the facility. This piped distribution system consists of a central supply area where manifold, bulk, or compressors are located; control equipment; and piping that extends to points in the facility at which the gas is to be utilized (Fig. 14—10). Seamless type K or L copper or brass pipe is used in the medical oxygen piping system. These pipelines must not be supported by other piping, as a safety precaution in the event that the supporting piping may be hot or may develop maintenance problems with damage to the oxygen piping occurring during the repairs. Pipe hooks or straps of the proper strength are necessary. Fittings used in copper tubing must be wrought copper, brass, or bronze made especially for solder or brazed connections. Piping is usually connected by welding. Fittings for oxygen systems should be free of corrosion or rust, and the pipes should be free of lacquer, paint, varnish, or any coating.

The system should be cleaned before it is put into use to remove any materials that may have collected in the pipes. After cleaning, each section of the pipeline should be pressure-tested, using oil-free dry air or nitrogen at 1 1/2 times the maximum working pressure (approximately 75 psi) of the pipeline system. This pressure is maintained for 24 hours. After the 24-hour test is completed, the entire system should be pressurized with oxygen and all of the outlets opened, starting with the one nearest the source and progressing to the outlet farthest away from the source. The oxygen should flow from the outlets until the test gas is completely purged from the system. Each outlet must be analyzed to see that 100% oxygen is present. Whenever any piping changes are made in the system, these pressure and priority checks must be repeated. Some states are now requiring periodic oxygen purity checks, even though the gas delivery system has not been modified in the interval. The Joint Commission on Accreditation of Healthcare Organizations (JCAHO) requires that hospitals have a program of preventive maintenance with periodic inspections of the oxygen-piping system. These in-

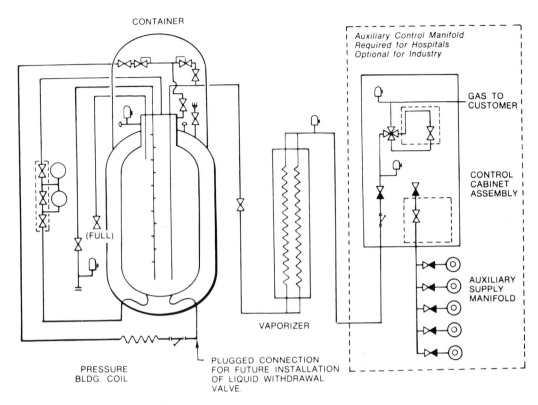

Figure 14—10. Flow diagram of a customer station. (Compressed Gas Association)

spections must be documented, with any corrective action taken noted.

CYLINDERS

MANUFACTURE

The Department of Transportation (DOT) establishes regulations and specifications for the manufacture, marking, testing, and transportation of cylinders in the United States. This was formerly the responsibility of the Interstate Commerce Commission (ICC). DOT establishes what type of material is to be used in the construction of cylinders and the method of fabrication. High-pressure oxygen cylinders must be made of seamless steel, meeting certain chemical and physical requirements. Other cylinders may be formed of seamless, drawn, welded, or brazed tubing. In addition to these requirements, DOT also specifies the maximum wall stress permissible at which the cylinder may be used.

MARKINGS

All cylinders must carry certain easily recognized identifying marks that are stamped into the steel (Fig. 14—11). The marks must include the number of the specification by which the cylinder was manufactured, the authorized service pressure, a serial number, and the data of manufacture. There must also be symbols identifying the original owner of the cylinder, the manufacturer, and the independent agency that performed the tests required at the time of manufacture. Sometimes tare weights (i.e., the weight of the cylinder full, making allowance for the weight of the cylinder), water capacities, and the elastic expansion value of the cylinder are also included, if the cylinder will be used to hold liquefied gas.

Most cylinders used in the United States are marked either DOT or ICC to indicate that they conformed to the specifications in force at the time of the original test by the manufacturer. Some older cylinders, however, may be marked BE, indicating they were made to specifications prepared by the

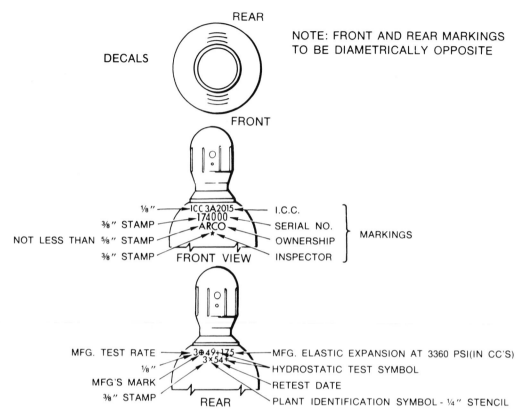

Figure 14—11. Permanent cylinder markings required for Interstate Commerce Commission (ICC) or Board of Transportation Commission for Canada (BTC) specifications. (Compressed Gas Association)

Bureau of Explosives. In Canada, cylinders may be marked CRC (Canadian Rail Commission), BTC (Board of Transport Commission for Canada), or CTC (Canadian Transportation Commission) to indicate that they conform to the Canadian specifications. Cylinders carrying any other markings are considered to be foreign; they may be filled in the United States, but only for export, and the cylinder must have been hydrostatically tested within the past 5 years.

Following the letters ICC or DOT will be a combination of numbers and letters indicating the manufacture and testing specifications of that particular cylinder. These may be 3A, 3AA, 4B, 8AL, or any combination thereof. Each indicates a separate set of specifications for chemical composition, tensile strength, elongation of metals used, and method of fabrication. They also indicate the type of final acceptance test used, various inspections to be performed by an independent agency, and the cylinder service pressure limitation.

Cylinders marked 3A, 4B, and ICC8 are made of relatively low-strength steels and, as a result, have thicker sidewalls that make the cylinder heavier. Cylinders marked 3AA, 4BA, and DOT or ICC8AL are made of lighter-strength steel and are lighter in weight, but cylinder cuts, gouges, or corrosion are more serious hazards. The thicker side-wall cylinder is made either of manganese or carbon, compared with the alloy steel of the thinner-walled cylinder.

The serial number on a cylinder identifies it as part of a given lot produced for a specific owner and is the basis for a historical record of the life of the cylinder. It is part of the data recorded each time the cylinder is visually or hydrostatically retested, making possible a comparison of retested results and a subsequent evaluation of the rate of deterioration of the cylinder. The serial number is also important as a source of identification for any cylinder involved in an accident.

The ownership symbol or letters, used to identify the company or individual for whom the cylinder was originally made, are registered with the Bureau of Explosives. Regulations state that a container of compressed gas cannot be shipped unless it was charged by or with the consent of the owner, and it is important that the filler or distributor know if he is legally permitted to fill and ship the cylinder in filled condition. Because cylinders may change owners, the mark on the cylinder may not be positive proof of ownership; any distributor should require proof of ownership before filling a cylinder.

Each cylinder is marked in generally the same way. Markings on the front of the cylinder include the DOT or ICC mark, serial number, ownership, and inspector symbol. On the rear of the cylinder are found the manufacturer's mark, test date and elastic expansion values, the hydrostatic test symbol, the retest date, and the plant identification symbol. The original elastic expansion value of the cylinder, measured in cubic centimeters, is not required by DOT; however, it is of value in providing a reference for subsequent retests.

There are two other important marks on every cylinder. Some cylinders are made from seamless tubing by forge-welding the bottom closure in a spinning process. The spinning process requires a high degree of manual skill to make sure the cylinders are tightly closed, and these cylinders must be tested for tightness, using dry air. The letters SPIN are then marked into the shoulder of the cylinder.

Other manufacturers, as a final step in the process, drill and plug and bottom closure of the cylinders with pipe-threaded plugs. This type of closure can develop leaks from service impacts, and because the plugs are not visible when the cylinder is in an upright position, the shoulder of these cylinders is marked PLUG so that the bottom closure will be checked at each filling.

TESTING

Hydrostatic testing and retesting of cylinders is required by DOT. The most common method is the water-jacket volumetric expansion test, standard in the compressed gas industry for testing high-pressure gas cylinders (i.e., those of over 900 psig). This method is used to determine elastic expansion, which is directly related to the wall thickness of the cylinder. An increase in the elastic expansion will indicate a reduction in average wall thickness (Fig. 14–12).

In the water-jacket test the cylinder is suspended in a vessel of water. As pressure is applied to the interior of the cylinder, a volume of water is forced from the jacket. As the pressure is released from the interior of the cylinder, some of the originally displaced water returns to the jacket. The volume of water that is originally displaced represents the total expansion of the cylinder, and the final displaced volume represents the permanent expansion. Total expansion minus permanent expansion results in the elastic expansion value, giving a definite measure of the average wall thickness of the cylinder at a given pressure.

To determine if the cylinder is still usable, the percentage of permanent expansion is then calculated by dividing 100 times the permanent expansion by the total expansion. If that percentage exceeds the allowable DOT specifications, the cylinder must be rejected. Some cylinders may originally have been tested for the specific purpose of being used for oxygen, and, at a later date, the retesting will no longer permit the cylinder to be filled to that capacity. Such a cylinder may be used for other gases for which the maximum pressure of a full cylinder is less.

There are several other acceptable but less commonly used cylinder tests. In the *direct expansion method*, expansion is determined by compressing a volume of water into the cylinder, but compensation for water compressibility and temperature are factors that must be taken into account. The *proof pressure method* may be used when DOT regulations do not require the determination of total and permanent volumetric expansion. The *pressure recession method* is practically obsolete.

The frequency and type of periodic cylinder testing are regulated by DOT, depending upon the specification to which the cylinder was manufactured and the gas for which it is to be used. Records showing the results of inspection must be maintained by the owner until the cylinder comes due for retest or additional inspection. The cylinder is inspected externally for signs of damage or corrosion and internally for signs of corrosion (Fig. 14–13). When corrosion is severe, there will usually be large quantities of loose scale in the bottom of the cylinder. The loose scale should be removed and the cylinder hydrostatically retested to be sure it is safe for continued service. Light rusting of the interior sidewalls when there is no localized corrosion and very little scale in the bottom of the cylinder is not normally considered a cause for removal from service.

The hammer or dead-ring test should be performed on all cylinders every time they are refilled. Striking the cylinder lightly on the side should pro-

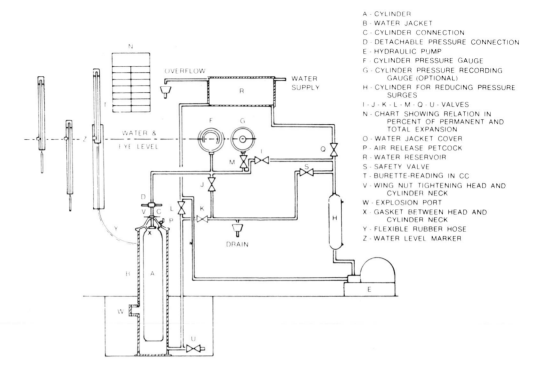

A - CYLINDER
B - WATER JACKET
C - CYLINDER CONNECTION
D - DETACHABLE PRESSURE CONNECTION
E - HYDRAULIC PUMP
F - CYLINDER PRESSURE GAUGE
G - CYLINDER PRESSURE RECORDING
    GAUGE (OPTIONAL)
H - CYLINDER FOR REDUCING PRESSURE
    SURGES
I - J - K - L - M - Q - U - VALVES
N - CHART SHOWING RELATION IN
    PERCENT OF PERMANENT AND
    TOTAL EXPANSION
O - WATER JACKET COVER
P - AIR RELEASE PETCOCK
R - WATER RESERVOIR
S - SAFETY VALVE
T - BURETTE-READING IN CC
V - WING NUT TIGHTENING HEAD AND
    CYLINDER NECK
W - EXPLOSION PORT
X - GASKET BETWEEN HEAD AND
    CYLINDER NECK
Y - FLEXIBLE RUBBER HOSE
Z - WATER LEVEL MARKER

Figure 14—12. The water jacket leveling burette method of testing cylinders consists essentially of enclosing the cylinder in a water jacket and measuring the volume of water forced from the jacket upon application of pressure to the interior of the cylinder, and the volume remaining displaced upon release of the pressure. These volumes represent the total and permanent expansions of the cylinder, respectively. To measure them accurately, a movable burette calibrated in cubic centimeters is positioned to maintain the water level at a uniform height when taking readings. (Modified from Compressed Gas Association: Handbook of Compressed Gases. New York, Reinhold, 1967)

duce a clean, ringing tone that lasts for 2 to 3 seconds. If the tone is flat or fades almost immediately, it indicates that the cylinder may have suffered fire damage, is severely corroded on the inside, or contains a contaminant such as water or oil, in which case the cylinder should not be refilled until a complete inspection can be made.

Cylinders were originally made of low-yield tensile steel, and excessive corrosion could be detected with the hydrostatic test when the permanent expansion exceeded 10% of the total expansion. Later, around 1937, alloy steels were introduced in the manufacture of cylinders, and the specified 10% expansion limit was weakened. There could be a considerable amount of corrosion in the cylinder before the 10% permanent expansion test would show that the cylinder should be rejected.

During World War II, a 10% increase in cylinder filling pressure was authorized with no change in the test pressure of the safety device setting. Following this emergency measure, regulations were established authorizing the continued practice of 110% filling, provided the wall-stress limitations were based on the water-jacket hydrostatic test and that the unbacked frangible disk safety device was used. If the elastic expansion reading at minimum pressure did not exceed DOT specifications, the cylinder could then be examined internally and externally for objectionable defects and stamped with a plus (+) sign following the test date to signify that the cylinder had been filled to 110% of the service pressure marking.

Cylinders that are made to the specifications of 3A and 3AA must be hydrostatically retested every 5 or 10 years at a pressure that is equal to five-thirds of the service pressure. Originally, the test was used to prove that the stress at service pressure

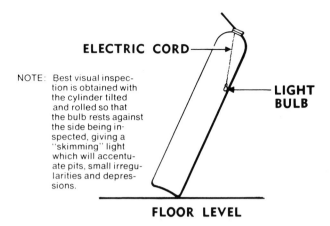

NOTE: Best visual inspection is obtained with the cylinder tilted and rolled so that the bulb rests against the side being inspected, giving a "skimming" light which will accentuate pits, small irregularities and depressions.

Figure 14—13. Method for internal inspection of a cylinder with a drop light. (Compressed Gas Association)

would not exceed five-thirds of the yield strength of the steel. It was later found, however, that data used in this retest could also be used to determine loss of wall thickness caused by wear and corrosion. The test, therefore, justified increasing the filling pressures of these cylinders to 110% of the service pressure, and DOT extended the 5-year retest period for 3A and 3AA cylinders to 10 years, provided the cylinders were used with only certain gases and were under specific inspection and retest procedures. Such cylinders are stamped with a five-pointed star. Only cylinders under 35 years of age qualify for the retest permission, unless special permits have been obtained for older cylinders. The specifications of the various cylinders are listed in Figure 14—14; the color coding index is found in Table 14—2.

Table 14—2 Color Markings

INTENDED GAS	COLOR
Oxygen (O_2)	Green
Carbon dioxide (CO_2)	Gray
Nitrous oxide (N_2O)	Blue
Cyclopropane ($CH_2)_3$	Orange or chrome
Helium (He)	Brown
Ethylene (C_2H_4)	Red
Carbon dioxide and oxygen (CO_2/O_2)	Gray and green
Helium and oxygen (He/O_2)	Brown and green
Nitrogen (N_2)	Black
Air	Yellow
Mixtures of nitrogen and oxygen	Black and green

SAFETY

The term *laws, regulations,* and *standards,* used in dealing with medical gases, on the surface, may appear synonymous. However, although the intent of the law, regulation, or standard may be aimed at accomplishing the same objective, their enforcement, initiation, and penalties may vary widely. Consequently, it is important to be able to distinguish among these terms.

LAWS

A law requires the approval of some legislative body of the federal, state, or local government. This body of officials may be the United States Congress, a state assembly, or possibly a local city council. These laws may establish an agency within the government to enact the regulations, or they may state specifically what is to be governed and to what extent.

When an agency is appointed to promulgate the regulations, such action is usually referred to as *enabling* legislation. This means that the passage of a law establishes an agency that is enabled, or given the power, to write regulations.

REGULATIONS

Regulations do not require legislative approval for enforcement, but they have the same effect as law and are subject to penalties whenever there are violations. Federal, state, and local governments may delegate the writing and enforcement of laws to other persons or agencies, such as the state fire marshal or the local boards of standards and appeals.

STANDARDS

A standard is quite different from a law or regulation in that it may not have the effect of law. Standards may be prepared by technical agencies, by industry, or by any group of experienced persons who establish a recognized acceptable procedure for a common purpose, such as safety.

Standards are intended to be followed voluntarily; however, they are frequently adopted by an enforcement agency; under their regulatory powers, the standard may change from a strictly voluntary guideline to a law that is subject to the penalties under which the law was enacted. An example is Standard 50 of the NFPA, which provides for the installation of bulk oxygen systems at consumer sites (see Fig. 14—6). This standard was developed by the Atmospheric Gases Committee of the Com-

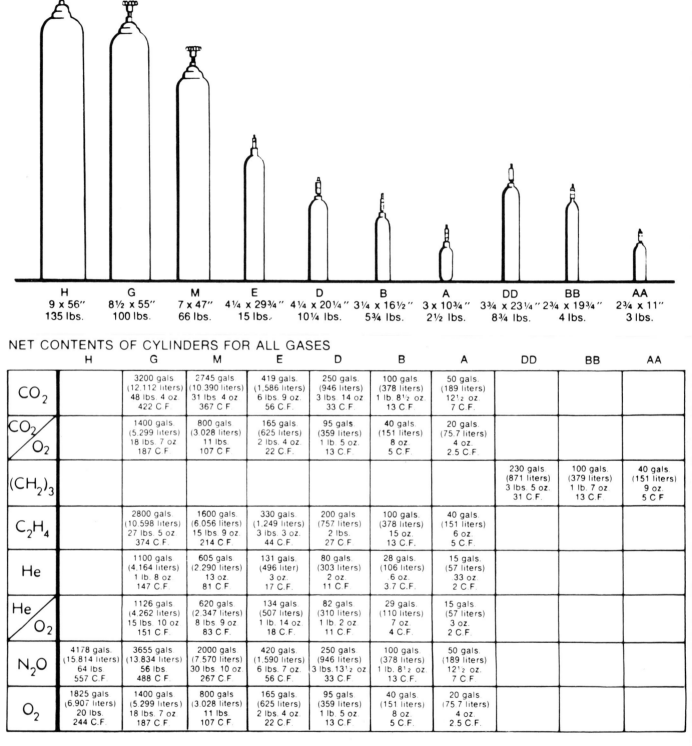

	H	G	M	E	D	B	A
	9 x 56" 135 lbs.	8½ x 55" 100 lbs.	7 x 47" 66 lbs.	4¼ x 29¾" 15 lbs.	4¼ x 20¼" 10¼ lbs.	3¼ x 16½" 5¾ lbs.	3 x 10¾" 2½ lbs.

	DD	BB	AA
	3¾ x 23¼" 8¾ lbs.	2¾ x 19¾" 4 lbs.	2¾ x 11" 3 lbs.

NET CONTENTS OF CYLINDERS FOR ALL GASES

	H	G	M	E	D	B	A	DD	BB	AA
CO_2		3200 gals. (12.112 liters) 48 lbs. 4 oz. 422 C.F.	2745 gals. (10.390 liters) 31 lbs. 4 oz. 367 C.F.	419 gals. (1,586 liters) 6 lbs. 9 oz. 56 C.F.	250 gals. (946 liters) 3 lbs. 14 oz 33 C.F.	100 gals. (378 liters) 1 lb. 8½ oz. 13 C.F.	50 gals. (189 liters) 12½ oz. 7 C.F.			
CO_2/O_2		1400 gals. (5.299 liters) 18 lbs. 7 oz 187 C.F.	800 gals. (3.028 liters) 11 lbs. 107 C.F.	165 gals. (625 liters) 2 lbs. 4 oz. 22 C.F.	95 gals. (359 liters) 1 lb. 5 oz. 13 C.F.	40 gals. (151 liters) 8 oz. 5 C.F.	20 gals. (75.7 liters) 4 oz. 2.5 C.F.			
$(CH_2)_3$								230 gals. (871 liters) 3 lbs. 5 oz. 31 C.F.	100 gals. (379 liters) 1 lb. 7 oz. 13 C.F.	40 gals. (151 liters) 9 oz. 5 C.F
C_2H_4		2800 gals. (10.598 liters) 27 lbs. 5 oz. 374 C.F.	1600 gals. (6.056 liters) 15 lbs. 9 oz. 214 C.F.	330 gals. (1,249 liters) 3 lbs. 3 oz. 44 C.F.	200 gals (757 liters) 2 lbs. 27 C.F.	100 gals. (378 liters) 15 oz. 13 C.F.	40 gals. (151 liters) 6 oz. 5 C.F.			
He		1100 gals. (4.164 liters) 1 lb. 8 oz 147 C.F.	605 gals. (2.290 liters) 13 oz. 81 C.F.	131 gals. (496 liter) 3 oz. 17 C.F.	80 gals. (303 liters) 2 oz. 11 C.F.	28 gals. (106 liters) .6 oz. 3.7 C.F.	15 gals. (57 liters) 33 oz. 2 C.F.			
He/O_2		1126 gals. (4.262 liters) 15 lbs. 10 oz 151 C.F.	620 gals. (2.347 liters) 8 lbs. 9 oz. 83 C.F.	134 gals. (507 liters) 1 lb. 14 oz. 18 C.F.	82 gals. (310 liters) 1 lb. 2 oz. 11 C.F.	29 gals. (110 liters) 7 oz. 4 C.F.	15 gals (57 liters) 3 oz. 2 C.F.			
N_2O	4178 gals. (15.814 liters) 64 lbs. 557 C.F.	3655 gals. (13.834 liters) 56 lbs. 488 C.F.	2000 gals. (7.570 liters) 30 lbs. 10 oz. 267 C.F.	420 gals. (1,590 liters) 6 lbs. 7 oz. 56 C.F.	250 gals. (946 liters) 3 lbs.13½ oz. 33 C.F.	100 gals. (378 liters) 1 lb. 8½ oz. 13 C.F.	50 gals. (189 liters) 12½ oz. 7 C.F.			
O_2	1825 gals. (6.907 liters) 20 lbs. 244 C.F.	1400 gals. (5.299 liters) 18 lbs. 7 oz. 187 C.F	800 gals. (3.028 liters) 11 lbs. 107 C.F.	165 gals. (625 liters) 2 lbs. 4 oz. 22 C.F.	95 gals. (359 liters) 1 lb. 5 oz. 13 C.F.	40 gals. (151 liters) 8 oz. 5 C.F.	20 gals (75.7 liters) 4 oz. 2.5 C.F.			

Figure 14—14. Listing of dimensions and weights of empty cylinders, as well as the net contents of cylinders for all gases listed. The approximate dimensions and weights of empty cylinders include the valves. Note that tank sizes AA through E have flush-type valves and the larger tanks (M through H) have diameter-indexed valves. (Modified from Garrett DF, Donaldson WP: Physical Principles of Respiratory Therapy Equipment. Madison, Wisconsin, Ohio Medical Products, 1975)

pressed Gas Association to promote uniform safety. It is important that the gas industry, as well as the users of such products, effectively control the standards by which they operate. If they do not accomplish this with effective and up-to-date standards, it becomes necessary for governmental agencies to enforce the standards. The important implication is that persons who are governed by these controls can and do have a large voice in the writing of standards, a lesser voice in writing regulations, and often little or no voice in the writing or changing of laws. Therefore, it is essential that respiratory care workers do an effective job in governing themselves, or unnecessary restrictions may be placed on their activities.

REGULATORY AGENCIES

The regulations of the federal agencies, mentioned earlier, not only establish the rules for the transportation of compressed gases and cryogenic liquids, but also govern their packaging, marking, labeling, and shipping-paper preparation. There are severe penalties for failure to comply with these regulations, and they are enforced by field inspectors from the DOT and the BE. (One important distinction here is that the BE is not a government agency but rather an agency of the Association of American Railroads. Their inspectors do not have the police powers of the government inspectors and are not making inspections on behalf of the federal government.)

Many states, such as Oregon, Washington, and California, have adopted the federal regulations to govern the shipment of compressed gases and cryogenic liquids within the state. These states administer the regulations within the state through the state highway patrol, the Public Service Commission, the Public Utilities Commission, or the state fire marshal, depending on the state involved.

In addition to the aforementioned agencies that govern the transportation of compressed gases and cryogenic liquids are the regulations covered in the *Postal Manual* of the US Postal Service. These regulations cover domestic and international mail shipment and, generally, place the responsibility for the shipment on the mailer.

The shipment of compressed gases and cryogenic liquids must conform to the requirements of the DOT. These regulations apply to the qualifications of drivers, the driving of motor vehicles, the parts and accessories necessary for safe operation, the hours of service of the drivers, and the inspec-

tion, maintenance, and transportation of hazardous materials.

The Food and Drug Administration (FDA) of the Department of Health and Human Services has for some time regulated the commodities used in the food, drug, and cosmetic industries. In 1962, however, certain changes were made in the Federal Food, Drug, and Cosmetic (FD & C) Act, and for the first time a drug was defined as being anything that is listed in the *US Pharmacopeia* or the *National Formulary*. This list, at present, includes oxygen, nitrous oxide, cyclopropane, carbon dioxide, helium, ethylene, and mixtures of these gases, and it is anticipated that air for human respiration and nitrogen will eventually be added. This 1962 amendment to the FD & C Act also required that all producers or repackagers of drugs must register with the FDA, with heavy penalties for failure to comply. The significance of this amendment is that anyone who is filling, refilling, or "trans-filling" cylinders (i.e., filling one cylinder from another) must comply with these regulations. The FDA has field inspectors that evaluate establishments periodically for compliance with these regulations.

In 1966, the FDA also issued regulations for the labeling of certain hazardous substances that might cause substantial personal injury or illness to anyone handling them. These regulations appeared under the Federal Hazardous Substances Labeling Act.

In addition to the federal and state laws and regulations, many counties and municipalities have zoning laws, fire prevention codes, pressure-vessel regulations, hazardous-materials storage and transport rules, and so on. Furthermore, there are bridge, tunnel, and turnpike regulations that govern the transportation of compressed gases and cryogenic liquids over these facilities. These regulations are usually enforced by the state under the turnpike authority or the bridge authority.

The Occupational Safety and Health Act of 1970 (OSHA), sometimes referred to as the Williams–Steiger Act, was developed by the occupational Safety and Health Administration of the Department of Labor in response to governmental recognition of the need for further reducing the incidence of occupational injury. The rate of occupationally related disabling injuries in the United States has been on an increase since about 1964. Under the provisions of this law, it is the duty of every employer to furnish each of his employees with a place of employment that is free from recognized hazards that are causing, or are likely to cause, serious physical harm or death to his employee. The basic concept in the Williams–Steiger Act is that the individual states will assume the responsibility for occupational safety and health standards. These standards, however, must be approved through the Department of Labor and are subject to modifications and monitoring by OSHA.

Some of the OSHA standards were established before the beginning of this act. Existing standards and regulations from the NFPA, National Electric Code, American National Standards Institute (ANSI), and others have been adopted by OSHA. These standards are enforced through a program of inspections. Compliance officers, trained by OSHA, have greater authority than that of almost any other enforcement officer. These compliance officers make inspections according to a priority schedule. Fatalities are given first priority, followed by serious injuries, employee complaints, high-risk target industries, and routine inspections. OSHA seeks to provide freedom from occupationally related injuries for all workers. It is true that inspections and citations are a necessary part of the program; however, safety promotion through employee training and awareness, improvement, and management is stressed.

WARNING AND ALARM SYSTEMS

The NFPA recommends that audible and visual signals and pressure gauges be installed in the office or working area of the person who is to be responsible for the maintenance of any bulk oxygen system, and that a second alarm be located in an area where continuous monitoring of the system can take place. The second system may be located at the telephone switchboard, security office, or other location where responsible persons can monitor the system 24 hours a day. The system should be provided with an audible and visual alarm that will indicate that the oxygen supply has changed over to the reservoir system. A separate alarm system should be located in areas of vital life support, such as the recovery room, and the coronary or intensive care units, that would indicate the amount of pressure located in the lines. Again, these alarm systems should be both visual and audible, and preferably located at the nurses' stations or other locations near these areas.

FIRE SAFETY

According to the NFPA, a fire requires the presence of combustible or flammable material, an atmosphere containing oxygen or other oxidizing agents, and a source of ignition for it to occur. Any of the mixtures of breathing gases that are routinely used in respiratory therapy will support combustion. Materials that are combustible and flammable in air will ignite more easily and will burn more vigorously in an oxygen-enriched atmosphere; materials that are not normally considered to be combustible in air may be considered combustible in an oxygen-enriched atmosphere.

Many combustible materials may be found near a patient receiving respiratory therapy, including oils, skin lotions, facial tissues, clothing, bed linen, oxygen tent canopies, rubber and plastic articles, suction and oxygen tubing, cyclopropane, ether, alcohols, and acetone. Another material that is highly flammable, even in air, is cellulose nitrate (nitrocellulose)–based plastic, this may be found in such articles as eyeglass frames, mechanical pens and pencils, combs, and toothbrushes. Toys are occasionally made of this plastic.

Another hazard exists when high-pressure oxygen equipment becomes contaminated with oil, grease, or other combustible materials. These contaminants will ignite readily, burn much more rapidly in the presence of high oxygen concentrations, and make it easier to ignite less combustible materials with which they may come in contact.

In the presence of an oxygen-enriched atmosphere, sources that a person may not ordinarily consider hazardous may become significant. These include open flames, smoking, electric heaters, the discharge of a cardiac defibrillator, arcing and excessive temperatures in electrical equipment, and defective electrical equipment. Under normal conditions the energy content of a static discharge will not be a source of ignition for a fire, as long as the static discharge does not occur in the presence of items that are easily ignited, such as ether, cyclopropane, alcohols, acetone, oils, and grease. However, a static discharge in a hyperbaric chamber containing oxygen under pressure greater than ambient would be extremely hazardous (see Chap. 16).

Another potential fire safety hazard is from *adiabatic compression*. The rapid filling of an oxygen line from one pressure level to another will result in an increase in temperature of the oxygen gas within the line. To prevent this potential hazard, the lines should be pressurized slowly to minimize the temperature rise.

Compressed gas cylinders are heavy and bulky and are a potential hazard if they are not handled properly. Those cylinders that are supplied with a cap should have it kept in place until the cylinder is ready to be used. Carriers specifically designed

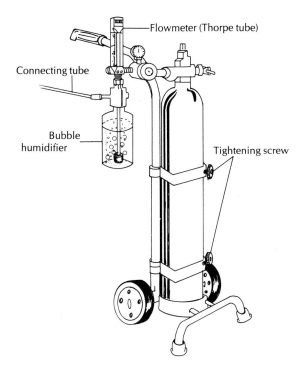

Figure 14—15. E size oxygen cylinder mounted in small wheeled stand. (Reproduced with permission from Eubanks DH, Bone RC: Comprehensive Respiratory Care, 2nd ed. St. Louis, CV Mosby, 1990)

for cylinder use are the only ones that should be used for moving the cylinder about, and a cylinder should be secured to a nonmovable object at all times when it is not being transported (e.g., Fig. 14–15).

Improper maintenance, handling, or assembly of oxygen equipment may be another cause for personal injury, property damage, or fire. Care should be exercised that electrical equipment be in proper working order, with adequate grounding. Every effort should be made to eliminate any source of ignition during the administration of oxygen. Smoking materials should be removed from patients receiving therapy and their visitors, and the patient should be advised of the potential fire hazards. Precautionary signs that are readable from a distance of 5 ft are to be placed in conspicuous places at the site of administration as well as in aisles or walkways leading to such an area. They are to be approximately 8 × 11 in. in size and must also be attached to the doorway of the room in which oxygen administration is taking place.

COLOR-MARKING AND PRECAUTIONARY LABELING

Compressed gases that are intended for medical use and are supplied in cylinders should be clearly identifiable for the type of gas that the cylinder contains. Because there is no existing United States standard for color marking of gas cylinders, the compressed gas industry has, for about 30 years, adhered to the *Simplified Practice Recommendation for Color Marking for Anesthetic Gas Cylinders* of the US Department of Commerce.

Standard Z48.1 of the American National Standards Institute (ANSI) states that the only absolute way to determine the content of any compressed gas cylinder is by means of the chemical name or other commonly accepted name that is marked legibly on the exterior of the cylinder. Furthermore, the standard states that the marking should be done by means of stenciling, stamping, or labeling, and should not be readily removable. Certain precautionary information that is relative to the handling, storage, and use of the material should also be on the label. As stated previously, the FDA requires that specific warning statements be included in the labeling of any containers of gases that are intended for medical use.

A secondary way of guarding against use of the wrong gas is by means of the standardized valve outlet connections (discussed in the next section). As a third means of guarding against inadvertently administering the wrong gas, the compressed gas industry uses color to designate certain cylinders for use with specific gases that are intended for medical use. Because of the variations in color tones, chemical changes in the paint pigments, various lighting effects, and the differences in color perception by personnel, the color marking of the cylinders is not considered a reliable means for identification of the content of the cylinder (see Table 14–2 for usual color markings).

STANDARDIZED VALVE OUTLET CONNECTIONS

A secondary way of guarding against the inadvertent use of the wrong gas is by means of the standardized valve outlet connections. Following World War I, efforts were made to standardize the valve threads on cylinders because of the difficulties that arose, both in industry and the military, owing to the multiplicity of connections that were then in use. Marginal progress was made in this area through the Gas Cylinder Valve Thread Committee

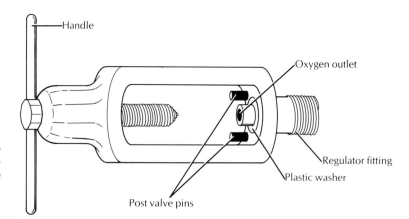

Figure 14—16. Yoke connector used to attach regulator to cylinder post valve. (Reproduced with permission from Eubanks DH, Bone RC: Comprehensive Respiratory Care, 2nd ed. St. Louis, CV Mosby, 1990)

of the Compressed Gas Manufacturers' Association, Inc. During the interwar years, several compressed-gas manufacturers achieved virtual standardization; much of the progress in this area was due to the Federal Specifications Board. Although many manufacturers achieved standardization within their companies, these were not fully coordinated with other related standards.

In October 1945, the standards association representing Great Britain, Canada, and the United States met in Ottawa to consider standardization of valve threads. In January 1946, an agreement was reached that resulted in final approval of a considerable number of additional gas cylinder valve threads; these data were included in the *National Bureau of Standards' Handbook H-28*. In January 1949, the Compressed Gas Manufacturers' Association, Inc., changed its name, and its Valve Thread Standardization Committee became known as the Valve Standards Committee of the Compressed Gas Association, Inc. Between 1946 and 1949, much progress was made in the area of standardization for valve threads, and in 1949 uniform standards were accepted by the American Standards Association and the Canadian Standards Association. The American Standard Compressed Gas Cylinder Valve Outlet and Inlet Connections (ANSI) are the OSHA standard for cylinder valves.

The standard is for large cylinders (sizes M through G), and the threaded outlets are separated into four basic divisions: internal, external, right-hand, and left-hand. Within each of the four divisions are further variations made by changing the diameter (see the following), as well as the pitch of the threads. As far as possible, the assignment of the different connections to the different gases has been made to prevent the interchange of connections that may result in a catastrophe.

Cylinder sizes E and smaller have what is known as a *Pin Index Safety System*. As early as the spring of 1940, various medical societies, as well as the manufacturers of medical gases, determined that a system should be developed that would prevent the possibility of interchanging the medical gas cylinders that are equipped with flush-type valves. Various methods were studied, but the

Figure 14—17. The pin index safety system. The drawing shows details of the hole positions in a flush-type valve, in accordance with standards set by the Compressed Gas Association. The yoke with its matching pins is not shown. (Modified from Garrett DF, Donaldson WP: Physical Principles of Respiratory Therapy Equipment. Madison, Wisconsin, Ohio Medical Products, 1975)

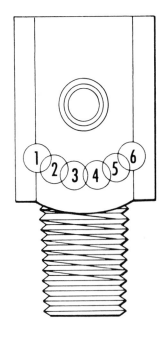

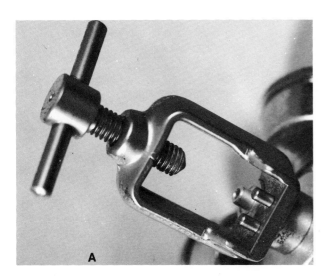
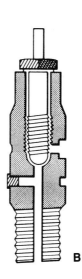
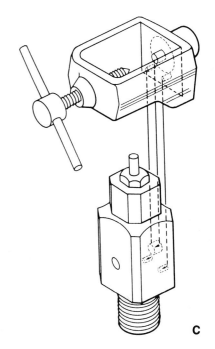

Figure 14—18. (*A*) Yoke connector used with small gas cylinders. (Reproduced with permission from Spearman CB, Sheldon RL, Egan EF: Egan's Fundamentals of Respiratory Therapy, 4th ed. St. Louis, CV Mosby, 1982) (*B*) Cross-section of direct-acting high-pressure (yoke-type) cylinder valve. (*C*) Diagram of yoke connector showing regulator inlet and pin safety system. (Barnes TA: Respiratory Care Practice. Chicago, Year Book Medical Publishers, 1988)

present pin-index safety system (PISS) has been adopted as an international standard. The system is designed to prevent the improper attachment of any regulator to a cylinder for which it was not intended. This is accomplished by the placement of two pins on the regulator yoke (Fig. 14–16), so arranged that only the correct gas cylinder valve (Fig. 14–17) will fit onto them. The specific gas is assigned a combination of pins that coincides with the yoke attachment on the regulator (Fig. 14–18 and Table 14–3).

A system was developed by the Compressed Gas Association to provide a standard for noninterchangeable connections with individual gas lines of medical gas-administering equipment that operate at pressures of 200 psig or less. This system is known as the *Diameter Index Safety System* (DISS) and is used on such low-pressure outlets as regulators and connectors for anesthesia, resuscitation, and respiratory therapy apparatus. This noninterchangeability of gas connections is achieved by a series of increasing and decreasing diameters in the connector, as well as by variations in thread size.

Each of the connections of the DISS consists of three parts: body, nipple, and nut (Fig. 14–19). To achieve the noninterchangeability between the different connections, the two diameters on each part vary in opposite directions, such that as one diameter increases, the other will decrease. Thus only the

Table 14—3 Pin Index System

INTENDED GAS	PIN COMBINATION
Oxygen	2 and 5
Carbon dioxide/oxygen (CO_2 7% or under)	2 and 6
Helium/oxygen (He 80% and under)	2 and 4
Ethylene	1 and 3
Nitrous oxide	3 and 5
Cyclopropane	3 and 6
Helium/oxygen (He over 80%)	4 and 6
Carbon dioxide/oxygen (CO_2 over 7%)	1 and 6
Air for human respiration	1 and 5

Body   Nipple

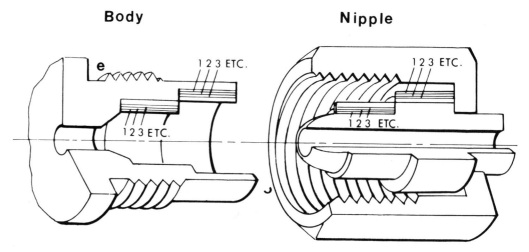

Figure 14—19. The diameter index safety system standard low-pressure connection for medical gases, compressed air, and suction. The small bore in the body mates with the small diameter of the nipple, and the large bore in the body mates with the large diameter of the nipple (Compressed Gas Association)

Figure 14—20. Comparison of safety systems used for compressed gases. Note that the DISS connections are for outlets having reduced pressures (less than 200 psig), whereas the American Standard connection is shown for a large cylinder and the PISS connection is shown for a small cylinder. (Reproduced with permission from Spearman CB, Sheldon RL, Egan DF: Egan's Fundamentals of Respiratory Therapy, 4th ed. St. Louis, CV Mosby, 1982)

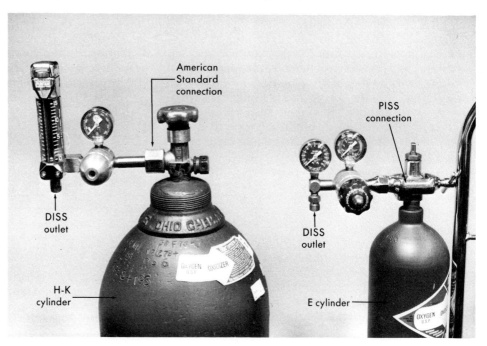

Table 14—4 K Factors (L/psi) to Calculate
Duration of Cylinder Flow

| | CYLINDER SIZE | | | |
GAS	D	E	G	H and K
O_2, O_2/N_2, air	0.16	0.28	2.41	3.14
O_2/CO_2	0.20	0.35	2.94	3.84
He/O_2	0.14	0.23	1.93	2.50

(Chatburn R, Lough M: Handbook of Respiratory Care, 2nd ed. Chicago, Year Book Medical Publishers, 1990, used with permission)

properly mated and intended parts will fit together. In Figure 14–20 the uses and interrelationships of the DISS, PISS, and American Standard connection systems are illustrated.

USE-TIME OF HIGH-PRESSURE GAS CYLINDERS AND LIQUID OXYGEN SOURCES

The use time of a high-pressure gas cylinder is related to its gauge pressure in the following manner:

$$\text{Duration of flow (min)} = \frac{K \times \text{gauge pressure (psi)}}{\text{Flow rate (L/min)}}$$

where K is a factor relating gas volume to pressure drop in the cylinder. K factors (expressed as L/psi) for various gases and gas mixtures are presented in Table 14–4.

The approximate amount of time remaining in various cylinders at various flow rates, as a function of their "full–empty" gauge readings, is found in Table 14–5.

For example, consider a high-pressure K cylinder containing 6900 L, 85% (5865 L) of which is usable. If the prescription is for 2 L/min continuously, then 2 L/min × 60-minute hours × 24-hour days × 30-day months means that 86,400 L/month will be needed to supply the patient. This will require 15 K cylinders per month.

Oxygen in liquid form takes only a fraction of the space required for oxygen in the gaseous form. Liquid oxygen is frequently ordered by physicians because of two features specific to the system: (1) for high-volume users (e.g., the patient's prescription requires more than 4 L/min, the liquid oxygen system can best meet these demands; and (2) a portable unit can be filled from the reservoir. This "ox-

Table 14—5 Approximate Number of Hours of Flow

| | CYLINDER TYPE | | | | | | | |
| | Full | | 3/4 Full | | 1/2 Full | | 1/4 Full | |
FLOW RATE (L/min)	E	H	E	H	E	H	E	H
2	5.1	56	3.8	42	2.5	28	1.3	14
4	2.5	28	1.8	21	1.2	14	0.6	7
6	1.7	18.5	1.3	13.7	0.9	9.2	0.4	4.5
8	1.2	14	0.9	10.5	0.6	7	0.3	3.5
10	1.0	11	0.7	8.2	0.5	5.5	0.2	2.7
12	0.8	9.2	0.6	6.7	0.4	4.5	0.2	2.2
15	0.6	7.2	0.4	5.5	0.3	3.5	0.1	1.7

(Chatburn R, Lough M: Handbook of Respiratory Care, 2nd ed. Chicago, Year Book Medical Publishers, 1990, used with permission)

ygen walker" provides a compact and extremely lightweight source for oxygen so that patient compliance with rehabilitative exercise regimens can be successful and a greater degree of mobility can be enjoyed by the patient.

If the patient is using 2 L/min of oxygen continuously, then in the foregoing example, 86,400 L/month will be needed to fill prescription (1 lb of liquid oxygen equals 342 L). The typical reservoir capacity is 70 lb, or 23,900 L; at 2 L/min, this will last 200 hours, or more than 8 days. The average portable capacity is 3 lb, or 1026 L; at 2 L/min, this will last 8 hours.

In conclusion, the safe usage of medical gases requires an understanding of the nature of the gases on the part of those individuals handling them Accidents happen through carelessness and, perhaps, because those who are involved in the accident do not understand the potential dangers when the regulations are not followed. Every effort should be made to ensure the safety of patients, employees, and visitors in medical institutions.

REFERENCES

1. Adriani J: The Chemistry and Physics of Anesthesia, 2nd ed. Springfield, Ill, Charles C Thomas, 1962
2. Compressed Gas Association: Handbook of Compressed Gases. New York, Reinhold, 1967
3. National Fire Protection Association: Respiratory Therapy, NFPA, no. 56B. Boston, 1973
4. Chatburn R, Lough M: Handbook of Respiratory Care, 2nd ed. Chicago, Year Book Medical Publishers, 1990

BIBLIOGRAPHY

Adriani J: The Chemistry and Physics of Anesthesia, 2nd ed. Springfield, Ill, Charles C Thomas, 1962

Broberner RH: Roi's Principles of Chemistry, 10th ed. St Louis, CV Mosby, 1967

Brooks SM: Integrated Basic Science, 3rd ed. St Louis, CV Mosby, 1970

Compressed Gas Association: Handbook of Compressed Gases. New York, Reinhold, 1966

Compressed Gas Association: Pamphlet P-12, Safe Handling of Cryogenic Liquids. New York, 1980

Compressed Gas Association: Pamphlet C-7, Precautionary Labeling & Marking of Compressed Gas Containers. New York, 1983

Compressed Gas Association: Pamphlet G-4, Oxygen. Arlington, Va, 1984

Ent WL, Kitson FK: Filling procedures for compressed gases, including liquefied gases. Paper presented at the Distributor Safety Seminar. New York, Compressed Gas Association, 1973

Garrett DF et al: Physical Principles of Respiratory Therapy Equipment. Madison, Wis, Ohio Medical Products, 1975

Gilbert DL: Cosmic and geophysical aspects of the respiratory gases. In Fenn WO, Rahn H (eds): Handbook of Physiology, Sect 3: Respiration, Vol 1. Washington, DC, American Physiological Society, 1964

Introduction: oxygen and life. Anesthesiology 37:100–111, 1972

Harris NC et al: Introductory Applied Physics, 2nd ed. New York, McGraw-Hill, 1963

Macintosh R et al: Physics for the Anesthetist, 3rd ed. Philadelphia, FA Davis, 1963

National Fire Protection Association: Manual for the Home Use of Respiratory Therapy. NFPA, no. 56HM. Boston, 1973

National Fire Protection Association: Bulk Oxygen Systems. NFPA no. 50. Boston, 1974

National Fire Protection Association: Fire Hazards in Oxygen-Enriched Atmospheres. NFPA, no. 53M. Boston, 1974

National Fire Protection Association: Respiratory Therapy. NFPA no. 56B. Boston, 1973

National Fire Protection Association: Standards for the Use of Inhalation Anesthetics. NFPA, no. 56A. Boston, 1973

US Pharacopoeal Convention: Pharmacopoeia of the United States of America, 18th ed. Easton, Pa, Mack Publishing, 1975

Pinney GG: OSHA, state and local employee safety standards. Paper presented at the Distributor Safety Seminar, New York, Compressed Gas Association, 1973

Scott RB: Cryogenic Engineering. Clinton, Mass, D Van Nostrand, 1966

Senesky JS: Gas mixtures. Paper presented at the Distributor Safety Seminar. New York, Compressed Gas Association, 1973

Shaner RL: Production of Industrial Gases from the Air. Union Carbide Corporation, Linde Division, New York, 1969

Scanlon CL, Spearman CB, Sheldon RL (eds): Egan's Fundamentals of Respiratory Care. CV Mosby Co, St Louis, 1990

Smith AL: Principles of Microbiology, 7th ed. St Louis, CV Mosby, 1973

Swope RL et al: Compressed gas containers. Paper presented at the Distributor Safety Seminar. New York, Compressed Gas Association, 1973

Tribolet R, Willoughby TE: Cryogenic-liquid containers. Paper presented at the Distributor Safety Seminar. New York, Compressed Gas Association, 1973

Vance RW, Duke W: Applied Cryogenic Engineering. New York, John Wiley & Sons, 1962

Van Volen L: The history and stability of atmospheric oxygen. Science 171:439–443, 1971

Willoughby TE: Safety laws, regulations, and standards. Paper presented at the Distributor Safety Seminar. New York, Compressed Gas Association, 1973

Young JA, Crocker D: Principles and Practice of Inhalation Therapy. Chicago, Year Book Medical Publishers, 1970

FIFTEEN

Oxygen as a Drug: Clinical Properties, Benefits, Modes, and Hazards of Administration

Gene G. Ryerson
A. Jay Block

CHEMICAL PROPERTIES

Oxygen is a colorless, odorless, and tasteless gas that is essential for life of the human organism. The atmosphere contains 20.95% oxygen. This percentage of the total atmospheric pressure remains constant at higher altitudes as atmospheric pressure decreases. In both the free and combined forms, oxygen is one of the most plentiful chemical elements on earth. Oxygen makes up 89% of the weight of water; nearly half of the weight of rocks and minerals is oxygen.

An atom of oxygen has an atomic number of 8. Therefore, its structure contains eight nuclear protons and eight orbital electrons. The extremely stable isotope ^{16}O has eight nuclear neutrons, resulting in an atomic weight of 16. Medical oxygen consists mainly of this isotope. In nature, however, the oxygen atom exists in three stable isotropic forms: ^{16}O, ^{17}O, and ^{18}O, which occur in the approximate ratios of $1000 : 3.7 : 20$, respectively.[18] The electron configuration of an oxygen atom allows electrons in the other orbit to be shared with another atom (Fig. 15–1). This outer orbit also allows room for two additional electrons, which accounts for the negative valence of 2. Two oxygen atoms combine to form molecular oxygen (O_2), with a molecular weight of 32. Molecules made of three oxygen atoms constitute the gas ozone (O_3). This allotropic form of oxygen results from the action of an electrical discharge or ultraviolet light on oxygen. Oxygen is extremely reactive and combines with many elements, resulting in a class of compounds called oxides.

The methods used to measure oxygen concentrations that are delivered to patients are based on physicochemical properties of the oxygen molecule.[27] Oxygen possesses unique paramagnetic susceptibility. When placed in a magnetic field, oxygen alters the configuration of the field. Nonparamagnetic gases, such as ozone, carbon dioxide, and nitrogen, are displaced out of the magnetic field. This special property of oxygen is due to its unpaired electron structure, and it forms the basis for *paramagnetic analyzers*. Bedside instruments can measure oxygen concentrations of 0.1% to 100%.

The *polarographic* property of oxygen is the basis for several electrochemical methods of measuring oxygen.[27] Electric cells are designed to analyze low concentrations of oxygen in either gas or liquid mixtures. The oxygen molecule will result in a flow of electrons, thereby producing an electric current. The electric cells are surrounded by an oxygen-permeable membrane when dissolved oxygen is being measured in blood. Miniature electrochemical analyzers have been designed to measure oxygen tension in blood vessels.

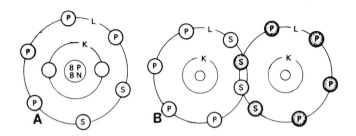

Figure 15—1. Atomic structure of oxygen. *(A)* An atom of oxygen: The nucleus contains eight protons and eight neutrons; the electron configuration is composed of an inner *(K)* orbit of two electrons and an outer *(L)* orbit of six electrons. *(B)* A molecule of oxygen (two atoms). Note the sharing of the s electrons in the L orbit filling the capacity of that orbit.

Mass spectrometry utilizes the ionization property of gases. In an ionization chamber, gas molecules, including those of oxygen, are converted to positive ions by the loss of electrons. The gases are then separated according to the molecular mass of their ions.[44] The extremely rapid response time of spectrometers allows continuous, breath-by-breath oxygen analysis.

The primary commercial means of manufacturing oxygen is by liquefaction, followed by fractional distillation of air (see Chap. 14). This method utilizes differences in boiling points. A cooling process condenses air from the gaseous to the liquid state. As the temperature is slowly raised, nitrogen and inert gases evaporate before the boiling point of oxygen is reached. At atmospheric pressure, this boiling point of oxygen is $-183°F$ ($-119.4°C$). Liquid oxygen is then coverted under high pressure to the gaseous state. Oxygen is stored in steel cylinders under a pressure of about 2000 lb/in.^{2} (psi). Characteristics of the most commonly used cylinders are listed in Table 15–1. The most frequently used are D, E, G, and H cylinders. Since emergency portable oxygen and anesthetic gases are most often stored in E cylinders. Because various gases are stored in cylinders, color coding is used for easy identification (Table 15–2). If oxygen is to remain in the liquid state, it must be stored at atmospheric pressure at a temperature below its boiling point.

ADVERSE EFFECTS OF OXYGEN THERAPY

The potential complications of exposing patients to increased oxygen tensions can be divided into categories: (1) adverse physiologic effects and (2) oxygen-induced toxic effects in tissues. Physiologic effects are generally less severe and more readily reversible and may develop with a modest increase in inspired oxygen. Examples of adverse physiologic effects are depression of ventilatory drive, depression of cardiac output, and constriction of most systemic arterials. In contrast to this systemic vasoconstriction, the pulmonary vessels dilate. This effect is helpful in patients if hypoxia from lung disease is associated with pulmonary hypertension.

All human organs are potentially susceptible to the toxic effects of hyperoxia. However, in adults who are breathing oxygen-enriched mixtures at atmospheric pressure, lung injury predominates (Table 15–3).

HYPOVENTILATION

In certain clinical situtations, the ventilatory drive that results from carbon dioxide stimulation of the respiratory centers is blunted. Depression of the ventilatory drive is an unpredictable side effect. Normal humans tolerate this adverse effect well, whereas in the presence of chronic respiratory fail-

Table 15—1 Common Oxygen Cylinders

CYLINDER SIZE	EMPTY WEIGHT (lb)	OXYGEN VOLUME* (ft³)	OXYGEN VOLUME* (L)	AMOUNT OF OXYGEN AVAILABLE IN HOURS (APPROXIMATE), FLOW RATE 2 L/min (hr)
D	10.25	12.6	356.0	3
E	15	22.0	622.0	5
G	100	186.0	5260.0	43
H–K	135	244.0	6900.0	56

* Measured at 70° F and 14.7 lb/in. absolute.

Table 15–2 Color Codes of Compressed Gas Cylinders

GAS	UNITED STATES	ISO*
Oxygen (O_2)	Green	White
Air	Yellow	White and black
Carbon dioxide (CO_2)	Gray	Gray
Nitrous oxide (N_2O)	Blue	Blue
Cyclopropane (C_3H_6)	Orange	Orange
Helium (He)	Brown	Brown
Ethylene (C_2H_4)	Red	Violet
Carbon dioxide and oxygen (CO_2–O_2)	Gray and green	White and gray
Helium and oxygen (He–O_2)	Brown and green	White and brown

* International Standards Organizations recommendation for single color code for all cylinders.

ure, hypercapnia, or impairment of the respiratory centers, carbon dioxide narcosis may develop. Hypoventilation is of particular importance in patients with severe chronic obstructive pulmonary disease (COPD) when carbon dioxide retention develops gradually over months. Patients so affected appear to have a depression of the normal responsiveness of the respiratory centers to carbon dioxide, whereas the carotid body peripheral chemoreceptors remain sensitive to hypoxemia. Therefore, relief of hypoxemia removes the stimulus to breathing, leading to further alveolar hypoventilation. A sometimes unavoidable factor in carbon dioxide retention in patients with respiratory failure is the injudicious administration of excessive oxygen.

Table 15–3 Manifestations of Oxygen Toxicity

ALTERED PHYSIOLOGY

  Pulmonary
    Hypoventilation
    Absorption atelectasis
    Pulmonary vasodilatation
    Decreased mucociliary clearance
    Decreased macrophage function
  Extrapulmonary
    Suppressed erythropoiesis
    Decreased cardiac output
    Systemic vasoconstriction

PULMONARY TISSUE INJURY SYNDROMES

  Tracheobronchitis
  Adult respiratory distress syndrome
  Bronchopulmonary dysplasia

Once carbon dioxide retention develops after oxygen administration, under no circumstances should oxygen be withdrawn. Without supplemental oxygen, dangerous hypoxemia can occur. High air-flow oxygen enrichment (HAFOE) therapy, e.g., with a Venturi wash, may be helpful (see discussion later in this chapter). If spontaneous inhalation remains depressed, artificial ventilation may be necessary.

ABSORPTION ATELECTASIS

Alveolar collapse may develop during inhalation of high oxygen concentrations. Nitrogen, an inert gas that is relatively insoluble in blood, maintains a residual volume in an alveolus: If oxygen replaces nitrogen, the gas volume within the alveolus is reduced because oxygen is rapidly absorbed into the blood. This is particularly likely in alveoli with low ventilation/perfusion ratios (perfusion in excess of ventilation). In pulmonary diseases that involve narrowing or obstruction of airways (e.g., retention of mucus), alveolar collapse may result within minutes after breathing pure oxygen.[42] Consequently, absorption atelectasis reduces the vital capacity and increases the shunting of blood through the lung.

NORMOBARIC PULMONARY OXYGEN TOXICITY

Oxygen tissue injury is a real clinical concern, especially in patients who require the delivery of continuous high concentrations of supplemental oxygen. These patients must receive sufficient oxygen to prevent tissue hypoxia, despite the danger that oxygen toxicity can worsen pulmonary function.

Clinical and Pathologic Findings

The manifestations of lung toxicity can be separated into three clinical entities: tracheobronchitis, adult respiratory distress syndrome (ARDS), and bronchopulmonary dysplasia, which is primarily a neonatal disorder.[12] It is not certain whether these syndromes are a progression of oxygen injury or are actually unique disorders. The earliest clinical findings in normal human volunteers after breathing 100% oxygen for 6 hours are cough and substernal chest pain.[37] This acute tracheobronchitis appears to result from an irritant effect of oxygen, which is transitory and tolerated by most patients. Bronchoscopic studies performed as early as 3 hours after breathing 90% to 95% oxygen have shown depressed tracheociliary and mucus clearance.[37] Pulmonary function, however, generally remains unchanged until after 24 hours of oxygen breathing. At this point, the vital capacity progressively decreases. This diminution appears to be the best objective index for the development of pulmonary oxygen toxicity.[10] Determination of vital capacity, however, is a difficult maneuver to perform if the patient is unable to cooperate or has some type of mechanical limitation. The chest roentgenogram in these early stages usually remains normal, except for decreased lung volumes.

After 1 to 4 days of continued ±100% oxygen exposure, patients develop progressive dyspnea, increasing hypoxemia, a productive cough, and a widened alveolar–arterial oxygen gradient. At this point, diffuse, patchy infiltrates first appear on the chest roentgenogram (Fig. 15-2). Physical examination for the first time may show abnormalities of basilar crackles.

In both humans and well-studied animal models, the pathologic pulmonary changes of hyperoxia are divided into an early exudative phase and a later proliferative phase.[22] Within 24 to 48 hours of oxygen exposure, exudative morphologic changes appear, with the development of interstitial, perivascular, and intra-alveolar edema; hemorrhage; an influx of polymorphonuclear leukocytes; variable loss of type I alveolar pneumonocytes; and necrosis of pulmonary capillary endothelium.

After more than 72 hours of continued exposure and if the patient survives the acute phase, the proliferative phase begins, with reabsorption of early exudates and thickening of the alveolar septa. The relatively oxygen-resistant type II pneumonocytes hypertrophy and increase in number. However, these surfactant-producing cells show signs of intracellular damage. Once this proliferative phase has been reached, total recovery is unlikely, and residual scarring is permanent, with variable loss of lung function. The resulting clinical pattern is similar to that of pulmonary fibrosis. These chronic changes in the newborn are referred to as *bronchopulmonary dysplasia*.[10,31] Lung toxicity resulting

Figure 15–2. *(A)* An AP roentgenogram of a patient exposed to 100% oxygen for 5 days. There is an alveolar-filling pattern in the lower half of the right lung and at the left base. These findings are consistent with oxygen toxicity. *(B)* In response to appropriate therapy the oxygen exposure was reduced to safe levels. The patient was eventually weaned from oxygen, and his roentgenogram at 6 weeks (shown here) had returned to normal.

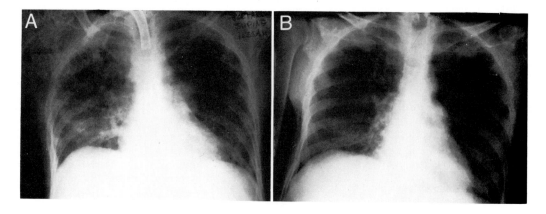

from the administration of oxygen to infants with respiratory distress syndrome (RDS) appears to be a major contributing factor for this disorder. Possibly, the newborn lung is more susceptible to the effects of oxygen toxicity.

High oxygen tensions also decrease the ability of alveolar macrophages to kill bacteria. The combination of decreased tracheobronchial clearance and impaired alveolar macrophage function may be responsible, at least in part, for the increased susceptibility to pulmonary infection observed in patients who are breathing high concentrations of oxygen.

Level of Exposure

The major determinants of hyperoxic lung injury are the partial pressure of oxygen in the inspired air ($P_{I}O_2$) and the duration of exposure.[10] Although a high percentage of oxygen ($F_{I}O_2$) is an important factor, this by itself is not toxic as long as the partial pressure is significantly low.

Astronauts, for example, have tolerated many days of 100% oxygen, but at a barometric pressure one-third that of atmospheric (about 250 mmHg). *The partial pressure of inspired oxygen ($P_{I}O_2$) is the best guide of effective exposure.* The $P_{I}O_2$ is given by the equation $P_{I}O_2 = (P_B - 47) \times F_{I}O_2$, where PB is barometric pressure mmHg, 47 is the partial pressure of water vapor at body temperature in mmHg, and $F_{I}O_2$ is the inspired oxygen concentration expressed as a decimal fraction. The $P_{I}O_2$ is often stated in terms of *atmospheres of oxygen* as shown by the equation:

$$\text{Atmospheres } O_2 = \frac{P_{I}O_2}{760}$$

where 760 represents atmospheric pressure at sea level.

Pulmonary oxygen toxicity is a consequence of direct exposure of the lung parenchyma to excessive oxygen tension. Experimental studies in animals have demonstrated that the elevated alveolar oxygen concentration ($P_{A}O_2$) is the prime factor causing pulmonary oxygen toxicity, not the level of oxygen tension in systemic arterial blood (PaO_2).

The duration of exposure necessary to produce pulmonary oxygen toxicity is directly related to the $P_{I}O_2$. In normal humans, there appears to be a threshold of 0.5 atm of oxygen or an $F_{I}O_2$ of 0.50 at sea level, below which clinically apparent oxygen toxicity has not been reported. Despite variations in human susceptibility, there is little or no identifiable lung injury to humans exposed to 700 torr (approximately 100% oxygen at 1 atm) for nearly 24 hours.

Host Tolerance

Certain factors have been reported to potentiate the development of pulmonary oxygen toxicity, whereas others modify the syndrome.[8] Most experimental studies, however; have been conducted in animal models; therefore; they may not apply to humans. At present, prophylactic measures, including use of various drugs, have not been subjected to clinical evaluation and, consequently, are of no practical value. One notable exception is intermittent exposure to oxygen, which has been shown to delay the onset of pulmonary oxygen toxicity. If it is possible to reduce the $F_{I}O_2$ for short periods, every few hours during an exposure to a high oxygen tension, the duration of high-tension exposure can be extended with a lessening of detrimental effects. In most clinical situations, this is not practical; however, intermittent therapy could be considered if high oxygen tensions are used to aid in the absorption of trapped body air, such as is found in a pneumothorax.

Another possible beneficial agent used in the prevention of oxygen toxicity is the antioxidant vitamin E. Preliminary results in premature newborns who have received high fractional concentrations of inspired oxygen suggest that this vitamin may delay the onset of bronchopulmonary dysplasia.[11] This is a unique circumstance, however, in that newborns are vitamin E–deficient. Because vitamin E deficiency is rarely encountered in adults, these results cannot be extended to older age groups.

Several factors appear to accelerate lung oxygen injury (Table 15–4). Corticosteroids, sometimes used to treat critically ill patients, have had no beneficial effects in pulmonary oxygen toxicity. In fact, animal studies suggest that they may actually accelerate oxygen-induced lung damage.

Table 15—4   Factors That Increase Susceptibility to Oxygen Toxicity

Adrenergic stimulation	Paraquat
Bleomycin	Premature birth
Corticosteroids	Protein deficiency
Hyperthermia	Vitamin E deficiency
Hyperthyroidism	

Biochemical Mechanisms

The precise mechanisms of oxygen toxicity have not been well characterized in humans. The most widely accepted theory is that biologically active oxygen radicals induced by hyperoxia participate in this cytotoxic process.[8,14]

Oxygen radicals are formed intracellularly by one of the many oxidase systems that donate an electron to oxygen. These oxygen metabolites, including superoxide, activated hydroxyl radical, hydrogen peroxide, and singlet oxygen, are all considered possible agents of hyperoxic tissue damage. These free radicals act to inhibit or inactivate sulfhydryl enzymes, disrupt DNA, or interact with membrane lipids, with resultant loss of membrane integrity. Superoxide is probably the radical most responsible for the biochemical alterations that result in the morphologic changes of oxygen toxicity (Fig. 15–3).[14]

Several natural cellular mechanisms are present in cells to protect themselves from oxidant damage. The three most important are superoxide dismutase, the sulfhydryl compounds, and the antioxidant vitamins C and E. *Superoxide dismutase is an enzyme the sole function of which appears to be the inactivation of superoxide.* The most abundant sulfhydryl compound is glutathione, which acts to reduce compounds oxidized by oxygen or to

be oxidized itself, thereby acting as a scavenger of oxygen radicals. During prolonged hyperoxia, the production of activated oxygen molecules may overwhelm natural antioxidant defenses, thereby allowing toxic morphologic changes in the lung to proceed unchecked.

Treatment

There is no specific therapy for pulmonary oxygen toxicity. The emphasis should be on prevention by adequate monitoring of the FiO_2, employing the lowest level that allows adequate tissue oxygenation. One must be aware, however, of the relative dangers of hypoxia and hyperoxia. A patient should never be allowed to be exposed to hazardous levels of hypoxia because of the fear of producing oxygen toxicity. There is no evidence that a high FiO_2 causes any clinically significant damage when used for brief periods (e.g., during surgery or bronchoscopy). Clinical oxygen toxicity is a problem in the setting of prolonged severe respiratory failure. In these situations in which hyperoxic therapy is essential for managing an adult or neonatal patient, pulmonary oxygen toxicity can be avoided only by reducing the duration of exposure to high partial pressures of oxygen. This may be accomplished with use of other techniques to improve gas exchange, such as positive end-expiratory pressure (PEEP), mobilization of secretions, and decreasing bronchospasm.

HYPERBARIC OXYGEN TOXICITY

Under hyperbaric conditions, 100% oxygen accelerates the development of pulmonary oxygen toxicity (see Chap. 16). Exposure to pure oxygen at 2-atm pressure results in the onset of dyspnea within about 8 hours. Vital capacity will begin to decrease after several hours (Fig. 15–4). However, the major toxicity of oxygen at a partial pressure greater than 2 atm is a characteristic central nervous system syndrome. This often appears as the first symptom in a hyperbaric environment.[15] Early manifestations are diverse and include muscular twitching, nausea, vertigo, paresthesias, and mood changes. Any of these minor symptoms may be rapidly followed by a grand mal seizure. If oxygen exposure is terminated at the onset of convulsions, there is usually no evidence of residual brain damage. Of course, physical trauma, especially in a debilitated patient, is a real danger during the seizure. The appearance of this syndrome is related to both the partial pressure of arterial oxygen and the duration

Figure 15-3. Chemical mechanism of oxygen toxicity: free radical theory. (Drawn with suggestions by Dr. Edward R. Block)

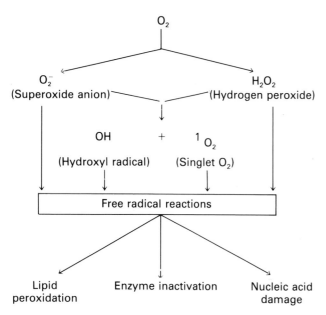

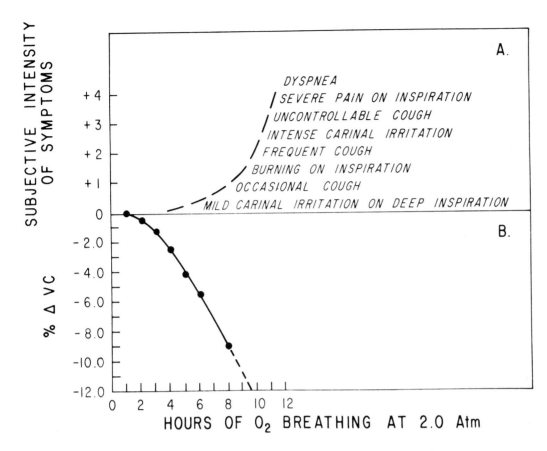

Figure 15—4. The early clinical stage of oxygen toxicity. *(A)* Progression from mild (1+) to severe (4+) symptoms over the first 12 hours of exposure to 2.0 atm of oxygen. *(B)* Percentage of reduction of vital capacity (%ΔVC) with respect to time.

of exposure. The symptoms may appear in fewer than 2 hours at 3 atm or within a few minutes at 6 atm of oxygen. The mechanism of this toxicity appears to be complex.

RETROLENTAL FIBROPLASIA

If excessive oxygen is administered to a premature newborn infant, immature retinal vessels constrict and endothelial cells are damaged.[23,31] Subsequent abnormalities, including disorganized vascular proliferation and retinal destruction, appear between the 3rd and 6th week of life. These changes may progress to retinal detachment and blindness. The amount of retinal destruction depends on the degree of immaturity of the newborn, the length of exposure, and importantly, the arterial PO₂. It is not clear what the exact limits of oxygen tolerance are for the newborn retina; however, if the inspired ox-

ygen concentration is adjusted to maintain the arterial PO₂ between 60 and 100 torr (the range of normal for the newborn), the risk of retrolental fibroplasia is minimized.[23,31]

Retinal injury can also occur in adults after exposure to 100% oxygen. This is especially true under hyperbaric conditions. Patients with previous retinal disease (i.e., a history of retinal detachment causing compromised retinal circulation) are especially vulnerable.

MODES OF OXYGEN DELIVERY

The many delivery devices available for supplemental oxygen can be divided into two major groups.[38] A *low-flow oxygen system* is an apparatus the oxygen flow of which is not intended to provide the total inspiratory requirements of the patient.

Table 15—5   Oxygen Concentrations for Delivery Systems*

SYSTEM	O_2 FLOW RATE (L/min)	F_IO_2 RANGE
Nasal cannula	1	0.21–0.24
	2	0.23–0.28
	3	0.27–0.34
	4	0.31–0.38
	5–6	0.32–0.44
Venturi masks	4–6 (total flow = 105)†	0.24
	4–6 (total flow = 45)	0.28
	8–10 (total flow = 45)	0.35
	8–10 (total flow = 33)	0.40
	8–12 (total flow = 33)	0.50
Simple masks	5–6	0.30–0.45
	7–8	0.40–0.60
Masks with reservoirs	5	0.35–0.50
Partial rebreathing	7	0.35–0.75
	10	0.65–1.00
Nonrebreathing	4–10	0.40–1.00

* Values listed in this table are approximate.

† Values for total gas delivered are for the Accurox Venturi Mask.

Each tidal volume contains a variable amount of room air. Accordingly, the inspired oxygen concentration is variable and is influenced by the patient's ventilatory pattern. A *nasal cannula* is an example of a low-flow oxygen system. This remains true even if the oxygen source for the apparatus is set at a high flow rate.

On the other hand, a *high-flow system* has a reservoir and a total gas flow that supplies the entire inspired volume. The patient's ventilatory pattern has no effect on the inspired oxygen concentration. Under most circumstances, a *Venturi mask* falls into the high-flow category. In the intubated patient attached to a ventilator, a designated F_IO_2 at a level that ranges from that of room air to 100% can be prescribed. Because of the ventilator reservoir and flow rates, this is also a high-flow oxygen system.

Several factors must be considered before selecting the technique for administering supplemental oxygen to patients. The desired range of the fractional oxygen concentration limits the type of the apparatus. If there is a danger of reducing the respiratory drive, especially in patients with hypercapnia, low-concentration, controlled oxygen therapy is warranted.

Commonly used methods of delivering oxygen in nonintubated patients will be described in the following sections (Table 15-5).

NASAL CANNULA AND PRONGS

Low concentrations of inspired oxygen can be provided by nasal cannula or prongs, which are generally inexpensive, well-tolerated by patients, and are among the most commonly used oxygen therapy devices. This simple system delivers 100% oxygen through two prongs inserted 1 cm into each anterior naris (Fig. 15–5A). The cannulas are made of unobtrusive, soft plastic and are generally comfortable for long-term use. The nasal passages should be patent. Mouth breathing does not, however, significantly affect the final oxygen concentration since inspired ambient airflow in the oral pharynx entrains oxygen from the nasopharynx. The prongs must also be positioned properly because a malposition can reduce the F_IO_2.

Because this is a low-flow oxygen system, the final concentration of oxygen received by the patient depends on a mixture of ambient air and oxygen and, therefore, is sensitive to changes in tidal volume and ventilatory pattern. If the tidal volume is large, the F_IO_2 will be low; if the tidal volume is small, the F_IO_2 will be higher. A child will receive a higher F_IO_2 with nasal prongs than will an adult given the same oxygen flow rate. This flow rate system does not provide a low concentration of oxygen if the patient is hypoventilating. On the other hand, a hyperventilating, dyspneic patient may receive a

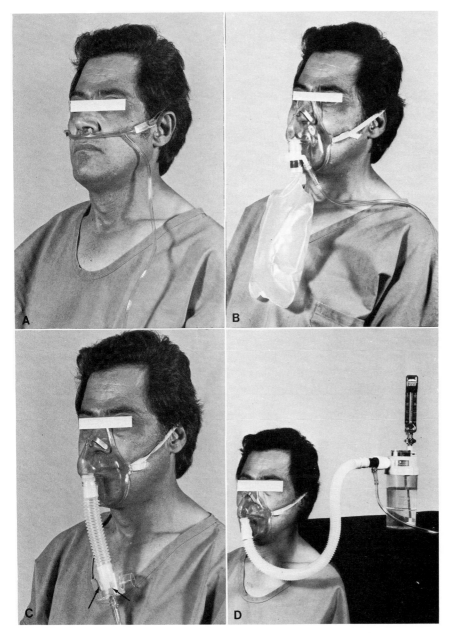

Figure 15–5. *(A)* Nasal prongs. The patient is receiving 100% oxygen at a low flow rate (i.e., 2 l/min.). *(B)* Tight-fitting mask with reservoir bag. The patient is breathing 100% oxygen delivered by the thin tubing to both the mask and a reservoir bag. Note the mask contains two one-way expiratory valves to permit exhalation without F_IO_2 dilution. The reservoir bag supports high flow rates. *(C)* Venturi mask. The source gas entering the thin tubing is 100% oxygen but is diluted down to a fixed F_IO_2 (i.e., 24, 28, 35, 40%) by the air as it enters the specially constructed openings (arrows) of the Venturi system. This unit is equipped with a humidification port as well. *(D)* High airflow oxygen enrichment with nebulization. Gas (air/O_2) at a high flow rate is provided from a Venturi-type nebulizer. Low flow-rate oxygen can be delivered through a side port, producing oxygen enrichment in the wide-bore tubing with resultant oxygen levels between 22% and 40% F_IO_2.

reduced F_IO_2 because of increased dilution with ambient air. Therefore, if nasal prongs are selected for oxygen supplementation, the arterial PO_2 must be monitored frequently to measure the therapeutic effect. Alternatively, oxygenation may be followed with an oximeter.

Generally, flow rates of 1–4 l/min are used, with the desired F_IO_2 ranging from about 24% to 40%. Higher flow rates by nasal cannula (i.e., 7–8 l/min) should be avoided because they cause crusting of secretions and drying of the nasal mucosa. Despite these various practical limitations, nasal prongs have many valuable uses:

- For long-term domiciliary oxygen requirements.

- For patients without hypercapnia who require supplemental oxygen up to an F_IO_2 of 40%.
- For patients who require low concentrations of controlled oxygen but who cannot tolerate mask devices

VENTURI MASKS

A technique based on the Bernoulli principle is one of the most accurate methods of delivering a prescribed dose of oxygen. These masks are engineered to provide controlled oxygen by flowing 100% oxygen through a narrowed orifice, resulting in a high-velocity stream that creates a "subatmospheric" pressure after leaving the orifice. This, in turn, entrains room air through multiple open side ports at the base of the mask. Primarily, by altering the orifice size, the F_IO_2 can be varied (Fig. 15–5C, 15–6). Above a minimum oxygen flow, the flow rate can be altered without causing a substantial change in the ratio of oxygen to entrained room air. Venturi masks can provide a range of specific oxygen concentrations from 24 to 50%. These masks are accurate to within 1% to 2% of the stated concentration imprinted on the base of the mask.[16] As a result of the entrainment of large quantities of air, a large volume of enriched gas is delivered to the patient. Therefore, the pattern and volume of the patient's ventilation will not affect the specific inspired oxygen concentration delivered by these masks.

Venturi masks have many clinical uses, and their value has been well proved. They are particularly efficacious in treating hypoxic–hypercapnic respiratory failure when there is a danger of respiratory depression from excessive inspired oxygen concentrations. Furthermore, the 40% Venturi mask is particularly useful in patients who are in no danger of respiratory depression, but who require prolonged oxygen treatment at nontoxic oxygen concentrations. There are several disadvantages from this mask: a feeling of claustrophobia, especially in an anxious, dyspneic patient; the removal of the mask by patients so that they may ingest meals or expectorate; and discomfort. Also, because this system requires high-flow rates of oxygen, it is relatively expensive and not practical for extended home use.

OPEN FACE MASK

Simple open face masks cover the nose and mouth and deliver oxygen concentrations up to 60%. Oxygen flow rates of 5–6 l/min are required so that the patient does not accumulate carbon dioxide within the mask. Open face masks do not allow precise inspired oxygen concentrations and are impractical in situations requiring controlled oxygen therapy. If the mask is designed to fit the patient's face tightly, the amount of ambient air dilution with each inspiration will be lower; therefore, a higher inspired oxygen concentration will be achieved. One of the main uses of simple masks is humidification of aerosol therapy with oxygen. A disadvantage is that the F_IO_2 is variable and depends on the ventilatory pattern.[17] Other limitations are similar to those of all face masks, including discomfort and frequent removal.

PARTIAL REBREATHING MASK

To deliver more than 60% oxygen to a nonintubated patient, a reservoir bag must be added to a tight-fitting mask. If there are no one-way valves between the mask and the bag, this is referred to as a partial rebreathing mask. However, this name is misleading because the bag serves as an oxygen reservoir, not as a carbon dioxide reservoir. An oxygen flow rate of approximately 5–6 l/min must be applied so that the bag does not completely collapse during inhalation; then only a small portion of early exhaled gas will enter the bag as it is reinflated. This

Figure 15–6. Air flow diagram with Venturi mask. Arrows indicate direction of flow.

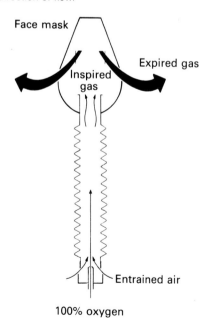

Face mask

Expired gas

Inspired gas

Entrained air

100% oxygen

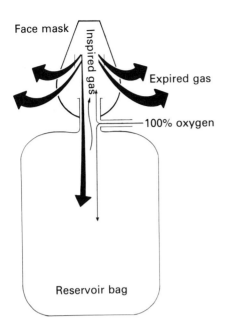

Figure 15—7. Air flow diagram with partial rebreathing mask. Arrows indicate direction of flow.

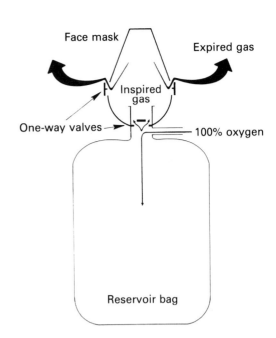

Figure 15—8. Air flow diagram with nonrebreathing mask. Arrows indicate direction of flow. Note one-way valve.

early exhaled gas, which originates primarily from dead space, contains very low amounts of carbon dioxide (Fig. 15–7). The rebreathing mask can provide adjustable inspired oxygen concentrations up to about 80%. Because minimal room air enters the system, the FIO_2 is fairly predictable, even if the patient's ventilatory pattern exceeds the flow rate of the oxygen source. This method is best suited for short-term support of a patient who requires a high FIO_2.

NONREBREATHING MASK

The nonrebreathing mask differs from the partial rebreathing mask in that one-way valves allow the patient to inhale only from the reservoir bag and exhale through separate valves on the side of the mask (see Fig. 15–5B, 15–8). If the mask has a tight seal over the face, it is designed to deliver 90% to 100% oxygen. Those masks that fit tightly are used less commonly because of discomfort.

INDICATIONS FOR SHORT-TERM OXYGEN THERAPY

The primary goal of oxygen therapy is to supply adequate oxygen to tissues for metabolic functions. Under most circumstances the PaO_2 is used as a guide for oxygen deficiency at the tissue level. However, PaO_2 is just one of many variables of oxygen delivery. Tissue oxygenation depends on several other critical factors: the transport of oxygen by hemoglobin, cardiac output, and the cellular uptake of oxygen. There is an important difference between hypoxemia and hypoxia. *Hypoxemia* is a reduction of oxygen tension in arterial blood below the range of normal for age; *hypoxia* is deficiency of oxygen at the tissue level.[3,39] Hence, hypoxemia is one of the causes of hypoxia and only one of the variables of oxygen delivery. Tissue hypoxia can occur in the absence of hypoxemia.

ARTERIAL HYPOXEMIA

Arterial hypoxemia should be demonstrated and quantified before oxygen therapy is initiated, unless an emergency situation prevents measurement. The absolute level of hypoxemia at which supplemental oxygen is indicated for all patients is debatable. There is general agreement that an arterial PO_2 less than 45 mmHg requires urgent treatment. However, on a physiologic basis, many patients receive supplemental oxygen at an arterial PO_2 of 60 mmHg or less. Below this level, oxygen saturation rapidly drops for small decreases in arterial oxygen tension (Fig. 15–9).

In contrast, an arterial PO_2 higher than 60

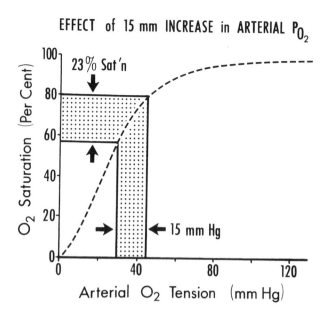

EFFECT of 15 mm INCREASE in ARTERIAL P$_{O_2}$

Figure 15—9. Hemoglobin dissociation curve illustrating large increase in oxygen saturation for modest increase in arterial oxygen tension in the hypoxic patient who starts out on the steep portion of the curve. (Block AJ: Management of pulmonary insufficiency. In The Acute Cardiac Emergency. Mt. Kisco, New York, Futura Publishing, 1972. Reproduced with permission)

mmHg may indicate a need for oxygen therapy in certain unstable patients with acute conditions, such as pneumonia, pulmonary embolism, or myocardial infarction. An arterial oxygen tension above 70 mmHg will permit some changes in PaO$_2$ caused by sudden deterioration in gas exchange, without significant changes in oxygen saturation. The arterial oxygen tension that is minimally acceptable for each patient will be influenced by oxygen delivery, patient tolerance, and symptoms of hypoxia.

Arterial hypoxemia is the reason that most patients need supplemental oxygen. As reviewed in Chapters 8 and 10, there are four pathophysiologic mechanisms for hypoxemia: alveolar hypoventilation, a diffusion defect, ventilation-perfusion mismatching, and right-to-left intrapulmonary or cardiac shunt. Although more than one mechanism may be operative in a given patient with respiratory failure, one disorder often predominates. The most common cause of hypoxemia in lung disease is mismatching of ventilation and perfusion. The next most frequent abnormality is intrapulmonary right-to-left shunts secondary to such diseases as pneumonia, atelectasis, or ARDS. These two common physiologic mechanisms of hypoxemia can be dis-

tinguished rapidly by noting the effect caused by increasing the inspired oxygen concentration (Fig. 15–10). The arterial PO$_2$ increases readily in patients with ventilation–perfusion mismatching. In patients with right-to-left shunts, the arterial PO$_2$ does not improve significantly. Even increasing the inspired oxygen concentration to 100% will increase the arterial PO$_2$ by only a few mmHg in severe shunting.

The goal of acute oxygen therapy is to provide a PaO$_2$ sufficient to assure adequate tissue oxygenation, without causing side effects such as oxygen toxicity or depression of overall ventilation. A division of patients with acute respiratory failure into two categories on the basis of arterial blood gas abnormalities is helpful: (1) hypoxemia with concomitant hypercapnia and (2) hypoxemia without concomitant hypercapnia.

Hypoxemia with Hypercapnia

Hypoxemia with hypercapnia is a particularly common type of respiratory failure in patients with chronic bronchitis and emphysema. The hypoxemia associated with episodes of decompensation results from both ventilation–perfusion mismatching and alveolar hypoventilation.

Acceptable levels of PaO$_2$ can be achieved by treating these patients with minimally elevated inspired oxygen concentrations. This improvement results because ventilation-perfusion mismatching (and not right-to-left shunting) is a major cause of hypoxemia (see Fig. 15–10). In addition, these patients are frequently less responsive to the respiratory stimulus of an elevated PaCO$_2$. Therefore, they depend on the effects of hypoxia on peripheral chemoreceptors to preserve nonvoluntary respiratory control. This hypoxic respiratory drive is functional when the PaO$_2$ is less than 60 mmHg.[13] Controlled low-dose oxygen, the cornerstone of therapy for most hypoxemic patients, corrects hypoxemia without depressing the hypoxic drive.[4,5] Furthermore, at a PaO$_2$ of 60 mmHg, hemoglobin is approximately 90% saturated with oxygen. Since the upper portion of the oxyhemoglobin dissociation curve plateaus beyond this point, additional increases in PaO$_2$ only minimally increase hemoglobin saturation. Thus, in acute respiratory failure secondary to COPD, the appropriate objective is to elevate the PaO$_2$ to the range of 50 to 60 mmHg. This permits adequate tissue delivery of oxygen, without depressing overall ventilation. Small increments of inspired oxygen can be delivered by nasal prongs at a low-flow rate or by a Venturi

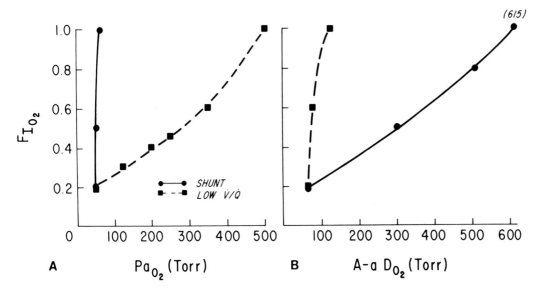

Figure 15—10. *(A)* The effects of increasing fractional inspired oxygen (F_IO_2) on arterial oxygen tension (PaO_2) in patients with shunt and low ventilation-perfusion relationships ($\dot{V}/\dot{Q}$). A patient with a 50% shunt has a change in arterial oxygen tension from 50 to 60 torr. By contrast, a patient with low $\dot{V}/\dot{Q}$ has a change in arterial oxygen tension from 50 to more than 500 torr. *(B)* The effects of increasing F_IO_2 on alveolar-arterial oxygen difference (A-aDO_2) in these two patients. In a patient with a shunt, raising the F_IO_2 serves to markedly widen to A-aDO_2. By contrast, in a patient with low $\dot{V}/\dot{Q}$ there is little widening of this gradient.

Figure 15—11. Regression lines for different inspired percentages of oxygen. (F_IO_2). Each line gives the expected arterial oxygen tension and applied F_IO_2. The relationship was obtained with patients in acute respiratory failure (*dashed lines*) and stable patients (*solid lines*). If a patient with chronic obstructive pulmonary disease presents with a certain arterial PO_2 on room air (*horizontal axis*), the resulting arterial $PO_{2'}$ after supplemental oxygen (*vertical axis*) can be predicted for an applied F_IO_2. (Bone RC: Arch Intern Med 140:1018, 1980. Reproduced with permission.)

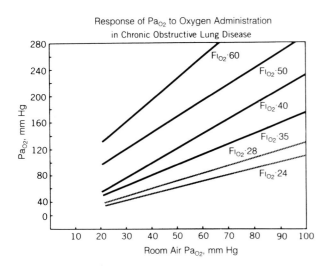

mask. If a Venturi mask is used arterial PO_2 can be reasonably predicted.[5] For example, on a 24% Venturi mask, arterial PO_2 rises 8 to 10 mmHg (Fig. 15–11). Although low concentrations of oxygen are used to produce an acceptable arterial oxygen level, other therapy is directed at reversing the factors that precipitated respiratory failure, such as bronchospasm or superimposed infection. In most patients, intubation or mechanical ventilation can be avoided.[13]

Hypoxemia Without Hypercapnia

Noncardiogenic pulmonary edema or ARDS is characterized by a diffuse lung injury that results in increased capillary permeability and lung edema.[36] As a consequence of alveolar flooding and atelectasis, an intrapulmonary shunt ensues. Large numbers of alveoli are perfused, but not ventilated. As expected, the hypoxemia responds poorly to supplemental oxygen. In contrast, elimination of carbon dioxide usually is not a problem during the early stages of ARDS. Most patients exhibit hypoxemia with a normal or low carbon dioxide level. Therefore, supplemental oxygen administration is not concerned with suppression of the ventilatory drive. The dilemma, instead, is that the continuous high inspired oxygen concentrations necessary to raise the blood oxygen to a minimally acceptable level increase the risk of pulmonary oxygen toxicity. If the PaO_2 cannot be raised to at least 60 mmHg with nontoxic supplemental oxygen therapy, maneuvers such as mechanical ventilation with PEEP must be initiated. The PEEP appears to reestablish the patency of airways and alveoli by increasing lung volume. Therefore, ventilation of gas exchange units within the lung improves, resulting in a decrease in shunting and improvement in PaO_2. Consequently, inspired oxygen tensions can be lowered to a nontoxic range.

TISSUE HYPOXIA WITHOUT HYPOXEMIA

Tissue hypoxia can exist in the absence of arterial hypoxemia. In most of these instances, oxygen therapy is not helpful in correcting tissue hypoxia. Some common uses of oxygen therapy in this area are controversial, such as administration of high concentrations of oxygen to athletes to facilitate performance. In contrast, benefits are well established in a few disorders, such as carbon monoxide poisoning. If a high concentration of oxygen is used, it must be supplied for brief periods to avoid oxygen toxicity. The indications for oxygen therapy in several hypoxic clinical situations will be reviewed.

Anemic Hypoxia. In acute hemorrhage or severe anemia, tissue hypoxia may occur because of the reduced oxygen-carrying capacity of blood. Primary treatment should be directed at increasing the hemoglobin level. However, increased inspired oxygen tension is palliative until blood transfusions are available.

The major benefit of oxygen therapy is to increase the oxygen content of blood. Since hemoglobin is near maximum saturation at a PaO_2 greater than 100 mmHg, the primary benefit of further arterial oxygen elevation relates to dissolved oxygen in plasma. If the PaO_2 is raised to approximately 600 mmHg, nearly 2.0 mL of oxygen is dissolved in each 100 mL of blood. This form of oxygen can, to a small but important degree, enhance oxygen delivery to tissues. (see Chap. 16)

Circulatory Hypoxia. Oxygen therapy is generally recommended for patients with hypotension and congestive heart failure. Usually, arterial oxygen tension is reduced; however, even in the face of a normal arterial PO_2, inadequate tissue perfusion may result in tissue hypoxia. The mixed venous oxygen tension has been proposed as another index of measuring tissue oxygenation (see Chap. 10). An increased inspired oxygen concentration is useful as palliative therapy until circulatory abnormalities can be corrected.

Cyanide Poisoning. Cyanide, a rapid-acting poison, is an example of agents that will cause cytotoxic hypoxia. Cyanide is a component of nitroprusside, an antihypertensive agent. It reacts readily with the trivalent iron of cytochrome oxidase in mitochondria of cells. Cellular respiration is inhibited. Oxygen alone has only slightly beneficial effects in cyanide poisoning. However, oxygen may potentiate specific treatment and, therefore, high concentrations should be used.[21]

Carbon Monoxide Poisoning. In this condition, oxygen therapy is more than palliative —it is the definitive treatment to reverse carboxyhemoglobinemia. Carbon monoxide binds to hemoglobin with an affinity greater than 210 times that of oxygen. The PaO_2 remains relatively normal, but tissue hypoxia is present because of reduced oxygen saturation and content. Furthermore, carboxyhemoglobin causes a left shift in the oxygen–hemoglobin dissociation curve, further decreasing oxygen available to tissues. The immediate therapy is administration of as high a concentration of oxygen as possible. The half-life of carboxyhemoglobin is longer than 5 hours when room air is breathed, compared with fewer than 90 minutes when 100% oxygen is breathed. In severe cases of carbon monoxide poisoning hyperbaric oxygen therapy may be indicated[20] (see Chap. 16).

Acute Myocardial Infarction (also see Chap. 33). Supplemental oxygen is routinely given to most patients with acute myocardial infarction.[41] There is no doubt about the efficacy of oxygen if the patient exhibits hypoxemia, a relatively common finding in myocardial infarction. In this situation, the reduced PaO_2 associated with a diminished cardiac output interferes with oxygen delivery. There is, however, some controversy about oxygen therapy in uncomplicated acute myocardial infarction without hypoxemia. In a controlled study, mortality, incidence of arrhythmias, and the use of analgesics were the same, with or without oxygen.[33]

In contrast, other reports of both human and animal studies demonstrate the advantage of oxygen. With use of a technique of ST-T segment mapping to indicate infarct size, early oxygen therapy in the absence of hypoxemia appears to reduce the extent of the myocardial infarction.[24,25] These studies emphasize that high concentrations of oxygen should be used as soon as possible after acute myocardial infarction. Therefore, routine administration of oxygen to patients with acute myocardial infarction and a normal PaO_2 is supported by most studies.

LONG-TERM THERAPY

Continuous low-flow oxygen has emerged as an important aspect of outpatient respiratory therapy regimens, especially for managing patients with advanced COPD. Supplemental oxygen is supplied by both portable and stationary systems to selected patients with manifestations of sustained hypoxemia. Reports have shown that long-term oxygen therapy can improve exercise tolerance, decrease symptoms, return patients to ambulatory status, and prolong survival in patients with COPD.[1,2]

EFFECTS OF LONG-TERM OXYGEN THERAPY

The definitive advantages of long-term oxygen therapy were proved in two hallmark studies reported in the early 1980s: The Nocturnal Oxygen Therapy Trial (NOTT) and the Medical Research Council (MRC) Working Party in the United Kingdom.[35] The NOTT study of advance COPD patients was to determine whether or not 12 hrs/day of oxygen (including the hours of sleep) might be just as effective as continuous oxygen in terms of survival, neuropsychiatric function, and physiologic indicators, including reduction in pulmonary hypertension. In this multicenter project, 203 patients were randomly allocated to either 12- or 24-hr/day oxygen groups. Patients entered this study only if they had clinically stable COPD with an FEV_1/FVC of less than 0.6 and a resting arterial PO_2 of 55 mmHg or less, or an arterial PO_2 less than 60 mmHg, with associated evidence of tissue hypoxia such as polycythemia, cor pulmonale, or electrocardiographic evidence of right ventricular hypertrophy.

Randomization resulted in close matching of the two groups, and the compliance to the oxygen treatment regimen was close to expected. The nocturnal group averaged 11.8 hours of oxygen per day, whereas the continuous group averaged 19.4 hr/day. The results revealed that continuous oxygen therapy is associated with a better survival than nocturnal therapy (Fig. 15–12). In addition, the continuous group required fewer hospitalizations during the 2 years of observation.

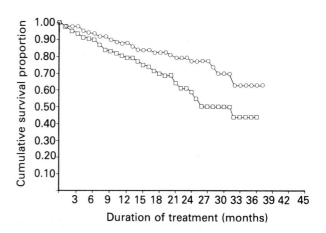

Figure 15—12. Overall mortality of continuous oxygen therapy versus nocturnal oxygen therapy. Vertical axis is fraction of patients surviving; horizontal axis is time for randomization or duration of treatment. Open circles represent continuous oxygen; squares represent nocturnal oxygen. (From Nocturnal Oxygen Therapy Trial Group: Ann Intern Med 93:391, 1980. Reproduced with permission.)

The British Medical Research Council Study compared the benefits of no oxygen therapy versus 15 hours of oxygen a day, including the hours of sleep in 87 patients with severe hypoxic COPD. This randomized trial showed a significant improvement in mortality after oxygen was administered for 500 days, and these benefits continued for up to 5 years. The conclusion of both the NOTT and MRC studies was that long-term oxygen therapy improves the survival rate in hypoxic patients with COPD and that the more continuous the therapy, the better the survival.

Comprehensive neuropsychiatric studies on COPD patients treated with extended oxygen therapy reveal significant changes after correction of hypoxemia. These improvements include intelligence, motor coordination, memory, and visual motor ability. Psychologic studies indicate that patients become more independent, less concerned with social problems, and better equipped to handle emotional stress. The relief of cerebral hypoxemia is postulated as the cause of this improved function.

Polycythemia is an adaptive response to chronic hypoxemia regularly found in high-altitude dwellers. However, the polycythemic response in hypoxemic COPD patients is unpredictable and appears to be inhibited by superimposed infections, iron deficiency, carbon dioxide retention, and congestive heart failure. If, however, secondary polycythemia develops in COPD patients, long-term oxygen therapy has been beneficial in reversing this compensatory mechanism.[28]

Pulmonary artery resistance and pressure increase in patients with COPD after induced hypoxemia and correlate inversely with the level of arterial saturation.[6] The pulmonary hypertension in these patients is partly related to the vasoconstrictor response to the reduce arterial PO_2. Studies have shown that the pulmonary artery pressure is favorably affected with correction of arterial hypoxemia by domiciliary oxygen given over extended periods. The NOTT study suggests that more than 15 hours of oxygen administration per day, but not 12 hr/day, can be effective in lowering pulmonary artery pressure. This response appears to correlate with survival. A long-term oxygen therapy trial in France reported that 15–18 hr/day of oxygen can reverse the progression of pulmonary arterial hypertension in a significant proportion of patients.[43]

SELECTION OF PATIENTS AND DURATION OF TREATMENT

Long-term oxygen therapy has been most widely applied to patients with COPD, although the indications are certainly not confined to this disease.[29,32] Conditions covered under most current reimbursement guidelines include other primary lung diseases such as diffuse interstitial lung disease, cystic fibrosis, bronchiectasis, and pulmonary neoplasm. Whatever the underlying illness, arterial hypoxemia or tissue hypoxia must be documented. Candidates should have persistent resting hypoxemia, with an arterial PO_2 of 55 mmHg or less when breathing room air. The patient should be under optimal medical management, including treatment of bronchospasm, pneumonia, heart failure, and discontinuance of cigarette smoking. A single abnormal arterial blood gas measurement should not be the sole criterion for prescribing home oxygen. Some COPD patients with less severe arterial hypoxemia (PaO2 of 55 to 59 mmHg) are also candidates, but these patients must exhibit one or more manifestations of tissue hypoxia (Table 15–6).[30]

Some patients with severe COPD, as well as patients with pulmonary fibrosis and a resting arterial PO_2 of 60 mmHg, desaturate during exercise. In this group of patients, exercise capacity can improve when portable low-flow oxygen is given. Before oxygen is prescribed, documentation of exercise desaturation by arterial blood gas measurements or oximetry is required. Dyspnea alone is not an indication for supplemental oxygen.

Table 15—6 Blood Gas Criteria for Prescribing Home Oxygen Therapy*

One of the following criteria is met
  PaO2 ≤ 55 mmHg
  Oxygen saturation ≤ 88%
  PaO2 ≤ 59 mmHg with clinical evidence of at least one of the following:
      Pulmonary hypertension
      Right ventricular hypertrophy
      Cor pulmonale
      Erythrocytosis (hematocrit ≥ 55%)

* Established by the Health Care Financing Administration.

The arterial oxygen saturation also decreases to very low values during sleep in some patients with COPD. In some persons, cor pulmonale apparently is potentiated by disordered breathing during sleep, with frequent nocturnal apneic or hypopneic episodes.[6] Some patients do not meet the criteria for continuous oxygen therapy on the basis of their arterial PO_2 while awake, yet might benefit from oxygen while asleep. If cor pulmonale is present disproportionately to awake arterial blood gas findings, desaturation during sleep should be suspected. Confirmation can be obtained by monitoring oxygen saturation during sleep.

The presence of carbon dioxide retention with chronic respiratory acidosis is not a contraindication to instituting long-term oxygen therapy; however, oxygen therapy should first be monitored in the hospital so that the oxygen flow can be adjusted and the effect on the patient's hypercapnia determined. Moreover, the patient must be informed and reliable concerning the dangers of high flow rates. At prolonged low rates of flow that have been used in long-term oxygen therapy, a gradual rise in carbon dioxide tension does occur, but this hypercapnia has been well tolerated by most patients.

TECHNIQUES OF LONG-TERM OXYGEN ADMINISTRATION

Oxygen is most often administered at home with a nasal cannula at a predetermined low flow rate, usually 2 L/min. In patients with advanced COPD; however, this flow rate dose may vary in the same patient depending on the ventilatory pattern. Mild increases in oxygen flows may be necessary during exercise or sleep. In the nocturnal oxygen trial, 1 L/min *more* oxygen was provided during exercise and sleep than during the rest of the day.[28] Goals of extended oxygen therapy include improvement in the quality of life, allowance of an ambulatory existence, and, for some, prolonged survival. To accomplish this, both stationary and portable systems have been developed to provide practical, relatively inexpensive sources of oxygen. Portable systems allow the patient to be ambulatory and away from a large reservoir for up to 8 hours. Oxygen sources for home use are provided by conventional high-pressure oxygen cylinders, low-pressure liquid oxygen, or devices that concentrate oxygen from ambient air.[26,29,32]

Compressed Gas

Large oxygen tanks, usually of the H-K size, are preferable to smaller high-pressure oxygen cylinders because of the relative cost. Disadvantages of tanks include the need for frequent change of the tanks, and their heavy weight and the possible torpedo hazard. Either the tank or the valve apparatus is a potential projectile, given sufficient damage to the valve end of the tank. Long extension tubing can be attached that will allow a patient some mobility within the home. Small portable tanks, containing nearly a 3-hour supply of oxygen at a flow of 2 L/min, are also widely available. These cylinders, some of aluminum construction, can be transfilled from a large reservoir tank at home. Transfilling must be done carefully because of the fire hazard that can result if any petroleum product lubricant is applied to the transfilling connectors.

Liquid Oxygen Systems

The low-pressure liquid oxygen system comprises a reservoir canister and a light-weight, readily transfillable portable device. Oxygen liquefies when its temperature is decreased to −183° F (−119.4°C). The resulting volume of oxygen is less than 0.2% of an equivalent amount of oxygen at atmospheric pressure and temperature. Liquid oxygen is stored in a low-pressure, vacuum-insulated reservoir canister that usually contains about 40 lb of oxygen. This reservoir can provide a continuous flow of 2 L/min for 4-1/2 days.

Portable units that weigh about 11 lb can supply enough oxygen to last about 8 hours at a flow rate of 2 L/min. The low pressure of the liquid oxygen systems allows lightweight construction of these portable units. This type of system allows the patient to be ambulatory and away from the reservoir for extended periods. Liquid oxygen is more expensive than compressed gas therapy, and most reservoirs require filling about twice a week.

Concentrators

The most recent development in home oxygen therapy is the oxygen enricher or oxygen concentrator. Ambient air is pumped through either banks of molecular sieves or a semipermeable membrane, which then preferentially separates oxygen from nitrogen. These devices can operate on household electricity and can deliver about 90% oxygen at a flow rate of 2 L/min. The oxygen concentrators are initially expensive and are not portable. Small

Table 15—7   Characteristics of Three Oxygen Conservation Methods

	TRANSTRACHEAL	RESERVOIR CANNULA	DEMAND DELIVERY
Mechanism of conservation	Reduces dead space, some storage	O₂ storage during exhalation	Inspiratory-only delivery
Advantages	Unobtrusive, may have better compliance	Disposable, least subject to mechanical failure	Maintains O₂ savings ratio over usual delivery ranges
Oxygen savings	2 : 1 to 3 : 1	2 : 1 to 4 : 1	3 : 1 to 7 : 1
Necessity for humidification	Unnecessary	Unnecessary	Unnecessary
Obtrusiveness	Least obtrusive	Most obtrusive	Same as steady-flow
Disadvantages	Catheter kinks, dislodges, plugs with mucus; surgical complications (e.g., infection, subcutaneous emphysema)	Most obtrusive	Most subject to mechanical failure

(Tiep BL: Oxygen conservation and oxygen-conserving devices in chronic lung disease. Chest 92:25, 1987, reproduced with permission)

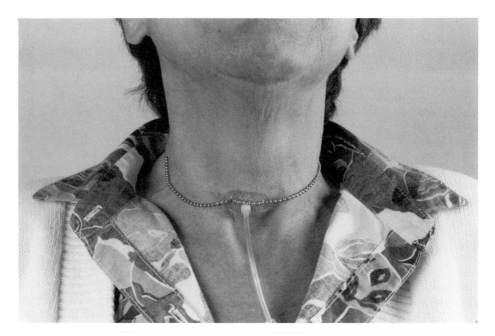

Figure 15–13. Transtracheal oxygen therapy (TTO$_2$T) device. (Courtesy of Transtracheal Systems, Denver, Colorado)

high-pressure tanks cannot be filled from these devices. However, this system is inexpensive for long-term use and convenient for continuous oxygen therapy. A 50-ft tube can allow ambulation in the home. A separate portable system may be necessary if the patient leaves his or her home. Disadvantages of the system are the added expense of electricity and the possibility of electrical outage. Patients should be advised to have a separate source of oxygen, such as a compressed oxygen tank, in the event of an electrical failure.

Oxygen-Conserving Devices (Table 15–7)

The high cost of long-term oxygen therapy necessitated methods to improve the efficiency of oxygen administration. The conventional continuous low-flow nasal cannula wastes oxygen during expiration and to the anatomic dead space. Patients with COPD spend 60% to 70% of the respiratory cycle in expiration. An additional 15% to 20% of oxygen is lost to dead space. Furthermore, the delivered volume (and thus concentration) of oxygen drops as the respiratory rate rises. Three types of oxygen-conserving devices are currently available: transtracheal oxygen delivery (tracheal catheter), reservoir cannula, and a pulse-dose demand valve.[40]

Transtracheal Oxygen Delivery. Oxygen is delivered into the trachea through a small plastic catheter (Fig. 15–13). This catheter is introduced by a transtracheal puncture and is directed toward the carina. Storing oxygen in the trachea reduces oxygen waste. Transtracheal catheters are used with standard oxygen equipment. Studies have shown greater than 50% oxygen savings. An additional advantage is that the catheter is hidden from view by a scarf.[9] Complications, other than clogging of the catheter by mucus, are few and primarily result from the transtracheal puncture itself.[7]

Reservoir Oxygen Delivery Systems. Reservoir devices allow oxygen to be stored during expiration and to be available to the patient at the beginning of inhalation. With these reservoirs a lower oxygen flow rate is required to achieve adequate oxygen saturation in the blood. Two reservoir configurations are presently available: the mustache-configured nasal prongs* (Fig. 15–14) and a pendant* (Fig. 15–15).[19] Reservoir nasal cannulae have been reported to produce up to 72% oxygen savings at low-flow rates. Disadvantages of reservoir systems include not only the conspicuous appearance, but

---

* Supplied by Oxymizer, Chad Therapeutics, Woodland Hills, California.

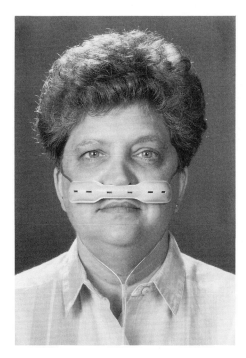

Figure 15—14. A mustache-configured reservoir oxygen delivery system. (Courtesy of CHAD Therapeutics, Inc., Chatsworth, California)

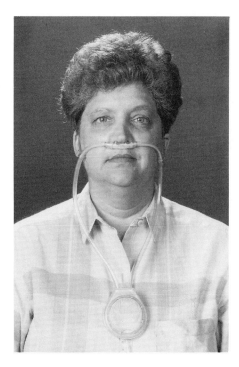

Figure 15—15. A pendant reservoir oxygen conserving device. (Courtesy of CHAD Therapeutics, Inc., Chatsworth, California)

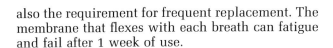

also the requirement for frequent replacement. The membrane that flexes with each breath can fatigue and fail after 1 week of use.

Pulse-Dose Demand-Valve Delivery Systems. Demand oxygen-conserving devices deliver oxygen only when the patient inhales, thus conserving oxygen when he or she exhales. Demand devices function by opening a solenoid valve at the onset of inspiration, allowing pressurized oxygen to flow to the patient. Commercially available systems differ in the type of sensor that detects the onset of inspiration through a standard nasal cannula. Devices operate using either electronic, fluidic, or combined electronic–fluidic sensors. The major advantage of demand-valve devices is the elimination of the need to adjust oxygen flow when a patient's respiratory rate changes. This is especially relevant for advance COPD patients during exercise. The oxygen flow must increase in the same proportion as the patient's respiratory rate. Disadvantages of the demand systems include cost, mechanical failure, and problems with sensing if the cannula becomes clogged.

REFERENCES

1. Anthonisen NR: Home oxygen therapy in chronic obstructive pulmonary disease. Clin Chest Med 7:673, 1986
2. Anthonisen NR: Long-term oxygen therapy. Ann Intern Med 99:519, 1983
3. Anthonisen NR: Hypoxemia and O_2 therapy. Am Rev Respir Dis 126:729, 1982
4. Bone RC: Acute respiratory failure and chronic obstructive lung disease: Recent advances. Med Clin North Am 65:563, 1981
5. Bone RC, Pierce AK, Johnson RL: Controlled oxygen administration in acute respiratory failure in chronic obstructive pulmonary disease: A reappraisal. Am J Med 65:896, 1978
6. Boysen AG, Block AJ, Wynne JW et al: Nocturnal pulmonary hypertension in patients with chronic obstructive pulmonary disease. Chest 76:536, 1979
7. Christopher KL, Spofford BT, Petrun MD et al: A program for transtracheal oxygen delivery. Ann Intern Med 107:802, 1987
8. Bryan CL, Jenkinson SG: Oxygen toxicity. Clin Chest Med 9:141, 1988
9. Claiborne RA, Paynter DE, Dutt AK et al: Evaluation of the use of an oxygen conservation device in long-term oxygen therapy. Am Rev Respir Dis 136:1095, 1987
10. Deneke SM, Fanburg BL: Normobaric oxygen toxicity of the lung. N Engl J Med 303:76, 1980

11. Edwards DK, Dyer WM, Northway WH Jr: Twelve years' experience with bronchopulmonary dysplasia. Pediatrics 59:839, 1977
12. Fisher AB: Oxygen therapy: Side effects and toxicity. Am Rev Respir Dis 122(Part 2):61, 1980
13. Fulmer JD, Snider GL: National Conference on Oxygen Therapy. Chest 86:236, 1984
14. Jackson RM: Molecular, pharmacologic, and clinical aspects of oxygen-induced lung injury. Clin Chest Med 11:73, 1990
15. Gabb G, Robin ED: Hyperbaric oxygen, a therapy in search of diseases. Chest 92:1074, 1987
16. Gibson RL, Comer PB, Beckham RW et al: Actual tracheal oxygen concentrations with commonly used oxygen equipment. Anesthesiology 44:71, 1976
17. Goldstein RS, Young J, Rebuck AS: Effect of breathing pattern on oxygen concentration received from standard face masks. Lancet 2:1188, 1982
18. Grant WJ: Medical Gases: Their Properties and Uses. Chicago, Year Book Medical Publishers, 1978
19. Hoffman LA: Patient response to transtracheal oxygen delivery. Am Rev Respir Dis 135:153, 1987
20. Ilano AL, Raffin TA: Management of carbon monoxide poisoning. Chest 97:165, 1990
21. Isom GE, Way JL: Effect of O_2 on cyanide intoxication: Reactivation of cyanide-inhibited glucose metabolism. J Pharmacol Exp Ther 189:235, 1974
22. Jackson RM: Pulmonary oxygen toxicity. Chest 88:900,1985
23. James LS, Lanman JT (eds): History of oxygen therapy and retrolental fibroplasia. Pediatrics 57(suppl):591, 1976
24. Madias JE, Madias NE, Hood WB Jr: Precordial ST segment mapping: Effects of oxygen inhalation on ischemic injury in patients with acute myocardial infarction. Circulation 53:411, 1976
25. Maroko PR, Radvany P, Braunwald E et al: Reduction of infarct size by oxygen inhalation following acute coronary occlusion. Circulation 52:360, 1975
26. McDonald GJ: Long-term oxygen therapy delivery systems. Respir Care 28:898, 1983
27. McPherson SP: Respiratory Therapy Equipment. St Louis, CV Mosby, 1977
28. Nocturnal Oxygen Therapy Trial Group: Continuous or nocturnal oxygen therapy in hypoxemic chronic obstructive lung disease. Ann Intern Med 93:391, 1980
29. Petty TL: Practical tips on prescribing home oxygen therapy. Postgrad Med 84:83, 1988
30. Petty TL, Snider GL: Further recommendations for prescribing and supplying long-term oxygen therapy. Am Rev Respir Dis 138:745, 1988
31. Phibbs RH: Oxygen therapy: A continuing hazard to the premature infant. Anesthesiology 47:486, 1977
32. Pingleton SK: Home oxygen therapy for ambulant COPD patients. J Respir Dis 3:35, 1982
33. Rawles JM, Kenmure ACF: Controlled trial of oxygen in uncomplicated myocardial infarction. Br Med J 1:1121, 1976
34. Redding JS, McAlfee DD, Parham AM: Oxygen concentrations received from commonly used delivery systems. South Med J 71:169, 1978
35. Report of the Medical Research Council Working Party: Long-term domiciliary oxygen therapy in chronic hypoxic cor pulmonale complicating chronic bronchitis and emphysema. Lancet 1:681, 1981
36. Rinaldo JE, Rogers RM: Adult respiratory distress syndrome: Changing concepts of lung injury and repair. N Engl J Med 306:900, 1982
37. Sackner MA, Landa J, Hirsch J et al: Pulmonary effects of oxygen breathing: A 6-hour study in normal men. Ann Intern Med 82:40, 1975
38. Shapiro BA, Harrison RA, Walton JR: Clinical Applications of Respiratory Care. Chicago, Year Book Medical Publishers, 1982
39. Snider GL, Rinaldo JE: Oxygen therapy: Oxygen therapy in medical patients hospitalized outside of the intensive care unit. Am Rev Respir Dis 122(Part 2):29, 1980
40. Tiep BL: Oxygen conservation and oxygen-conserving devices in chronic lung disease. Chest 92:263, 1987
41. Valencia A, Burgess JR: Arterial hypoxemia following acute myocardial infarction. Circulation 40:641, 1969
42. Wagner PD, Laravuso RB, Uhl RB et al: Continuous distribution of ventilation–perfusion ratios in normal subjects breathing air and 100% O_2. J Clin Invest 54:54, 1974
43. Weitzenblum E, Santegeaw A, Elrhart M et al: Long-term oxygen therapy can reverse the progression of pulmonary hypertension in patients with chronic obstructive pulmonary disease. Am Rev Respir Dis 131:493, 1985
44. Wilson RS, Laver MB: Oxygen analysis: Advances in methodology. Anesthesiology 37:112, 1972

BIBLIOGRAPHY

Chemical Properties

Grant WJ: Medical Gases: Their Properties and Uses. Chicago, Year Book Medical Publishers, 1978

McPherson SP: Respiratory Therapy Equipment. St Louis, CV Mosby, 1977

Adverse Effects of Oxygen Therapy

Fisher AB: Oxygen therapy: Side effects and toxicity. Am Rev Respir Dis 122(Part 2):61, 1980

Indications for Acute Oxygen Therapy

Snider GL, Rinaldo JE: Oxygen therapy in medical patients hospitalized outside of the intensive care unit. Am Rev Respir Dis 122(Part 2):29, 1980

Chronic Oxygen Therapy

Anthonisen NR: Home oxygen therapy in chronic obstructive pulmonary disease. Clin Chest Med 7:673, 1986

Petty TL: Practical tips on prescribing home oxygen therapy. Postgrad Med 84:83, 1988

Pingleton SK: Home oxygen therapy for ambulant COPD patients. J Respir Dis 3:35, 1982

Modes of Oxygen Delivery

Shapiro BA, Harrison RTA, Walton JR: Clinical Application of Blood Gases. Chicago, Year Book Medical Publishers, 1982

Oxygen Conserving Devices

Christopher KL: A program for transtracheal oxygen delivery. Ann Intern Med 107:802, 1987

Tiep BL: Oxygen conservation and oxygen-conserving devices in chronic lung disease. Chest 92:263, 1987

General

Fulmer JD, Snider GL: National Conference on Oxygen Therapy. Chest 86:236, 1984

SIXTEEN

Hyperbaric Oxygen Therapy

David A. Desautels

Hyperbaric oxygen (HBO) therapy is the administration of oxygen at pressures greater than atmospheric. Patients are placed inside a cylindric vessel, known as a hyperbaric, recompression, or decompression chamber, and the pressure is increased. The pressure level to which the chamber is taken is prescribed by treatment schedules designed for each sanctioned disease. Many uses have been proposed, some with questionable scientific basis, to establish credibility within the medical community. The Committee on Hyperbaric Oxygenation of the Undersea and Hyperbaric Medical Society set up three categories of disorders and diseases relative to HBO therapy: (1) disorders currently accepted for HBO therapy, (2) special considerations, and (3) investigational[1] (Table 16–1).

The first concern of hyperbaric oxygen therapy in diving disorders is to reduce the bubble size of intracorporeal oxygen and nitrogen. This is accomplished by increasing chamber pressure to the prescribed depth of 60 to 165 ft of sea water (FSW). This function may be used for a disorder as benign as skin "bends" or as critical as air embolism. The secondary purpose of hyperbaric oxygen therapy is to increase the nitrogen gradient to remove nitrogen from the tissue and to provide therapeutic oxygen to the ischemic areas caused by bubbles.

At increased pressures, the patient's physiology is altered and phenomena relative to increased pressure or increased oxygen tension, or both, can provide therapeutic results. In disorders for which the primary purpose is to provide increased pressure, hyperbaric oxygen therapy is considered the primary mode of therapy. These disorders are *decompression illness* and *air embolism*.

In disorders treated primarily to increase tissue oxygenation, hyperbaric oxygen therapy is considered adjunctive. An exception to this is that of *carbon monoxide* and *cyanide poisoning* for which hyperbaric oxygen therapy is considered the primary mode of therapy, but the purpose is to provide increased oxygen tension at the cellular level.

Hyperbaric oxygen therapy is a realtively new discipline for the respiratory care practitioner. It requires a firm background in the gas laws, the mechanical aspects of respiratory care, and the nuances of medicine; thus, the field is a "natural" for the respiratory care practitioner. In caring for patients from pediatric to geriatric ages, from quite healthy to critically ill, the hyperbaric technologist is unique, combining an industrial equipment orientation with that of a compassionate health care provider.

Despite controversy in the medical community, hyperbaric oxygen therapy is increasing in popularity. With more and more chambers being installed, many respiratory care practitioners are becoming involved in this exciting and highly technical field.

Table 16—1 Indications for Hyperbaric Oxygen Therapy: Approved Uses

Air or gas embolism
Carbon monoxide poisoning and smoke inhalation
Carbon monoxide complicated by cyanide poisoning
Clostridial myonecrosis (gas gangrene)
Crush injury, compartment syndrome, and other acute traumatic ischemias
Decompression sickness
Enhancement of healing in selected problem wounds
Exceptional blood loss (anemia)
Necrotizing soft tissue infections (subcutaneous tissue, muscle fascia)
Osteomyelitis (refractory)
Radiation tissue damage (osteoradionecrosis)
Skin grafts and flaps (compromised)
Thermal burns

(Hyperbaric Oxygen Therapy: A Committee Report. Undersea and Hyperbaric Medical Society, Inc., Bethesda, MD, 1989)

HISTORY

The history of hyperbaric medicine was preceded by a long and tumultuous history in diving, linked more often than not to military triumphs. Aristotle writes of Alexander the Great using a diving bell at the siege of Tyre in 332 B.C. In peacetime, it was used as early as 1531 to raise the *Caligua*, sunk in the Lake of Nemi. In this recovery, Demarchi was able to stay underwater for 1 full hour. Sir Edmund Halley (1656–1742), astronomer of comet fame, dove in the Thames River for 1 hour in a barrel to a depth of 60 ft. He could stay underwater for the full hour because he used two barrels, one for observation and the other to deliver fresh air to the diver at depth. (A brilliant young scientist, he was appointed to the Royal Society. Halley actually paid the cost of the publication of Sir Isaac Newton's famous *Principia*.)

It was not until 1662 that a British physician named Henshaw made a "domicilium," a chamber in which he used high pressure for acute diseases and low pressure for chronic diseases. This, of course, preceded Priestley's discovery of oxygen in 1775. However, Paul Bert is considered the "father of pressure physiology." Born in 1883 to well-to-do parents, he worked on such subjects as nitrous oxide/oxygen anesthesia under pressure, oxygen toxicity, and plant growth under pressure. His classic work, *La Pression Barometrique* is still considered the cornerstone of hyperbaric medicine. In the

United States, HBO therapy began in Philadelphia, then "progressed" to Cunningham's hotel, a five-story treatment facility built in Kansas City in 1928. It was not until 1960 that HBO received a more scientific beginning, with its use in treating gas gangrene and supporting life without blood in anemic patients.

Monoplace chambers were used for clinical therapy only after 1960. The first real clinical use of monoplace chambers was in radiation therapy. It had been demonstrated that some tissue was more radiosensitive under pressure; therefore, radiation therapy was delivered through acrylic hyperbaric chambers.

PHYSICS AND PHYSIOLOGY

As its name implies, HBO therapy is based on the principle of increased pressure and its effect on human physiologic function. The weight of a column of air, reaching from sea level to the outer reaches of space, constitutes the barometric pressure at sea level. Hyperbaric pressure is an extension of that sea level pressure, with 100% oxygen or air under pressure in the HBO chamber. In normal practice, we do not measure sea level pressure or gauge pressure. However, if we are to be accurate in our calculations, we must use absolute pressure, which includes atmospheric pressure and gauge pressure. In respiratory care, we usually measure pressures in centimeters water (cmH_2O), therefore the atmospheric pressure to add to the gauge pressure would be 1033.6 cmH_2O. For each addition of 1033.6 cmH_2O we add 1 atmosphere.

Hyperbaric pressure is the weight of air and water, often measured in feet of sea water, as it extends beneath sea level. Pressure increases are significant because of the added pressure provided by the weight of sea water (Table 16–2). The analogy of going beneath the sea is accurate even if we

Table 16—2 Depth Equivalents in Feet of Sea Water

0 FSW =	0 psig =	14.7 psia =	1 ATA
33 FSW =	14.7 psig =	29.4 psia =	2 ATA
66 FSW =	29.4 psig =	44.1 psia =	3 ATA
99 FSW =	44.1 psig =	58.8 psia =	4 ATA
132 FSW =	58.8 psig =	73.5 psia =	5 ATA
165 FSW =	73.5 psig =	88.2 psia =	6 ATA

FSW, feet of sea water equivalent; psig, pounds per square inch, gauge; psia, pounds per square inch, absolute; ATA, atmospheres, absolute.

remain in a dry environment, such as a hyperbaric chamber. To explain the physics and physiologic principles involved in hyperbaric medicine we will liken it to diving beneath the sea. Progressing through a simulated "dive," we will separate the dive into three processes: the descent, the changes at depth, and the ascent. The pertinent physics and physiologic principles at each stage of the "dive" will be described for clarity. We will discuss the dive from the perspective of the patient and what he or she will experience.

DESCENT

The patient begins the dive by entering the hyperbaric chamber (with an attendant if in a multiplace chamber), and the door is closed. Gas added to this closed environment increases pressure. As the gas enters, noise is created from the turbulent motion of gas rushing into the chamber. Noise levels greater than 90 dB can be measured; protection is provided by muffling the gas as it enters and by ear protection devices. As gas rushes into the chamber, the addition of gas molecules into this closed space creates heat from the Joule-Thomson effect, or friction of molecules colliding. This heat buildup can be uncomfortable to the patient during compression. The rate of compression and amount of ventilation provided can make the temperature more comfortable for the patient. Once the pressure reaches about 8 to 10 ft of sea water (FSW), the pressure differential in any air-filled space in the body can cause barotrauma. The airspaces in the body, such as the lungs, sinuses, middle ears, and even teeth (if improperly filled) must all be pressurized at the same pressure or pain will result.

According to Boyle's law, if the temperature is held constant, the volume will vary inversely with the pressure. This means that if pressure surrounding the patient is doubled, the volume in any airspace will be halved. This is the reason all body airspaces must communicate to the body surface for equilibration in HBO therapy. The middle ear communicates to the surrounding atmosphere by the eustachian tube. This flattened tube acts as a valve, requiring a maneuver called a Toinby maneuver (versus a Valsalva maneuver, which pressurizes the body from the glottis down) to pressurize air behind the tympanic membrane. If pressure is not equalized, the eardrum will be flexed inward to try to fill the space with a volume to equalize the pressure, causing pain. Failure to equalize pressure can result in rupture of the eardrum if descent is continued without equilibration. Unconscious patients who do not have the ability to communicate their discomfort on descent should receive myringotomies or have pressure equalization (PE) tubes placed to prevent eardrum tear. The same pressure effect applies to sinuses, lungs, or airspaces attached to the body (such as a tooth with a filling that has an air pocket beneath it). Failure to equalize pressure in these spaces can cause pain and damage from the body's attempt to reduce the volume by filling the space with body fluids.

As an example, if a diver swims down underwater holding his breath, as he approaches 33 FSW (2 atmosphere, absolute [ATA]) lung volume will halve. Should he continue his descent to depths greater than 132 FSW still holding his breath, the lung is compressed to one-fifth its total volume, or roughly residual volume. Once residual volume is exceeded, pulmonary edema fluids will try to fill the lung. This sets a theoretical depth limit to breath-holding dives; however, some divers can exceed this limit because of their total lung capacity/residual volume ratio. Additionally, all apparatus entering a hyperbaric chamber should be considered sources of potential danger, for the same pressure–volume principles apply. These might include sphygmomanometer cuffs, IV bottles (use only IV solutions in plastic bottles), IV drip chambers, endotracheal tube cuffs, gastric tube cuffs, arterial line pressure bags, ventilation circuits, vials, syringes, medicine bottles, or any device with a closed airspace.

Other interesting phenomena that occur at increased pressure relate to increased gas density: sound travels faster in a dense medium, therefore the voice changes as depth increases; breathing comes more labored; under extreme pressure mitosis stops because cytokinesis cannot occur; cilia do not regenerate; red cells change shape; the peripheral platelet count decreases; and lactic acid increases, causing a leftward shift of the P_{50}.

AT DEPTH

At increased depth, oxygen partial pressure is increased. This increased oxygen partial pressure will suppress the action of the carotid and aortic bodies; suppress respiratory sensitivity to carbon dioxide; decrease the "alveolar splinting effect" played by nitrogen; vasoconstrict blood vessels, thereby decreasing blood flow to the brain, coronary arteries, and eyes; and cause bradycardia. Once hemoglobin is fully saturated, the only increase in oxygen content that can occur is that of dissolved oxygen. *Under hyperbaric conditions, 2 vol% of oxygen are added, in a linear fashion, for each additional atmosphere compressed.* Breathing 100% oxygen at 2.4 ata (45 FSW), a PaO_2 of 1707 mmHg or 5.3 vol% of physically dissolved oxygen will occur.

In carbon monoxide intoxication, this physically dissolved oxygen can sustain life until the carbon monoxide unloads from the hemoglobin.

Oxygen under pressure at depth is not without hazards. Like any drug, oxygen can be toxic at increased concentrations. Oxygen under pressure can be toxic in two ways: pulmonary and cerebral.[2]

Pulmonary oxygen toxicity, known as the *Lorrain–Smith effect*, is caused by exposure to oxygen at concentrations greater than 40% for extended periods. Hyperbaric oxygen therapy patients are exposed to high-concentration oxygen therapy for short intervals on a daily basis; this exposure is dose-related and cumulative. Patients are observed on a daily basis for progressive symptoms, such as tickling cough, symptoms of carinal irritation and burning, uncontrollable cough, dyspnea, decreased tidal volume, tracheobronchitis, or atelectasis. Even attendants working in the hyperbaric chamber should be aware of the potential for diminishing vital capacity (5% to 10% after 4.5 hours at 2 ATA), diffusing capacity, compliance (15% after 6 hours at 2 ATA), PO_2 during exercise, and widening of $A-aDO_2$ (after 6 hours at 2 ATA). Most symptoms return to normal after 12 hours at normobaric pressures. No treatment is required other than removal from high-concentration oxygen.

Cerebral oxygen toxicity, known as the *Paul Bert effect*, is encountered any time 100% oxygen is breathed at pressures greater than 2 ATA. Cerebral oxygen toxicity is dose-related; therefore, as depth increases, the time to onset of symptoms becomes shorter. Because the therapeutic effect of hyperbaric medicine is from high oxygen partial pressures and because most therapy schedules in multiplace chambers go to 2 to 3 ATA, a solution for this problem is necessary. The solution is to use an oxygen/air-breathing schedule that allows the patient to breath air every 20 minutes (so called "air breaks") (Fig. 16–1). After a 5-minute air-breathing period, another oxygen-breathing cycle of 20 minutes is conducted. Any sign that the patient is becoming toxic is a signal to switch the patient from oxygen to air. Symptoms of cerebral oxygen toxicity include nausea, eye twitch, excitation, rigid tonic phase, unconsciousness, clonic contractions, amnesia, hiccups, headache, aphasia, weakness, and eventually grand mal seizures. To prevent oxygen toxicity, one should maintain body temperature, normal metabolic state, and decrease work. Treatment is not necessary, as symptoms cease as soon as the hyperbaric oxygen therapy is discontinued.

On occasion, a patient is taken to depths equivalent to 165 FSW. At this depth, because of the toxic effects of oxygen, alternative gas mixtures such as air, nitrogen–oxygen (nitrox), or helium–oxygen (heliox) are breathed. These gas mixtures each create their own unique problems. The mixtures used the most are air and nitrox (50:50). By Dalton's law, each gas exerts its own pressure proportional to the percentage of the total gas that it represents. In air, nitrogen exerts 80% of the partial pressure and in nitrox 50%. This "inert" gas is not so inert at extreme depths. In his book *The Silent World*, Cousteau popularized the term "l'ivresse des grandes profondres" or "rapture of the deep" to describe the narcotic effect of nitrogen at great depths. According to the Meyer Overton theory, this anesthetic effect of nitrogen, or any inert gas, is that the narcotic potency is equal to the solubility of the agent in lipids. The inert gas gains access to the nervous system by virtue of lipid solubility. There is some evidence that carbon dioxide retention potentiates the onset of nitrogen narcosis. Varying the inert gas can occasionally reduce the potential for narcosis; however, complications of decompression can result from indiscriminate alteration of the inert gases. The effects of nitrogen or inert gas narcosis require only one circulation of blood through the system to affect the patient because of the vascular nature of the central nervous system (CNS). The greatest effects are noted within 2 minutes of reaching depth, and any detrimental symptoms will be no worse after 30 minutes. Symptoms of inert gas narcosis include euphoria, a false sense of well-being, and paranoia. Symptoms occur in stages (Table 16–3).

Reasoning ability is affected the most, followed closely by a decrease in reaction time. The least affected ability is mechanical dexterity and motor skills (Table 16–4). Emotionally stable individuals are better able to cope with nitrogen narcosis and, once given a task, can carry it out. However, if the task should change, the individual is not able to think it through to a new solution.

This is why medical decisions should be made outside the chamber. Mistakes are easily made at depth under the influence of nitrogen narcosis. Strong-willed individuals are better able to cope with nitrogen narcosis, and, in fact, this may be an additive factor along with anxiety, fatigue, rapid descent, and carbon dioxide retention. Training for

DECOMPRESSION SICKNESS

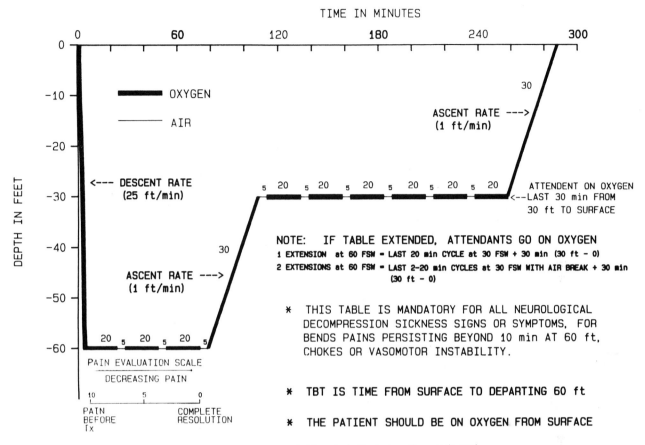

Figure 16—1. United States Navy Treatment Table 6: Time is indicated on the x axis and depth on the y axis. Oxygen-breathing periods are represented by bold lines on the x axis, whereas air is represented by thin lines.

Table 16—3   Stages of Narcosis

Stage 1: 100–200 ft, primary nerve centers affected, mild feeling of drunkenness, light-headed, loss of fine discrimination, euphoria

Stage 2: 200–250 ft, secondary nerve centers affected, inhibitions released, poor judgment, slow reflexes, peripheral numbness

Stage 3: 250–300 ft, lower nerve centers affected, relaxation and lapsing into total submission, pronounced numbness, decreased coordination, drowsiness

Stage 4: 300–400 ft, progressive depression, sensory problems, impairment of neuromuscular coordination

(Bennert PB: The Aetiology of Compressed Air Intoxication and Inert Gas Narcosis, London, Pergamon Press, 1966)

multiplace chamber attendants must include a deep dive to determine their ability to work at depth. Recovery from symptoms is rapid and there are no ill effects.

ASCENT

The ascent is the most dangerous part of the dive. The patient is cautioned to breath normally, and ascent is carried out in a slow, controlled manner. Deviation from this can cause tragedy. As Boyle's law affects volume on descent, so also does it affect ascent. If the patient has breathed compressed air at depth, additional molecules are packed into the lungs. Should the patient hold his breath, lock his

Table 16—4 The Effects of Nitrogen Narcosis on Body Function

	DECREMENT AT	
	100 ft	400 ft
Reasoning ability decreased	33.46%	61.6%
Reaction time decreased	20.85%	
Mechanical dexterity decreased	7.9 %	

(Kiessling RJ, Maag CH: Performance impairment as a function of nitrogen narcosis. J Appl Psychol 46: 91–95, 1962)

glottis, have laryngospasm, or panic in any way during a rapid uncontrolled ascent, there is a possibility of overdistending or stretching the lung until it tears. This is most acute as the patient nears the surface, because this is the zone of greatest pressure change.

An ascent of only 1 ft, *while holding the breath*, will increase the pressure in the lungs by 31 cmH$_2$O and its volume by 1/33. If volume expansion is allowed to inflate the lung, without any splinting, the lung will tear. Think of a balloon held between the hands while inflating it. Pressure can get very high before the balloon bursts; however, if the balloon is inflated without being held, it will expand to bursting with little pressure in it. From this analogy, we know that it takes a rise of only 4 to 8 ft to tear the lung.

A tear in the lung can cause free air to dissect along connective tissue lines and to appear in any one of three places: the pleura, as a pneumothorax; the mediastinum, as a pneumomediastinum and, subsequently, subcutaneous emphysema; or the blood vessels, to appear as air embolism.

A pneumothorax will present as chest pain or dyspnea, or both. Should a pneumothorax occur at depth in the multiplace chamber, pressure is increased in the chamber until the patient can breath easily. The patient is placed on the affected side until a surgeon can insert a chest tube. In a multiplace chamber, treatment of the pneumothorax is necessary before ascent can continue.

Treatment of a pneumothorax that develops inside a monoplace chamber necessitates removal of the patient from the chamber, while a tube thoracotomy is performed. The chest tube is attached to a one-way Heimlich valve to prevent air entry into the thorax when monoplace chamber therapy is resumed.

When air enters the mediastinum or subcutaneous tissue in the neck area, the symptoms will be crepitus, chest pain, difficulty swallowing, or change in voice, or a combination thereof. Treatment is usually not necessary. However, the patient should be closely watched for a potential air embolism, which can often accompany this phenomenon.

On the other hand, when air gets into a blood vessel in the form of an air embolism, it is a true medical emergency that is treated immediately with compression to 165 FSW to shrink the bubble size. Immediate diagnosis and action are essential to survival. The first thing to be done for the patient is to place him or her head down and on the left lateral side in the hope that this will cause bubbles to rise to the feet instead of the brain. Symptoms of an air embolism include tunnel vision, acute loss of consciousness, respiratory distress, seizure, paralysis, convulsion, or death by coronary or cerebral occlusion. More objective signs that may be seen include air bubbles in retinal vessels, pallor of the tongue, marbling of skin, hemoptysis, focal or generalized convulsions, and neurologic abnormalities. Treatment by recompression (see Fig. 16–1) will usually reverse symptoms if treatment is immediate; any delay in beginning therapy reduces the chance of complete recovery.

Decompression illness is usually not a risk for patients undergoing hyperbaric oxygen therapy because of the oxygen inhaled. The possibility of decompression illness occurs when one breathes an inert gas for an extended period at increased pressure. Attendants who accompany the patients in multiplace chambers are at risk because they breathe air during their depth exposure.

According to Henry's law, the solubility of gas in a liquid at a given temperature is proportional to the partial pressure of the gas above the solution. This defines only the relative quantity of gas entering solution, related to gas partial pressure, not the absolute amount in physical solution. The absolute amount of dissolved gas is determined by a solubility coefficient that varies with the gas. This means that at increased pressures, tissues will absorb increasing amounts of gas in an attempt to equilibrate with the gas tension in the blood. The equilibration takes a finite period, depending upon the pressure differential and vascularity of the tissue.

Thus, when the attendant is decompressed, the tissue will have the increased pressure, rather than the blood. As pressure around the body decreases, the tissue pressure gradient increases to a point at which an excessive gas tension is created and gas (usually nitrogen) will come out of solution and cause a bubble. This is similar to opening a carbonated beverage quickly. The bubbles formed in this manner will press on nerve endings and cause symptoms known as decompression illness or "bends." Symptoms are graded into four forms, depending upon the location of the bubble:

Type I: Pain only symptoms—bubbles in joints
Type II: Neurologic symptoms
> Spinal cord symptoms: paresthesia, paralysis, balance, incontinence, seizures, visual disturbance, headache
> Brain symptoms: unconsciousness, paralysis, visual disturbances
> Pulmonary symptoms: dyspnea, substernal pain, nonproductive cough with cyanosis (called "chokes")
Type III: Vestibular symptoms—bubbles in inner ear
Type IV: Orthopedic symptoms—long-term bubbles in long bones

First aid for decompression illness is to provide oxygen and fluids and to position the victim as though for air embolism, because the neurologic symptoms of one are indistinguishable from those of the other, and precautions must be taken against the potential for air embolism. Treatment is prompt recompression and then decompression according to prescribed treatment tables (see Fig. 16–1). Response to treatment in the hyperbaric chamber is subjective; therefore, it is not advisable for the patient to take any analgesics before arrival and during treatment. The ability to detect symptoms can dictate the course of his or her therapy.

The proper use of decompression tables removes most, but not all, risks inherent in hyperbaric exposures. The variability in human physiology can add risk to the process of decompression. It is known that age, temperature, fitness, obesity, trauma, smoking, fatigue, drugs (such as alcohol), dehydration, and being female can increase the risk of decompression illness. It is also known that having once had decompression illness predisposes the patient to developing it again. Therefore, prevention is the cornerstone of proper decompression practices. Close supervision of all hyperbaric chamber dives must be in a professional manner to avoid subjecting patients or attendants to decompression illness. Adjustments in decompression schedules must be made for the amount of work, temperature, and rate of ascent.

Any of the foregoing complications of therapy can occur, and each must be explained to the patient on the informed consent. However, with proper precautions, training, quality controls, and procedure standards, hyperbaric oxygen therapy is a routine procedure.

CHAMBERS

Hyperbaric chambers are of two general types: multiplace (more than one occupant) or monoplace (single occupant). Multiplace chambers may have one or more compartments, which are interconnected. The National Fire Protection Association (NFPA) classifies chambers as follows:

Class A: Human, multiple occupancy
Class B: Human, single occupancy
Class C: Nonhuman

Chambers are constructed from steel or acrylic according to the American Society of Mechanical Engineers—Pressure Vessels for Human Occupancy (ASME-PVHO-1) standards. The ASME certifies pressure vessels that are stationary, whereas the Department of Transportation (DOT) certifies vessels that cross state lines. Each must be hydrostatically tested upon manufacture. The DOT vessels are tested every 5 years thereafter. The ASME vessels are identified by the method of manufacture and the fact that they have a drain valve installed on them.

As in any enclosed space in which oxygen or compressed air is introduced, fire hazard is a primary consideration. If any electricity is delivered into the chamber, it must have explosion-proof connectors and lighting; for the most part, electricity is not provided inside chambers. If it is, any electrical connection made inside the chamber must be completed before the chamber is compressed and not disconnected during the dive. Electrical and mechanical penetrations can be made for both multiplace and monoplace chambers so that monitoring is provided. Pressure transducers must be vented and calibrated before the door is closed.

Multiplace chambers (Fig. 16–2) are pressure vessels that may have more than one compartment, although not always (Fig. 16–3), which allow personnel to enter and leave the main treatment compartment at will. A multiplace chamber is large enough to accommodate one or more patients, plus

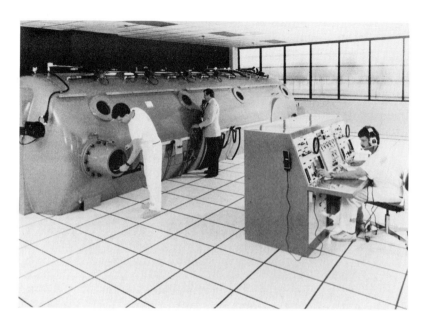

Figure 16—2. A multiplace HBO chamber.

an attendant. It has an additional compartment attached that serves as a lock through which additional personnel or supplies are compressed to the depth of the patient. Hyperbaric chambers are used in the commercial diving industry as well as in medicine. The major difference is the mode of use; most commercial diving chambers are closed-circuit systems (the chamber is sealed and only metabolic oxygen is added to the chamber as needed, while a CO_2 scrubber removes the CO_2). On the other hand, medical chambers are generally used as open-circuit systems (air ventilating the chamber is exhausted from the chamber).

Monoplace chambers (Fig. 16—4) resemble the "iron lungs" of yesteryear, which accommodate only one patient at a time. They have no additional compartment or direct access to the patient under pressure. However, with careful forethought and special devices, critical patients are treated in monoplace chambers, and one can monitor anything that can be monitored in a multiplace chamber. Because of the ease of installation, ease of operation, smaller space requirements, and expense considerations, use of monoplace chambers has proliferated.

Monoplace chambers are simple to operate and

Figure 16—3. A hybrid HBO chamber.

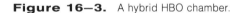

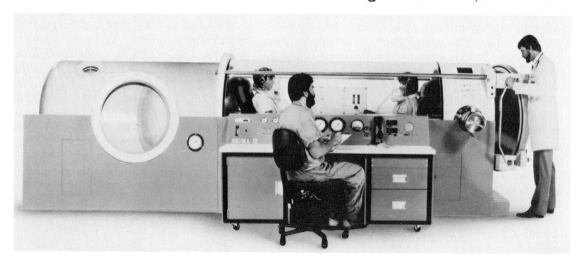

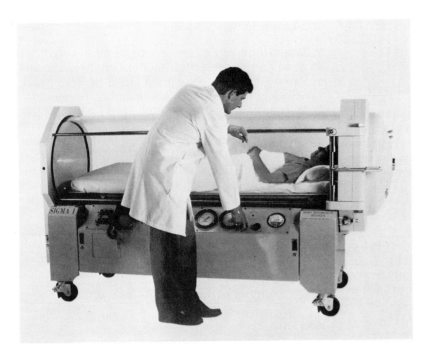

Figure 16–4. A monoplace HBO chamber.

quite comfortable for the patient (unless he or she is claustrophobic). The rate of descent and ascent is controlled, and the patient is completely visible during the operation. This allows the patient to see his or her surroundings and, in routine care, the patient can watch television, listen to the radio, and such. No electrical or battery-operated devices can be used inside a monoplace chamber. However, cables penetrating the chamber can measure ECG, temperature, respiration, pressure, and any other parameter that needs measuring. Transcutaneous oxygen should not be measured because of the electrical voltage carried to the measurement site by the sensing electrode. The patient is grounded to the gurney tray, and all jewelry must be removed to avoid scratching the acrylic hull.

In a monoplace chamber a one-way valve is placed into the intravenous system as it enters the hull of the chamber to prevent exsanguination, and special pumps and high-pressure tubing are used. Should the patient need defibrillation, the patient is removed completely from the chamber and quickly moved to an area away from the chamber. All the patient's clothing is removed before placing the paddles and defibrillating the patient. In the event of seizure or cardiac arrest, the patient is vented to the surface by the emergency ascent valve (button).

CHAMBER SYSTEMS

Materials, connecting piping, portholes, and electrical and support equipment must also meet the standards of ASME–PVHO-1, as well as National Fire Protection Association (NFPA) 99, Compressed Gas Association (CGA) (air purity), American National Standards Institute (ANSI), United States Coast Guard (USCG), Occupational Safety and Hazard Association (OSHA), and Joint Commission of Accreditation of Health Organizations (JCAHO) (pending).

CONSTRUCTION

The hyperbaric chamber is usually cylindrical, lying flat or on end, but it can be spherical. It must be constructed in accordance with the ASME–PVHO-1 Standards, grounded, and any pipe or fitting that attaches to the structure must be of compatible material. Metallic surfaces are painted with inorganic zinc or high-quality epoxy or an equivalent, which is flame-resistant to prevent corrosion and deterioration. The multiplace chamber's interior is fitted with bunks, a medical suction system, communication equipment, and breathing apparatus for all occupants.

An in-chamber ventilator is available for the patient who needs ventilation, i.e., CO_2 removal, during HBO treatment.

Pressurization and Depressurization System

The pressurization–depressurization apparatus encompasses ancillary equipment, such as the compressor system, receiver, and valves to pressurize or depressurize the chamber(s), which may consist of the main compartment, lock compartment, or medical lock in the multiplace system.

Breathing Gas System

The breathing apparatus delivers air, oxygen, or any gas mixture to the personnel inside the chamber. This system can also include compressors, booster pumps, cylinders, and oxygen administration systems such as flowmeters, masks, and hoods (see Equipment section).

Fire Detection and Protection System

The fire detection–protection system is of prime importance in HBO therapy. Only by always being on guard for fire can one avoid these catastrophic events. In the multiplace chamber, the fire system consists of a deluge system, fire detection system, fire hoses, and a pump to increase regular water pressure to that required by the increased pressure of the system. Manual backup systems are required for this essential system. Monoplace chambers do not usually have these fire suppression systems.

Electrical Systems

The electrical systems are for support services, outside the chamber. Electricity is usually not supplied inside; however, some chambers use explosion-proof connections and lights. Emergency electrical backup is required to maintain support during power failures; this may be as simple as a battery or as complex as the hospital emergency power-generating system.

Communication Systems

Communication must have open systems from inside to outside the chamber. To ensure that all conversations inside the chamber are heard, it must also have an emergency backup, even if this consists of a writing pad or a previously agreed upon set of hand signals.

Air-Conditioning Systems

Air-conditioning systems are required if a chamber is used in the saturation mode. Otherwise, a safe internal environment is maintained by periodic or continuous venting of the chamber (monoplace chambers vent at a rate of 200–400 L/min). Multiplace chambers operated in the closed-circuit mode are not vented. Oxygen consumed by the occupants is replaced, whereas carbon dioxide is absorbed with a carbon dioxide scrubber. In the open-circuit mode, multiplace chambers are vented for high carbon dioxide, high oxygen (multiplace chamber only), temperature, and comfort (Table 16–5).

In an open-system chamber, carbon dioxide buildup is determined by the resting minute volume (RMV) of the occupants. The normal ventilation rate is given by the following formula:

$$\text{Number of occupants} \times 12.5 \text{ ft}^3/\text{min.}$$

SAFETY

Emergencies

Emergencies can involve the chamber system or patient. Virtually any medical emergency that can occur may happen inside a hyperbaric chamber. We will discuss only those situations unique to the hyperbaric chamber.

The most dreaded of all hyperbaric chamber emergencies is fire. In monoplace chambers, a fire is catastrophic; therefore, the only answer is pre-

Table 16–5 Ventilation Schedule for One Resting Patient and Active Attendant[3]

DEPTH (FT)	VENTILATION FOR OXYGEN (SCFM)	VENTILATION FOR AIR (PATIENT BREATHING OXYGEN) (SCFM)
10	16	9
20	20	10
30	24	12
40	28	13
50	31	15
60	35	17
80		21
100		24
120		29
140		31
165		36

SCFM, standard cubic feet per minute.

vention. Three factors must be present to cause a fire: burnable materials, proper oxygen concentration, and an ignition source. In hyperbaric chambers, especially the monoplace chamber, the oxygen concentration is high enough to cause just about any material to burn. Therefore, all burnable materials and ignition sources are removed. Close attention must be paid to all clothing that personnel wear inside the chamber (cotton or fire retardant cloth—no nylon), dressings containing petroleum-based lubricants, and battery-operated or electrical systems inside, unless they are contained in a unit that is nitrogen purged. The oxygen-breathing systems must be scavenged to the outside.

In multiplace chambers, oxygen concentration is maintained at minimal levels to reduce the fire hazards by venting the chamber at regular intervals to maintain oxygen levels below 24% referenced to the surface. The NFPA Code 99 addresses hyperbaric chamber environments and sets standards to avoid fire.

Because of these standards, personnel have survived multiplace fires in recent years. Fire burn is not the only hazard in multiplace chamber fires. The most acute hazard is inhalation of toxic fumes. Therefore, the procedure for a fire in a multiplace chamber would have the inside attendant first put a full-face mask supplied by air for himself and then care for the patient. After that is accomplished, the sprinkler system is tripped or a hose is used. The outside operator may trip the sprinkler system, while the inside attendant is putting on the mask, and turn off the oxygen supply. Halon 301 fire-extinguishing gas can also be used, as it does not harm chamber personnel.

Another feared accident in the multiplace chamber is an explosive decompression. The proper procedure here is to remain far away from the port while the chamber is decompressing and, then, once the surface pressure is reached, seal the port with a port plug and prepare for recompression to treat the potential decompression illness that results. One standard that hyperbaric chambers must meet is hydrostatic testing. Hydrostatic testing is done by filling the chamber with water and increasing the pressure to 25% above working pressure, then measuring the expansion and contraction of the chamber. The vessel must return to within 10% of its original size. Unlike DOT-certified cylinders, those certified by ASME do not have to be tested on a regular basis. The ASME-certified cylinders are identified by the drain valve on their ventral side.

A fire that occurs in the area surrounding the chamber while occupants are inside is also a critical problem. Codes require that sprinklers be installed in rooms housing hyperbaric chambers. However, difficult decisions must be made about the safety of the chamber occupants and the outside operators when a fire breaks out in an area. All attempts should be made to bring the occupants safely to the surface before evacuation procedures are started.

Gas purity can also be a problem. If chamber air becomes fouled, a separate freestanding backup air-breathing system can be used, which is also always available for fires.

Occupational Safety

Occupational safety considerations are necessary to assure the health and safety of chamber personnel. Such workers are at risk for decompression illness and occupational accidents such as the difficult positioning while carrying patients through small hatches, lifting patients to cots when normal bed-transfer mechanisms do not work, high sound levels, infections related to high humidity in enclosed spaces, ear problems, and various hazards from devices that can explode or implode (e.g., the LifePac portable defibrillator implodes at 100-ft depth).

EQUIPMENT

Monoplace chambers are compressed with oxygen; therefore, the patient breathes chamber oxygen, unencumbered by any breathing device, throughout the therapy period (unless ventilatory support is required). Multiplace chambers, on the other hand, are compressed with air; therefore, the patient must always breathe through some respiratory device to receive the therapeutic effect of oxygen.

In the multiplace chamber, the patient receives 100% oxygen delivered by a tightly fitting demand-valve oxygen mask, special hood, T-tube, or ventilator. Each of these devices must scavenge the exhaled gas and exhaust it outside the chamber to maintain low levels of oxygen concentration in the chamber environment. Aviator masks with demand valves attached for inhalation and exhalation are the best type of oxygen delivery systems for patients who can tolerate them. Hoods, which can be more comfortable for patients with orofacial complications, are of two types: one is taped to the chest, the other has a closure around the neck. Each has an inlet and outlet. The inlet is baffled for deflection of incoming gas; the outlet has holes in the adapter to protect against the scavenging system grabbing the patient's cheek. Gas to the patient can be cooled by putting the delivery hose through an ice bucket or by placing ice in the nebulizer. Patients with tracheostomies, endotracheal tubes, and laryngectomies function well with a T-tube setup. However, the attendant must remember the effect of pressure changes on the cuff. Ventilators should be volume cycled,[3] and supply pressure should be 50 psi above ambient. Exhaled gas must be scavenged to the outside of the chamber. Other respira-

tory devices used are a full-face mask and gas mixture breathing devices.

Other equipment used inside multiplace hyperbaric chambers include diagnostic equipment such as stethoscopes, blood pressure cuffs, safety pins, reflex hammers, and monitoring equipment such as ECG and pressure recorders. Emergency equipment must be available inside the chamber or close by, including special trays for thoracentesis, minor procedures, vascular cut-down, thoracotomy/chest tubes, lumbar puncture, tracheostomy, and cardiovascular procedures (Table 16–6).

Table 16—6 Equipment Available Inside or Near Chamber

HYGIENE EQUIPMENT

  Emesis basins
  Urinals
  Bedpan
  Kleenex box
  Chux

SUCTION EQUIPMENT

  Red rubber Robinson suction catheters
  T-connector
  Yankaur suction tube
  Suction kit with glove
  Suction connecting tubing
  Suction canister
  Suction machine
  5 in 1 connector
  Saline for tracheal irrigation

RESUSCITATION EQUIPMENT (RESPIRATORY)

  Self-inflating resuscitator (complete)
  Ventilator
  Laryngoscope
  MacIntosh blades 3 and 4
  Miller blade 6
  McGill forceps
  ET tubes
      3.0, 4.0, 4.5, 5.0, 5.5, 6.0, 6.5, 7.0, 7.5, 8.0, 8.5
  Wire guide
  Mapelson with tubing
  Light bulb for Miller blade

BANDAGE EQUIPMENT

  4 × 4s
  2″ cloth tape
  1″ cloth tape
  ½″ cloth tape

SAFETY EQUIPMENT

  Ear protectors

IV EQUIPMENT

  Tourniquets
  35-mL syringe
  12-mL syringe
  6-mL syringe
  3-mL syringe
  1-mL syringe
  Blood tubes
      Red top
      Purple top
  Needles
      14 g
      16 g
      19 g
      23 g

CARDIAC EQUIPMENT

  Blood pressure cuff
  Stethoscope
  ECG cables
  ECG lead wires
  ECG electrodes
  Redux paste for defibrillator

MEDICATIONS

  Decongestant
  Sterile water, 30 mL
  Sodium bicarbonate, 50 mEq
  Epinephrine 1 : 100
  Calcium chloride, 100 mg
  Potassium chloride, 20 mg
  Dextrose 50%, 50 mL
  Atropine 0.5 mg/5 mL
  Lidocaine 2 g/10 mL
  Lidocaine 100 mg/5 mL

MISCELLANEOUS EQUIPMENT

  Screw clamp
  Needle holder

HYPERBARIC OXYGEN THERAPY

Hyperbaric oxygen therapy is used for primary and adjunctive care (see Table 16–1). It is used as a primary mode of therapy in diving accidents (*decompression illness* and *arterial gas embolism*) because of the mechanical effect of bubble reduction from the increased pressure and, secondarily, for the therapeutic effects of hyperoxygenation. Hyperoxygenation increases the inert gas gradient for off-gassing and repair of ischemic tissue. Tissues off-gas at a rate of 5 mL/sec, whereas the cardiac system off-gasses at a rate of 1 mL/sec in the hyperbaric environment.

The rationale for the high-pressure oxygen utilized in hyperbaric oxygen is multifaceted. In *carbon monoxide* intoxication and *smoke inhalation*, the dissolved oxygen corrects cellular hypoxia, while oxygen, bound to hemoglobin, speeds carbon monoxide elimination and reduces cerebral and intercranial pressure. In *gas gangrene*, the high concentrations of oxygen shut down α-toxin production and, in high enough doses (1500 mmHg), are bactericidal. In *wound healing*, repair will not occur if the PO_2 is less than 30 torr. Therefore, oxygen enhances fibroblastic proliferation, improves collagen synthesis, and improves capillary budding in avascular areas. In *osteomyelitis* and *osteoradionecrosis,* oxygen stimulates osteogenesis and fibroblastic activity, as well as increasing collagen production and neovascularization. In addition, oxygen affects microorganisms present by augmenting antibiotic action and improving phagocytic killing.

In *crush injuries* of the extremities, HBO therapy is used to produce vasoconstriction and is helpful in treating the edema associated with the injury. Tissue oxygenation is maintained and, indeed, improved by this technique, despite the vasoconstriction so induced.

TREATMENT SCHEDULES

Each disease has a recommended therapy schedule that uses oxygen most effectively. In the multiplace chamber, the patient receives high-concentration oxygen through a demand-valve mask, hood, or T-tube. In monoplace chambers, the patient breathes the ambient chamber environment. Therefore, multiplace and monoplace chambers each have their own set of treatment schedules. Monoplace chambers use lower pressure, without air-breathing cycles, for shorter duration, whereas multiplace chambers use higher pressure, with air-breathing cycles interspersed to reduce the oxygen toxicity potential. The disease entity being treated dictates the depth, duration, and number of treatments. Most treatment schedules are empirical; however, many have a long history of success.

Special gas mixtures can be used for the treatment of patients with decompression illness or air embolism. This may even lead to a *saturation dive,* in which the occupants of the chamber remain at the increased pressure long enough to bring their inert breathing-gas mixtures into equilibrium with the tissue. This might take many hours; however, it takes longer to surface from the decompression of a saturation dive (usually 7 to 10 days). If a saturation dive is performed, the logistics become extensive. At increased pressure, nitrogen is added to the system to decrease the oxygen tension to near atmospheric levels; otherwise the attendant inside the chamber will experience oxygen toxicity symptoms and will have significant decreases in vital capacity for extended periods.

STAFFING

A hyperbaric facility must be operated under the medical direction of a physician, preferably one who has hyperbaric medicine training and is interested in its growth and development. Staff members who function as chamber operators, attendants, and supervisors can be from many diverse areas of the medical community. They should be able to demonstrate competence in the technical aspects of HBO therapy, and they must maintain their skill through regularly scheduled training programs. A minimum number of personnel required to be in attendance should be defined for each treatment facility. For multiplace chambers a physician, operator, attendant, and supervisor should be the minimum. However, attendant team size can vary with the condition of the patient. Additional personnel are helpful to serve as timekeepers, recordkeepers, and messengers, as cases warrant. These personnel can be on call until they are needed.

NURSING CARE

Many aspects of hyperbaric nursing care are unique. We only consider these aspects here; it is not our intent to teach nursing practice.

Patients treated inside a hyperbaric chamber can be healthy young adults who have just made a mistake diving and now have "the bends," or they can be badly traumatized patients who will require the constant supervision of a critical care nurse, respiratory therapist, and physician inside the chamber with them. Alternatively, they may be prepared and placed inside a monoplace chamber in which they are isolated until they reach the surface again. Any one of these patients, at any time, can have a crisis that requires extraordinary measures at a moment's notice. It is important for the personnel treating these patients to be constantly vigilant and prepared. The first treatment requires special instructions and patient preparation, including the removal of petroleum-based cosmetics and dressings, watches, nylon clothing, jewelry, burnable materials, devices that cause sparks, or any devices that trap air. All patients should sign an informed consent concerning the potential hazards of HBO treatments, and attempts should be made to reduce the anxiety level. The patient is then reinstructed on how to clear the ears. He or she should be told of the expected temperature changes (hot on descent, cold on ascent), noise, and pressure changes, and how to deal with them. Any untoward noises (such as venting, cylinder movement, or alarms) that might occur during the treatment should be announced to the patient before their occurrence. During changes in depth, the attendant must change the air in all air-filled spaces such as endotracheal cuff tubes, urinary bladder tubes, and gastric tubes. In monoplace chambers these balloons are filled with saline so that pressure changes do not affect them.

The attendant in a multiplace chamber should assure a good mask fit on the patient throughout the dive and should be proficient in administering a neurologic examination. Talking should be minimized during therapy to assure proper oxygenation. On ascent, air passages should be rechecked for patency.

In the monoplace hyperbaric environment, patient care is no different from that at the surface except that access to assistance and equipment is limited. Only a few situations pose special problems inside the chamber; a little forethought can lessen these.

A quick ascent to the surface can jeopardize the health of a normally healthy attendant working inside a multiplace chamber. Before any decision is made to bring occupants to the surface, all alternative methods should be considered and the decompression schedule carefully calculated.

SUMMARY

Hyperbaric oxygen therapy administered in either monoplace or multiplace chambers is a technical modality appropriate for the respiratory care practitioner's armamentarium. Although controlled studies of the efficacy of HBO therapy are still in progress, education in the physics and physiology of hyperbaric medicine should be basic to the field of respiratory care. Growth of the respiratory care practitioner in hyperbaric medicine should be firmly established in the basic tenets of quality patient care, as established by the Undersea and Hyperbaric Medical Society.

REFERENCES

1. Hyperbaric Oxygen Therapy: A Committee Report. Undersea and Hyperbaric Medical Society, Inc., Bethseda, MD, 1989
2. Jenkinson SG: Oxygen toxicity. J Int Care Med 3: 137, 1988
3. Blanch PB, Desautels DA, Gallagher TJ: Mechanical ventilator function under hyperbaric conditions. (Submitted for publication)
4. Wells M: NOAA/UHMS Diving Physician Course Manual. Miami, FL, 1988

SEVENTEEN

Applied Humidity and Aerosol Therapy

Jeffrey J. Ward
H. F. Helmholz, Jr.

This chapter will describe the rationale for, and use of, humidity, aerosols, and related equipment in patient care. The theoretical background may overwhelm those who hope to master the entire science. However, competency in patient care is attainable. Unfortunately, there is a lack of solid scientific basis for some forms of humidity and aerosol therapy. Therefore, the objective of this chapter is to review the literature on the current status of therapy and equipment for humidity and aerosol production to allow respiratory care providers to better evaluate their use of equipment.

Administration of aerosolized medications to the airways is a primary medical treatment. Humidification of inspired gases and addition of bland fluids is also part of current respiratory care procedures. Medical gases for use in therapy and mechanical ventilation require humidification. Chest physical therapy for secretion removal commonly follows airway hydration, before bronchial drainage and chest percussion or vibration.

ANATOMY AND PHYSIOLOGY OF THE MUCOCILIARY SYSTEM

The airways of the respiratory system provide passage of gases to and from the alveoli. The upper airways (nasal, oral, pharyngeal, and bronchial) condition the inspired gas by warming and addi-

tion of water molecules. These surfaces also provide a complex system for clearing the airways of solids and substances dissolved in solution.

The embryologic origin of the lungs is the primitive foregut. The airway-lining cells are epithelial and have some secretory function. These cells line the nasal passages to the terminal bronchioles (Fig. 17–1A, B). The cell population is pseudostratified ciliated columnar epithelium, attached to a basement membrane (Fig. 17–2). The cell shape changes to cuboidal in the alveolated respiratory bronchioles. Each ciliated cell has approximately 200 cilia. These 6-μm long hairlike projections beat synchronously at about 1000 strokes per minute to propel the mucous layer at 10–15 mm/min, from the terminal airways toward the pharynx (Fig. 17–3). The beating cilia are synchronized in a metachronal, wavelike fashion, similar to the "wave" cheer of fans at a sports stadium.

Bronchial secretions are produced by the goblet cells of the columnar epithelium and glands in the bronchial submucosa. Goblet cells lie in a 1 : 5 ratio among ciliated cells. In chronic states of irritation, such as bronchitis and cystic fibrosis, increased numbers of submucosal glands and goblet cells develop. The glands have mucus- and serous-secreting cells and a network of tubules and ducts. They are innervated by parasympathetic branches of the autonomic nervous system and are affected by parasympathetic blocking agents (e.g., atropine)

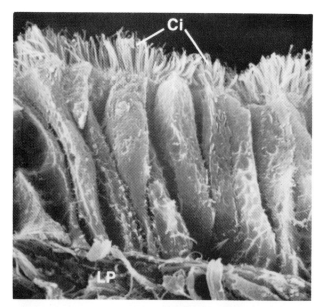

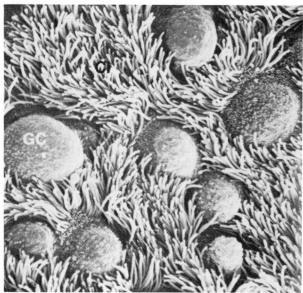

Figure 17—1. Scanning electron micrographs of the bronchial epithelium (A) Cross-sectional view: columnar epithelial cells with cilia (Ci) and lamina propria (LP). (B) Lower-power view from above: ciliated cells interspersed with goblet cells (Gc). (Kessel RG, Karoon RH: Tissues and Organs. A Text-Atlas of Scanning Electron Microscopy, p 210. San Francisco, WH Freeman & Co, 1979. Reproduced with permission)

cause disruption of the normal mucociliary transport system, which provide a basis for rationally selecting candidates for humidity and aerosol therapy (Table 17–1). Inhaled substances, congenital disorders, and pathologic conditions can interfere with normal ciliary activity.[44,72,119,120]

Sputum (secretion from the lower respiratory tract) is a nonhomogeneous, proteinaceous material consisting mainly of glycoproteins–mucopolysaccharides, or mucins. The substance forms long, interconnected fibrous molecules in a gel. Both viscous and elastic components of sputum can be modified by factors such as intermolecular charge and by the presence of other products such as DNA from leukocyte breakdown. The Lucas–Douglas model of in vivo sputum proposes a two-layer system. The less viscous portion, next to the airway wall, is termed the *sol* layer; above that is the *gel* layer. Apparently, the tips of the cilia just touch the gel layer, which is propelled cephalad. During conditions of significant dehydration or in those bypassing the normal "air-conditioning" system, the lack of adequate humidity can lead to drying and disruption of the sol–gel system. In addition, cellular components (such as eosinophils) and differing electrolyte concentrations can alter the viscosity and function of this protective system.[120] The exact

Table 17—1 Factors That Affect Transport of Mucus

DISORDERS THAT PRODUCE EXCESSIVE OR ABNORMAL MUCUS

Cystic fibrosis
Pneumonias (bacterial and viral)
Bronchitis (acute or chronic)
Bronchiectasis
Asthma
Airway burns
Pulmonary neoplasms

CAUSES OF RETARDED CILIARY ACTIVITY

Dehydration (see text)
Alcoholism
Immotile cilia syndrome and Kartagener's syndrome
Tobacco smoke
Trauma/defoliation (e.g., suctioning)
Tacheobronchial infections causing defoliation
Oxygen toxicity
Nitrous oxide and sulfur dioxide
Aspirin or other prostaglandin inhibitors
Alcohol and other depressant drugs
Local and general anesthetics

that reduce secretions and by vagal stimulation that increases activity. Normally, secretion of mucus from all sites amounts to approximately 60–90 mL/day. The exact source of each layer is unclear.[20]

There are several pathologic conditions that

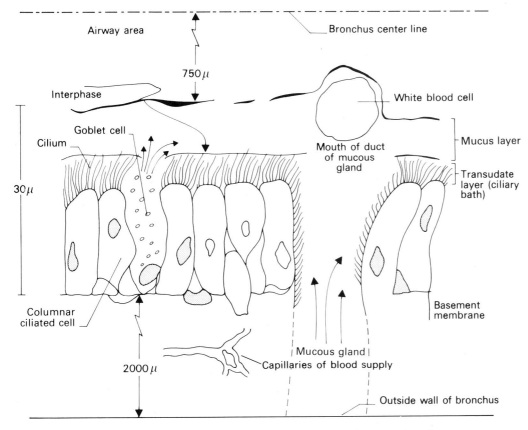

Figure 17–2. Drawing of surface of typical ciliated epithelium. (Adapted from Denton R, Hwang SH, Litt M: Chemical engineering aspects of obstructive lung disease. Chem Eng Progr 62:12, 1966. Reproduced with permission)

Figure 17–3. Drawing of cilium at each phase of beat cycle (metachronal movement). (Adapted from Denton R, Hwang SH, Litt M: Chemical engineering aspects of obstructive lung disease. Chem Eng Progr 62:12, 1966. Reproduced with permission)

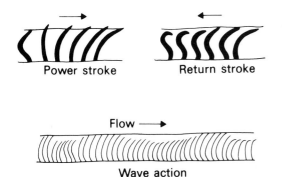

moisture level needed to preserve ciliary activity remains controversial and will be reviewed following the discussion of the related physics.

PHYSICAL PRINCIPLES OF HUMIDIFICATION

Temperature is determining in relation to humidification. It is theory that molecules of a substance are motionless (i.e., there is no kinetic activity) at absolute zero on the Kelvin scale (or −273° K on the Celsius [centigrade] scale) (Table 17–2 gives a temperature conversion chart). *Critical temperature* is defined as the energy level of a substance above which the molecules can exist only as a gas. At or below the critical temperature, substances can be liquefied by compression. Above the critical temperature, compression will not liquefy a gas.

Critical pressure is the vapor pressure of a substance at its critical temperature. It is the pressure

Table 17—2 Relation of Temperature to Water Content and Vapor Pressure (in Saturated Gas)

TEMPERATURE		CONTENT		VAPOR PRESSURE	
C	F	mg/L	mmol/L	mmHg	kPa
0	32	4.85	0.2694	4.58	0.6106
5	41	6.8	0.3777	6.54	0.8719
10	50	9.40	0.5222	9.20	1.2265
15	59	12.83	0.7127	12.79	1.7051
16	60.8	13.64	0.7578	13.62	1.8158
17	62.6	14.47	0.8039	14.51	1.9344
18	64.4	15.36	0.8534	15.46	2.0611
19	66.2	16.31	0.9061	16.45	2.1934
20	68.0	17.30	0.9611	17.51	2.3344
21	69.8	18.35	1.0194	18.62	2.4424
22	71.6	19.42	1.0789	19.79	2.6384
23	73.4	20.58	1.1433	21.02	2.8024
24	75.2	21.78	1.2100	22.32	2.9757
25	77.0	23.04	1.2800	23.69	3.1584
26	78.8	24.36	1.3533	25.13	3.3503
27	80.6	25.75	1.4305	26.65	3.5530
28	82.4	27.22	1.5122	28.25	3.7663
29	84.2	28.75	1.5972	29.94	3.9916
30	86.0	30.35	1.6861	31.71	4.2276
31	87.8	32.01	1.7783	33.58	4.4769
32	89.6	33.76	1.8755	35.53	4.7369
33	91.4	35.61	1.9783	37.59	5.0115
34	93.2	37.57	2.0872	39.75	5.2995
35	95.0	39.60	2.2000	42.02	5.6021
36	96.8	41.70	2.3167	44.40	5.9184
37	98.6	43.90	2.4389	46.90	6.2527
38	100.4	46.19	2.5611	49.51	6.6006
39	102.2	48.59	2.6994	52.26	6.9673
40	104.0	51.10	2.8389	55.13	7.3499
41	105.8	53.7	2.9833	58.14	7.7512
42	107.6	56.5	3.1500	61.30	8.1725
43	109.4	59.5	3.3056	64.59	8.6111
44	111.2	62.5	3.4722	68.05	9.0724
45	113.0	65.6	3.6444	71.66	9.5536
50	122.0	83.2	4.6222	92.3	12.3054
55	131.0	104.6	5.8111	117.85	15.7117
60	140.0	130.5	7.2500	149.19	19.8900
100	212	598	33.2222	760	101.3232
121	249.8	1156	64.2222	1530	203.9796 (autoclave)
374	705.2	400	22.2223	165,452.0	22,058.0 (crit. temp.)

required to liquefy a gas at its critical temperature, or that which is exerted by a liquid at its critical temperature.

Example: Carbon dioxide has a critical temperature of 31.1° C (304.1° K). Room temperatures may reach this temperature, hence, CO_2 gas would exist. In a pressur-

ized cylinder of CO_2, where the pressure will be near the critical pressure of 73 atmospheres or 547 psia, the contents will be a gas above 31.1° C and a liquid below that temperature. Even when room temperature is below 25° F (31.7° C), CO_2 will boil, hence, the CO_2 will be a gas above the liquid because it is at, or above, the boiling temperature at that pressure.

The *boiling point* of a substance is that temperature at which the escaping tendency of the molecules (kinetic energy) equals the confining pressure of 1 atm. At boiling point, the substance will change completely to a gas (boil), although heat must be added. The boiling temperature will rise when the total pressure rises, and it will fall when the total pressure decreases.

Vapor pressure is the pressure at which a liquid will boil at any given temperature; all liquid becomes a gas. A *vapor* is the molecular form of a substance below its boiling temperature, dispersed in a true gas (e.g., water in molecular form in air). Vapor will be present only if a true gas is also present. At a specific temperature, the vapor pressure of a liquid designates the escaping tendency of those molecules to produce an equal pressure of vapor in a gas phase, at equilibrium. Whenever ambient pressure is equal to or below a substances vapor pressure, it boils, producing a gas.

Water vapor pressure designates the partial pressure effect exerted by water vapor in a gas sample. The pressures are presented in Table 17–2. Of note is the vapor pressure level at body temperature (37° C, 310° K), which is 47 mmHg or 6.27 kPa). Because water vapor is not a true gas, when the partial pressure of humid gases are calculated, the water vapor pressure (P_{H_2O}) must be subtracted from the barometric pressure, before it is multiplied by the fraction of gas in a sample. *Dalton's law* describes the relationship of partial pressure of each gas in a composite sample, exerting a partial pressure, proportional to its concentration in the sample (FiO_2), and dependent upon the total barometric pressure (P_B). Water vapor can be thought of as a "contaminant," non-gas, yet exerting a real pressure (P_{H_2O}).

Partial pressure of "wet" inspired oxygen (PiO_2)
$$= FiO_2 \ (P_B - P_{H_2O})$$

Example: At sea level the barometric pressure is 760 mmHg (normal sea level), water vapor pressure at normal body temperature is 47 mmHg, and the fraction of oxygen in room air is 0.21. This calculation illustrates the situation of gases after being brought into the body and warmed and humidified by normal upper airways.

$$P_B = P_{H_2O} + PO_2 + PN_2$$
$$760 = 47 + 149.73 + 563 \ (\text{if no } CO_2 \text{ in inspired air})$$

$$PiO_2 = FiO_2 \ (P_B - P_{H_2O})$$
$$PiO_2 = (760 - 47) \ 0.21 = 149.73 \text{ mmHg } (19.93 \text{ kPa})$$

Humidity is the term to describe water vapor in environmental gases. *Absolute humidity* refers to the mass (weight) of water (vapor) in a given volume of gas. The most common unit for this measurement in respiratory care is milligrams of water in 1 L of gas–vapor mixture. Temperature determines the amount of water that can be "held" in a volume of gas and the vapor pressure created. Gas containing this maximum is described as *saturated* gas. Table 17–2 indicates these amounts and vapor pressures in saturated gas for a range of temperatures. Figure 17–4 depicts the same data in graphic form and identifies body humidity (the content or partial pressure of saturated gas at body temperature).

> *Example:* Air we breathe at "room" temperature of 20° C or 293° K has an absolute humidity of approximately 9 mg H_2O. This is less than the maximum 17.3 mg/L, as air is usually not maximally saturated, except during the most humid weather. At body temperature (37° C or 310° K) air has an absolute humidity of 43.9 mg/L. The body's water content normally guarantees complete saturation of gas with water vapor in alveoli. Body humidity is then 43.9 mg/L or 47 mmHg partial pressure of water (P_{H_2O}).

Relative humidity is used to describe the actual content of water vapor compared with the potential amount that could be held, at the same temperature and at equilibrium. This ratio is usually expressed as a percentage.

> *Example:* The room air described in the previous example, with an absolute humidity of 9 mg/L at 22° C (293° K), would then be compared with the saturated content of 17.3 mg/L.

$$\frac{\text{Water content in gas (measured)}}{\text{Water content in gas (capacity)}} \times 100$$
$$= \text{Relative humidity (\%)}$$

Note: gas sample must be compared with capacity level at the same temperature.

$$\frac{9 \text{ mg/L}}{17.3 \text{ mg/L}} \times 100$$
$$= 52\% \text{ relative humidity at } 20° C$$

By algebraic manipulation, the content of a gas sample can be calculated, knowing the

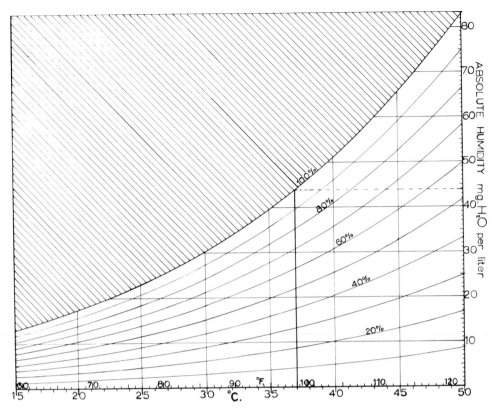

Figure 17—4. Nomogram demonstrating the water content of air over a range of temperatures. Temperature is displayed on the horizontal axis, water content (mg H₂O/L) on the vertical axis, and percentages of saturation as relative humidity on the curved isopleths. The bold vertical line arising from 98.6°F (37° C) identifies the water content at various levels of percentage (%) body humidity.

relative humidity and the capacity at that temperature (see Table 17–2).

$$\text{Content} = \frac{\text{capacity} \times \text{relative humidity}}{100}$$

$$= \frac{17.3 \text{ mg/L} \times 52}{100} = 9 \text{ mg/L}$$

Water vapor capacity is often used to describe the absolute humidity of a gas sample when saturated at a given temperature. This term would be consistent with maximum water content levels at specific temperatures (see Table 17–2).

Dew point is the temperature to which a gas–vapor mixture must be cooled before "dew" condenses on the vessel containing the sample (i.e., the temperature at which the content provides full saturation). High humidity levels will correlate with higher dew-point temperatures. Accordingly, with high ambient humidity, condensation will occur more rapidly on an iced beverage glass than on one at room temperature. By looking at Table 17–2, one

can see that if the dew point occurs at 37° C, the sample was maximally saturated and had a water content of 43.9 mg/L and a vapor pressure of 47 mmHg.

Body humidity is a variation of relative humidity, but the temperature is specified to that of the patient (or assumed to be 37° C) and with full water saturation of the sample. Similar to relative humidity it is expressed as the ratio (percentage) of absolute humidity and capacity at body temperature (normally 43.9 mg/L); therefore, it is 100% relative humidity at body conditions.

Example: The percentage body humidity of room-temperature air with a water vapor content of 9 mg/L (with a relative humidity of 52% at 20° C) is calculated as follows:

$$\% \text{ body humidity} = \frac{9 \text{ mg/L}}{43.9 \text{ mg/L}} \times 100 = 21\%$$

Humidity deficit, as used for respiratory care,

describes the condition of insufficient water to provide 100% body humidity. One can speak of a humidity deficit of any gas sample taken into the body that is not saturated at body temperature, even though saturated at a lower temperature. In theory, it is an index of how much water the mucosal surfaces of the upper airway must "provide" to the inspired gas.

Example: The humidity deficit for each liter of gas with 9 mg/L or 21% body humidity is as follows:

Body "capacity"   43.9 mg/L
Ambient content − 9.0 mg/L
Humidity deficit   34.9 mg/L

Another way of expressing humidity deficit is the percentage difference from 100% (from the previous example):

100%
− 21%
79% humidity deficit

If the patient had a minute ventilation of 10 L/min, the total humidity deficit for 1 minute would be:

34.9 mg/L
× 10   L/min
349.0 mg/min

If the subject continued to breathe for a 24-hour period, the total deficit would be

349 mg/min
× 1440 min/day
502,560 mg/day   or 502.5 g/day

Heat capacity or *specific heat* is that amount of heat energy required to raise a unit weight of a substance 1° C. The specific heat of water (commonly measured in calories per gram per degree Celsius [$cal \cdot g^{-1} \cdot C^{-1}$]) is considered to be 1.0.

The *heat of vaporization* is the heat energy required to change a unit mass of liquid to a gas at the same temperature. Figure 17–5 plots total calories added versus absolute temperature. From point *A* to *B*, a solid is heated to its melting point. Along *BC*, the solid is changed into a liquid. Line *CD* corresponds to the heating of a liquid to the boiling point. Along line *DE*, the liquid is changing to a gas at a constant temperature. The amount of heat to accomplish this is the heat of vaporization. At point *E*, only gas exists. Line *EF* corresponds to further gas heating. For water, it requires 539 calories to convert 1 g of water to 1 g of steam at 100° C (373° K). Water requires more heat in changing from liquid to vapor than does any other substance familiar to man. The heat of vaporization is greater for water at temperatures below 100° C. The heat loss from the respiratory tract because of water evaporation is likewise significant at 579 cal/g/

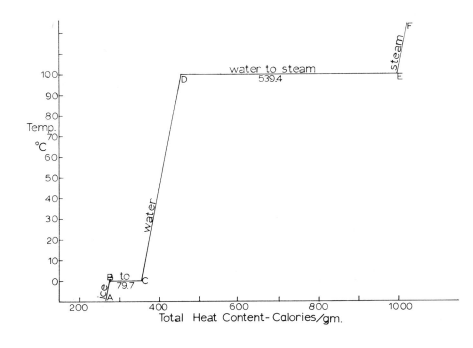

Figure 17–5. Behavior of a system for which temperature is plotted as a function of the total amount of heat added (refer to text for details).

H_2O. Under normal conditions, approximately 250 mL of water and 350 kcal of heat are lost from the lungs each day. Most of this heat loss is due to heat of vaporization, not heating the air itself. No humidifier can produce 100% relative humidity at the temperature of the gas and water unless heat is also provided. The three major factors that influence this process are temperature, the area of contact between the water and gas, and the time allowed for gas–water contact. The rate at which an equilibrium (between vapor concentration and water) is approached depends on the amount of heat available.

Example: The heating and humidification of 10 L of dry oxygen in contact with water (all at 20° C; 293° K) will require 342.8 calories (1434.48 joules) to bring it to 100% body temperature

$$10 \text{ L of } O_2 \text{ weighs } 13.31 \text{ g}$$

It has a heat capacity of 0.2178 cal (0.911 joules)/1° C. Just to raise the gas temperature to 37° C will require:

$$13.31 \times (37 - 20) \times 0.2178$$
$$= 49.28 \text{ cal (206.24 joules)}$$

However, the heating will cause the volume to increase to 10.58 L and addition of water vapor to enlarge to 11.28 L. The 43.9 mg H_2O/L (495.08 mg) will be required and additional heat will be needed to raise this water to 37° C.

$$0.49508 \times 17 \times 1 = 8.42 \text{ cal (35.22 joules)}$$

The amount of heat required to change water at 37° C to a vapor at 37° C is 575.8 cal (2409.7 joules)/g.

$$0.49508 \times 575.8 = 285.07 \text{ (1193 joules)}$$

In summary, the total energy needed is

$$
\begin{array}{r}
49.28 \\
8.42 \\
+ 285.07 \\
\hline
342.8 \quad \text{cal (1434.48 joules)}
\end{array}
$$

If only the gas were to supply this energy, it would have to enter at 118.25° C above the 20° C, or 138.25° C. If only the water supplied the energy, it would have to be at 692.4° C above the 20° C or 712° C. However if a 100-mL reservoir of water were available, a temperature of only 40.26° C would be needed. One can see that this is the most efficient way to provide this energy. To some extent, the human airway functions to provide an efficient gas–water interface. The greater this area, the greater number of escaping molecules. If heat energy is available, the rapid escape will continue; if not, the greater surface area will increase the rate of temperature drop, decreasing molecular escape.

The *isothermic saturation boundary* is a point in the airway at which inspired gases reach the 100% body humidity level. Some researchers specify this area to be just below the tracheal carina (assuming normal conditions).[29] Endotracheal intubation would shift the isothermic boundary deeper into the bronchial tree, as would inspiration of "bone-dry" medical gases through an endotracheal tube.[89]

RATIONALE FOR SUPPLEMENTAL HUMIDITY

In the 1950s, Ingelstedt found that the minimum temperature in the subglottic space during nasal breathing was 32.2° C. During expiration the maximum temperature averaged 36.4° C, and at the nose 33.2° C. The relative humidity for both was 98% to 99%.[55] During the 1960s, other investigators confirmed the earlier work and showed that during expiration, water condenses on the tracheal surfaces and latent heat and water are held until the next inspiration.[29] During anesthesia, a minimal need of 15 mg/L was found to prevent cilia and mucosal damage, and investigators suggested an optimal level of 25–28 mg/L.[13] More recent research has found that during quiet breathing of room air (at 26° C and 35% relative humidity) gas was heated to 32° C in the upper trachea and increased to 35° C in the subsegmental bronchi.[70] The temperature differential was 10° to 11° C between inspired and expired gas, regardless of the proportion of mouth or nose breathing.

These data do not support the notion that 37° C and 100% saturation are mandatory for inspired gas in the upper airways. Electron microscopic evidence of airway damage was detected after inhalation of gas at 35° C and 100% relative humidity for 3 to 24 hours. Pulmonary surfactant also showed a decrease in surface tension, presumably owing to condensed water from overhumidification.[112] This information appears to contrast with somewhat arbitrary recommendations, passed down from a variety of respiratory care texts, that suggest that humidity deficit should be prevented, or corrected, by providing inspired gas at 100% body humidity (i.e., 37° C and water content of 43.9 mg/L). In summary, recent data suggests that if the normal airways are bypassed, the lower level of humidity would be in the area of 24–27 mg/L, and the upper level 32–34 mg/L.[14,102]

Manufacturers of humidification devices tend to follow standards set down by organizations such as the American National Standards Institute (ANSI). The following are excerpts from their publications.

> 3.1.1.1 The minimum level of 10 mg/L was felt to be the lowest acceptable humidity level necessary to minimize mucosal damage under a wide variety of environments. In addition 10 mg/L will provide approximately 50% relative humidity at 72° F ambient conditions, enhancing the dissipation of static electricity in order to prevent fires.[3]
>
> 3.1.1.2 The devices covered in this standard are for subjects who have a tracheostomy or endotracheal tube. Humidifier output of 30 mg/L was felt to be the minimum amount of moisture necessary to prevent crusting of secretions and mucosal damage. The user must decide on the appropriate device for applications other than those in which the upper airway has been bypassed.

It should be noted that the standard refers to the output at humidifier, not at the patient-entry point. Tubing that conducts gas to the patient is not always heated. This cooling will decrease the temperature, lower humidity levels, and cause condensation.[3]

A lucid application of research data and suggested standards for patient care suggests matching the humidification system to the inspiratory conditions at the entry point of the respiratory system. If levels of heat and humidity are below normal levels, then supplementation should occur to prevent a humidity deficit (Table 17–3).

APPLICATION OF MEDICAL GASES TO THE NOSE

When medical gases are applied to the nose, normal room air conditions should be duplicated with gas a 22° C at 50% relative humidity. This would include nasal oxygen masks, low-flow nasal cannulas, demand nasal cannulas, or oxygen enclosures (continuous high-flow oxygen cannulas may require a higher relative humidity). The moisture level of the room air will be a factor, as the patient significantly dilutes the oxygen with this environmental gas. Although an adequate level has not been defined, some have suggested that supplemental humidity not be required if the flows are 4 L/min or less.[2] There is no solid guideline on this point.[27]

APPLICATION OF MEDICAL GASES TO THE NOSE AND MOUTH

Gases entering the respiratory system at the oropharynx should range from 29° to 32° C at 100% relative humidity. This applies to facial mask-type medical gas appliances, such as partial or nonrebreathing oxygen masks. The only exception is the Venturi mask. This device entrains most of the inspired gas from the room. The room ambient humidity is added to the dry medical gas, and humidification by a artificial device is usually unnecessary.

Table 17–3 Summary of Current Humidification Recommendations for Respiratory Care Applications

ENTRY POINT OF SYSTEM	EXAMPLE	GOAL OF HUMIDIFICATION INSPIRED AIR SYSTEMS
Nasalpharynx	Low-flow cannula Nasal mask	22° C at 50% relative humidity
Oropharynx	Facial masks Nasal catheter	29–32° C at 100% relative humidity
Trachea	Mechanical ventilators Tracheostomy collar	32–34° C at 95–100% relative humidity

APPLICATION OF MEDICAL GASES THROUGH "ARTIFICAL" AIRWAYS

Inspired gases that bypass the normal anatomic airways should be delivered at 32° to 34° C at approximately 95% to 100% relative humidity (water content minimum of 24–27 mg/L).[14]

SPECIAL APPLICATIONS OF HUMIDITY THERAPY

The aforementioned approaches may need modification for patients with abnormal airway reactivity (i.e., asthmatics), increased need for moisture in the upper airway (i.e., laryngotracheobronchitis or croup), and those patients who have abnormalities in pulmonary secretions or their clearance. (Not following the foregoing plan may result in thickened secretions, and increased humidity will be required.) Some patients in the asthmatic population have documented increases in airway resistance when they hyperventilate, as with exercise, breathe during sleep, or breathe very cold air.[15,106,116] Breathing inspired air that is humidified to a water vapor content of 20 mg/L at 23° C "blunts" the obstructive response, and breathing gases at 100% body humidity (43.9 mg/L) can eliminate bronchospasm. Asthmatics who exercise when swimming do not show exercise-induced bronchospasm. It is suggested that there is less thermal stress by preventing heat loss in the form of latent heat of vaporization, preventing the shifting of the isothermic saturation boundary deeper into the airways. Local stimulation of mucosal mast cells is believed to be the cause of the bronchospasm.[116] Worsening of asthma in the nighttime hours may also operate on a similar scheme, in that airway cooling occurs as a result of total body temperature decrease.[15]

Supplemental humidification of inspired gas for nonintubated patients with pathologic secretion production or retention requires an analysis of the specific problem. Patients with acute or chronic bronchitis do not need further irritation of their airways. This is also true in patients with cystic fibrosis. Children with tracheolaryngobronchitis (croup) may benefit from supplemental humidity to lessen airway resistance caused by topical irritation and mucosal crusting in the upper airway.[50]

Application of heated humidified breathing gases for victims of significant hypothermia has been advocated, especially if the patient is breathing through an artificial airway. This method of rewarming is quite effective and simple compared with other invasive techniques.[4]

EQUIPMENT TO PROVIDE HUMIDITY THERAPY

Classification of humidification equipment traditionally has been based on a description of the physical method or technique. Problems in classification arise because devices that produce aerosol normally produce humidity (water vapor). However the reverse is less often true (i.e., most humidifiers generate only water vapor). A general classification developed by Klein and co-workers is used in the following review.[58]

HUMIDITY GENERATORS

Heat and Moisture Exchangers

The heat and moisture exchanger (HME) is based on a mechanical replication of the body's anatomic humidification system. With the artificial "nose/mouth/pharynx," exhaled heat and moisture are collected and made available to warm and humidify the following inspiration. A scarf wrapped around the nose and mouth on a cold winter day is a common application of the HME used in respiratory care. The HMEs under discussion are primarily used with patients who are intubated or tracheostomized. Although used in Europe for some years, commercial HMEs have only seen increased use in United States hospitals since the early 1980s.

The method of operation applies basic physical principles. Expired gas at body temperature and fully saturated with water vapor exits the patient and enters the HME. As gas enters the device, water condenses on the inner surfaces, and the latent heat that has kept water in a vaporized state is released, causing warming (Fig. 17–6). This is inferior to the body's system in that the HME is not "self"-heated and warmed as are the mucosal tissues. During inspiration, the collected heat and moisture is transferred to the gas passing through. Dry inspired air will progressively cool the HME; the cooling is essential to recycle the surfaces to be able to condense the next breath of expired air. The temperature gradient across the HME, therefore, is an index of its efficiency or output. The higher the temperature of gas exiting a HME, the greater the level of humidification it can provide.[93]

When researchers studied certain animals, they were surprised to find that exhaled air was less than body temperature and below 100% saturation. When the camel is deprived of water its nose becomes hygroscopic, in that it can extract more water than would be collected from condensation alone.[100] This effect is said to hold water in a non-

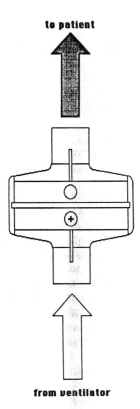

to patient

from ventilator

Figure 17—6. Diagram of a heat—moisture exchanger (HME).

condensed state, which lessens evaporative cooling, thereby improving output. Surfaces covered with various salts or ordinary filter paper possess this quality. The term *hygroscopic condenser humidifier* has appeared in the trade and medical literature to describe such units.[71]

The following are physical variables that affect the performance of all types of heat—moisture exchangers:

- Temperature and humidity level in the inspired air
- The level of inspiratory and expiratory flows: more rapid flows offer reduced time to reach equilibrium and absorb or deposit moisture
- The size of a device's internal interface will limit the capability of the unit i.e., greater surface allows more heat and moisture contact. (In addition, this volume is considered "dead space," or expired gas that is rebreathed)
- Good thermal conductivity of the exchanging material and poor conductivity of the housing

Clinical Application and Performance. The application of these units is to humidify dry inspired gases for patients with artificial airways, who are breathing room air or dry medical gas or are being mechanically ventilated. These HMEs are supplied with inlet—outlet fittings (15/22 mm) to connect ventilator and airway. The use of the HME is an alternative because of its simplicity, safety (lack of electrical or thermal hazard), portability (transport), and reduced cost compared with standard heated humidifiers. Some units may be useful for spontaneously breathing patients with permanent tracheostomy. A gauze pad "ascot" may be a simple system. Cold weather or problems with thick pulmonary secretions may suggest a need for a portable supplemental humidity device.

Performance standards have not been set specifically for HMEs. When used with mechanical ventilators or anesthesia machines, HMEs can be compared with standards for conventional heated-water systems. Laboratory testing of HME outputs shows values from 10 to 28 mg/L, with temperatures about 30° C (over the adult range of inspiratory flows and minute ventilation).[9,34,71,113,115] It appears that those using "hygroscopic" elements do perform better than HMEs without that design.

Table 17—4 summarizes factors that affect the clinical use of HMEs in patient application.

Product Descriptions and Characteristics. Several currently available HMEs are pictured in Figure 17—7. Table 17—5 provides a composite to identify dimensions, element material, dead space, and moisture output. These data are the result of numerous laboratory evaluations.[9,34,63,102]

The HMEs offer a number of potential advantages in respiratory care applications.

- Simplicity of design, setup and maintenance (e.g., transport or short-term ventilation)
- Low cost ($2.00–$6.00 for single-patient use units)
- Freedom from electrical and thermal hazard
- Relative freedom from under- or overhydration

These advantages should be considered with the knowledge that patients who are dehydrated, hypothermic, or have pulmonary abnormalities (that may lead to or result in retained secretions) are *not* ideal candidates for HMEs.[68] In addition, certain units with substantial internal dead space may be contraindicated for patients who have difficulty weaning because of ventilatory demands.

Table 17—4 Summary of Clinical Factors for Heat—Moisture Exchangers [9,11,34,63,68,71]

1. Gas leakage: There have been reports of leaks in some units that could result in significant loss of ventilation. Leakage is suggested to be less than 30 mL/min at 30 cmH$_2$O and to withstand pressures of 100 cmH$_2$O.
2. Resistance through or pressure drop across the HME: To minimize inspiratory effort during spontaneous breathing, the pressure drop is suggested to be less than 3 cmH$_2$O for flows of 50 L/min. With long-term use, elements absorb water and resistance to flow increases, resulting in increased work of breathing.
3. Weight of the HME: Low weight is favored as it tends to reduce traction on the airway.
4. Internal volume: The space for gas compression will affect the dead space as well as the potential compressible volume loss. It should be as low as possible without compromising output. For neonatal or pediatric application, dead space should be minimal.
5. Output of particulate matter and microbiologic safety: There should be no effluent particles from the moisture exchange elements. HME manufacturers have claimed that these units can trap bacteria or are bacteriostatic, reducing the autocontamination of patient circuits. There have been reports of dust or fungicide exiting from HMEs. Studies have shown mixed results in the effectiveness of the HME to prevent patient contamination of ventilators.
6. Failure of the HME to adequately maintain patient's airway hydration: Scientific comparison trials are not clear. For short-term use, no demonstrated difference could be found. Changes in the patient's status that could relate to secretion retention or changes in sputum characteristics may suggest use of a heated humidifier.

Whether a HME can modify bacterial contamination during mechanical ventilation is controversial.[11]

Bubbler Humidifiers (Unheated)

"Bubbler" humidifiers pass medical gases through a diffuser to break the gas into small bubbles that increase their humidity levels as they rise in a vessel of water (Fig. 17—8). Various substances are used for the diffuser, including, mesh, sintered metal, and plastic foam. The content of water will be greatest if the bubbles are very small and the water container is tall, to allow maximum time for water—gas contact. Humidifiers of this type are most efficient at low flows (e.g., 1.5–5 L/min), as increasing flow causes evaporative cooling of the water. As has been mentioned, lower temperatures reduce the potential content of water vapor in the gas. These units typically are physically unable to humidify dry medical gas much beyond 40% body humidity, when normally operated at room temperature.

Clinical Application and Performance. Traditionally, bubblers have been used with low-flow (less than 15 L/min) medical gas administration devices such as nasal cannulas, simple (nonreservoir) masks, and reservoir masks. Gas exits the bubbler through small-bore tubing. Recently, there has been a trend to eliminate the bubbler from such devices, with statements that they are only "cosmetic" and not necessary with oxygen flows producing 30% concentrations.[2,36,61] Such discussions, lack of solid scientific rationale, and pressure of cost-containment have all contributed to a reduced utilization of these devices. Improved criteria based on good patient-oriented research appears to be needed in this area. The potential for improved product design may be part of the scientific effort.

Although scientific assessment of bubbler humidifiers has been sparse, two laboratory studies have produced similar results. Klein and co-workers found outputs to range from 38% to 48% body humidity when flows were 2.5 L/min. When flow was increased to 10 L/min, the percentage body humidity fell to 26% to 34%.[58] Darin and associates reviewed prefilled (single-patient use) bubblers, with comparable results. At 2 L/min, units ranged from 39% to 46.6%, and decreased to 33% to 35% body humidity at 8 L/min. They concluded that the major factors determining performance are the design of the diffuser and the level of medical gas flow. Darin's group suggested that improved engineering design could increase vapor output and noted that bubblers reach their peak efficiency within 15 minutes of use, then decrease to a plateau level as the temperature decreases.[15]

Therapeutic gases delivered to the nose—mouth (e.g., by nasal cannula or mask) should minimally match average room air conditions. (American National Standards Z-79.9 suggests 22° C at 50% relative humidity or 19.43 mg/L.) However, meeting this level may not be necessary, as nasal cannula breathers inspire a large portion of room air with their oxygen. Continuous nasal cannula breathers may require a higher humidity level if, at higher flows, the prongs cause significant drying of nasal mucosa. Patients breathing with a nasal or facial mask tend to warm and humidify gas with their expired air.

Figure 17—9 and Table 17—6 provide a summary of performance data for a variety of permanent and single-patient use unheated bubbler humidifiers.

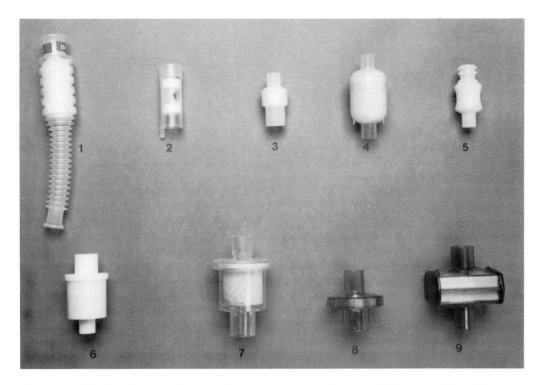

Figure 17—7. Commercially available heat–moisture exchangers. (1) Engstrom Edith, (2) Portex Humid-Vent, (3) Portex, (4) Mallinckrodt, (5) American Hospital Supply Humid-Air, (6) Siemens 152, (7) Siemens 150, (8) Vitalograph, (9) Pall Conserve.

Table 17—5   Heat—Moisture Exchangers (HME)

BRAND/DEVICE	WEIGHT(g)	VOLUME(mL) (DEAD SPACE)	ELEMENT	COMPLIANCE (mL/cmH$_2$O)	OUTPUT (mg/L)
Dameca	44	62	Corrugated aluminum	0.062	16
Portex Humid-Vent	9	10	Corrugated paper	0.01	21
Terumo Breath Aid	14	11.5	Aluminum and fabric disks	0.01	14
Airlife* Humid Air	11.1	40.5	Synthetic felt	—	24
Siemens-Elma Servo 150	40.5	92	Cellulose Sponge and felt	0.09	25
Engstrom* Edith	18.4	89	Polypropylene fiber	—	26
Vitalograph	67	30	Stainless steel screens	0.03	16
Mallinckrodt*	16	60.8	Porous plastic foam	—	21
Pall* Conserve	47.2	98	Ceramic fiber	—	23

Unless otherwise noted: (Data from Emergency Care Research Institute: Heat moisture exchangers. Health Devices 12:155, 1983. Conditions for output measurement: tidal volume 0.666 L, frequency 10/min, and inspiratory flow 40 L/min.
* (Data from Branson RD, Hurst JM: Laboratory evaluation of seven airway heat and moisture exchangers, Respir Care 32:741, 1987) Conditions for output measurement: tidal volume 0.75 L, frequency 12/min, and inspiratory flow 40 L/min.

In clinical practice, a few technical problems can occur. Because small-bore tubing is used to carry the medical gases, there is potential for blockage by (liquid) water collecting in low spots. Because of the unheated system, condensation is not the cause, but more likely, the water jars spilling into the output tube. At very high flows, the churning action of the bubbling can displace water into the tubing. Confirmation that lines are clear and that there is flow through the appliance should be part of the initial and ongoing check of patients using such systems. Small-bore tubing from bubblers may also be kinked or compressed by bed rails and such. Bubbler humidifiers have gravity or spring-loaded pressure valves to vent off pressures that could rupture units if not relieved, which will alert operators to the problem.

Because bubblers are water reservoirs, they can support the growth of *Pseudomonas aeruginosa.* They have been linked to respiratory nosocomial infections with this pathogen.[45]

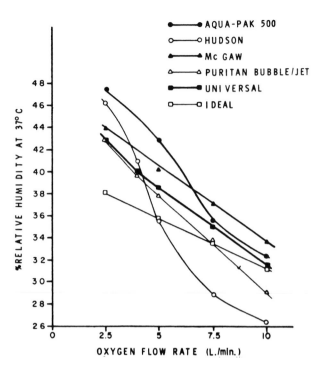

Figure 17—9. Humidity output (percentage body humidity) of six unheated bubbler humidifiers with increasing flow of oxygen. (Klein EF, Shah DA, Shah, NJ, Modell JH, Dasautels D: Performance characteristics of conventional and prototype humidifiers and nebulizers. Chest 64:690, 1973. Reproduced with permission)

Figure 17—8. Section of a bubbler humidifier. These devices are commonly used with low-flow oxygen appliances (e.g., cannula, masks, and such). A weighted pressure pop-off is shown at the top of the housing.

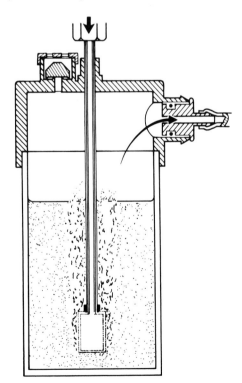

Heated "Mainstream" Humidifiers

Rational and Clinical Usage. Heated humidifiers are used to condition dry inspired gases for patients who have artificial airways in place, are being mechanically ventilated, or are in oxygen hoods. By physically adding heat, these units can potentially replicate the heat and humidity levels that normal airways would provide. The term *mainstream* indicates that the patient's entire source of inspired gas is conveyed through the humidifier.

Suggested capabilities are provided by ANSI Z-79.9, which recommends a water output level of 30 mg/L (100% relative humidity at 86° F [30° C]).[3] The Emergency Care Research Institute recommends 37 mg/L (85% relative humidity at 90° F [32.5° C]).[32,33] As has been mentioned, there is no unanimous agreement among clinicians on the

Table 17—6 Water Vapor Content and Relative Humidity for Unheated Prefilled Bubble Humidifiers

BRAND	OXYGEN FLOW	H₂O VAPOR CONTENT (mg/L)	RELATIVE HUMIDITY (%) AT 37°C [BODY HUMIDITY]
Aerwey 300	2	17.2	39.1
	4	16	36.4
	6	15.6	35.5
	8	14.6	33.2
Aquapak 301	2	17.6	40
	4	17.7	40.3
	6	16.9	38.4
	8	14.9	34
McGaw 250	2	20.4	46.6
	4	18.4	41.9
	6	16.9	38.4
Travenol 500	2	20.4	46.4
	4	19.5	44.4
	6	16.2	36.9
	8	15.7	35.7

(Data from Darin J, Broadwell J, MacDonell R: An evaluation of water–vapor output from four brands of unheated prefilled bubble humidifers. Respir Care 27:41, 1981)

minimum safe humidity output for treatment of patients with *normal* airways.

Almost all heated units have the capability of humidifying gas to 100% body humidity. They can be considered the standard device for mechanical ventilator-breathing circuits and for application of high-flow gas systems (e.g., continuous positive airway pressure [CPAP]), medical gases for asthmatics, and delivery of gas to infant oxygen hoods. Some units have limits to the total flow that can be brought to 100% body humidity. Heated humidifiers are stressed at high-flow conditions. Flows of 60–100 L/min may be required for high-flow systems (e.g., oxygen blender or Down's flow generator). Heated humidifiers must also be considered the devices of choice for patients with bypassed upper airway who have secretion problems. Patients with abnormal thickening of mucus, mucous plugs, or crusting of endotracheal or tracheostomy tubes can have their humidity deficit corrected. A history of lung disease that typically presents with secretion abnormalities may indicate that a heated humidifier be placed prophylactically, instead of a device (e.g., HME) with less moisture capability.

Category Descriptions and Performance. Classification of mainstream humidifiers is based on terms depicting the basic design. The following categories are based on those used by the ECRI.

1. Pass-over
2. Bubble-through (also referred to as "cascade")
3. Pass-over wick (gas may pass "through" wicks)

All three designs provide humidification by heating water–gas, while providing an interface for their contact. Units may also be described as servocontrolled or non-servocontrolled. This refers to some method of regulating the heating elements. Servocontrolled humidifiers have some type of thermister (electronic thermometer) that works with a microprocessor to maintain a specific temperature. The thermister probe is usually located in the inspiratory circuit near the patient connection. Whether or not humidifiers use heated wires in the inspiratory/expiratory tubing may offer another descriptive category.

Heated humidifiers must function over a wide range of clinical uses, accommodating both low- and high-flow situations. Additional capabilities suggested for safe clinical use are presented in Table 17–7.

Pass-Over Humidifier. This design of humidifier simply passes gas over a reservoir of heated water (Fig. 17–10A). Escaping molecules of water vapor are taken up by the gas. Currently,

Table 17—7   Suggested Heated Humidifier Capabilities

1. Overtemperature protection: Gas temperature at the patient should not be settable above 40° C. It is recommended that heaters must have power interrupted when the temperature at the thermister exceeds 40° C, and audible and visual alerts/alarms be activated. If a servocontrolled unit's probe is inadvertently omitted, the device should not create a thermal hazard. Humidifiers that are in a warmup status or have gas flow interrupted should not be allowed to overheat. Exposed surfaces should not be too hot to touch, or they should have a warning label if over 50° C.
2. Warmup time: Humidifiers should reach operating temperature in an appropriate time and stabilize at the desired level.
3. Electromagnetic interference (EMI): EMI from adjacent electrical equipment should not affect humidifier function. Units should not be affected or cause electrical hazard by water spills.
4. Misassembly: It should not be possible to reassemble a humidifier system in a way that could lead to a hazardous patient situation. The direction for correct gas flow should be indicated on the device.
5. Water level visibility: The water level in the humidifier or the remote reservoir should be visible in lighting conditions typical of an intensive care unit.
6. Pressure integrity: Humidifiers are recommended to withstand a ventilation pressure of 100 cmH$_2$O.
7. Internal compliance or compressible volume loss: To deliver accurate tidal volumes over a range of ventilating pressures, humidifier compliance should be less than the compliance of that of the intended patient. Neonatal application would suggest a level of 1 mL/cmH$_2$O. The compliance should also remain stable as water levels vary.
8. Resistance or pressure drop: The pressure caused by resistance to flow through a humidifier should be less than 5 cmH$_2$O at 50 L/min. When spontaneously breathing patients attempt inspiration at low flows, the pressure across the systems should be less than 0.5 cmH$_2$O.

(Summarized from Emergency Care Research Institute: Heated humidifiers. Health Devices 16:223, 1987)

Figure 17—10. Pass-over humidifiers: (*A*) section of generic "pass-over" humidifier; (*B*) section of Bear VH-820 humidifier (Courtesy of Bear Medical Systems Inc., Riverside, Calif)

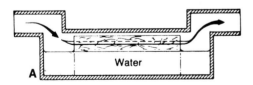

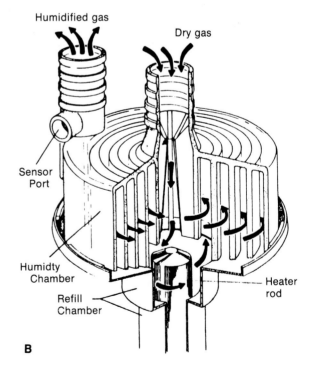

there are three examples used clinically; the "stock" humidifiers available with the Emerson 3-PV and 3-MV mechanical ventilators, the Bear VH-820 (see Figs. 17–10B and 17–11A), and the Inspiron Vapor-Phase Plus.

The Emerson resembles a food pressure cooker and has been termed a "hot pot." Copper mesh in the proximal inspiratory tubing enhances the efficiency of the device. Clinically oriented laboratory testing has shown that the Emerson pass-over humidifier is limited to water outputs less than 30 mg/L when used during mechanical ventilation. However, the resistance to gas flow was quite low (1 cmH2O) when used over a clinical range of flows.[85]

The Bear humidifier (Bear Medical Systems, Inc.) uses spiral vanes that increase the pass-over surface area for water–gas contact, without a substantial increase in compliance or resistance (see Figs. 17–10B and 17–11A). This servocontrolled, heated-wire humidifier's relevant clinical data is presented in Table 17–8.

The pass-over design is slightly different in the Vapor-Phase Plus shown in Figure 17–11E (Inspiron Inc.). A hydrophobic filter separates the heated water and gas. Water is "vaporized" below the filter and is then picked up by the mainstream gas flow. This single-patient humidifier is available as a servocontrolled and continuous-feed system. (Relevant product information is found in Table 17–8.)

Bubble-Through "Cascade." This style of device is a more efficient design of the bubbler hu-

Figure 17–11. Commercially available heated humidifiers: (a) Bear VH-820, Bear Medical Systems, Inc.; (b) Bird, Bird Products; (c) Fisher & Paykel MR450 and (d) MR600, Fisher & Paykel/ American Pharmaseal Co.; (d) Inspiron Vapor-Phase Plus, Inspiron Corp. Omnicare, Inc.; (f) Puritan-Bennett Cascade II, Puritan Bennett Corp.; (g) RCI Conchatherm III, Respiratory Care, Inc. (h) Saratoga SCT, Marquest Medical Products Inc.; (i) Travenol HLC-37S, Travenol/Americal Pharmaseal Co. (Courtesy ECRI from Health Devices 16:228–229, 1987)

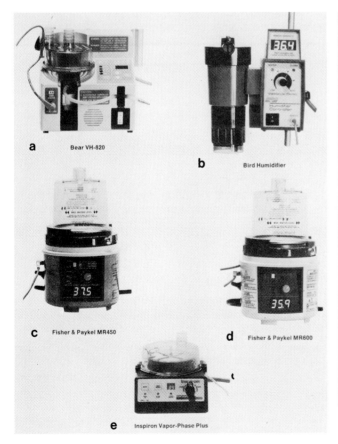

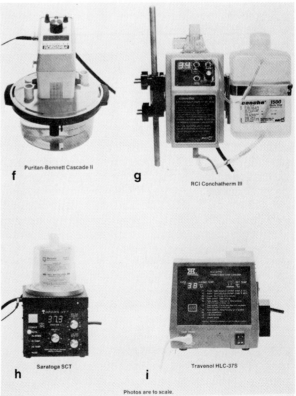

Table 17—8 Summary of Heated Humidifiers

BRAND	HUMIDIFICATION METHOD	SERVO CONTROL	HEATED WIRE	HUMIDIFICATION CHAMBER H$_2$O VOL (ml)	ALARMS
Bear VH-820	Pass-over vanes	Yes	NA	5–10	High/low temp Probe disconnect Wire disconnect Overfill/depleted
Inspiron Vapor-phase	Pass-over filter	NA	NA	10	High temp Probe failure
Cascade II	Bubble-through	Yes	NA	900	High temp
Bird	Pass-over wick	NA	NA	20	High temp Probe disconnect Module disconnect
Fisher & Paykel 450 wick	Pass-over	Yes	NA	Adult 280 Pediatric 230	High/low temp Probe disconnect
600	Pass-over	Yes	Yes	"	Above plus heated wire disconnect
RCI Chonchatherm	Pass-over wick	Yes	NA	Adult 182 Pediatric 72	High/low temp Probe disconnect
Saratoga SCT	Pass-over wick	Yes	Yes	300	Low/high temp probe and heated Wire disconnect Power failure
Travenol HLC-37S	Pass-over wick	Yes	NA	75	High/low temp Probe disconnect Feed system fail

(Data from Emergency Care Research Institute: Heated humidifiers, Health Devices 16:223, 1987)

midifier. Besides being heated, the area for gas–water interface is increased by use of a large diffuser tower (see Figs. 17–11F and 17–12). The Bennett Cascade I was developed in the late 1960s; a servocontrolled and alarmed unit followed with the Cascade II in the 1970s. The alarm functions alert to overtemperature at the sensor and sensor failure or disconnect. A continuous-feed water system can be used. In the tower of each humidifier, a small hole allows the ventilator to sense a pressure differential caused by the patient's inspiratory effort. In the past it was assumed that no bacterial aerosol was emitted when using a cascade humidifier. Recently, this has been disputed.[92] A summary of the Cascade II is presented in Table 17–8.

Bubble-Through Wick. Several humidifiers utilize a submerged paper or composite (e.g., Gortex) wick through which the mainstream flow must pass. The saturated wicks may be vertical or horizontal and provide the surface for imparting water

Figure 17—12. Section of a "cascade" humidifier.

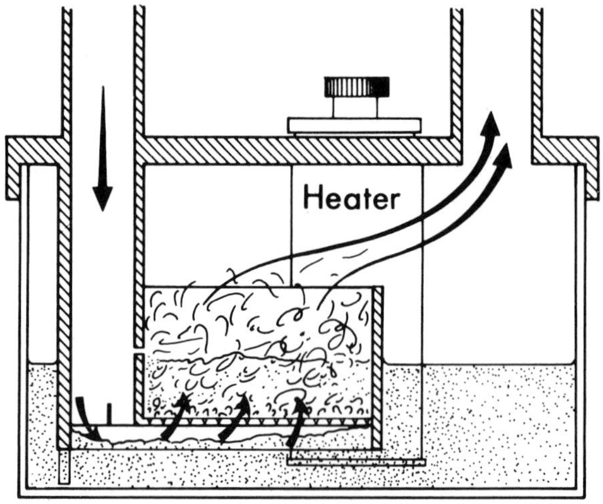

vapor to gas. The Bird Wick humidifier, (see Figs. 17–11B and 17–13), Bird Corporation; Conchatherm (see Fig. 17–11G), Respiratory Care Inc.; Travenol HLC-37S (see Fig. 17–11I) and Fisher Paykel MR450/MR600 (see Fig. 17–11C, D), American Pharmaseal Co.; and Saratoga SCT (see Fig. 17–11H), Marquest Products Inc., are current designs using this principle. All wick humidifiers use a servothermostat, except the Bird. The Fisher and Paykel (model MR600/630) and Saratoga units have capabilities for heated wires in the patient tubing.

These humidifiers have alarm systems that warn of overtemperature, probe disconnect, and low temperature. Servohumidifiers tend to overheat if, during warm-up, the temperature probe is not placed in the breathing circuit. However, in most of the humidifiers an alarm will be activated. Non-servo units will give overheated gas if the operator sets the temperature too high or if gas flow is substantially reduced. The advantage of the heated wire feature appears to be primarily convenience, in that with reduced condensation, ventilator water traps need less maintenance. Humidifiers without heated wires have acceptable output. Safety may also be a factor when using small tubing in breathing circuits (e.g., neonatal ventilation) or when ventilator checks cannot be done regularly. Water collecting in low spots in the circuits can increase resistance to flow and create a PEEP-like effect to airway pressure. Heated wire humidifiers appear to offer the best output performance, with low gas flow, found in pediatric ventilation.

Figure 17–13. Section of a Bird Wick Humidifier. (Courtesy of Bird Products Corp., Palm Springs, Calif)

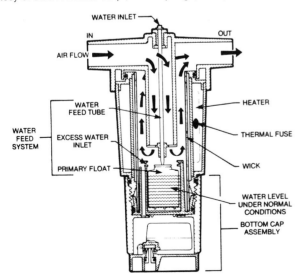

The Bird humidifier is a non-servocontrolled unit that uses a vertical paper wick (see Fig. 17–13). It has a reusable chamber, which connects to the power module, and remote continuous water feed. Its alarm functions include probe disconnect, overtemperature (40° C), and humidification module disconnect. Table 17–8 presents a summary of other pertinent technical data.

The Fisher & Paykel is a servocontrolled unit with disposable wick and reusable humidification chamber (see Fig. 17–11C, D). The model 450 is the basic unit. Model 600 uses only heated-wire operation and model 630 has the option for use (disposable or reusable). A continuous water-feed system has been added to these humidifiers. (A summary of data can be found in Table 17–8.)

The Conchatherm III is a servocontrolled unit with some operator requirement (see Fig. 17–11G). It has relative rather than specific temperature controls. The system includes a remote continuous water-feed but requires RCI-packaged sterile water (see Table 17–8 for information on this humidifier).

The Saratoga SCT is a servocontrolled device with disposable heated wire and humidification chamber (see Fig. 17–11H). A remote continuous feed is provided. Alarm functions include independently adjustable high and low temperature, probe and/or heated-wire disconnect, and power failure (see Table 17–8 for other specifications).

The Travenol HLC-37S is a servocontrolled humidifier with disposable heated wire system (see Fig. 17–11I). A remote continuous feed is incorporated. The unit will alarm at high and low temperatures, probe disconnect, and depletion of the water reservoir (see Table 17–8 for additional data on this humidifier).

PATIENT ASSESSMENT AND EQUIPMENT TROUBLESHOOTING

As each major type of humidity generator has been discussed, the rational and patient application have been reviewed. The practice of applying humidity to dry gases appears to be benign. However, either inappropriate choice of device, operator error, or malfunction may result in potential harm to the patient.

After a patient has been placed on some type of humidification system, the respiratory care practitioner should evaluate the effectiveness of maintaining the airway. Chest auscultation should alert one to increased retention of mucus (rhonchi) and to atelectatic lung zones (crackles).

Evaluating the character of the sputum after cough or suctioning can help assess whether there is adequate hydration of the airway. If the artificial airway frequently requires clearing because of crusting of mucus, the appropriateness of that system should be reevaluated. Patients without an artificial airway may also provide subjective information if poor humidification of nose or facial medical gas systems causes uncomfortable drying.

Respiratory care practitioners should constantly be attentive to condensate in breathing circuits. Water traps may not be completely effective. Mechanically ventilated patients commonly become colonized quite rapidly with organisms found in the sputum. Changing circuits or removing condensate is not a benign event and may lead to nosocomial pneumonia when care is not exercised.[23,24] This potentially infected waste should be drained away from the patient to prevent inadvertent passage into the tracheobronchial tree.

Circuit gas leaks in the humidifier portion of a breathing circuit may interfere with sufficient pressurization and lead to hypoventilation. Ventilators should be checked before patient use to confirm a leak-free system. Low-pressure or volume alarms should provide an ongoing clinical evaluation.

Malfunctions or misassembly of continuous water-feed systems are potentially hazardous if the units flood the inspiratory circuit. Heated humidifiers that overheat can cause airway burns. The most common cause, other than malfunction, is omission of the servoprobe or operation when mainstream gas flows are quite variable. Recent sophistication of heater alarm systems reduces this hazard. However, operator error in non-servo systems can occur. Manufacturer's information should be available for individual humidifiers on troubleshooting procedures. Readers desiring a more detailed analysis of heated humidifiers may consult recent consumer reviews.[32,33]

AEROSOL THERAPY

PHYSICAL PRINCIPLES RELATED TO AEROSOL THERAPY

A complete review of this topic is well beyond the clinical scope of this chapter. However, respiratory care practitioners may be required to evaluate equipment and apply devices to specific conditions. Therefore, a general background in terminology, physical characteristics, and methods of describing aerosols will be reviewed.

An *aerosol* is defined as a suspension of solid or liquid particles in gas. Particles may vary in shape, density, and size, all of which can affect their physical behavior. Such physical characteristics determine the depth of travel into the respiratory tract and tendency to be deposited.

In nature, smoke, dust, and fog are examples of aerosols. The following table gives approximate sizes of environmental aerosols.

MATERIALS	DIMENSION RANGE (μm)
Sand grains	200–2000
Pollens	10–100
Fungal spores	0.5–100
Tobacco smoke	0.2–2
Viruses	28 nm–0.2 μm

Aerosols can be made by condensation of water vapor into the liquid state and comminution of solid or liquid substances by shattering particles into a suspension. The latter method is frequently used in respiratory care. There are several techniques to accomplish the shattering effect, which will be examined later in this chapter.

Because the size of particles is critical to their distribution in the respiratory tract, scientists have devised a number of terms and techniques to help characterize the aerosol.

Manufacturers often develop aerosol-generating devices that target a certain particle size. In reality, most therapeutic aerosols are composed of a range of particle sizes and are called *heterodisperse* aerosols. *Monodisperse* aerosols have a narrow range of diameters and are used more for research application.

During aerosol therapy, water or drugs are deposited in or on the respiratory tract surfaces. When the density is constant, the volume of substance in an aerosol particle is proportional to its size. Specifically, the volume of a particle is directly proportional to the cube of the radius:

$$\text{Aerosol volume} = \frac{4}{3} \times \pi \times \text{radius}^3$$

The implication of this is significant to therapy. Because of the foregoing relationship, many small particles must be deposited in the same area to equal one large particle. Particles below 1 μm have so little mass, hence volume, that they provide little deposition in the lung.[66] The surface area of an aerosol particle = π × diameter^2. The surface area/volume ratio increases as particles become smaller and their inertia becomes less. They tend to deposit less by impaction and to settle more slowly during breath-holding.

The mass median aerodynamic diameter (MMAD) assists in describing size distribution. This concept is used to describe a specific particle that has 50% of its fellow particles heavier and 50% lighter. (This assumes that the distribution follows a typical "bell-shaped" probability distribution.)

Some aerosol generators do not follow this distribution. Propellant-powered metered-dose inhalers have several peaks, and a number of clinical aerosols have a log-normal distribution. A plot of the latter giving mass mean diameter is provided in Figure 17–14. However, large particles constitute most of the mass.

Count median diameter (CMD) and *geometric mean diameter* (GMD) are both indices used to reflect a "typical" particle, in that 50% of the other particles are larger and 50% smaller. The difference between the CMD and the MMD is demonstrated in Figure 17–14. It is possible that about 1% of the large aerosol particles account for the difference between the two mean levels, in that it takes only a few large particles to increase the mass or volume exponentially.

Figure 17–14. Log-normal distribution of aerosol particle diameter plotted against fraction of particles per increment in diameter. Because of the "skewed nature of log-normal distribution, *mode, median,* and *mean* do not coincide. (Reproduced with permission, Lourenco RV, Cotromanes E: Clinical aerosols I: Characterization of aerosols and their diagnostic use. Arch Intern Med 142:2163, 1982)

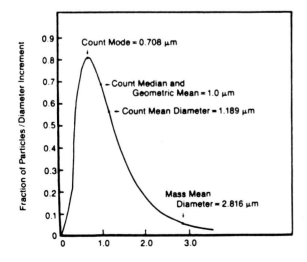

The *aerodynamic mass diameter* (AD) is a measurement that helps correlate a particle's size with properties that would cause it to settle with gravity. An aerosol is assigned a particle diameter (spherical), with a specific density, that has a settling velocity identical with that of a reference particle. Therefore, size, shape, and density factors may differ, but if a particle settles out at a specific point it is assigned that aerodynamic mass diameter.

Most therapeutic aerosols have aerodynamic diameters between 1 and 10 μm. This size range is sufficiently stable, and particles larger than 1 μm are large enough to carry sufficient volumes of water or drug. Particles of 0.01 to 1-μm diameter are so stable that they fail to deposit on lung surfaces and are exhaled.

Aerosol particles can either shrink through evaporation or grow in size as they travel. An increase in size by condensation of water vapor is termed *hygroscopic property.* The specific substance (i.e., drug), water, and salinity, as well as the ambient humidity and temperature, influence this. The humidity level, in turn, is crucially dependent on the collective surface area of the gas—liquid interface. A 1-μm diameter aerosol particle is estimated to completely evaporate in 0.5 seconds, if warmed from 20° C to 37° C in transit from room to body temperature.[66]

Unfortunately, manufacturers and evaluators of aerosol equipment have not yet agreed upon a set of standards to describe their physical characteristics. Recently, there has been more interest in research in small-volume medication nebulizers and their comparative performance. However, similar data on large-reservoir and disposable jet nebulizers are not easily available.

FACTORS INFLUENCING DEPOSITION OF AEROSOLS IN THE LUNG

Inertial impaction describes deposition of particles by collision with surfaces. This would most commonly occur as particles negotiate their way through the first ten airway generations. Aerosols experience turbulent gas flows and abrupt airway bends, such as at bifurcations. With increased velocities from high inspiratory flows (>30 L/min), particles tend to deposit in the upper airway. Finally, the size or mass of the particle will affect the tendency for impaction. Particles in the 5- to 10-μm range tend to deposit before they reach bronchioles of 2-mm diameter.

Gravitational sedimentation is the term to describe deposition of particles as they reach a velocity too slow to maintain travel. This time-dependent mechanism is believed to affect particles down to 1 μm in diameter. Deposition occurs in the last five or six airway generations. A patient's breath-holding time is the most significant factor in promoting deposition by sedimentation. A parallel physical mechanism that promotes deposition is that caused by *Brownian motion*. Random motion of aerosol particles by carrier gas molecules can cause fallout of the aerosol. This may be of only theoretical interest, as the particles are quite small (0.5 μm).

Actual measurements of penetration and deposition of aerosols in the lung zones have documented the combined effects of inertial impaction and sedimentation. There is some variation in the literature on specifics, but, in general, a patient's breathing pattern and the particle size are the major factors. Table 17–9 compares particle size with mean percentage of deposition, by lung zone.

When using either a pressurized metered-dose inhaler (MDI) or jet nebulizer, deposition in the lung is only 10% to 12%. Metered-dose inhalers and jet nebulizers differ in their amount of deposition elsewhere as follows:[64,79,120,121]

	MDI (%)	X̄ (%)	JET (%)	X̄ (%)
Deposited in the lung	9–11	10	4–18	12
Pharynx and stomach	80–84		2	
Remaining in device	5–10		66	
Exhaled	1		20	

The following is a summary of clinical and physical research findings:

1. Variations in breathing patterns provide a crucial factor in altering deposition of aerosols. Some studies are based on fixed tidal volume, inspiratory flow, and frequency of breathing; others are based on spontaneously breathing human subjects. There have been conflicting data on deposition of aerosolized drugs when subjects inhaled at various levels of their vital capacity.[91] Proper education and self-administration techniques in dispensing MDI aerosol is critical and will be reviewed later in this section of the chapter.

2. Breathing through the nose tends to deposit particles larger than 5 to 10 μm in the upper airways. Breathing through the open mouth results in greater deposition of 5- to 10-μm diameter particles in the oropharynx and the first six airway generations.

3. Maximum deposition occurs with reduced inspiratory flows (<30 L/min), large tidal volumes, and 10-second breath-holding time.[79,80]

4. Particles in the 1- to 4-μm range tend to deposit in the lung periphery.[73,107] Optimal alveolar deposition requires particle sizes of 1 to 2 μm.[79]

5. The size and condition of the conducting airways will influence aerosol deposition.[30,97]

Table 17–9 Deposition of Aerosol Particles in Lung Zones

PARTICLE SIZE (μm)	MEAN % DEPOSITION			
	Mouth	Naso pharynx	Trachea to Term Bronchiole	Bronchiole to Alveoli
1.0	0	3.6	2.7	25
2.0	0	40.6	5.1	34.6
3.0	5	55.2	7.1	30.8
4.0	10	65.4	8.4	23.8
6.0	30	80.0	9.0	10.3
10.0	65	99.2	0.7	0.2
12.0	75	—	—	—
14.0	85	—	—	—
>16.0	100	—	—	—

(Data from Rau JL: Humidity and aerosol therapy. In Barnes T (ed): Respiratory Care Practice, p 164. Chicago, Year Book Medical, 1988)

RATIONALE AND USE FOR AEROSOL THERAPY

Deposition of Topical Drugs and Diagnostic Agents in the Lung

There is a long record of aerosol therapy. Ancients began the practice of inhaling the smoke from various buring medicinal plants.[120] There is a growing list of medications currently being prescribed for administration in aerosol form. Table 17–10 lists major categories, with examples of drug groups and general usage. The advantages of the aerosol route include the following:

- Smaller dosage required versus systemic therapy
- Usually has rapid therapeutic effect
- Side effects are usually reduced (especially extrapulmonary ones)
- Inhalational route normally is easily accessible
- Administration is often simple (i.e., patient self-administered)

Aerosol therapy is one of the main forms of delivering drugs for prophylaxis or treatment of asthma and the bronchospasm seen with chronic bronchitis.[77] The medication groups most frequently prescribed are the β-agonist bronchodilators, corticosteroids, and cromolyn sodium. Therapy may be as simple as a self-administered MDI on an as-needed basis or before exercise. Aerosol therapy may also be involved in a complex medical regimen that includes parenteral medications.

The emergency treatment of acute exacerbations of asthma involves an aerosol β-agonist as the first drug of choice.[95] Parenteral sympathomimetics are reserved for use in asthmatics whose initial response to inhaled medications is poor.[118] This signals the need for hospitalization and allows additional treatment beyond the emergency room.

Aerosols of adrenergic agonists cause fewer untoward effects, such as tremor, tachycardia, palpitations, and the like, than equivalent doses of oral or intravenous medications. This is also true for the cholinergic blocking drug ipratropium, reducing atropine-like effects. Similarly, inhaled topical steroids act effectively in the lung, decreasing the risk of serious complications of long-term systemic steroid therapy.[65]

Cromolyn sodium is also a major aerosolized drug for asthma. However, its role in treatment is strictly for prophylaxis; it is contraindicated and of no value for urgent therapy.

Table 17—10 Major Categories of Inhalational Aerosol Drugs Currently Prescribed

DRUG CATEGORY	GENERIC/TRADE EXAMPLES	USE TO TREAT
Bronchodilators		
Sympathomimetic	Albuterol/Ventolin	Bronchospasm
Parasympatholytic	Ipratropium bromide/Atrovent	Bronchospasm
Antiasthmatic	Cromolyn sodium/Intal	Prophylaxis for bronchospasm
Corticosteroids	Flunisolide/Aerobid	Anti-inflamatory with asthma
Decongestant/ vasoconstrictor	Racemic epinephrine/ Vaponephrin	Vasoconstriction of mucosal surfaces
Mucolytic	Acetylcysteine/Mucomyst	Secretion retention
Antimicrobial		
Antibacterial	Gentamicin	Topical treatment of lung infections
Antifungal	Nystatin	
Antiviral	Ribavirin/Virazol	
Antiprotozoan	Pentamidine isethionate/Nebu-Pent	
Surface active	50% ethyl alcohol	Pulmonary edema
Anesthetic agents	Lidocaine/Xylocaine	Preintubation

The bronchial target areas for these drugs require particles in the 2- to 5-μm range. Selection of a device and the administration technique will be reviewed subsequently.

Topical vasoconstriction delivered by aerosol therapy has been used in the treatment of tracheitis, tracheolaryngobronchitis (croup), and intubation/bronchoscopy. Aerosols in the 7- to 15-μm range are desirable to treat the upper airway.[5,86]

Results from administration of aerosolized antimicrobial agents have generally been inferior to systemic administration. There have been reports of treatment of gram-negative infections in cystic fibrosis, but little evidence of real therapeutic value.[67,69] Aerosol medications are now being used in therapy for respiratory syncytial virus (RSV) and prophylaxis and treatment of *Pneumocystis* pneumonia.[21,28] Topical treatment of pneumonia in alveoli requires aerosol particles to be in the 1- to 2-μm range.

Mucolytic drugs are used to aid the expectoration of mucus that cannot be hydrated or liquefied by simpler methods.[114]

Aerosols are also used in diagnostic procedures. Radioactively tagged aerosols can be inhaled to examine their lung distribution by γ-detectors. Technetium-99m–labeled albumin (or sulfur colloid) and neutralized indium-133m chloride are agents used (clearance of agents demonstrates mucociliary activity). Bronchial provocation agents such as methacholine and histamine are used to determine if asymptomatic subjects demonstrate increased bronchial reactivity to the bronchospastic agents.[120]

In the past, attempts were made to aerosolize pulmonary surfactant for neonates with respiratory distress syndrome. However, enthusiasm for that approach has been reduced in favor of direct instillation into the airway.[62]

Hydration of Pulmonary Secretions

Although there is no overwhelming scientific evidence to support them, periodic treatments with bland aerosols of water or saline continue to be used in respiratory care.[52] Inhalation of water–saline aerosols isotonic or hypertonic has been shown to increase mucociliary clearance in chronic bronchitic patients and is used for sputum induction.[17,82] Studies show that only a small amount of water actually is deposited on the airways.[120] In objective studies, it is difficult to control variables such as cough, bronchial drainage, concomitant bronchodilator therapy, and type of disease. It is

unclear whether clinical improvements are due to just the liquefaction of mucus, stimulation of a vagally mediated production of mucus, or stimulation of cough receptors increasing expectoration. Aerosol therapy may be considered as supportive to more definitive methods of secretion mobilization through systemic hydration and chest physical therapy procedures, including effective coughing. Several scientific reviews have suggested that inhalation of water aerosols should be reevaluated for its therapeutic value.[41,51,114]

Aerosolized alcohol has a controversial role in the treatment of airway-obstruction foam in pulmonary edema. Ethyl alcohol (50%) denatures the surfactant and modifies the surface tension of the edema fluid, thus decreasing the tendency for frothing of secretions.[67]

HUMIDIFICATION OF MEDICAL GASES FOR INHALATION

Before the development of effective heated humidifiers for large flows of medical gases, both ultrasonic and cool/heated nebulizers were used. The rationale was to use devices that had the capability of adding enough water to oxygen or air to reach 100% body humidity levels. A major use was with mechanical ventilators. Currently, it is unusual to see either type of device used for this application. However, it is common to find them used for patients with artificial airways or for those breathing by mouth–nose. The Briggs "T" piece, face mask/tent, and tracheostomy collars are frequently coupled with large-bore tubing and nebulizers. This practice of using all-purpose nebulizers appears to be based on tradition, reduced cost (compared with heated humidifiers and an oxygen blender), and flexible oxygen administration. Patients receiving oxygen by such systems may not present a need for aerosol therapy (i.e., retained secretions). Although a relatively safe practice, there are risks of microbial infection, overhydration, bronchoconstriction, and impairment of mucus transport. Any aerosol particle is potentially a bronchoconstrictive agent to asthmatics. It is prudent to recommend that this group, as well as others (e.g., patients with cystic fibrosis) who exhibit increases in airway resistance, be placed on humidification systems.

Facilitation of Sputum Induction

Sputum induction for microbiologic or cytologic examination is based on the empiric evidence that patients are more able to have a productive cough after aerosol therapy. Agents such as water, normal saline, or hypertonic saline mixtures probably activate) vagal pathways and augment production of mucus.[17,82] More acutely, the irritant effects of the aerosol produces a profound stimulation to cough. Traditionally, ultrasonic or high-output pneumatic nebulizers have been used for this purpose.[114]

Treatment of Upper Airway Inflammation

Pediatric patients with croup and patients with postextubation laryngospasm have traditionally been treated with "cool mist" aerosols. The mist tent has been used for croup because of the difficulty with placement of masks on young children. However, its clinical value has been difficult to document.[50,114] In addition, some feel that it is a hostile environment that can cause chilling of the child, bacterial contamination, and poor visibility and access to the patient. Use of topical aerosols such as racemic epinephrine for croup has an established role in treatment.[5]

There have been little clinical data to support use of bland aerosols to treat postextubation laryngeal edema. Whether the high-humidity environment versus the aerosol deposition on the upper airway produces a positive effect has not been investigated.

In the past, children with cystic fibrosis were treated with mist tents while sleeping. This was abandoned after documentation of its ineffectiveness in delivering bland mists to the entire tracheobronchial tree. With nose breathing, at rest, deposition was localized to the upper airway.[114]

HAZARDS RELATED TO AEROSOL THERAPY

Although specific problems with each type of aerosol generator will be described as they are discussed, the following is a review of the generic hazards.

Untoward Responses to Aerosol Drugs

Depending on the type of drug administered by aerosol methods, side effects can occur. Practitioners monitoring patients should be aware of the following side effects for the major categories of aerosolizable drug:

Bronchodilators
  Sympathomimetic (e.g., epinephrine)—tachycardia, blood pressure changes, palpitations, central nervous system effects (headache, ner-
vousness, irritability, anxiety, and insomnia), muscle tremor, nausea, increase in glucose, acute drop in arterial oxygen tension
  Parasympatholytic (e.g., atropine)—dryness of mouth and skin, tachycardia, blurred vision, dysphagia, dysphonia, difficulty with micturition, and mental confusion or excitement
Antiasthmatic (e.g., cromolyn sodium)—bronchospasm, hoarseness, and dry mouth
Mucolytic (e.g., acetylcysteine)—bronchospasm, bronchorrhea, and nausea
Corticosteroids (e.g., triamcinolone)—upper airway fungal infections with *Candida* or *Aspergillus*, throat irritation, dry mouth and coughing
Antimicrobial agents—anaphylactic sensitivity reactions and others specific to the drug

Bronchospasm. Patients with hypersensitive airways have a tendency to develop increased airway resistance when aerosols are inspired. Certain substances are particularly irritating, such as acetylcysteine, cromolyn sodium (powder), hypertonic saline, and antimicrobial agents. Pretreatment or simultaneous treatment with a rapid-acting sympathomimetic bronchodilating drug is often indicated. Aerosols of sterile water, normal saline, and bronchodilators have caused problems, especially when administered by high-output ultrasonic nebulizers.[38] Paradoxic response to inhaled bronchodilators does occur but is an uncommon finding.[104]

Infectious Contamination. Bacterial contamination of pneumatic or ultrasonic aerosol systems can occur as a result of cross-contamination or autoinfection. This was a significant problem in the 1960s before use of ethylene oxide gas sterilization procedures (for heat-sensitive equipment). Large-volume nebulizers pose the greatest risk. Gram-negative bacteria appear to be the most common infecting agents. Hands of workers changing water supplies, reflux of contaminated condensate, and contaminated water supplies have all been implicated.[22,24]

Airway Burns. Airway burns have occurred when immersion or bottom plate nebulizer heaters are improperly set, are defective and "run wild," or if the reservoir runs out of water and heats inspired gas directly. Airway temperatures over 44°C can potentially burn mucosal surfaces.

Sound Levels. Sound levels of pneumatic nebulizers may cause hearing loss in infants when used with enclosures such as hoods or incubators. The American Academy of Pediatrics Committee on Environmental Hazards recommends a level below 58 dB.[1] Such levels are exceeded by several mainstream nebulizers, even with 60 cm of tubing leading to the enclosure.[6]

Overhydration and Excessive Salt Loads. Patients receiving long-duration or continuous aerosol therapy from high-output nebulizers may be subjected to fluid or sodium chloride overload. A positive water balance can occur with intubated patients because of abolition of the normal insensitive water loss. Patients at greatest risk are in the neonatal or pediatric group and those with renal failure. Monitoring of urine output, body weight, electrolyte concentrations, and consistency of pulmonary secretions can indicate problems in this area.[108]

AEROSOL-GENERATING EQUIPMENT

METERED-DOSE INHALERS

Metered-dose inhalers (MDIs) are glass, ceramic, or metal canisters containing drug in the form of a suspension of crystals or in solution, with a propellant (Fig. 17–15). Chlorofluorocarbons or other propellants provide the positive pressure to activate the nebulization process. The vapor pressure of the propellants is high, 3003 mmHg (400 kPa) being required to keep them as liquids. When the device is actuated by pressing the nozzle down, the contents of a small metering chamber are released. There is a rapid initial vaporization of the liquid fluorocarbon, termed "flashing," as the gas–liquid traverses the orifice. The propellant becomes a gas, leaving the drug suspended as droplets. The mass median aerodynamic diameter at the orifice is in the 35-μm or larger range. Particle size is reduced as the aerosol moves from the actuator orifice, but after 10 cm little size reduction occurs.[49,54,66,79] Mass median aerodynamic diameters 10 cm from the orifice range from 1.4 to 4.3 μm.[35,54]

The size of the aerosol particles emitted is dependent primarily upon the preparation of drug and condition of the propellant. The dimension of the nozzle plays a smaller role.[66] Most MDIs elaborate their contents in a fairly monodisperse pattern.

Aerosol delivery to the patient involves additional effects. Temperature affects the internal pressure of the propellant; with cooler-than-normal room temperatures, the lowered pressure tends to produce larger particles. The drug tends to concen-

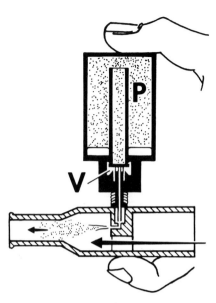

Figure 17–15. Sectional diagram of a gas-propelled hand nebulizer or metered-dose inhaler (MDI) for delivery of medication. (*V*) indicates the actuator valve (*P*) is the fluid–vapor mixture containing the propellant and medication.

trate as more propellant vaporizes to fill the canister's dead space. However, this effect is apparently balanced by the fact that most actuator valves decrease their dose through use. There is also a tendency for low doses to be emitted if the units are not used for several days. Shaking and actuation once or twice is then advocated.[66]

Because of the small size and ease of operation of MDIs, they are routinely prescribed for patients' self-administration. The advantage is greater portability and availability than compressor-driven devices. This access also leads to problems of potential abuse, with increase in side effects and loss of effectiveness.[25] Total bronchodilator dosages by MDIs are lower, by approximately four to ten times, than those of a jet hand-held nebulizer.[121] A typical dose of two puffs may be conservative and suboptimal in bronchodilating effect.[78,95] Severe acute asthma frequently requires larger doses of aerosol medication because of the high inspiratory flows, low tidal volumes, and already narrowed peripheral airways.[96]

Metered-dose inhalers are also being used with increasing frequency in the hospital setting. Patients with stable asthma appear to obtain the same therapeutic effect from bronchodilators administered by MDIs versus jet nebulizers.[57,94,96,110] During the initial acute phase of asthma, however, hand-held nebulizers can be superior to MDIs.[75] There is also interest in the potential cost savings of in-hospital aerosol therapy by using MDIs.[18,56] Under either circumstance, therapy should include proper patient education and monitoring of the self-administration technique.

Metered-dose inhalers have been evaluated in circuits of mechanical ventilators.[46,51] There are several types of adaptors that facilitate actuating the MDI, some by insertion at the endotracheal tube swivel connector. Although the endotracheal tube provides a considerable barrier to aerosol penetration, one study has shown comparable bronchodilation with the MDI and a small-volume jet nebulizer.[46]

Bronchodilator responsiveness can also be evaluated with MDIs in the pulmonary function laboratory.[16]

The major problem in clinical use is in proper patient education and technique. Even after appropriate education, some patients fail to master the skill or revert to incorrect technique.[105,110] It is estimated that 10% to 20% of patients fail to receive optimal aerosol deposition because of poor technique;[25] Most of this group are the very young and the elderly.[105] This has resulted in the development of a good deal of patient education literature, training effort, and inhalational aids.[80] The major problem relates to timing inhalation with canister actuation. Other issues related to "aiming" into the mouth, placement in the mouth, and failing to shake or clean the MDI. The proper technique for a cooperative adult is as follows:

1. Remove MDI, shake vigorously (actuate if MDI has not been used in several days)
2. Exhale to resting level
3. Holding the canister, nozzle down, place mouthpiece 3 to 5 cm from the open mouth or place mouthpiece in mouth with open lips
4. Begin inspiration. Actuate inhaler as inhalation begins
5. Inspire deeply, slowly for about 5 seconds
6. Hold breath for approximately 10 seconds (or, if less, as long as possible)
7. Wait 3 minutes before taking a second dose*
8. Repeat

* The ideal time may be longer or there may be no benefit in waiting beyond 3 minutes. (Patients with episodic wheezing and poor control of symptoms derive greater benefit in delay than those with stable asthma.[83])

Inhalational aids for MDIs come in a variety of designs, falling into three major categories: extension tubes (spacers), extension tube–chambers with valves, and collapsible bags (Fig. 17–16). The tubes provide a reservoir for the bolus of the aerosol to be held prior to the beginning of inhalation. One-way–valved MDI aids simply trap the particles until the patient can evacuate them.

The goals of spacers and chambers are to eliminate the need for precise timing of canister actuation with inhalation, to assist in the aiming of the MDI outlet, to optimize particle size, and to promote low-flow inspiration. Spacers provide a distance for particles to evaporate and impact on internal walls. Particle shrinkage is related to the tube or chamber volume; impaction is relatively independent of volume or configuration of the device.[35,47,99,110]

The MDI adjuncts appear to be of most benefit to children and elderly patients. Dyspneic asthmatic children tend to inhale rapidly and to have difficulty holding their breath. Ideally, inspiratory flows should be 10–20 L/min or less to better deposit aerosols of the 1- to 5-μm range.[31] Some MDI adjuncts provide an audible "biofeedback" guide to inspiratory flow (e.g., Inspirese). It is reasonable to expect that MDI aids are effective when used properly, and some drug manufacturers supply a unit with the MDI. The MDI aids probably do not substantially enhance the efficacy of an aerosol delivery for a patient who uses correct technique. They do appear to help a standard MDI to be more effective if otherwise used poorly.[111] Some reservoir chambers may not provide adequate inspiratory volume for adults because they are limited to 600 to 700 mL. Inspired volumes should be larger than the tidal volume. Deposition increases directly with increased volumes; doubling the tidal volume results in approximately a 20% increase.[81] Volumes of tube spacers vary from 60 to 150 mL. After MDI activation into a chamber, particles do coalesce; therefore, inhaling puffs one at a time improves the delivery of smaller-diameter particles inhaled.[90]

The act of gargling after inhalation reduces side effects from pharyngeal absorption of sympathetic bronchodilators or topical corticosteroids.[65,87]

Spacers cost 10 to 30 dollars; patient compliance may not be aided by the bulky size of some units or by a reluctance to use them in public.

Technical problems with MDIs are few. Temperature, shaking the canister, and positioning have been discussed. Soap-and-water cleaning of the actuator orifice should be done according to the manufacturer's recommendations. Cross-contami-

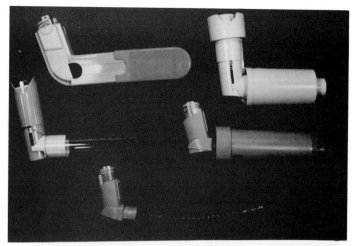

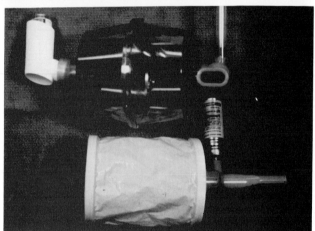

Figure 17—16. Commercially available examples of metered-dose inhaler administration "aids": (*A*) tube extensions; (*B*) chambers.

nation is not an issue for this single-patient item.

There is a danger for aspiration of coins or other purse or pocket articles that may get into uncovered MDI mouthpieces.

Freon propellants can cause life-threatening cardiac dysrhythmias. However, blood levels of fluorocarbons with therapeutic nebulizers are too small to have any adverse effects.[49] Because of environmental issues, manufacturers are evaluating systems that do not rely on freon propellant.

SMALL-VOLUME JET NEBULIZERS

Small-volume medication nebulizers have been used to dispense medication for some time. Early glass hand-bulb units were "baffled" versions of basic atomizers (Figs. 17–17 and 17–18A). Today there are a variety of contemporary devices that utilize the same principles, with various techniques and levels of sophistication of baffling. These "jet" nebulizers utilize the Venturi application of the

Figure 17—17. Sectional diagram of an atomizer. Pressurized air is applied at the point indicated by an *arrow*. This may be applied by a hand bulb. Common applications are administration of a local anesthetic for tracheal intubation, endoscopy, or otolaryngology.

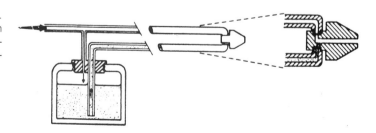

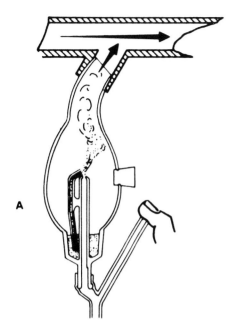

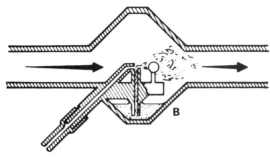

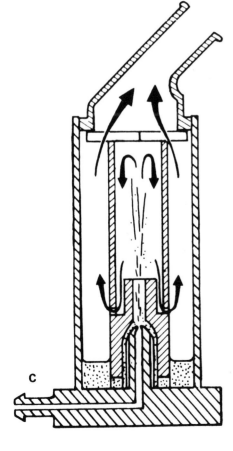

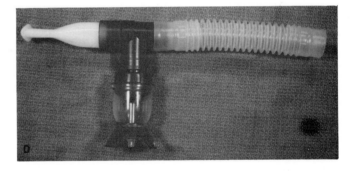

Figure 17—18. Sectional diagrams and photograph of medication nebulizers: (A) Vintage glass "side-stream" unit, with "wye" gas actuator; (B) bird-type "mainstream" medication nebulizer; (C) Dautrebande design of baffeling system used in contemporary medication nebulizer (R.E. Reynolds Co.); (D) Photograph of nebulizer for sidestream applications (Courtesy of Marquest Medical Products, Inc.)

Bernoulli theorem. A high-pressure gas source is passed through a constriction. The gas jet is positioned at an intersection of a tube that is immersed in a fluid. The constriction increases gas velocity and decreases lateral pressure. Liquid is "drawn up" by the subatmospheric pressure and immediately shattered into small particles. The flow of gas and aerosols is directed at surfaces; hence, particles too large for therapeutic use will impact and be retained in the liquid reservoir (Figs. 17–18*A,B*) Dautrebande was known for his early work with sophisticated baffling systems, which can still be seen in contemporary nebulizers (see Fig. 17–18*C*).[120]

Clinical Application

Jet medication nebulizers are used as simple hand-held devices powered either by portable compressors or hospital gas supplies (see Fig. 17–18). They have been used extensively for administration of bronchodilators and other drugs, and appear to be the device of choice for administration of β-adrenergic drugs in the initial phase of acute asthma.[75] The nebulizer is simply placed in the vertical section of a breathing "T," with mouthpiece on one side and aerosol reservoir tubing on the other (see Fig. 17–18*D*). The reservoir appears to increase the amount of aerosol in these systems, documented by in vitro evaluation.[84]

Some systems use a "wye," with one-way valves allowing undirectional patient gas flow (Fig. 17–19). The one-way valves apparently act as baffles to remove larger particles. Some systems utilize a tubing reservoir, making a bolus of medication available upon immediate inhalation. These nebulizing systems have been used for topical administration of pentamidine isethionate for treatment or prophylaxis of *Pneumocystis carinii* pneumonia.[21,74] The goal of this therapy is to deposit the drug in alveolar zones, requiring particles with mass median diameters of 1 to 2 μm. With normal inspiration, there is preferential distribution of gas particles to dependent lung zones. This has apparently resulted in relapses of pneumonia in the upper lobes. More homogenous aerosol deposition may be achieved if patients periodically initiate inspiration from residual volume, are recumbent, or breathe at higher frequencies.[21]

Mouthpiece breathing is more efficient compared with face masks, which increase waste. Patients may control the flow of gas to the nebulizer, so nebulization will occur only during inspiration by use of a finger-operated "y-piece."

These nebulizers have been incorporated into breathing circuits of intermittent positive-pressure breathing (IPPB) machines. The benefit of this combination is for the patient incapable of adequate depth of inhalation or of synchronizing breathing with nebulization. IPPB does not improve aerosol delivery for patients with adequate inspiratory volumes.[39] Medication nebulizers have also been placed in mechanical ventilator circuits.

Performance

Most small-volume nebulizers produce total fluid outputs of 1 to 2 mL/min. Aerosol particle diameters range from 1 to 5 μm (mass median aerodynamic diameter). Table 17–11 gives approximate comparisons of particle size for various brands of nebulizer. (*Note:* Differing methods of particle measurement makes direct model comparisons difficult.)

Aerosol size is directly proportional to compressed gas flow. Most nebulizers will give the smallest particle size when a minimum of 6 L/min is used. Unfortunately, domiciliary use is fre-

Figure 17—19. Medication nebulizer with one-way valves (for unidirectional gas flow), tubing reservoir, and expiratory particle filter. (Courtesy of Marquest Medical Products)

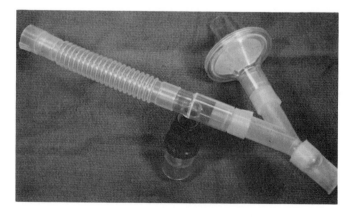

Table 17—11 Performance and Features of Jet Medication Nebulizers

BRAND	MMAD* (μm)	GSD	RESERVOIR	EXPIRATORY FILTER	INLET FLOWS	REF.
Aerotech II (Cadema)	2.0	+2.5*	No	Optional	10–15 L/min	21
Centimist (Marquist Medical Products)	1.1	±2.2	Yes	No	9 L/min	21
Fan Jet (Marquist Medical Products)	4.3	±2.5	No	Optional	7 L/min	21
Respigard II (Marquest Medical Products)	0.93	±1.8	Yes	Yes	7 L/min	21
Ultra Vent (Mallinckrodt)	0.25	±2.0	No	Yes	11–14 L/min	21
DeVilbiss 40 (DeVilbiss Co.)	6.0	±1.8	No	No		91
Raindrop	7.9	+2.3	No	No		37
Air Shields Jet	6.0	±2.5	No	No		91
Acorn	4.8	±2.0	No	No		37

* MMAD, Mass median aerodynamic diameter. (*Note:* Data collected from a variety of sources. Conditions and measurement technology differences make direct comparisons difficult.)

quently carried out with small-capacity compressors that cannot develop such flows with the resistance of the nebulizer jet. If flows of 6 L/min are used, medication diluent volumes can be increased from the often listed 2 mL up to 4 to 6 mL. The combination of high flows and larger volumes is recommended to ensure the highest output, smallest particle size, and reasonably short treatment time.[21]

Problems and Patient Evaluation

Like MDIs, small-volume jet nebulizers are simple devices. Failure to produce mist is usually caused by interruption in gas flow, clogged fluid pick-up tube, or clogged jet orifice. Most manufacturers of reusable nebulizers suggest cleaning and air-drying between use. Nebulizers are a source for circuit leaks in mechanical ventilators, as well as for microbial contamination.[22]

Effectiveness of bronchodilation can be determined by evaluating patients before and after therapy. Auscultation of the chest can provide a guide to improvement of airflow and level of wheezing. Before-versus-after comparison of peak flow or the forced expiratory volume at 1 second (FEV_1) pro-

vide good indices of change. Patient cooperation is often a major variable outside the pulmonary function laboratory. However, a FEV_1 improvement of 10% to 15% is considered "significant" effectiveness. The following example illustrates the calculation:

$$\text{Proportion of improvement} = \frac{\text{Posttherapy } FEV_1 - \text{Baseline } FEV_1}{\text{Baseline } FEV_1}$$

For example:

Baseline FEV_1 1.9 L
Posttherapy FEV_1 2.3 L

$$\frac{2.3 - 1.9}{1.9} = \frac{0.4}{1.9} = 0.21 \text{ or } 21\%$$

Effectiveness of bronchodilator therapy in mechanically ventilated patients can be evaluated by noting increase in passive expiratory flows at specific recoil pressures or a reduction in peak pressures when volume-preset devices are used.[42]

SMALL-PARTICLE AEROSOL GENERATOR

Administration of the antiviral medication ribavirin (Virazole) has been advocated for treating specific groups of infants infected with respiratory syncytial virus (RSV). Most healthy infants can deal with this common infection. However, in children with congenital heart diseases, immunodeficiency, or bronchopulmonary dysplasia, RSV can cause life-threatening pneumonia and bronchiolitis.[48]

Ribavirin is supplied as a lyophilized crystalline powder that is reconstituted with sterile water. The aerosolizable solution's concentration is 20 mg/mL. The drug manufacturer provides an administration device called a "small-particle aerosol generator" (SPAG; Fig. 17–20). The jet-type aerosol generator reduces 50 psig line pressure to 26 psig and allows regulation of flow to a nebulizer and drying chamber. The flow to the nebulizer should be 7 L/min and no less than 15 L/min total airflow, with use of the drying chamber flowmeter. The particle diameter is nearly monodisperse, with aerosols in the 1.2- to 1.4-μm range.[12] Treatment with the medication proceeds over several consecutive days, depending on the severity of symptoms. The SPAG will provide a retained dose of ribavirin of about 2.25–3 mg/kg of body weight when given for 18 to 24 hours.[59] The drug is poorly absorbed by the lung. High alveolar levels appear to interfere with viral replication. Administration through the SPAG can be performed using a head hood, aerosol mask, mist tent, or mechanical ventilator (Fig. 17–21). When a head hood is used, about 66% of the drug is delivered to the patient chamber.[12] Initially, there were problems with the ventilator route. However, with minor modification, appropriate attention to filtering exhaled air and pressure pop-off valves should prevent problems.[28,40]

Figure 17–20. Sectional diagram of small-particle aerosol generator (SPAG) for administration of ribavirin aerosol. (Courtesy of ICN Pharmaceuticals, Inc.)

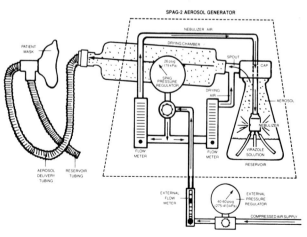

SPINHALER AND ROTAHALER

In the early 1970s, the antiasthma drug cromolyn was introduced along with a solid particle administration device—the spinhaler (Fig. 17–22). The drug was combined with lactose particles that had better "ballistic qualities" than cromolyn itself. The drug is contained in a gelatin capsule and is placed in a small cup. A system allows piercing the capsule, and propellers driven by the patient's inspiratory flow help disperse the medication. The spinhaler must be held with the barrel level to aid in the capsule evacuation.

Manufacturers of cromolyn sodium now also produce the medication in a liquid for jet nebulization and for use in an MDI. Young children may have found the device hard to operate, but there was no problem of timing the inspiration with actuation as in a MDI. Some patients may fail to follow instructions and exhale into the system; moisture in expired air can clog it. Repeated capsule piercing can allow the gelatin capsule to break up and be aspirated.

Recently a device similar to the spinhaler has been introduced for administration of powdered albuterol for bronchodilation. This device, termed a "rotahaler," appears to be an option for the patient who cannot use MDIs or jet nebulizer systems. Bronchodilation appears to be equivalent to the MDI when proper technique is not a factor.[10]

LARGE-VOLUME PNEUMATIC NEBULIZERS

Rationale and Clinical Use

Since the development of "inhalation therapy," mainstream nebulizers have been used to aerosolize liquids, primarily water or physiologic saline solutions. The lack of objective evidence to guide their application has been apparent following several scientific conferences.[2,8,67,107,114] The following is a list of indications for the use of mainstream nebulizers in *current practice*:

- Humidification of medical gases for patients with artificial airways
- Treatment of upper airway inflammation
- Sputum induction

Category Descriptions and Performance

Pneumatically driven nebulizers can be categorized by the physical technique of producing aerosol. *Jet nebulizers utilize the Venturi application* of the

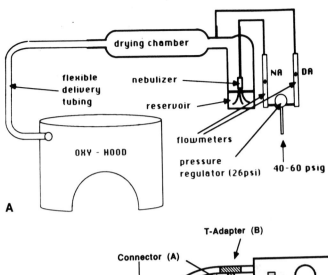

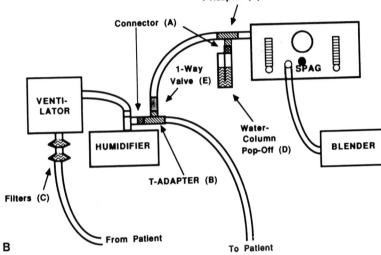

Figure 17–21. (A) Diagram of typical system for pediatric administration of ribavirin aerosol with SPAG and head hood. (Byron PR, Phillips EM, Kuhn R: Ribavirin administration by inhalation: Aerosol-generating factors controlling drug delivery to the lung. Respir Care 33:1011, 1988. Reproduced with permission) (B) Diagram of SPAG aerosol administration in combination with mechanical ventilation.

Bernoulli theorem. A high-pressure gas source is passed through a constriction that ends at the intersection of a tube that is immersed in water (Fig. 17–23). Water is "drawn up" by the subatmospheric pressure at the jet. Liquid impacts with the high-velocity gas and is projected against surfaces that "baffle" larger particles. Immersion or bottom plate heating units offer the option of heating the water reservoirs.

Babbington nebulizers use a similar mechanism. Instead of a jet, gas is directed into a glass sphere that is continuously coated with liquid (Fig. 17–24). Gas exits from a slit in the sphere, rupturing the water film, and projecting particles toward the impactor/baffle. Small aliquots of water are elevated to a drip chamber above the sphere by rising bubbles. A portion of the source gas is routed to a tube in the water reservoir and carries water between rising gas bubbles.

During the aerosol-generating process, both jet and Babbington devices have the option of entraining room air. By governing the size of openings in

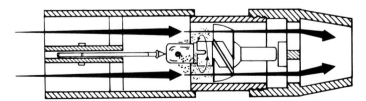

Figure 17–22. Sectional diagram of a spinning powder aerosol dispenser for cromolyn sodium or spinhaler. Subatmospheric pressure from the patients inspiration causes vanes to rotate and medication from a capsule to be evacuated and propelled to the airways.

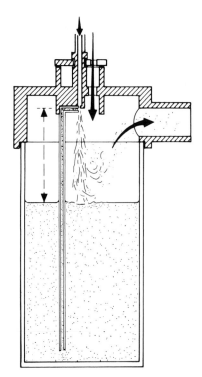

Figure 17–23. Sectional diagram of an "all-purpose" pneumatic jet nebulizer (refer to the text for operational details).

Figure 17–24. Sectional diagram of a "solospere" nebulizer illustrating the Babbington principle (refer to the text for operational details).

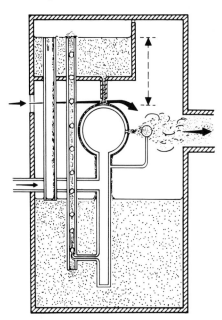

the housings, an FIO_2 from 0.3 to 1.0 can be selected (if powered by pure oxygen). Most units can be connected directly to 50-psig gas sources or run from flowmeters through DISS fittings. Respiratory care practitioners should be familiar with the gas output capabilities of pneumatic nebulizers at various FIO_2. Besides the FIO_2 setting, the flow output must meet or exceed the patient's demands, to ensure consistent oxygen levels. Large holes in masks and open-circuit design will permit additional dilution by the patient. This will lower the FIO_2 and prevent accurate correlation with blood or oximetric measurements. Table 17–12 lists air/oxygen mixing ratios for a range of FIO_2. The following example will illustrate calculation of the total flow output:

> **Example:** A mainstream nebulizer is set at 40% dilution and is being driven with 15 L/min of oxygen. What is the total flow to the patient?
>
> Air/O_2 ratio for FIO_2 of 0.4 = 3.17/1
> 3.17 × 15 = 48 L/min of entrained air
> + 15 L/min of oxygen
> = 63 L/min total flow

Table 17–12   Air/Oxygen Mixing Ratios

FIO_2	AIR/OXYGEN
0.24	25.30/1
0.25	18.75/1
0.30	7.78/1
0.35	4.64/1
0.40	3.17/1
0.45	2.29/1
0.50	1.72/1
0.55	1.32/1
0.60	1.02/1
0.65	0.79/1
0.70	0.61/1
0.75	0.46/1
0.80	0.34/1
0.85	0.23/1
0.90	0.14/1
0.95	0.07/1

The following equation can be used to calculate any air/O_2 ratio:

$\dot{V}O_2$ = flow of oxygen (set at 1 L/min since air/O_2 ratio X/1)
$\dot{V}_{air}$ = flow of room air
$\dot{V}_{Tot}$ = total flow of gas = $\dot{V}O_2$ + $\dot{V}_{air}$
$\dot{V}_{Tot}$ (FIO_2) = $\dot{V}O_2$ + 0.21($\dot{V}_{air}$)
e.g.: for a FIO_2 of 0.40
$\dot{V}_{Tot}(0.4)$ = $\dot{V}O_2$ + 0.21($\dot{V}_{air}$)
($\dot{V}_{air}$ + 1)0.4 = 1 + 0.21($\dot{V}_{air}$)
$0.4\dot{V}_{air}$ + 0.4 = 1 + $.21\dot{V}_{air}$
$0.19\dot{V}_{air}$ = 0.6
$\dot{V}_{air}$ = 3.16 L/min   Therefore, the air/O_2 ratio = 3.16/1

As the FIO_2 is increased, the air/O_2 ratio decreases, causing the total flow to be reduced.

Example: The all-purpose nebulizer, when selected to deliver 70% oxygen, produces the following total output:

$$\text{Air/O}_2 \text{ ratio for FIO}_2 \text{ of } 0.70 = 0.61/1$$
$$0.61 \times 15 = 9.15 \text{ L/min of entrained air}$$
$$+ 15 \text{ L/min of oxygen}$$
$$= 21.15 \text{ L/min total flow}$$

When set on the 100% mode, most manufacturers have limited the inlet orifice to allow about 15 L/min of source gas, which is the total output. Severely dyspneic patients may require up to 60–90 L/min. By not having their inspiratory needs met, they will inspire the necessary volume of room air. Sound decision making will be impaired when blood oxygen levels are correlated to incorrect FIO_2s.

Mainstream jet nebulizer water output (vapor and particulate) is most dependent upon whether the units are heated or cool. The scientific literature is incomplete for water output and aerosol particle size. Most units generate aerosols in the 1- to 10-μm range. Water output is about 0.5–5 mL/min, but will vary with temperature, gas flow, and length of tubing from the nebulizer. However, because these units are designed to deposit particles throughout the airways, particle size is not as significant as it is for medication nebulizers.[19] Levels of relative humidity or body humidity have been reviewed for both heated and unheated units. Tables 17–13 and 17–14 list performance data for Babbington and pneumatic jet nebulizers.

Babbington pneumatic nebulizers are available in three models: solosphere, hydrosphere, and maxicool. The solosphere has the option for a clip-on bottom heater and is used clinically for face masks or tents, T-piece, and tracheostomy collars. It can be connected to source gas through a flowmeter or run directly from 50 psig. The latter two are high-output devices designed for aerosol enclosures (tents). All three have multiposition air entrainment attached to one arm of the housing, to regulate FIO_2 when run on source oxygen.

When run on 50 psig, the hydrosphere and maxicool units are used with closed or open-top "croup" tents. Their high-output flows can flush out heat and carbon dioxide from tents and commonly do not require a refrigeration unit to maintain an environment below ambient temperature. With lower-driving gas flows (i.e., from a flowmeter), the hydrosphere or maxicool can be used for applications similar to an ultrasonic nebulizer (e.g., sputum induction).

Pneumatic Nebulizers in Mist Tent Applications

Mist tents that utilize jet nebulizers commonly incorporate an adjunct cooling apparatus. By convention, most systems attempt to reduce the intratent temperature 5° to 15° F below room temperature. The Air-Shields Croupette uses ice to cool the aerosol. The Ohmeda Ohio Pediatric Aerosol Tent incorporates a Freon refrigeration unit, with fan, to cool tent contents. Mistogen's CAM-2 Tent uses a Freon refrigeration device to cool water that circulates in a "radiatorlike" cooling panel. That company's CAM-3 uses a thermoelectric system, utilizing the Peltier effect. Electric current passing through a semiconductor of dissimilar metals augments heat absorption and release. Warm air is circulated through the heat-transfer module, which returns cool air to the tent and exhausts warm air.

Hazards and Troubleshooting Pneumatic Nebulizers

The following briefly describe problems associated with mainstream pneumatic nebulizers:

Table 17–13 Specifications for Babbington Design Pneumatic Nebulizers

UNIT	RANGE OF OUTPUT FLOW	WATER OUTPUT	PARTICLE SIZE (MASS MEDIAN DIAM.)
Solosphere	15–63 L/min		
Hydrosphere	15–135 L/min		3.6–4.4 μm
Maxicool	30–257 L/min	2–7 mL/min	

Table 17—14   Humidity Output of Jet Mainstream Nebulizers*

BRAND	OUTPUT PERCENT BODY HUMIDITY HEATED/UNHEATED	RESERVOIR VOLUME (mL)	FiO₂ SETTINGS
Ohmeda			
Ohio Deluxe	125/80‡	800	0.4, 0.6, 1.0
High Output	NA	2500	(no indicators)
Puritan-Bennett			
All Purpose	87/70†	375	0.4, 0.7, 1.0 (0.35–1.0 newer models)
Bird Inline Micronebulizer	105/70‡	500	(no dilutional settings)
Mistogen HV-12	NA	2000	0.35–0.7
RCI-Aquapak	NA	440, 760, 1070, and 2200	0.28, 0.35, 0.4, 0.6, 0.8, and 0.98
RCI-Conchapak	—	1650	0.35, 0.4, 0.6, 0.8, and 0.98
Seamless Hosp. U-Mid	76/62†	500	0.35, 0.4, 0.6, 0.7, and 1.0
Corpak	—	465 765	0.28, 0.3, 0.4, 0.6, 0.8, and 1.0
Medical Moulding	NA	400	0.28, 0.35, 0.4, 0.6, 0.8, and 1.0
Mistyox		800	
Inspiron	93/73‡	500	0.35, 0.4, 0.5, 0.7, and 1.0
Travenol	95/61†	1000	0.28, 0.3, 0.35, 0.4, 0.5, 0.7, and 1.0
American Hospital Airlife	—	500, 750, and 1000	0.28, 0.35, 0.4, 0.6, and 0.98

* Manufacturers' data unless noted.
† (Data from Hill TV, Sorbell. JG: Humidity outputs of large-reservoir nebulizers. Respir Care 32:255, 1987)
‡ (Klein EF, Shah DA, Shah NJ, Modell JH, Desautels D: Performance characteristics of conventional and prototype humidifiers and nebulizers. Chest 64:690, 1973)

1. Airway burns have occurred with use of heated nebulizers. Most systems do not have sophisticated servosystems such as heated humidifiers. Immersion, bottom plate, or other styles of heaters can be improperly set or become defective. Temperatures over 44° C can potentially burn airway surfaces. Units that run out of water can quickly heat to unsafe temperatures. Measurement of gas temperature near the airway should be done to ensure safe operation.

2. Bronchospasm occurs as a response to aerosol particles irritating hyperreactive airways. Hypertonic saline solutions, by design, are irritating. Switching patients to humidification devices and pretreatment with a bronchodilator are two options to consider.

3. Sound levels of pneumatic nebulizers may cause hearing loss in infants when used with enclosures such as oxygen hoods or incubators. The American Academy of Pediatrics Committee on Environmental Hazards recommends a level below 58 dB. Such a level is exceeded by a number of mainstream nebulizers with up to 60 cm of large-bore tubing leading to the enclosure.[6]

4. Use of aerosol nebulization systems can be linked to nosocomial infections by either acting as a bacterial reservoir or by direct inoculation of microorganisms. Outbreaks of both pneumonia and sepsis caused by *Pseudomonas*, *Serratia*, *Legionella*, and other organisms have been documented in heated and cool pneumatic nebulizers.[98]

5. Overhydration and excessive salt loads are potential hazards, primarily to neonatal

and pediatric patients receiving long-duration or continuous aerosol therapy.[108]

ULTRASONIC NEBULIZERS

Clinical Application

The ultrasonic nebulizer came into clinical practice in the United States during the 1960s. Although different from the pneumatic devices in nebulization mechanism, they are frequently used interchangeably for delivering bland mists, medications, and hypertonic solutions for sputum induction. Manufacturers have created units for limited application of medicated aerosols and for uses similar to those of mainstream nebulizers. In addition, large-output ultrasonics are also available to apply by mask, face tent, Briggs adaptor, and so on. Mist tents may also be incorporated with ultrasonics. They have also been placed in breathing circuits of mechanical ventilators or IPPB devices. Ultrasonics were touted as the device of choice to apply aerosol to distal airways of the lung by virtue of their high-density, small, and uniform particle size, as well as substantial water output. In theory high-output deposition of saline–water should aid therapy to mobilize thick, tenacious pulmonary secretions. Documentation of improvement from such adjunctive treatment (i.e., used with chest physical therapy, adequate hydration, and such) is not adequate.

The ability to target a certain lung zone by delivering a particle size is quite dependent upon the operating conditions of the nebulizer. Diameter and length of tubing, valves, and patient's breathing pattern are also significant variables. Most texts give a particle dimension of approximately 3 μm for ultrasonics. The mass median diameters of commercial units can range from 0.93 to over 10 μm. Clinical documentation for medication administration has been more abundant than for bland mist therapy. However, most clinically oriented in vitro studies demonstrate that ultrasonic medication nebulizers produce particles only slightly smaller than their pneumatic counterparts.[67,91,114] One advantage of these nebulizers is the lower level of particles smaller than 2 μm, which tend to be so stable that many are exhaled undeposited. Other reports suggest there is little in vivo effect in distribution between particles with diameters of 1.4 or 5.5 μm when inhaled by stable asthmatic patients.[73]

Nebulization by these units is by application of vibrational energy to liquids. Electrical energy is first converted to "sound waves" of acoustic energy. This effect, termed *piezoelectric*, involves vibrating planes of crystal material (quartz–barium titanate) and similar substances. If submerged in shallow depths of water, crystal movement create surface waves. The frequencies, lower than those used for aerosol therapy, are employed in cleaning jewelry and surgical instruments. When the energy density in the liquid phase is large enough, the oscillation waves "crest." This causes a rupturing of filaments, which break into droplets. The mass median diameter of droplets has been shown to be predictable, when the vibratory frequency or wavelength is known.[7]

To generate therapeutic aerosols, the frequency is increased above 800,000 cycles/sec (Hertz, Hz) and the acoustic beam is focused on the fluid. Water couplant is commonly placed between the transducer and the substance being nebulized (Fig. 17–25). Instead of crests, "ultrasonic fountains" are created. An aerosol is emitted adjacent to the bases and along the cylindrical column. The diameter of the fog formation area appears to be a function of frequency and acoustic energy density. Larger fountains, therefore greater output, can be created by increasing the power to the crystal, whereas the frequency remains in the 0.8- to 2.5 million-Hz (MHz) range. However, there appears to be a pla-

Figure 17–25. Sectional diagram of an ultrasonic nebulizer. The aerosol-producing geyser is formed by acoustic energy supplied by a vibrating crystal, shown at the bottom of the device.

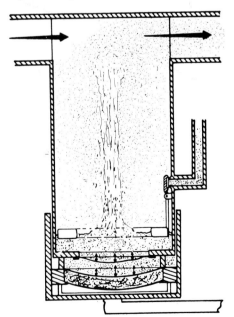

teau at which greater power fails to produce higher output. The physics tend to be complex and involve surface tension, liquid density, and viscosity, in addition to frequency and power.[7]

Another approach is used by a Swedish-designed nebulizer that drips water (by drop or up to 0.3 mL/min) on an unsubmerged transducer. The droplets explode in a high-intensity airborne field.

Unlike pneumatic aerosol generators that use their source gas to propel particles to the patient, ultrasonic nebulizers production must be evacuated from the transducer cup. Auxiliary oxygen flows or low-flow blowers are used on commercial units. Mainstream gas from a mechanical-ventilating device may also be used. The density and mass median diameter is affected by the total flow versus the aerosol production. Low-flow gases tend to produce dense mists of small particles; larger particles are forced back into the geyser. Higher flows produce lower-density mists with larger particles being carried.

Product Description and Performance

Ultrasonic nebulizers can be grouped into two major categories: small-output units for medication administration (Fig. 17–26) and large-output nebulizers for bland mist therapy. Because the clinical setup and measuring procedures vary greatly, there is substantial variation in the literature on particle size output.

Current examples of ultrasonic medication units include the Pulmosonic (DeVilbiss Health Care Division), which has a "fluid" output of approximately 0.5 mL/min, and with which a mass median particle size of 4.2 or 5.4 μm has been re-ported.[21] The device is designed for portable or home application. The Portosonic (DeVilbiss Health Care Division) is similar to the former unit, except that the mass median diameter is reported to be 1.6 μm. Both ultrasonics run on a continuous-flow mode. The Fisoneb (Fisons Corp.) produces particles by pressing a trigger. The mass median diameter of the particle is approximately 5 μm.[21]

Large-volume nebulizers typically have mist outputs of from 3–6 mL/min, depending on the power setting. This would provide body humidity levels of 100% g for gas flows of 68–136 L/min.[58]

Patient Assessment and Troubleshooting

The most common untoward patient response from an ultrasonic nebulizer is some evidence of increased airway reactivity. Signs or symptoms include dyspnea, tachypnea, chest pain, or wheezing. This occurs more frequently when sterile water is used instead of normal saline or bronchodilator drugs. Other problems include overhydration or increased sodium loading. These side effects are of greatest concern when using large-volume nebulizers and when dealing with neonatal or pediatric patients and patients with kidney disorders. If used with mist tents, ultrasonic nebulizers may best be used with open-top tents or auxiliary cooling devices. In contrast with pneumatic aerosol generators, ultrasonic nebulizers add heat.

Studies of ultrasonic nebulizers have shown that reservoirs rapidly become contaminated, which may lead to direct airway inoculation. The most common contaminating bacteria are *Bacillus*, *Staphylococcus*, *Pseudomonas*, and *Enterobacter* species. A high percentage of devices (33%) in in-

Figure 17–26. Commercial small-volume medication nebulizer.

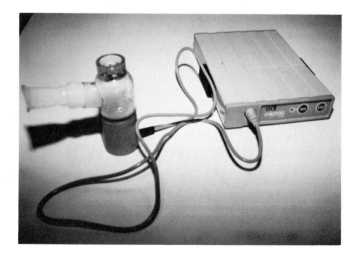

tensive care units become contaminated by gram-negative microbes from background air.[98]

If ultrasonic nebulizers fail to produce mist during operation, several problems can occur that may be remedied at the bedside. Because of high-output capabilities, water can collect at bends or low spots in the tubing, causing blockage. Large-output units commonly have continuous-feed water supplies. Malfunction can flood out the geyser or allow too little water into the nebulization chamber. Other problems are unit-specific and may involve water levels in the couplant chamber, blown fuses or circuit breakers, and vibrational frequency levels out of adjustment.

The possibility also exists for medication to undergo chemical breakdown. Increase in concentration of medication can also occur as solvent evaporates more rapidly than the solute. A prudent protocol involves periodically discarding the remaining nebulizer solutions of saline or medication during prolonged therapy and the addition of fresh solutions.[7]

Acknowledgment: *The authors would like to thank Robert Demers for his contribution in the areas of heat and moisture exchangers, metered close inhalers, and ribavirin aerosol administration.*

REFERENCES

1. American Academy of Pediatrics Committee on Environmental Hazards: Noise pollution neonatal aspects. Pediatrics 54:476, 1974
2. American College of Chest Physicians—National Heart, Lung, and Blood Institute: National conference on oxygen therapy. Respir Care 29:922, 1984
3. American National Standards Institute Inc.: American national standards for humidifiers and nebulizers for medical use. ANSI Z79:9, 1979
4. Anderson S, Herbring BG, Widman B: Accidental profound hypothermia. Br J Anaesth 42:653, 1970
5. Barker GA: Current management of croup and epiglottitis. Pediatr Clin North Am 26:565, 1979
6. Beckham RW, Mishoe SC: Sound levels inside incubators and oxygen hoods used with nebulizers and humidifiers. Respir Care 27:33, 1982
7. Boucher RM, Kreuter J: The fundamentals of the ultrasonic atomization of medicated solutions. Ann Allergy 26:591, 1968
8. Brain J: Aerosol and humidity therapy. Am Rev Respir Dis 122:17, 1980
9. Branson RD, Hurst JM: Laboratory evaluation of seven airway heat and moisture exchangers. Respir Care 32:741, 1987
10. Bronsky E, Bucholtz GA, Busse WW et al: Comparison of inhaled albuterol powder and aerosol in asthma. J Allergy Clin Immunol 79:741, 1987
11. Bygdeman D, von Euler C, Nystrom B: Moisture exchangers do not prevent patient contamination of ventilators. Acta Anaesthesiol Scand 28:591, 1984
12. Byron PR, Phillip EM, Kuhn R: Ribavirin administration by inhalation: Aerosol-generation factors controlling drug delivery to the lung. Respir Care 33:1011, 1988
13. Chanlon J, Loew D, Malbranche J: Effect of dry anesthetic gases on tracheobronchial epithelium. Anesthesiology 37:338, 1972
14. Chatburn RL, Primiano FP: A rational basis for humidity therapy. Respir Care 32:249, 1987
15. Chen WY, Horton DJ: Airway cooling and nocturnal asthma. Chest 81:675, 1982
16. Cissik JH, Bode FR, Smith JA: Double-blind crossover study of five bronchodilator medications and two delivery methods in stable asthma. Chest 90:489, 1986
17. Clarke SW, Lopez-Vidriero MT, Pavia D et al: The effect of sodium 2-mercaptoethane sulfonate and hypertonic saline aerosols on bronchial clearance in chronic bronchitis. Br J Clin Pharmacol 7:39, 1979
18. Clausen JL: Self-administration of bronchodilators: Cost effective? [Editorial] Chest 91:475, 1987
19. Clay MM, Pavia D, Newman SP et al: Assessment of jet nebulisers for lung aerosol therapy. Lancet 2:592, 1983
20. Comroe JH: Physiology of Respiration, 2nd ed. Chicago, Year Book Medical, 1974
21. Corkery KJ, Luce JM, Montgomery AB: Aerosolized pentamidine for treatment and prophylaxis of *Pneumocystis carinii* pneumonia: An update. Respir Care 33:676, 1988
22. Craven DE, Lichtenberg DA, Goularte TA et al: Contaminated medication nebulizers in mechanical ventilator circuits: A source of bacterial aerosols. Am J Med 77:834, 1984
23. Craven DE, Goularte TA, Make BJ: Contaminated condensate in mechanical ventilator circuits: A risk factor for nosocomial pneumonia. Am Rev Respir Dis 129:625, 1984
24. Craven DE, Steger KA: Pathogenesis and prevention of nosocomial pneumonia in the mechanically ventilated patient. Respir Care 34:85, 1989
25. Crompton GK: Problems patients have using pressurized aerosol inhalers. Eur J Respir Dis 63(Suppl):119, 1982
26. Darin J: The need for rational criteria for the use of unheated bubbler humidifiers [editorial]. Respir Care 27:945, 1982
27. Darin JD, Broadwell J, MacDonell R: An evaluation of water–vapor output from four brands of unheated prefilled bubble humidifiers. Respir Care 27:41, 1982
28. Demers RR, Parker J, Frankel LR, Smith DW: Administration of ribavirin to neonatal and pediatric patients during mechanical ventilation. Respir Care 31:1188, 1986
29. Dery R: The evolution of heat and moisture in the respiratory tract during anesthesia with a non-rebreathing system. Can Anaesth Soc J 20:296, 1973
30. Dolovich MB, Sanchis J, Rossmand C, Newhouse MT: Aerosol penetration: A sensitive index of peripheral airways obstruction. J Appl Physiol 40:486, 1976
31. Dolovich MB, Ruffin RE, Roberts R, Newhouse MT: Optimal delivery of aerosols from metered dose inhalers. Chest 80(Suppl 6):911, 1981

32. Emergency Care Research Institute: Evaluation: Heated nebulizers. Health Devices 6:3, 1976

33. Emergency Care Research Institute. Heated humidifiers. Health Devices 16:223, 1987

34. Emergency Care Research Institute: Heat moisture exchangers. Health Devices 12:155, 1983

35. Eriksson NE, Haglind K, Hidinger KG: A new inhalation technique for Freon aerosols: Terbutaline aerosol with a tube extension in a 2-day cross-over comparison with salbutanol aerosol. Allergy 35:617, 1980

36. Estey W: Subjective effects of dry versus humidified low flow oxygen. Respir Care 25:1143, 1980

37. Ferron GA, Kerrebijn KF, Weber J: Properties of aerosols produced with three nebulizers. Am Rev Respir Dis 114:899, 1976

38. Flick MR, Moody LE, Block AJ: Effect of ultrasonic nebulization on arterial oxygen saturation in chronic obstructive pulmonary disease. Chest 71:366, 1977

39. Fowler WS, Helmholz HF, Miller RD: Treatment of pulmonary emphysema with aerosolized bronchodilator drugs and intermittent positive-pressure breathing. Mayo Clin Proc 28:743, 1953

40. Frankel LR, Wilson CW, Demers RR et al: A technique for the administration of ribavirin to mechanically ventilated infants with severe respiratory syncytial virus infection. Crit Care Med 15:1051, 1987

41. Gawley TH, Dundee JW: Attempts to reduce respiratory complications following upper abdominal operations. Br J Anaesth 53:1073, 1981

42. Gay PC, Rodarte JR, Tayyab M, Hubmayr RD: Evaluation of bronchodilator responsiveness in mechanically ventilated patients. Am Rev Respir Dis 136:880, 1987

43. Gedeon B, Lindholm CE: The foam nose—a new disposable heat and moisture exchanger. Acta Anaesthesiol. Scand 23:34, 1979

44. Gerrity TR, et al: The effect of aspirin on lung mucociliary clearance. N Engl J Med 308:139, 1983

45. Goodison RR. Pseudomonas cross-infection due to contaminated humidifier water. Br Med J 281:1288, 1980

46. Gutierrez CJ, Nelson R: Short-term bronchodilation in mechanically ventilated patients, patients receiving metaproterenol via small volume nebulizer or metered-dose-inhaler. A pilot study. Respir Care 33:910, 1988

47. Haesoon L, Evans HE: Evaluation of inhalation aids of metered dose inhalers in asthmatic children. Chest 91:366, 1987

48. Hall CB, Powell KR, McDonald NE et al: Respiratory syncytial viral infection in children with compromised immune function. N Engl J Med 315:77, 1986

49. Hayton WL: Propellant-powered nebulizers. J Am Pharm Assoc 16:201, 1976

50. Henry R: Moist air in the treatment of laryngotracheitis. Arch Dis Child 58:577, 1983

51. Hess D, Beener C, Watson KK: An evaluation of the effectiveness of metered dose inhaler use with mechanical ventilation. Respir Care 33:910, 1988

52. Hess D: The open forum: Reflections on unanswered questions about aerosol therapy delivery techniques [Editorial]. Respir Care 33:19, 1988

53. Hill TV, Sorbello JG: Humidity outputs of large-reservoir nebulizers. Respir Care 32:255, 1987

54. Hiller C: Aerodynamic size distribution of metered-dose bronchodilator aerosols. Am Rev Resp Dis 118:311, 1978

55. Ingelstedt S: Studies on the conditioning of air in the respiratory tract. Acta Otolaryngol Suppl 131:1, 1956

56. Jasper AC, Mohsenifar Z, Kahan S et al: Cost–benefit comparison of aerosol bronchodilator delivery methods in hospitalized patients. Chest 91:614, 1987

57. Jenkins SC, Heaton RW, Fulton TJ, Moxham J: Comparison of domiciliary nebulized salbutamol and salbutamol from a metered-dose inhaler in stable chronic airflow limitation. Chest 91:804, 1987

58. Klein EF, Shah DA, Shah NJ et al: Performance characteristics of conventional and prototype humidifiers and nebulizers. Chest 64:690, 1973

59. Knight V, Wilson SZ, Wyde PR et al: Small particle aerosols of amantadine and ribavirin in the treatment of influenza. In Ribavirin: A Broad Spectrum Antiviral Agent. London, Academic Press, 1980

60. Konig P: Spacer devices used with metered-dose inhalers. Chest 88:276, 1985

61. Lasky MS: Bubble humidifiers are useful—fact or myth? [Letter] Respir Care 27:735, 1982

62. Lawson EE: Exogenous surfactant therapy to prevent respiratory distress syndrome. J Pediatr 110:492, 1987

63. Leigh JM, White MG: A new condenser humidifier. Anaesthesia 39:492, 1984

64. Lewis RA, Fleming JS: Fractional deposition from a jet nebulizer: How it differs from a metered dose inhaler. Br J Dis Chest 79:361, 1985

65. Li JT, Reed CE: Proper use of aerosol corticosteroids to control asthma. Mayo Clin Proc 64:205, 1989

66. Lourenco RV, Cotromanes E: Clinical aerosols I: Characterization of aerosols and their diagnostic use. Arch Intern Med 142:2163, 1982

67. Lourenco RV, Cotromanes E: Clinical aerosols II: Therapeutic aerosols. Arch Intern Med 142:2299, 1982

68. MacIntyre NR, Anderson HR, Silver RM: Pulmonary function in mechanically ventilated patients during 24 hours use of a hygroscopic condenser humidifier. Chest 5:560, 1983

69. MacLusky I, Levison H, Gold R, McLaughlin J: Inhaled antibiotics in cystic fibrosis: Is there a therapeutic effect? J Pediatr 108:861, 1986

70. McFadden ER Jr et al: Thermal mapping of the airways in humans. J Appl Physiol 2:564, 1985

71. Mebius C: A comparative evaluation of disposable humidifiers. Acta Anaesthesiol Scand 27:403, 1983

72. Miller RD, Divertie MB: Kartagener's syndrome. Chest 62:130, 1972

73. Mitchell DM, Solomon MA, Tolfree SE et al: Effect of particle size of bronchodilator aerosols on lung distribution and pulmonary function in patients with chronic asthma. Thorax 42:457, 1987

74. Montgomery AB, Debs RJ, Luce JM et al: Selective delivery of pentamidine to the lung by aerosol. Am Rev Respir Dis 137:477, 1988

75. Morley TF, Marozsan E, Zappasodi SJ et al: Comparison of beta-adrenergic agents delivered by nebulizer vs. metered dose inhaler with Inspirease in hospitalized asthmatic patients. Chest 94:1205, 1988

76. Morrow PE: Aerosol characterization and deposition. Am Rev Respir Dis 110:88, 1974

77. Newhouse MT, Dolovich MB: Current concepts:

Control of asthma by aerosols. N Engl J Med 315:871, 1986

78. Newhouse M, Dolovich MB: Aerosol therapy: Nebulizer vs. metered dose inhaler. Chest 91:799, 1987

79. Newman SP, Clarke SW: Therapeutic aerosols: Physical and practical considerations [Editorial]. Thorax 38:881, 1983

80. Newman SP, Clarke SW: Proper use of metered dose inhalers [editorial]. Chest 86:342, 1984

81. Pavia D, Thompson M, Shannon HS: Aerosol inhalation and depth of deposition in the human lung: The effect of airway obstruction and tidal volume inhaled. Arch Environ Health 32:131, 1977

82. Pavia D, Thomson ML, Clarke SW: Enhanced clearance of secretions from the human lung after the administration of hypertonic saline aerosol. Am Rev Respir Dis 117:199, 1978

83. Pedersen S: The importance of a pause between inhalation of two puffs of terbutaline from a pressurized aerosol with tube spacer. J Allergy Clin Immunol 77:505, 1986

84. Pisut F: Comparison of medication delivery by T-nebulizer with expiratory reservoir and without reservoir. Respir Care 33:916, 1988

85. Poulton TJ, Downs JB: Humidification of rapidly flowing gas. Crit Care Med 9:59, 1981

86. Postma DS, Jones RO, Pillsbury HC: Severe hospitalized croup: Treatment trends and prognosis. Laryngoscope 94:1170, 1984

87. Poulton TJ: Humidification hazard [Letter]. Chest 85:583, 1984

88. Prahl P, Jensen T: Decreased adrenocortical suppression utilizing the Nebuhaler for inhalation of steroid aerosols. Clin Allergy 17:393, 1987

89. Primiano FP Jr, Montague FW Jr, Saidel GM: Measurement system for water vapor and temperature dynamics. J Appl Physiol 56:1679, 1984

90. Rachelefsky GS, Clark AR, Goldenhursh M et al: Multi-shot metered dose inhaler (MDI) and reservoir devices [Abstract]. J Allergy Clin Immunol 81:315, 1988

91. Rau, JL: Humidity and aerosol therapy. In: Barnes T (ed): Respiratory Care Practice, p 164. Chicago, Year Book Medical, 1988

92. Rhame FS, Streifel A, McComb C, Boyle M: Bubbling humidifiers produce microaerosols which can carry bacteria. Infect Control 7:403, 1986

93. Revenas B, Lindholm CE: Temperature variations heat and moisture exchanges. Acta Anaesthesiol Scand 24:237, 1980

94. Rivlin J, Mindorff C, Reilly P, Levinson H: Pulmonary response to a bronchodilator delivered from three inhalation devices. J Pediatr 104:470, 1984

95. Rossing TH, Fanta CH, McFadden ER: Effect of outpatient treatment of asthma with beta agonist on the response to sympathomimetics in an emergency room. Am J Med 75:781, 1983

96. Ruffin RE, Montgomery JM, Newhouse MT: Site of beta-adrenergic receptors in the respiratory tract: Use of fenoterol administered by two methods. Chest 74:256, 1978

97. Ruffin RE, Kenworthy MC, Newhouse MT: Response of asthmatic patients to fenoterol inhalation: A method of quantifying the airway bronchodilator dose. Clin Pharmacol Ther 23:338, 1978

98. Rutala WA, Weber DJ: Environmental issues and nosocomial infection. In: Farber BF (ed): Infection Control in Intensive Care, p 131. New York, Churchill Livingstone, 1987

99. Sakner MA, Kim CS: Auxiliary MDI aerosol delivery systems. Chest 885:161S, 1985

100. Schmidt-Nielsen K: Countercurrent systems in animals. Sci Am 244:118, 1981

101. Shanks CA: The effects of inspiration of gases saturated with water vapor on heat and moisture exchange during endotracheal intubation. Br J Anaesth 45:887, 1973

102. Shelly M, Bethune DW, Latimer RD: A comparison of fine heat moisture exchanges. Anaesthesia 41:527, 1986

103. Shelly MP, Lloyd GM, Pack GR: A review of the mechanism and methods of humidification of inspired gases. Intensive Care Med 14:1, 1988

104. Shepherd KE, Johnson DC: Bronchodilator testing: An analysis of paradoxical responses. Respir Care 33:667, 1988

105. Shim C: Inhalation aids of metered dose inhalers. Chest 91:315, 1987

106. Strauss RH et al: Influence of heat and humidity on the airway obstruction induced by exercise in asthma. J Clin Invest 61:433, 1978

107. Swift DL: Aerosols and humidity therapy: Generation and respiratory deposition. Am Rev Respir Dis 122(Suppl):71, 1980

108. Tamer MA, Modell JH, Rieffel CN: Hyponatremia secondary to ultrasonic aerosol therapy in the newborn infant. J Pediatr 77:1051, 1970

109. Thompson A, Traver GA: Comparison of three methods of administering a self-propelled bronchodilator. Am Rev Respir Dis 125:140, 1982

110. Tobin MT, Jenouri G, Danta I et al: Response to a bronchodilator drug administered by a new reservoir aerosol delivery system and review of the auxiliary delivery systems. Am Rev Respir Dis 126:670, 1982

111. Toogood JH, baskerville J, Jennings B et al: Use of spacers to facilitate inhaled corticosteroids in treatment of asthma. Am Rev Respir Dis 129:723, 1984

112. Tsuda T, Noguchi H, Takaumi Y, Aochi O: Optimum humidification of air administered to a tracheostomy in dogs: Scanning electron microscopy and surfactant studies. Br J Anaesth 49:965, 1977

113. Walker AKY, Bethune DW: A comparative study of condenser humidifiers. Anaesthesia 31:1086, 1976

114. Wanner A, Rao A: Clinical indications for and effects of bland, mucolytic and antimicrobial aerosols. Am Rev Respir Dis 122:79, 1980

115. Weeks DB, Ramsey FM: Laboratory investigation of six artificial noses for use during endotracheal anesthesia. Anesth Analg 62:758, 1983

116. Wells RE, Walker JEC, Hickler RB: Effects of cold air on respiratory airflow resistance in patients with respiratory-tract disease. N Engl J Med 263:268, 1960

117. Weinstein RE et al: Effects of humidification on exercise-induced asthma [Abstract]. Allergy Clin Immunol 57:250, 1976

118. Williams S, Seaton A: Intravenous or inhaled salbutamol in severe acute asthma? Thorax 32:555, 1977

119. Wilton LJ, Teichtahl H, Temple-Smith PD, de Kretser DM: Kartagener's syndrome with motile cilia and immotile spermatozoa: Axonemal ultrastructure and function. Am Rev Respir Dis 134:1233, 1986

120. Ziment I: Respiratory Pharmacology and Therapeutics. Philadelphia, WB Saunders, 1978
121. Ziment I: Bronchodilator aerosol therapy: How to make an efficacious treatment more reliable. Respir Ther 12:59, 1982

BIBLIOGRAPHY

Brain JD: Aerosol and humidity therapy. In O'Donohue WJ (ed): Current Advances in Respiratory Care. Park Ridge, Ill, American College of Chest Physicians, 1984

Chatburn RL, Primiano PR: A rational basis for humidity therapy [Editorial]. Respir Care 32:249, 1987

Corkery KJ, Luce JM, Montgomery AB: Aerosolized pentamidine for treatment and prophylaxis of *Pneumocystis carinii* pneumonia. Respir Care 33:676, 1988

Emergency Care Research Institute: Heated humidifiers. Health Devices 16:223, 1987

Emergency Care Research Institute: Heat moisture exchangers 12:155, 1983

Lourenco RV, Cotromanes E: Clinical aerosols I: Characterization of aerosols and their diagnostic use. Arch Intern Med 142:2163, 1982

Lourenco RV, Cotromanes E: Clinical aerosols II: Therapeutic aerosols. Arch Intern Med 142:2299, 1982

Newhouse MT, Dolovich MB: Current concepts: Control of asthma by aerosols. N Engl J Med 315:871, 1986

Newman SP, Clarke SW: Therapeutic aerosols: Physical and practical considerations [Editorial]. Thorax 38:881, 1983

Op't Holt, T: Aerosol generators and humidifiers. In Barnes TA (ed): Respiratory Care Practice, p 356. Chicago, Year Book Medical, 1988

Rau JL: Humidity and aerosol therapy. In Barnes TA (ed): Respiratory Care Practice, p 164. Chicago, Year Book Medical, 1988

Shelly MP, Lloyd GM, Pack GR: A review of the mechanism and methods of humidification of inspired gases. Intensive Care Med 14:1, 1988

Ziment I: Respiratory Pharmacology and Therapeutics. Philadelphia, WB Saunders, 1978

EIGHTEEN

Infectious Disease Aspects of Respiratory Therapy

John A. Washington

Pulmonary infections may be due to a variety of microorganisms, including bacteria, mycobacteria, chlamydiae, mycoplasmas, fungi, parasites, and viruses, that may be acquired either in the community or in the hospital. Initial management of the patient with pulmonary infection, therefore, requires an understanding of various host factors, including age, sex, and occupation; underlying diseases or conditions; medications; sexual practices and preferences; place of acquisition of the infection (i.e., community, hospital, or nursing home); circumstances surrounding onset of infection, such as the season of the year, recent travel or environmental exposures; and the type of presentation, including the mode of onset of illness and its rate of progression.

MICROBIAL CLASSIFICATION AND PATHOGENICITY

There are many approaches to the classification of microorganisms. First, they may be classified according to their structural characteristics as (1) *viruses*, which are the smallest infectious agents, have the simplest structure, and are obligate intracellular parasites; (2) *prokaryotes*, which lack a nuclear membrane enclosing chromosomal material, do not reproduce by mitosis, and include bacteria, chlamydiae, mycoplasmas, rickettsiae, and spiro-chetes; and (3) *eukaryotes*, which have chromosomes enclosed within a membrane, reproduce by mitosis, and include fungi and protozoa.

Bacteria have a rigid, relatively thick cell wall external to a cytoplasmic membrane that encloses their nuclear bodies, ribosomes, and a variety of small molecular structures, inorganic ions, and enzymes. The thickness of the bacterial cell wall is a major determinant of the Gram stain reaction in that the crystal violet–iodine complex is retained by the relatively thick cell wall of gram-positive (purple) bacteria, but not by the thin cell wall of gram-negative (red) bacteria. Bacteria are further categorized morphologically as bacilli or cocci, and as aerobic, facultatively anaerobic, or anaerobic, according to their requirements for growth in air (aerobic), in the absence of oxygen (anaerobic), or their ability to grow under either condition (facultatively anaerobic). Chlamydiae and rickettsiae are obligate intracellular bacteria.

Fungi include yeast and filamentous (mold) forms and differ structurally from bacteria not only in having a nuclear membrane and in their mode of reproduction, but also by the presence of sterols in their cytoplasmic membranes and chitin in their cell walls. The protozoa, by contrast, share many structural properties with human cells.

Viruses contain a central core of DNA or RNA that is surrounded by a protein coat (capsid), which protects the viral nucleic acid from physical or chemical inactivation and facilitates attachment of the virus to the host cell. Other than their simple organization, viruses differ from prokaryotes or eukaryotes in their mode of reproduction in that, after their invasion of the host cell, viruses use the cell's machinery to synthesize their separate components and then assemble them into complete viral particles.

A second approach to classification of disease-producing microorganisms is according to whether they are (1) extracellular parasites that produce infection by multiplying outside cells and are usually killed when ingested by phagocytes; (2) facultative intracellular parasites that can be ingested, although not killed, by phagocytes; or (3) obligate intracellular parasites that can multiply only within cells. Examples of the first category are *Streptococcus pneumoniae*, *Staphylococcus aureus*, *Escherichia coli*, *Pseudomonas aeruginosa*, and *Haemophilus influenzae*. Examples of the second category are mycobacteria (other than *Mycobacterium leprae*), *Legionella*, *Nocardia*, and fungi, such as *Candida*, *Cryptococcus*, and *Coccidioides*. Obligate intracellular parasites include chlamydiae, rickettsiae, and viruses.

Microorganisms are sometimes classified as *saprophytic* (i.e., they can exist independently of a living host) or *parasitic*, (i.e., their survival depends on living cells or tissue). Parasitic microorganisms may be commensals that coexist harmlessly with host cells or pathogens that damage host cells. The separation between commensals and pathogens has now become quite blurred in this era of immunocompromised patients, in that microorganisms previously thought to be harmless commensals (e.g., coagulase-negative staphylococci) have been found to be pathogenic in patients with impaired host defenses.

INDIGENOUS MICROBIAL FLORA

Many microorganisms are normally present on the skin and mucous membranes and, therefore, represent indigenous or commensal flora (Table 18–1). The oropharynx, for example, normally harbors over 200 bacterial species in quantities of up to 10^8 bacteria per milliliter of saliva. Certain components of the indigenous flora vary because of occupational exposure. For example, *Staphylococcus aureus* is found in the nares of approximately 30% of the normal, healthy population; however, it may be found in the nares of up to 70% of hospitalized patients and health care personnel. Carriage of

S. aureus on the hands is also significantly higher in health care personnel. Although not normally present on the skin, gram-negative bacilli, such as *Pseudomonas aeruginosa* and *Klebsiella pneumoniae*, may be transiently present on the skin. The transient carriage of such pathogenic microorganisms on the skin of health care personnel constitutes an important mechanism for nosocomial spread of infection within hospitals and underscores the importance of handwashing between treating each patient to limit the transmission of infectious agents.

The composition of indigenous flora can also be influenced by disease, environment, and antimicrobial agents. For example, enteric bacilli seldom constitute the indigenous flora of the oropharynx; however, they are frequently found in this site in chronic alcoholics and in seriously ill and debilitated intensive care unit patients, regardless of whether such patients are receiving ventilatory assistance or antimicrobial therapy. Antimicrobial therapy may suppress the susceptible indigenous flora and allow colonization by pathogenic antibiotic-resistant microorganisms. Experimental data derived from animals have shown that a reduction in the normal gut flora facilitates colonization by pathogenic bacteria, such as *Salmonella*, *Pseudomonas*, or *Enterobacter*. Although the mechanism by which the indigenous flora of the gut plays a role in colonization resistance is unclear, selective decontamination regimens with antibiotics that spare the anaerobic bacterial flora of the gut have shown some success in preventing gram-negative infections in seriously ill intensive care unit patients, as well as during maximal immunosuppression of patients undergoing bone marrow transplantation.

The most common lower respiratory pathogens are listed in Table 18–2.

MICROBIAL PATHOGENICITY

The first requirement for microbial pathogenicity is the microorganism's ability to adhere to epithelial surfaces. This process occurs through rather specific surface interactions involving *adhesins*, which are microbial surface molecules or organelles that bind to a receptor with complementary substrate molecules. Many bacteria, for example, possess fimbriae, which are filamentous structures that serve as adhesins that may be host-specific or specific for certain epithelial surfaces. For example, the meningococcus adheres by means of its fimbriae to nasopharyngeal cells more than to buccal

Table 18—1 Microorganisms Encountered on Healthy Human Body Surfaces*

ORGANISM	SKIN	CONJUNCTIVA	UPPER RESPIRATORY TRACT	MOUTH	TERMINAL ILEUM, CECUM, LARGE INTESTINE	GENITOURINARY TRACT		
						External Genitalia	Anterior Urethra	Vagina
Bacteria								
Actinomyces			+	+	±			
Bacteroides			+	++	++	+	+	+
Bifidobacteria				+	++			
Clostridia	±			±	++		±	±
Corynebacteria	++	+	+	+	+	+	+	+
Enterobacteriaceae	±		±	±	++	+	+	±
Eubacteria	±		±	+	++			±
Fusobacteria			+	++	+	+	+	±
Haemophili		±	++	+				+†
Lactobacilli				+	+		±	++
Neisseriae		±	++	+			±	±
Propionibacteria	++	+	+	±	±			+
Staphylococci	++	+	+	+	±	++	+	+
Streptococci								
Enterococcal			±	+	+	+	+	+
Pyogenic			±	±				± to ++‡
Viridans	±	±	±	++	+	+	+	+
Cocci, anaerobic								
Gram-positive	+	±	+	++	++	+	±	+
Gram-negative			+	++	+		±	+
Chlamydiae							±	±
Mycoplasmas			+	+			+	+
Spirochetes		+		±	+			
Fungi								
Aspergillus	±	±		+				
Candida	±	±	+	++	+			+
Cephalosporium	±	±	±					±
Cryptococcus	±			±				
Fusarium	±	±		±				
Penicillium	+	±		+				
Rhodotorula	±	±		+				

(Washington JA: Laboratory Procedures in Clinical Microbiology, 2nd ed, pp 2–3. Springer-Verlag, Mayo Foundation, 1985)
* ±, irregular or infrequent; +, common; ++, prominent.
† *Gardnerella vaginalis.*
‡ Group B.

or urethral cells. Pneumococci that are associated with otitis media adhere firmly to pharyngeal cells, whereas *P. aeruginosa* adheres more to nasal and tracheal cells than to buccal cells.

Once attached to an epithelial cell surface, the microorganism may multiply on the surface without invading the cell and produce disease by elaborating a soluble toxin that is absorbed by the cell to produce local or distant damage. Examples of such pathogens include *Corynebacterium diphtheriae*, which causes diphtheria, and *Bordetella pertussis*, which causes whooping cough.

Alternatively, microorganisms can multiply and cause disease by penetrating and damaging the cell, passing through the cell to the submucosa, and perhaps, spreading to other parts of the body, or, as with viruses, utilizing the cell's machinery to reproduce themselves before damaging the cell.

Table 18—2 Common Lower Respiratory Pathogens

CLASS	PATHOGENS
Viruses	Influenza A
	Influenza B
	Adenoviruses
	Respiratory syncytial virus
	Parainfluenza viruses
Bacteria	*Streptococcus pneumoniae*
	Staphylococcus aureus
	Haemophilus influenzae
	Enterobacteriaceae
	Klebsiella pneumoniae
	Pseudomonas aeruginosa
	Legionella sp
	Mycoplasma pneumoniae
	Chlamydia sp
Fungi	*Coccidioides immitis*
	Histoplasma capsulatum
	Blastomyces dermatitidis
	Aspergillus sp
	Cryptococcus neoformans
	Candida sp
Protozoa	*Pneumocystis carinii**

* Taxonomy uncertain.

HOST DEFENSE MECHANISMS

The first line of host defense against microorganisms is the skin, which provides a mechanical barrier, except where its continuity is broken. An intact mucosal epithelial surface, including that of the conducting airways of the lung, is also important to host defense, but constitutes an appreciably less difficult barrier than does the skin. No bacteria are known to penetrate the intact skin. In fact, the acidic pH of normal skin, along with long-chain fatty acids that are located in sebaceous glands and have antibacterial activity, prevent the survival of pathogenic bacteria on the skin for any length of time. Moreover, many of the bacteria that make up the indigenous flora of the skin and mucous membranes produce bacteriocins, which are toxins directed at other bacteria. Nonetheless, because pathogenic microorganisms may survive transiently on the skin, the skin does serve as an important vehicle for transmission of infection, and careful handwashing, especially by health care workers, is an important control measure to prevent the transmission of infection.

An important internal defense mechanism is the inflammatory response. Once microorganisms penetrate the mechanical barrier of the skin or mucous membrane, they stimulate an inflammatory response, which consists of a variety of phagocytic cells, including neutrophils, monocytes, lymphocytes, and tissue macrophages. The functions of these cells is to ingest and destroy invading microorganisms, as well as to remove microbial and host debris and dispose of inflammation-producing toxins. Macrophages are normally present in the alveoli, in the interalveolar and peribronchial tissue, and near the surfaces of airways in the lungs. Pulmonary macrophages, therefore, are uniquely situated to interact with microorganisms and other particulate matter that have penetrated the normal mechanical barriers.

Many microorganisms resist phagocytosis by means of surface components, such as a capsule or a specific cell wall antigen. In such cases, plasma proteins may contain specific antibody that interacts with a plasma component (complement) that promotes phagocytosis.

Antibodies or immunoglobulins (Ig) are normally present in the body and bind to numerous foreign substances (antigens) that the host may encounter over a lifetime. Antibodies mediate humoral immunity and are intended to eliminate or destroy an antigen. Antibody is formed after a latent period of several days when the host is first exposed to an antigen (primary response). Antibody, predominantly IgM, increases exponentially, peaks in 1 or 2 weeks, and then decreases; however, reexposure to the same antigen provokes a secondary response in which the amount of antibody produced is substantially greater than that in the primary response and is predominantly of the IgG class.

Antibodies promote (1) *opsonization,* whereby microorganisms become coated with antibody and complement and are prepared for ingestion by phagocytic cells; (2) *activation of the complement system* that causes lysis of cells; (3) *neutralization of toxins;* (4) *prevention of bacterial adherence* to epithelial cells; and (5) *neutralization of viral infectivity,* whereby viruses are prevented from attaching to cells.

Lymphocytes play a major role in the immune response in several ways. Lymphocytes are divided into two classes, B and T cells, according to their tissue of differentiation (bone marrow and thymus). The B lymphocytes synthesize immunoglobulins following exposure to specific antigens and are precursors of plasma cells, which are the major cells involved in antibody production. T lymphocytes have a number of functions in immunity. Some T lymphocytes enhance the immune response, whereas others suppress it. In general, however, cell-mediated immunity (CMI) is effected by T lymphocytes and contributes to host defenses against a variety of intracellular parasites, such as *Legionella, Mycobacterium, Chlamydia, Histoplasma,* and cytomegalovirus (CMV). Immunity to such infections cannot be transferred from immunized to nonimmunized hosts by serum containing antibodies directed against the microorganisms causing these infections, rather it may be transferred by lymphocytes from an immunized host to a nonimmunized host.

In brief, an antigen interacting with a macrophage is taken up by the macrophage, processed, and presented to B lymphocytes that are activated to synthesize antibody and to T lymphocytes that are stimulated to produce other factors responsible for CMI. At the same time, however, T lymphocytes may generate inhibitory or suppressor factors or cells, so that, ultimately, immunity represents a highly complex and as yet incompletely understood process representing a balance between activation and regulation.

PATHOGENESIS OF PNEUMONIA

Host defenses that are specific to the respiratory tract include not only humoral- and cell-mediated immunity but also the ciliated and squamous epithelium in the nasopharynx, anatomic barriers such as the epiglottis and larynx, mucociliary clearance, coughing, bronchoconstriction, and secretory IgA.

The nasal ciliated epithelium overlies a submucosa with abundant plasma cells and secretes fluid containing predominantly IgA immunoglobulins, which may diminish bacterial attachment. Immunoglobulin A is also present in high concentrations in the large airways. At the alveolar level neither mucous-secreting cells nor ciliated epithelium is present, and microbial clearance depends on humoral and cellular factors. In addition, *surfactant,* which is excreted by pneumocytes in the alveoli, may inactivate certain bacteria. Immunoglobulins and complement opsonize bacteria and prepare them for ingestion by alveolar macrophages. Cell-mediated immunity is of particular importance for control of intracellular microorganisms, including mycobacteria, *Legionella, Listeria monocytogenes, Pneumocystis carinii,* and cytomegalovirus.

From the foregoing, it should be obvious that alteration of mechanical barriers, depressed cough reflex, immunoglobulin defects, complement deficiencies, and immunosuppression can predispose to pulmonary infection. Many factors contribute to the development of pneumonia, including those that are (1) host-specific, such as smoking, alcoholism, obesity, underlying disease (diabetes, chronic obstructive pulmonary disease, prior viral illness, acidosis, trauma, altered consciousness), and immunosuppression (hematologic malignancy, AIDS); (2) invasive procedures, such as surgery, nasogastric and endotracheal intubation, and tracheostomy; and (3) medications, such as antimicrobial agents, corticosteroids, cytotoxic agents, antacids or histamine type 2 receptor antagonists, and central nervous system depressants.

Microorganisms usually reach the lung by inhalation or, far less frequently, through the bloodstream from another infected site. Inhaled or aspirated microorganisms may originate from the oropharynx (endogenous) or from aerosols created exogenously, either from the environment or from other persons who are coughing or sneezing nearby.

As previously discussed, the oropharynx harbors a wide variety of bacterial species and a multitude of bacteria overall. This microbial flora is acquired shortly after birth and varies slightly in its composition from person to person. It may also vary because of interpersonal transmission from other family members or in other settings of close interpersonal contact, such as day care centers and convalescent hospitals. Certain bacterial species have a predisposition for adherence to specific sites such as tooth surfaces, the tongue, or the buccal mucosa. Thus, potentially pathogenic bacteria must not only effectively compete with the indigenous flora of the oropharynx but also overcome local physical, chemical, and immunologic factors.

In seriously ill hospitalized patients, the oropharynx often becomes colonized with gram-negative bacilli, such as *E. coli, K. pneumoniae,* or *P. aeruginosa.* The mechanisms by which such colonization occurs is complex and incompletely understood. One interesting observation is that colonization of the stomach may precede oropharyngeal colonization, as the result of enteral feedings or the administration of antacids or histamine type 2 receptor antagonists that decrease gastric acidity and allow bacterial overgrowth to occur. Another observation is that antimicrobial therapy eradicates the largely susceptible indigenous flora of the oropharynx and allows it to be replaced by antibiotic-resistant "opportunistic" bacteria. Other potential mechanisms include transmission of pathogenic microorganisms from contaminated sources, such as respiratory equipment, hands of health care workers, and uncooked vegetables and fruits.

Whatever the mechanisms, oropharyngeal colonization with potentially pathogenic bacteria constitutes a major risk factor for the development of pneumonia. It should be emphasized, however, that because we normally aspirate small amounts of oropharyngeal secretions during sleep, factors such as the number of microorganisms aspirated, their pathogenicity, and the integrity of multiple host defense mechanisms are important determinants of whether infection results.

Intubation poses a number of unique risk factors for the development of pneumonia.[1] The endotracheal tube reduces the natural warming and humidification of inspired air; bypasses the normal mechanical host defense barriers; acts as a foreign body that causes local inflammation and alters bacterial colonization; causes obstruction and secondary infection of the paranasal sinuses; traumatizes the tracheal epithelium, causing decreased bacterial clearance; reduces the cough reflex and increases the need for suctioning to clear secretions; allows bacterial access to the trachea; and alters swallowing, oral hygiene, and nutritional status. The nasogastric tube also causes local trauma to and inflammation in surrounding tissues, acts as a foreign body, serves as a conduit for bacteria from the stomach to the pharynx, and prevents closure of the lower esophageal sphincter, which increases the reflux of gastric bacteria. For all of these reasons, the incidence of nosocomial pneumonia is about four times greater in the intubated patient than in the nonintubated patient.

The intubated patient is often connected to a mechanical ventilator with nebulization equipment that may become contaminated with bacteria and, thereby, poses risks for the development of pneumonia, depending on the size of the aerosol particles, the concentration of bacteria, and whether the aerosol is delivered directly through an endotracheal or tracheostomy tube.[1] Only particles smaller than 4 μm in size will reach the terminal bronchioles and alveoli. Large-volume nebulizers with large (>500-mL) reservoirs and ultrasonic nebulizers pose the greatest risk of contamination and, therefore, of colonizing the patient with gram-negative bacilli. Although in-line nebulizers have small-volume reservoirs, contamination occurs frequently within 24 hours of use. Craven and Driks[1] have listed the possible sources of contamination of nebulizers as follows: (1) oxygen, (2) room air, (3) hands of hospital personnel, (4) use of contaminated water to fill the reservoir, (5) reflux of contaminated material into the reservoir, and (6) inadequate sterilization or disinfection of the equipment. In contrast with equipment for nebulizers, cascade humidifiers used in volume ventilators do not generate microaerosols and, thereby, substantially reduce the risk of colonization of the patient.

ETIOLOGIC AGENTS OF PULMONARY INFECTION

Although the microbial etiologies of pneumonias are quite diverse, age, underlying disease or condition, and place of acquisition of the infection are helpful in assessing therapeutic approaches to the patient. For example, respiratory syncytial virus, *Chlamydia trachomatis*, *Streptococcus pneumoniae*, and *Haemophilus influenzae* are the most frequent causes of pneumonia in 2-week to 6-month-old infants, whereas *S. pneumoniae*, *H. influenzae*, and adenoviruses are the most frequent causes of pneumonia in 7-month to 5-year-old children, and *S. pneumoniae*, adenoviruses, and *Mycoplasma pneumoniae* are the most frequent causes of pneumonia in children over 5 years of age.[2]

For patients older than 15 years of age, *S. pneumoniae* remains the most frequent cause of community-acquired pneumonia; however, its incidence appears to have diminished from 60% to 70% in the 1960s and 1970s to only 30% to 40% in more recent studies.[3] *Staphylococcus aureus*, *H. influenzae*, and enteric gram-negative bacilli, *P. aeruginosa*, *Legionella*, and anaerobic bacteria have become more frequently associated with community-acquired pneumonias in adults, either because they were missed in earlier studies because methods were not available for their recovery (e.g., *Legionella*) or because the populations that constitute the "community" changed. An aging population, changing life styles, increasing outpatient management of patients with serious underlying diseases and conditions, and evolving antibiotic-resistance patterns have all contributed to a changing spectrum of the microorganisms that cause community-acquired pneumonia.

The place of acquisition of pneumonia is another important variable in determining its etiology. In some settings, for example, *Mycobacterium tuberculosis* may be a frequent cause of community-acquired pneumonia. For example, in one recent report of community-acquired pneumonia in patients over 20 years of age in France,[4] *M. tuberculosis* was the cause in 10%, *S. pneumoniae* accounted for 26%, *S. aureus* for 12%, and a variety of other microorganisms for the rest. The spectrum of microorganisms causing hospital-acquired (nosocomial) pneumonias differs from that causing community-acquired pneumonia and is predominantly gram-negative bacillary, including especially *P. aeruginosa, E. coli, K. pneumoniae,* and *Enterobacter* species.

Legionellosis may result from inhalation of dust from excavation sites or from aerosols from contaminated cooling towers, shower heads, and respiratory therapy humidification reservoirs.

Blastomyces dermatitidis, Coccidioides immitis, and *Histoplasma capsulatum* are found in soil in the mold (mycelial) form and produce spores that may be inhaled and cause, in most instances, asymptomatic infection in individuals present in endemic areas. Individuals who have not previously encountered the fungus (such as Minnesotans vacationing in Arizona) and who encounter unusually large concentrations of the fungus may develop clinically apparent infection (in this example, coccidioidomycosis). Thus, travel history is an important component of a careful history.

DIAGNOSTIC TECHNIQUES FOR LOWER RESPIRATORY INFECTIONS

Diagnosis is suggested by the patient's age, clinical presentation, underlying disease, environmental and historical factors, and radiographic and laboratory tests. Definitive diagnosis depends on the detection or isolation of an etiologic agent from lower respiratory secretions or on the detection of antibodies specific for a particular etiologic agent. A variety of diagnostic techniques are available and are recommended by the American College of Chest Physicians and the American Society for Microbiology.[5]

Because of the number and variety of microorganisms that are normally present in the oropharynx, culture of specimens collected through the oropharynx are more difficult to interpret than are those obtained by bypassing this site. Normally, the tracheobronchial tree below the level of the larynx is sterile or only minimally colonized with bacteria so that specimens taken directly from lung tissue or by methods designed to minimize contamination by oropharyngeal flora facilitate diagnosis. Exceptions to these rules are microorganisms that usually represent pathogens, regardless of their source and whether that source is contaminated by other microorganisms. Among the usually pathogenic microorganisms are *M. tuberculosis, B. dermatitidis, C. immitis, H. capsulatum, M. pneumoniae,* respiratory viruses, and *Legionella.*

The procedure selected for obtaining specimens for the diagnosis of lower respiratory infection depends on the suspected diagnosis or disease, underlying diseases or conditions, prior antimicrobial therapy, and the availability of technical expertise for performing invasive procedures.[5] Communication between the clinician and the pathologist or microbiologist is important, especially when unusual pathogens are being considered and when special laboratory procedures are required. In certain instances, such as with bronchoalveolar lavage (BAL) and open-lung biopsy, it is desirable for the clinician and the pathologist or microbiologist to establish protocols to ensure that specimens are routinely examined carefully for the most likely pathogen.

SPECIMEN TYPES AND COLLECTION

Expectorated Sputum

Expectorated sputum is the specimen most frequently collected for diagnosis of pneumonia; however, its value remains highly controversial because of the difficulties involved in obtaining lower respiratory secretions that are uncontaminated by upper respiratory flora and, therefore, in interpreting results of cultures. Sputum for Gram stain and culture generally should be obtained from patients who have pneumonia or acute airways infection; however, it is important to instruct the patient to remove any dentures and to rinse or gargle the mouth with water before attempting to expectorate, into a specimen container, a specimen resulting from a deep cough. When asked simply to spit into a jar, most patients will usually oblige by providing a sample of saliva, the bacteriology of which is well established in the literature, and culture of which provides no clinically useful information.

The expectoration of sputum requires, among other things, an alert, cooperative patient who may have to try several times to produce a satisfactory specimen. One method used in many laboratories today to assess the suitability of sputum for bacterial culture is to examine the specimen microscopically for the presence of squamous epithelial cells. Squamous epithelial cells live in the oropharynx so that their presence in large numbers means that the specimen is substantially contaminated with oropharyngeal secretions (spit) and, therefore, is not suitable for bacterial culture. The absence of alveolar macrophages or bronchial epithelial cells microscopically indicates the absence of any lower respiratory secretions whatsoever in the specimen. Under these circumstances, the laboratory should reject the specimen as being unacceptable for culture and request that another specimen be collected. Because the recovery of mycobacteria (e.g., *M. tuberculosis*) and certain fungi (e.g., *H. capsulatum*) is clinically significant, regardless of the quality of the specimen, rejection of specimens for mycobacterial and fungal cultures on the basis of microscopic examination is inappropriate; however, there is no disputing the fact that mycobacteria and fungi are far more likely to be recovered from specimens consisting predominantly of lower respiratory secretions than from those consisting predominantly of upper respiratory secretions.

Given all of the problems associated with collection of a valid sputum specimen, it should not be surprising that in some hospitals the responsibility for patient instruction and collection of specimens lies with the respiratory therapist.

For the diagnosis of bacterial pneumonia, it is generally sufficient to obtain a single sputum specimen; however, for the diagnosis of mycobacterial or deep fungal infections, it is recommended that specimens be obtained on three to five successive mornings. Formerly, it was routine practice to collect and pool specimens over a 24-hour period for mycobacterial culture; however, this practice has been abandoned because overgrowth by normal oropharyngeal flora interfered with the recovery of mycobacteria from cultures.

In some instances, patients with pneumonia do not have a productive cough, and a productive cough is induced by having these patients inhale an aerosol or hypertonic salt solution. Such *sputum induction* is helpful in the diagnosis of mycobacterial, deep fungal, and, in aquired immune deficiency syndrome (AIDS) patients, *Pneumocystis* pneumonias.

Invasive Techniques

There is a wide variety of invasive techniques, ranging from nasotracheal suctioning to open-lung biopsy, that are considered for use in patients who are able to produce sputum (spontaneous or induced), whose sputum examination provides equivocal or inconclusive results, or whose condition either fails to improve or worsens following the initiation of antimicrobial therapy. When performed skillfully, nasotracheal suction can be used to obtain sputum; however, when repeated attempts must be made to get the catheter into the trachea, oropharyngeal secretions are greatly stimulated, and it becomes nearly impossible not to contaminate the specimen.

In some instances *transtracheal aspiration* is useful for the detection of bacterial pathogens and, especially, for anaerobic bacteria because this method bypasses the oropharynx, which is heavily contaminated with such bacteria. The procedure requires technical expertise and is contraindicated for patients with severe hemoptysis, bleeding disorder, inability to cooperate, severe hypoxemia, and recent antimicrobial therapy. Because the procedure carries a considerable amount of discomfort for, and some risk to, the patient, its use has been largely replaced by bronchoscopy procedures.

In the intubated patient, lower respiratory secretions often are contaminated by oral flora from upper respiratory secretions that pool around and leak past the cuff of the endotracheal tube; therefore, the distinction between bacterial colonization and infection becomes difficult. The finding of many bacteria (one to ten per oil immersion field; oif), many polymorphonuclear leukocytes ($\geq$25 per high-power field; hpf), many intracellular bacteria (1% to 5% of polymorphonuclear leukocytes), along with the presence of elastin fibers microscopically, is highly suggestive of infection.[6] Although there is some evidence that quantitative cultures of endotracheal aspirates may be helpful in distinguishing between bacterial colonization and infection, microscopic examination appears to be the more accurate means of making this distinction.

Bronchoscopy is often used in patients with chronic or refractory infections and in immunocompromised patients for whom a diagnosis cannot be made from an expectorated or induced sputum specimen. There are two special procedures that warrant mention. The first is bronchoscopy with a protected catheter brush consisting of a double-lumen, distally occluded brush catheter. The catheter is inserted through the bronchoscope channel to an area of infection, and the inner protected brush catheter is then advanced through the outer cannula; the distally occluding propylene glycol tip is jettisoned, and the brush is extended beyond the catheter tip into the area of the infection. Once the specimen has been obtained, the brush is retracted into the inner catheter and the entire catheter is withdrawn from the bronchoscope. The brush is then transected with a sterile scissors and placed into 1 mL of sterile lactated Ringer solution (without preservative) for transport to the laboratory. The protected brush catheter is intended to minimize contamination of the lower respiratory tract by upper respiratory flora that is carried into the lower respiratory tract by the bronchoscope.

When quantitative culture of the brush is performed, it is often possible to distinguish between contamination and infection. Once again, because the recovery of mycobacteria and deep fungi in any quantity is significant and because selective techniques are used for the recovery of mycobacteria and fungi in cultures, use of the protected brush catheter is usually limited to the diagnosis of bacterial infection.

A second, special bronchoscopy procedure is *bronchoalveolar lavage* (BAL), whereby the tip of the bronchoscope is wedged into an infected bronchus and isotonic saline is instilled into the bronchus, aspirated, and collected in a suction trap. Several instillations are usually collected to obtain 40 to 70 mL of lavage fluid. The fluid is then concentrated by centrifugation and the concentrate used for microscopic examination and culture. Although quantitative culture of BAL fluid is helpful in distinguishing between bacterial colonization and infection, the procedure of BAL is usually performed to diagnose opportunistic infections caused by microorganisms other than bacteria, such as mycobacteria, fungi, *P. carinii*, and viruses. Either the protected brush catheter or BAL may be helpful in the diagnosis of pneumonia in the intubated patient.

In a few instances, the aforementioned invasive procedures will still be nondiagnostic and an *open-lung biopsy* is performed for definitive diagnosis. Obviously, this procedure involves general anesthesia, a chest incision, and the risk of postoperative complications, such as pneumothorax, hemorrhage, or infection. Use of the open-lung biopsy appears to be declining as a result of the increasing use and diagnostic yield of BAL.

PREVENTION OF INFECTION

Because of the high morbidity and, in the case of nosocomial pneumonia, mortality of pneumonia, prevention represents the major component of any program for control of pneumonia. Prevention may focus on three areas: host defenses, colonization, and aspiration. Immunization (e.g., pneumococcal and influenza vaccine), therapy and control of underlying diseases or conditions, and nutritional support contribute to or enhance host defenses. A variety of experimental approaches to stimulate CMI are under investigation and may be helpful in preventing pneumonia in the immunocompromised patient in the future.

Measures to prevent colonization by potentially pathogenic microorganisms take many forms. One form is environmental control, including handwashing, isolation procedures, control of contamination of equipment; maintenance of an acidic gastric pH; and, perhaps in the future, measures that prevent microbial adhesion to mucous membranes and foreign objects.

Measures to prevent aspiration include the avoidance of central nervous systems depressants and, perhaps in the future, novel intubation devices that minimize aspiration of pharyngeal flora into the lung.

Of the three areas just described for prevention of pneumonia, that of colonization and environmental control is most germane to respiratory therapy. An ongoing assessment of the effectiveness of environmental and colonization control falls within the purview of a nosocomial infection control program, the essential components of which are (1) an effective surveillance program designed to establish and maintain a data base that describes the endemic infection rates of nosocomial infection and, thereby, allows recognition of epidemic occurrences; (2) establishment of a series of regulations and policies to reduce the risk of nosocomial infection; and (3) maintenance of a continuing education program.[7] Ordinarily, these functions are the responsibility of an infection-control practitioner who works with a hospital epidemiologist, both of whom are responsible to the hospital's infection-control committee, which develops guidelines, regulations, or policies that ideally are designed to foster habits and attitudes that lead to reduced nosocomial infections.

HANDWASHING

The fact that disease-producing microorganisms are frequently present on the hands of health care personnel has been recognized for over a century. Transfer of microorganisms between patient and the hands of health care personnel is well documented, and personnel hands have been shown to be a major vector of transmission of bacterial, fungal, and viral infections in burn units, intensive care units, and a variety of other hospital settings. The risk of skin and postoperative wound infections has also been related to general handwashing practices. Although plain soap appears to be sufficient to reduce fecal–oral transmission, antiseptic products may have added benefits in reducing nosocomial infections.[8] Evidence of the benefits of handwashing notwithstanding, the major difficulty remains compliance with handwashing policies on busy wards or intensive care units in which the architect's plans failed to include a conveniently located sink.

ISOLATION

Isolation procedures have been used in hospitals for many years to prevent the spread of potentially communicable diseases. The procedures recommended by the Centers for Disease Control (CDC) are either category-specific or disease-specific.[9] The category-specific precautions include seven catego-

ries: strict isolation, contact isolation, respiratory isolation, tuberculosis isolation, enteric precautions, drainage–secretion precautions, and blood–body fluid precautions. Because these precautions are to be followed by all health care workers, their purposes and specifications are summarized in Table 18–3.

Disease-specific precautions have the advantages of being individualized for each disease and of minimizing unnecessary precautions; however, such precautions require more diagnostic information, skill, and responsibility to assign precautions. Some modifications of the category-based precautions may be made at the discretion of the hospital epidemiologist and are often necessary in intensive care units, particularly for private rooms.

The advent of the acquired immunodeficiency syndrome (AIDS) has raised several important is-

Table 18–3 Category-Specific Isolation Precautions*

CATEGORY	INDICATIONS	PRECAUTIONS
Strict isolation	Pharyngeal diphtheria, viral hemorrhagic fevers, varicella (chickenpox), zoster infections in immunocompromised host or when disseminated	Private room Gown, mask, gloves Handwashing
Contact isolation	(1) Acute respiratory infections in children; (2) neonates with gonococcal conjunctivitis, herpes simplex infection, staphylococcal skin infections; (3) group A streptococcal endometritis, pneumonia, skin infection; (4) cutaneous diphtheria, colonization with multiple, variable resistant bacteria, staphylococcal pneumonia, major skin infections, pediculosis, scabies, rubella	Private room Gown, gloves for direct contact Handwashing
Respiratory isolation	*H. influenzae* epiglottitis, meningitis, or pneumonia in children; serious meningococcal disease (pneumonia, meningitis, septicemia), mumps, pertussis	Private room Mask Handwashing
Tuberculosis isolation	Pulmonary/laryngeal tuberculosis	Private room Mask Handwashing
Enteric precautions	Infectious diarrhea caused by *Campylobacter, Salmonella, Shigella, Yersinia, Vibrio, Entamoeba, Giardia,* viruses	Private room if patient hygiene poor Gloves for direct contact with stool Handwashing
Drainage–secretion precautions	Purulence, drainage, secretions	Private room Gown, gloves for direct contact Handwashing
Blood–body fluid precautions	Hepatitis B, non-A, non-B hepatitis, HIV, Creutzfeld-Jakob disease, syphilis (1^0 and 2^0), malaria, babesiosis	Private room Gown, gloves for direct contact Handwashing

(Based on Garner J, Simmons, BP: Isolation precautions. In Bennett JV, Brachman PS (eds): Hospital Infections, 2nd ed, pp 143–150. Boston, Little, Brown & Co, 1986)
* See text for discussion of universal blood and body fluid precautions.

sues affecting isolation precautions and the management of human immunodeficiency virus (HIV) infections in the hospital. Persons infected with HIV may be asymptomatic or may manifest a variety of clinical conditions, of which AIDS is the most severe form. Although HIV has been isolated from blood, vaginal secretions, semen, saliva, tears, urine, cerebrospinal fluid, breast milk, and amniotic fluid, transmission of HIV has been linked only to blood and blood products, semen, vaginal secretions, and possibly breast milk. It occurs through (1) sexual contact; (2) parenteral (intravenous) exposure, including transfusion of blood or blood products, sharing of needles and syringes with illicit drug use, occupational needlestick injuries, and contact of blood with mucous membranes or skin lesions; and (3) perinatal exposure. The major risk groups for contacting HIV infection have remained fairly constant since AIDS was first recognized and include homosexual males, intravenous drug abusers, heterosexuals with sexual contact with persons infected with HIV or in major risk groups for HIV infection, and recipients of transfusion of blood or blood products. A small percentage of persons infected with HIV have no known or definable source of infection.

To date, most health care workers infected with HIV have belonged to the recognized risk groups, and the risk of infection among health care workers owing to occupational exposure is extremely small. Studies conducted by the CDC and at several major medical centers, for example, indicate the risk of HIV infection following injury with a needle contaminated with the blood of an HIV-infected patient to be less than 0.5%, compared with a 6% to 30% risk of hepatitis B (HBV) infection following an injury from a needle contaminated with the blood of a patient with HBV infection. The reason is that HIV is present at concentrations of only 10^0 to 10^2 tissue culture infectious doses (TCID)/mL of blood, whereas HBV is present at concentrations of 10^8–10^9 TCID/mL of blood.

Persons who become infected with HIV usually develop antibodies within 6 to 12 weeks after infection. These antibodies, which are not protective but rather indicate infection with HIV, can be detected by an enzyme immunoassay (EIA). Although EIAs are highly sensitive and highly specific, false-negative results may occur during the first several weeks of infection before detectable antibody appears. Conversely, the presence of nonspecific and cross-reactive antibodies may cause a false-positive EIA result. Consequently, positive results of EIA must be regarded with caution and require confirmation with a more specific antibody test, such as the Western blot. As with any test, the sensitivity, specificity, false-negative and false-positive rates of the HIV EIA will vary according to the population being tested and the incidence and prevalence of HIV in such populations. Thus, it is customary to retest any serum sample found to yield a positive EIA result for HIV antibody and, then, to perform a confirmatory test on any sample that has been repeatedly positive by the EIA method. Currently, neither the EIA nor the Western blot is a stat test with a turnaround time of less than 1 hour. Because a high proportion of persons infected with HIV will go on to develop AIDS, because of the highly uniform mortality of AIDS patients and, therefore, because of the enormous socioeconomic implications of a positive HIV antibody test, hospitals must develop policies for HIV testing, including circumstances under which testing should be performed in a health care setting, methods for obtaining informed consent for testing and for providing counseling, systems for handling results, and maintaining confidentiality of the patient's HIV status.

Against this background, hospitals need to balance the need for appropriate precautions to prevent transmission of HIV with the need to ensure confidentiality of the results of HIV testing. Because it is not always possible to know a patient's HIV status, it is probably most reasonable for health care workers to use protective barriers consistently to prevent exposure to blood and body fluids or secretions, commonly referred to as universal blood and body fluid precautions or, simply, *universal precautions*. This approach has been recommended by the CDC and is mandated by the Occupational Health and Safety Administration (OSHA). With universal precautions, all patients are regarded as potentially infected with HIV or other blood-borne infectious agents, and the use of barriers and other protective measures becomes routine to prevent exposure of blood and body fluids to the skin and mucous membranes. These precautions should apply to *all* health care workers for *all* patients, including those seen in emergency rooms and other outpatient settings. Thus, universal precautions actually encompass most of the category-specific precautions listed in Table 18–3.

More specific guidelines for the care of patients are as follows:[10]

1. Gloves should be worn for direct contact with blood, body fluids and secretions, wounds, and for handling all items or surfaces that are contaminated with blood,

body fluids, or secretions. Gloves should be worn for venipuncture and for handling vascular access lines or intravascular monitoring devices.

2. Gloves should be changed between patients, when they are torn, or whenever a perforation occurs, as with a needlestick injury. Hands should be washed whenever gloves are removed.

3. Hands should be washed immediately whenever contamination with blood or body fluids or secretions occurs.

4. Masks and protective eyewear or face shields should be worn during procedures in which splattering, splashing, or generation of droplets of blood, body fluids, or secretions is likely to occur.

5. Gowns or aprons should be worn under conditions described in item 4.

6. Precautions should be taken when handling needles and sharp instruments. Used disposable needles and syringes, scalpels, and other sharp items should be placed into puncture-resistant containers for disposal. Used needles should not be bent, broken, recapped, or cut.

7. Mouthpieces, resuscitation bags, and other ventilatory devices should be available to minimize the need for mouth-to-mouth resuscitation.

8. All blood and body fluid specimens should be placed into a sturdy, leakproof container (e.g., ziplock bag) for transport to the laboratory. The laboratory requisition form should be placed outside this container to minimize contamination.

9. Health care workers with exudative skin lesions should refrain from patient care activities.

DISINFECTION AND STERILIZATION

Disinfection means the removal of microorganisms capable of causing infection; *sterilization* means the elimination of all viable microorganisms. The principal difference between the two is, for all practical purposes, the elimination of bacterial spores by sterilization, but not by disinfection. In either case, the elimination of microorganisms does not take place instantaneously, but rather occurs over time in the form of a straight-line killing curve. The number of microorganisms killed is proportional to the number that is initially present. Thus, a particular process may be disinfecting or sterilizing, depending on the exposure time.

There are many physical and chemical methods available for disinfection and sterilization. Moist heat under pressure (autoclaving) and ethylene oxide gas are the principal sterilization methods in use today. In the autoclave, killing of organisms is achieved at high temperatures (121° C), using steam at 2 atm of pressure. Ethylene oxide (ETO) is a gas that is widely used to sterilize many heat-sensitive products. This technique is particularly useful in respiratory therapy, with its wide use of plastic products. Under specified conditions and use, chemical germicides that are ordinarily used as disinfectants may be used for sterilization purposes.

Disinfectants are usually classified in three levels: high, intermediate, and low. A high-level disinfectant is effective against bacterial spores (sporicidal), vegetative bacteria, tubercle bacilli (tuberculocidal), fungi, and viruses. Intermediate-level disinfectants may, but do not necessarily, exert some sporicidal activity. They do exert tuberculocidal, bactericidal, fungicidal, and limited virucidal activity. Hepatitis B and human immunodeficiency viruses (HBV and HIV, respectively) are inactivated by several intermediate- to high-level disinfectants, including aqueous glutaraldehyde, stabilized hydrogen peroxide, aqueous formaldehyde, iodophors, and chlorine compounds.

In all instances, proper physical cleaning of any item is an absolute prerequisite for disinfection because blood, mucus, feces, or soil may shield microorganisms from the disinfectant or sterilant or may actually inactivate the disinfectant or sterilant. Moreover, it is essential to follow carefully the manufacturer's instructions for use of the disinfectant and for its suitability for the purposes intended. The selection and final concentration of disinfectant will depend on the surface to be disinfected.

Household bleach in a 1:10 to 1:100 dilution (made up fresh on a daily basis) may be used for surface decontamination; however, bleach may be corrosive to metallic surfaces and, as with other disinfectants, is less effective if serum, blood, or other proteinanceous materials are not first removed by cleaning with detergent. Low-level quaternary ammonium compounds should not be used for disinfection purposes, and phenolics should not be used on HIV- or HBV-contaminated medical devices. For blood spills, the blood should be absorbed with disposable towels; the spill site is then cleaned of all visible blood with a detergent, and finally wiped down with disposable towels soaked with an intermediate- to high-level disinfectant. All disposable materials used in the decontamination process should be placed into a biohazard container.

Unfortunately, there are numerous disinfectant products on the market today, and there is no longer a federal testing program to validate manufacturers' claims of efficacy when the product is registered with the Environmental Protection Agency (EPA). Therefore, caution must be exercised in the selection of products.

DECONTAMINATION OF VENTILATION EQUIPMENT

A number of approaches have been used to minimize or prevent contamination of ventilatory equipment. All modern respiratory therapy departments have space provided for cleaning and disinfecting various pieces of therapy equipment. Separate "dirty" (contaminated) and "clean" (noncontaminated) areas will be provided, where disassembly, washing, sterilization, rinsing and drying, repackaging, and labeling functions will be served. The primary approach has been that of replacement of solutions and critical equipment at specified intervals, since "in-use" disinfection is impractical. Thus, reservoirs should be completely emptied and refilled before use with sterile water (not tap water) every 8 to 24 hours, with special care to avoid contamination by microorganisms on hands and to prevent reflux of ventilator tubing condensate that may be contaminated with gram-negative bacilli.[1,11]

The CDC guidelines strongly recommend replacing Venturi wall nebulizers with sterilized or disinfected units every 24 hours and moderately recommend that other nebulizers be replaced with sterilized or disinfected units every 24 hours;[12] however, Craven and Driks recommend removal of the nebulizer from the circuit, rinsing with sterile water, and air-drying between treatments, rather than replacing nebulizers every 24 hours.[1] The CDC guidelines also strongly recommend replacing ventilatory circuits, including tubing and exhalation valve, every 24 hours;[12] however, given results of studies at the Boston City Hospital that showed that bacterial contamination levels in the inspiratory phase gas and tubing did not differ between 24 and 48 hours, Craven and Driks recommend changing ventilatory circuits every 48 hours.[1]

After considering the principles of sterilization and disinfection discussed in the previous section, it should be apparent that all reusable equipment must first be cleaned to remove any blood, secretions, or other proteinaceous material before sterilization or disinfection procedures are undertaken.

Coolant chambers of ultrasonic nebulizers cannot be disinfected adequately and should be sterilized with ethylene oxide or be in contact with a high-level disinfectant for at least 30 minutes.[12] Sterilization or disinfection of the internal machinery of ventilatory equipment should not be routinely performed and may be necessary only after potential contamination with a highly dangerous microbial agent such as Lassa fever virus.[12]

Endotracheal suction through an endotracheal tube or tracheostomy should be considered a sterile procedure that requires the use of sterile equipment and aseptic technique. Care must be taken not to contaminate the sterile suction catheter with the ungloved hand, bed linen or clothing, or other nonsterile surfaces. Suction collection tubing (up to the canister) should always be changed between patients and undergo sterilization or high-level disinfection.[12] A sterile suction catheter should be used for each series of suctioning, defined as a single suction or repeated suctioning with only brief intervening periods to clear or flush the catheter.[12] The major objective of recommended procedures for tracheal suctioning is to prevent cross-contamination, because patients with endotracheal tubes or tracheostomies are at high risk of developing hospital-acquired pneumonia.

INFUSION THERAPY

Although not directly related to lower respiratory infection, infusion therapy[13] for blood or blood products, drugs, fluids, or nutrition is used in many seriously ill patients. Approximately one-third of nosocomial bloodstream infections (bacteremias and fungemias) are infusion related. The sources of the infection are (1) infected cannulas (i.e., devices used for temporary vascular access, including plastic catheters used for hyperalimentation, hemodynamic monitoring, and hemodialysis) and, albeit much less frequently, (2) contaminated infusates. Infection of cannulas is generally due to introduction of microorganisms from the skin of the patient or from the hands of the person inserting or manipulating the cannula. Bacteria adhere to irregularities in the surface of the cannula and form a biofilm consisting of polysaccharides. Within this biofilm, bacteria multiply that are resistant to high concentrations of antibiotics and phagocytosis.

The frequency of cannula-associated infection varies widely and is often related to the care exercised during insertion and the length of time the cannula is left in place. Contaminated infusate may result from the introduction of microorganisms during preparation and administration in the hospital. Contamination of intra-arterial infusions used for hemodynamic pressure monitoring and with the transducer chamber dome has caused sporadic epidemics of bacteremias in hospitals. Proper sterilization of the chamber or the use of disposable chamber domes should reduce this risk. Infections have also resulted from multiple-use bronchodilator medication vials or containers.

Prevention of infusion-related sepsis depends on careful handwashing before cannula insertion, the use of sterile gloves and aseptic technique when inserting cannulas into high-risk patients; or when inserting high-risk cannulas, the daily surveillance of all intravascular lines, limiting the use of lines for hemodynamic monitoring to 4 days, exercising care when compounding parenteral admixtures, and routinely replacing the entire delivery system every 48 hours.[13]

REFERENCES

1. Craven DE, Driks MR: Nosocomial pneumonia in the intubated patient. Semin Respir Infect 2:20–33, 1987
2. Klein JO: Emerging perspectives in management and prevention of infections of the respiratory tract in infants and children. Am J Med 78 (Suppl 6B):38–44, 1985
3. Garibaldi RA: Epidemiology of community-acquired respiratory tract infections in adults: Incidence, etiology, and impact. Am J Med 78 (Suppl 6B):32–37, 1985
4. Lévy M, Dromer F, Brion N, Leturdu F, Carbon C: Community-acquired pneumonia: Importance of initial noninvasive bacteriologic and radiographic investigations. Chest 92:43–48, 1988
5. Bartlett JG, Ryan KJ, Smith TF, Wilson WR: Cumitech 7A: Laboratory diagnosis of lower respiratory infections. Washington JA (coordinating ed), pp 1–18. Washington, American Society for Microbiology, 1987
6. Salata RA, Lederman MM, Shlaes DM et al: Diagnosis of nosocomial pneumonia in intubated, intensive unit patients. Am Rev Respir Dis 135:426–432, 1987
7. Ponce de Leon RS: Organizing for infection control. In Wenzel RP (ed): Prevention and Control of Nosocomial Infections, pp 56–69. Baltimore, Williams & Wilkins, 1987
8. Larson E: A causative link between handwashing and risk of infection? Examination of the evidence. Infect Control Hosp Epidemiol 9:28–36, 1988
9. Garner J, Simmons BP: Isolation precautions. In Bennett JV, Brachman PS (eds): Hospital Infections, 2nd ed, pp 143–150. Boston, Little, Brown & Company, 1986
10. Technical Panel on Infections Within Hospitals: Management of HIV Infection in the Hospital. Chicago, American Hospital Association, 1988
11. Sanford JP: Lower respiratory infections. In Bennett JV, Brachman PS (eds): Hospital Infections, 2nd ed, pp 385–422. Boston, Little, Brown & Company, 1986
12. Simmons BP, Wong ES: CDC guidelines for the prevention of nosocomial pneumonia. Am J Infect Control 11:230–243, 1983
13. Maki DG: Infections due to infusion therapy. In Bennett JV, Brachman PS (eds): Hospital Infections, 2nd ed, pp 561–580. Boston, Little, Brown & Company, 1986

BIBLIOGRAPHY

Townsend TR Jr: Infection in the ICU: How to protect yourself and others. J Crit Illness 2:29–37, 1987

Washington JA: Techniques for noninvasive diagnosis of lower respiratory tract infections. J Crit Illness 3:97–103, 1988

NINETEEN

Drugs Used in Respiratory Therapy

Irwin Ziment

Many of the drugs used to treat disorders of the lungs can be administered by nebulization or by instillation into the respiratory tract. Drugs given directly are not always prescribed by physicians in precise dosages and concentrations. The actual administration of the medication is performed by a nurse or a respiratory therapist or by the patient himself. A ridiculous legalistic quibble occasionally is voiced, expressing doubts on the legal propriety of respiratory therapists mixing and delivering prescribed drugs. Since, obviously, the patient can be instructed in safe self-therapy, there can be no serious questioning of the trained therapist's capability as a provider of pharmacologic therapy in the hospital setting. Indeed, the educated therapist generally knows more about respiratory aerosol pharmacology than does the average physician or nurse; in fact, it would be reasonable to expect the nonspecialist physician to consult with a therapist about the details of aerosol drug administration.

Relatively few drugs are used in aerosol therapy, and it is essential for therapists to be completely familiar with the pharmacology of these agents and to know the indications and contraindications for their use, as well as the complications that may arise during their administration. The main emphasis herein will be placed on drugs commonly given by aerosolization, and comparatively less detail will be provided for the other drugs used to treat respiratory disease. Many drugs given by inhalation can also be given orally, and, in the fu-

ture, probably more developments will occur in the latter field because oral therapy is cheaper and easier to administer. The well-educated respiratory therapist, therefore, should maintain a strong interest in all respiratory pharmacologic preparations, not simply those given by nebulization.

AEROSOL THERAPY

The use of inhalational drug therapy developed empirically, and numerous controversies about the value of such therapy still exist. Prescribers and providers of aerosols should recognize the advantages and limitations of aerosol therapy technique.

ADVANTAGES OF AEROSOL THERAPY

The main disadvantage of delivering a drug by aerosol is that relatively small quantities of the drug can be given, with maximal pulmonary effect and minimal extrapulmonary side effects. The onset of action usually is rapid, and repeated therapy with small doses can be given at relatively frequent intervals, according to the patient's needs, with little risk of toxicity. The use of aerosols may be preferable in situations for which oral or intravenous medications are difficult to give because of the unavailability of these routes. Certain drugs are specifically designed for aerosolization and cannot be given by other means.

411

DISADVANTAGES OF AEROSOL THERAPY

The major problem in inhalation treatment is that, unless the trachea is intubated, patients must be able to cooperate by breathing deeply in coordination with the administration of the aerosol by mouthpiece or mask. Oral therapy with a pill or liquid is usually much simpler because no expensive or cumbersome equipment is required. In contrast, aerosol therapy necessitates nebulizers of various degrees of complexity, which makes the modality expensive; moreover, in most hospitals skilled personnel are required to operate and to maintain the more complex pieces of machinery, such as positive-pressure respirators. Domiciliary equipment suffers from dual disadvantages: Difficulty in operation and maintenance may discourage patients from using the more expensive machines, yet accessibility of ready relief from simple nebulizers may result in overuse of potent drugs. Much money can be spent on domiciliary nebulization devices that are not indicated and are probably not used correctly by patients, who would do just as well with oral medications or simple, inexpensive humidifiers. An additional concern about aerosol therapy is based on the experience of Great Britain in the 1960s: The death rate from asthma in children greatly increased because of overuse of metered aerosol bronchodilators.[1] However, a recent increase in many countries of deaths from asthma does not appear to be related to the use of inhaled drugs.[2]

Thus, aerosol therapy suffers from disadvantages that include overuse, underuse, and misuse of the prescribed medications. Furthermore, even when drugs are administered appropriately, there is a lack of knowledge about what the appropriate dosage of most inhalational agents should be. More precise dosing would be attained if clinicians prescribed drugs in milligrams, rather than in milliliters or in percentage strengths of solutions. Not only are drugs prescribed imprecisely, but many physicians and therapists fail to appreciate that the dose delivered can be extremely variable. The cooperative patient given an aerosol through a mouthpiece by intermittent positive-pressure breathing (IPPB) probably retains only 5% to 10% of the prescribed amount of the drug in the respiratory tract, whereas more efficient aerosolizing devices can result in much larger doses being delivered, for example, by metered units with spacers.

The problem of *droplet size* is still a controversial topic, and it is difficult to know if any one of the conventional nebulizing units offers significant advantages over its competitors.[3] The less effective equipment delivers droplets of larger diameter, which are deposited mainly in the mouth and upper airways. Many patients treated with bronchodilator aerosols provided by such equipment may actually obtain the bronchospasmolytic effect as a result of systemic absorption of the drug through the oropharyngeal or gastric mucosa. Similarly, the very dyspneic asthmatic patient who is unable to take a deep breath and hold it may resort to excessive use of the nebulizer because pharmacologic relief is derived only from systemic absorption of large amounts of drug deposited in the mouth. Furthermore, the hypoxemic asthmatic may become even more hypoxemic after aerosolizing drugs such as isoproterenol, since systemic absorption causes vasodilation of pulmonary vessels disproportionate to the bronchodilatation achieved, resulting in an increased shunt through poorly ventilated areas of the lung.

There are other disadvantages to administering drugs as aerosols. Many patients find that the taste and the oropharyngeal irritation of the droplets cause gagging and nausea, whereas the irritant effect of the aerosol on reactive airways can cause deterioration in respiratory variables (e.g., oxygen transport, dynamic compliance) and may result in bronchospasm. The latter problem is likely to arise with any pharmacologic aerosol and, consequently, incorporation of a bronchodilator drug with other classes of drugs may be necessary when giving treatment. Unfortunately, bronchodilators are not entirely compatible with all other inhalational drugs; many inhalational drugs are alkaline, whereas bronchodilators are acidic and undergo fairly rapid breakdown in an alkaline medium.

A further disadvantage of aerosol therapy is that the nebulizer readily becomes contaminated with microorganisms. Thus, inhalational apparatus is a potential source of serious nosocomial infections. This fact is so well known that elaborate precautions are taken, including the use of disposable equipment and the employment of complex cleaning and sterilizing protocols in hospitals. The expense of such methods constitutes a major factor in the relatively poor cost-effectiveness benefits of aerosol therapy. Moreover, the more complex and "effective" an aerosol generator may be, the more expensive it is to keep clean and in good working order.

ADVANTAGES OF AEROSOL THERAPY

1. Topical administration results in rapid therapeutic effect.

2. Only a small total dose of potent drug need be nebulized.
3. Minimal extrapulmonary side effects are produced.
4. Individual dosage titration is possible.
5. The respiratory route is always available for drug delivery.
6. Certain drugs (e.g., cromolyn) cannot be given by other routes.
7. Humidification and bland droplet therapy are essential for tracheostomized and intubated patients; they are soothing and probably beneficial for most patients with respiratory disease.
8. Administration of aerosol therapy in the hospital involves the respiratory therapist, with the attendant benefits of skilled attention to the respiratory tract.
9. Patients develop faith in nebulizers and derive psychological benefits from their use.
10. Aerosol therapy may provide patients with an oral–inhalational substitute for smoking.

DISADVANTAGES OF AEROSOL THERAPY

1. Special, expensive equipment is often required.
2. Patients must be able to cooperate in taking synchronized deep breaths (unless intubated).
3. Precise drug dosage is usually not achieved; underdosage and overdosage are readily produced.
4. Only a small proportion of a nebulized drug is retained in the lung.
5. Oropharyngeal deposition of an aerosol results in appreciable systemic absorption.
6. Oropharyngeal irritation by the aerosol can result in gagging, nausea, vomiting, or aerophagia.
7. Tracheobronchial irritation by the aerosol can result in bronchospasm, coughing (thus limiting the inhaled dose), and possibly tracheobronchitis.
8. The inhalational adjuvants may cause detrimental side effects (e.g., oxygen, Freon).
9. Nebulizers readily become dirty, thus losing effectiveness, and possibly become sources of infection.
10. Aerosol therapy results in unreasonable complexity (involving patient, equipment, and personnel factors) that is greatly reduced if oral administration is used instead.

PHARMACOLOGY OF RESPIRATORY DRUGS

The most important and frequently administered drugs in aerosol therapy are agents used to improve mucociliary clearance (mucokinetic agents) and agents used to relieve bronchospasm. Relatively few other categories of drugs are given by nebulization; they include antiasthmatic agents, mucosal vasoconstrictors, local anesthetics, and antibiotics. The major drugs in these categories will be considered in this chapter.

MUCOKINETIC AGENTS

Drugs in this category include mucolytics, expectorants, and other agents found in "cough medicines" (Table 9–1). The most important mucokinetic agent is actually water.

The end result of successful mucokinetic therapy is usually seen in a sputum receptacle by the bedside or in the suction bottle in an intensive care unit. Sputum is a complex fluid consisting of mucoprotein (including mucopolysaccharides), electrolytes, water, cellular debris, and, with expectorated specimens, oropharyngeal secretions (i.e., saliva, food particles, and bacteria).

The respiratory tract secretions originate from two major sources (Fig. 19–1): the goblet cells that produce a gelatinous secretion, mainly in response to irritation; and the bronchial glands that secrete a more watery solution and are under vagal control. Infected sputum contains, in addition, DNA, which is liberated from polymorphonuclear (white) blood cells and bacteria. This material gives a yellow or green color to the secretions, which it renders highly viscous.

The normal mucous blanket has two layers: the more watery sol layer in which the cilia beat, and the superficial viscous gel layer. The ciliary activity serves to waft the gel layer proximally up the respiratory tract against gravity. Problems with sputum expectoration occur when there is increased production of viscous secretions in airways having damaged cilia and impaired architecture which interferes with effective coughing.

Although pharmacologic agents can alter the consistency of mucus, subsequent mucokinesis requires the presence of an effective cough; other-

Table 19—1   Important Aerosol Mucokinetic Drugs

DRUG	USUAL AEROSOL DOSAGE	COMMENTS
N-acetyl-L-cysteine (10–20%) (Mucomyst)	2–5 mL q6hr	Breaks disulfide bonds, causes mucolysis. Malodorous and may cause bronchospasm. Solution should be diluted with an equal volume of isotonic saline or sodium bicarbonate.
Sodium bicarbonate (1.4–7.5%)	2–5 mL q6hr Range: 1–10 mL q2–8hr	Surfactant in low concentrations, bronchorrheic in higher concentrations. May be combined with other drugs for immediate use.
Sodium chloride (0.45–20%)	2–5 mL q6hr Range: 1–10 mL q2–8hr	Hypotonic solution used for patients on sodium restriction. Hypertonic solutions stimulate cough and may have mucolytic effect; particularly useful for inducing sputum production. Normal saline is a standard diluting agent.
Propylene glycol (2–25%)	2–5 mL q4hr Range: 1–10 mL q1–8hr	Soothing demulcent for tracheobronchitis (2% solution). Stabilizes droplets; used with therapeutic aerosols to improve distal deposition. Effective for cough induction (15% or stronger solution).

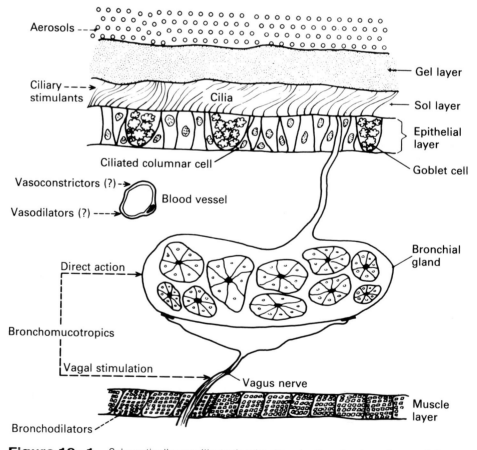

Figure 19—1.   Schematic diagram illustrating the sites of action of various classes of pharmacologic agents within the wall and lumina of the respiratory tract.

wise, loosened, hypoviscous secretions can gravitate down the airways, causing the patient to "drown in his secretions." If a patient is unable or unwilling to cough, then postural drainage or, alternatively, tracheobronchial suctioning will be required. Thus, effective mucokinesis requires more than active drug therapy, and pharmacologic agents contribute only the first half of the process: Physical therapy is equally or, at times, more important.[4]

Mucokinetic Drugs Suitable for Aerosolization

Water. The addition of water to mucus results in decreased viscosity of sputum. If relatively large quantities of water are added, the sputum is simply diluted; however, smaller amounts of water can become incorporated into mucus to reduce the adhesiveness of gelatinous secretions. In the case of retained secretions within the respiratory tract, mucokinesis may be improved by the addition of water to a depleted sol layer, since this allows the cilia to beat more effectively, thereby contributing to the proximal propulsion of the viscous gel layer.

▌ FACTORS INVOLVED IN MUCOKINESIS

Natural
- Respiratory tract secretions of adequate amount and consistency
- Maintenance of appropriate sol–gel relationship
- Ciliary activity and coordination
- Patent airways and adequate airflow
- Muscular coordination with laryngeal activity and effective cough

Pharmacologic
- Hypoviscosity agents and diluents
- Bronchorrheics
- Bronchomucotropic agents
- Mucolytics
- Detergents and surfactants
- Bronchodilators
- Mucosal constrictors

Mechanical
- Cough stimulation (*e.g.,* IPPB, pharyngeal catheter)
- Postural drainage
- Physical therapy (*e.g.,* percussion–vibration, rocking bed)
- Suctioning
- Psychic stimulation, encouragement, and teaching of patient

There is considerable question whether water provided in the form of an aerosol or as humidity (e.g., in "croup tents") has a significant effect on mucociliary clearance;[5,6] certainly, the nebulization of 2 mL of water (resulting in the actual deposition of less than 0.2 mL in the respiratory tract) may do no more than add an imperceptible amount of fluid to the gel layer coating of the tracheobronchial tree.[7] In contrast, secretion of a watery fluid by the bronchial glands may serve to replenish the sol layer from below and, thereby, to loosen adherent inspissated secretions from attachment to the ciliated epithelium.

A further criticism of plain water as a topical inhalational agent is that the low osmolality of the fluid may cause it to be absorbed by the respiratory mucosa with an adverse effect on airway flow mechanics. However, it is not certain that aerosols of plain water have this effect in practice, because droplets that are aerosolized into the lungs may rapidly evaporate to smaller sizes and may not deposit at all.[8] Consequently, plain water is not favored as a mucokinetic for nebulization therapy, although it does have a valuable prophylactic effect in preventing dehydration of the secretions in the upper airway during normal respiration. Thus, plain water in inhalational therapy subserves a "demulcent," soothing effect, rather than acting as a mucokinetic; it should be given as humidification therapy or as hot or cold mists.

Saline. Various concentrations of sodium chloride (NaCl) in water are used in aerosol therapy, either as primary drugs or as diluents or carriers for other drugs.

Normal saline (0.9% NaCl, which is isotonic with tissue fluids) is generally favored as a "bland" aerosol solution.

Half-normal saline (0.45% NaCl, hypotonic saline) is sometimes preferred, particularly for use in ultrasonic nebulization. The aerosol droplets of half-normal saline are thought to undergo some evaporative concentration when they reach the warmth of the respiratory tract; thus, the droplets that impact are almost isotonic.[9]

Hypertonic saline (e.g., 1.8%–15% NaCl) offers a theoretically more effective form of mucokinetic therapy. Deposition of hypertonic droplets on the respiratory mucosa results in the osmotic attraction of fluid from the mucosal blood vessels and tissues into the airway. Thus a "bronchorrhea" is induced, and the watery solution helps to dilute the respiratory tract secretions and to increase their bulk, thereby augmenting expectoration. Moreover, there is evidence that hypertonic saline has a direct effect on mucoprotein–DNA complexes, and by reducing the cohesive intramolecular forces the salt helps to decrease the viscous properties of the mucoid fluid.

Hypertonic saline is most useful as a sputum-inducing agent. An aerosol of 3% to 15% sodium chloride is an effective stimulus to expectoration in patients who have little spontaneous sputum production, and such mixtures are recommended for use when induced sputum specimens are needed for cytologic and microbiologic studies. Recently, the delivery of hypertonic saline by ultrasonic nebulization has proved very effective in inducing sputum for the diagnosis of *Pneumocystis carinii* infection.

Although various concentrations of sodium chloride can be used without significant untoward effects in inhalation therapy, certain precautions should be taken. For purposes of irrigation or instillation into the tracheobronchial tree, normal saline and perhaps half-normal saline are favored because they are relatively nonirritating to the airways. If hypertonic saline is used, not more than 10 mL/day should be given for no more than a few days; excessive use is not only irritating to the respiratory tract, but patients who cannot handle the sodium load may develop edema, heart failure, or hypertension. Improved results may be obtained by using a heated aerosol, or by adding 10% to 20% propylene glycol to the saline.

Sodium Bicarbonate. For many years, solutions of sodium bicarbonate ($NaHCO_3$) have been used as surgical irrigating fluids and for cleaning tracheostomy tubes. The salt was introduced into inhalation therapy in Alevaire: This product contained 2% sodium bicarbonate in combination with 0.125% tyloxapol (a "wetting" agent or "detergent") and 5% glycerin (used as a hygroscopic agent for stabilizing droplets and for "soothing" the respiratory mucosa). There is no satisfactory evidence that Alevaire was more successful than hypertonic sodium bicarbonate alone;[10] consequently, it is no longer marketed. Bicarbonate solutions can be given by aerosolization or by direct instillation; the higher concentrations may be somewhat irritating.

The success of sodium bicarbonate seems to be related partly to its alkaline pH (whereas sodium chloride is provided as an acidic solution), and sputum may be less adherent in an alkaline medium.[11] The hypertonic solutions also have a bronchorrheic effect, and possibly a direct salt effect, that helps disrupt some of the complex molecular bonds in mucus.

A minor disadvantage of sodium bicarbonate is that added bronchodilators (which have an acid pH) undergo more rapid breakdown in the alkaline solution. However, if a bronchodilator is added to a solution of sodium bicarbonate immediately before nebulization, effective therapy without adverse effects can be achieved, although the material that is subsequently expectorated or suctioned from the respiratory tract may be colored pink because of the presence of breakdown products (adrenochromes) of the catecholamine. Sodium bicarbonate makes a particularly suitable diluent for acetylcysteine because this mucolytic agent is more effective in an alkaline medium.

Acetylcysteine. Acetylcysteine (N-acetyl-L-cysteine sodium salt; Mucomyst) is the most powerful mucolytic agent in use in inhalation therapy. Like its parent compound, the amino acid cysteine, acetylcysteine contains a thiol group, and the free sulfhydryl radical of this group is a strong reducing agent that ruptures the disulfide bridges that serve to give stability to the mucoprotein network of molecules in mucus. Agents that break down these disulfide bonds produce the most effective mucolysis in laboratory studies.[12] The most powerful thiol compound is dithiothreitol, which is too toxic to be used therapeutically but is valuable as a laboratory mucolytic. Interestingly, the main constituent of garlic, which is a traditional expectorant, is the compound S-allyl-L-cysteine sulfoxide (also known as alliin); however, this agent does not have the mucolytic properties of acetylcysteine.

It has not been clearly demonstrated that nebulization of thiol compounds in small amounts can produce the same degree of mucolysis as that seen in test tube experiments. Indeed, the well-documented effect of acetylcysteine as a mucokinetic agent may depend more on the irritative qualities of the compound, which may thus simply induce bronchorrhea and stimulate coughing, thereby increasing expectoration. Acetylcysteine should be used as the 10% or 20% solution with the addition of an equal volume of sodium chloride or, preferably, sodium bicarbonate.

Once a bottle of the agent has been opened, it must be stored in a refrigerator; it should be used within a few days, as its potency rapidly declines.

Acetylcysteine is an irritant to the respiratory tract: it can cause mucosal changes and may induce bronchospasm. In addition, it can inhibit ciliary activity. These side effects may be obviated by pretreating with an aerosol bronchodilator or by using the combined product, Mucomyst with isoproterenol, which is 10% acetylcysteine with 0.05% isoproterenol.

Acetylcysteine has a sulfurous odor and an unpleasant taste, and on nebulization can irritate the oropharynx and may induce gagging and nausea or vomiting. However, the drug has no serious toxicity and, indeed, can be given with a fair degree of safety orally or even intravenously. In Europe and South America, oral acetylcysteine is a very popular mucolytic because their product is tasteless and odorless and does not cause irritation of the airways. Acetylcysteine by the oral or intravenous route is a specific antidote for the treatment of poisoning by acetaminophen. The drug provides cysteine, which is converted in the liver into glutathione, and this scavenger agent removes the toxic metabolites of acetaminophen. It is of interest that acetylcysteine may become more important as a free-radical scavenger. Through this mechanism, the drug may help prevent pollutant damage to the lungs, and it may help if given in the early stage of adult respiratory distress syndrome (ARDS).

Enzymes. Currently, enzymes are out of favor in respiratory therapy. They are irritating to the respiratory tract and can induce bronchospasm; more prolonged use may result in tracheobronchitis. Many patients develop febrile and hypersensitivity responses to enzymes; these may include rashes, asthma, pulmonary infiltrates, and fever.

Deoxyribonuclease (pancreatic dornase; Dornavac) is obtained from beef pancreas. It can break down DNA, and, therefore, was advised for treatment of patients with thick, purulent secretions. Dornavac is no longer available in the United States.

Trypsin has an antifibrin digestive effect. It was formerly used to treat fibropurulent exudates in the lung. The drug is no longer marketed.

Streptokinase and *streptodornase* were sometimes used in a combined preparation for inhalation. However, the use of these enzymes is no longer promoted.

Hygroscopic Agents. Several agents are incorporated into proprietary aerosols as soothing demulcents or as droplet-stabilizing adjuvants. Propylene glycol is probably the best of these agents and can be used with sodium chloride as a sputum-inducing aerosol. Glycerol (glycerin) is more irritating and cannot be recommended.

Alcohol. Many respiratory therapists believe alcohol is a useful mucokinetic agent. However, alcohol is an irritant, and any increase in respiratory tract secretions that follows nebulization with this agent probably results from bronchorrhea. Prolonged use of this drug causes tracheobronchitis, and, because alcohol also inhibits ciliary activity, the adverse effects of injudicious use might actually be seen in the form of mucus retention. One must not assume that the mucokinetic effect of an irritant agent is necessarily beneficial; after all, cigarette smoking is a prime means for stimulating mucus production, but obviously smoking should not be encouraged. Likewise, alcohol should not be used as a means of improving expectoration.

The main use for ethyl alcohol in respiratory therapy is in managing foaming pulmonary edema. Alcohol, as a vapor or droplets, acts to reduce the stability of the edema bubbles and, thereby, results in rapid dispersion of the foam.[13] The alcohol can be used in the form of vodka diluted with one or two parts water.

Other Mucokinetic Agents. Various other drugs are advised for use in loosening respiratory tract secretions (Table 19–2). Some of these are controversial, and others are not used or are used only in other countries. Those that are unavailable in the United States will not be discussed in detail.

Tergemist. Tergemist was formerly promoted in the United States. It contained 0.125% sodium ethasulfate (a "wetting" agent) and 0.1% potassium iodide.

Traditional Remedies. Traditional household inhalational remedies have never become popular in modern hospital practice. Agents such as menthol, eucalyptus, camphor, and benzoin are still popular as home remedies, and years of apparently satisfactory experience suggest that steam, rendered aromatic by the addition of one of these essential volatile oils, may be an effective, inexpensive, and pleasant mucokinetic. Many such agents are available as proprietary products (e.g., Vick's Vaporub and Friar's Balsam).[14]

L-Arginine. L-Arginine can reportedly reduce the viscosity of sputum in patients with mucoviscidosis (fibrocystic disease). It is thought that this amino acid combines with calcium, thereby reducing covalent bonding in mucoprotein. Aside from an increased amount of calcium in the respiratory tract secretions in mucoviscidosis, no basic abnormalities have been clearly identified to be the cause of the highly viscous mucus that characterizes this disease.[15] No recent corroboration of the value of L-arginine has appeared.

Table 19—2 Classification of Mucokinetic Drugs

CLASS	ACTION	EXAMPLES
Drugs that increase the depth of the sol layer	1. Topical diluents	1. Hydrating agents (e.g., water,* electrolyte solutions*)
	2. Stimulators of respiratory mucosa a. Irritants	2. Bronchorrheics a. Smoke,* aromatic vapors,* ultrasonic particles,* alcohol*
	b. Hyperosmolar solutions	b. Hypertonic drug or salt solutions*
	3. Stimulators of mucous secretion	3. Bronchomucotropics (e.g., iodide)
	4. Stimulators of gastropulmonary vagal reflex	4. Expectorants (e.g., ipecac, guaifenesin)
Drugs that alter the consistency of the gel layer	1. Topical diluents	1. Hydrating agents (e.g., water,* electrolyte solutions*)
	2. Break down (lyse) protein or DNA a. Thiol (split disulfide bonds) b. Decomplexing agents (break mucoprotein–DNA complexes)	2. True mucolytics a. Acetylcysteine b. Hypertonic salt solutions,* alkalis
	c. Enzymes (digest protein) d. Activators of natural proteases e. Reducing agents f. Amides g. Calcium binders	c. Proteases (e.g., dornase) d. Iodides, electrolyte solutions* e. Ascorbic acid† copper*† f. Urea*† g. L-Arginine*† chelating agents, hypertonic saline*
	3. Normalize biochemical production of mucus a. Mucoregulators (alter mucoprotein synthesis)	a. Bromhexine,† ambroxol,† S-carboxymethyl-cysteine,†sobrerol,† stepronin†
	b. Antimicrobials (decrease DNA production) c. Nonspecific 4. Thicken watery sputum	b. Antibiotics c. Glucocorticosteroids 4. Mucospissics a. Anticholinergic agents (e.g., atropine) b. Some antibiotics (e.g., tetracycline*) c. Glucocorticosteroids
Drugs that decrease the adhesiveness of the gel layer	1. Wetting agents 2. Surfactant	1. Sodium ethasulfate,*† water* 2. Tyloxapol,*† sodium bicarbonate,* glycerine,* propylene glycol*
Agents that improve airway patency	1. Bronchodilators 2. Anti-inflammatory agents 3. Mucosal constrictors 4. Ciliary stimulants	1. Sympathomimetics,* methylxanthines 2. Glucocorticosteroids 3. Phenylephrine* 4. Sympathomimetics*

* Usually given by inhalational route.
† Not available in the United States.

Noninhalational Mucokinetic Drugs

Most of the noninhalational drugs are given orally and are generally classified as expectorants. Boyd and others give evidence to suggest that these agents stimulate afferent receptors in the stomach.[16] These postulated receptors result in a vagal reflex that may relay through a "mucokinetic" medullary center, which possibly lies between the respiratory center and the vomiting center. The efferent arc of the reflex is thought to be provided by vagal fibers to the lungs; similar vagal fibers supply the stomach. Strong stimulation of this reflex results in vomiting; the act of vomiting includes salivation and sometimes expectoration. A lesser stimulus by a subemetic dose of a vagal stimulant does not cause vomiting, but does result in increased expectoration, presumably by activating the bronchial glands (i.e., the gastropulmonary mucokinetic vagal reflex). The submucous glands are under vagal control, and a suitable stimulus results in the output of a watery secretion.[17]

Certain drugs are preferentially concentrated by the bronchial glands, which are then stimulated to secrete. These drugs attain their effect after being absorbed by the stomach into the bloodstream, after which they reach the bronchial glands from the supplying blood vessels. Some agents, when secreted into the respiratory fluid, have a direct or indirect mucolytic effect on the mucoproteins.

In the following section, the more important oral mucokinetic drugs will be discussed briefly (Table 19–3).

Potassium Iodide. For many years, a saturated solution of potassium iodide (SSKI) has been favored as a mucokinetic agent. There are several ways in which iodides may have an effect.

1. The drug stimulates the gastropulmonary mucokinetic vagal reflex, thereby activating the submucosal bronchial glands. Excessive dosage with potassium iodide causes nausea and vomiting.
2. The bronchial glands selectively concentrate circulating iodide, which then stimulates the glands to secrete. This is termed a "bronchomucotropic" effect.[6] The salivary, nasal, and lacrimal glands act similarly, and iodotherapy may cause salivation, rhinorrhea, and lacrimation. The stimulus to the salivary glands can be so great that

they actually enlarge to produce a mumpslike appearance. Moreover, iodide concentrated in and then secreted by the salivary glands results in a characteristic metallic taste of the secretions, which patients often notice.

3. There is evidence that iodides stimulate natural proteolytic enzymes in the respiratory secretions, thereby enhancing the digestive breakdown of mucoprotein.[18] Thus, iodide can have a direct mucolytic effect.
4. There is some evidence that potassium iodide can stimulate ciliary activity, thereby improving mucociliary clearance.[19]
5. Iodide may have an anti-inflammatory effect, thus aiding in the resolution of conditions such as bronchitis, pneumonitis, and asthma.[20]

Iodide is usually administered as a saturated solution of the potassium salt (SSKI), 5 to 10 drops in a glass of water; as many as 20 to 30 drops may be given in this way three or four times a day. Unfortunately, iodide may cause an acneiform eruption, and many patients develop rashes while taking the drug; it should be used with particular care in adolescents prone to acne. Long-term administration of the drug may affect thyroid function; therefore, the TSH and T_4 tests for thyroid function should be checked after the first 2 or 3 months of therapy. Hypothyroidism coexisting in patients

Table 19–3 Some Oral Mucokinetic Agents

AGENT	USUAL ADULT DOSAGE	NOTES
Water	Variable	Essential
Potassium iodide (SSKI)	5–20 drops (500–2000 mg) 3 or 4 times a day	One of most effective mucokinetics. Toxicity: rashes, metallic taste, parotid swelling, lacrimation, rhinorrhea, nausea, thyroid suppression
Iodopropylidene glycerol (Organidin)	60–120 mg 2–4 times a day	Much less toxicity than SSKI
Syrup of ipecac	0.5–2 mL 3 times a day	One of more effective agents; may cause nausea and vomiting
Ammonium chloride	0.3–1 g 3 times a day	Probably effective; nauseating
Guaifenesin (glyceryl guaiacolate)	400 mg 4–6 times a day	Probably ineffective if less than 2400 mg/day is used. Toxicity: nausea, vomiting, drowsiness
Terpin hydrate	300 mg 4 times a day	Probably ineffective
Bromhexine	8–16 mg 3 times a day	Not available in the United states
Ambroxol	0.5–1 g 2–3 times a day	Not available in the United States
S-Carboxymethylcysteine	375–750 mg 4 times a day	Not available in the United States
Acetylcysteine	200 mg 3 times a day	Oral form not available in the United States
Sobrerol	400 mg 2 times a day	Not available in the United States

with chronic obstructive disease is not always clinically apparent, and thyroid function tests should always be performed at the first suspicion of hypothyroidism in patients taking protracted courses of iodide medication.

An organic iodide, Organidin, has been shown to be of benefit in the management of chronic mucus stasis. The recommended oral dose is 120 mg twice a day.

If oral therapy was contraindicated, *sodium iodide* was once given intravenously. This product has recently been taken off the market.

Syrup of Ipecac. Syrup of ipecac is best known as an emetic agent. However, it has long been used, in small doses, as a mucokinetic agent. The appropriate dose for adults is 0.5 to 2 mL three to four times daily; at this low dosage nausea should not be a problem.

Salts. Various salt solutions are suitable for oral use as vagal stimulants. Thus, concentrated solutions of sodium chloride, ammonium chloride, sodium citrate, and similar salts are used on their own or incorporated into proprietary expectorant mixtures. Any osmotic cathartic, used for its effect on the bowel, may also have a beneficial effect on respiratory tract fluid by means of the postulated gastropulmonary mucokinetic vagal reflex. Each of these agents may be contraindicated in patients with electrolyte problems, particularly subjects who retain sodium.

Guaifenesin. Guaifenesin was formerly called glyceryl guaiacolate. It is still one of the most popular expectorants, being present in proprietary "cough medicines" such as Robitussin. The drug is derived from creosote, which was formerly used as an expectorant.

There is evidence that guaifenesin acts both as a vagal stimulant and by direct stimulation of the bronchial glands. The drug is absorbed from the stomach and is concentrated by the bronchial glands, which rapidly secrete it into the respiratory tract. The recommended dose for adults is 100 to 200 mg four times daily, but it is doubtful whether this dosage has any beneficial effect.[21] The drug is also present in bronchodilator mixtures such as Bronkotabs and Quibron, but the amount is less than 100 mg/dose, which is unlikely to have any mucokinetic effect. A more appropriate dosage would be 500 to 1000 mg, but such amounts may produce vomiting and can cause cerebral depression.

Terpin Hydrate. Terpin hydrate is a volatile oil derivative of turpentine, and it supposedly has similar actions to those of guaifenesin. However, the conventional dosage of 5 mL (85 mg) is probably without effect, and the drug should be regarded simply as a flavoring agent for use with other "cough medications."

Bromhexine. Bromhexine (Bisolvon) is used in Europe, where it has gained a reputation of being one of the most successful oral mucokinetic agents.[22] Evidence suggests that bromhexine acts on the bronchial glands to increase their secretions, thereby causing an augmented volume of sputum of decreased viscosity in bronchitic patients. The drug may also have a mucolytic action, since it can produce depolymerization of mucopolysaccharides in vitro. A derivative of bromhexine, *ambroxol*, appears to be a potent stimulator of surfactant production, and it has been used in the management of neonatal respiratory distress syndrome.

S-Carboxymethylcysteine. S-Carboxymethylcysteine (Mucodyne) is an oral mucokinetic that has recently been introduced in Europe. Although it is related to acetylcysteine, the molecular structure is such that its thiol group is not free (*i.e.*, it is "blocked"), and thus the molecule cannot directly rupture disulfide bonds. It is thought that this agent acts directly on the bronchial glands to induce secretion of an increased amount of sialomucins, thereby producing fluid of relatively low viscosity; this action has been called a mucoregulator effect. Interestingly, this drug is closely related to alliin, the parent compound of garlic, which is also believed to be an effective oral mucokinetic agent, probably because it has mucoregulator properties (Fig. 19–2).

Miscellaneous Oral Mucokinetic Drugs. Other orally administered drugs are credited with mucokinetic properties, although substantiation is needed. Among the more popular of such agents are *anise, camphor, pine syrup, licorice, paregoric* (camphorated tincture of opium), *senega, squill,* and *tolu balsam.* Many of these agents are still incorporated into proprietary "cough medicines."

Garlic has already been discussed, and this spice is credited with expectorant effects in several national pharmacopeias. Some evidence suggests that various foods and spices favored in folk medicine do have a mucokinetic effect, as does chicken soup.[6,23] Because agents such as pepper, mustard, and horseradish can cause lacrimation and rhinor-

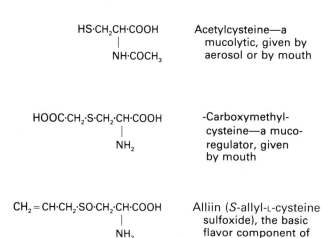

HS·CH$_2$CH·COOH
  |
  NH·COCH$_3$

Acetylcysteine—a mucolytic, given by aerosol or by mouth

HOOC·CH$_2$·S·CH$_2$·CH·COOH
        |
        NH$_2$

-Carboxymethyl-cysteine—a muco-regulator, given by mouth

CH$_2$ = CH·CH$_2$·SO·CH$_2$·CH·COOH
              |
              NH$_2$

Alliin (*S*-allyl-L-cysteine sulfoxide), the basic flavor component of garlic—a probable mucoregulator

Figure 19—2. Chemistry of some related cysteine derivatives with mucokinetic properties.

rhea, not surprisingly they can cause an appreciable augmentation of tracheobronchial secretions; perhaps vagal stimulation is involved.

Parasympathomimetic drugs are powerful stimulants of the bronchial glands. However, although they can produce mucokinesis, they may also cause bronchospasm and other harmful parasympathetic effects. Apparently, no cholinergic drug has been found suitable as a therapeutic mucokinetic agent. In contrast, antiparasympathomimetic drugs, such as atropine, have an antimucokinetic action and can cause drying of the respiratory tract mucosa when given systemically in large doses. Aerosol preparations, including ipratropium (Atrovent) do not cause this adverse effect.

BRONCHODILATORS AND ANTIASTHMA DRUGS

Most drugs used to manage bronchospasm act on the biochemical mechanisms that control bronchial muscle tone. A critical factor in the complex cascade is the "second messenger," cyclic 3′,5′-adenosine monophosphate (cAMP), which serves to reverse bronchospasm (Fig. 19–3 and Table 19–4). Intracellular levels of cAMP are increased by either of two mechanisms: stimulation of the enzyme *adenylate cyclase* catalyzes the conversion of the precursor adenosine triphosphate (ATP) to form cAMP; and inhibition of the enzyme *phosphodiesterase* prevents the rapid breakdown of cAMP to

inactive metabolites. The major bronchodilators have their effect on one or the other of these two mechanisms.[24]

Catecholamines and similar sympathomimetics stimulate adenylate cyclase, whereas *methylxanthines* are phosphodiesterase inhibitors. At present, only the catecholamines and related compounds are routinely given by both oral and inhalational routes.

Cyclic-AMP is also important in allergic asthma, as increased intracellular concentrations of this messenger inhibit antigen-induced release of mediators, such as histamine and slow-reacting substance of anaphylaxis, that induce the pathophysiologic response. The release of these mediators is enhanced by cholinergic (*i.e.*, vagal) stimuli that may cause increased concentrations of intracellular cyclic 3′,5′-guanosine monophosphate (3′,5′-GMP); this is a further messenger, which, in effect, has an action opposite that of cAMP and results in bronchospasm.[25] These mediators, in turn, control prostaglandin and leukotriene formation from arachidonic acid, and it is these products that modulate the biochemical processes involved in bronchospasm, mucosal inflammation, and mucus production.

SYMPATHOMIMETIC DRUGS

The natural hormonal transmitters of the sympathetic nervous system are norepinephine and epinephrine. These hormones are chemically related to cathechol and are known as catecholamines; they are also classified as sympathomimetic agents, adrenergic agents, or adrenoreceptor stimulators. These chemicals have various categories of effects on autonomic function, and these effects are subdivided into α-, β_1-, and β_2-properties, depending on the anatomic sites of the various receptors that are stimulated. The bronchial muscle receptors are termed β_2-adrenergic receptors, and stimulation of these activates the adenylate cyclase mechanism, leading to cAMP production and resulting bronchodilatation.

Stimulation of β_1-receptors of the heart and blood vessels results in undesired side effects, including tachycardia, possible arrhythmias, and blood pressure changes. Blood vessels are supplied with β_2-receptors; stimulation results in vasodilation. The blood vessels of the respiratory mucosa are also supplied with α-receptors, the stimulation of which causes vasoconstriction, which may be valuable in treating bronchospasm, especially that associated with edema and cellular infiltrates as a

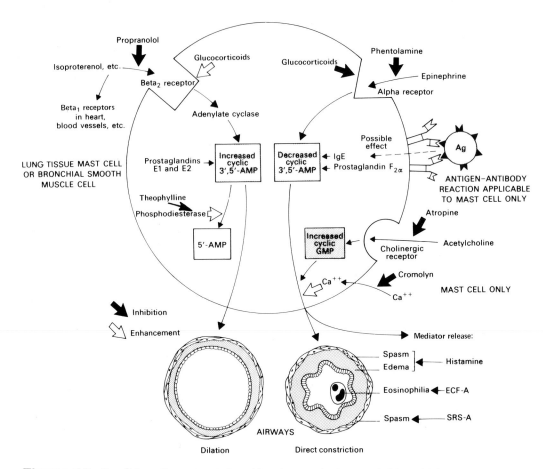

Figure 19—3. Schematic representation of the pharmacologic control of bronchial tone and allergen-induced release of chemical mediators. Cholinergic or α-adrenergic stimulation in the presence of β-adrenergic blockade results in bronchial constriction directly, as well as enhanced release of mediators from lung tissue. The biochemical sequence is known to be more complex than is illustrated; it involves the arachidonic acid cascade that activates the release of leukotrienes, prostaglandins, and other groups of mediators. The slow-reacting substance of anaphylaxis (SRS-A) is made up of several leukotrienes.

Table 19—4 Pharmacology of Autonomic Modulation*

EXAMPLE OF REACTANT	SITE OF ACTION	CYCLIC NUCLEOTIDE EFFECT	MAST-CELL MEDIATOR RELEASE	BRONCHIAL END-ORGAN RESPONSE	EXAMPLE OF BLOCKER
Isoproterenol	β-adrenergic receptor–adenylate cyclase stimulation	↑ cAMP	Inhibited	Bronchodilatation	Propranolol
Norepinephrine	α-adrenergic receptor–ATPase (?) stimulation	↓ cAMP	Enhanced	Bronchodilatation	Phentolamine
Theophylline	Phosphodiesterase inhibition	↑ cAMP	Inhibited	Bronchodilatation	Calmodulin (?)
Acetylcholine	Cholinergic receptor–guanylate cyclase stimulation	↑ cGMP (?)	Enhanced	Bronchoconstriction	Atropine

* This is a simplified examination of an extremely complex and evolving area in cyclic nucleotide research.

result of inflammation. A further sympathomimetic effect, which is unwanted, is stimulation of the nervous system, causing nervousness, sleeplessness, and tremor; this effect is inevitable with large doses of drugs that are potent β_2-stimulators.

Epinephrine is the prototype of the catecholamines. It has α-, β_1-, and β_2- effects and thus, in addition to being a very effective bronchodilator, has unwanted cardiovascular and nervous system side effects. Epinephrine also has the powerful β-effect of releasing glucose from the liver (glycogenolysis). The molecule of epinephrine contains hydroxyl groupings in the 3 and 4 positions of the benzene nucleus and, accordingly, is susceptible to degradation by at least two different enzyme systems.

1. In the bowel wall, and to some extent in the liver, are enzymes that degrade epinephrine and related catecholamines by mechanisms such as sulfatization. Consequently, epinephrine and isoproterenol are relatively ineffective as bronchodilators when given orally.
2. In various tissues, including the lungs, the enzyme catechol-O-methyltransferase (COMT) causes inactivation of the 3,4-hydroxysympathomimetics by O-methylation.

The amino group of the ethylamine side-chain is responsible for the α- and β-stimulatory properties of the catecholamines. The addition of alkyl substitution radicals in the amino group leads to a progressive increase in β_2-activity, with a corresponding decrease in β_1- and α-potency. The amino group is deaminated by monoamine oxidase (MAO) during metabolic breakdown. As a result of these metabolic processes, the catecholamines are finally excreted in the urine as ethereal sulfates, glucuronides, and vanillylmandelic acid (VMA).

Although the activities of the various catecholamines and derivatives used in therapeutics have been carefully evaluated, their effects are complex because they not only have multiple sites of action, but also their primary actions are complicated by reflex responses in the intact animal. Therefore, it is difficult to compare the bronchodilator potency of the various sympathomimetics and to determine the comparative β_2-receptor selectivity of these agents. The therapeutic response to an agent is also affected somewhat by the route of administration, but generally the best bronchodilator/side effect ratio is obtained by aerosolization rather than by oral administration.

In the following section, the various sympathomimetic agents best suited for respiratory therapy are described. Most, but not all, of these drugs can be given by inhalational administration. Norepinephrine, which has an unsubstituted amino group, is a powerful α-receptor stimulator and also has strong β_1-effects; however, clinically it has no β_2-activity and is not a bronchodilator, although it is a potent pressor agent. A tentative classification of adrenergic receptors is given in Table 19–5.

Sympathomimetic Drugs Suitable for Aerosolization

Numerous individual products are available, with multiple formulation of the older bronchodilators epinephrine (which is marketed over-the-counter) and isoproterenol (which requires a prescription). For home use, almost all patients use metered-dose inhalers, but inhalant solutions for updraft delivery are often used in hospitals and for occasional outpatients. Currently, most products do not contain sulfites, because this preservative can induce bronchospasm in the rare patient whose asthma is triggered by sulfites and related chemicals.

Epinephrine. Epinephrine (adrenaline) is a natural sympathomimetic hormone that has been recognized as a bronchodilator for more than 80 years. It is rarely used in modern respiratory therapy because of its marked β_1-effects, although it remains popular for self-therapy because it is available without prescription. For inhalational therapy, a 1 : 100 solution is used; this solution is too concentrated for subcutaneous administration (Tables 19–6, 19–7, and 19–8).

Racepinephrine. Racemic epinephrine (Micronefrin, Vaponefrin) is obtained synthetically; it is a racemic mixture of *dextro-* and *levo-* epinephrine, whereas the natural hormone exists only in the *levo* form. The racemic mixture is claimed to have adequate β_2-potency, with less β_1- and α-activity than epinephrine. Although the manufacturers suggest that racepinephrine is a more suitable drug for use in respiratory therapy, no adequate controlled comparison of the two drugs has been reported.

The presence of α-receptor activity makes racepinephrine a useful drug when mucosal congestion requires treatment. The drug has been recommended for aerosolization in managing croup and

Table 19—5 Classification of Adrenergic Receptors

	α	β_1	β_2
Distribution of receptors			
Airways			
Muscle	Yes	No	Yes
Blood vessels	Yes	Yes	No
Heart	Yes	Yes	Few
Systemic blood vessels	No (?)	No (?)	Yes (?)
Central nervous system	?	?	Yes (?)
Result of receptor stimulation			
Bronchial muscle	Weak contraction	No effect	Relaxation
Bronchial glands	Stimulation (?)	Stimulation (?)	Stimulation
Cilia	?	?	Stimulation
Blood vessels (general)	Constriction	?	Dilation
Cardiac muscle	Excitation	Stimulation	Slight stimulation
Skeletal muscle	?	?	Excitation
Central nervous system	?	?	Excitation
Liver and muscle	Glycogenolysis	?	Glycogenolysis
Adipose tissue	?	Lipolysis	No effect
Uterus	Excitation	?	Inhibition
Physiologic effects*			
Bronchospasm	Slight increase	No effect	Decrease
Respiratory tract secretions	Slight increase (?)	Slight increase (?)	Increase
Cough	?	No effect	Decrease
Airway resistance	Decrease (?)	No effect	Decrease
Heart rate	Reflex slowing (may cause ectopy)	Increase	No effect
Blood pressure			
Weak stimulus	May increase	Varies	Varies
Strong stimulus	Increase	May decrease	Varies
Skeletal muscle	No effect (?)	No effect (?)	Tremor
Pupils	Dilation	?	?
Central nervous system	?	?	Stimulation
Uterus	Contraction	?	Tocoylsis

* The effect on human adrenergic receptors depends on factors such as route of administration, total dose given, time at which measurement is made, and reflex responses, among other variables.

epiglottitis, but the validity of favorable reports is questionable. Clinical experience has shown that the drug is a useful bronchodilator, although in recent years it has become relatively obsolescent.

Isoproterenol. Isoproterenol (isoprenaline, Isuprel) was once the most popular inhalational bronchodilator. The drug is a synthetic derivative and appears to be one of the most potent β_2-stimulators. Oral preparations are available, but absorption is unreliable; intravenous administration in asthmatic patients may be effective, but there is a risk of dangerous inotropic and chronotropic cardiac stimulation.

The marked β_1-activity of isoproterenol makes it a less than ideal bronchodilator, and its inhalational use may be complicated by unwanted effects on the heart and blood pressure. Moreover, since the drug has no α-effect (see Table 19–6), its unopposed β_2-effect causes vasodilatation in the pulmonary vasculature. This may result in mucosal congestion, and the increased blood flow leads to rapid systemic absorption of the drug, with resulting shortening in the length of the bronchodilator response and increased risk of extrapulmonary side effects. A further problem is that systemic absorption can cause pulmonary vasodilatation in poorly ventilated lung areas, which increases the shunt

Table 19—6 Structure and Actions of Common Bronchodilator Catecholamines and Derivatives*

	2	3	4	5	β	α	NH	α (Vasoconstriction)	β_1 (Cardiac Stimulation)	β_2 (Bronchodilatation, Nervous System Stimulation, Vasodilatation)	Persistence of Effect of Aerosol (hr)
Epinephrine	H	OH	OH	H	OH	H	CH_3	+++	++++	+++	1–2
R-Epinephrine	H	OH	OH	H	OH	H	CH_3	++(+)	+++(+)	++(+)	1–2
Isoproterenol	H	OH	OH	H	OH	H	$CH(CH_3)_2$		++++	++++(+)	1–2
Isoetharine	H	OH	OH	H	OH	C_2H_5	$CH(CH_3)_2$		+(+)	+++(+)	2–4
Ethylnorepinephrine	H	OH	OH	H	OH	C_2H_5	H	++	++	++(+)	2–4
Metaproterenol	H	OH	H	OH	OH	H	$CH(CH_3)_2$		+(+)	+++(+)	3–5
Terbutaline	H	OH	H	OH	OH	H	$C(CH_3)_3$		+(+)	+++(+)	4–7
Colterol†	H	OH	OH	H	OH	H	$C(CH_3)_3$		+(+)	+++(+)	4–7
Albuterol	H	CH_2OH	OH	H	OH	H	$C(CH_3)_3$		+(+)	++++(+)	4–5
Pirbuterol	(N)	CH_2OH	OH	H	OH	H	$C(CH_3)_3$		+(+)	++++(+)	4–6
Ephedrine	H	H	H	H	OH	CH	CH_3		++(+)	+++	4–6
Fenoterol	H	OH	H	OH	OH	H	$(C_9H_{11}O)$		+(+)	++++(+)	5–8

* The relative effects are not established accurately and, therefore, the above information is only approximate. The actual result obtained depends on the total dose given, the route and rate of administration, the presence of disease and other drugs, and factors such as tachyphylaxis. The measured response will also vary with time, as initial pharmacologic effects result in reflex adjustments. Consequently, the actual findings at any time in a given patient may show major departures from this schema.
† Marketed as the prodrug bitolterol.

effect in the lungs, and this may be manifested as a fall in the PaO_2.

Isoproterenol, when given by nebulization, is one of the shortest-acting bronchodilators. Patients with severe asthma frequently have to take inhalations of the drug every 1 to 2 hours and, by so doing, they run the risk of inducing *tachyphylaxis*. This is a phenomenon whereby responsiveness to the bronchodilating effects of a drug becomes progressively smaller, although β_1-effectiveness may be maintained. As a result, the patients who overuse the aerosol may develop cardiac side effects, including tachycardia, tachyarrhythmias, and even myocardial necrosis. These adverse effects are particularly dangerous in patients who have underlying heart disease or blood pressure problems, and the concomitant presence of hypoxemia may increase the danger of a fatal arrhythmia or a cardiovascular catastrophe.[1]

When the drug is given by updraft nebulizer, the therapist should watch for evidence of toxicity. The patient may complain of palpitations, anxiety, flushing, or tinnitus or may experience faintness or a throbbing headache. The pulse should be checked during and after therapy and, in patients at particular risk, monitoring of the electrocardiogram and blood pressure is advisable. Rinsing the mouth and throat may decrease systemic absorption through the oropharyngeal and gastric mucosa and may reduce the incidence of unwanted β_1-complications. Overuse and overdosage with isoproterenol must always be avoided.

The main value of isoproterenol aerosol is in the pulmonary function laboratory, where it can be used to evaluate the reversibility of obstructive airway disease. However, it can also be useful for occasional aerosol therapy for younger asthmatics with no cardiovascular abnormalities.

An attempt has been made to enhance the usefulness of isoproterenol by including phenyl-

Table 19—7   Metered Aerosol Bronchodilators

DRUG	DOSES PER CARTRIDGE (APPROXIMATE NO.)	AMOUNT OF DRUG DELIVERY PER INHALATION (MG)
EPINEPHRINE		
Asthma Haler (Norcliffe-Thayer)	300	0.16
Bronitin Mist (Whitehall)	300, 400	0.16
Bronkaid Mist (Winthrop)	300, 450	0.25
Bronkaid Mist Suspension (Winthrop)	200	0.16
Medihaler-EPi (Riker)	300	0.16
Primatene Mist (Whitehall)	300, 450	0.22
Primatene Mist Suspension (Whitehall)	200	0.16
ISOPROTERENOL		
Isoproterenol (generic)	300	0.125
Isuprel Mistometer (Winthrop)	200, 300	0.131
Medihaler-Iso (Riker)	300, 450	0.080
Norisodrine Aerotrol (Abbott)	350	0.120
ISOPROTERENOL–PHENYLEPHRINE		
Duo-Medihaler (Riker)	300, 450	
Isoproterenol		0.137
Phenylephrine		0.126
ISOETHARINE		
Bronkometer (Winthrop)	200, 400	0.340
METAPROTERENOL		
Alupent (Boehringer)	200	0.65
Metaprel (Sandoz)	200	0.65
ALBUTEROL (SALBUTAMOL)		
Proventil (Schering)	200	0.09
Ventolin (Glaxo)	200	0.09
TERBUTALINE		
Brethaire (Geigy)	300	0.20
BITOLTEROL		
Tornalate (Winthrop)	300	0.37
PIRBUTEROL		
Maxair (3M Riker)	300	0.20
FENOTEROL		
(Berotec-Boehringer)	300	0.16

Table 19—8 Bronchodilator Inhalant Solutions Available for Updraft Aerosolization Using Simple Nebulizer, IPPB, or Compressor

DRUG	CONCENTRATION (%)	INITIAL DOSAGES*	
		Hand Nebulizer No. of Inhalations	Updraft or Compressor (mL)†
EPINEPHRINE			
Adrenalin (Parke-Davis)	1	2–3	0.25–0.7
RACEMIC EPINEPHRINE			
(Racepinephrine)			
Asthma Nephrin (Norclift-Thayer)§	2.25	1–3	0.4–0.8
Vaponefrin (Fisons)§	2.25	2–6	0.25–0.7
ISOPROTERENOL‡			
Aerolone (Lilly)	0.25	6–12	0.3–1
Dispos-a-Med (Parke-Davis)	0.25, 0.5	6–12	0.25–1
Isuprel (Winthrop)	0.5	5–15	0.5
Isuprel (Winthrop)	1	3–17	0.25
Vap-Iso (Fisons)	0.5	5–15	0.5
ISOETHARINE‡			
Arm-a-Med (Armour)	0.062–0.25		2–4
Bronkosol (Winthrop)	1	3–7	0.25–1
Bronkosol Unit Dose (Winthrop)	0.25	3–7	2
Dispos-a-Med (Parke-Davis)	0.5, 1		0.25–1
METAPROTERENOL			
Alupent (Boehringer)	5	5–15	0.2–0.3
Alupent Unit Dose (Boehringer)	0.4, 0.6		2.5
Arm-a-Med (Armour)	0.4, 0.6		2.5
ALBUTEROL			
Proventil (Schering)	0.5		0.25–0.5
Proventil Unit Dose (Schering)	0.083		3
Ventolin (Glaxo)	0.5		0.25–0.5

* These dosages are based on manufacturers' recommendations and illustrate the imprecision in prescribing that exists.
† The recommended amount can be diluted with 1–3 mL saline. Prepackaged unit-dose preparations are available with various diluents.
‡ Generic preparations are marketed in various concentrations. Each manufacturer's information should be used in determining dosages.
§ Available without prescription.

ephrine in the product (e.g., as Duo-Medihaler). The strong α-effect of phenylephrine may counteract the vasodilator effect of isoproterenol on the respiratory mucosa, thereby reducing the systemic absorption of the drug. This may serve to prevent some of the cardiac effect, while prolonging the lo-cal bronchodilator effect in the lungs. The pharma-cologic principles on which this combination ther-apy is based appear to be reasonable. A further possible advantage of the combination is that the aerosol is less likely to cause a fall in PaO$_2$, thus suggesting that the combination of drugs in the

Duo-Medihaler offers a more suitable bronchodilator preparation than does isoproterenol alone for patients with hypoxemia.

The appropriate dosages of isoproterenol preparations are given in Tables 19–7 and 19–8.

Isoetharine. The catecholamine isoetharine is available as a proprietary aerosol, which formerly also contained phenylephrine. Isoetharine differs from isoproterenol in having an ethyl group on the α-carbon atom, and, as a result, it has somewhat less of a β_2-effect than does isoproterenol, and much less β_1-activity (see Table 19–6). The addition of phenylephrine, which is a powerful α-receptor stimulator, may have served to reduce mucosal vasodilatation and to prolong the bronchodilator effect of the isoetharine. However, proof of these possible benefits was lacking, and phenylephrine was removed from the formulation.

Isoetharine was formerly very popular as a metered preparation (Bronkometer), as well as for updraft delivery (Bronkosol). In bronchospastic patients who are hypoxemic and who have tachycardia and underlying coronary artery disease, isoetharine is much less likely to cause serious cardiac side effects than is isoproterenol.

Recommended dosages of isoetharine are provided in Tables 19–7 and 19–8.

Metaproterenol. Metaproterenol (orciprenaline, Alupent, Metaprel) is available as a metered aerosol and as an inhalant solution. It is chemically related to isoproterenol, but the hydroxy groups, which occupy the 3 and 4 positions in the benzene nucleus of isoproterenol, are in the 3 and 5 (*meta*) positions (see Table 19–6). This configuration renders metaproterenol immune to sulfatization in the bowel; therefore, it is effective when given orally. The molecule is not inactivated by COMT; consequently, the drug has a more sustained bronchodilator effect.

When used by aerosol, metaproterenol causes few side effects; it is far less likely to cause tachycardia than is isoproterenol. The effect of the aerosol usually lasts 3 to 4 hours or more, and it is usually required four times daily.[26] Dosages of the aerosol are listed in Tables 19–7 and 19–8.

Terbutaline. Terbutaline (Brethine, Bricanyl) is available as a metered-dose inhaler, but the inhalant solution has had a delayed arrival in the United States. The drug is long-lasting, but causes more tremor than other bronchodilators.[27,28] Aerosol dosages are listed in Tables 19–7 and 19–8, but there is

no justification for giving the subcutaneous form by aerosol, since other authorized aerosol bronchodilators are preferable.

Albuterol. Albuterol (salbutamol, Proventil, Ventolin) is available as a metered-dose inhaler and as an inhalant solution. It is very similar to terbutaline, but appears to be more potent; it is somewhat shorter acting and may have a greater tendency to cause hypoxemia. Albuterol resembles terbutaline in having a tertiary butyl substitution in the amino group; therefore, it has similar β_2-selective properties. The drug is protected from sulfatization and from COMT, because the hydroxyl group in position 3 of the catechol nucleus has been replaced by a CH_2OH group that interferes with the activity of these enzymes.[29]

Bitolterol. The only new bronchodilator developed in the United States was introduced as a metered-dose inhaler. The product is a prodrug, bitolterol (Tornalate), which is converted into the active drug colterol (see Table 19–6) in the body by esterases that are found in the blood and tissues. These enzymes are found in particularly large quantities in the lungs, and conversion of the aerosol to colterol occurs within a few minutes. However, the resulting delayed onset of bronchodilatation is unacceptable to some patients. The slow release of colterol from bitolterol can produce bronchodilatation lasting 6 to 8 hours after a single dose. In structure, colterol is similar to terbutaline, and its effects and side effects appear to be similar.

Pirbuterol. The European drug pirbuterol was recently introduced in the United States as a metered-dose inhaler (Maxair). In structure it is related to albuterol, but carbon atom 2 of the benzene ring is replaced by a nitrogen atom in pirbuterol, which is thus a sympathomimetic pyridine derivative rather than a benzene derivative. It appears to be comparable in most respects with albuterol, although it may have a slightly slower onset of action and a more prolonged effect.[30]

Fenoterol. This agent is hydroxyphenylorciprenaline (orciprenaline is the European name for metaproterenol). It is claimed to be longer acting and to have a more selective effect on β_2-receptors than does metaproterenol.[31] However, although it has long been marketed in Europe (as Berotec), its introduction into the United States market has been repeatedly delayed. In New Zealand, the drug's safety has recently been questioned.

Noninhalational Sympathomimetic Drugs

Several inhalational drugs for treating bronchospasm are also commonly given by alternative routes of administration. A few sympathomimetics are not suitable at all for inhalation, and these will also be considered in this section.

Epinephrine. Epinephrine is available as the hydrochloride and as the bitartrate; there are no significant differences between these preparations. In status asthmaticus 0.1 to 0.5 mL of the 1:1000 aqueous solution can be given subcutaneously and repeated after half an hour if necessary. An aqueous solution for intramuscular administration (Sus-Phrine) has a longer persisting effect that lasts up to 8 hours. If the response is not satisfactory, further reliance on this drug is probably not warranted, and other forms of treatment should be initiated. A 1:5000 solution in oil is available for intramuscular injection: 0.2 to 1.0 mL can be given and may have an appreciable effect for 8 to 16 hours.

Isoproterenol. Isoproterenol is rarely given by the noninhalational route for the treatment of asthma. An oral preparation is available, but absorption is erratic. Sublingual tablets are effective, although it is difficult to regulate the dose when using this route of absorption. The drug has been given intravenously to adequately oxygenated young patients with status asthmaticus, who are less susceptible to its cardiotoxicity.

Metaproterenol. This drug is only about 40% absorbed in the bowel, but effective bronchodilatation usually lasts at least 3 to 4 hours, and as long as 6 hours or more. It is advisable to start with a dosage of 10 mg every 6 to 8 hours, in adults, and then to increase the dosage every few days to reach an optimal schedule; this is likely to be 20 mg every 4 to 6 hours. Generally, side effects are not severe, but nervousness, tremor, and palpitations may occur. Maintenance therapy with oral metaproterenol can be effective for many months or years.

Metaproterenol is marketed as Alupent and Metaprel. It is available for oral intake as 10-mg and 20-mg tablets and as a syrup containing 10 mg of the drug per 5 mL. No subcutaneous or intravenous forms are available in the United States, and it is unlikely that such preparations will be introduced. The drug is approved for use in children, but particular caution is needed when giving it to those under 6 years of age.

Terbutaline. This drug is the longest active bronchodilator currently available, with an effect that may persist for more than 7 to 8 hours.[27] However, this relative potency is accompanied by a relatively high incidence of side effects; tremor is the most troublesome complaint and is particularly likely to be a problem in older patients. The drug is not yet recommended for use in children under 12, for whom its safety needs to be proved.

Terbutaline is available as Brethine and Bricanyl, which are marketed as injectable solutions for subcutaneous use and as 2.5-mg and 5-mg tablets. Initially one 2.5-mg tablet should be taken every 8 hours; if the effect is inadequate, but the drug is well tolerated, then the 5-mg tablet can be taken as often as every 6 hours. The subcutaneous injection preparations contain 1 mg/mL of solution; the usual adult dose is 0.25 mg, which can be repeated if necessary in 15 to 30 minutes. It had been hoped that this product would be better tolerated than subcutaneous epinephrine; unfortunately, terbutaline causes equivalent side effects, although its bronchodilator action does persist longer.[32]

Albuterol. Albuterol is available as rapidly acting tablets and a syrup; more recently, it was formulated as a slow-release oral tablet that need be given only twice a day. In some countries it is given intravenously, but this route is not approved in the United States. The available products are Proventil syrup and tablets (2 and 4 mg), slow-release tablets (4-mg Repetabs), and Ventolin syrup and tablets. With its various formulations, albuterol currently is the most widely used bronchodilator.

Ephedrine. Ephedrine is the longest-established oral agent for treating bronchospasm; curiously, it has not proved to be suitable for inhalational use. The drug is a strong stimulator of β_2-receptors, but also has a marked effect on β_1- and α-receptors.

The oral dose of 15 to 50 mg (given three or four times daily, according to individual needs of the bronchospastic patient) usually causes some stimulation of the central nervous system. Several proprietary preparations are marketed containing ephedrine and theophylline with a tranquilizer. Some of these are available without prescription, but their use cannot in general be condoned.

Ephedrine has other disadvantages: it can cause urinary retention in men with prostatic hypertrophy and is ineffective in severe asthma. Moreover, the long-term effectiveness of this drug cannot be relied on, since tachyphylaxis readily develops, apparently because ephedrine works, in part, by releasing catecholamines from neuronal storage vesicles, which eventually become depleted.

Other Sympathomimetic Bronchodilator Drugs. The pharmaceutical industry keeps searching for the ideal bronchodilator: a potent, moderately long-acting drug with few side effects when given in the therapeutic dosage range. It must be suitable for aerosol, oral, or parenteral administration, and predictable dose–response effects must be achieved. Thus far, no contender for the title has appeared. Several potentially useful bronchodilators have been reported, including rimiterol, carbuterol, salmefamol, hexoprenaline, reproterol, clenbuterol, salmeterol, ibuterol, and broxaterol.

NONSYMPATHOMIMETIC BRONCHODILATORS AND ANTIASTHMA DRUGS

Several nonsympathomimetic drugs have been used to manage bronchospasm. These agents can be classified as phosphodiesterase inhibitors (methylxanthines); mucosal constrictors; antiallergy agents; immunosuppressives; prostaglandins; and a miscellaneous group.

The important drugs in these categories will be discussed in the following section. Some of the agents are suitable for inhalational administration, although most are not given by this means.

Methylxanthines

Methylxanthines are important to respiratory therapy; theophylline and aminophylline are of major value in treating bronchospasm, although they are not inhalational agents. The methylxanthines are phosphodiesterase inhibitors; they increase the availability of cAMP by inhibiting its breakdown by the intracellular enzyme phosphodiesterase. Although tea, coffee, chocolate, and cola beverages all owe their characteristic taste and properties to their content of methylxanthine, they do not have any significant inhibitory effect on phosphodiesterase and, thus, are not of pharmacologic value for bronchospasm. Presumably, theophylline has additional biochemical effects that cause bronchodilation, including adenosine antagonism. However, the methylxanthine enprofylline has potent bronchodilator properties, although it does not antagonize adenosine. At present, the mechanism of action of theophylline remains controversial.

Theophylline. *Properties.* The major pharmacologic use of theophylline and a few related compounds is in treating bronchospasm. Theophylline is a potent bronchodilator and has numerous less impressive, but generally beneficial, effects.[6] Therapeutic doses can produce cardiac stimulation, resulting in a slightly increased heart rate, but arrhythmias may occur with larger therapeutic doses. Cardiac performance and left ventricular output may be improved in patients with heart failure, but in normal persons cardiac output is not significantly affected. Generally, theophylline appears to be a vasodilator, and it may cause a useful decrease in vascular resistance in pulmonary and coronary arterial vessels. However, the drug is believed to be a vasoconstrictor of the cerebrovascular supply and, indeed, theophylline was formerly used to treat hypertensive and migraine headaches. This is difficult to reconcile with the experience, particularly of pediatricians, that theophylline can cause headaches. An additional possible benefit of theophylline is its diuretic effect.

Theophylline has no beneficial effect on the gastrointestinal tract; on the contrary, therapeutic levels may cause adverse reactions, including increased gastric acid secretion, which results in indigestion, vomiting, gastric irritation, and reflux; abdominal pain, diarrhea, and even gastric bleeding may result. Certain oral products are better tolerated than others, but the symptoms are related to the concentration of the drug in the blood rather than to the direct irritative effect of the preparation in the bowel.

Stimulation of the nervous system is produced by the methylxanthines, which accounts for their popularity in beverages. Normal serum levels of theophylline may produce anxiety and tremulousness in susceptible patients, whereas excessive levels may result in potentially lethal seizures.

Dosage. A partial bronchodilator response may be produced by a serum level of theophylline of about 5 μg/mL (0.5 mg/dL), whereas a full response is usual with a serum level of 10–20 μg/mL. However, some patients require higher levels (20–25 μg/mL), and, although such concentrations are potentially dangerous, there are patients who tolerate these levels without signs of toxicity. Thus, in practice, the therapeutic range for theophylline is 5–25 μg/mL (Table 19–9).

The clearance of theophylline from the body occurs mainly as a result of enzymatic degradation in the liver. Any condition that impairs hepatic function will decrease the clearance rate; hepatocellular failure, hypoxia, and venous congestion

Table 19–9 Correlations of Serum Levels of Theophylline with Responses

SERUM LEVEL (μg/mL)	CORRESPONDING BRONCHODILATOR EFFECT	CORRESPONDING POSSIBLE SIDE EFFECTS
5	Partial	Side effects unusual
10	Moderate	Vague discomfort
15	Usually optimal	Gastrointestinal problems
20	Usually maximal	Anxiety, tremor
25	These levels are required for	Tachycardia
30	occasional patients	Arrhythmias
40+	This level is never therapeutic	Convulsions

have all been shown to prolong the presence of the drug in the body. Stimulation of liver enzymes can increase the clearance rate, and this can result from the effects of constituents in cigarette smoke, smog, and barbecued protein; certain drugs, such as phenytoin, barbiturates, and marijuana, also increase theophylline clearance. Generally, children clear theophylline more rapidly than do adults, and in very old patients clearance rates may be decreased. Dosages for theophylline depend on many factors,[33] and guidelines for reaching therapeutic serum levels are suggested in Table 19–10.

Numerous brand and generic preparations of theophylline have been marketed. In recent years, long-acting products have become extremely popular because they result in smoother bronchodilatation and encourage better compliance. Currently, slow-release products that need to be given only once a day are being evaluated and seem to be particularly useful for controlling nocturnal asthma.

Table 19–10 Theophylline and Aminophylline Dosages

	THEOPHYLLINE	AMINOPHYLLINE
LOADING	mg/kg	mg/kg
Initial		
Average	5	6
Range	2.5–7.5	3–9
MAINTENANCE	mg/kg/6 hr	mg/kg/hr
Average adult		
Nonsmoker	2.4	0.5
Smoker	4.2	0.9
Neonate	0.6	0.12
Young child	2.4–4.8	0.5–1.0
Geriatric	2.1–3.6	0.26–0.50

ADJUSTMENTS	Increase Dosage By (%)		Decrease Dosage By (%)
Cigarette smoking	30–50	Liver failure	50
Marijuana smoking	20–50	Cimetidine therapy	30–50
Phenytoin use	20–50	Heart failure	20–50
Rifampin use	20–50	Cor pulmonale	20–50
High-protein diet	10–20	Ciprofloxacin use	20–50
Barbecued food	10–20	Allopurinol use	25
Smog exposure	10–20	Propranolol use	20–50
Barbiturate use	10–20	Hypoxemia	10–30
Carbamazepine use	10–20	High-carbohydrate diet	?
		Viral upper respiratory infection	?
		Macrolide antibiotic therapy	25
		Oral contraceptive use	25

The main preparations are listed in Table 19–11. Combination products with ephedrine cannot be recommended, although very mild bronchospasm may respond adequately to such preparations.

Aminophylline. A major disadvantage of theophylline is that it is relatively insoluble in water. This is why this hazardous drug is not suitable for inhalation; the solution would be too dilute to be effective. Long ago, it was discovered that theophylline is 20 times more soluble in the ammoniacal solvent ethylenediamine; the resulting solution is aminophylline. Ethylenediamine is not inert; one benefit is that it can stimulate the respiratory center and, thereby, correct some cases of Cheyne-Stokes breathing.

The average dosage of aminophylline is 5–7 mg/kg as a loading dose, to be given over 15 to 30 minutes intravenously; this is followed by 0.5 mg/kg/hr given as a continuous intravenous drip. A smaller loading dose is needed if the patient has recently taken a theophylline preparation. In contrast, some patients with status asthmaticus (particularly young smokers) need and tolerate a larger dose.[33] If in doubt of the appropriate maintenance dosage, one should obtain a serum theophylline level for guidance.

Aminophylline has the same side effects as theophylline, as well as some individualistic ones. Although aminophylline is available for oral use as tablets, theophylline preparations seem to be better tolerated and are generally preferred. Rectal preparations of aminophylline are available but are rarely used because they irritate the mucosa and are unreliably absorbed. Inhalational aerosols of aminophylline may provoke bronchospasm and, in

Table 19–11   Examples of Theophylline and Derivatives

ROUTE OF ADMINISTRATION OF THEOPHYLLINE AND DERIVATIVES	AVAILABLE FORMULATIONS	RANGE OF CONTENTS IN MARKETED PREPARATIONS
THEOPHYLLINE 100%*		
Oral	(a) Liquids, syrups, elixirs, suspension	100–250 mg/15 mL
	(b) Quick-release tablets, capsules	80–300 mg
	(c) Slow-release tablets, capsules	60–500 mg
Rectal	No longer available	
Aerosol	No longer available	
AMINOPHYLLINE (THEOPHYLLINE ETHYLENEDIAMINE) 79–84%*		
Injection	(a) Intravenous	250 mg/10 mL
	(b) Intramuscular	500 mg/2 mL
Oral	(a) Tablets	100, 200 mg
	(b) Slow-release tablets	225–300 mg
	(c) Elixirs, liquids	100–315 mg/15 mL
Rectal	Solutions, suppositories	250–500 mg/unit
DYPHYLLINE (HYPHYLLINE, DIHYDROXYPROPYL THEOPHYLLINE) 70%*		
Oral	(a) Liquids, elixirs	100–300 mg/15 mL
	(b) Tablets	200, 400 mg
	(c) Slow-release tablets	400 mg
Injection	Intramuscular	250 mg/mL
Aerosol	Not approved	
CHOLINE THEOPHYLLINATE (OXTRIPHYLLINE) 64%*		
Oral	(a) Tablets	100, 200 mg
	(b) Elixir, syrup	50, 100 mg/5 mL
	(c) Sustained action tablet	400, 600 mg

* Content of theophylline.

practice, nebulization is not of therapeutic value. The ethylenediamine component of aminophylline presents one additional, poorly recognized hazard; it is a potent sensitizing agent and, occasionally, sensitive people develop skin reactions after administration of the drug. Of greater concern is that, rarely, bronchospasm may be induced by ethylenediamine when the drug is given intravenously.

Intravenous administration of aminophylline has resulted in a number of deaths, usually caused by rapid infusion of the drug; hazards can be avoided by injecting the drug slowly or by giving it as a continuous infusion. The explanation for the fatal reaction is unknown, but both hypotensive and hypertensive cardiac failure and arrhythmias have been invoked. Similarly, fatalities have occurred after the administration of excessive dosages of aminophylline per rectum (as suppositories or solutions) to young children.

Dyphylline. Dyphylline (hyphylline, Dilor, Lufyllin) is the only substituted derivative of theophylline; it has only 70% of the effect of theophylline. It can be given intramuscularly because, unlike other theophylline preparations, it is very soluble and does not cause tissue irritation. Dyphylline is also available as tablets and liquid for oral administration, the recommended adult dosage being 400 to 800 mg four to six times daily. Of interest is the suggestion that the drug is suitable for intravenous use in acute asthma.[34] There is some evidence to suggest it could be a useful inhalational agent for treating bronchospasm.[35]

Oxtriphylline. Oxtriphylline (Choledyl) is the choline salt of theophylline, but claims that it is better absorbed in the gastrointestinal tract, with less irritation, are not convincing enough to support its use. The appropriate dose for adults is 400 mg four times daily; 400 mg provides the equivalent of 250 mg of theophylline, since oxtriphylline has only 64% anhydrous theophylline content. It is also available as 400- and 600-mg sustained-release tablets.

Mucosal Vasoconstrictors

Mucosal vasoconstrictors have α-receptor-stimulating properties. Drugs in this category are mainly used to treat the swollen nasal mucosa, but several of them are used in inhalation therapy. Their main value in the respiratory tract is in decreasing vascular engorgement and the accompanying edema of the mucosa and, also, in delaying absorption and dispersion of topical bronchodilator drugs. Several agents are available, but the most important one is phenylephrine.

Phenylephrine. Phenylephrine (Neo-Synephrine) is the most popular nasal decongestant. It may be reasonable to administer 0.5 to 2 mL of 0.25% phenylephrine by nebulization into the tracheobronchial tree in managing inflammatory conditions such as bronchitis, tracheobronchitis, or postextubation tracheitis. There is no evidence that rebound congestion occurs in the lung after use of phenylephrine, although this problem may arise in the nasal mucosa after treatment with nose drops or spray. In suitable cases, the drug may be added to a bronchodilator for pulmonary aerosol therapy.

Antiallergy Agents

Since asthma is not infrequently allergic in its etiology, one would expect that *antihistamines* and other popular agents for treating allergic rhinitis would be valuable in managing asthma. However, the antihistamines are rarely beneficial in adult asthmatics, although they may be useful adjuvants in children. Perhaps some of these drugs would be of greater value if given by inhalation, but investigations have failed to establish the value of topical antihistamines in respiratory therapy.[36]

The main antiallergy drugs for asthma are the corticosteroids and cromolyn. These drugs, and some less important ones, will be discussed.

Corticosteroids. The adrenal cortex secretes various natural hormones, including cortisol (hydrocortisone) and cortisone; the pharmaceutical industry has produced an additional bewildering array of synthetic corticosteroids (Table 19–12). These drugs have an extraordinary variety of effects and are used to treat innumerable diseases, even though the mechanism by which they help is not always understood. In respiratory medicine the corticosteroids are mainly used to manage allergic diseases, but they are of particular value in severe asthma.

The beneficial actions of corticosteroids in asthma have not been fully worked out, but the following important actions are involved: inhibition of antibody formation, thereby preventing antigen–antibody reactions; inhibition of formation or storage of messenger agents such as histamine, which are involved in the asthmatic response; and inhibition of various cellular mechanisms involved in bronchoconstriction by a nonspecific anti-in-

Table 19—12 "Older" Corticosteroid Preparations

GENERIC NAME	TRADE NAMES	TOPICAL ANTI-ALLERGY POTENCY	APPROXIMATE EQUIVALENT DOSE (ORAL) (MG)	USUAL DOSAGE (ORAL OR IV) (MG/DAY)	NOTES
SHORT-ACTING (PLASMA HALF-LIFE LESS THAN 2 HRS)					Short-acting agents have more sodium-retaining potency
Hydrocortisone (cortisol)	Cortef, Solu-Cortef	1	20	80–120	Hydrocortisone has been given by inhalation in doses up to 30 mg/day; this is not recommended
Cortisone	Cortone	0.8	25	100–150	Used for replacement therapy in adrenal insufficiency
INTERMEDIATE-ACTING (PLASMA HALF-LIFE 1–4 HRS)					
Prednisone	Meticorten, Deltasone	3.5	5	5–80	Standard oral drug
Prednisolone	Meticortelone, Delta-Cortef	4	5	5–80	Oral drug; may be indicated if patient has liver insufficiency
Methylprednisolone	Medrol, Solu-Medrol	5	4	4–80	Parenteral alternative to hydrocortisone; may cause less electrolyte disturbance
Triamcinolone	Aristocort, Kenalog	5	4	4–80	Triamcinolone diacetate (Aristocorte Forte has been given to prevent asthma) (e.g., 3–48 mg IM once a week)

flammatory action. Additionally, there is evidence that corticosteroids potentiate sympathomimetic agents, probably by acting directly on the β_2-receptors, and can cause muscle relaxation, probably by acting to increase the intracellular concentration of cAMP. Thus, the anti-inflammatory steroids (glucocorticoids) can be of value not only in preventing asthma, but also in managing status asthmaticus of any etiology.

Unfortunately, the glucocorticoids can cause numerous long-term side effects that are dramatically serious. They may result in a constellation of bodily changes, known as cushingism; these unpleasant features include excessive weight gain, truncal obesity, hirsuitism, acne, ecchymoses, striae, plethora, and edema. The more dangerous side effects include psychosis, hypertension, impairment of ability to fight infection, diabetes, cataracts, glaucoma, sodium retention, potassium loss, osteoporosis, and stunted growth; in some patients, peptic ulcer disease may be induced. Moreover, once a patient becomes dependent on steroid therapy, withdrawal of the drug may be difficult; the patient feels ill, and the disease exacerbates if dos-

age is lowered too quickly. Evidence of inadequate adrenal and pituitary function may also appear.

Corticosteroid preparations are given intravenously in the treatment of severe asthma (status asthmaticus), and oral preparations are used for long-term therapy. In recent years, metered-dose inhaler preparations of steroids have become important, but they are not suitable for administration by updraft aerosolization (Table 19–13).

Whenever steroid therapy is used, the systemic drug should be gradually reduced in dosage to the lowest that is effective, or an aerosol preparation should be substituted. However, systemic doses must not be changed rapidly to aerosol management because there is a danger of precipitating steroid-deficiency problems in a dependent patient.

Beclomethasone (Vanceril, Beclovent) is marketed as a metered inhaler that delivers 50 µg/puff. Investigations suggest that up to 2 mg/day may be given without significant adrenal gland suppression or other serious side effects. Responsive patients seem to do well on much smaller doses, and steroid-dependent patients have been successfully transferred from oral preparations, which cause

Table 19—13   Corticosteroid Preparations Suitable for Aerosol Administration

GENERIC NAME	TRADE NAMES	TOPICAL ANTIALLERGY POTENCY*	DOSE PER PUFF OF METERED CARTRIDGE (MG)	AEROSOL DOSAGE (ADULT) (MG/DAY)
Beclomethasone dipropionate	Beclovent, Vanceril Beconase,† Vancenase†	20–500	0.042	0.12–0.84 0.17–0.34†
Betamethasone valerate	Bextasol	25–360	Not available	0.6–0.8
Dexamethasone sodium phosphate	Decadron Respihaler,† Decadron Turbinaire	30	0.084	0.33–1
Flunisolide	AeroBid, Nasalide†		0.25; 0.025†	2–4; 15–0.20†
Triamcinolone acetonide	Azmacort	5–100	0.1	0.8–1.6

* Compared with hydrocortisone having a potency of 1.
† Nasal products.

cushingism, to the relative safety of beclomethasone aerosol therapy. Aerosolized steroids may produce oropharyngeal candidiasis in some patients; this is generally not severe and is easily treated.

Beclomethasone may be effective enough if it is administered only once or twice a day. It is very effective topically and is poorly absorbed; thus it does not produce systemic effects. For individual patients, it is uncertain how many administrations a day will be needed, but, initially, the aerosol is used four times daily, two to four puffs at a time. A more concentrated formulation is available in Europe, and can be given as two to four puffs twice a day when high doses are required.

Dexamethasone (Decadron) was the first metered preparation of a corticosteroid available for inhalation in the United States. The drug has lost popularity because effective dosages for asthmatic patients seem to lead to appreciable systemic absorption with resultant side effects. A metered preparation is also available for aerosol therapy of the nasal mucosa, and this may be valuable in treating allergic or perennial (vasomotor) rhinitis; however, irritation and dryness of the mucosa often occur, and nasal septal perforation has been reported.

Triamcinolone (Aristocort, Kenalog) is available as a metered-dose inhaler, with a builtin spacer (Azmacort): the usual dose is two to four inhalations three or four times a day as a micronized preparation of the acetonide. The long-acting depot preparation (Aristocort Forte) is sometimes given as a weekly injection in the prophylaxis of asthma. The appropriate dosage has not been defined, and the overall benefit of this treatment requires evaluation.

Flunisolide (Aerobid) is a fluorinated steroid that has a more prolonged action; therefore, it can be given twice a day, using two to four puffs of the metered-dose inhaler. The aerosol has a very unpleasant taste; hence, it is advisable to use it with a spacer to decrease oral deposition.

Hydrocortisone (cortisol) is a valuable corticosteroid for general use in many diseases. It can be given orally and systemically and also as a cream and by injection into joints. The usual oral dose is 10–80 mg/day, and the intravenous dose for conditions such as status asthmaticus is 250 to 500 mg initially, followed by 100 to 250 mg every 3 hours.

Hydrocortisone has been given as an inhalational aerosol to asthmatic patients, but it offers no advantage in this type of therapy, because considerable systemic absorption occurs.

Cortisone is occasionally used to treat asthma, but the drug is primarily of value in replacement therapy for patients with adrenocortical insufficiency. There is no reason for using this drug in respiratory therapy.

Prednisone and *prednisolone* are similar synthetic drugs that are suitable for oral maintenance therapy in asthma and in many other diseases. These two drugs are similar to hydrocortisone, but they are about four times as potent. The maintenance dose is 5–20 mg/day; cushingism can develop with prolonged use. Many asthmatic patients do well on alternate-day dosage; this form of therapy markedly decreases the incidence of unwanted side effects.

Methylprednisolone (Solu-Medrol) is the favored intravenous preparation; it is also available for oral use (Medrol). It has less salt-retaining effect than prednisolone.

Phenobarbital increases the rate of metabolism of steroids such as prednisone and dexamethasone.[37] If an asthmatic patient being maintained on one of these drugs is started on a preparation that contains a barbiturate, the steroid dose may need to be increased. Extra caution is therefore required if barbiturates are given to asthmatic patients receiving steroid therapy. In contrast, the macrolide antibiotics, such as erythromycin, appear to potentiate steroids, and oleandomycin (TAO) may act specifically to enhance the effect of oral methylprednisolone.

Cromolyn Sodium. An old asthma remedy, khellin, was the source of a chromone derivative that was called disodium cromoglycate in England; it was subsequently introduced into the United States as cromolyn sodium (Aarane, Intal—but only Intal is currently marketed). Initially, it was packaged in capsules, and a special spinhaler was needed to release the powder when an inhalation was taken from the device. The content of cromolyn in each capsule is 20 mg. More recently, a metered-dose inhalant product has replaced the powder; each activation releases 0.8 mg. An inhalant solution is marketed; this contains 20 mg/2-mL ampule, and can be given by updraft aerosolization.

Cromolyn is not a bronchodilator, and, in fact, inhalation may cause reactive airways to develop bronchospasm. Cromolyn is of prophylactic value only and can be used instead of corticosteroids in some asthmatic patients who are steroid-dependent. Cromolyn is also effective in preventing exercise-induced bronchospasm. Patients must recognize that the drug will not relieve acute attacks of bronchospasm. Cromolyn is particularly valuable for the prevention and treatment of allergic rhinitis.

The drug is believed to act by interfering with the antigen–antibody effect on tissue mast cells (so-called stabilization of mast cells). In the allergic patient, this results in a decreased release of messengers, such as histamine. The mechanism by which cromolyn prevents exercise-induced asthma has not been fully elucidated. Cromolyn may also be of benefit in some types of cough, as it may inhibit the activity of nerves involved in the tussive reflex.

Cromolyn is usually given as two to four puffs or one ampule of the inhalant solution four times daily for the first 2 to 3 weeks and, if a beneficial effect is obtained, the dosage may be reduced. Some asthmatics do well with only one or two treatments a day. Several days or even weeks of therapy may be needed before the benefits of cromolyn become manifest. Prophylactic bronchodilator therapy may be needed before each inhalation of cromolyn to prevent reactive bronchospasm. The use of cromolyn in less severe asthma may be very effective. In more severe disease, the drug may allow the dosage of concomitant steroid therapy to be reduced.

As shown in Figure 19–3, cromolyn may have a basic action on calcium flux: By interfering with the entry of calcium into the cell, subsequent reactions resulting in release of mediators are prevented.[38] Other new drugs that interfere with calcium flux are of minor value in asthma, especially that induced by exercise—for example, *verapamil* and *nifedipine*.[39] A related compound, *nedocromil*, has been introduced in Europe; it may be more effective than cromolyn for treating allergic rhinitis. Another related antiasthma agent of interest is the mast cell-stabilizing drug *ketotifen*;[40] this oral drug is currently available in many countries, but its value has not been clearly determined.

Immunosuppressive Drugs. Many drugs, including corticosteroids, are used to suppress immunologic reactions, and such therapy is mandatory for patients with transplanted organs to prevent rejection reactions. Several of these drugs are also of value in immunologic diseases such as periarteritis or rheumatoid arthritis, and a number of these agents have been tried for asthmatics (e.g., chloroquine, chlorambucil, 6–mercaptopurine, thioguanosine, and azathioprine). However, these immunosuppressive drugs do not seem to have been of major benefit in the treatment of asthma. Recently, it has been reported that methotrexate can be of considerable value for reducing the steroid requirements necessitated by severe asthma.[41]

Prostaglandins. The body produces a series of potent natural hormones called prostaglandins, since the prostate gland is a particularly rich source. The agent identified as prostaglandin F (PGF) is a potent bronchoconstrictor (especially $PGF_2\alpha$), whereas prostaglandins E (PGE_1 and PGE_2) are potent bronchodilators. Aerosolization of PGE_1 has reportedly resulted in 10 to 100 times as much bronchodilation as the same weight of isoproterenol. These agents appear to cause increased cAMP activity, but the mechanism involved is uncertain. Prostaglandins of the E series may eventually find a role in respiratory therapy, although no progress has been made during the past few years.

Anticholinergic Agents.   One of the earliest forms of treatment for bronchospasm was provided by derivatives of plants such as *Datura*; a good example is the jimson weed or thornapple, *D. stramonium*. These solanaceous plants contain a number of anticholinergic agents, including atropine, scopolamine, and *l*-hyoscyamine. Extracts from various parts of the plant have been used, including stramonium cigarettes or powders, which release the active drug in the smoke created by slowly burning them.[42] Asthmatic patients around the world have long used these herbal preparations—for example, Asthmador cigarettes.

Atropine is *dl*-hyoscyamine, and it is the best known anticholinergic drug. It is a potent inhibitor of the neurotransmitter acetylcholine at the cholinergic receptor sites of the parasympathetic postganglionic system. This type of cholinergic stimulation is classically caused by muscarine, the agent in poisonous mushrooms; therefore, atropine is classified as an antimuscarinic drug. The muscarinic parasympathetic sites of relevance in the lung are the vagal nerve efferents to the bronchial muscles and the bronchial glands; stimulation results in bronchospasm and mucous secretion, respectively. This is achieved by nebulizing about 0.1 to 0.2 mL of the 1% solution.

Atropine sulfate is a tertiary ammonium compound, that is readily absorbed to cause systemic responses, although these reactions after aerosol administration use much less than those resulting from systemic administration. Major side effects are dry mouth and tachycardia; these problems can be severely exacerbated if sympathomimetic drugs are given concurrently. Drying of respiratory secretions is not usual after atropine aerosolization in asthmatic patients, and the drug is particularly well tolerated in bronchitis.[43] The appropriate aerosol dosage is 0.1–0.5 mL of the 1% solution.

Ipratropium (Atrovent) is a quaternary ammonium derivative of atropine. It is particularly effective in COPD, but can be of value in asthma. It appears to be a very effective, relatively long-lasting aerosol bronchodilator, with less potential for cardiac side effects than atropine.[44] The aerosol is well tolerated in the usual dose of three to four puffs three or four times a day; larger doses may be more effective and are equally well tolerated. It can be given with sympathomimetic aerosol bronchodilator therapy to potentiate an inadequate response. There is some evidence that ipratropium is of benefit in allergic rhinitis and possibly for the common cold.[45] Other anticholinergic agents that are of possible value for bronchospasm are scopolamine and glycopyrrolate[51a] (Table 19–14).

Miscellaneous Agents.   Other agents have reportedly been effective in some cases of asthma, but further studies are needed to establish the validity of these reports.

Phentolamine is a blocker of α-receptors and thus has a similar action to β_2-stimulators. This drug has been given orally and by inhalation and has reportedly prevented exercise-induced asthma. Other α-blockers may have a similar effect in some patients with bronchospasm.

Table 19—14   Anticholinergic Agents For Bronchospasm

DRUG	AEROSOL DOSE	SPEED OF ONSET (MIN)	PEAK EFFECT (MIN)	DURATION (HR)
ATROPINE SOLUTION				
Sulfate (1%)	0.025–0.075 mg/kg	15–30	30–170	3–5
Methonitrate	1–1.5 mg	15–30	40–60	4–6
IPRATROPIUM				
(Atrovent MDI)	20–40 μg	3–30	90–120	3–6
SCOPOLAMINE	(not by aerosol)	10–30	60–120	2
GLYCOPYRROLATE SOLUTION				
(Robinul)	100–1200 μg	15–30	30–45	2–8

Ascorbic acid (vitamin C), the controversial agent advocated by some for the prevention of colds, does have definite effects on the respiratory tract. In addition to being a component of the mucolytic preparation Gumox (which contained copper sulfate, sodium percarbonate, and ascorbic acid), ascorbic acid has been shown to inhibit histamine-induced bronchospasm. However, no convincing evidence justifies its use for the prevention or treatment of colds or asthma.

Pituitary extract (both anterior and posterior lobe hormones) is used in England in various combination inhalants that also include drugs such as atropine, papaverine, and epinephrine; all of these constituents allegedly act synergistically as bronchodilators.

Marijuana has a long history of use in therapeutics and has been studied to determine what effect it has on the pulmonary function of asthmatic patients. Without doubt, smoked marijuana and oral ingestion of its principal psychoactive ingredient tetrahydrocannabinol (THC) both produce bronchodilation. Although the effect is not as great as that of isoproterenol, the decrease in airway resistance lasts longer.[46] Unfortunately, this proven value of marijuana cannot be taken as an endorsement of its use by asthmatic patients, since the smoke may lead to the development of bronchitis.

Erythromycin is an antibiotic often used to treat pulmonary infections. Erythromycin estolate can lead to improved asthmatic symptoms in patients receiving corticosteroid therapy. The related macrolide antibiotic *triacetyloleandomycin* (TAO), which is more toxic, may be more effective as a potentiator of the action of methylprednisolone in asthma.

ANTIBIOTICS

At various times the support for the inhalational use of antibiotics and other antimicrobic agents waxes, but generally there seems to be waning enthusiasm. Relatively little evidence suggests that the topical administration of antibiotics into the respiratory tract is of value in established infections, whereas there is an abundance of proof in favor of systemic therapy. There is a valid argument for giving small doses of antibiotics topically if the agents are very expensive or very toxic, because the relatively small amount required by aerosolization can reduce both the dose and the danger. However, there is no reason to give inexpensive or relatively safe antibiotics by this route; thus, agents such as penicillin, tetracyclines, erythromycin, sulfonamides, and similar antimicrobics should not be given by inhalation. Furthermore, inhalational administration of antibiotics carries risks of inducing hypersensitization and of causing bronchospasm and mucosal irritation.

Antibiotic drugs may be given by nebulization, although this is a relatively clumsy form of therapy; direct instillation may be preferable.[47] In all cases, reactive bronchospasm must be guarded against by giving a bronchodilator. Some practitioners advocate nebulization or instillation of topical antibiotics to treat sinus or nasal infections, and topical antimicrobic treatment is used to manage tracheostomy wounds that are colonized or infected.

Table 19–15 summarizes the available data on topical antimicrobial therapy for respiratory tract colonization or infection. The dosage ranges provided for most agents show a huge spread, reflecting the uncertainty about whether or not most of these drugs are truly effective.

Miscellaneous Antimicrobial Agents. Other antibiotic and sterilizing agents have been given in respiratory therapy. However, proof of their efficacy is generally inadequate, and because most agents can be given by other routes in clearly established dosage regimens, the uncertainties of dosage and the unreliability of effect mean that inhalational administration constitutes an experimental approach.

Iodides are known to have an antifungal effect, and sodium iodide as a 1% to 2% solution has been used to treat pulmonary aspergilloma by means of an endobronchial drip. Whether nebulization therapy with sodium or potassium iodide would be valuable in treating other fungal problems in the lungs remains to be determined.

Pentamidine has been given by aerosol for the treatment and for prophylaxis of *Pneumocystis carinii* pneumonia in patients with AIDS. Although good results have been reported, it is still unclear what dosages and methods of aerosolization are optimal. Thus, therapy may require about 4 mg/kg of the drug nebulized for 30 to 75 minutes every day for 18 to 21 days, using an ultrasonic nebulizer that produces particles of 2 to 3 μm in diameter.[48] For prophylaxis, a smaller dose given once every 2 to 4 weeks may suffice. A special nebulizer system is used when delivering this agent; it has one-way valves that lead expired air to a filtering device, which prevents exhalation of medication into the work place (Respirgard II Nebulizer system). At the time of writing the Centers for Disease Control (CDC) is investigating reports on asthmatic reac-

Table 19—15 Topical Antimicrobial Agents in Respiratory Therapy

AGENT	ANTIMICROBIAL SPECTRUM	USUAL DOSAGE RANGE*
Amikacin	Gram-negative bacteria	Uncertain
Amphotericin B	Fungal infections	1–20 mg
Bacitracin	Staphylococci	5,000–20,000 units
Carbenicillin	*Pseudomonas* sp.	125–1000 mg
Cephalosporins	Not recommended for use	
Colistin	Gram-negative bacteria	2–300 mg
Gentamicin	Gram-negative bacteria	5–120 mg
Kanamycin	Gram-negative bacteria†	25–300 mg
Neomycin	Gram-negative bacteria	25–400 mg
Nystatin	*Candida, Aspergillus* spp.	25,000–50,000 units
Penicillins	Not recommended for use	
Pentamidine	*Pneumocystis carinii*	50–600 mg‡
Polymyxin	Gram-negative bacteria	5–50 mg
Tobramycin	Gram-negative bacteria	50 mg

* Dosages are poorly established. The drug should be dissolved in 2 mL of saline and each dose administered two to four times daily after initial bronchodilator therapy.
† Not suitable for *Pseudomonas*.
‡ Treatments given in large dosage daily for treatment, and in small dosage once every 1–2 weeks for prophylaxis.

tions in health workers who administer pentamidine.

Acetic acid has been claimed to be a useful sterilizing agent for use in respiratory therapy. A solution of 0.25% acetic acid can be used as a decontaminating fluid for nebulizers; nebulization of 10 mL through the equipment effectively eliminates gram-negative bacterial contaminants. Some workers have nebulized 0.25% acetic acid into the lung; apparently the agent is well tolerated and can kill colonizing bacteria. Whether or not topical acetic acid should be used prophylactically in tracheostomized or intubated patients remains to be determined.

Copper and other metals can suppress the growth of many bacteria in water by an "oligodynamic" bactericidal effect. Copper mesh has been used by some workers as a prophylactic measure; the material is left in nebulizers and humidifiers that are at risk of being contaminated. The subsequent nebulization of the solution (which probably contains ionic copper) does not appear harmful to the lungs; however, there is insufficient evidence to endorse this form of nebulization therapy for its prophylactic or therapeutic value.

The antiviral medication ribavirin (Virazole) has been used with success in respiratory syncytial virus infections involving children with congenital heart disease, immunodeficiency, or bronchopulmonary dysplasia. A special medication nebulizer, known as an SPAG (Small Particle Aerosol Generator) device is used to administer the drug (see Figs. 17–20 and 17–21).

LOCAL ANESTHETICS

The popularity of fiberoptic bronchoscopy has resulted in increased use of topical local anesthesia in the respiratory tract. Various methods of administration are used, including direct application of the agent to the upper respiratory tract and ultrasonic nebulization or direct instillation into the larynx, trachea, and lower airways. Anesthesia can also be produced by injection, carefully placed to cause blockade of the glossopharyngeal nerve and its recurrent branch.

Local anesthetics may cause initial bronchospasm, but generally no significant adverse effect seems to be produced on pulmonary function. These drugs may also inhibit mucociliary activity, although low concentrations of some agents have allegedly improved ciliary action. Certain agents may have a bacteriostatic effect, and specimens of secretions taken for culture after exposure to local anesthetics may not yield their full microbial content.[49] However, this does not seem to be a major concern in practice.

Cocaine. Cocaine is favored by some endoscopists because it is potent as an anesthetic, it suppresses cough, and its vasoconstrictive action limits absorption. The dosage used varies, but 5 mL of a 10% solution should be diluted to give a 2% to 4% concentration, which can be safely used. The dose given should not exceed 3.3 mg/kg [i.e., 225 mg for a 150-lb (70-kg) adult].

Lidocaine. Lidocaine (Xylocaine) is used most frequently in bronchoscopy. The drug is one of the safest of the local anesthetics and can be given in concentrations varying form 1% to 20%. It is usually given as a 4% solution by machine nebulizaton, as an ultrasonically generated aerosol, or by direct instillation, with a total dose of 10 to 20 mL. Epinephrine in concentrations of 1:250,000 to 1:50,000 may be added; this helps to prevent instrument-induced bronchospasm and constricts the mucosal vessels, thereby decreasing the systemic absorption of the lidocaine. Additionally, the presence of epinephrine may prevent or stop bleeding during instrumentation of friable mucosa.

Lidocaine has acted as a bronchodilator in some asthmatic patients when given by aerosol or intravenously.[50] The drug may also be valuable in some cases of intractable cough caused by persisting damage to the tracheobronchial tree.

Dyclonine. Dyclonine (Dyclone) has been recommended for topical airway anesthesia. Up to 30 mL of a 1% solution can be given by ultrasonic nebulization or direct instillation. However, this drug may be less safe and less effective than lidocaine.

Miscellaneous Local Anesthetics. Other local anesthetics are used mainly as topical preparations for endoscopic procedures and in bronchography. Some of these agents, besides lidocaine, have been given intravenously to suppress cough.

Local anesthetics are also used in various oral "cough medications," such as tablets that dissolve in the oropharynx; the mucosal anesthesia may interrupt irritative cough reflexes. Some agents are taken systemically for their cough-suppressing effects. *Benzonatate* (Tessalon), chemically related to the local anesthetic tetracaine, may owe part of its antitussive activity to its action on cough receptors in the lung. In contrast, most cough suppressants (other than dextromethorphan) are narcotics, re-

lated to morphine; they act centrally, and thus many of them cause some respiratory center depression.

AEROSOL PROPELLANTS

The metered aerosol bronchodilator preparations have become very popular, although there is some controversy about the safety of the devices generally and the propellants particularly. Moreover, there is a major concern that release of the propellants into the environment can deplete the ozone layer that protects the world from overheating. Many propellants are being withdrawn from use because of this fear.

Most propellants used in the United States are encompassed by the trade name Freon (the corresponding product in England is Arcton). Freon consists of a number of haloalkanes (fluoroalkanes), which are fluorocarbon derivatives of methane and ethane. The important agents in use are FC 11 (trichloromonofluoromethane), FC 12 (dichlorodifluoromethane), and, to a lesser extent, FC 113 (trichlorotrifluoroethane). These gaseous agents are liquefied by pressure, and metered cartridges contain the active bronchodilator as a suspended powder or solution in the liquid Freon. When the product is released from the cartridge, the Freon becomes gaseous, and a cloud of droplets of the bronchodilator is created.

Aviado has performed extensive work on the toxicity of propellants, and he classifies them as follows.[51]

Class 1: low-pressure propellants of high toxicity that cause tachycardia and hypotension. Included in this class are FC 11 and FC 113.

Class 2: low-pressure propellants of intermediate toxicity that influence either circulation or respiration, or both.

Class 3: high-pressure propellants of low toxicity that cause bronchoconstriction. FC 12 is in this class.

Class 4: high-pressure propellants of low toxicity.

The propellants in Freon do have definite toxic potential. FC 11 (CCl_3F) is the most potent agent in class 1 and also has respiratory-depressant action. FC 12 (CCl_2F_2) is the most potent drug in its class, and, in addition to causing bronchoconstriction, can cause respiratory depression, tachycardia, and hypotension.

The most toxic propellant is FC 11, which is believed by some workers to cause fatal cardiac side effects in patients who use metered bronchodilator aerosols excessively. Patients who do overuse inhalers in this way may suffer equally or more from the concomitant overdosage of the bronchodilator. In practice, there is no clinical evidence that the propellants are harmful to patients who use metered-dose inhalers to treat bronchospasm.

THE ADMINISTRATION OF RESPIRATORY DRUGS

Physicians generally have greater familiarity and security with the administration of oral and intravenous drugs than they do with inhalational drugs. Accordingly, oral and intravenous drugs are prescribed with relative accuracy and appropriateness, whereas inhalational drugs do not receive the same consideration from most physicians. Respiratory therapists and nurses who administer therapy carry a considerable responsibility when they receive a physician's order, since the prescription must be interpreted and monitored with active awareness of the desired effects and the possible side effects.

DOSAGES OF DRUGS

The appropriate dosages for inhalational drugs are, in fact, quite variable because many factors influence the effectiveness of the different agents. The reliability and efficiency of the equipment and the cooperation of the patient profoundly influence the amount of drug deposited in the lungs.[23] The response to an individual dosage varies in each patient, particularly when catecholamines are given, because tachyphylaxis or converse effects may obviate the expected result. Side effects are very variable and may be related to the gaseous vehicle, the diluent, or the droplets, rather than to the drug itself.

For all these reasons, therapists should not be overly surprised or concerned when a physician prescribes an "inappropriate," excessive amount of drug. If the physician, for some reason, is unwilling to change the prescription when the error is brought to his attention, the therapist or nurse can administer the drug but should carefully monitor the patient for any adverse response; if evidence of toxicity appears, then the treatment can be stopped

short before all the prescribed amount of the drug is given, and the fact should be recorded in the patient's chart. Similarly, when an "appropriate" recommended dosage is prescribed, the patient should nevertheless be monitored for an idiosyncratic or individualistic adverse response.

EVALUATION OF THERAPY

Unfortunately, the recognition of "adverse effects" is not cut and dried. Thus, when a bronchodilator is used, an increased pulse rate from 70 to 110 may be tolerable, whereas an increase from 110 to 125 may not. Similarly, it is difficult to recognize a meaningful change in blood pressure, because observations are not easy to make and changes in systolic and diastolic values may vary independently. Thus, epinephrine in small doses may cause a small increase in systolic pressure with a fall or no change in diastolic pressure, whereas larger doses (such as probably cannot be attained with inhalation therapy) result in more marked changes in both values. The individual physician should request the therapist to check blood pressure before, during, and after bronchodilator administration in those selected patients in whom these changes may be detrimental. However, it is unreasonable to expect a therapist to worry about the effect on the blood pressure in every patient who takes an aerosolized sympathomimetic.

Rational aerosol therapy requires a recognition of the therapeutic objectives, skillful administration of appropriate dosages, and accurate assessment of the effects of treatment. In most patients, bedside pulmonary function evaluations of vital capacity, peak flow rate, or forced expiratory volumes can be used to assess bronchodilator responsiveness. The patient's subjective feelings, volume of sputum production, and monitoring of the pulse and auscultatory findings in the lungs should be routinely evaluated to determine whether desired effects or undesired side effects have been obtained. The patient's subjective response is often the best indicator of adverse effects, and more objective measurements may be less helpful.

When a mucokinetic drug is given, it is the therapist's responsibility to ensure that a therapeutic response occurs. Thus, relying uncritically on the drug alone is inadequate; the patient must be encouraged to cough and to expectorate, and some chest percussion, postural drainage, and even suctioning may be needed to facilitate the process. The therapist should record the amount of sputum produced and note the color and consistency.

ADMINISTRATION OF AEROSOLIZED DRUGS

When bronchodilator therapy is initiated for the hospitalized patient, it is conventional to prescribe treatment by means of a respirator if the patient requires ventilatory support, or IPPB if the patient is very dyspneic, and then to follow with simple air-driven nebulizer therapy once the patient improves. With any of these techniques, much of the drug in the nebulizer may be lost in the apparatus or in the air, unless a special delivery device is used. Most studies suggest that aerosolization by means of a gas-driven nebulizer results in deposition of 5% to 10% of the drug in the lungs, whereas an equal amount might be deposited in the mouth and swallowed, thereby resulting in systemic effects. However, different techniques of drug delivery may produce greater or lesser aerosol deposition in the lungs and oropharynx; therefore, the effect of any prescribed dose can vary. Similarly, if the drug is nebulized through an endotracheal tube, more drug is deposited in the lungs, whereas none enters the gastrointestinal tract.

When a metered aerosol is used, the amount deposited in the respiratory tract is extremely variable and is related to the competency of the patient's technique. Indeed, it is all too common to see patients who exhale while nebulizing the aerosol, thereby assuring that none of the drug gets into the body. With the best technique, it is unlikely that more than 30% of the "puff" of aerosol is deposited in the lungs, and the average patient is more likely to deposit closer to 10% of the metered dose. As shown in Table 19–16, manufacturers generally advise that about ten times as much drug should be measured into a nebulizer as is released by a standard treatment using the metered product.[23] This results in a much larger dose being nebulized into the lungs than is obtained with the standard two to four puffs from a metered-dose inhaler (Table 19–16).

Therapists should become very familiar with the appropriate technique to be used with each aerosol device (see list following), and the last day or two of a respiratory patient's stay in hospital should be used to teach and to supervise the patient in the correct technique to be used following discharge home. Different metered dispensers should be used in different ways depending on their individual design. In all cases, the patient must inhale the sprayed drug deeply and then hold his breath to encourage maximal deposition. If side effects are troublesome, then rinsing out the mouth and throat with water may help remove the excess drug, the systemic absorption of which may add to the side effects. Further important concerns are that the patient should be instructed to keep the nebulizing unit clean and that overuse of the aerosol should be avoided.

Multiple drugs are often prescribed in respiratory therapy; fortunately, most agents are compatible when mixed in the nebulizer. However, bronchodilators are relatively unstable, which is why they are stored in dark bottles and maintained at an acid pH. When the drugs are placed in a nebulizer and exposed to light and oxygen, they slowly break down to reddish-brown adrenochromes. Although these products are probably not harmful, their presence suggests that the mixture has diminished bronchodilator activity and thus should be discarded. Patients' secretions may be stained pink by a bronchodilator, and this should not cause alarm to them, their physicians, or therapists.

TECHNIQUE FOR USING METERED AEROSOL DEVICES

1. Shake the canister several times.
2. Hold upside down, with mouthpiece held either between closed lips or about ½ to 1 in. away from wide-open mouth. (The latter technique may be better, but most patients feel less comfortable using this method.)
3. Exhale normally but not forcefully.
4. Inhale deeply and release a puff of bronchodilator.
5. Hold breath for several seconds before exhaling. (*Note:* If an aerosol steroid is used, exhale through the nose to deposit steroid on the nasal mucosa, thereby treating any nasal allergy that may be present.)
6. Breathe normally, and wait for up to 5 minutes to evaluate response.
7. Repeat with one, two, or three more inhalations over the next 20 minutes, if needed and if tolerated.
8. Rinse out mouth after each inhalation of drug to prevent oral absorption if side effects are a problem.
9. Do not overuse any preparation; if more than 16 inhalations a day are needed, then a different treatment regimen or a change in drug is advisable.
10. Keep the dispensing unit clean by occasionaly rinsing it in warm water.

Table 19—16 Comparative Dosages Achieved Using Metered and Inhalant Solution Preparations of Bronchodilators

	METERED DEVICE		INHALANT SOLUTION			Probable Amount Deposited in Lungs (i.e., 10%) (mg)
	Dose per Puff (mg)	Dose Delivered with Three Puffs (mg)	Potency of Solution (%)	Usual Dose (mL)	Usual Dose (mg)	
EPINEPHRINE						
Medihaler-Epi	0.16	0.48				0.048
Primatene Mist	0.22	0.66				0.066
Vaponephrin			2.25	0.25	6	0.6
ISOETHARINE						
Bronkometer	0.34	1				0.034
Bronkosol Solution			1	0.5	5	0.5
Bronkosol Unit-Dose			0.25	2	5	0.5
ISOPROTERENOL						
Medihaler-Iso	0.08	0.24				0.024
Isuprel Mistometer	0.13	0.39				0.039
Isuprel Solution			1	0.5	5	0.5
METAPROTERENOL						
Alupent Inhaler	0.65	2				0.20
Alupent Solution			5	0.3	15	1.5
Alupent Unit Doses			0.4, 0.6	2.5	10, 15	1, 1.5
ALBUTEROL						
Proventil Inhaler	0.09	0.27				0.027
Ventolin Inhaler	0.09	0.27				0.027
Ventolin Solution			0.5	0.5	2.5	0.25
Proventil Unit-Dose			0.083	3	2.5	0.25
TERBUTALINE						
Brethaire Inhaler	0.20	0.60				0.06
Bricanyl Solution			0.1	2	2	0.2

Note: The probable amounts of each drug deposited varies considerably depending on whether a jet nebulizer or metered cartridge is used. The figures provided are based on typical recommended dosages.

ADMINISTRATION OF NONAEROSOLIZED DRUGS

When drugs are given intravenously, the major respiratory agents can be mixed without any apparent adverse effects. Thus, saline, dextrose, aminophylline, corticosteroids, and sodium iodide are all compatible. However, some antibiotics may be incompatible with various drugs, and they should be given through an independent setup.

Most oral drugs used in respiratory therapy are compatible with one another and are often administered in combination preparations. Alcoholic elixirs are potentially hazardous when given to alcoholics and are contraindicated if the patient is on disulfiram (Antabuse) or a similar type of drug. Epinephrine, when given subcutaneously (and perhaps when given by inhalation), may interact with various drugs (e.g., with monoamine oxidase inhibitors) to cause hypertension and excitability; with digitalis glycosides to cause cardiac arrhythmias; or with hypotensive drugs to cause the reverse effect of hypertension. Epinephrine may also interfere with the action of insulin and oral antidiabetic agents, since catecholamines tend to cause a rise in blood sugar level.

It is of interest that certain drugs can be administered by the intratracheal route, particularly in emergencies such as a cardiac arrest. Drugs such as naloxone, diazepam, lidocaine, epinephrine, and atropine are readily absorbed when given by this route in amounts similar to the standard intravenous dosage.[52]

APPENDIX: DOSAGES OF INHALATIONAL DRUGS

VOLUMES

The amount of solution delivered from an uncalibrated dropper is very variable and depends on the characteristics of the dropper, the method of use, and the nature of the solution. One drop approximates 1 minim of an aqueous solution, or 0.5 minim of an alcoholic solution, or 2 minims of a viscous solution. There are about 15 minims (or 15 drops of an aqueous solution) in 1 mL of water.

For practical purposes the following approximate conversion table can be used for dilute aqueous solutions.

    1 minim = 1 drop
    15 minims = 1 mL (1 cc) = 1 g
    60 minims = 1 teaspoonful = 4 mL (approx)
    240 minims = 1 tablespoonful = 15 mL (approx)
    480 minims = 30 mL = 30 g = 1 oz

Abbreviations

    ml = milliliter (1000 mL = 1 liter [L])
    cc = cubic centimeter
    mg = milligram (1000 mg = 1 gram)
    g = gram (1000 g = 1 kilogram [kg])
    1000 micrograms (μg or mcg) = 1 mg
    1,000,000 micrograms = 1 g

Apothecary versus Avoirdupois. Because these two systems of weights and measures differ, *pints* and *pounds* (lb) should not be used as pharmacologic units. The apothecary pint contains 16 oz, but there are only 12 oz to the pound in the apothecary scale, whereas there are 16 oz to the pound in the avoirdupois scale.

PERCENTAGES

Inhalational solutions are commonly labeled according to a percentage or ratio scale. The following scales may be used.

    Weight-in-weight (w/w; e.g., g/100 g)
    Weight-in-volume (w/v; e.g., g/100 mL)
    Volume-in-volume (v/v; e.g., mL/100 ml)

Most frequently, a w/v percentage is used.

    1% = 1 : 100 = 1 g/100 mL = 1 g/dL
    (i.e., 1000 mg/100 mL or 10 mg/mL)

    5% = 5 : 100 = 5 g/100 mL
    (i.e., 5000 mg/100 mL or 50 mg/mL)

    Thus, 0.1% = 1 : 1000 = 0.1 g/100 mL
    (i.e., 100 mg/100 mL or 1 mg/mL)

Various expressions can be used, for example,

    0.5% = 5 : 1000 or 1 : 200
        = 1 g/200 mL, or 0.5 g/100 mL, or 500 mg/
        100 mL, or 500 mg/dL, or 5 mg/mL, or 5
        g/L.

Example: A mixture of 0.25 mL of 1 : 200 isoproterenol in 2.5 mL of water contains

    0.25 mL of 0.5% isoproterenol
    = 0.25 mL of a solution containing 1 g
    isoproterenol in 200 mL (or 5 mg/mL)
    = $\frac{0.25}{200} \times 1000$ mg = 1.25 mg.

Thus, the mixture contains 1.25 mg (1250 μg) of isoproterenol in 2.75-mL solution. If this solution is nebulized by IPPB, about 10% will be retained in the lungs, providing about 0.125 mg (125 μg) of isoproterenol. This is similar to the amount delivered by one activation of a metered aerosol of isoproterenol.

REFERENCES

1. Stolley PD: Asthma mortality: Why the United States was spared an epidemic of deaths due to asthma. Am Rev Respir Dis 105:883, 1972

2. Kirn TF: Asthma mortality rate raises questions, emphasizes need to determine facts of situation. JAMA 260:455, 1988

3. Wood M: Production of therapeutic aerosols. Respir Ther 5:19, 1975

4. Miller WF: Aerosol therapy is acute and chronic respiratory disease. Arch Intern Med 131:148, 1973

5. Gibson LE: Use of water vapor in the treatment of lower respiratory disease. Am Rev Respir Dis 110(6, Part 2):100, 1974

6. Ziment I: Hydration, humidification and mucokinetic therapy. In Weiss EB, Segal MS, Stein M (eds): Bronchial Asthma. Mechanisms and Therapeutics, 2nd ed, Chap 64. Boston, Little, Brown & Company, 1985

7. Parks CR, Woodrum DE, Graham CB et al: Effect of water nebulization on normal canine pulmonary mucociliary clearance. Am Rev Respir Dis 104:99, 1971

8. Morrow PE: Aerosol characterization and deposition. Am Rev Respir Dis 110(6 Part 2):88, 1974

9. Muir DCF: Clinical Aspects of Inhaled Particles, Chaps 1 and 9. Philadelphia, FA Davis, 1972

10. Barton AD: Aerosolized detergents and mucolytic agents in the treatment of stable chronic obstructive pulmonary disease. Am Rev Respir Dis 110(6, Part 2):104, 1974

11. Lieberman J: Measurement of sputum viscosity in a coneplate viscometer. II. An evaluation of mucolytic agents in vitro. Am Rev Respir Dis 97:662, 1968

12. Hirsch SR, Zastrow JE, Kory RC: Sputum liquefying agents: A comparative in vitro study. J Lab Clin Med 74:346, 1969

13. Obenour RA, Saltzman HA, Sierer HO, Green JL: Effects of surface-active aerosols and pulmonary congestion on lung compliance and resistance. Circulation 27:888, 1963

14. Boyd EM, Sheppard EP: Friar's balsam and respiratory tract fluid. Am J Dis Child 111:630, 1966

15. Solomons CC, Cotton EK, Dubois R: The use of buffered L-arginine in the treatment of cystic fibrosis. Pediatrics 47:384, 1971

16. Boyd EM: A review of studies on the pharmacology of the expectorants and inhalants. Int J Clin Pharmacol Ther Toxicol 3:55, 1970

17. Ziment I: What to expect from expectorants. JAMA 236:193, 1976

18. Lieberman J, Kurnick NB: The induction of proteolysis in purulent sputum by iodides. J Clin Invest 43:1892, 1964

19. Carson S, Goldhamer R et al: Mucus transport in the respiratory tract. Am Rev Respir Dis 98(2):86, 1966

20. Siegal S: The asthma-suppressive action of potassium iodide. J Allergy 35:252, 1964

21. Hirsch SR, Viernes PF, Kory RC: The expectorant effect of glyceryl guaiacolate in patients with chronic bronchitis. Chest 63:9, 1973

22. Editorial: Bromhexine. Lancet 1:1058, 1971

23. Ziment I: Pharmacologic therapy of COPD. In Hodgkin JE, Petty TL (eds). Chronic Obstructive Pulmonary Disease. Current Concepts, Chap 7. Philadelphia, WB Saunders, 1987

24. Paterson JW, Woolcock AJ, Shenfield GM: Bronchodilator drugs. Am Rev Respir Dis 120:1149, 1979

25. Reed CE: Basic mechanisms of asthma. Role of inflamation. Chest 94:175, 1988

26. Beck GJ: Controlled clinical trial of a new dosage form of metaproterenol. Ann Allergy 44:19, 1980

27. Roth MJ, Wilson ALF, Novey HS: A comparative study of the aerosolized bronchodilators, isoproterenol, metaproterenol and terbutaline in asthma. Ann Allergy 38:16, 1977

28. Sackner MA, Greeneltch N, Silva G et al: Bronchodilator effects of terbutaline and epinephrine in obstructive lung disease. Clin Pharmacol Ther 16:499, 1974

29. Light RW, Taylor RW, George RB: Albuterol and isoproterenol in bronchial asthma. Arch Intern Med 139:636, 1979

30. Ence TJ, Tashkin DP, Ho D et al: Acute bronchial and cardiovascular effects of oral pirbuterol and metaproterenol. Ann Allergy 43:29, 1979

31. Huhti E, Poukkula A: Clinical comparison of fenoterol and albuterol administered by inhalation. Chest 73:348, 1978

32. Amory DW, Burnham SC, Cheney FW: Comparison of the cardiopulmonary effects of subcutaneously administered epinephrine and terbutaline in patients with reversible airway obstruction. Chest 67:279, 1975

33. Hendeles L, Weinberger M: Theophylline, a "state of the art" review. Pharmacotherapy 3:2, 1983

34. Lawyer CH, Bardana EJ, Rodgers R, Gerber N: Utilization of intravenous dihydroxypropyltheophylline (dyphylline) in an aminophylline-sensitive patient, and its pharmacokinetic comparison with theophylline. J Allergy Clin Immunol 65:353, 1980

35. Hirshman CA et al: Dyphylline aerosol attenuates antigen-induced bronchoscontriction in experimental canine asthma. Chest 78:420, 1981

36. Meltzer EO: To use or not to use antihistamines in patients with asthma. Ann Allergy 64:183, 1990

37. Brooks SM, Werk EE, Ackerman SJ et al: Adverse effects of phenobarbital on corticosteroid metabolism in patients with bronchial asthma. N Engl J Med 286:1125, 1972

38. Ahmed T, D'Brot J, Abraham W: The role of calcium antagonists in bronchial reactivity. J Allergy Clin Immunol 81:133, 1988

39. Patel KR: Calcium antagonists in exercise-induced asthma. Br Med J 282:932, 1981

40. Tanser AR, Elmes J: A controlled trial of ketotifen in exercise-induced asthma. Br J Dis Chest 74:398, 1980

41. Mullarkey MF, Blumenstein BA, Andrade WP et al: Methotrexate in the treatment of corticosteroid-dependent asthma. N Engl J Med 318:603, 1988

42. Charpin D, Orehek J, Velardocchio JM: Bronchodilator effects of antiasthmatic cigarette smoke (Datura stramonium). Thorax 34:259, 1979

43. Marini JJ, Lakshminarayan S: The effect of atropine inhalation in "irreversible" chronic bronchitis. Chest 77:591, 1980

44. Bergofsky EH: Role of ipratropium in treating airway obstruction. Hosp Ther (July), p 51, 1988

45. Borum P: Nasal disorders and anticholinergic therapy. Postgrad Med J 61(Suppl 1):61, 1987

46. Tashkin DP et al: Bronchial effects of aerosolized delta 9-tetrahydrocannabinol in healthy and asthmatic subjects. Am Rev Respir Dis 115:57, 1977

47. Klastersky J, Carpentier-Meunier F, Kahan-Coppens L et al: Endotracheally administered antibiotics for gram-negative bronchopneumonia. Chest 75:586, 1979
48. Girard P-M, Couderc L-J, Farinotti R et al: Ultrasonic nebulised pentamidine for pneumocystis pneumonia. Lancet 1:1165, 1988
49. Ravin CE, Latimer JM, Matsen JM: In vitro effects of lidocaine on anaerobic respiratory pathogens and strains of *Haemophilus influenzae*. Chest 72:439, 1977
50. Weiss EB, Patwardhan AV: The response to lidocaine in bronchial asthma. Chest 72:429, 1977
51. Aviado DM: Toxicity of propellants. Drug Res 18:365, 1974
52. Editorial: Intratracheal drugs. Lancet 1:743, 1988

BIBLIOGRAPHY

General Reviews of Drugs Used in Respiratory Therapy

AMA Drug Evaluations, 6th ed. Chicago, American Medical Association, 1986

Barnes PJ, Rodger IW, Thomson NC (eds): Asthma: Basic Mechanisms and Clinical Management. London, Academic Press, 1988

Dautrebande L: Physiological and pharacologic characteristics of liquid aerosols. Physiol Rev 32:214, 1952 (A classic account of aerosol therapy, with an extraordinary range of information.)

Gilman AG, Goodman LS, Rall TW, Murad F (eds): The Pharmacologic Basis of Therapeutics. New York, Macmillan, 1985 (The chapters on the autonomic nervous system and bronchodilators are extremely good.)

Kay AB (ed): Asthma, Clinical Pharmacology and Therapeutic Progress. Oxford, Blackwell Scientific Publications, 1986

Martindale: The Extra Pharmacopoeia, 29th ed. London, The Pharmaceutical Press, 1989 (This compendium provides an extraordinary amount of information, including traditional and international drugs.)

Ziment I: Respiratory Pharmacology and Therapeutics. Philadelphia, WB Saunders, 1978 (A comprehensive practical guide to drugs used in inhalation therapy and pulmonary medicine.)

Ziment I: Pharmacologic Therapy of COPD. In Hodgkin JE, Petty TL (eds): Chronic Obstructive Pulmonary Disease. Current Concepts, Chap 7. Philadelphia, WB Saunders, 1987

Ziment I, Popa V (eds): Clinics of Chest Medicine. Respiratory Pharmacology. Philadelphia, WB Saunders, 1986

Mucokinesis

Respiratory Tract Secretions and Mucociliary Clearance

Boyd EM: Respiratory Tract Fluid. Springfield Ill, Charles C Thomas, 1975 (This book gives a comprehensive review of Boyd's considerable research on sputum and the agents that affect the material.)

Dulfano MJ (ed): Sputum Fundamentals and Clinical Pathology. Springfield, Ill, Charles C Thomas, 1973 (This book provides an encyclopedic account of sputum and its structure, examination, properties, and management.)

Okeson GC, Divertie MB: Cilia and bronchial clearance: The effects of pharmacologic agents and disease. Mayo Clin Proc 45:361, 1970

Mucokinetic Agents

Barton AD: Aerosolized detergents and mucolytic agents in the treatment of stable chronic obstructive pulmonary disease. Am Rev Respir Dis 110(6, Part 2):104, 1974

Braga PC, Allegra L (eds): Drugs in Bronchial Mucology. New York, Raven Press, 1989

Boyd EM: Expectorants and respiratory tract fluid. Pharmacol Rev 6:521, 1954

Boyd EM: A review of studies on the pharmacology of the expectorants and inhalants. Int J Clin Pharmacol Ther Toxicol 3:55, 1970

Gunn JA: The action of expectorants. Br Med J 4:972, 1927

Lish, PM, Salem H: Expectorants. In Salem H, Aviado DM (eds): International Encyclopedia of Pharamacology and Therapeutics, Vol 3, Sec 27. New York, Pergamon Press, 1970

Marin R, Litt M, Marriott C: The effect of mucolytic agents on the rheologic and transport properties of canine tracheal mucus. Am Rev Respir Dis 121:495, 1980

Richardson PS, Phipps RH: The anatomy, physiology, pharmacology and pathology of tracheobroncial mucus secretion and the use of expectorant drugs in human disease. Pharmacol Ther B 3:441, 1978

Ziment I: Mucokinetic agents. In Hollinger MA (ed): Current Topics in Pulmonary Pharmacology and Toxicology, Vol. 3, Chap 5. New York, Elsevier Science Publishing, 1987

General

Buckle DR, Smith H (eds): Development of Anti-Asthma Drugs. London, Butterworth & Co, 1984

Gershwin ME (ed): Bronchial Asthma: Principles of Diagnosis and Treatment, 2nd ed. Orlando, Grune & Stratton, 1986

Jenne JW, Murphy S (eds): Drug Therapy for Asthma, Research and Clinical Practice, New York, Marcel Dekker, 1987

Mason RH (ed): Asthma, Part-Two. Semin Respir Med 8:H4, April 1987

Middleton E, Reed CE, Ellis EF et al (eds): Allergy, Principles and Practice, 3rd ed. St Louis, CV Mosby, 1988 (Volume I has excellent accounts on pharmacology.)

Weiss EB, Segal MS, Stein M (eds): Bronchial Asthma: Mechanisms and Therapeutics, 2nd ed. Boston, Little, Brown & Co, 1985

Sympathomimetic Agents

Brittain RT, Dean CM, Jack D: Sympathomimetic bronchodilator drugs. Pharmacol Ther B 2:423, 1976

Clark TJH, Cochrane GM (eds): Bronchodilator Therapy. The Basis of Asthma and Chronic Obstructive Airways Disease Management. Auckland, ADIS Press, 1984

McFadden RR: Aerosolized bronchodilators and steroids in the treatment of airway obstruction in adults. Am Rev Respir Dis 122(5, Part 2):89, 1980

Nelson HS: Adrenergics in asthma: Where we stand today. J Respir Dis 7:43, 1986

Popa V: Beta-adrenergic drugs. Clin Chest Med 7:313, 1986

Svensson L-A: Development of β_2-adrenoceptor agonist bronchodilator prodrugs. In Hollinger MA (ed): Current Topics in Pulmonary Pharmacology and Toxicology, Vol 3, Chap 1. New York, Elsevier Science Publishing, 1987

Ziment I: How to select an appropriate respiratory drug. Geriatrics 36:89, 1981

Methylxanthines

Anderson KE, Persson CGA (eds): Anti-Asthma Xanthines and Adenosine, p 19. New York, Excerpta Medica Current Clinical Practice Series, 1985

Cummiskey JM, Popa V: Theophyllines—a review. J Asthma 21:243, 1984

Hendeles L, Massanari M, Weinberger M: Theophylline. In Middleton E, Reed CE, Ellis EF, Adkinson NF, Yunginger JW (eds): Allergy. Principles and Practice, 3rd ed, Chap 30. St Louis, CV Mosby, 1988

Jenne JW (ed): Rationale for the use of theophylline in COPD: Bronchodilation and beyond. Chest 92(Suppl) July 1987

Littenberg B: Aminophylline treatment in severe acute asthma. A meta-analysis. JAMA 259:1678, 1988

Turner-Warwick M, Levy J (eds): New Perspectives in Theophylline Therapy. London, The Royal Society of Medicine, 1984

Mediators

Barnes PJ: Neutral control of human airways in health and disease. Am Rev Respir Dis 134:1289, 1986

Kay AB (ed): Asthma. Clinical Pharmacology and Therapeutic Progress. Oxford, Blackwell Scientific, 1986

Anticholinergics

Bergofsky EH (ed): Cholinergic pathway in obstructive airways disease. Am J Med 81(5A):1986

Gross NJ, Skorodin MS: Anticholinergic antimuscarinic bronchodilators. Am Rev Respir Dis 129:856, 1984

Gross NJ: Drug therapy: Ipratropium bromide. N Engl J Med 319:486, 1988

Mann JS: Anticholinergic drugs in the treatment of airways disease. Rev J Dis Chest 79:209, 1985

Ziment I, Au JP: Anticholinergic agents. Clin Chest Med 7:355, 1986

Antibiotics

Corkery KJ, Luce JM, Montgomery AB: Aerosolized pentamidine for treatment and prophylaxis of *Pneumocystis carinii* pneumonia: An update. Respir Care 33:676, 1988

Hodson ME: Antibiotic treatment, aerosol therapy. Chest 94(Suppl):156S, 1988

Newman SP, Woodman G, Clarke SW: Deposition of carbenicillin aerosols in cystic fibrosis: Effects of nebuliser system and breathing pattern. Thorax 43:318, 1988

Wanner A, Rao A: Clinical indications for and effects of bland, mucolytic, and antimicrobial aerosols. Am Rev Respir Dis 122(5, Part 2):79, 1980

Williams MH: Steroid and antibiotic aerosols. Am Rev Respir Dis 110(6, Part 2):122, 1974

Additives

Tiersten S: RT pharmacology: Where has it been and where is it going? Respir Ther 4:23, 1974

Wood M, Ziment I: Additives and combinations. Respir Ther 4:19, 1974

Aerosol Therapy

Clarke SW, Pavia D (eds): Aerosols and the Lung: Clinical and Experimental Aspects. London, Butterworth & Co., 1984

Dautrebaude L: Microaerosols. New York, Academic Press, 1962

Dolovich MB, Newhouse MT: Aerosols: Generation, methods of administration, and therapeutic applications in asthma. In Middleton E, Reed CE, Ellis EF, Adkinson NF, Yunginger JW (eds): Allergy, Principles and Practice, 3rd ed, Chap 25. St Louis, CV Mosby, 1988

Newhouse M, Dolovich M: Aerosol therapy of asthma: Principles and application. Respiration 50(Suppl 2):123, 1986

Wilson A: Aerosol dynamics and delivery systems. In Jenne JW, Murphy S (eds): Drug Therapy for Asthma. Research and Clinical Practice, Chap 11. New York, Marcel Dekker, 1987

Corticosteroids

Clark TJH (ed): Steroids in asthma: A reappraisal in the light of inhalation therapy. Auckland, ADIS Press, 1983

Fanta CH: Corticosteroid therapy in asthma: The double-edged sword. J Respir Dis 8:75, Nov. 1987

Morris HG: Mechanism and action and therapeutic role of corticosteroids in asthma. J Allergy Clin Immunol 75:1, 1985

Spector SL: The use of corticosteroids in the treatment of asthma. Chest 87S:73S, 1985

Ziment I: Steroids. Clin Chest Med 7:341, 1986

Cromolyn

Altounyan REC: Review of clinical activity and mode of action of sodium cromoglycate. Clin Allergy 10:481, 1980

Konig P: The role of cromolyn sodium in the treatment of asthma. Pract Cardiol 13:89, Feb. 1987

Symposium. Changing concepts in asthma: Mechanisms and therapy. J Respir Dis (Suppl.) 8:1987

TWENTY

Airway Management

David J. Plevak
Jeffrey J. Ward

A focus of this chapter is to review the equipment and techniques necessary to manage the airway of critically ill patients, but it also includes a discussion of airway management for patients requiring long-term ventilatory support. Ensuring adequate ventilation and oxygenation is crucial. A brief interval of hypoxia can result in loss of consciousness, impairment of brain function, or death. The intent of this chapter is to provide the reader with information necessary to begin to master the art of airway management. Facility comes only after much practice in the laboratory and in controlled clinical settings. It is only after such training that certification be granted and unsupervised clinical performance allowed. The chapter will begin with a review of normal anatomy. Artificial airways and adjunct equipment will be presented, including the indications and rationale for their use. Finally, the specific procedures of airway management: suctioning, endotracheal intubation, tracheotomy, and tracheostomy care will be discussed. The potential complications associated with airway management will be outlined so that they might be anticipated and avoided.

AIRWAY ANATOMY

A sound background in the anatomy of the upper airway is essential for respiratory care. Clinical situations arise when anatomic structures are not visible or are obscured, and the practitioner must rely on mental images of spatial relationships. When a patient develops an obstructed airway, a knowledge of upper airway anatomy illustrates the application of proper head and neck maneuvers designed to attain airway patency. During a difficult intubation, the larynx may not be visible. The practitioner may have to rely on the relationships of adjacent structures to properly place the endotracheal tube. Adult and neonatal airway anatomy will be reviewed together to emphasize differences.

The nose, pharynx, and trachea function to warm, filter, and humidify inspired air. Figure 20–1A shows a sagittal section of the entire adult upper airway. Anatomically the pharynx is divided into three major zones: the nasopharynx, oropharynx, and laryngopharynx or hypopharynx. These zones include several specialized structures that will be individually reviewed.

The nose includes the external nose (which protrudes from the face) and the nasal cavity or internal nose. The external orifices of the nose are the nostrils or nares. The nasal cavity is divided into two chambers (fossae) by a cartilaginous septum. The floor is formed by the hard and soft palate. Each fossa has three turbinates (conchae) that project downward from the lateral surfaces to increase the air–tissue surface area. The nasal cavity opens into the nasopharynx through divided posterior choanae. Squamous ciliated columnar epithelial and secretory cells line the structure, which is

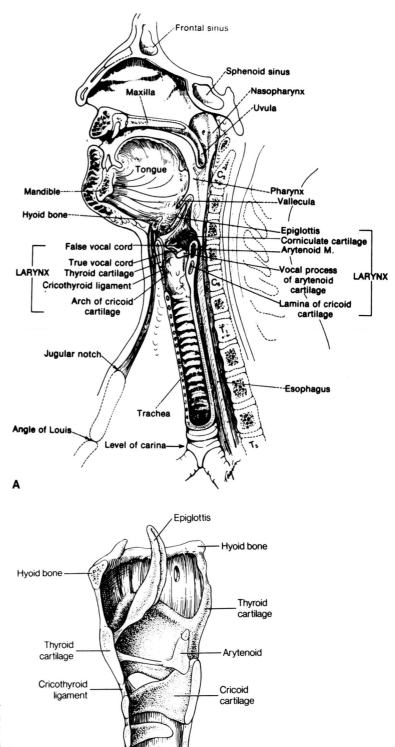

Figure 20–1. (*A*) Normal adult upper airway (sagittal section). (McCabe BF: Pathologic principles. In Wilkins EW (ed): MGH Textbook of Emergency Medicine, 2nd ed. Baltimore, Williams & Wilkins, © 1987, with permission) (*B*) Detailed view of the adult larynx. (Finucane BT, Santora AH (eds): Principles of Airway Management. Philadelphia, FA Davis, 1988, with permission)

highly innervated. Besides sensory capabilities, receptors evoke sneezing in response to irritating odors, chemicals, or particles (e.g., smoke or pepper). The human nose can differentiate over 4000 different odors.

Openings in the lateral and posterior nasal walls communicate with sinuses and the nasolacrimal duct. During normal breathing, the nose and nasopharynx account for approximately 50% of the total airway resistance. Access to this area may be made more difficult by a deviated septum, mucosal edema, nasal polyps, or trauma. Insertion of airways or catheters into the nasal cavity should be done in a horizontal direction following the floor of the nasal cavity. This will usually avoid painful trauma to the turbinates.

The nasopharynx begins at the posterior choana and reaches downward to the soft palate. The posterior wall is the location of the pharyngeal tonsils (adenoids). The eustachian tube empties into the nasopharynx. Because the nasopharynx accepts drainage from the sinuses and the eustachian tube, the presence of an artificial airway (e.g., nasopharyngeal airway) may lead to colonization or infection of adjacent structures. Otitis media and sinusitis may result.

The oropharynx begins at the distal tip of the uvula and extends past the tongue to the tip of the epiglottis. The uvula is a posterior extension of the soft palate and is a useful visual landmark. The palatine tonsils are located between the tissue folds of the palatoglossal and palatopharyngeal arches. The tonsils are collections of lymphoid tissue. The tongue occupies a large portion of the oral cavity. It is attached anteriorly to the hyoid bone and to the mandible, palate, and pharyngeal wall. It functions to provide speech, taste, swallowing, and also frequently causes obstruction of the pharynx. This occurs commonly in the unconscious patient, when the oropharyngeal musculature becomes relaxed. Motor innervation of the tongue includes the lingual, glossopharyngeal, and hypoglossal nerves.

The larynx is a group of specialized cartilaginous structures (see Fig. 20–1B). They connect the lower part of the pharynx with the trachea and are about 5-cm long in the adult male (slightly shorter in the female). The adult larynx is located at the level of cervical vertebrae between C-3 through C-6. The cartilage skeleton consists of nine cartilages, three paired and three single.

The zone of the hypopharynx begins superiorly with the tip of the epiglottic cartilage and continues inferiorly to include the cricoid cartilage. It includes the area from the anterior larynx and base of the tongue to the cervical vertebra posteriorly. The epiglottis functions as a valve to guard the airway from fluids or food, especially during swallowing. The upper portion moves freely and is a well-known landmark for intubation. With a straight blade laryngoscope, the epiglottis is manipulated anteriorly to allow visualization of the glottis. The base of the epiglottis is attached to the thyroid cartilage near the epiglottic vallecula. The tip of a curved blade laryngoscope is placed in this space (epiglottic vallecula), just below the tongue, during intubation. The epiglottis may become acutely inflamed and edematous. Acute epiglottitis is most frequently caused by *Haemophilus influenza* and can be a life-threatening emergency.

The three sets of paired cartilages in the larynx are the arytenoids ("ladle"), corniculates ("horned"), and cuneiforms ("wedge-shaped"). The corniculates are superior to the pyramid-shaped arytenoids. These and the cuneiforms support the aryepiglottic and interarytenoid folds. These folds form the aditus or entrance of the larynx. Muscles and ligaments connect cartilages to interior vocal structures to allow movement of speech. Their value to the respiratory care practitioner is in the form of a visual landmark to the laryngeal opening.

The largest single cartilage in the larynx is the thyroid. It is a shield-shaped cartilage with horn-like cornua on its inferior and superior aspects. The anterior portion of the thyroid cartilage is known as the "Adam's apple" and is more pronounced in adult men. The cricoid cartilage articulates through the cricothyroid ligament with the thyroid cartilage. The cricoid is unique in that its cartilage forms a ring that provides a firm posterior border for the larynx at this level. Inferiorly, the cricoid cartilage is attached to the first tracheal ring. The cricoid is a "signet ring"–shaped structure, with the larger portion anterior to the esophagus.

Entering the interior cavity of the larynx would reveal the glottis or the opening between the vestibular folds or false vocal cords. When contracted, these folds allow breath holding against positive pressure, such as coughing or a Valsalva maneuver. The laryngeal area above the true vocal cords is termed the vestibules and below, the ventricles. The true cords lie just inferior to the false cords, and the zone below them is termed the infraglottic cavity. The vocal folds consist of a vocal ligament and the vocalis muscle. This is the narrowest part of the adult airway. These folds are readily moved aside by expired air, such as during speech, and resist inspiratory flow when opposed. Relative to surface anatomy, the vocal cords lie at midlevel of the thyroid cartilage.

The thyroid, cricoid, and most of the arytenoid cartilages are made of hyaline cartilage. These can benignly calcify at approximately 60 years of age. The remaining cartilages and the vocal processes of the arytenoids are made of elastic cartilage. Most of the interior surfaces of the larynx are lined with nonkeratinizing stratified squamous epithelium. The laryngeal ventricles and infraglottic areas are lined with pseudostratified columnar ciliated epithelium.

There is a complex system of musculature for the laryngeal structures. They can be separated into two groups: those that protect the airway by sphincteric contraction, and those that adjust the larynx and cords during breathing and phonation. Upper airway muscle tone may be compromised when patients are unconscious.

Innervation and blood supply to the larynx is provided by the superior and inferior laryngeal nerves and arteries. The superior laryngeal nerves arise from the vagus. They provide motor, sensory, and secretory innervation to small widespread mucous glands in the larynx. The inferior laryngeal nerves are terminal branches of the recurrent laryngeal nerves that also arise from the vagus. The left-sided recurrent laryngeal nerve approaches the larynx after dipping below the aortic arch. On the right, connection is more direct, with the nerve looping around the subclavian artery. Both nerves innervate all of the intrinsic muscles, except the cricothyroid. Neoplasm, vascular disease, or surgery in the periaortic area can cause left-sided fold or cord dysfunction. At first, a paralyzed side of the vocal cords would bow outward and could not be abducted or adducted. The voice would sound different and hoarse because the two cords could not properly oppose. Over time, the paralyzed cord might gradually move closer to the midline with the aid of the still-innervated cricothyroid muscle.

The *trachea* is a tubular structure with a flattened posterior surface. In the adult its length is approximately 12 to 15 cm. It is 1.8 to 2.5 cm in diameter. The anterior and lateral surfaces are supported by 16 to 20 C-shaped cartilage rings. The trachealis muscle forms the posterior wall of the trachea. During cough, the latter area invaginates to decrease the cross-sectional area to 18%, allowing linear airflow velocities of up to 500 miles/hr. At approximately the level of the fourth or fifth thoracic vertebra, the trachea bifurcates into right and left mainstem bronchi at the *carina*. In the adult the right side's branching angle is more vertical, approximately 25° from midline. The left angles about 45° from midline. Because of this configuration, aspiration of foreign bodies, liquids, and intubations are more likely to occur on the right.

NEONATAL AND PEDIATRIC CONSIDERATIONS

Structures of the airway in the newborn appear to facilitate feeding and breathing. The newborn's tongue is relatively larger, the entire larynx is located more cephalad, and the hyoid bone and thyroid cartilage lie closer together when compared with an adult (Fig. 20-2). The epiglottis is U-shaped and stiff. The relative size of the infant's head is much larger than that of an adult, and the weight of the head can cause the cervical spine to assume a flexed position. This can precipitate airway obstruction. The vocal cords are more concave than an adult's and have an anteroinferior incline. The trachea of the newborn is short, and the narrowest part of the airway is at the level of the cricoid cartilage. Newborns are obligatory nose breathers, reserving eating for the mouth. This allows them to breath and nurse simultaneously.[30]

Intubation is sometimes more difficult in the infant owing to a bulky tongue. In addition, the size of the epiglottis usually necessitates direct instrumentation with the laryngoscope blade. Passage of a tube through the larynx is sometimes difficult because the angle of the vocal cords may hinder its advance. Trauma to the mucosal tissue surrounded by the cricoid cartilage can result in edema and significant reduction in cross-sectional area. This may result in postextubation stridor. The shorter

Figure 20-2. Anatomic comparison of infant (left) and adult (right) larynx. Refer to text for details. (Eckenhoff JE: Some anatomic considerations of the infant larynx influencing endotracheal anesthesia. Anesthesiology 12:401, 1951, with permission)

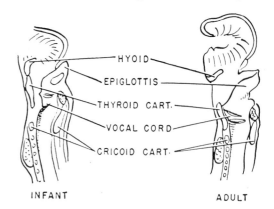

INFANT   ADULT

trachea provides a greater chance for unilateral endobronchial intubation.[30] The angle of the tracheal bifurcation in children totals approximately 80°. The right bronchial angle is 31 ± 5°, whereas the left bronchial angle is 49 ± 7°.[49] Left bronchial intubations are more common in children than in adults.

Congenital anatomic abnormalities such as stenosis or atresia of the choanae usually result in respiratory distress for obligate nose breathers. This rare lesion can be diagnosed by the inability to pass a catheter through the nasopharynx. Radiographic examination can provide the definitive diagnosis. Obstructing lesions of the nasopharynx that produce stridor accompany a number of congenital craniofacial dysmorphologies.

Instability of the trachea (tracheomalacia) is a rare congenital abnormality of the trachea. During cough the walls of the trachea move back and forth, producing a harsh barking cough. Other tracheal problems include compression extrinsically by vascular anomalies and tracheoesophageal fistulas or atresia.

EMERGENCY AIRWAY MANAGEMENT

The American Heart Association (AHA) and the American Red Cross have both done much to train lay and medical personnel in techniques to manage the airway during resuscitation. The following information coincides with the most current published standards.

MANUAL TECHNIQUES

Head-Tilt/Chin-Lift

During initial assessment of the victim of cardiopulmonary arrest, the rescuer shakes the victim and shouts to determine unresponsiveness. Unconsciousness would predispose the airway to lack of muscular tone and obstruction by pharyngeal structures. In addition, the arrested individual may be in a body position that compromises the airway. Of major importance to successful resuscitation is opening the airway. The basic initial manual technique is termed the "head-tilt/chin-lift" maneuver (Fig. 20–3). This is performed by placing the most cephalad hand on the victim's forehead and applying enough pressure with the palm to tilt the head back into the "sniffing" position (Fig. 20–4A, B). This posture of the head and neck provides a minimal angle between the pharyngeal and tracheal planes. The second component of this action is to

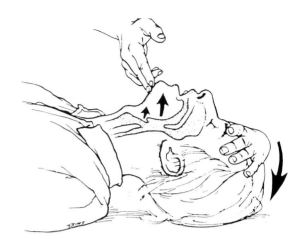

Figure 20–3. Manual opening of the adult airway using the head-tilt/head-lift. (Reproduced, with permission, © Instructor's Manual for Basic Life Support, 1987. Copyright American Heart Association)

use the first two fingers of the remaining hand to lift up the bony portion of the mandible near the chin (the thumb should not be used). This brings the tongue forward, preventing it from blocking the posterior oropharynx. The maneuver also supports the jaw and helps to hold the head-tilt positioning. The teeth will be close to occlusion but open enough for mouth-to-mouth ventilation to occur. Loose dentures tend to be supportive in this maneuver but should be removed if they prove to be obstacles in maintaining the airway. Victims with facial trauma, inability to open the mouth, or inability to provide a leakproof mouth-to-mouth seal may require that the rescuer perform mouth-to-nose ventilation. The mouth is then held closed but may need to be manually opened to allow exhalation. Rescue breathing for patients with a permanent tracheal stoma must occur by mouth-to-stoma ventilation. Patients who have received a laryngectomy cannot be ventilated in the standard fashion, as there is no longer a connection between trachea and mouth.

Jaw-Thrust/Head-Tilt

The "jaw-thrust/head-tilt" maneuver is a variant on the head-tilt/chin-lift (Fig. 20–5). It is recommended for use in opening the "difficult airway" and has also been termed the "triple airway maneuver." It can also be applied without the head-tilt for suspected or confirmed neck injuries, in that it opens the airway without extension of the cervical spine.

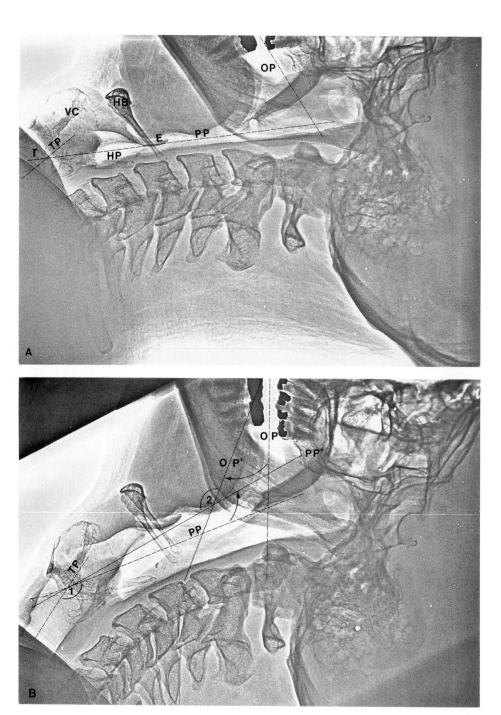

Figure 20—4. Xeroradiographs of the adult airway. (*A*) A supine posture neutral position, causing the tongue to obstruct the posterior pharyngeal plane (along line PP). (*B*) The "sniffing position" showing minimal angulation between pharyngeal and tracheal planes. This facilitates intubation: T, trachea; TP, tracheal plane; VC, vocal cords; HP, hypopharynx; HB, hyoid bone; E, epiglottis; PP, pharyngeal plane; PP', pharyngeal plane with forward head tilt; OP, oral plane; OP', oral plane in sniffing position.

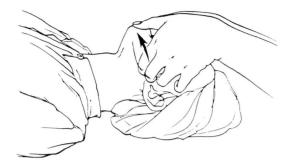

Figure 20—5. The jaw-thrust maneuver without head tilt. (Reproduced, with permission, © Instructors Manual for Basic Life Support, 1987. Copyright American Heart Association)

To perform the jaw thrust the rescuer positions both elbows on a surface, on either side of the victim's head. The fingers grasp the mandible at the angle and lift to displace the jaw forward. The thumbs are often employed to retract the victim's lower lip to allow mouth-to-mouth breathing. (This requires that the cheek be used to seal the nostrils of the victim.) The jaw thrust alone can be successful in opening the airway. To also incorporate the head-tilt, the rescuer simply tilts the head backward. For the victim with suspected spinal trauma, the head should be supported and movement prevented. If the jaw thrust alone is not successful in opening the airway, the head should be tilted back slightly. Although the jaw-thrust maneuvers are difficult to perform and are fatiguing, they are quite effective.

Tongue—Jaw Lift

The tongue—jaw lift is recommended to visually check for foreign body obstruction in adults, children, and infants (Fig. 20—6). This mandibular displacement is also very effective in providing an airway. However, the rescuer risks being bitten unless the victim remains unconscious or is edentulous. The thumb is placed in the mouth inside the lower incisors. The fingers grasp the chin, and the hand pulls upward. This position facilitates visual location of an obstructing substance or object and allows sweeping (clearing) of the airway with the fingers of the opposite hand.

Pediatric Considerations

The aforementioned techniques are also used for pediatric airway management. The head-tilt/chin-lift is employed, with special care taken to prevent

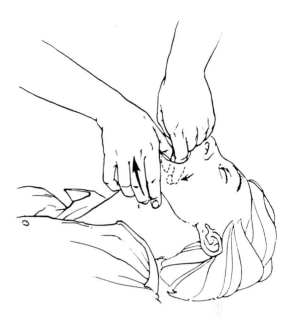

Figure 20—6. The tongue—jaw lift used in combination with a finger sweep maneuver performed on an unconscious victim of foreign body obstruction. (Reproduced, with permission, © Instructor's Manual for Basic Life Support, 1987. Copyright American Heart Association)

overextension of the head or to prevent the soft parts of the underchin from occluding the airway (Fig. 20—7A). The jaw-thrust, with or without head tilt, is performed as in the adult (see Fig. 21—7B). The tongue—jaw lift is also used on unconscious children and infants who have complete airway obstruction. The AHA suggests it be combined with direct removal of a visualized object or "blind" sweeping of the posterior pharynx (adult and child only).

MANUAL METHODS TO CLEAR AN OBSTRUCTED AIRWAY

Even though manual techniques for airway opening are performed correctly, blockage of the upper airway may still prevent successful ventilation. A victim who aspirates foreign materials, including food, toys, teeth, or other objects, should be encouraged to clear the object by coughing it up while he or she is conscious. Physical signs of hypoxia, increased dyspnea, and ineffective cough are signals for intervention. With complete obstruction the victim will be unable to breathe, speak, or cough. The universal distress signal for a conscious victim is the clutching of the neck between thumb and fingers. Unconscious victims will not respond to

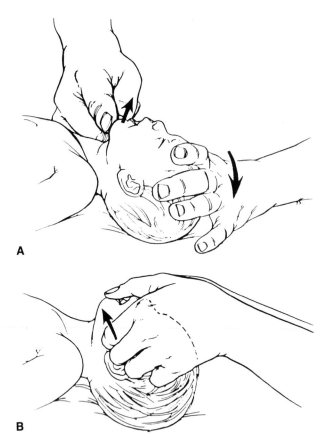

A

B

Figure 20—7. Infant airway maneuvers. (A) Head-tilt/ chin-lift and (B) jaw-thrust. (Reproduced, with permission, © Instructor's Manual for Basic Life Support, 1987. Copyright American Heart Association)

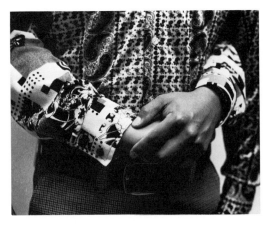

Figure 20—8. The Heimlich maneuver, used to expel aspirated food or other objects from the trachea and oropharynx. The technique is discussed in detail in the text.

repeated attempts to ventilate if a foreign body is obstructing the airway. The rescuer will not see the chest rise upon mouth-to-mouth breathing or feel air freely move into the victim. This blockage will continue in spite of airway repositioning or altering the type of airway opening techniques.

The *Heimlich maneuver* or subdiaphragmatic abdominal thrust is recommended for relieving foreign body airway obstruction in adults and children. (It is not recommended for infants.) The technique provides an artificial cough by compressing abdominal viscera against the diaphragm. If the victim is upright, the rescuer should wrap his or her arms around the victim's waist and compress by pulling upward against the abdomen (Fig. 20–8). The rescuer's arms should be under the victim's. The location for compression is below the xiphoid

process, or the lower rib margins, and above the navel. The fist of one hand (thumb side against the abdomen) is grasped by the opposite hand. Each compression should be brisk and a separate distinct movement. Compressions may need to be repeated six to ten times. Without successful removal of the obstruction, further CPR efforts are in vain.

Conscious obstructed victims who are in the later stages of pregnancy or who are markedly obese should have the point of compression moved from the abdomen to the middle sternum. Chest thrusts are used instead of a upward thrusting movement. The action is directed backward, toward the rescuer, like a horizontal "bear hug."

A version of the Heimlich maneuver can be performed on an unconscious victim in the supine posture. The rescuer straddles the victim and places the heel of one hand against the victim's abdomen. The hand position is in the midline slightly above the navel and well below the tip of the xiphoid process. The second hand is placed directly on top of the first. The thrust should be quick and directed upward and centered toward the midabdomen. This procedure is recommended for adults and children but not infants.

In concept, the Heimlich maneuvers can move a bolus out of the airway and permit a conscious victim to completely clear the object by coughing. In the unconscious victim, the tongue–jaw lift is then used to permit visualization and manual removal. If no object is seen, a blind finger sweep is recommended for adults and children but not in-

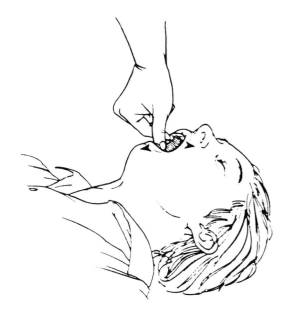

Figure 20–9. The crossed-finger technique for opening the mouth. (Reproduced, with permission, © Instructor's Manual for Basic Life Support, 1987. Copyright American Heart Association)

fants. If the rescuer is unable to open the mouth in performing the tongue–jaw lift, the crossed-finger technique is suggested (Fig. 20–9). The index finger and thumb are crossed and, by applying opening pressure, act as levers to pry the teeth apart. The index finger of the opposite hand can then be inserted into the throat in a hooking motion.

Pediatric Considerations

In infants, foreign-body obstruction is common. Toys, coins, or food, such as hot dogs, candies, peanuts and fruits (grapes), may be aspirated. In a partial obstruction, infants should be observed, supported with oxygen, and transported for definitive diagnosis or care to an emergency or operating room. If the obstruction is significant enough to compromise consciousness, ventilation, or oxygenation, a combination of back-blows and chest-thrusts is recommended. To deliver back-blows, the infant's head is supported by the thumb and forefinger and the anterior chest placed on the forearm. The infant is held prone with a head-down angle. The thigh of the rescuer may be used as support. The blows are directed to the midscapular area with the heel of the hand. Four blows should

be delivered firmly and slowly over 3 to 5 seconds. While continuing to support the head and neck, the infant should be "sandwiched" by the opposite hand/arm and turned into a supine head-down position. Chest thrusts are then provided by the first two fingers to the midsternum. The thrusts are similar to cardiac compressions but delivered at a slower rate (four in 3 to 5 seconds). The tongue–jaw lift is used to check for a foreign body and to assist removal if any is visualized.

ASSESSING BREATHLESSNESS AND RESCUE BREATHING

After successful opening of the airway, the rescuer must determine whether there is spontaneous respiration or whether rescue breathing is required. The AHA suggests (1) looking for chest wall movement, (2) listening for sounds of air movement, and (3) feeling for exhaled air with the cheek. If all three are present, then the airway needs to be maintained. When only chest wall movements (without air movements) are seen, an obstructed airway may be present. The rescuer must then reposition the airway or use an alternative manual technique. That being unsuccessful, the previously mentioned maneuvers (e.g., the Heimlich) are indicated.

Next, rescue breathing by mouth-to-mouth, mouth-to-nose, or mouth-to-stoma ventilation should be initiated with two breaths, each delivered in 1 to 1.5 seconds. For an average-sized adult, the volume should be between 0.8 L and 1.2 L. Children and infants require proportionally less volume. Exhaled air given with excessive pressure tends to inflate the stomach. Breathing can continue at 12 breaths/min for an adult and 20/min for children and infants.

When possible practitioners should take protective measures when performing airway maneuvers. Devices are available that act as a barrier to the patient's body secretions and blood; these include rubber gloves, eye shields, and valved or filtered face masks.

SUMMARY

Figure 20–10 reviews the AHA standards for cardiopulmonary resuscitation (CPR), including an obstructed airway protocol. Readers are urged to complete a AHA– or Red Cross–sponsored course with an opportunity to master techniques on manikins designed for such practice. A complete discussion of CPR is found in Chapter 34.

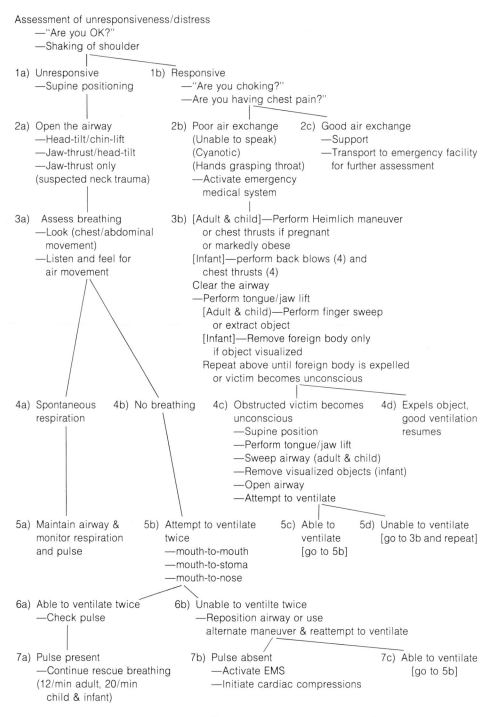

Figure 20—10. Decision-making flow sheet to deal with airway management, including foreign body obstruction.

MECHANICAL ADJUNCT TO AIRWAY MANAGEMENT

FACE MASKS

The face mask enables CPR rescuers or respiratory care or anesthesia personnel to form a seal around the patient's airway, apply medical gases, and administer positive-pressure ventilation. "Anesthesia"-type face masks are commonly used in conjunction with an anesthesia bag/circuit or self-inflating resuscitators. Their purpose is to provide a leak-proof interface between the patient and the gas source. Manufacturers have produced several sizes and styles of masks to allow "fitting" a variety of patients. Both permanent and disposable models are available (Fig. 20–11). A good mask fit is essential to ventilate the patient with positive pressure and to prevent dilution of inspired gases with room air in spontaneously breathing patients.

Masks are composed of three parts: the seal, the body, and the connector. Mask *seals* are commonly made of a cushion composed of covered foam or an inflatable rim. A rubber or plastic flange, which is an extension of the mask body and is not inflated, may also be used. The *body* of the mask provides it with a rigid structure. There is some effort made to keep the internal "dead" space of the mask body to a minimum. Average adult-sized masks have dead space volumes of 75 to 110 mL.[28] The smallest mask that fits properly minimizes dead space and is usually easier to hold on the patient's face. The mask seals rest on the nasal and maxillary bones; muscles in the cheeks help seal the area between the maxilla and mandible. The following facial features often present a difficulty in achieving a tight mask–face fit:

- "Hawk-like" or flat noses
- Receding lower jaws (micrognathia) and other forms of maxillofacial dysmorphology
- Bushy beards
- Maxillofacial trauma
- Facial burns
- Edentulous patients
- Drainage tubes placed through the nose
- Patients with poor facial muscle tone or "saggy" cheeks

Success with the aforementioned patients is increased by experimenting with a variety of mask shapes and styles. The vertical dimension of the face shortens in the edentulous patient. Insertion of an oral airway will increase that distance by lowering the mandible.[28]

The *connector* in a mask allows fitting of a 22-mm (outside diameter) valve-bag or other breathing device. Masks for anesthetic practice often have metal clips for attachment to a set of head straps. The use of such straps increases the risk of aspiration when emesis occurs; consequently, patient selection is of importance.

The skill of holding a face mask and providing a tight seal must be combined with airway positioning as discussed earlier. The most common method uses one hand and allows the other to ventilate by bag device. Figure 20–12 illustrates the hand place-

Figure 20–11. Assortment of mask styles and sizes to provide manual ventilation to adults and infants.

Figure 20–12. One-handed technique to apply a mask to the airway. Notice placement of the fingers under the mandible and maintenance of head extension.

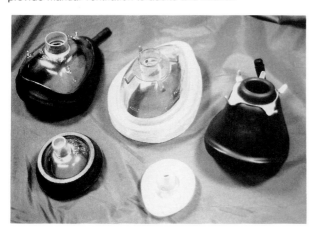

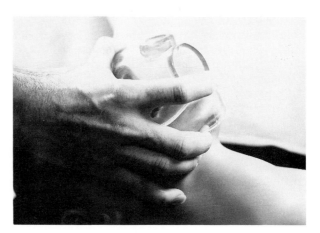

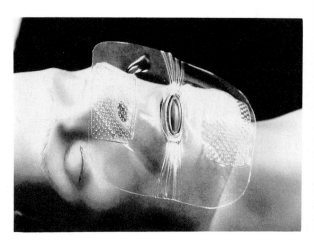

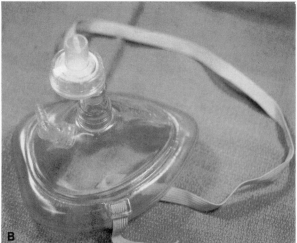

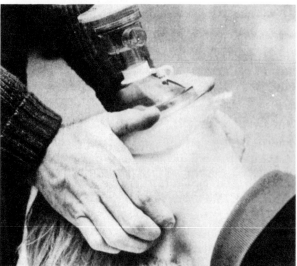

Figure 20—13. Mouth-to-mask ventilation devices. (A) Microshield mask with duckbill valve (not visible). (B) Pocket mask with valve. (C) Mouth-to-mask ventilation in position using two-handed technique. (Hess D, Ness C, Oppel A, Rhoads K: Evaluation of mouth-to-mask ventilation devices. Respir Care 34:191, 1989.)

ment. The thumb and forefinger grasp the body of the mask around the connector. The "ridge" of the mandible is grasped by the ring-finger's distal phalanges. The little finger is placed under the angle of the mandible. As the head is held in the position of extension used in the jaw-lift/head-tilt, these fingers squeeze the mask to the face.

An alternative method is often reserved for the difficult airway and resembles the jaw-lift/head-tilt position or triple-airway maneuver (see Fig. 20–13C). Both thumbs are placed on the body of the mask, on either side of the connector. The distal portions of the two index fingers grasp the underportion of the angle of the jaw. A second practitioner is then required if manual ventilation is necessary.

Problems associated with mask usage includes pressure damage to the eyes (e.g., corneal abrasion) and facial nerves, contact or allergic dermatitis, and aspiration. Proper mask sizing, style, and holding technique should prevent pressure trauma. If sustained use of a mask is required, removal and readjustment will prevent pressure trauma. Use of positive-pressure ventilation increases the potential for gastric insufflation and regurgitation. Masks with clear bodies allow this to be more easily noticed, so that the mask can be removed immediately and suctioning initiated.

Mouth-to-mask ventilation devices have recently been developed as substitutes for direct mouth-to-mouth contact. This is largely related to the acquired immunodeficiency syndrome (AIDS) epidemic. The United States Centers for Disease Control (CDC) now recommends that a "protective barrier" be used between rescuer and victim.[17] A plastic shield and "duckbill" one-way valve is shown in Figure 20–13A. This "CPR Microshield" valve flange is inserted into the mouth, and the shield is held flush with the patient's lips. The airway is then manually positioned and the nares pinched closed under the mask. In theory, no expired air or material can pass through the valve to the rescuer. Mouth-to-mask devices with masks similar to those use for anesthesia are also available (see Figs. 20–13B and 20–13C). Many of these devices have the added protection of a bacterial filter, in addition to a one-way valve. Clinical evaluation has shown that these masks are an acceptable alternative, but they give slightly smaller volumes than comparable mouth-to-mouth ventilations.[43]

NASAL MASKS

Masks applied to the nose are used for nasal continuous positive airway pressure (CPAP) and for mechanical nasal ventilation. The CPAP mask acts as a pneumatic internal splint to maintain an open airway in patients with obstructive sleep apnea.[71] Nasal masks can serve as an alternative to tracheostomy in providing a means of mechanical ventilation to patients with neuromuscular weakness or restrictive lung or chest wall disorders. Commonly, these masks are custom-molded with silicon rubber material.[47,51] A more detailed discussion on these topics will be found in Chapters 13 (Sleep-Disordered Breathing) and 21 to 23. Nasal CPAP prongs are airway appliances used as alternatives to intu-

Figure 20–14. Nasal prongs to provide continuous positive airway pressure (CPAP) to neonatal patients.

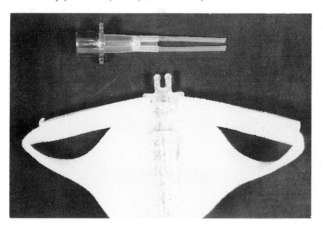

bation in neonates (Fig. 20–14). A discussion of this device can be found in Chapter 29.

MANUAL RESUSCITATION BAGS AND DEMAND VALVES

Manual resuscitation bags and demand valves provide medical gases under positive pressure to the sealed airway (i.e., face mask, endotracheal tube, or tracheostomy). Manual resuscitators are available in a variety of sizes and styles, and many have the capability of providing positive end-expiratory pressure (PEEP). These devices are reviewed in detail in Chapter 28.

ORAL (OROPHARYNGEAL) AIRWAYS

An oral airway is indicated when manual positioning of the airway must be interrupted and when airway patency requires a mechanical "splint." This device also facilitates suctioning of the airway and can aid in preventing occlusion of an oral endotracheal tube by biting. When in place, the distal curved portion of the device lifts the posterior aspects of the tongue, elevating the epiglottis and adjacent tissue away from the pharyngeal wall. Standards for the design of these airways were provided by the American National Standards Institute (ANSI). Their recommended dimensions and manufacturing tolerances are presented in Table 20–1.[3] Recently, the American Society for Testing and Materials (ASTM) has become the dominant agency to recommend standards for these airways and other anesthesia and respiratory care equipment. Currently, the ASTM's F-29 committee is working on a draft to update these standards.[5]

When properly positioned, the oropharyngeal airway can stimulate gag and vomit reflexes and should not be used in patients who are conscious. Placement does not guarantee an open airway; the jaw-lift may still be required.

The basic design of the oral airway is quite simple, consisting of a flange, bite portion, and air channel. The flange prevents the airway from falling back into the mouth. The bite portion fits between the teeth. It, and the air channel, can be tubular (Guedel style, Fig. 20–15A) or open-sided (Berman and Connell styles, see Fig. 20–15B). The open-sided construction has the greatest potential for causing trauma because of its rigidity and relatively thin edges (ANSI recommends a minimum radius of curvature of 0.5 mm); however, it usually provides easier passage of a suction catheter.[32]

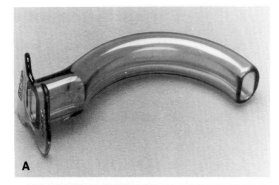

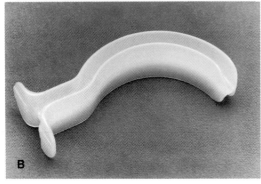

Figure 20—15. Oropharyngeal airways: (*A*) Guedel-style; (*B*) Connel style.

Whichever design is chosen, it must be firm enough that the patient cannot close the channel by biting and must provide a channel for passage of a suction catheter. Manufacturers provide a variety of sizes to fit the anatomic sizes of all patients, from infant through adult.

Table 20—1 Dimensions and Tolerances of Oropharyngeal Airways

NOMINAL SIZE OF AIRWAY	LENGTH (mm)	TOLERANCE LENGTH (mm)
3.0	30	2.5
3.5	35	2.5
4.0	40	2.5
4.5	45	2.5
5.0	50	2.5
5.5	55	2.5
6.0	60	2.5
6.5	65	2.5
7.0	70	2.5–5.0
8.0	80	5.0
9.0	90	5.0
10.0	100	5.0
11.0	110	5.0
12.0	120	5.0

(American National Standards Institute: American national standards for oropharyngeal airways (ANSI Z79.3-1974). New York, ANSI. 1974, with permission)

Insertion of the airway may be accomplished by one of two methods. The practitioner should stand at the patient's head and separate the teeth with the crossed-finger technique previously discussed. Figure 20–16A shows the airway being inserted 180° from the final position. This avoids displacing the tongue backward and blocking the hypopharynx. Once the tip has passed the uvula, it is rotated 180°. This places the distal tip posterior to the tongue (see Fig. 20–16B). An alternate

Figure 20—16. (*A*) Insertion of an oropharyngeal airway should be initiated in the "upside-down" position. As the airway is advanced, it is rotated so the distal portion supports the posterior pharynx. (*B*) Airway shown in position.

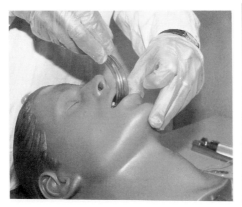
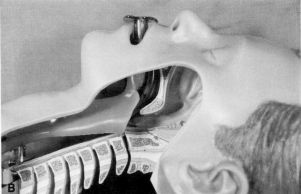

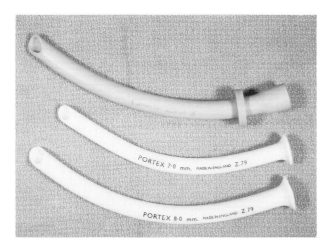

Figure 20–17. Nasopharyngeal airways.

method uses a tongue depressor to move that structure forward so that the airway can be placed without rotation.

Problems in using the oropharyngeal airway are few, other than stimulation of the gag reflex. Users must be aware that patients can cause ulceration of the tongue and hard palate if adults "chew" or infants suckle the airway.[91] Therefore, the oral cavity should be periodically inspected. In such situations a padded bite-block may be indicated to protect teeth and lips from trauma.

NASAL (NASOPHARYNGEAL) AIRWAY

The nasopharyngeal airway is an alternative to the oral airway that provides similar functions (Fig. 20–17). This airway offers advantages in the following situations:

- In facilitating or reducing the discomfort associated with nasotracheal suctioning
- When performing fiberoptic bronchoscopy (in nonintubated patients)
- In providing a patent airway when access to the oral cavity is limited (e.g., facial trauma)
- In providing a more tolerable and effective alternative to the oral airway in the conscious or semiconscious patient[91]

Insertion begins with lubrication of the entire tube with a water-soluble preparation (e.g., K–Y Jelly). The nasopharyngeal airway is held so the built-in curve will follow the curvature of the anatomy (Fig. 20–18A).

The tube's tip should be advanced so it follows the floor of the nasopharynx, avoiding the nasal turbinates. The length for proper insertion can be estimated as the distance from the tragus of the ear to the nares plus 1 in.,[20] or from the meatus of the ear to the nares.[61] If resistance is encountered upon insertion, the opposite naris should be accessed. When properly positioned, the distal portion of the tube lies just above the epiglottis, protecting the posterior pharynx from obstruction (see Fig. 21–18B).

Potential problems in using the nasopharyngeal airway include bleeding (epistaxis), infection (otitis media and sinusitis), obstruction by blood or mucus, and laryngospasm (if the tube touches the epiglottis or vocal cords). The latter problem can occur if the tube slips inward or is too long. Besides the conical flange on the tube, a safety pin may be applied at the proximal end to prevent distal movement into the trachea or esophagus.

Figure 20–18. Placement of a nasopharyngeal airway. (*A*) Insertion showing the tip being inserted parallel to the floor of the nasal cavity; (*B*) airway in position.

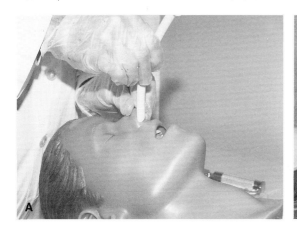
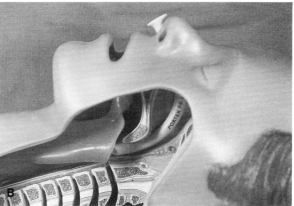

ESOPHAGEAL OBTURATOR AIRWAY AND ESOPHAGOGASTRIC AIRWAY

It has been estimated that approximately 70% of cardiac arrest victims in the field can be managed with oropharyngeal airway, head-tilt, and mask–mask ventilation. Of the remaining 30%, approximately one-half are managed by direct tracheal intubation and the rest by esophageal intubation devices.[63] The esophageal obturator airway (EOA); Fig. 20–19A) and esophagogastric tube airway (EGTA; see Fig. 20–19B) were originally developed for prehospital or "field" airway management by emergency medical technicians and paramedics. Although it is not normally placed in the hospital setting, patients may present to the emergency room with the EOAs in place. Intubation should then occur before removal of esophageal airway.

The basic purpose of the EOA is occlusion of the esophagus, protecting the trachea from vomiting and aspiration while permitting ventilation through the pharynx and trachea.[27] Ventilation takes place through holes in the proximal (oral) aspect of the tube. Proponents of EOAs suggest that intubation occurs easily and rapidly and accelerates the transport of victims to a hospital. However, controversy continues over whether the EOA (or its variations) should be used in preference to tracheal intubation.[78,98]

The basic esophageal obturator airway consists of a cuffed 37-cm long tube with sealed distal tip that is placed in the esophagus. Sizing limits this device to adult use. It is placed by "blind" insertion, with the tip following the contour of the posterior pharynx. Its placement requires minimal movement of the neck. However, because of the esophageal placement there is significant discomfort and reflex retching if the patient is conscious. Just above midtube are multiple holes that allow gas to enter the hypopharynx. The esophageal tube

Figure 20–19. Esophageal obturator airways. (*A*) Esophageal obturator airway (EOA) and (*B*) esophageogastric tube airway (ETGA) (McCabe BF: Prehospital medical care. In Wilkins EW (ed): MGH Textbook of Emergency Medicine, 3rd ed. Baltimore, © Williams & Wilkins, 1989, with permission)

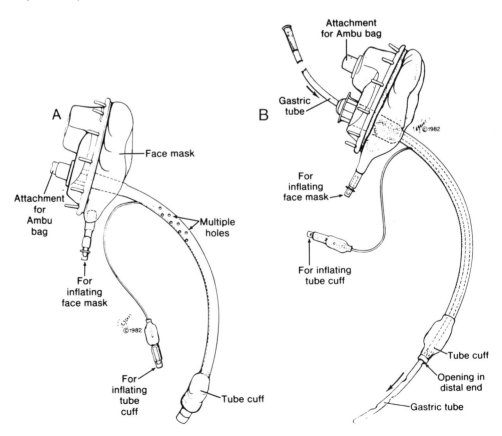

is fitted to a mask with an inflatable cushion. Positive-pressure ventilation is applied to the outer tube connector through bag- or demand-valve resuscitators. With the distal cuff inflated to 35 mL and with face mask sealed, gas exits the holes and should enter only the lungs.[44]

Experience has shown that upon removal of the esophageal tube in the hospital, patients commonly vomit.[57] To address this concern, the ETGA was developed (see Fig. 20–19B) The ETGA allows passage of a gastric tube through the esophageal tube lumen into the esophagus and stomach. The breathing port attachment was moved to the upper portion of the mask. This modification of the EOA allowed ventilation plus decompression, as well as suction of gastric contents, before tube removal.

Clinical use of the EOA and ETGA occurred before objective assessment of their efficacy. One field report indicated that performance of the EOA is comparable with endotracheal intubation when an oxygen-pressured delivery system is used.[41] Other researchers report less favorable findings.[6,85] The blind insertion of either airway does not assure placement in the esophagus. Unrecognized inadvertent insertion in the trachea results in the most serious and lethal complication of these devices (asphyxiation). Esophageal rupture or trauma and gastric rupture have also been reported.[1,42]

ESOPHAGOTRACHEAL COMBITUBE AND PHARYNGOTRACHEAL LUMEN AIRWAY

The esophagotracheal combitube (ETC) and pharyngotracheal lumen airway (PTLA) are modifications of the esophageal obturator designed for prehospital use. Both propose to offer solution to the problems of adequate face–mask seal and inadvertent tracheal intubation. The tracheal combitube (Fig. 20–20A) is a double-lumen device: one channel resembles an EOA (with distal stopper); the other resembles an open tracheal tube. The tubes are separated by a partition wall, and the combined outer diameter is 13 mm. There are distal and proximal cuffs or balloons, each with pilot tubes for separate inflation. The distal balloon is designed to seal in the esophagus (intended location) or trachea if inadvertent placement occurs. The proximal or pharyngeal balloon replaces the mask of the EOA.

Figure 20–20. (A) Esophagotracheal combitube. (B) Insertion procedure: intubation of either the esophagus or trachea will facilitate ventilation. (Frass M, Frenzer R, Rauscha F, Weber H, Pacher R, Leithner C: Evaluation of esophageal combitube in cardiopulmonary resuscitation. Crit Care Med 15:609, 1986, © Williams & Wilkins, with permission)

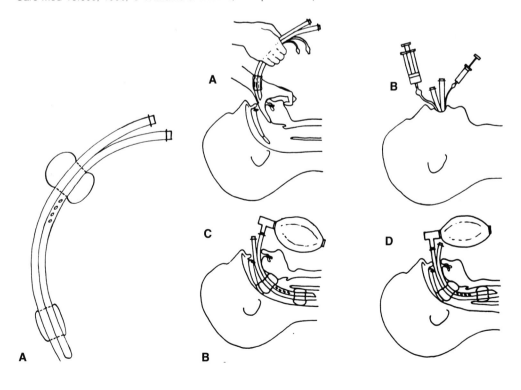

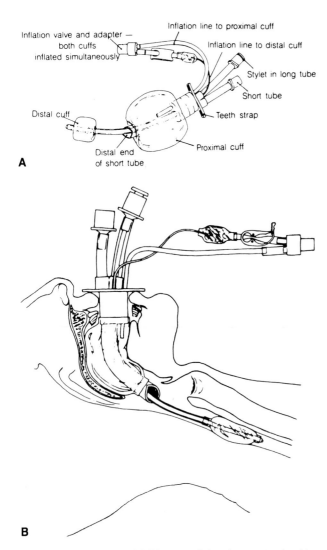

Figure 20—21. (A) Diagram of the pharyngotracheal lumen airway (PTL). (B) Representation of the PTL airway in position. (Niemann JT, Myers R, Scarberry EN: The pharyngotracheal lumen airway: preliminary investigation of a new adjunct. Ann Emerg Med 13:591, 1984. With permission)

When the ETC is inserted (blindly until a printed ring-mark lies at the teeth) the pharyngeal cuff seals the mouth and nose cavities. A group of holes are found in the esophageal tube between the two balloons[35] (see Fig. 20–20B).

These newer designs allowed the tube to provide tracheal ventilation regardless of esophageal or tracheal positioning. When properly placed in the esophagus, tracheal ventilation occurs through the perforations in the esophageal tube, much like an EOA. If the esophageal tube is placed in the trachea, there will be absence of breath sounds and

gastric distention instead. The ventilator device can then be switched to the tracheal tube connector. Even if the rescuer does not realize a patient is being ventilated by a "false" lumen, spontaneously breathing patients can breathe through the unused lumen. In-hospital evaluation of the combitube has been favorable but limited.[35]

The PTLA is quite similar in purpose and design to the tracheal combitube (Fig. 20–21A). However, instead of dual tubes of similar length, the PTLA has a short tube (21 cm) and, passing through that, a long tube (31 cm). Both tubes have inflatable cuffs; the distal cuff seals the esophagus and the proximal cuff seals the pharynx. The latter cuff is applied at the end of the short tube, and the former midway down the long tube. Like the combitube, the long tube can provide ventilation if inadvertently placed in the trachea (see Fig. 20–21B). An additional advantage of the combitube and pharyngotracheal airways is their apparent ability to protect the trachea from aspiration of upper airway hemorrhage.[8]

The PTLA is advanced blindly until the "teeth strap" is at the level of the incisors. A removable stylet provides rigidity for this process. Both cuffs are then inflated. The rescuer ventilates through the short tube and determines if the chest rises and bilateral breath sounds can be auscultated. If that is not the case, the trachea has been intubated. The stylet in the long tube is then removed and ventilation is applied to that tube connector. In this condition, the PTLA approximates an endotracheal tube. Limited animal and human simulation testing has shown this device to be a promising alternative to tracheal intubation in out-of-hospital airway management. The combitube and PTLA may have some advantage over the EOA and EGTA in patients for whom there is difficulty with face mask seal or when airway hemorrhage is present.[8,63] However, if a patient does not display clinical signs of improvement with any of the aforementioned airways, the stomach should be decompressed and endotracheal intubation attempted. Intubation should be performed with an EOA or EGTA in place; the combitube and PTLA must be removed before that procedure.

TRACHEAL TUBES

The term *tracheal tube* will often be used in this chapter to describe a tube placed through the larynx, either orally or nasally, that is positioned in the trachea. Synonyms are endotracheal, intratracheal, or tracheal catheter.

Basic Design

Although there are numerous specialty tubes, the basic design of the tracheal tube has been standardized. The ASTM provides voluntary standards through its F-29 subcommittee. A division subcommittee works on airways, laryngoscopes, and bronchoscopes. (*Note:* Formerly direction came from the ANSI Z-79.) Standardization helps those using airways by reducing variations among manufacturers and inappropriate materials.[2,5]

The components of the endotracheal tube with standardizations of the ASTM are as follows (Fig. 20–22A and B):

Connector. A tapered fitting inserts into the tube's proximal end. The opposite end is a 15-mm outside diameter fitting that permits connection to a resuscitator bag, anesthesia device, or mechanical ventilator.

Tube Body. Tubes are made to have a curvature radius of 14 ± 2 cm. The internal diameters (ID) are used to size tubes of 6 mm (ID) or larger and are printed on the tube. Outside diameter marking is optional. Those that are smaller than 6 mm must have both the outside and inside diameter listed (ID/OD). The appropriate length is determined by

Figure 20–22. (*A*) A cuffed endotracheal tube. (*B*) Diagram illustrating basic design features and dimensional zones. (ASTM: Standards for cuffed and uncuffed tracheal tubes (F 2290201). Philadelphia, © American Society for Testing and Materials, 1989, with permission.)

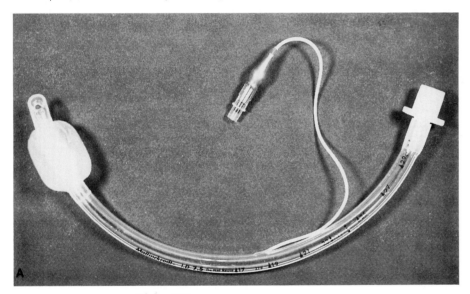

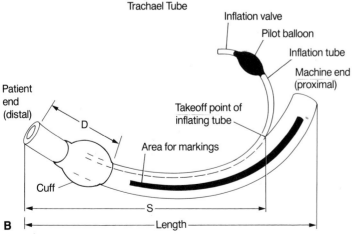

the internal diameter. Tubes can be purchased either "precut" or in a longer form (with a minimum length). The latter tubes are then cut once in place so that the proximal end does not protrude extensively. Other markings include the length (measured from the patient end), whether it is intended for single-use only, and "F29" if it meets ASTM standards. Radiopaque markers are placed the length of the tube or at the patient end. This helps locate the intratracheal position on a chest radiograph.[5]

Tracheal Tube Cuff. A donut-shaped sleeve, when inflated seals the trachea, permitting positive-pressure ventilation and preventing aspiration. When inflated, the cuff should not traumatize the adjacent tissue or herniate so as to block the distal tip. (*Note:* Tubes intended for pediatric patients [prepubescence] are uncuffed.)

Inflating System. The cuff is inflated through a small-bore inflation tube. It lies within the wall of the endotracheal tube in the "inserted portion," but diverges from the body of the tube. The take-off point varies with the tube length. An air-filled syringe is inserted into an inflation valve. Air cannot exit or enter unless a spring-loaded valve is actuated. The external pilot balloon indicates the general inflation state of the hidden cuff by allowing the operator to feel for air pressure. The intracuff pressure may be measured with an inline manometer.

Distal Tip. The patient end of tracheal tubes has a bevel angle of 38° from midline. Traditionally, oral tubes have had bevels facing left (when the concave aspect is up in the "intubating position"). Nasal tubes have had the bevel facing either direction.

A Magill-type tracheal tube has only a distal opening in the tip. The Murphy-type tracheal tube has a small hole opposite the bevel. The size and location of the Murphy eye are specified by the ASTM F-29 committee. This "side port" can allow ventilation if the tip becomes occluded by the tracheal wall, blood clots, or sputum.[5]

Endo/Nasotracheal Tube Materials

Early endotracheal tubes were made of "natural" or synthetic rubber, with cuffs composed of latex. Several of the additives used in the manufacture of these tubes, or chemicals later absorbed, had the potential to be toxic to airway tissue. Currently, the ASTM recommends that materials be tested by *implantation testing*—laboratory analysis of the material's effect on living tissue. Small slivers of the tube material are placed in the muscle of laboratory animals (rabbits). To validate the test, known toxic and known tissue-inert materials are used as controls. The sites are inspected grossly and microscopically after 7 days. Tissue necrosis signals toxic problems. Those materials causing no damage are recommended for patient use. The printing of "F29" on a tracheal tube indicates that it has passed the (ASTM) implantation-testing specifications. Other test methods (e.g., cell culture) may also be used if demonstrated to yield comparable results. Besides a response to chemical components, a reaction to the outer texture of the tube material can occur. The reasons for this effect are less well understood but apparently involve the roughness of the tube's surface.[5]

Currently the following materials are used for endotracheal tubes: natural rubber, synthetic rubber, polyvinyl chloride (PVC), silicone rubber (polysiloxane), and polyethylene. Manufacturers use a variety of accelerators (catalysts), curing agents, plasticizers, stabilizers, antioxidants, fillers, and other additives. The relative merits and problems of the generic materials are listed in Table 20–2. Each manufacturer may customize the material with various additives, altering the rigidity and slipperiness. Tubes are more rigid at room temperatures and quickly soften at body temperature. Exposure to temperatures below freezing can permanently alter materials.[25] Tracheostomy tubes are also constructed of these materials. Tubes of other materials will be reviewed later in this chapter.

An ideal material for tracheal tubes should be nontoxic, soft enough to allow conformation to anatomic pressure points, yet firm enough to resist kinking and permit insertion. The outer surfaces of tubes should be "microscopically" smooth to avoid tissue abrasion. Lastly, the materials used should resist surface bacterial adhesion.[89]

Tube Size

Manufacturers provide a range of outside diameters to fit differing sizes of upper airway structure. Tube diameters for infants and adults are listed in Table 20–3. In adults, generally, the largest diameter tube that fits through the patient's glottis should be used. Nasal intubation usually requires a tube one-half-size smaller, as it must pass through the nose–nasopharynx.

One of the major concerns in clinical care is the potential for airway tubes to increase the resistance

Table 20–2 Materials Used for Manufacture of Tracheal and Tracheostomy Tubes

MATERIAL	ADVANTAGES	PROBLEMS
Natural rubber		• Additives potentially toxic • Tendency to kink • Does not conform to body contours well • Difficult to pass a suction catheter • Degraded by petroleum-based lubricants
Silicone rubber (Silastic polysiloxane)	• Flexible • Conforms well to body contours • Relatively "slick" surface, reducing the tendency of secretions and catheters to adhere	• Overly flexible. May interfere with intubation and necessitate a stylet
Polyvinyl chloride (PVC)	• Soft, smooth nonirritating surface • Reduced tendency to kink at body temperature; tends to mold to body contours • Most widely used substance	• Heat labile • Must be gas sterilized and purged of ETO • Highly flammable with laser therapy
Teflon (polytetrafluoroethylene)	• Can be sterilized by autoclave or boiling • Slippery, nonwettable, nonadhesive surface	• Rigid • Rough surface • Expensive
Polyethylene	• Minimal tissue toxicity	• Low-density polyethylene is flexible, and high-density is rigid

Table 20–3 Recommended Sizes for Tracheal Tubes and Suction Catheters In Newborn and Pediatric Patients

AGE	INTERNAL DIAMETER (mm)	SUCTION (Fr)
Newborn	2.5–3	6
6 mo	3.5	8
18 mo	4.0	8
3 yr	4.5	8
5 yr	5.0	10
6 yr	5.5	10
8 yr	6.0	10
12 yr	6.5	10
16 yr	7.0	10
Adult(female)	8.0–8.5	12
Adult(male)	8.5–9.0	14

(National Conference Steering Committee: Standards for cardiopulmonary resuscitation and emergency cardiac care. JAMA 227:852, 1974. With permission)

to airflow. A greater pressure will be required by the patient (or ventilating device). As a result, the work of breathing will be increased. The differential pressure required to move air through a tube varies, depending on the type of flow conditions. Under laminar flow conditions, the pressure drop down a straight tube follows *Poiseuille's law*:

$$\text{Pressure gradient } (\Delta P) = \frac{8 \times L \times \mu \times \dot{V}}{\pi\, r^4}$$

or

$$\text{"Laminar" resistance } (R) = \frac{\Delta P}{\dot{V}} = \frac{8 \times L \times \mu}{\pi\, r^4}$$

It should be noted that the pressure gradient (ΔP) is linearly related to the flow ($\dot{V}$), *tube length* (L), and viscosity (μ) but inversely proportional to the fourth power of the radius (r).

Rohrer's equation also relates pressure drop to flow. Under laminar conditions the following relationship exists:

$$\text{Pressure gradient } (\Delta P) = K_1 \times \dot{V}$$

K_1 refers to a constant of linear resistance.

For the foregoing equations to best approximate clinical conditions, the tube must be long enough for the establishment of fully developed *laminar* flow. The distance from the entry point is termed the entrance length (*Le*), defined by the following equation.

Length (*Le*) to develop laminar flow = $K^1 \times Re \times D$

K^1 is a constant, D is tube diameter, and *Re* is the Reynolds number.

The *Reynolds number* is a dimensionless number that compares inertial with viscous forces in flowing fluid. It can predict whether flow conditions would be laminar or turbulent; this is relevant because turbulent flows exist in clinical applications. The pressure gradient increases linearly as flow increases, until turbulent flow occurs. Reynolds numbers are laminar if less than 2300 and turbulent if greater than 2500. The following equation defines the Reynolds number:[39]

$$Re = \frac{4 \times \gamma \times \dot{V}}{\pi \times \mu \times D}$$

where μ is viscosity, γ is density, D is the diameter, and $\dot{V}$ is flow.[39] The pressure gradient for fully developed turbulent conditions is described by the following equation:

$$Pressure\ gradient = \Delta P = \frac{8f \times (L/D) \times \dot{V}^2}{\pi \times D^4}$$

The pressure drop is directly related to f, a friction factor (which depends on the Reynolds number and surface roughness), tube length/diameter, and flow squared, but is inversely related to the fourth power of the diameter.

Rohrer's equation describing the pressure drop for *turbulent* flow conditions is as follows:

$$Pressure\ gradient = \Delta P = K_2 \times \dot{V}^2$$

K_2 is the coefficient of nonlinear resistance. It is suggested that under clinical conditions, both laminar and turbulent flows exist. An estimate of the pressure drop is described by summing the two Rohrer equations:

$$Pressure\ gradient = \Delta P = (K_1 \times \dot{V}) + (K_2 \times \dot{V}^2)$$

Most bench tests on tracheal tubes indicate nonlinear flow patterns for breathing conditions that simulate clinical conditions.[13,26,96] Tracheal tubes are not long enough to allow laminar conditions to fully develop. Therefore, Poiseuille's law underestimates the pressure gradient.

Depending on tube size, gas flow, and experimental design, resistance or work of breathing data

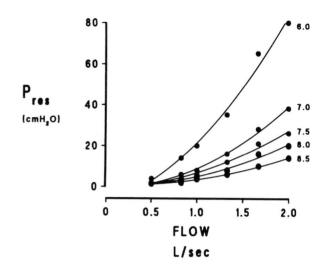

Figure 20–23. Graphic illustration of the pressure gradient or resistive pressure (P_{res}) required to maintain constant flows through varying diameter endotracheal tubes (Wright PE, Marini JJ, Bernard GR: In vitro versus in vivo comparison of endotracheal tube airflow resistance. Am Rev Respir Dis 140:10, 1989, with permission)

will vary. In general, data from in vitro studies indicate that resistance will increase 25% to 100% for each 1-mm decrease in internal tube diameter.[13] Figure 20–23 demonstrates the effect of tube size on the pressure gradient at differing (constant) flows. Figure 20–24 illustrates the effect of changes in tube diameter on work of breathing at differing tidal volume and breathing frequencies.

Patients seldom breathe at constant gas flows; rather, their flow patterns are oscillatory. The *Womersley number* predicts turbulent flow during oscillatory patterns and can be used like the Reynolds number. The physics become more complex when tube curvature and internal surface roughness are also considered. The pressure gradient must increase to maintain flow if there is a bend in a tube. This becomes significant because tubes deform in the body, and the tracheostomy tube has its 90° bend. Secretions will increase the *Moody friction factor*, which is an index of the roughness of the internal lumen.[39]

In vivo studies have demonstrated that airway resistance values will be greater than when measured in vitro. All tubes contribute significantly to distortion of bedside measurements of pulmonary mechanics such as dynamic compliance and airways resistance.[99] In summary, artificial airways require a greater pressure gradient than natural airways, which increases with smaller tubes, longer tubes, and increasing flow.

In addition to the reduced work of breathing, a larger-diameter tube also increases the safety and ease of suctioning. Finally, with a larger tube, the volume of air injected into the cuff can be reduced. If either very small volumes or excessively large volumes are required to produce a seal, there tends to be a change from the usual low-pressure cuff design to that of high pressure. Excessive pressure can lead to ischemic damage to the tracheal mucosa as well as to cartilage erosion. In adults, the regions of the arytenoid and cricoid cartilages are particularly affected.

An empiric rule of thumb is to use an outside diameter (OD) of two-thirds the estimated tracheal diameter. Adult endotracheal tube diameters generally range from approximately 5 to 10 mm ID. Neo-

natal and pediatric anatomies require sizes in the 2.5 to 5.0-mm ID range. Refer to Table 20–3 for age-based diameter estimates for adult and neonatal or pediatric use.

Tube Length

The length of tracheal tubes must be considered for proper placement. Adult nasal tubes require an additional 2 to 4 cm in length over those used orally. The average distance from the nose to midtrachea is approximately 25 cm in a normal adult. The distance from the incisors to the midtrachea is about 21 to 23 cm with oral tubes.

Manufacturers either provide tubes "uncut," with a minimum length recommended by the ASTM, or at a precut length (Table 20–4). The concern is to follow anatomic increases in the diameter

Figure 20–24. (A) Work of breathing through endotracheal tubes of varying diameters and at differing minute ventilation. (Shapiro M, Wilson RK, Gregorio C, Bloom K: Work of breathing through different-sized endotracheal tubes. Crit Care Med 14:1028, 1986, with permission) (B) Work of breathing for varying tidal volumes and respiratory frequencies, showing increase as the internal endotracheal tube diameter decreases. R, ventilatory rate; V_T, tidal volume. (Reprinted with permission from the International Anesthesia Research Society from Boulder AR, Beatty PC, Kay B: The extra work of breathing through adult endotracheal tubes. Anesth Analg 65:853, 1986)

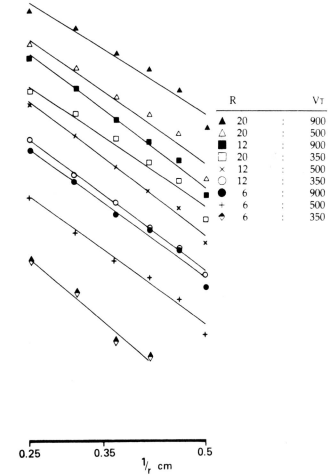

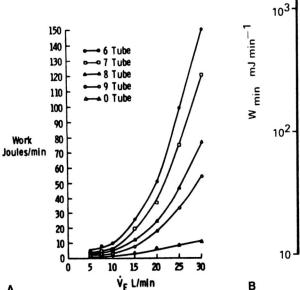

dimension with appropriate increases in length. A tube that is too short cannot have the cuff placed below the vocal cords in the midtrachea; a tube that is too long is more likely to be accidently advanced into a mainstem bronchus.

Tube Cuffs

Before the 1970s, cuffs for endotracheal and tracheostomy tubes were of the low-volume/high-pressure design, and use was limited to short-term intraoperative application. Previously, rare tracheal and laryngeal lesions, such as tracheal stenosis, had begun to be reported in high numbers in the late 1960s.[53] This increase in problems paralleled the increase in the numbers of intensive care units and the acceptance of positive pressure as the method of ventilation (which required an artificial airway). To apply a softer seal to the tracheal wall, clinicians began ''prestretching'' cuffs before their use.[38] Later, manufacturers began producing tubes with a low-pressure design.

The sealing function of the tube's cuff is a threat to the trachea. The pressure applied to the wall causes the following effects:

SHORT-TERM

- Destruction of ciliated epithelium that interferes with mucus transport postextubation.
- Pressure necrosis of mucosal and deep tracheal wall tissue
- Dilatation and rupture of the trachea

LONG-TERM

- Fibrous tracheal stenosis, tracheomalacia, and development of a tracheal zone with poor mucus transport

It is currently accepted that high-pressure cuffs should not be considered for prolonged use. Cuff-to-tracheal wall pressures above 60 cmH$_2$O (8 kPa) destroy columnar epithelial tissue if sustained over 15 minutes.[9,10] When an endotracheal tube is properly sized in the trachea, intracuff pressure should approximate cuff-to-tracheal wall pressure. Pressure on the tracheal wall will become excessive in low-pressure designs when the cuff has to be stretched to fill the trachea (i.e., the tube is too small for the patient). To prevent ischemic damage, the cuff-to-tracheal wall pressure should not exceed tissue capillary perfusion pressure. That pressure is estimated to be 20 to 30 mmHg (2.67 to 4.0

Table 20—4 Tracheal Tube Internal Diameters and Lengths

NOMINAL SIZE (mm)	TOLERANCE (mm)	MINIMUM TUBE LENGTH (cm)	PRECUT LENGTH (cm)
2.5	0.15	14	11
3.0	0.15	16	12
3.5	0.15	18	13
4.0	0.15	20	14
4.5	0.15	22	15
5.0	0.15	24	16
5.5	0.15	27	17
6.0	0.15	28	19
6.5	0.20	29	21
7.0	0.20	30	23
7.5	0.20	31	24
8.0	0.20	32	25
8.5	0.20	32	26
9.0	0.20	32	27
9.5	0.20	32	28
10.0	0.20	32	28

(American Society for Testing and Materials: Standard for cuffed and uncuffed tracheal tubes (F290201). Philadelphia, ASTM, 1989)

kPa) but can be lower with hypotension. In addition, pressure points can develop between cuff and trachea, as the trachea is not circular in cross-section. (Normal variations include C-shaped, D-shaped, elliptic, and triangular.)

When using low-pressure cuffs, the practitioner should attempt to ''just seal'' the airway at pressures below those causing ischemic damage. Intracuff pressure to seal in the trachea can be simulated with artificial tracheas and pressure manometers (Fig. 20—25).

Ideally, the peak intracuff pressures can be maintained at 25 to 27 cmH$_2$O (3.3 to 3.6 kPa) or less.[9,10,53] Manufacturers have developed pressure-relief valves, or large pilot balloon reservoirs to reduce the potential for high intracuff pressures. Operators using the minimum-seal technique auscultate the area above the tracheal cuff for sounds of air movement around the cuff. The smallest amount of air that will just limit airflow around the cuff is injected. Cuff location may move to larger-diameter parts of the trachea with head extension or flexion. This migration can be minimized with the use of tracheal tube stabilizer systems.[7,21]

Manufacturers produce a variety of cuff designs. Cuffs may be circular or cylindrical, large or small in diameter, long or short, of thin- or thick-

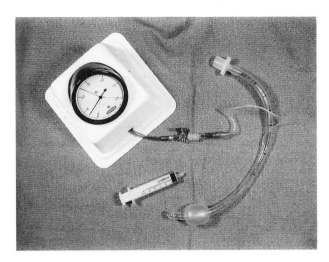

Figure 20—25. An aneroid pressure gauge and stopcock to monitor intracuff pressure.

In spite of contemporary designs and materials, silent aspiration continues to be a problem.[9,65] Aspiration of gastrointestinal material occurs in approximately 30% to 40% of mechanically ventilated patients.[24] Endotracheal tubes bypass the natural defenses of the pharynx. This impairs ciliary activity, interferes with effective cough mechanics, and increases oropharyngeal colonization, which can lead to nosocomial pneumonia. Pneumonias of this type have a significant mortality (55%) in hospitalized, mechanically ventilated patients.[23,24]

SPECIALIZED TRACHEAL TUBES

Foam-cuffed or Kamen–Wilkenson endotracheal tubes differ from standard tubes only in the cuff design (Fig. 20–27). The sealing pressure relies on "recoil forces" of the covered internal foam. Unlike standard cuffs, the cuff self-inflates when the pilot tube is opened to the atmosphere. Active aspiration of air is required so that intubation or extubation can occur. Respiratory care practitioners and nurses must be alert to these differences. Injection of air can turn the device into a high-pressure system. The cuff is spacious and can seal the large trachea. Potential difficulties in using foam-cuffed tubes include air leak with positive airway pressures in excess of 45 to 50 cmH$_2$O (6.0 to 6.67 kPa). Also, cuffs can become soggy and resist complete deflation prior to extubation. Foam-cuffed tubes are an excellent choice for air transport, as they adapt to atmospheric pressure changes. In unpressurized

walled materials, and air or foam filled. Thin-walled, large-diameter cuffs tend to form thin folds against tracheal mucosa. This allows minimal pressure to seal and reduces fluid aspiration through cuff folds. However, intubation and extubation may be more difficult with a cuff that has a "bulky" design when deflated (Fig. 20–26).[53] The ASTM recommends that the endotracheal tube lumen should resist compression from the inflated tube cuff. Nitrous oxide can diffuse into the closed gas space of a tracheal cuff. This results in an increase of intracuff volume and pressure.[90]

Figure 20—26. Endotracheal tube cuff designs demonstrating "trim" and "bulky" cuffs. (A) Tubes with cuffs inflated to therapeutic levels. (B) The same tubes with cuffs completely evacuated of air.

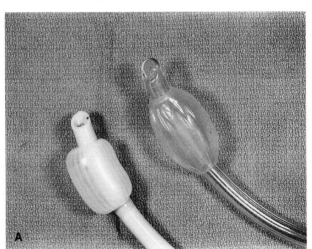

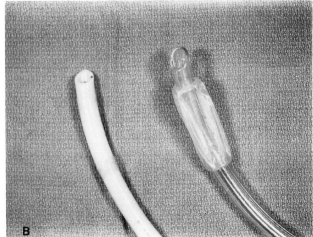

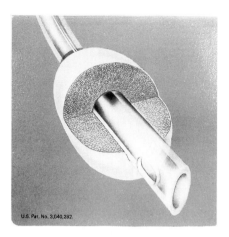

Figure 20—27. Diagram of the Bivona Fome-Cuff endotracheal tube. (Courtesy Bivona, Inc. Gary, Indiana)

aircraft or under loss of pressure, cuff volumes will decrease with increased altitude. With descent, cuff volumes would increase according to Boyle's law (pressure is inversely related to volume).

The "Lindholm anatomic tube" was developed to better fit the curve angle into the trachea (Fig. 20–28). This tube appears to lessen tracheal damage at the cricoid cartilage area but does not spare the arytenoid and tracheal region from injury.[31]

Spiral-embedded tubes have the advantage of withstanding kinking and collapse from external pressure (Fig. 20–29). However, they have excessive flexibility in their longitudinal axis, similar to a long spring (e.g., "Slinky"). A stiffening guidewire or stylet is required for intubation.

The double-lumen endobronchial tube is used to isolate each lung (Fig. 20–30). One-lung anesthesia, lung lavage, and independent lung mechanical

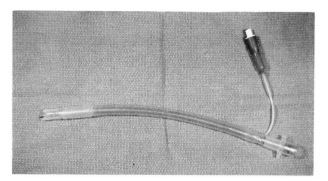

Figure 20—29. A metal spiral-embedded endotracheal tube.

ventilation utilize this type of tube. Older designs such as the rubber Carlens tube have been replaced with contemporary designs (e.g., the Robert-Shaw tube). Either the right or left mainstem bronchus may be intubated, with use of a tracheal and endobronchial cuffs. Care must be taken not to occlude either right or left segmental bronchi to the upper lobes. Ventilation occurs through two separate lumina.[14]

The "Univent" tube incorporates a directable bronchus-blocking cuff to isolate a lung. The blocker cuff can be advanced or retracted on its separate tube, having both pilot and suction channels.[57]

Pediatric Considerations

Uncuffed oral and nasal endotracheal tubes are generally used in neonatal and pediatric practice (Fig. 20–31). As the cricoid cartilage ring poses the

Figure 20—30. A double-lumen endotracheal tube. The distal tip with cuff is designed for left endobronchial intubation, and the proximal cuff seals the trachea above the carina. This system facilitates independent ventilation of right or left lung.

Figure 20—28. The anatomic-shaped Lindholm endotracheal tube.

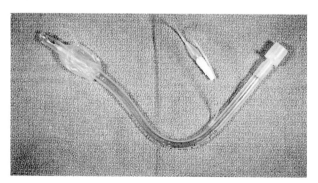

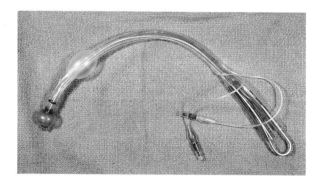

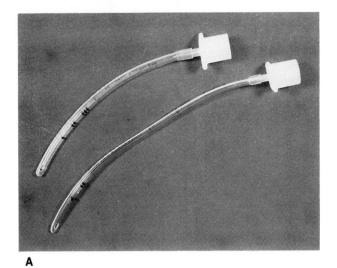

A

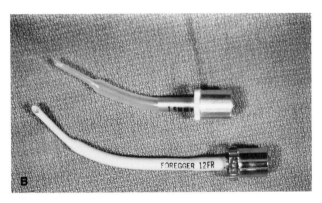

B

Figure 20–31. Pediatric endotracheal tubes. (*A*) Uncuffed, (*B*) Cole-style tubes.

narrowest point in the upper airway for prepubescent children (below the age of 8), an uncuffed tube of appropriate size should provide an adequate seal. Because the mucosa in this area is prone to trauma, a small leak is required. The following formulas can provide approximate clinical guides for uncuffed tube selection:

INSIDE DIAMETER (mm)

- Premature neonates: 2.5–3.0 mm
- Normal neonate: 3.5 mm
- Infants and children:
- $\dfrac{18 + \text{age (years)}}{4}$

Note: If a cuffed tube is used, it should be one-half-size smaller than calculated.

LENGTH (cm)

- Oral endotracheal tube length in children and neonates: $\dfrac{\text{age}}{2} + 12$[52]
- Nasal tracheal tube length in neonates: $0.16 \times \text{height (cm)} + 4.5 \text{ cm}$[58]

Some length recommendations are based on outside airway measurements or other body dimensions.[19,37] Endotracheal tubes have a black safety line that, if placed at the level of the vocal cords, ensures that the tip will be in the midtracheal region.

The Cole tube differs in that the distal 25% of its length is smaller than the proximal portion (see Fig. 20–31). The advantages are the increased proximal tube diameter and the fact that the "shoulder" area of narrowing abuts against the larynx, preventing accidental distal movement. However, pressure on glottic structures can result in necrosis.

High-frequency ventilation techniques have prompted the design of a specialized uncuffed tube. A jet delivery tube opens into the main lumen at a distance of 2 to 6 cm proximal to the end. In addition, a pressure monitoring channel opens 1 cm from the distal tube tip.[40]

Stylets and Changing Tubes

Stylets are malleable metal wires that can be inserted through the ventilating lumen of oral endotracheal tubes. The wire provides internal support and allows alteration of the tube's natural curvature. Although not a routinely used device, the stylet should be available for the difficult intubation. Users should confirm that the wire does not extend beyond the distal tip of the tube. Stylets should be lightly lubricated with a water-soluble product.

"Tube changers" are long hollow or solid plastic tubes that facilitate removal and replacement of endotracheal tubes. Suction catheters can also function for this purpose. The changer is inserted through the existing endotracheal tube, the patient is extubated without removing the tube changer, and the new tube is then slipped over the changer. A battery-powered lighted stylet ("light wand") is also available for intubation or changing tubes (see Fig. 20–50).[72]

Laryngoscopes

A laryngoscope is used to manipulate the structures in the upper airway to permit direct visualization and insertion of an endotracheal tube into the

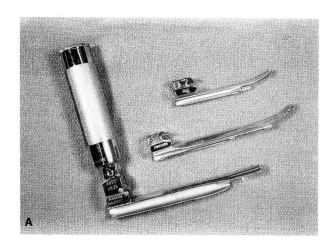
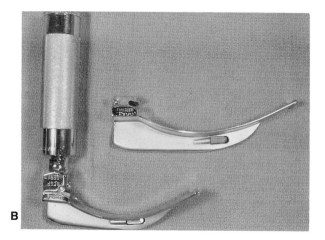

Figure 20—32. Laryngoscope handle and blades. (*A*) straight blades; (*B*) curved (McIntosh) blades.

glottis. The scope consists of a handle and blade with distal light (Fig. 20–32). The instruments are commonly made of plated metal, but disposable plastic laryngoscopes are also available. Batteries are contained inside the handle, which has an electrical contact point at the blade connection. Further discussion of laryngoscopes occurs later in this chapter.

TRACHEOSTOMY TUBES

Tracheostomy tubes provide an airway directly through the anterior neck into the tracheal lumen. Tracheostomy tube placement is generally indicated for long-term mechanical ventilation, chronic secretion management, and as an emergency airway. (A more complete discussion on the rationale and problems of tracheostomy care will follow in this chapter.) The tubes are available in a variety of sizes, styles, and materials. The standard clinical tracheostomy tube has a neck flange, tube body (extra- and intratracheal portions), and cuff (Fig. 20–33A). Tracheostomy tubes may also be uncuffed (see Fig. 20–33B), have removable inner cannulas (see Fig. 20–33C), and fenestrations (openings) to allow ventilation through the larynx (see Fig. 20–33D). A removable obturator permits easier insertion through the stoma.

Dimensions

Table 20–5 lists dimensions for standard tracheostomy tubes. In contrast with the inside-diameter sizing of endotracheal tubes, several systems describe the outside diameter for tracheostomy tubes. Anatomic variations of neck length, location, and diameter of the tracheostomy incision are factors that affect tube sizing for patients. Surgeons hope to limit the damaged area in the trachea by avoiding large stoma sites and excessively large tubes. In general, 10-mm OD (approximately 7-mm ID) tubes are optimal for adult women and 11-mm OD (approximately 8-mm ID) for men. French sizing is based on the circumference of the outer surface of

Table 20—5 Tracheostomy Tube Size and Conversion

OUTSIDE DIAMETER (mm)	FRENCH	JACKSON	APPROXIMATE INTERNAL DIAMETER (mm)
4.3	13	00	2.5
5.0	15	0	3.0
5.5	16.5	1	3.5
6.0	18	2	4.0
7.0	21	3	4.5–5.0
8.0	24	4	5.5
9.0	27	5	6.0–6.5
10.0	30	6	7.0
11.0	33	7	7.5–8.0
12.0	36	8	8.5
13.0	39	9	9.0–9.5
14.0	42	10	10.0
15.0	45	11	10.5–11.0
16.0	48	12	11.5

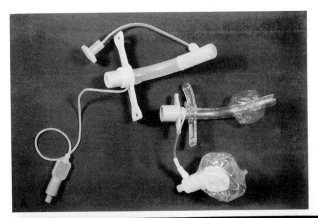

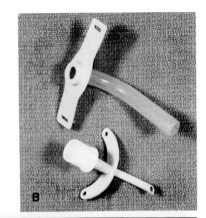

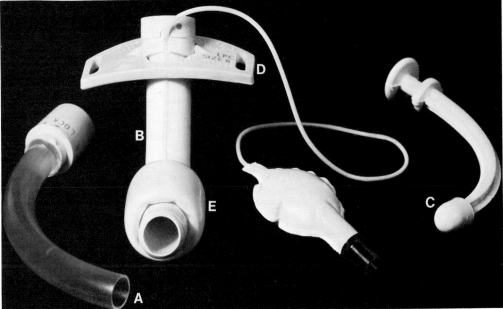

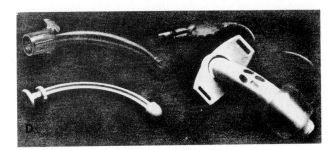

Figure 20—33. Tracheostomy tubes (A) standard disposable cuffed tracheostomy tube; (B) adult and pediatric uncuffed tracheostomy tubes; (C) tracheostomy tube, with removable inner cannula (on left) and obturator (right); (D) fenestrated tracheostomy tube, with inner cannula and obturator.

the tube. The following formula allows conversion to French sizing:

$$\text{French (mm)} = 3 \times \text{outside diameter (mm)}$$

The lengths of tubes have been standardized, but extralong tubes are available. These are helpful in morbidly obese patients. The intratracheal part of the tube should be straight and somewhat flexible. A desirable tube has a smooth curvature, with a small radius between intra- and extratracheal limbs. This permits an entrance of close to 90°, lessening pressure on the longitudinal aspect of the tracheal stoma. Once in the trachea, the tube sides or tip should not produce pressure points on the tracheal wall. In addition to the tracheal wall, the esophagus and major blood vessels are at risk for erosion. The flange should permit gentle yet firm fixation of the tube. Excessive movement of the tube increases the potential for lesions, especially at the stoma level. Some tubes have adjustable flanges to change the extratracheal dimension.[4]

Materials

Contemporary disposable tracheostomy tubes are composed of synthetic materials similar to endotracheal tubes. In addition, manufacturers produce tracheostomy tubes made of silver (or silver plate), nylon, and Teflon. These materials are considered for permanent tracheostomy and are more rigid than rubber or synthetics. Their inability to flex with the trachea can cause pressure necrosis. Oxides from metal tubes tend to cause tissue irritation and increased mucus production. However, the advantage is the ability to be sterilized by boiling or autoclaving. Cuffs are less commonly used on these materials but can be applied. High-pressure cuffs generally have been replaced with high-compliance, low-pressure designs. Cuffs that are thin-walled and that hug the tube when deflated are easier to insert or remove from a narrow stoma. The previously mentioned Kamen-Wilkinson Fome-Cuff is also available with tracheostomy tubes.

Special Purpose Tracheostomy Tubes

Laryngectomy tubes are shorter than standard tracheostomy tubes from the outer neck skin to the trachea. Rigid, three-piece tubes are generally used, although synthetic rubber tubes are available. Removal of the larynx obviates the need for cuffs on laryngectomy tubes.

Armored wire spiral-lined tubes are used to prevent compression from kinking in patients with short, bulky necks.

Fenestrated ("windowed") tracheostomy tubes allow selective opening of a channel to permit use of the natural airway above the tracheostomy tube (see Fig. 20–33D). Removal of an inner cannula gives access to a 6 to 8- by 8 to 10-mm orifice. The standard tracheal opening is plugged and the cuff deflated, allowing air movement through the vocal cords. Patients who use this device should have fairly good control of their airway and adequate spontaneous ventilation. Patients who again require ventilation or protection from aspiration can have the inner cannula reinserted and cuff inflated. Although manufacturers produce precut fenestrations, only 50% of patients have an anatomic structure that can be accommodated. Patients with measured distances of 34 mm or more from skin to anterior trachea generally do not fit standard tubes; custom fenestrations may be created in both metal and plastic tubes.[15,88] The ASTM has adopted standards for pediatric tracheostomy tubes.[4]

Speaking tracheostomy tubes have a separate pilot tube that directs compressed gas to an exit point just above the cuff (Fig. 20–34A, B). with practice, the patient can coordinate speech. Being able to again vocalize is a delight for most patients, especially those who have long been ventilator-dependent. Clinicians will be required to set inlet flows to the patient's needs. Automated devices can synchronize gas flow to the talking port during the expiratory phase of mechanical ventilation.[45] This is necessary for use by patients unable to operate the gas flow Y-piece. Operators should not confuse the cuff and talking tubes, to avoid blowing up the cuff in-situ. Special valves are also available for use with standard tubes with cuffs deflated (e.g., Passy-Muir Inc. and Olympic Medical; Fig. 20–35A, B).

The Montgomery tracheal T-tube was developed to act as a flexible internal stent in supporting the tracheal wall (Fig. 20–36A, B). The upper limb of the T fits into the trachea; the remaining limb fits through the surgical opening. A stopper may be placed in its outer orifice. Placement is performed by manipulation of a curved hemostat, analogous to putting on trousers one leg at a time. The tube is made of silicone plastic and is available in a number of sizes. Emergency resuscitation of a patient with a T-tube should be attempted with the outer cannula occluded, using mask–bag-valve to ventilate the nose and mouth.[62]

Tracheostomy "buttons" or stoma cannulas extend through the anterior neck to the tracheal wall (Fig. 20–37). The purpose of these devices is to prevent stoma closure and allow access to the trachea for suctioning or emergency ventilation. There is no intratracheal cannula. Usually, there is an in-

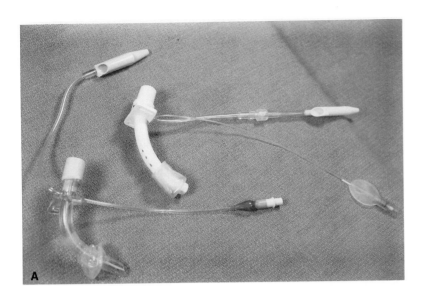

Figure 20—34. Speaking tracheostomy tubes. (*A*) Two speaking tubes. (*B*) Diagram of airflow directed toward the vocal cords when the Y-tube is occluded. (Safar P, Grenvik A: Speaking cuffed tracheostomy tube. Crit Care Med 3:23, 1975, © Williams & Wilkins, with permission)

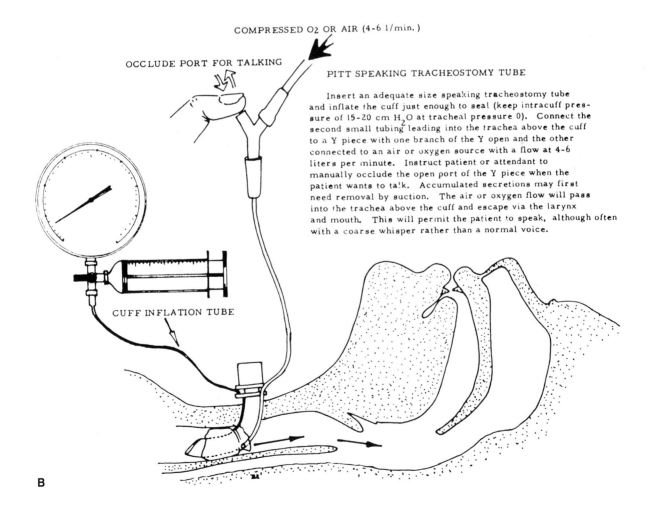

COMPRESSED O2 OR AIR (4-6 1/min.)

OCCLUDE PORT FOR TALKING

PITT SPEAKING TRACHEOSTOMY TUBE

Insert an adequate size speaking tracheostomy tube and inflate the cuff just enough to seal (keep intracuff pressure of 15-20 cm H_2O at tracheal pressure 0). Connect the second small tubing leading into the trachea above the cuff to a Y piece with one branch of the Y open and the other connected to an air or oxygen source with a flow at 4-6 liters per minute. Instruct patient or attendant to manually occlude the open port of the Y piece when the patient wants to talk. Accumulated secretions may first need removal by suction. The air or oxygen flow will pass into the trachea above the cuff and escape via the larynx and mouth. This will permit the patient to speak, although often with a coarse whisper rather than a normal voice.

CUFF INFLATION TUBE

B

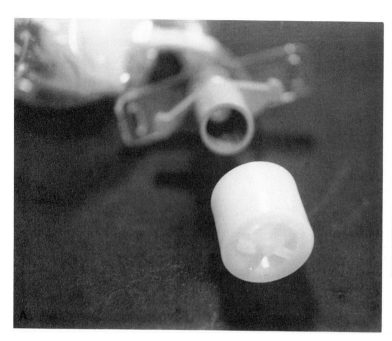
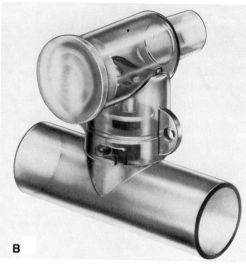

Figure 20–35. Valves to facilitate speech with tracheostomy tubes. (*A*) Passy-Muir valve; (*B*) an Olympic Trach-Talk valve.

ternal structure made of plastic "petals" or "washers" to gently retain the tube at the posterior stoma wall. Units can be made of rigid Teflon, such as shown in Figure 20–37*A* (Olympic Medical), or flexible silicon–rubber, as shown in Figure 20–37 *B*, *C* (Kistner and Montgomery).[48,62] One-way valves may be added to allow inspiration through the tube, permitting vocalization on exhalation. Pa-

tient sizing requires measurement of distances from the neck to the posterior stoma; manufacturers make both standard and custom lengths.[55] In these patients, emergency access to the trachea can also be obtained by cricothyrotomy. A review of this technique will be found later in this chapter in the discussion of the difficult intubation.

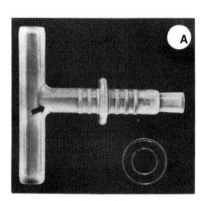
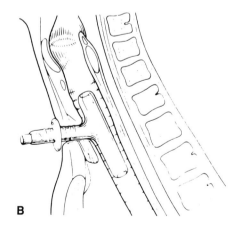

Figure 20–36. Montgomery T-tube. (*A*) Montgomery tracheal tube; (*B*) Montgomery tube in position. (Montgomery WW: Current modifications of the salivary bypass tube and tracheal tube. Ann Otol Rhinol Laryology 95:121, 1986; with permission)

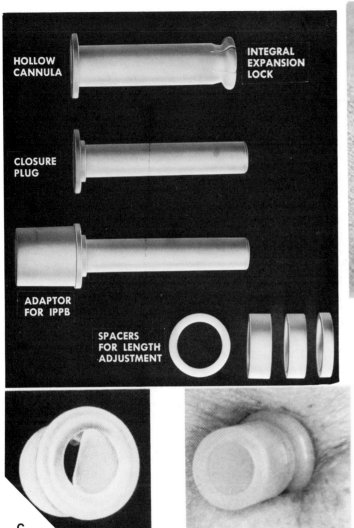

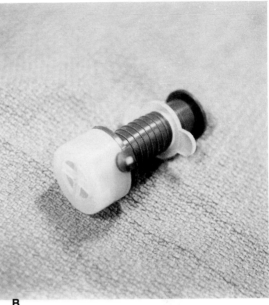

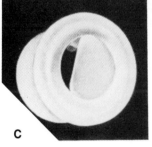

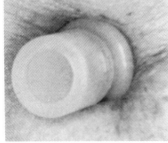

Figure 20–37. Tracheal stoma appliances. (A) Olympic tracheostomy button; (B) Kistner "valved" tracheostomy button; (C) Montgomery "valved" tracheostomy button. (Montgomery WW: Current modifications of the salivary bypass tube and tracheal tube. Ann Otol Rhinol Laryngol 95:121, 1986; with permission)

TRACHEAL INTUBATION

INDICATIONS FOR TRACHEAL INTUBATION

Not all situations requiring airway management call for endotracheal intubation. In fact, less aggressive measures, such as those previously described, may result in an improved clinical condition in which airway support is no longer required. Even when the decision to intubate has been made, intelligent "preintubation" airway management permits a more controlled atmosphere in which tracheal intubation can take place.

Indications for intubation are not always clear-cut and should be made on an individual basis for each patient. Table 20–6 lists many of these indications.

To assure the patency of the airway in certain situations, a tracheal tube may need to be placed. Respiratory depression, a depressed gag reflex, depressed cough, and relaxation of the posterior pharynx can occur (e.g., anesthesia, head trauma, etc.), and if the airway is not protected, can lead to aspiration. Anatomic abnormalities such as paralyzed vocal cords or external compression of the airway from hematoma or cervical tumor can also result in an inability to assure patency of the airway. Not

Table 20—6 Potential Indications for Intubation

To ensure a patent (unobstructed) airway
To protect from potential regurgitation and aspiration
To provide a conduit for the application of positive-pressure ventilation
To provide a conduit for suctioning
General anesthesia

---

only does the tracheal tube provide a conduit through which a patient can receive mechanical ventilatory support, it also allows the practitioner to institute various expiratory maneuvers, such as positive end-expiratory pressure (PEEP) or continuous positive airway pressure (CPAP). The tracheal tube provides a conduit for repeated suctioning of airway secretions in those patients who are producing copious quantities of sputum. Tracheal intubation is required during certain operative procedures, such as those in which the patients have either full stomachs or intestinal obstruction, intrathoracic procedures, operations in the prone position, and intracranial operations. Tracheal intubation should probably be performed whenever muscle relaxants are used, since these medications render the protective airway reflexes incapable of functioning.

ETHICS

Intubation of some patients may not improve outcome because of the prognosis of the underlying disease. Identifying such patients is an important task facing the physician in charge. A decision not to intubate might be made after medical, legal, and ethical–religious issues have been addressed and the patient and responsible relatives have been given the opportunity to express their desires (see Chap. 5). To help resolve ethical questions related to the appropriateness of tracheal intubation, an institutional ethics committee may be of help in providing advice and support for the care providers, the patients, and their families.[29]

CREDENTIALING

Because tracheal intubation is invasive and potentially associated with complications, only trained personnel should be allowed to perform the procedure. Institutions should credential personnel who perform intubation, with consideration given to

formal training, on-the-job experience, and continued medical education.

EVALUATION OF THE PATIENT

To predict the ease or difficulty of tracheal intubation, a thorough evaluation is necessary. Occasionally, despite evaluation, a patient may present unexpected problems; thus, a failed intubation attempt must always be anticipated even when the initial evaluation does not suggest potential difficulty. Any disease or anatomic defect (either acquired or congenital) that interferes with the mobility of the cervical spine or the mandible, or that alters the soft tissues of the nares, oral cavity, or neck may create difficulties for the respiratory care practitioner who is attempting tracheal intubation.

Medical History

In addition to a thorough physical evaluation, an accurate history can be an indicator of a potential difficulty. One should search the patient's history for documentation of previous intubations and whether these intubations were associated with difficulty. A medical history might alert the intubationist to potential difficulties if it includes certain congenital anatomic defects. These might include mandibular hypoplasia (e.g., Pierre Robin and Treacher Collins-Franceschetti syndromes), maxillary hypoplasia (e.g., Apert's disease), a deficiency in number of cervical vertebrae (e.g., Klippel-Feil syndrome), and macroglossia (e.g., Beckwith-Wiedemann syndrome). In addition, certain acquired anatomic defects might suggest a potentially difficult intubation, including tracheal stenosis, retropharyngeal abscess, epiglottitis, and rheumatoid arthritis (which may affect mobility of the cervical spine, temporal mandibular joint, or the arytenoid cartilages). Patients should be questioned about recent food or liquid ingestion because pulmonary aspiration of gastric material is more likely in these patients. Patients should also be asked about dental appliances; these should be removed before intubation to avoid obstruction of the airway and aspiration. A history of blood-clotting disturbances or nasal polyps would be important information for the intubationist considering nasal intubation.

Global Assessment

A global assessment is a quick evaluation of the patient's level of consciousness, vital signs (blood pressure, pulse, respirations), and overall severity of illness. The patient who has lost consciousness or the ability to spontaneously breathe, or who is hemodynamically unstable may require more immediate and special considerations when performing tracheal intubation. Depending on the results of this global assessment, further evaluation may need to be abbreviated or particular aspects emphasized.

Nasal Examination

When nasotracheal intubation is being considered, each naris should be assessed for patency, and the nasal septum should be examined for deviation. The naris that allows the most unhindered approach should be used for tracheal tube introduction.

Oral Cavity

Prior to intubation, the oral cavity should be inspected for foreign bodies; if found, they should be removed. Any existing teeth are inspected. Long, protruding teeth may limit the opening of the oral cavity. Any loose teeth should be identified and possibly removed by trained dental personnel if time permits.[54]

Tongue

A large tongue may present great difficulties to the intubationist, because this structure must be manipulated to directly view the larynx. If on inspection of the oral cavity, the tongue obstructs the view of the uvula, the patient should be asked to flatten the tongue by saying "ah." If the uvula still cannot be visualized, a difficult oral intubation should be anticipated[80,60] (Fig. 20–38).

Temporomandibular Joint

Temporomandibular joint function can be assessed by the insertion of adult fingers into the oral cavity. With fingers extended and placed into the oral cavity at its midline, three normal adult-sized fingers should be accommodated (Fig. 20–39). Patients capable of accommodating two or fewer fingers have some limitation of their temporomandibular joint and may be more difficult to intubate orally.

Mandible

Recognition of severe forms of mandibular hypoplasia, as in Pierre Robin syndrome, is not difficult. However, more subtle hypoplasia may be identified by placing fingers horizontally beneath the chin. The distance from the hyoid bone to the mandibu-

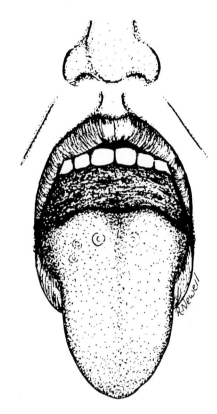

Figure 20—38. Inspection of the oral cavity showing obstructed view; uvula not visualized. (Mollampati SR, Gatt SP, Gugino LD, Sukumar PD, et al: A clinical sign to predict difficult intubation. Can J Anaesth 32:429, 1985; with permission)

lar symphysis is about three fingerbreadths in the normal adult (Fig. 20–40.) If two or fewer adult fingerbreadths are accommodated, the mandible is considered to be hypoplastic and intubation may be difficult.

Cervical Spine

Patients with short and immobile necks are more difficult to intubate. Factors that limit neck (cervical spine) mobility include obesity, cervical radiation therapy, previous cervical surgery, and other cervical deficiencies. Mobility of the cervical spine is assessed by measuring the distance from the lower border of the mandible and the thyroid notch at full neck extension; this distance should be greater than four fingerbreadths in the adult[64] (Fig. 20–41). With a thorough evaluation, potential intubation problems usually should be uncovered; however, there will always exist situations for which difficulty in intubation arises without good

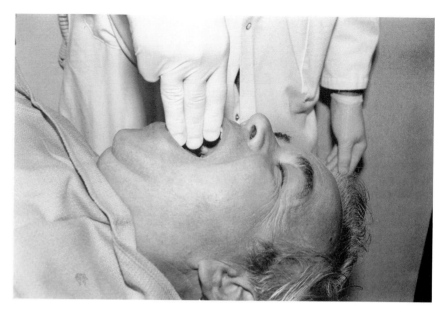

Figure 20—39. Accommodation of three fingerbreadths into the oral cavity, indicating adequate temporomandibular joint mobility.

explanation. Accordingly, the intubationist should always be prepared for the unexpected.

ROUTE FOR INTUBATION

Once a decision has been made to intubate a patient, the clinician must choose an appropriate route from which the tracheal tube is inserted into the trachea. The three main routes for tracheal intubation include:

1. Oral
2. Nasal
3. Transtracheal (to be discussed under tracheostomy)

Figure 20—40. Adequate mandibular length is indicated by a three-fingerbreadth distance from the hyoid bone to the mandibular symphysis.

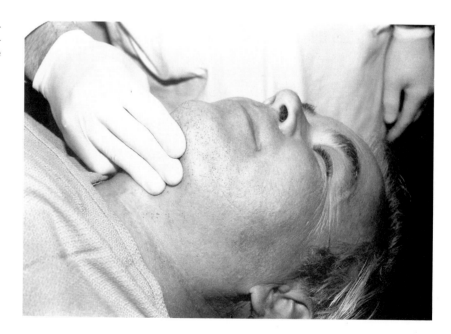

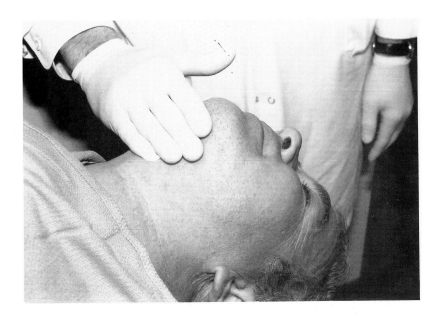

Figure 20—41. Adequate cervical spine mobility is indicated by a four-fingerbreadth distance from the mandibular symphysis to the thyroid notch at full neck extension.

Oral Tracheal route

In most instances, tracheal intubation can be accomplished most expediently through the oral route. Because the vocal cords are usually visualized during oral tracheal intubation, the tube can be placed with greater assurance. Oral tracheal tubes are less likely to kink than nasal tracheal tubes; this might result in less airflow resistance and, also, less obstruction to the passage of the suction catheter or fibroptic bronchoscope. In addition, the oral route can usually accommodate a tube 0.5 to 1 mm wider than the nasal route and, for this reason, may lessen airflow resistance and facilitate suctioning.

Potential disadvantages of oral tracheal intubation include the activation of the gag reflex, which may require higher doses of sedatives for patient tolerance. Oral hygiene is more difficult to maintain with an oral tube, since the swallowing mechanism is interfered with and oral pharyngeal secretions are stimulated by the presence of the tube.

Nasal Route

Possible advantages of the nasal route include situations in which access to the mouth is difficult or impossible, as when patients have mandibular trismus, status epilepticus, or a fractured mandible. In addition, certain oral surgical procedures require unhindered oral access. The nasal tracheal route is usually better tolerated by the patient, especially those who require tracheal intubation for extended periods. The nasal tracheal tube is easier to stabilize after its placement and does not run the risk of being occluded by the patient biting on the tube.

Possible disadvantages to nasal tracheal intubation include potential tissue destruction and hemorrhage as the tube passes through the nares. In addition, there is the potential for the development of sinusitis after a patient has been intubated for several days.

EQUIPMENT

A checklist of necessary equipment for intubation is provided in Table 20–7.

Blades

There are two general types of laryngoscope blades, the straight blade and the curved blade (Fig. 20–42). Examples of the straight blade include the Miller, the Wis-Hipple, and the Flag. The primary example of the curved blade is the McIntosh. The curved blade (McIntosh) has a larger blade surface area for easier manipulation of the tongue; the larger blade also allows more room for passage of the tracheal tube. Because of the curved blade's placement in the vallecula during intubation, there is less stimulation of the highly innervated epiglot-

Table 20—7   Equipment Needed
for Intubation

Two laryngoscopes handles with a variety of straight and
 curved blades
Oral and nasopharyngeal airways
A variety of endotracheal tubes
Syringe
Lubricant
Suction devices
McGill forceps
Tape
Local anesthetic solution
Large-bore angiocath (12 gauge)
Endotracheal tube ties
Eye shields and rubber gloves
Pulse oximeter

tis and thus, at least potentially, less chance for laryngospasm. The straight blade (e.g., Miller) allows greater exposure of the glottic opening, thereby permitting visualization of the tube as it passes through the vocal cords, consequently, greater assurance of proper tube placement.

Equipment in the Pediatric Patient

Equipment of varied shapes and sizes is necessary to accommodate the variety of patients seen in a pediatric practice. Suction catheters, laryngoscope blades, tracheal tubes, stylets, facemasks, and so on

Figure 20—42. Miller (straight) blade (*top*) and McIntosh (curved) blade (*bottom*).

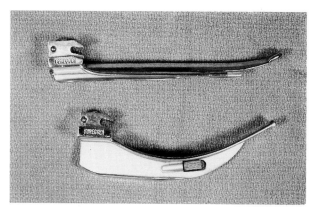

must be selected in an appropriate size to accommodate the patient. Estimates of the sizes of the equipment to be used should be made before therapeutic intervention; however, a variety of sizes of all equipment should be available, in the event that initial estimations prove inaccurate. A laryngoscope of appropriate size and shape is important in the pediatric patient. When using a blade that is too long for a particular patient for tracheal intubation, the tendency is to use it as a lever and pry the mouth open, with potential injury to the upper teeth and lip. A straight, rather than a curved, laryngoscope blade is preferred in the pediatric patient, for it allows easier manipulation of the epiglottis and better exposure of the larynx.

Equipment and Infection-Control Policy

Body secretions (blood, saliva, or other) of all patients should be treated as if they are contaminated. All contaminated equipment should be packaged in nonpenetrable bags and disposed of, if nonreusable, or transported to an area where cleaning of reusable equipment takes place. Reusable equipment is mechanically cleaned and then either gas sterilized with ethylene oxide, steam sterilized at 278° F for 10 minutes, or disinfected with 2% glutaraldehyde (a 45-minute soak in 2% glutaraldehyde is required to kill acid-fast bacilli; less time is required to kill viral organisms). To avoid the potential of contracting a transmissible disease, the practitioner should not come in contact with a patient's body secretions. Eye shields, rubber gloves, masks, and gowns may be necessary to avoid such exposure when performing endotracheal intubation.[66]

TRANSLARYNGEAL INTUBATION

PROCEDURE

Translaryngeal intubation may be performed by several different approaches. The choice of approach depends on the patient's clinical condition and, hence, the immediacy of the required intubation, the skill and the preference of the respiratory care practitioner, and the availability and skills of the supporting staff. The following techniques of translaryngeal intubation will be discussed: (1) awake oral intubation, (2) intubation under sedation, (3) intubation under general anesthesia, and (4) nasal intubation.

AWAKE ORAL INTUBATION

The awake oral intubation procedure is most appropriate for neonates and for patients who are unresponsive, who have recently ingested food, or in whom a preintubation evaluation has alerted one to the potential of a difficult intubation. A "first look" before the administration of sedative or anesthetic drugs is often desired in certain patients, such as patients with intestinal obstruction or trauma to the upper airway. In skillful hands, an awake intubation can be performed within a few seconds.

Despite the advantages of expediency, awake intubation is almost never ideal. In the patient who is not completely unconscious, awake intubation often provokes either vagal or sympathetic stimulation, with associated cardiac and bronchospastic effects. For the conscious patient, the experience of an awake intubaton can be traumatic. If time permits, administration of local anesthesia to the oral cavity, plus intravenous sedative drugs, may render the procedure more tolerable. As in all procedures for endotracheal intubation, the first task to perform is an equipment check (see Table 20–7). One should administer 100% oxygen through a bag and mask for 3 minutes prior to intubation. The availability of a suction apparatus is essential. The laryngoscope should be checked for proper functioning, as should the competency of the cuff of the tracheal tube. The tracheal tube should not be re-

moved from its sterile container until it is handed to the respiratory care practitioner at the time of the intubation. If lubrication jelly is applied to the distal end of the endotracheal tube, it should be done with sterile gauze, and then the endotracheal tube should be immediately replaced in its sterile container.

The patient is positioned supine; the neck is flexed to a moderate degree by placing a folded towel beneath the head. Next, the head is extended to achieve the sniff position. The three axes, those of the mouth, the pharynx, and the trachea are then aligned to permit direct visualization of the larynx (see Fig. 20–4).

In patients with depressed levels of consciousness (especially those with recent food ingestion or intestinal obstruction), a Sellick maneuver should be performed. An assistant applies thumb and index finger pressure at the level of the cricoid cartilage to compress the esophagus and prevent any gastric contents from being regurgitated and aspirated (Fig. 20–43).[83] The cricoid cartilage is the best location for esophageal compression because it is at this point that a cartilaginous ring completely surrounds the airway.

The respiratory care practitioner uses eye shields and gloves for protection from potentially infectious body secretions. A gown is worn if splashing of contaminated material is possible.

The laryngoscope is held with the left hand and

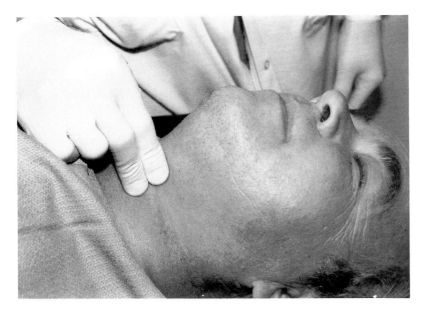

Figure 20—43. The Sellick maneuver is performed by having an assistant apply thumb, index finger, and middle finger pressure at the level of the cricoid ring.

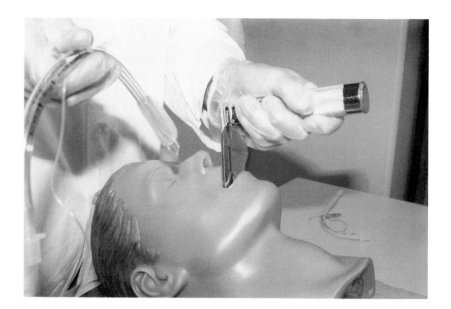

Figure 20—44. Intubation technique for oral tracheal intubation.

the blade is inserted to the right of the midline of the mouth (Figs. 20–44, 20–45). The tongue is elevated and moved to the left. As the blade is advanced, the epiglottis will come into view. When using a curved blade, its tip is placed in the valle-

Figure 20—45. Direct oral laryngoscopy with a Miller (straight) blade (Finucane BT, Santora AH: Principles of Airway Management. Philadelphia, FA Davis, 1988, with permission)

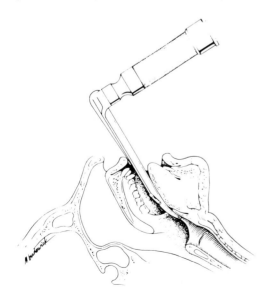

cula; when using a straight blade, the tip is placed beneath the epiglottis. Elevation in the direction of the laryngoscope handle should bring the larynx into full view.

The laryngoscope should never be used as a lever against the upper teeth. The tracheal tube is next inserted with the right hand from the right corner of the mouth. The distal end of the tracheal tube is visualized as it passes between the vocal chords into the glottic opening.

Immediately after intubation, the location of the tracheal tube is verified by an assistant listening over the epigastrium for any gurgling as positive pressure is applied to the tracheal tube. Gurgling indicates an esophageal intubation. If gurgling is heard, the tracheal tube should be left in place, the cuff inflated, and the application of positive pressure to the proximal end of the tube discontinued. A second tracheal tube should then be obtained and placed under direct visualization into the trachea. An assistant listens to both lung apices for breath sounds after a silent epigastrium has been verified.

The tracheal tube cuff is inflated to a volume that is required to just occlude any air leak around the endotracheal tube. After the endotracheal tube has been securely taped or tied into place, a chest x-ray is obtained to confirm that the tracheal tube tip lies in the middle portion of the trachea (near the level of the aortic knob). If the patient becomes hypoxic or if vital signs deteriorate immediately following tracheal intubation, one must strongly suspect misplacement of the tube and, under direct visualization with the use of a laryngoscope, establish that the tracheal tube traverses the glottic opening between the two vocal cords into the trachea.

Confirmation of tracheal intubation can also be obtained with use of a CO_2 monitor.[95] If a tracheal tube is correctly positioned in the trachea, the percentage of expired CO_2 should rise from almost 0% on inspiration to approximately 6% on expiration. If the endotracheal tube is placed in the esophagus, the percentage of CO_2 should rise and fall very little with respiration. Pulse oximetry is another useful monitoring device that may alert the respiratory care practitioner to the possibility of an esophageal or bronchial intubation by detecting hypoxemia.[101] However, the pulse oximeter is not as sensitive in detecting esophageal intubation as the CO_2 monitor, and will not alarm the practitioner until hypoxemia and possibly hypercarbic acidosis has occurred.

INTUBATION UNDER SEDATION

The items discussed for awake oral intubation also apply to patients receiving tracheal intubation under sedation. Sedative drugs, when properly administered, usually allow a more relaxed atmosphere and a more pleasant intubation experience for both patient and practitioner. Because sedative drugs take time to administer and titrate to effect, their use may be inappropriate in certain emergency situations. In addition, sedative drugs may have undesirable side effects, such as cardiovascular and respiratory depression, that would be particularly disadvantageous in an emergency situation. Hence, sedative drugs are usually reserved for those situations for which the expediency of tracheal intubation is not paramount.

The most reliable way to administer sedative drugs is by the intravenous route. The infusion of two drugs (one benzodiazepine and one narcotic) is a popular means of achieving sedation. Numerous different combinations of these two classes of drugs are used. Benzodiazepines produce sedation along with sleepiness and anterograde amnesia, usually with minimal respiratory depression and a mild decrease in blood pressure. Benzodiazepines can sometimes have unpredictable sedative effects and, occasionally, a paradoxical central nervous system stimulation occurs. Special caution should be used when sedating elderly and debilitated patients with benzodiazepines, as such patients can be sensitive to the respiratory depressive, cardiovascular depressive, and the sedative effects of the drug; also, the effects of the drug can be longer-lasting.

Diazepam (Valium) is one of the most popular benzodiazepines and the one that, until recently, has been used most frequently. The anterograde amnestic effect of diazepam begins about 1 to 2 minutes after intravenous injection; however, the sedative effect is quite variable. In some patients, as little as 0.07 mg/kg given intravenously can produce unconsciousness; in others, as much as 1 mg/kg given intravenously will produce little more than drowsiness. In adults, diazepam should be administered in incremental doses of 2.5 mg intravenously, with sedative, respiratory, and cardiovascular effects monitored carefully. The metabolites of diazepam (especially desmethyldiazepam) can accumulate after large or repeated doses and can cause prolonged effects of the drug.

Desmethyldiazepam is only slightly less potent than diazepam, and its plasma concentrations increase steadily over approximately the first 24 hours after injection of diazepam. This metabolite can contribute to a return of drowsiness after apparent recovery following diazepam administration.

Midazolam (Versed) is a newer benzodiazepam that has achieved recent popularity. This popularity results from the water-soluble nature of the drug, which causes less irritation and pain on intravenous injection. In addition, midazolam has a much shorter metabolic half-life (2 to 4 hours). However, as with diazepam, the effects of midazolam can be quite capricious and unpredictable. Midazolam is approximately two to four times more potent than diazepam; therefore, 0.5 to 1.0 mg increments of the drug should be used for sedation.

Opiates are often used in conjunction with benzodiazepines in preparing the patient for intubation. Opiates (narcotics) provide analgesia and also suppress the cough reflex. The side effects of opiates are primarily respiratory, but hypotension, bradycardia, nausea, and vomiting may also occur. The combination of benzodiazepines and narcotics can have a synergistic respiratory and cardiovascular depressive effect. Morphine is one of the most popular narcotics and has been used over the years for providing sedation. It is administered in incremental doses of 1 to 3 mg intravenously; its metabolic half-life is approximately 2 to 3 hours.

Fentanyl (Sublimaze) is a relatively new narcotic compound that has recently gained popularity. Fentanyl's possible advantage over morphine is that it is extremely lipid-soluble and, therefore, has a more rapid onset and shorter duration of action unless it is given in "anesthetic quantities" (i.e., greater than 500 μg/70 kg). Also, because of its lipid-solubility, fentanyl has more sedative properties than morphine. It is usually associated with less hypotension than morphine. In an adult, one hundred micrograms of fentanyl given slowly in combination with a benzodiazepine will usually provide adequate sedation, amnesia, and analgesia for intubation purposes, especially when used in conjunction with topical local anesthesia.

During the administration of sedative drugs, all patients should be monitored continuously, with close attention being paid to the patient's vital signs (pulse, blood pressure, and respirations). Additional helpful monitoring devices might include a precordial stethoscope, an electrocardiogram, and a pulse oximeter. Sedation is usually adequate for intubation purposes when the patient appears to be sleeping quietly, yet is responsive to verbal stimulation. If a patient becomes unresponsive to verbal stimulation or exhibits signs of impending airway obstruction (snoring or retractions), he or she should be regarded as being oversedated and should receive intubation on a more emergent basis. Of note is that the narcotic effects of sedative overdose can be reversed by the opiate antagonist naloxone, given 0.1 to 0.4 mg intravenously. It is anticipated that a benzodiazepine antagonist will be on the American market in the near future.

All sedative medication should be prescribed by a physician and administered only by licensed personnel who are fully familiar with the properties, side effects, and dosages of sedative medication. Life-sustaining equipment, including cardiac defibrillator, airway management equipment, and cardiac resuscitative medications, should be immediately available.

As an adjunct to sedative medication, a topical local anesthetic may be applied to the mucous membranes of the nose, mouth, and larynx with a nebulizer, a spray, soaked pledgets, nose drops, or viscous jelly. When using a local anesthetic solution, one must pay particular attention to the total dose of anesthetic administered. When these anesthetics are applied directly to the mucous membranes, rapid circulatory uptake can occur, with resultant systemic toxicity.[82] This toxicity can be evidenced in the early stages by perioral paresthesias, a metallic taste in the mouth, light-headedness, and tinnitus, and can progress to muscle twitching, tremors, convulsions, respiratory depression, hypotension, and, ultimately, cardiovascular collapse.[70] The local anesthetics most commonly used for topical application include lidocaine (2%, 4%, or 10% concentration), cocaine (4% concentration), and benzocaine (20% concentration). The dose of lidocaine, when administered alone, should not exceed 6.4 mg/kg.[22] The dose of cocaine, when used alone, should not exceed 200 mg in a 70-kg person.[70,81]

INTUBATION UNDER GENERAL ANESTHESIA

Only trained individuals should use general anesthetics to facilitate tracheal intubation. Excluding surgical patients, few patients require general anesthesia for intubation. In fact, if a patient needs to be restrained for intubation to the point of general anesthesia, then the need for intubation might need to be reexamined. However, there are certain circumstances in which it is necessary to call upon the skills of an anesthesiologist to afford translaryngeal intubation. These situations include intubation of the patient with cerebral or cervical spine injury, acute epiglottitis, and intubation of the patient who is totally uncooperative. All preintubation considerations as described in awake intubaton are necessary to consider for patients receiving general anesthesia. Certain additional considerations are necessary when using this approach, including obtaining monitoring equipment (i.e., electrocardiogram, blood pressure cuff, precordial stethoscope, pulse oximeter) and also anesthetic drugs or anesthetic-administration devices (volatile anesthetic vaporizers). The anesthetic drugs used to facilitate intubation can be categorized into three areas: (1) intravenous central nervous system (CNS) depressants, (2) volatile general anesthetics, and (3) muscle relaxants.

Thiopental sodium (Pentothal), the prototype intravenous CNS depressant, is an ultrashort-acting barbiturate. Its effects range from mild sedation to total loss of consciousness, depending on the dose and rate of administration. Thiopental has a rapid onset (approximately 30 seconds) and a short duration of action (approximately 5 minutes); consequently, it is ideal for short procedures such as intubation. It can significantly decrease blood pressure, especially in the critically ill and fluid-depleted patient. The average intubating dose is 2–5 mg/kg, depending upon the size, age, and general physical status of a patient.

The prototype volatile anesthetic still in use today is halothane. Tracheal intubation following anesthetic induction with a volatile agent is performed routinely in pediatric anesthesia practice for which, because of patient uncooperation or a paucity of venous access sites, intravenous induction is not easily accomplished. In addition, there are certain circumstances in both children and adults during which a loss of spontaneous ventilation, such as would occur with a rapid bolus of intravenous medication, might lead to total airway obstruction (e.g., acute epiglottitis). Under these circumstances the patient is allowed to spontaneously breathe the volatile agent until anesthetized, at which time the anesthetist assumes control of ventilation. To achieve tracheal intubation with halothane anesthesia alone, one must approach drug doses that can cause cardiovascular depression (e.g., bradycardia and hypotension). Hence, intravenous supplementation with sedative drugs and narcotics are sometimes used during volatile anesthetic induction to facilitate intubation. For halothane induction, the anesthetist begins with trace concentrations of the drug and gradually, over a 2- to 3-minute period, increases the inspired drug concentration to approximately 3%. Intubation is accomplished after the patient is apneic, there is a loss of eyelid reflex, and the pupils are centrally fixed.

The neuromuscular blocker most commonly used for intubation purposes is succinylcholine. This medication, like all muscle relaxants, is administered only after a patient is heavily sedated or anesthetized. Muscle relaxants provide no sedative or anesthetic effect. These drugs should never be prescribed for patients outside the operating room without close supervision by a physician who is familiar with their pharmacology and is capable of supporting the airway of a paralyzed patient. An intubating dose for succinylcholine is 1.5 mg/kg given intravenously. The onset of action is rapid (45 to 60 seconds) and the duration of effect is short (3 to 8 minutes), making it ideal for procedures such as intubation. Administration of succinylcholine to the infant and child can result in bradycardia. Atropine (0.01–0.02 mg/kg) should be given intravenously just before succinylcholine in all prepubertal children.

NASAL INTUBATION

Either naris may be chosen, depending on the history and examination, but the right naris is preferred because the bevel of most endotracheal tubes, when introduced through the right naris, will face the flat nasal septum, reducing damage to the turbinates. Topical anesthesia and vasoconstrictor drugs can be used to facilitate the passage of the tube through the nares, lessen the chance of hemorrhage, and make the procedure more comfortable for the patient. Two to three sprays of 0.25% to 0.50% phenylephrine can be used for vasoconstriction. When phenylephrine is dispensed by a plastic squeeze bottle, the bottle must be pointed upward when spraying; it is easy to overdose the patient with this sympathomimetic agent with the bottle

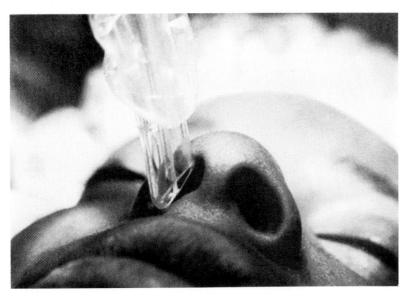

Figure 20—46. The head is positioned and a naris selected for nasal intubation. (Finucane BT, Santora AH: Principles of Airway Management. Philadelphia; FA Davis 1988, with permission)

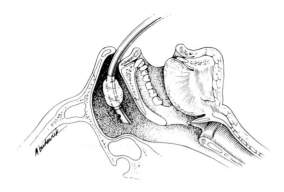

Figure 20—47. The endotracheal tube is passed through the nasopharynx during nasal intubation. (Finucane BT, Santora AH: Principles of Airway Management. Philadelphia, FA Davis, 1988, with permission)

pointing downward. Following administration of the vasoconstrictor, local anesthetic drugs can be applied to the nasal mucosa by means of soaked pledgets, spray, viscous jelly, or nose drops. The sequence of first administering the vasoconstrictor reduces the systemic uptake and the toxic manifestations of the local anesthetic.

The occiput is elevated about 10 cm with a pillow, and a generously lubricated nasotracheal tube is introduced into the selected naris (Fig. 20–46). Extension of the head lifts the epiglottis from the posterior pharyngeal wall. The tube is then advanced along the floor of the nose into the orophar-

ynx and aligned with the glottic opening by listening to the air passing through the tube in a spontaneously breathing patient (Fig. 20–47). The tube is advanced as long as breath sounds increase. If breath sounds diminish, the tube is withdrawn a few centimeters until breath sounds are maximal and then readvanced. Ideally, the tube is swiftly passed to the glottis at a time just prior to inspiration because the vocal cords are most open during inspiration. Nasotracheal intubation can be accomplished under direct vision by first inserting the tracheal tube through the nares and pharynx, holding the laryngoscope with the left hand, and advancing the tracheal tube with the right hand. If one cannot align the tracheal tube for introduction into the trachea, one can use a Magill forceps with the right hand while an assistant advances the nasotracheal tube at its entrance to the naris (Figs 20–48 and 20–49).

INTUBATION OF THE PEDIATRIC PATIENT

Intubation of the pediatric patient is, in some ways, similar to that of the adult patient. Areas in which techniques may differ will be emphasized. Awake intubation is usually carried out in neonates and infants up to 6 weeks of age. Beyond this age healthy infants are too vigorous, and consideration should be given to using sedative or anesthetic medication to afford patient cooperation. Nasal intubation is sometimes avoided in infants and chil-

Figure 20—48. A Magill forceps is used to align the nasotracheal tube for introduction into the trachea.

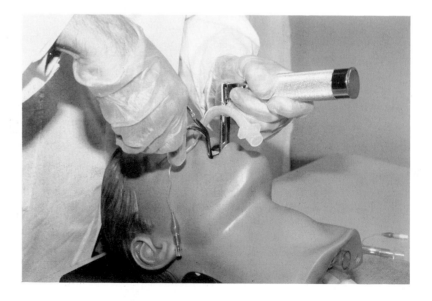

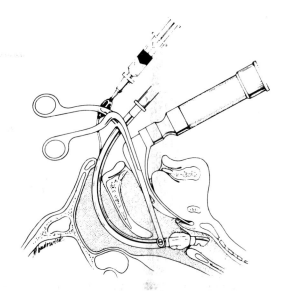

Figure 20—49. Nasotracheal intubation using a McIntosh (curved) blade and a Magill forceps. (Finucane BT, Santora AH: Principles of Airway Management. Philadelphia, FA Davis, 1988, with permission)

dren because adenoid hypertrophy can obstruct tube advancement in the nasopharynx and result in tissue obstruction and hemorrhage. Preoxygenation before intubation may be even more critical in the infant than in the adult because of several physiologic differences between infants and adults that predispose them to hypoxia. These differences include an increased oxygen consumption per kilogram of body weight, a reduced functional residual capacity, and a higher lung closing capacity.

It is important not to overextend the head when positioning for intubation, since this may contribute to complete airway obstruction in the infant. After passage of the tracheal tube and verification of tracheal intubation by maneuvers previously discussed, a mainstem bronchi is intentionally intubated to document the position of the carina; the endotracheal tube is then retrieved to a position in the midtrachea. When the tube has been satisfactorily positioned, 20 to 25 cmH$_2$O positive pressure is applied to the proximal end of the endotracheal tube. At this pressure, an audible gas leak should occur. If there is no leak or if the leak is excessive, the tracheal tube should be replaced by one of a more appropriate size. Of note is that during the process of intubation in a neonate or infant, vagal stimulation and bradycardia may occur; accordingly, intravenous atropine should be readily available for administration at an intravenous dose of 0.01–0.02 mg/kg.

DIFFICULT INTUBATION

Intubation difficulties may, at times, be anticipated by a preprocedural evaluation, with appropriate preparations made to obtain specialized equipment and to enlist the assistance of skilled colleagues. However, there are times when a difficult intubation is not anticipated and no good explanation for the difficulty can be found.

Difficult intubations can be divided into four categories: (1) limited access to the oropharynx, (2) poor visualization of the larynx, (3) diminished cross-sectional area of the pharynx or trachea, (4) and "unexplained reasons." Access to the oropharynx can be obstructed by occluded nares, protruding teeth, a large tongue, temporomandibular joint disease, and so forth. Visualization of the larynx can be obstructed by cervical spine immobility from arthritis, obesity, soft-tissue masses, or other abnormalities. The cross-sectional area of the larynx or trachea can be limited by laryngeal or tracheal stenosis (Table 20–8). Special equipment that may be useful during a difficult intubation includes endotracheal tubes of various sizes, specialized laryngoscope blades, stylets, tube changers, a light wand, a bronchoscope, and cricothyrotomy and tracheostomy equipment (Fig. 20–50).

There are specialized laryngoscope blades designed to facilitate difficult intubations. The Siker mirror blade may allow easier visualization of a more anterior larynx. The polio blade was designed for intubation at an obtuse angle, required for patients in iron lungs or body casts or those who have increased anteroposterior chest-wall dimensions.[33] A stylet is an elongated metal or plastic rod that is

Table 20—8 Conditions with Potential Intubation Difficulties

Limited access to the oropharynx
  Examples: Occluded nares
              Protruding teeth
              Large tongue
              Temporomandibular joint immobility
Poor visualization of the larynx
  Examples: Cervical spine immobility
              Soft-tissue mass
              Upper airway hemorrhage
Limited cross-sectional area of the larynx or trachea
  Examples: Laryngeal stenosis
              Tracheal stenosis
Unexplained and unanticipated difficulties despite a normal upper airway examination

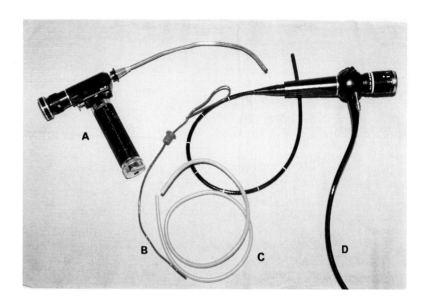

Figure 20—50. Equipment for difficult intubation. (*A*) light wand; (*B*) stylet; (*C*) fiberoptic laryngoscope, (*D*) fiberoptic bronchoscope.

inserted inside the tracheal tube to allow one to alter the natural curve of the tube. The stylet's purpose is to alter the shaft of the tube so that the tip can be maneuvered around structures that hinder direct vision of the larynx. A "tube changer" is an elongated hollow plastic tube that is usually used as a stent when changing endotracheal tubes in a previously intubated patient. This tube changer may also serve as a means of intubation when a difficulty is encountered, owing to its flexibility and ability to conform to different angles. After the trachea has been intubated with the tube changer, the endotracheal tube can be passed over it and the tube changer withdrawn. A light wand is a relatively new device that, like a tube changer, conforms to different angles to intubate the trachea. The advantage of the light wand is that a bright light at the tip transilluminates the trachea, verifying correct positioning.[100]

A fiberoptic bronchoscope can also be used to serve as a stent over which a tracheal tube can be inserted into the trachea. The tip of the bronchoscope can be maneuvered under fiberoptic vision to allow tracheal insertion. Digital insertion of the endotracheal tube or the retrowire intubation technique can be considered if specialized equipment is not available or has proved unsuccessful with several attempts. During a difficult intubation, one should call for assistance early to allow for help in monitoring the patient, readying available equipment, obtaining more specialized equipment, and serving as an advisor or additional intubator. The excitement surrounding a difficult intubation

occurs in an atmosphere in which professional egos are at risk. To avoid hazardous results for the patient, one should always be open to the advice of other practitioners. In the event that tracheal intubation cannot be accomplished and the airway cannot be maintained with mask ventilation, a cricothyrotomy should be considered. The purpose of the cricothyrotomy is to allow oxygen insufflation into the patient's airway to maintain oxygenation while further attempts at intubation are made or a tracheostomy is accomplished.

Cricothyrotomy does not allow for ventilation and carbon dioxide removal; hence, significant respiratory acidosis can occur when oxygen therapy is provided by this means alone. A catheter–needle combination (10 to 14 gauge) is directed caudally at a 45° angle and inserted into the midline of the cricothyroid membrane. During insertion, negative pressure is applied to the syringe. The entrance of air within the syringe signifies that the needle is in the trachea (Fig. 20–51). The catheter is then advanced over the needle into the trachea. The hub of the catheter is connected to an oxygen source. If a jet ventilator is available, the Luer-Lok of the jet ventilator can be connected to the catheter; if airway obstruction is not complete, some ventilation will take place. The Nu-Trake (Armstrong Industries, Inc.) is a sterile unit that combines a blade, needle, and cannula (Fig. 20–52). Potential complications of the placement and use of the cricothyrotomy include perforation of the esophagus, subcutaneous emphysema, pneumothorax, hemorrhage into the trachea, and infection.[86]

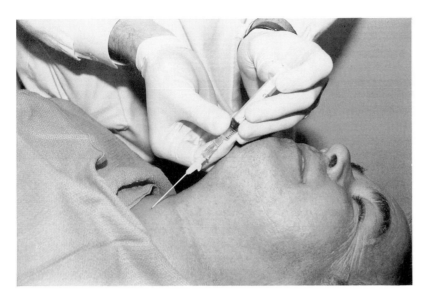

Figure 20—51. Cricothyrotomy being performed with an intravenous catheter.

PEDIATRIC AIRWAY EMERGENCIES

Pediatric airway emergencies frequently present as upper airway obstruction. The signs and symptoms of upper airway obstruction are extremely variable and are dependent upon the etiology in the site of obstruction. Supraglottic lesions tend to cause inspiratory stridor, whereas subglottic lesions cause both inspiratory and expiratory stridor. The diagnosis of obstruction caused by a foreign body is made by the history of a previously healthy child (usually younger than 5 years of age) who becomes acutely short of breath after either sucking on small foreign objects or eating while exercising. If foreign body airway obstruction results in com-

plete airway obstruction, back blows and chest thrusts are recommended as previously discussed. With incomplete airway obstruction, there may be time for x-ray confirmation and location of the object in the tracheobronchial tree. A bronchoscope can be used to retrieve the object.

Acute Epiglottitis

Acute epiglottitis results in supraglottic obstruction. It is caused by a bacterial infection (usually *Haemophilus influenzae*) and is characterized by rapid onset (less than 24 hours), sore throat, and significant fever (higher than 39°C). Acute epiglotti-

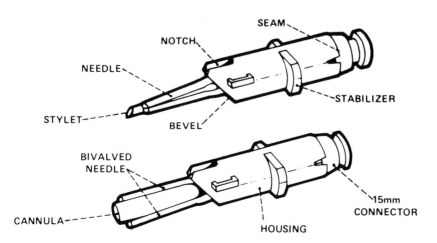

Figure 20—52. Nu-Trake cricothyrotomy device. (Bjoraker RG, Kumar NB, Brown AC: Evaluation of an emergency cricothyrotomy instrument. Crit Care Med 15:157, 1987; © Williams & Wilkins, with permission)

tis presents most commonly between the ages of 2 and 8 years. The child appears "toxic," adopts a sitting position to allow the drainage of saliva, and either has a muffled cough or no cough. Diagnosis is made on clinical grounds. Rarely is a lateral neck x-ray (exhibiting the swollen epiglottis) necessary or advisable. The patient's airway should be secured with endotracheal intubation, at which time the diagnosis can be confirmed by visualization of the "cherry-red," swollen epiglottis. This should occur ideally in the operating room under general anesthesia (see intubation under general anesthesia). Any premature examination of the airway for diagnostic or other purposes may precipitate complete airway obstruction.

Croup

Croup, or viral laryngotracheobronchitis, is usually the result of an infection from parainfluenza or respiratory syncytial virus. It normally affects children under the age of 3 years, develops gradually over several days, is characterized by a "barking" cough, and results in only mild temperature elevation. As the airway narrowing occurs subglottically, both inspiratory and expiratory stridor can be heard. The diagnosis of croup is made on clinical grounds. The diagnosis can be supported by a neck x-ray that shows subglottic narrowing ("steeple sign") (Fig. 20–53). Most children with this condition can be cared for at home with the aid of a humidifier. If hypoxia or signs of impending respiratory failure develop, the patient should be admitted to the hospital. Treatment consists of humidification with cool mist, oxygen, oral or intravenous fluids, and nebulized racemic epinephrine. Corticosteroid therapy is controversial, but, when used, dexamethasone is given at a dose of 4 mg intravenously. Endotracheal intubation is usually not necessary but should be considered if the patient shows signs of fatigue or remains hypoxic despite oxygen administration. Intubation in the operating room under general anesthesia is at times necessary, especially when the diagnosis of acute epiglottitis has not been completely excluded.

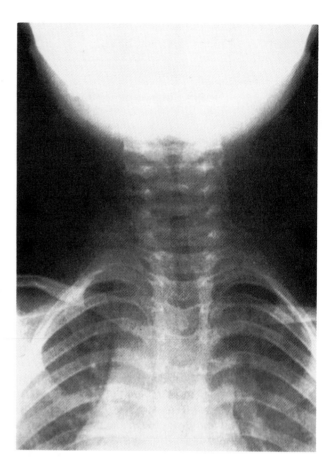

Figure 20–53. A neck radiograph showing subglottic narrowing (steeple sign). (Finucane BT, Santora AH: Principles of Airway Management. Philadelphia, FA Davis, 1988, with permission)

COMPLICATIONS OF TRACHEAL INTUBATION

The potential complications of tracheal intubation are numerous; Table 20–9 lists some of them.[92] The frequency of complications associated with tracheal intubation can be reduced. The incidence of fascial and oral trauma could be diminished by appropriate training and credentialing. Endotracheal tube displacement could be limited by a compulsive postintubation physical examination and by the application of certain monitoring techniques used to verify tracheal intubation (i.e., capnography). Tracheal injury might be reduced by adhering to established protocols for cuff inflation and by securing the endotracheal tube so that movement of the tube is minimized. Damage to the larynx might be reduced by placing appropriate limits on the duration of translaryngeal intubation. The risk of aspiration may be lowered by properly selecting a technique of tracheal intubation appropriate for the clinical situation (e.g., use of the Sellick maneuver for a patient with a full stomach) and by close mon-

Table 20—9 Complications of Tracheal Intubation

COMPLICATIONS DURING TUBE PLACEMENT

1. Facial trauma
2. Dental accidents
3. Nasal, oral, or pharyngeal soft-tissue injuries
4. Esophageal intubation
5. Laryngeal trauma
6. Laryngospasm
7. Intubation of the right mainstem bronchus
8. Pulmonary aspiration
9. Cardiac dysrhythmias
10. Cervical spine and cord injuries
11. Hypertension and tachycardia
12. Elevation of intracranial pressure

COMPLICATIONS FOLLOWING PLACEMENT OF A TRACHEAL TUBE

1. Sinusitis
2. Laryngeal injury
3. Subglottic edema
4. Tracheal injury
5. Dislocation of the tube
6. Reduction in mucociliary transport
7. Patient discomfort
8. Nosocomial infection

COMPLICATIONS OCCURRING AS A RESULT OF EXTUBATION

1. Laryngospasm
2. Regurgitation and aspiration
3. Sore throat
4. Postintubation croup

(Stauffer JL, Silvestri RC: Complications of endotracheal intubation, tracheostomy and artificial airways. Respir Care 27:417, 1982)

itoring after endotracheal extubation (a time when laryngeal reflexes are depressed). Nosocomial infection might be reduced by observing clean intubation techniques with prepackaged disposable equipment and by following established cleaning practices when using reusable equipment. Hypoxemia during intubation might be limited by preoxygenation, observation of proper technique to allow expedient intubation, and the use of monitoring devices (pulse oximetry) that might detect a fall in arterial oxygen saturation. Patient discomfort might be avoided by the appropriate use of sedative and local anesthetic agents.

TRACHEOSTOMY

Tracheostomy provides access to the airway in patients with upper airway obstruction. It also provides an alternative route to tracheal intubation for the patient who requires long-term mechanical respiratory support. A tracheostomy offers several advantages to the patient receiving mechanical ventilatory support. These include the following: (1) it spares direct laryngeal injury from a translaryngeal route; (2) it enhances patient comfort and patient mobility; (3) it facilitates nursing care, especially airway suctioning; (4) it facilitates transfer from the ICU setting; (5) with appropriate instrumentation, it allows the patient to speak; (6) it facilitates mouth care and can permit oral nourishment; (7) it provides a psychological benefit that is difficult to quantitate, but at times can be substantial and can greatly assist in patient recovery; and (8) because it is shorter and wider than a translaryngeal endotracheal tube, it offers less resistance to airflow.

Some potential complications of tracheostomy include (1) intraoperative and postoperative hemorrhage at the surgical site or as a result of erosion into the innominate vessels, (2) pneumothorax, (3) tracheoesophageal fistula, (4) tracheal stenosis, (5) infection, (6) displacement of the tracheostomy tube, (7) scar formation, and (8) inability to intubate the trachea (especially when performed on an emergency basis under suboptimal conditions) (Table 20—10).

Ideally, the tracheostomy should be performed by an experienced surgeon, with an anesthesiologist in attendance in the operating room or in a fully equipped intensive care setting. A decision on when a translaryngeal endotracheal tube might be removed and a tracheostomy performed should be based on individual patient factors. The National Association of Medical Directors of Respiratory Care (NAMDRC) has recently published guidelines for the performance of tracheostomy:

1. For anticipated need of the artificial airway up to 10 days, the translaryngeal route is preferred
2. For anticipated need of the artificial airway for longer than 21 days, tracheostomy is preferred
3. In circumstances in which the time anticipated for maintenance of an artificial airway is not clear, daily assessment is required to determine if conversion to tracheostomy is indicated

Table 20—10 Complications of Tracheostomy

SURGICAL COMPLICATIONS

1. Hemorrhage
2. Thyroid injury
3. Injury to laryngeal nerves
4. Air leaks (pneumothorax, subcutaneous emphysema, mediastinal emphysema)
5. Tracheoesophageal fistula
6. Cardiac arrest
7. Tracheostomy too high or too low

COMPLICATIONS WHILE TRACHEOSTOMY IS IN PLACE

1. Infection (sepsis, pneumonia, mediastinitis)
2. Hemorrhage (skin vessels or major artery)
3. Tracheal injury (inflammation, submucosal hemorrhage, ulceration, cartilage and mucosal necrosis)
4. Tracheal perforation and tracheoesophageal fistula
5. Tracheal web or pseudomembrane formation
6. Irritation of the carina
7. Self-decannulation
8. Air leak (pneumothorax subcutaneous emphysema)
9. Reduction of mucociliary transport, ineffective cough
10. Pneumonia
11. Pulmonary aspiration
12. Irritation of the carina
13. Mechanical problems with tube or cuff (obstruction, disconnection from ventilator)
14. Patient discomfort

COMPLICATIONS DURING AND AFTER DECANNULATION

1. Difficult decannulation (tight stoma)
2. Scar, granuloma, or keloid formation
3. Persistent open stoma
4. Dysphagia
5. Tracheal stenosis
6. Tracheomalacia
7. Tracheal web formation

(Stauffer JL, Silvestri RC: Complications of endotracheal intubation, tracheostomy and artificial airways. Respir Care 27:417, 1982, with permission)

4. The decision for conversion to tracheostomy should be made as early in the course of management as possible to minimize the duration of translaryngeal intubation. Once the decision is made, the procedure should be done without undue delay except in conditions such as life-threatening cardiopulmonary instability, uncorrected coagulopathy, or other mitigating circumstances.[8]

Following tracheostomy, the trachea is cannulated with a tracheostomy tube. Most tracheostomy tubes are equipped with an inner cannula, an outer cannula, an obturator, and an inflatable cuff. The outer cannula contacts the stoma and maintains airway patency. The inner cannula allows cleaning of the airway, as it is easily removed from its position inside the outer cannula. The obturator fills the lumen of the tube and aids during intubation of the stoma. After the tracheostomy tube is in place, the obturator is removed and the cuff is inflated.

During the first 24 hours following tracheostomy, the inner cannula should be removed every 4 hours. It should be cleaned with a tracheostomy brush and hydrogen peroxide and rinsed in sterile water before it is replaced. Tracheostomy tubes should be changed regularly (approximately every week) to allow inspection of the stoma and the tracheostomy tube. The first tube change following a tracheostomy should be performed by a surgeon unless the tracheostomy has been allowed to fully mature (more than 7 days have elapsed since the operation). The obturator should be readily available for tube reintroduction in case an unanticipated dislodgment occurs.

SUCTIONING

Suctioning of the upper airway (mouth to mainstem bronchi) may be required to remove saliva, pulmonary secretions, blood, or vomitus. Suctioning occurs when subatmospheric pressure is applied to a flexible catheter or rigid tube.

The nonflexible Yankauer suction is used to remove material from the oropharynx (Fig. 20–54). Catheters may be inserted directly into the nose and nasopharynx (nasotracheal suctioning) or through artificial airways. Normally, airway secretions are expectorated or swallowed. Loss of airway control, increased secretion production, inadequate cough, and thickened secretions may, individually or combined, overwhelm a patient. Loss of consciousness or inability to control the airway, or both, places patients at risk for secretion retention. Endotracheal or tracheostomy tubes compromise the ciliary escalator and effective cough.

Suctioning may be performed in conjunction with chest physical therapy procedures, such as bronchial drainage, percussion, hyperinflation, and assisted coughing. Secretions must be mobilized from peripheral bronchi to the trachea and mainstem bronchi for cough or suctioning to be effective. Suctioning is indicated when there are obvi-

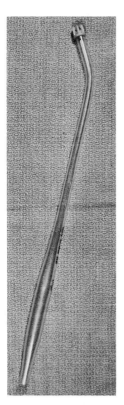

Figure 20—54. Yankaur rigid suction device.

ous rhonchi over the central airways, but also, it has been used prophylactically for ventilator and nonventilated patients to prevent secretion retention. Suctioning with an in-line trap is a method of sputum sampling for laboratory analysis.[50]

Although a necessary and seemingly benign procedure, tracheal aspiration can be very uncomfortable and potentially hazardous to patients. Table 20–11 lists potential complications of suction-

Table 20—11 Complications of Suctioning

Hypoxemia: decrease in arterial tension or saturation
Hemodynamic changes: either hypotension from vagal stimulation or hypertension from hypoxemia
Atelectasis: caused by excessively large catheters removing gas from lobar bronchi
Cardiac dysrhythmias of all types
Bronchoconstriction: caused by stimulation of bronchial smooth muscle
Increased intracranial pressure
Cardiac arrest and death
Microbiologic contamination
Tracheal tissue damage and hemoptysis

Table 20—12 Nonpatient Variables Affecting the Magnitude of Hypoxemia During Suctioning

Suction duration
Time interval between suctioning
Suction flow/pressure (vacuum) level
Suction catheter outside diameter versus endotracheal tube inner diameter
Duration of pre- and postoxygenation
Number of hyperinflations and size of inflation volumes
Concentration of oxygen supplied
Closed- or open-suction system

ing. Many of the side effects are the result of arterial desaturation. Arterial blood gas values provided the early documentation of the hypoxic effects.[93] Problems were most significant if the arterial oxygen tension (PaO_2) decreased below 65 mmHg. The ear–finger oximeter provides an instant evaluation of oxyhemoglobin saturation (SpO_2). Saturations below 90% are of potential concern.[77] Table 20–12 presents a listing of nonpatient variables that can contribute to hypoxemia during suctioning.

Damage to the airway mucosa associated with suctioning has long been recognized at autopsy or after bronchoscopic study.[67,79] Microbial contamination is also a hazard to both patient and health care workers. Airway colonization and nosocomial pneumonia are linked to suctioning procedures, primarily from transmission by workers' hands.[24] Direct hand contact with infected tracheal secretions has been linked to outbreaks of herpes simplex virus types 1 and 2, causing a digital infection known as herpetic witlow.

Gloving of both hands is now part of standard suctioning protocol, a recent result of awareness that all body secretions may serve as vectors for the transmission of certain diseases. (e.g., AIDS or hepatitis). Additional precautions, including eye shields, growns, and masks may be appropriate in instances in which splashing and aerosolization of secretions are possible.[36]

SUCTIONING EQUIPMENT

Vacuum Source

Wall vacuum is provided to hospital areas by a central pump and piping system. Portable electric and manually operated devices are also available. Central vacuum pumps can generate subatmospheric pressures to −25 in. Hg (−635 mmHg). Vacuum regulators reduce pressures to lower levels; most are adjustable from a range of zero to −200 mmHg. Regulators have on–off controls and vacuum pressure controls. A subatmospheric pressure setting of −100 mmHg is recommended; higher levels do not enhance secretion recovery.[93] Maximum suction flows depend on the level of vacuum and on the diameter and length of the catheter and connecting tubing. Suction flows commonly range from 10–30 L/min, but research has not determined an ideal level. The suction flow is the main factor that influences the amount of gas removed from the lungs, which can lead to hypoxemia. Bottle reservoirs collect suctioned materials, and valves protect the vacuum system from overflow. Older suction units created aerosols of potential microbial pathogens.[76]

Catheters

Standard suction catheters are available in a range of sizes and design of the distal tip. The outside diameter of the suction catheter should be less than one-half the inside diameter of the endotracheal tube; larger catheters increase the risk of atelectasis and hypoxemia. This can be determined by the following formula:

$$\text{Maximum diameter (french)} = \frac{\text{Inside diameter (mm)} \times 3}{2}$$

Older catheters were made of red rubber with an open end or "whistle-tip." Of note is an angle-tipped catheter, termed coudé, designed to facilitate entrance to the left mainstem bronchus. Contemporary devices are made of polyvinyl chloride and silicon rubber (Fig. 20–55). The ideal suction catheter tip design should efficiently clear secretions but subject the mucosa to minimal trauma. Trauma can occur when mucosa invaginates into the end and side hole(s) of the catheter. Mucosal surfaces are defoliated of cilia, and hemorrhagic erosion and edema result. An attempt to produce a minimally traumatic tip has resulted in a number of designs shown in Figure 20–56. In vitro and in vivo testing have demonstrated their relative superiority to older catheter designs.[18,46,79]

Adaptors have been developed to permit suctioning through an endotracheal or tracheostomy tube connector, which is advantageous for patients who have a critical oxygenation or ventilation status and may require PEEP.[12] This concept has been

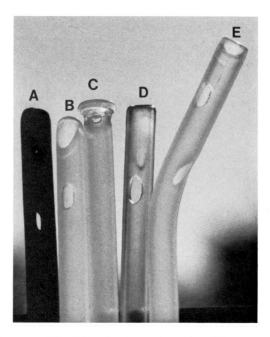

Figure 20—55. Suction catheter tips. (*A*) open-ended; (*B*) whistle-tip; (*C*) Argyle Aero-Flow; (*D*) modified whistle-tip; (*E*) Coudé.

Figure 20—56. Diagram of suction catheter tips to produce reduced trauma. (Chapman GA, Kim CS, Frankel J, Gazeroglu HB, Sackner MA: Evaluation of the safety and efficiency of a new suction catheter design. Respir Care 31:889, 1986; with permission)

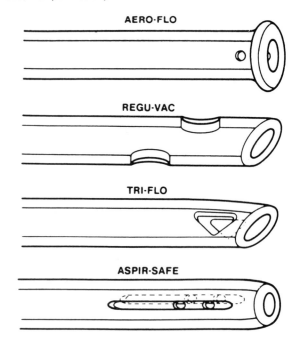

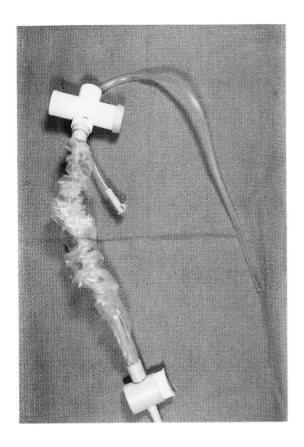

Figure 20—57. Continuous suction catheter system.

Table 20—13 Summary of Suctioning Protocol

A. Prepare equipment
  1. Vacuum system: pressure −100 mmHg (−13.3 kPa) or less
  2. Suction catheter: outside diameter less than half of inside diameter of endotracheal tube
B. Wash hands
C. Prepare patient
  1. Preoxygenate with 100% oxygen (unless contraindicated)
  2. Hyperinflate with six or more breaths of 1.5 times baseline tidal volume (unless contraindicated)
  3. Note baseline heart rate, ECG rhythm, and saturation by pulse oximeter (SpO_2)
D. Prepare suction catheter
  1. Glove both hands
  2. Moisten in sterile saline/water
  3. Lubricate with water-soluble material (nasotracheal suction only)
E. Suction
  1. Insert catheter full length or until an obstruction is reached
  2. Apply suction and gently withdraw the catheter
F. Provide postoxygenation and hyperinflation

advanced to involve closed-tracheal suction systems. A plastic sleeve envelops the catheter to prevent catheter contamination when not in use (Fig. 20–57).[16] However, initial study has not shown the closed system to have decreased rates of contamination when compared with single-use catheters.[75]

SUCTIONING PROTOCOL

Table 20–13 summarizes a general protocol for safe suctioning. Ideally it should be done by two health care workers, one to assure oxygenation and ventilation and the other to actually suction. The literature supports the practice of handwashing and preoxygenation before beginning the suctioning. Specific details of numbers of breaths or time of preoxygenation will depend on the condition of the patient. Many patients will be protected from hypoxemia if given approximately six breaths of 100% oxygen.

The use of hyperinflation has been controversial because some hemodynamically unstable patients experience decreased cardiac output, increase in intracranial pressure, and variations in arterial blood pressure with this technique.[94] Other researchers recommend increased volume of the breaths in the range of 1.5 times the size of the maintenance tidal volume of 12–14 mL/kg of lean body weight.[69,84] Delivery of the breaths may occur by anesthesia bag, self-inflating resuscitator, or mechanical ventilator (if the patient is being mechanically ventilated).[75] The resetting of FIO_2 on ventilators requires additional time to "purge" the internal reservoirs if the previous oxygen concentration was not 100%. Some ventilators have the ability to quickly flush gas from their systems. Operators must remember to return the oxygen concentration or volume settings to previous therapeutic levels.

The appropriate suction catheter should be moistened in a small tray of sterile water or saline. Prepackaged suctioning kits usually provide this device. For nasotracheal use the catheter may be lightly lubricated with water-soluble material. The catheter is then advanced into the patient's airway. Nasotracheal suctioning is technically more difficult because the catheter must be passed blindly into the trachea. A nasopharyngeal airway may be helpful in guiding the catheter horizontally until it lies just above the larynx and also in decreasing bacterial colonization of the airway when repeated introduction is indicated. Airflow sounds may be heard from the proximal catheter. When sounds are at their loudest, the patient can be asked to inspire as the catheter is advanced. Conscious patients will become hoarse, and speech will become whisperlike. The catheter is then passed further into the trachea. Stimulation of cough receptors is likely to occur. The major concern with nasotracheal suction is laryngospasm.

Suctioning through a tracheal tube or tracheostomy tube is much simpler. After traversing the tube's lumen, the catheter should be gently advanced its full length or until an obstruction is encountered. Suction is then applied. There is no current research on whether suction should be intermittent or continuous as the catheter is withdrawn.[34] Some authors suggest twirling the catheter between thumb and forefinger to circumferentially contact secretions. Suction should be applied for about 10 seconds or less. The ECG, pulse oximetry, or clinical signs may indicate hypoxemia or cardiovascular stress at shorter time intervals. Animal research indicates that the lowest PaO_2 appears to occur in the first 5 seconds.[74] Postoxygenation and hyperinflation with 100% oxygen should follow.

REFERENCES

1. Alder J, Dykan M: Gastric rupture: An unusual complication of the esophageal obturator airway. Ann Emerg Med 12:244, 1983
2. American National Standards Institute: Standards for cuffed oral and tracheal tubes for prolonged use. New York, ANSI, 1983
3. American National Standards Institute. American national standards for oropharyngeal airways, (ANSI 779.3-1974). New York, ANSI, 1974
4. American Society for Testing and Materials: Standard specifications for pediatric tracheostomy tubes (F927-86). Philadelphia, ASTM, 1986
5. American Society for Testing and Materials: Standards for cuffed and uncuffed tracheal tubes (F 290201). Philadelphia, ASTM, 1989
6. Averbach PS, Geehr EC: Inadequate oxygen and ventilation using the esophageal gastric tube airway in the prehospital setting. JAMA 250:3067, 1983
7. Badenhorst CH: Changes in tracheal cuff pressure during respiratory support. Crit Care Med April:300, 1987
8. Bartlett RL, Martin SD, Perina D, Raymond JI: The pharyngeo-tracheal lumen airway: An assessment of airway control in the setting of upper airway hemorrhage. Ann Emerg Med 16:343, 1987
9. Bernhard WN, Cottrell JE, Sivakumaran C et al: Adjustment of intracuff pressure to prevent aspiration. Anesthesiology 50:363, 1979
10. Bernhard WN, Yost L, Joynes D et al: Intracuff pressure in endotracheal and tracheostomy cuffs. Chest 87:720, 1985
11. Bjoraker DG, Kumar NB, Brown AC: Evaluations of an emergency cricothyrotomy instrument. Crit Care Med 15:157, 1987
12. Bodai Bi, Briggs SW, Goldstein M et al: Evaluation of the ability of the NeO_2 safe valve to minimize desaturation in neonates during suctioning. Respir Care 34:355, 1989
13. Bolder PM, Healy TE, Bolder AR et al: The extra work of breathing through adult endotracheal tubes. Anesth Analg 65:853, 1986
14. Burton NA, Watson DC, Brodsky JB, Mark JD: Advantages of a new polyvinyl chloride double-lumen tube in thoracic surgery. Ann Thorac Surg 36:78, 1983
15. Cane RD, Woodward C, Shapiro BA: Customizing fenestrated tracheostomy tubes—a bedside technique. Crit Care Med 10:880, 1982
16. Carlon GC, Fox SJ, Ackerman NJ: Evaluation of a closed-tracheal suction system. Crit Care Med 15:522, 1987
17. Centers for Disease Control: Recommendations for prevention of HIV transmission in health-care settings. MMWR 36:35, 1987
18. Chapman GA, Kim CS, Frankel J et al: Evaluation of the safety and efficiency of a new suction catheter design. Respir Care 31:889, 1986
19. Coldiron JS: Estimation of nasotracheal tube length in neonates. Pediatrics 41:823, 1968
20. Collins VJ: Principles of Anesthesiology. Philadelphia, Lea & Febiger, 1969
21. Conrardy PA, Goodman LR, Lainge F, Singer MM: Alteration of endotracheal tube position: Flexion and extension of the neck. Crit Care Med 4:8, 1976
22. Covino BG, Vassallo HG: General pharmacological and toxicological aspects of local anesthetic agents. In Covino BG, Vassallo HG (eds): Local Anesthetics, Mechanisms of Action and Clinical Use. New York, Grune & Stratton, 1976
23. Craven DE, Kunches LM, Kilinsky V et al: Risk factor for pneumonia and fatality in patients receiving continuous mechanical ventilation. Am Rev Respir Dis 133:792, 1986
24. Craven DE, Steger KA: Pathogenesis and prevention of nosocomial pneumonia in the mechanically ventilated patient. Respir Care 34:85, 1989
25. Dahlgren BE, Nilsson HG, Viklund B: Tracheal tubes in cold stress. Anaesthesia 43:683, 1988
26. Demers PR, Sullivan MJ, Paliotta J: Airflow resistance of endotracheal tubes. JAMA 237:1362, 1977
27. Don Michael TA, Gordon AS: The esophageal obturator airway: A new device in emergency cardiopulmonary resuscitation. Br Med J 281:1531, 1980
28. Dorsch JA, Dorsch SE: Understanding Anesthesia Equipment, 2nd ed. Baltimore, Williams & Wilkins, 1984
29. Dustan HP: (Ad Hoc Committee on Medical Ethics.) Ann Intern Med 101:129, 263, 1984
30. Eckenhoff JE: Some anatomic considerations of the infant larynx influencing endotracheal anesthesia. Anesthesiology 12:401, 1951
31. Eckerbom B, Lindholm CE, Alexopoulos C: Airway lesions caused by prolonged intubation with standard and with anatomically shaped tracheal tubes: A post-mortem study. Acta Anaesthesiol Scand 30:366, 1986

32. Emergency Care Research Institute: Artificial airways. Health Devices 7:67, 1978
33. Finucane BT, Santora AH: Difficult intubation. In Finucane BT, Santora AH, (eds): Principles of Airway Management. Philadelphia, FA Davis, 1988
34. Fluck RR: Suctioning—intermittent or continuous? [Editorial]. Respir Care 30:837, 1985
35. Frass M, Frenzer R, Rauscha F et al: Evaluation of esophageal tracheal combitube in cardiopulmonary resuscitation. Crit Care Med 15:609, 1986
36. Garner JG: Employee exposure and illnesses. In Farber BF (ed): Infection Control in Intensive Care. New York, Churchill Livingstone, 1987
37. Gillespie NA: Endotracheal anaesthesia in infants. Br J Anaesth 17:2, 1939
38. Grillo HC, Cooper JD, Geffin B, Pontopidden H: A low-pressure cuff for tracheostomy tubes to minimize tracheal injury: A comparative trial. J Thorac Cardiovasc Surg 62:898, 1971
39. Habib MP: Physiological implication of artificial airways. Chest 96:180, 1989
40. Hamilton LH, Londino JM, Linehan JH, Neu J: Pediatric endotracheal tube designed for high-frequency ventilation. Crit Care Med 12:988, 1984
41. Hammargren Y, Clinton JE, Ruiz E et al: A standard comparison of esophageal obturator airway and endotracheal tube ventilation in cardiac arrest. Ann Emerg Med 14:953, 1985
42. Harrison EE, Nord HJ, Beeman RW: Esophageal perforation following the use of the esophageal obturator airway. Ann Emerg Med 9:21, 1980
43. Hess D, Ness C, Oppel A, Rhoads K: Evaluation of mouth-to-mask ventilation devices. Respir Care 34:191, 1989
44. Hochbaum SR: Emergency airway management. Emerg Med Clin North Am 4:411, 1986
45. Honsinger MJ, Yorkston KM, Dowden PA: Communication options for intubated patients. Respir Manag 17:45, 1987
46. Jung RC, Gottlieb LS: Comparison of tracheobronchial suction catheters in humans. Chest 69:179, 1976
47. Kerby GR, Mayer LS, Pingleton SK: Nocturnal positive pressure ventilation via nasal mask. Am Rev Respir Dis 135:738, 1987
48. Kistner RL, Hanlon CR: A new tracheostomy tube in treatment of retained bronchial secretions. Arch Surg 81:259, 1960
49. Kubota Y, Toyoda Y, Nagata N et al: Tracheobronchial angles in infants and children. Anesthesiology 64:374, 1986
50. Larson RP, Ingalls-Severn KJ, Wright JR et al: Diagnosis of *Pneumocystis carinii* pneumonia by respiratory care practitioners: Advantages of a nasotracheal suctioning method over sputum induction. Respir Care 34:249, 1989
51. Leger P, Jennequin JJ, Gerard M, Robert D: Home positive pressure ventilation via nasal mask for patients with neuromuscular weakness or restrictive lung or chest-wall disease. Respir Care 34:73, 1989
52. Levin J: Endotracheal tubes in children. A formula for the lengths. Anaesthesia 13:40, 1958
53. Lindholm CE, Grenvik A: Tracheal tube and cuff problems. Int Anestheol Clin 20:103, 1981
54. Lockhart PB, Feldbau EV, Gabel RA et al: Dental complications during and after tracheal intubation. JAMA 112:480, 1986
55. Long J, West G: Evaluation of the Olympic Trach button as a precursor to tracheostomy removal. Respir Care 25:1242, 1980
56. Mace SE: Cricothyrotomy. Ann Emerg Med 6:309, 1988
57. MacGillivray RG: Evaluation of a new tracheal tube with a moveable bronchus blocker. Anaesthesia 43:687, 1988
58. Mattila MK, Heikel PE, Suutarinen T et al: Estimation of a suitable nasotracheal tube length for infants and children. Acta Anaesthesiol Scand 15:239, 1971
59. Meislin HW: The esophageal obturator airway: It works, but. . . Ann Emerg Med 9:171, 1980
60. Mollampati SR, Gatt SP, Gugino LD et al: A clinical sign to predict difficult tracheal intubation. Can J Anaesth 32:429, 1985
61. Monheim LM: General Anesthesia in Dental Practice, 3rd ed. St Louis, CV Mosby, 1968
62. Montgomery WW: Current modifications of the salivary bypass tube and tracheal T-tube. Ann Otol Rhinol Laryngol 95:121, 1986
63. Niemann JT, Rosborough JP, Myers R, Scarberry EN: The pharyngeo-tracheal lumen airway: Preliminary investigation of a new adjunct. Ann Emerg Med 13:591, 1984
64. Patil VU, Stehling LC, Zauder HL: Predicting the difficulty of intubation utilizing an intubation gauge. Anesthesiol Rev 10:32, 1983
65. Petring OV, Adelhoj B, Jensen BN et al: Prevention of silent aspiration due to leaks around cuffs of endotracheal tubes. Anesth Analg 65:777, 1986
66. Plevak DJ: Mayo Clinic Division of Intensive Care and Respiratory Therapy Infection Control Program Guidelines. 1988.
67. Plum F, Dunning MF: Techniques for minimizing trauma to the tracheobronchial tree after tracheostomy. N Engl J Med 254:193, 1956
68. Plummer AL, Gracey DR: Consensus conference on artificial airways in patients receiving mechanical ventilation. Chest 96:178, 1989
69. Preusser BA, Stone KS, Gonyon DS et al: Effects of two methods of preoxygenation on arterial pressure, cardiac output, peak airway pressure and postsuctioning hypoxia. Heart Lung 17:290, 1988
70. Raj PP, Winnie AP: Immediate reactions to local anesthetics. In Orlein FK, Cooperman LH (eds): Complications in Anesthesiology. Philadelphia, JB Lippincott, 1983
71. Rapport DM, Sorkin B, Garay SM et al: Reversal of the "pickwickian syndrome" by long-term use of nocturnal nasal-airway pressure. N Engl J Med 307:931, 1982
72. Rayburn RL: Light wand intubation. Anaesthesia 34:667, 1979
73. Riegel B, Forshee T: A review and critique of the literature on preoxygenation and suctioning. Heart Lung 14:507, 1985
74. Rindfleisch SH, Tyler ML: Duration of suctioning: An important variable. Respir Care 28:457, 1983
75. Ritz R, Scott LR, Coyl MB, Pierson DJ: Contamination of a multiple-use suction catheter in a closed-circuit system compared to contamination of a disposable, single-use suction catheter. Respir Care 31:1086, 1986

76. Robertshaw RG: Aerosol production by suction apparatus and methods of containment. J Hosp Infect 3:379, 1982

77. Rosen IM, Hillard EK: The effects of negative pressure during tracheal suction. Anesth Analg 41:50, 1962

78. Rosen P: The field airway controversy [Editorial]. J Emerg Med 2:305, 1985

79. Sackner MA, Landa JF, Greeneltch N, Robinson MJ: Pathogenesis and prevention of tracheobronchial damage with suction procedures. Chest 64:284, 1973

80. Samsoon GLT, Young JRB: Difficult tracheal intubation: A retrospective study. Anaesthesia 52:487, 1987

81. Scott DB, Cousins MJ: Clinical pharamacology of local anesthetic agents. In Cousins MJ, Bridenbaugh PO (eds): Neural Blockade. Philadelphia, JB Lippincott, 1980

82. Sellers WFS, Dye A, Harvey J: Systemic absorption of lidocaine ointment from tracheal tubes. Anaesthesia 40:483, 1985

83. Sellick BA: Cricoid pressure to control regurgitation of stomach contents during induction of anesthesia. Lancet 2:404, 1962

84. Skelley B, Deeren S, Powaser M: The effectiveness of two preoxygenation methods to prevent endotracheal suction induced hypoxemia. Heart Lung 9:316, 1980

85. Smith JP, Podai BL, Aobourg R et al: A field evaluation of the esophageal obturator airway. J Trauma 23:317, 1983

86. Smith RB, Schaer WB, Pfaeffle H: Percutaneous transtracheal ventilation for anesthesia and resuscitation. A review and report of complications. Can Anaesth Soc J 22:607, 1975

87. Smith RM: Anesthesia for Infants and Children, p. 58. St Louis, CV Mosby, 1959

88. Snyder GM: Individualized placement of tracheostomy tube fenestration and in-situ examination with fiberoptic laryngoscope. Respir Care 28:1294, 1983

89. Sottile FD, Marrie TJ, Prouch DS et al: Nosocomial pulmonary infection: Possible etiologic significance of bacterial adhesion to endotracheal tubes. Crit Care Med 14:265, 1986

90. Stanley TH: Nitrous oxide and pressure and volume of high and low pressure endotracheal tube cuffs in intubated patients. Anesthesiology 42:637, 1975

91. Stauffer JL, Petty TL: Cleft tongue and ulceration of hard palate: Complications of oral intubations. Chest 74:317, 1981

92. Stauffer JL, Silvestri RC: Complications of endotracheal intubation, tracheostomy, and artificial airways. Respir Care 27:417, 1982

93. Stone KS: Endotracheal suctioning in the critically ill. Crit Care Nurse Curr 7:5, 1989

94. Stone KS, Preusser B, Groch K, Karl J: The effect of lung hyperinflation on cardiopulmonary hemodynamics and post suctioning hypoxemia [Abstract]. Heart Lung 17:309, 1988

95. Takki S, Aromaa U, Kauste A. The validity and usefulness of the end-tidal PCO_2 during anesthesia. Ann Clin Res 4:278, 1972

96. Wall MA: Infant endotracheal tube resistance: Effects of changing length, diameter, and gas density. Crit Care Med 8:38, 1980

97. Wanner A, Zighelboim A, Sackner MA: Nasopharyngeal airway: A facilitated access to the trachea. Ann Intern Med 25:593, 1971

98. White RD: Controversies in out-of-hospital emergency airway control: Esophageal obstruction or endotracheal intubation? Ann Emerg Med 13:778, 1984

99. Wright PE, Marini JJ, Bernard GR: In vitro versus in vivo comparison of endotracheal tube airflow resistance. Am Rev Respir Dis 140:10, 1989

100. Yealy DM, Paris DM: Recent advances in airway management. Emerg Med Clin North Am 7:83, 1989

101. Yelderman M, New W: Evaluation of pulse oximetry. Anesthesiology 59:349, 1983

BIBLIOGRAPHY

American Heart Association: Healthcare Providers Manual for Basic Life Support. Dallas, AHA, 1988

Dorsch JA, Dorsch SE: Understanding Anesthesia Equipment, 2nd ed. Baltimore, Williams & Wilkins, 1984

Finucane BT, Santora AH: Principles of Airway Management. Philadelphia, FA Davis, 1988

Habib MP: Physiological implications of artificial airways. Chest 96:180, 1989

Hochbaum SR: Emegency airway management. Emerg Med Clin North Am 4:411, 1986

Selecky PA: Tracheostomy: A review of present day indications, complications and care. Heart Lung 3:272, 1974

Stauffer JL, Silvestri RC: Complications of endotracheal intubation, tracheostomy, and artificial airways. Respir Care 27:417, 1982

Tealy DM, Paris DM: Recent advances in airway management. Emerg Med Clin North Am 7:83, 1989

TWENTY-ONE

Mechanical Ventilation

David A. Desautels
Paul B. Blanch

Early references to ventilatory support appear in the Bible. Although other references to artificially supported ventilation are found over succeeding centuries, one of the most popular appears in a monograph published in 1796 entitled *An Attempt at an Historical Survey of Life-Saving Measures for Drowning Persons and Information on the Best Means by Which They Can Again be Brought Back to Life,* by Herholdt and Rafn.[1] This work discussed mouth-to-mouth ventilation and other mechanical or manual methods of moving air, including the insertion of the tip of a bellows-type apparatus into the victim's windpipe with rhythmical inflation of his lungs. Later, a publication by Emerson described positive-pressure breathing for the treatment of congestive heart failure and pulmonary edema.[2] Modern ventilatory support techniques, however, are an outgrowth of the tank-type respirator introduced by Drinker and Shaw in 1929 (see the Preface). Since then, new techniques and types of ventilatory support have rapidly appeared.

The first positive-pressure ventilators were pressure cycled or volume cycled. The pressure-cycled ventilator (PCV) was designed to terminate gas delivery when a predetermined pressure had been attained. Thus, the volume of gas delivered to the patient was related directly to lung compliance and inversely to airway resistance. Any leaks in the system reduced the amount of volume delivered to the patient. With large gas leaks the ventilators remained in prolonged inspiration because the pressure necessary for terminating flow could not be reached.

Operation of volume-cycled ventilators required selection of a desired volume, which was then delivered into the breathing circuit. However, no controls or alarms were built into early models of such ventilators to detect or to compensate for leaks in the system, and they could be disconnected accidentally from the patient without any visual or audible signs.

The popularization of intermittent positive-pressure breathing (IPPB) therapy in the 1950s and early 1960s aided the rapid development of numerous types of sophisticated mechanical ventilators, although the merits of IPPB therapy continue to be debated. Physicians soon recognized that ventilators that provided IPPB had substantial limitations during prolonged mechanical ventilation and, generally, where not suitable for long-term patient care.

Control of the inspired oxygen concentration was not possible initially. Many pressure-cycled ventilators had only two settings, which allegedly could deliver 40% and 100% oxygen. However, decreased compliance or increased airway resistance, which caused rapidly increased system pressure, altered the exact concentration of oxygen delivered at any given time, leading to excessive inspired oxygen concentrations and possible pulmonary oxygen toxicity. Systems that diluted oxygen with room air or mixed high-pressure sources of oxygen and compressed air in separate air–oxygen blenders were subsequently introduced.

Early ventilators lacked the necessary components to provide humidification. Tenacious secretions and mucus plugs often resulted from ventilation with dry gas, and mucociliary activity was depressed. Daily bronchoscopy to maintain the patency of airways was sometimes needed in patients supported with mechanical ventilation.

Subsequently, heated humidifiers that could produce up to 100% relative humidity at body temperature and high-efficiency nebulizers became commercially available. However, the clinician frequently had no reliable means of recognizing or controlling the exact level of humidification delivered to a patient. Underhumidification of respiratory gases or the delivery of an excessive water load were both possible. Also, a patient's airway could be burned with superheated mist, should a heating device malfunction.

Initially, mechanical ventilators had crude adjustments for pressure and volume that could not be controlled precisely, and clinicians frequently recommended that patients be ventilated through an uncuffed tracheostomy tube to prevent excessive tidal volume (VT) delivery. The danger of aspiration of gastric contents with uncuffed endotracheal and tracheostomy tubes soon became widely recognized. Later, control of the volume and pressure delivered to patients improved. Because known VT or predictable cycling pressures were difficult or impossible to attain with an uncuffed tube, cuffed tracheal tubes became widely used during prolonged mechanical ventilation. More recently, implant-tested, low-pressure cuffed tubes have allowed prolonged orotracheal or nasotracheal intubation in lieu of tracheostomy.

Early ventilators assisted or controlled respiration, but it was uncommon to find both modes available in a single unit. Subsequently, both assisted and controlled ventilation became available. As technology improved, ventilators that operated with pressure-cycled, time-cycled, or volume-cycled mechanisms could also be adjusted to change the inspiratory and expiratory pressure and flow patterns with variable gas flow rates, thereby allowing selection of a pattern of ventilation that was most advantageous to the patient. This increased flexibility allowed gas flow to be adjusted to compensate for the patient's pulmonary lesion, thereby improving the distribution of ventilation.

Indications for mechanical ventilation also changed. Early mechanical ventilators were used for patients who could not sustain spontaneous ventilation. Hypoxemia without carbon dioxide retention was treated by supplemental oxygen breathing rather than by mechanical ventilatory support.

As early as 1912, continuous positive airway pressure in spontaneously breathing patients undergoing thoracic surgical procedures was shown to improve ventilation and to decrease or eliminate cyanosis. By the 1930s, several reports attested to the efficacy of continuous positive-pressure breathing (CPPB), without mechanical ventilation, in treating pulmonary edema, pneumonia, and asthma. This therapy was later used successfully in respiratory distress syndrome of the newborn (hyaline membrane disease) by Gregory and his colleagues (continuous positive airway pressure [CPAP]).[3]

In 1969, positive end-expiratory pressure (PEEP) was combined with controlled mechanical ventilation and used to treat acute respiratory failure in adult patients (adult respiratory distress syndrome [ARDS]). Manipulation of airway pressure in this syndrome, characterized by hypoxemia, usually without carbon dioxide retention, improved ventilation/perfusion ($\dot{V}/\dot{Q}$) relationships and increased PaO_2 at the same or lower concentrations of inspired oxygen (FIO_2).

Intermittent mandatory ventilation (IMV) was introduced in 1971 (for infants) and 1973 (for adults) as a means of weaning patients from prolonged mechanical ventilatory support. Subsequently, IMV evolved into a technique of primary ventilatory care, combining the advantages of spontaneous breathing with those of conventional mechanical ventilation. The addition of PEEP/CPAP to IMV allowed clinicians to attack the problems of hypoxemia and carbon dioxide retention separately in a way that was not possible with conventional ventilators. Synchronized intermittent mandatory ventilation (SIMV) combined spontaneous breathing with periodic assisted or patient-triggered mechanical cycling and prevented superimposition of mechanical breaths on spontaneous ones. This technique, which was alleged to decrease the risk of pulmonary barotrauma, in comparison with IMV, was incorporated into the design of some later mechanical ventilators.

Other forms of treatment, such as inflation-hold (inspiratory pause) and synchronous or asynchronous independent lung ventilation, represent modifications of existing ventilation techniques. Such is not true with high-frequency positive-pressure ventilation (HFPPV), also known as high-frequency jet ventilation (HFJV), high-frequency ventilation

(HFV), and high-frequency oscillation (HFO). Introduced in one form in the late 1960s in Sweden, it took many years to become popular in the United States. The physical principles involved in high-frequency ventilation are as different as mechanical ventilation is from spontaneous breathing.

Currently, little is known about how and why HFPPV works, and only a few commercially produced, special-case and FDA-approved, primary high-frequency ventilators are available for purchase and use in adults. However, many investigators from the fields of medicine and engineering are engaged in research seeking to define the optimal characteristics of the technique, and such ventilators will soon be forthcoming.

Pressure support ventilation (PSV) first appeared in 1981 as "inspiratory assist" on the Engstrom Erica. Shortly thereafter, Siemens introduced the 900C, which featured "pressure support." Literature about this mode was sparse until 1985. Since that time, PSV has been incorporated into most commercially available mechanical ventilators, with the concept being accepted rapidly because patients seem to tolerate this modality very well.

Pressure control ventilation (PCV) was introduced in the 900C Servo by Siemens in 1981, along with pressure support. At the time, literature[4–7] seemed to indicate that neonates with hyaline membrane disease were most effectively ventilated with a constant-pressure, time-cycled, decelerating flow ventilator capable of inverse inspiratory/expiratory (I/E) ratios up to 4 : 1.

CLASSIFICATION OF MECHANICAL VENTILATORS

Classification of mechanical ventilators depends on the proposed function. In simplest terms, a ventilator functions as a substitute for the bellows action of the thoracic cage and diaphragm. To perform this function, the ventilator activity may be divided into separate categories (Table 21–1 and Fig. 21–1).

1. Inspiratory phase
2. Changeover from inspiratory to expiratory phase
3. Expiratory phase
4. Changeover from expiratory to inspiratory phase

Classification of mechanical ventilators has become difficult as manufacturers, responding to the demand from physicians and respiratory therapists, have developed increasingly complex units.

INSPIRATORY PHASE

During inspiration, a positive-pressure gradient causes gas to flow from the ventilator to the patient's lungs. Four factors to be considered during the inspiratory phase include the following:

- Gas flow rate
- Gas volume delivered
- Airway pressure
- Alveolar pressure

These variables are not independent of one another, and each will be affected by changes in the lungs, thorax, and connecting airways. A mechanical ventilator can maintain either constant gas flow or constant pressure, but not both at the same time. Therefore, ventilators may be classified as flow generators or pressure generators, depending on which of these two variables is held more steady.

Table 21—1 Ventilator Variables

INSPIRATORY PHASE

  Flow generator
  Constant
  Nonconstant
  Inflation hold

CHANGEOVER FROM INSPIRATORY TO EXPIRATORY PHASE

  Time-cycled
  Pressure-cycled
  Volume-cycled
  Flow-cycled
  Secondary limit

EXPIRATORY PHASE

  Retard pressure
  Subambient pressure
  Threshold pressure (PEEP, ZEEP, and so forth)

CHANGEOVER FROM EXPIRATORY TO INSPIRATORY PHASE

  Assistor
  Controller
  Assistor–controller
  Intermittent mandatory ventilation (IMV)
  Intermittent demand ventilation
  Synchronized intermittent mandatory ventilation (SIMV)

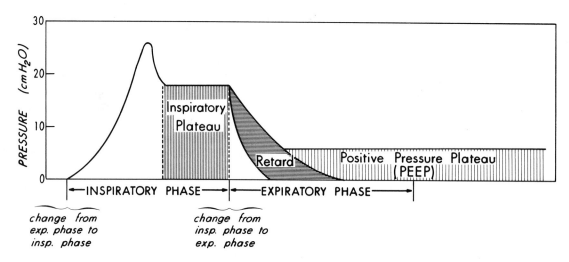

Figure 21—1. Phases of the mechanical ventilator cycle, with and without PEEP and retard.

Flow Generators

Constant-Flow Generator. Constant gas flow requires a high source pressure to maintain a large pressure gradient between ventilator and patient. The effects of alterations in airway resistance and pulmonary compliance on gas delivery are thus minimized. To accomplish this goal safely, constant-flow generators (Fig. 21–2) must have high internal resistance that protects the patient from the full impact of the pressure source.

An oxygen cylinder with an on–off switch between the cylinder and the patient's lungs is an example of a constant-flow generator. If a V_T of 500 mL were desired and the resistance of the cylinder valve was high enough to withstand a flow of 600 L/min, the desired V_T would be achieved in an inspiratory duration of 0.05 second. Such a system is not practical from a clinical standpoint. However, a reducing valve and a sophisticated on–off switch would make this device more efficient and safer.

As the operating pressure of a constant-flow generator is reduced, its characteristics become less and less "pure," and changes in the patient's resistance and compliance will alter the performance characteristics. If the operating pressure is reduced until it equals the pressure within the patient's lungs, the device (in theory) becomes a constant-pressure generator, albeit an entirely ineffective one.

The difficulty in classifying ventilators as either constant-flow or constant-pressure generators is obvious. The two classifications form the extremes on an entire spectrum of performance, and most ventilators fall somewhere in between. Generally, if the flow rate remains relatively constant throughout the inspiratory phase but the pressure varies significantly, a ventilator is classified as a constant-flow generator.

Figure 21—2. Characteristics of a constant-flow generator.

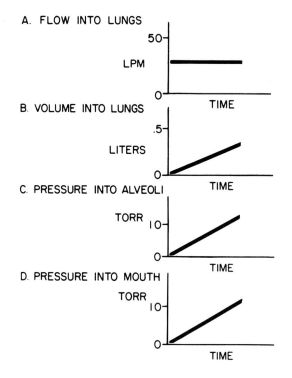

Various methods are used to develop constant gas flow in mechanical ventilators, and include

High-pressure gas sources with reducing valves
Compressors with or without reducing valves
Blowers
Pressure transformers
Gas injectors

Injectors are not, strictly speaking, constant-flow generators because they entrain varying amounts of auxiliary gas, depending on the source pressure and downstream resistance. In the early and middle portions of the inspiratory phase, gas flow is high and relatively constant; in the terminal phase, gas flow falls rapidly. Pressure is variable throughout.

Nonconstant-Flow Generator. A ventilator is classified as a nonconstant-flow generator (Fig. 21–3) when the flow rate changes, but the flow pattern delivered to the patient is the same during each inspiration, regardless of lung–thorax changes. The Emerson 3-PV ventilator is a nonconstant-flow generator that provides a sine wave flow pattern by means of an eccentric cam and piston.

Pressure Generators

Constant Pressure Ventilator. A constant-pressure generator (Fig. 21–4) maintains constant pressure in the patient-breathing circuit throughout inspiration, regardless of lung–thorax changes. It operates with low gas pressure and low internal resistance. Mapleson described a classic constant-pressure generator as a combination of bellows and

Figure 21—3. Characteristics of a nonconstant-flow generator.

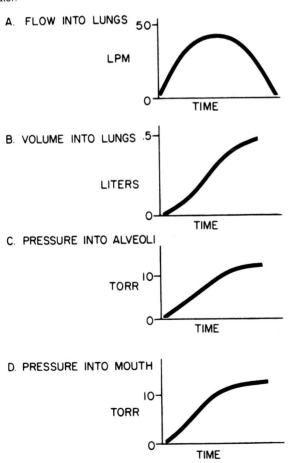

Figure 21—4. Characteristics of a constant-pressure generator.

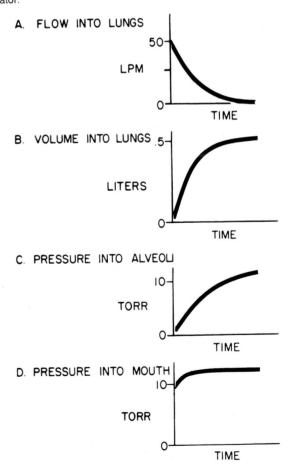

weight.[8] As the weight pushes the bellows down, the pressure output remains constant (the weight does not change). Complete occlusion of the outflow does not change the pressure or force per unit area.

Gas flow from a constant-pressure generator decreases exponentially until the patient and ventilator system pressures equalize. The rate at which equilibrium is attained depends on the compliance and resistance of both the patient and system because the pressure differential is not as great in a constant-pressure generator as it is in other types of ventilators. For example, when the patient compliance (C) is 0.05 L/cmH$_2$O), ventilator resistance is 5 cmH$_2$O/L/sec, and patient resistance is 5 cmH$_2$O/L/sec, the following relationship holds:

1. Patient resistance + ventilator resistance = total resistance (R)

(5 cmH$_2$O/L/sec) + 5 cmH$_2$O/L/sec)
= 10 cmH$_2$O/L/sec

2. The resultant time constant ($R \times C$) is

(10 cmH$_2$O/L/sec) × (0.05 L/cmH$_2$O) = 0.5 sec

In 0.5 second (one time constant) 63% of the V$_T$ will have been delivered. Because the approach of airway pressure to the ventilator-generated pressure is exponential, the two theoretically can never equalize and the preset V$_T$ cannot be delivered quantitatively. In practice, this discrepancy is not important, and a V$_T$ is generally considered complete (98.2%) within four time constants (or in this example 2 seconds).

A constant-pressure generator that employs pressure exceeding that necessary to deliver a desired V$_T$ to the patient deviates from the "ideal" and attains characteristics of a constant-flow generator. If generation pressure developed equals ten times that required to ventilate the patient, the ventilator would then be classified as a constant-flow generator.

Nonconstant-Pressure Ventilator. A ventilator is classified as a nonconstant-pressure generator (Fig. 21–5) if the pressure pattern remains constant from breath to breath, regardless of changes in lung characteristics.

INFLATION-HOLD (INSPIRATORY PLATEAU)

Strictly interpreted, an inflation-hold should be considered part of the inspiratory phase, since the

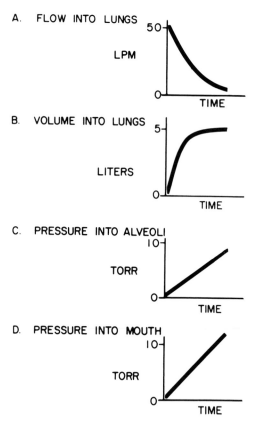

Figure 21–5. Characteristics of a nonconstant-pressure generator.

changeover from the inspiratory to the expiratory phase has not yet occurred (see Fig. 21–1). However, most ventilators that incorporate this mode into their design terminate gas flow during the inflation-hold. We have elected, therefore, to separate inflation-hold for purposes of classification. A few ventilators, such as the BABYbird and Bird Mark VI, continue to deliver gas into the circuit throughout this period (and also during the expiratory phase); hence, our decision is arbitrary. Once flow ceases, the delivered V$_T$ within the patient's lungs is retained, and, theoretically, better distribution of gas to areas of low $\dot{V}/\dot{Q}$ occurs. The duration of the inspiratory plateau usually is designated either in seconds or as a percentage of the total duration of the ventilatory cycle.

CHANGEOVER FROM INSPIRATORY TO EXPIRATORY PHASE

The changeover portion of the respiratory cycle is most familiar to clinicians. In 1958, Elam proposed that ventilators be classified into two primary categories: pressure-limited but volume-variable, and volume-limited but pressure-variable.[9] However, because leaks might develop within the ventilator circuit or other factors might alter the basic operational characteristics, Hunter (see Bibliography) proposed the terms *pressure preset* and *volume preset*. This classification eliminated the problem of determining whether the selected pressure or volume was actually delivered to the patient.

Mapleson introduced a third classification, which has become the most popular and includes the following categories:[8]

1. Time-cycled
2. Pressure-cycled
3. Volume-cycled
4. Flow-cycled

Table 21–2 lists the classifications of commonly used ventilators.

Time-Cycled Ventilators

Time-cycled ventilators terminate gas flow and change to the expiratory phase when a preselected interval has elapsed after the start of inspiration. At the designated time the exhalation valve opens (unless an inflation-hold is used), and the delivered V_T is vented to the ambient atmosphere. If gas flow is constant and the time interval precisely controlled, V_T can be predicted according to the relationship

$$\text{Volume} = \text{flow (volume/unit time)} \times \text{time}$$

This volume, however, is delivered into the circuit, not the patient. Changes in airway resistance and pulmonary or chest wall compliance may alter gas delivery to the patient and cause changes in airway pressure from one breath to the next.

In the United States, time-cycled ventilators have been used extensively to ventilate neonates. Several time-cycled ventilator models developed for older children and adults appear to be as versatile as volume-cycled ventilators in terms of pressure and flow capabilities.

Pressure-Cycled Ventilators

Pressure-cycled ventilators terminate the inspiratory phase when a preselected internal pressure has been achieved. The exhalation valve then opens, initiating the expiratory phase. If an inflation-hold is used, expiration is delayed.

Tidal volume and the time of delivery will vary according to airway resistance, pulmonary and chest wall compliance, and integrity of the ventilator circuit. A significant decrease in the gas delivered to the patient may occur either because of leaks within the ventilator circuit or increased resistance in the circuit or in the patient's airway. A large circuit leak prevents the buildup in pressure needed to terminate gas flow, but the gas does not reach the patient. In contrast, increased resistance, which may be caused by kinking of the circuit tubing or endotracheal tube or by mucus and secretions within the patient's airway, causes a rapid buildup in pressure, and premature cycling occurs before adequate V_T has been delivered. Some pressure-cycled ventilators (such as the Bird Mark 14) incorporate an auxiliary flow augmentation device. This mechanism is activated at a preselected time during the inspiratory phase so that even with significant leaks, V_T is maintained and cycling pressure is reached.

Adjustment to changes in the patient's compliance and resistance is limited with pressure-cycled ventilators; therefore, these ventilators are not usually adapted for use in intensive care. A general opinion prevails that the pressure and flow characteristics of these machines are insufficient to meet the requirements of a patient with acute respiratory failure, because a constant pattern of ventilation is difficult to achieve. However, some pressure-cycled ventilators (such as the Bird Mark 9 and 14) could provide pressure and flow equal to or in excess of that provided by most volume- or time-cycled ventilators currently available.

Pressure-cycled ventilators usually lack a system to deliver precisely controlled levels of oxygen and PEEP. They are used predominately for IPPB and home therapy.

Volume-Cycled Ventilators

Volume-cycled ventilators terminate the inspiratory phase when a preselected volume of gas has been delivered. As with pressure- and time-cycled ventilators, if an inflation-hold is used, the expiratory phase will be delayed. Current volume-cycled ventilators are manufactured with pressure-limiting valves, some fixed and others adjustable, that prevent excessive pressure from developing within the system if airway obstruction occurs. Without this pressure-limiting valve, excessive pressure may lead to pulmonary barotrauma.

Volume-cycled ventilators generally cannot compensate for significant air leak and may not in-

Table 21–2 Ventilator Classification

VENTILATOR	INSPIRATORY PHASE				CHANGE FROM INSPIRATORY TO EXPIRATORY					EXPIRATORY PHASE			CHANGE FROM INSPIRATORY TO EXPIRATORY				
	Flow Generator		Pressure Generator		Inspiratory Plateau	Time Cycle	Pressure Cycle	Volume Cycle	Flow Cycle	Retard	Sub-Ambient	PEEP	Assistor	CMV	Assistor CMV	IMV	SIMV
	Constant	Non-constant	Constant	Non-constant†													
Bear 1	X	X			X		2	X				X		X	X		X
Bear 2/3	X	X	3		X		2	X	3			X		X	X		X
Bear 5	X	X	3		X		2	X	3			X	X	X	X		X
Bear BP 200	X				X	X	2					X		X		2	
Bear Cub	X					X					X	X		X		X	
Bennett 7200a	X	X	2/3			X	2	X	3			X	X	X	X	X	X
Bennett MA-1	X						2			X		*	X	X	X	2	
Bird 6400ST	X	X	3		X	X	2	3		X	X	X	X	X	X	*	X
BABYbird	X					X	2				X	X		X		2	
IMVbird		X				X						*		X		X	
Emerson 3PV	X	X				X				*		*	*	X		X	
Emerson 3MV	X	X				X						X		2		X	
Hamilton Amadeus			3		X	X	2		3			X	X	X	X	2	X
Hamilton Veolar	X	X	2/3		X	X	2		3			X	X	X	X	2	X
Infant Star	X					X	2					X		X		X	
Monaghan 225	X					X	X					X		X			
Ohmeda Advent	X		2/3		X	X	2		3			X	X	X	X	X	X
Ohmeda CPU-1	X		3		X	X	X		3			X	X	X	X		X
Sechrist IV-100B	X					X					X	X		X		X	
Siemens 900C	X	X	2/3		X	X	2		3		X	X	X	X	X	2	X

X = Primary; 2 = alternative method of adjustment; 3 = during pressure-supported breaths only; * = optional; † = The Engstrom Model 300 (not discussed in this chapter) is the only ventilator with this type of pressure generator.

dicate its presence. Gas delivery from a piston stroke or compressible bellows (the most common mechanical devices used to deliver VT) continues unabated, even if the patient is disconnected from the circuit. A leak is usually detected by monitoring the exhaled VT. When the measured flow from the valve is substantially less than that delivered by the ventilator, a leak is present.

Physicians have been led to believe that volume-cycled ventilators maintain constant VT delivery to the patient, regardless of changes in resistance and compliance. This alleged characteristic is largely responsible for the popularity of these devices in critical care settings. Actually, the volume of gas received by the patient may vary considerably with volume-cycled ventilators. When the ventilator cycles, gas flows into both the circuit and the patient. How much is distributed to each depends on their relative compliance. If the patient's compliance decreases, a larger percentage of the tidal volume is lost within the circuit (expansion of the tubing and compression within the humidifier or nebulizer, water traps, bellows or cylinder, connectors, and so forth). Conversely, if the patient's com-

pliance improves, less gas is retained within the circuit.

The compliance/compression factor is variable, but a value of 4 mL/cmH$_2$O is representative. This means that 4 mL of gas is retained within the circuit for each cmH$_2$O of circuit pressure developed. In severe ARDS that requires high airway pressures to maintain adequate ventilation, several hundred milliliters of the total volume may be retained in the circuit rather than delivered to the patient (Fig. 21–6). Personnel who are monitoring the patient and ventilator may be unaware of this discrepancy, however, because a spirometer connected to the exhalation valve assembly records gas passing from both the patient and circuit. The sum of these is the volume that was delivered by the ventilator, but not necessarily to the patient. The latter can be determined only if exhaled gas is collected between the patient's airway and the Y-connector of the ventilator circuit, a technically difficult feat in some cases, or by interposing a respirometer in the same location.

Despite these problems, volume-cycled ventilators are popular in the ICU. They can provide high

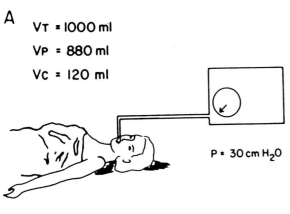

A
VT = 1000 ml
VP = 880 ml
Vc = 120 ml

P = 30 cm H$_2$O

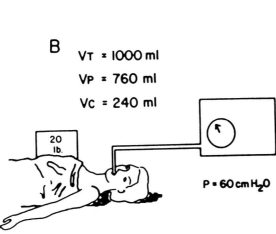

B
VT = 1000 ml
VP = 760 ml
Vc = 240 ml

20 lb.

P = 60 cm H$_2$O

Figure 21–6. Effect of changing patient compliance on ventilation. (*A*) A pressure of 30 cmH$_2$O delivers a tidal volume of 1000 mL, of which 880 mL reaches the patient and 120 mL is retained in the ventilator circuit. (*B*) The ventilator again delivers the 1000 mL tidal volume, but because of decreased patient compliance a pressure of 60 cmH$_2$O is needed, and only 760 mL reaches her, whereas 240 mL is lost to the circuit. In this example, circuit compliance/compression is 4 mL/cmH$_2$O. (VT = total volume delivered by ventilator; VP = patient volume; Vc = retained circuit volume; P = airway pressure.)

pressure and flow; oxygen delivery can be controlled accurately; the humidifiers are efficient; and many incorporate an alarm system to detect mechanical malfunctioning.

Flow-Cycled Ventilators

Flow-cycled ventilators terminate inspiration when gas flow falls below a critical level that is independent of airway pressure, V_T, or duration of inspiration. The best-known example in the United States is the Bennett PR-2 ventilator.

SECONDARY LIMIT

All commonly used mechanical ventilators have a maximum pressure capability. This limit may be incorporated into the basic design or added to the circuit in the form of a "pop-off" valve. Thus ventilators, whatever their primary cycling mechanism may be, are ultimately pressure-limited (whether or not they are also pressure-cycled). This feature is designed to protect the patient against possible excessive pressure buildup or V_T delivery that may occur inadvertently or through the carelessness of a respiratory care practitioner.

The pressure relief mechanism is adjustable in many ventilators, thereby adding to its protection effect. Commonly the relief valve is set 5 to 10 cmH_2O higher than the pressure that is required to ventilate the patient. The primary time- or volume-cycling mechanism will then be operative, and slight to moderate decreases in compliance will be compensated for by the additional available pressure. Significant decreases in compliance or increases in resistance, or both, will cause a buildup in pressure that exceeds the limit that has been set. The relief assembly is then activated, and the excess gas flow and pressure, which might otherwise injure the patient, is vented from the circuit. An alarm usually sounds at the same time to alert persons caring for the patient that something has gone wrong.

In some ventilators it is possible to remove or inactivate the pressure-limiting valve assembly and, thereby, develop a higher operational pressure. This temptation should be resisted because of the risk of injury to the patient and because ventilators generally are designed to operate efficiently within a preselected range of pressure.

EXPIRATORY PHASE

The expiratory phase begins when the exhalation valve opens. The valve may open immediately upon cessation of inspiration or later if an inflation-hold is interposed. Ventilator modulation of expiratory events has become increasingly important.

Because exhalation is usually passive, a longer time is required than for inhalation. However, this ratio (I/E ratio) should be individualized, particularly when an inflation-hold is deemed necessary.

Expiratory Retard

Observation of patients with chronic obstructive pulmonary disease (COPD), who use pursed-lip breathing to apparently prevent premature airway collapse and air trapping, has led to the design of systems that increase resistance or retardation to exhalation (Fig. see 21–1). More complete emptying of the lungs (decreased FRC) occurs, in contrast with PEEP, which characteristically increases FRC. At the termination of expiratory retardation, airway pressure returns to ambient before the next cycle.

All ventilator circuits produce a certain amount of retardation because of the intrinsic resistance to flow of the airway connectors, tubing, and the exhalation valve. The respiratory therapist must be aware of the normal expiratory flow pattern so that undesirable increases in retardation can be detected. The easiest method of detecting increased expiratory retardation is to note the rate at which the airway pressure manometer needle returns to baseline level from the peak after inflation. To be most accurate, one should measure the airway pressure as close as possible to the junction of the ventilator circuit and patient; otherwise, the pressure measurements may be altered by resistance of the ventilator, tubing and so forth.

The importance or desirability of the use of expiratory retard during mechanical ventilation of patients with COPD, acute asthmatic attacks, or the like is unknown. Some studies suggest that the importance attached to pursed–lip breathing has been exaggerated.

Subambient Pressure

The application of a subambient negative pressure to the ventilator circuit during the expiratory phase has been advocated primarily for two purposes: (1) to decrease mean airway (and, hence, mean intrathoracic) pressure, in order to enhance venous return and improve cardiac output; and (2) to offset the effects of excessive resistance that may result from an artificial airway. Reduction of circuit pressure in this way increases the pressure gradient across the tube from the patient end to the circuit end and, in theory, should enhance expiratory gas flow. How much practical importance may be attached to this maneuver is unclear. The use of subambient pressure has fallen from favor because of the difficulty in determining whether the reduced pressure is transmitted to the patient side of the airway. If this occurs, airway collapse and air trapping—the opposite of what is desired—will occur.

Positive End-Expiratory Pressure

Application of positive pressure to the airway during the expiratory phase (see Fig. 21–1) is a mainstay in the treatment of ARDS. The effects of this therapy presumably prevent terminal airway and alveolar collapse and improve overall $\dot{V}/\dot{Q}$ ratios, although some regional $\dot{V}/\dot{Q}$ relationships may actually worsen. Improvement in pulmonary compliance and arterial oxygenation is often significant and may allow a reduction of F_IO_2, a desirable goal to prevent absorption atelectasis and pulmonary oxygen toxicity.

Various techniques are used to generate PEEP. A simple method allows patient exhalation through tubing, the distal end of which is under water. The level of PEEP depends on the depth to which the tubing has been submerged. With other systems, the ventilator activates a valve assembly during exhalation. The valve closes when the desired expiratory positive pressure is reached, and any gas that has not been exhaled is held within the lungs and ventilator circuit. In some cases the valve used to create PEEP also has a high internal resistance, which gives an expiratory retard effect. An elevated mean intrathoracic pressure above that produced by PEEP may result. This can be important in reducing venous return in the patient with marginal intravascular volume or cardiovascular performance.

Before 1975, the recommended maximum level of PEEP was 10 to 15 cmH$_2$O; however, many patients with severe ARDS did not respond with improved oxygenation and decreased shunting at these levels. Subsequent reports attest that increased PEEP (40 cmH$_2$O or more) can be used in selected patients, combined with IMV. A reduced mortality with no increase in ventilator-related morbidity has been reported.

This therapy (termed "super-PEEP" by some) requires meticulous cardiopulmonary monitoring, including pulmonary arterial catheterization. Since some ventilators cannot attain such pressure, it must be generated by special devices such as the Emerson water column PEEP-exhalation valve assembly.

High-level PEEP is indicated for a small percentage of patients. Most persons who require PEEP respond adequately to the earlier recommended levels. For those who do not, however, a willingness on the part of clinicians and respiratory therapists to apply more aggressive therapy may be lifesaving.

CHANGEOVER FROM EXPIRATORY TO INSPIRATORY PHASE

Once the expiratory phase has been completed, a new inspiratory phase is initiated. This cycling may be performed either by the patient or by the ventilator.

Assist Ventilators

A ventilator that incorporates an assist (patient-triggered) mode must be equipped with a mechanism that detects the decrease in airway pressure caused by the patient's voluntary inspiratory activity. An adjustment control allows change of the pressure decrement (sensitivity) that triggers the inspiratory phase, thereby controlling the ventilator response time. Once the ventilator has initiated inspiration, it will deliver gas flow until the desired pressure, volume, or time has been reached. The ventilator-assist mechanism may be electronic, magnetic, fluidic, or pneumatic.

Control Ventilators

Control ventilators cycle automatically at a rate selected by the operator. The adjustment usually is made by a knob calibrated in breaths per minute. The ventilator will cycle regardless of the patient's need or desire for a breath, but guarantees a minimum level of minute ventilation in the apneic, sedated, or paralyzed patient, as long as the ventilator–patient connection is intact and no air leaks are present. Not all ventilators have single controls that set respiratory frequency per se. In some, inspiratory or expiratory timers are available, or controls that vary inspiratory flow rate and expiratory time.

Assist–Control Ventilators

Assist–control ventilators may operate in either mode individually or in both simultaneously (i.e., the ventilator will assist the patient's spontaneous respirations and will also cycle itself should the patient stop breathing or breathe so weakly that the ventilator cannot function as an assistor).

Intermittent Mandatory Ventilation

Ventilators with IMV capability allow the patient to breathe spontaneously, usually through an independent gas supply, but periodically (at a preselected rate and volume) cycle to give a "mandated" breath. Thus, a combination of spontaneous and controlled breaths is provided for the best overall pattern of ventilation in the individual patient. As with controlled ventilation, a minimum level of minute ventilation is provided. Various methods of administering IMV have been used, both "homemade" and factory installed. Most, however, operate with a gas reservoir directed into the inspiratory limb of the ventilator circuit through a unidirectional valve (Fig. 21–7). When the patient inspires, the valve opens, admitting gas from the reservoir; when the ventilator cycles, the valve closes, and gas flow proceeds normally. Gas provided for spontaneous breathing may flow either continuously or from a demand regulator that is activated by the patient.

INDICATIONS FOR MECHANICAL VENTILATION

The decision to institute mechanical ventilation is a serious one. Such therapy entails significant risks to the patient, and the potential benefits must be enough to justify these risks. Proper understanding of the ventilator, its limitations, and the physiologic effects it may produce will limit the untoward responses and complications.

A useful categorization of the indications for mechanical ventilation takes into account whether the lungs are primarily involved in the disease process, secondarily affected by other organ dysfunction, or are normal but compromised because of failure to breathe. The therapeutic implications in each type of disorder are quite different, although entities such as flail chest encompass more than one abnormality.

EXTRAPULMONARY FACTORS

Failure To Breathe

Failure to breathe may result from any disease process that involves the neuromuscular ventilatory

Figure 21–7. IMV circuitry. A demand regulator is substituted for the reservoir bag in some commercially available systems. Spontaneous ventilation is supported from the bag or regulator, while controlled breaths delivered intermittently from the ventilator close the unidirectional valve and are directed to the patient. (Reproduced with permission from Kirby RR: IMV held satisfactory alternative to assisted, controlled ventilation. Clin Trends Anesthesiol 6(4):14, 1976)

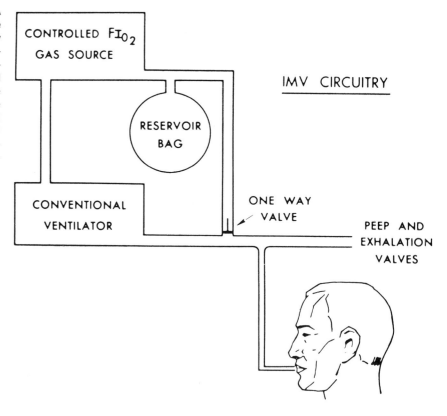

CONTROLLED FI$_{O_2}$ GAS SOURCE

IMV CIRCUITRY

RESERVOIR BAG

CONVENTIONAL VENTILATOR

ONE WAY VALVE

PEEP AND EXHALATION VALVES

axis. In the absence of preexisting pulmonary disease, the lung function is not compromised. If ventilation is supported by mechanical techniques, alveolocapillary gas exchange proceeds normally.

Nevertheless, secondary pulmonary involvement may occur. Patients who must be totally immobilized for long periods and require prolonged tracheal intubation or tracheostomy are increasingly susceptible to infection. They usually cannot mobilize their secretions or cough effectively. Frequent tracheal aspiration using aseptic techniques must be performed, and vigorous attempts should be made to provide good bronchial hygiene through postural drainage, change of position, and chest physiotherapy.

Neuromuscular Disease

Disease processes such as polimoyelitis, Guillain-Barré syndrome, myasthenia gravis, and organic phosphate poisoning produce respiratory insufficiency by preventing normal neuromuscular transmission and effector-organ responses. Respiratory paralysis may develop gradually, and the patient will be unable to maintain normal alveolar ventilation. The deterioration of arterial blood gas concentrations (hypoxemia when the patient breathes air, and hypercarbia) is a direct result of hypoventilation and is not caused by functional disorder of the lungs.

Many of the conditions are potentially reversible; the primary problem from a mechanical ventilatory standpoint is that weeks, and often months, of support must be provided before the patient can once again maintain his or her own ventilation. Physicians and respiratory therapists involved in the treatment of these patients must provide meticulous airway care. The threat of traumatic damage to the trachea by either endotracheal or tracheostomy tubes and their occlusive cuffs increases with the duration of mechanical ventilation.

Central Nervous System Disease

Diseases that originate in the brain or spinal cord (Chap. 35) are included as diseases of the CNS. Direct trauma that causes cerebral hemorrhage or transection of the spinal cord at a high cervical level is the most immediately life-threatening. If the patient survives the initial insult, however, prolonged mechanical ventilatory support, sometimes for the duration of his or her life, may be needed. A complication of brain trauma is neurogenic pulmonary edema, which may result from regional hy-

poxemia or hypoperfusion of the hypothalamic area at the base of the brain. Hence, an organic pulmonary lesion is superimposed on the functional derangement caused by the CNS lesion.

Other CNS disorders that lead to ventilatory abnormalities include bacterial and viral infectious processes, such as meningoencephalitis and tetanus. These conditions often are associated with initial tachypnea and hyperventilation, but if respiratory arrest and convulsions ensue, mechanical ventilation may be needed for prolonged periods.

More perplexing, and less common, are primary CNS disorders that result in alveolar hypoventilation. These may be present in premature infants who have no detectable organic lung disease and who experience long apneic periods. Tactile stimulation may initiate and sustain ventilation, otherwise, mechanical ventilation is needed. In older children and adults with this problem, hypoventilation occurs with sleep; as long as the person is awake, ventilation appears to be normal. This syndrome (primary idiopathic alveolar hypoventilation, or Ondine's curse) as yet has no explanation. However, in severe cases, tracheostomy and mechanical ventilation may be needed during the sleeping hours.

Finally, several neurologic disease processes of unknown etiologies progress slowly but eventually result in respiratory failure, including multiple sclerosis and amyotrophic lateral sclerosis. Clinical courses vary from patient to patient, but the long-term prognosis is now generally unfavorable.

Musculoskeletal Disease

The most common musculoskeletal derangement involves chest wall trauma with multiple rib fractures and subsequent disruption of ventilation (flail chest). In the past, patients with this lesion required mechanical ventilation for 20 days or longer before ventilation occurred without flail. Recent evidence shows that the flail of itself is not usually of pulmonary significance, but rather the underlying pulmonary injury, and that the total period of mechanical ventilation can be shortened significantly or even eliminated. Other disease entities in this category include kyphoscoliosis, muscular dystrophies, and dermatomyositis.

DISORDERS OF PULMONARY GAS EXCHANGE

Pulmonary gas exchange disorders collectively account for the largest number of patients who require mechanical ventilation in neonatal, pediatric, and adult intensive care units. These disorders are characterized by primary lung involvement rather than by extrapulmonary factors.

Respiratory Distress Syndrome of the Newborn

Respiratory distress syndrome of the newborn (RDS) is associated primarily with prematurity of the newborn infant and is characterized by atelectasis, decreased FRC, right-to-left intrapulmonic shunting, hypoxemia, and carbon dioxide retention. Mortality figures before 1969 were as high as 80% in mechanically ventilated infants. However, since the introduction of PEEP/CPAP, used either alone or in conjunction with mechanical ventilation, survival has improved substantially. The subject is discussed in detail in Chapter 28.

Adult Respiratory Distress Syndrome

A large number of seemingly unrelated disease processes are included in ARDS. Pulmonary involvement, however, is similar, suggesting that the pathologic response of the lung to various noxious stimuli is limited. The disease characteristics of ARDS are similar to those of RDS. However, the $PaCO_2$ usually is lower than normal. In fact, hypercapnia in a patient without chronic pulmonary disease is an ominous prognostic sign.

The signs and symptoms of ARDS frequently can be reversed with mechanical ventilation and PEEP. A clear-cut reduction in mortality, such as that seen in IRDS, has not been demonstrated, probably because many patients with ARDS have multiple complicating problems (CNS damage, renal and hepatic failure, long-bone fractures, sepsis, hemorrhage, and cardiac disease, among others). This subject is discussed in detail in Chapter 32.

Cardiac Disease

Disorders of gas exchange occur with some cardiovascular diseases and secondarily affect pulmonary function. Any condition that leads to left-sided heart failure and significant elevation of left ventricular end-diastolic pressure can result in pulmonary edema and decreased arterial oxygenation. Mechanical ventilation may be used to improve oxygenation and impede venous return, thereby reversing cardiac dilatation and allowing the heart to contract more effectively.

If heart failure has been long-standing or severe, pulmonary hypertension will occur, and permanent structural changes may lead to cor pulmonale. Mechanical ventilation may be needed, but the results are less dramatic and the prognosis is grave. This subject is discussed in detail in Chapter 33.

Pulmonary Embolism

Venous thromboemboli and fat embolization often result in hypoxemia because of reflex bronchospasm, permeability changes in the alveolar-capillary membrane, and pulmonary microvascular hypertension. Mechanical ventilation with PEEP is often associated with marked improvement in oxygenation. This subject is discussed in Chapter 36.

Miscellaneous Disorders

Mechanical ventilation is indicated postoperatively in patients whose ventilation remains depressed from the residual effects of anesthetic agents or muscle relaxants. Support is maintained only until these effects have dissipated and then may be discontinued rapidly.

Occasionally, mechanical ventilation is used for the patient who is at high risk for developing respiratory failure, although, when the decision is made, no direct evidence for failure may be present. The use of prophylactic intervention with mechanical ventilation in an attempt to abort or prevent respiratory failure has many adherents, but little objective evidence supporting its use has been published.

CRITERIA FOR VENTILATORY SUPPORT

Various criteria have been suggested to ascertain when to begin mechanical ventilation[10] (Table 21-3). When pulmonary function tests are used as a guide either to initiate or to terminate mechanical ventilation, physicians must remember that many factors are involved in the individual tests themselves (Table 21-4). Few reasons can be advanced to ventilate a patient with COPD solely on the basis of a $PaCO_2$ of 70 torr if his normal $PaCO_2$ is 60 to 70 torr. Conversely, an identical value in a previously healthy young adult suggests that ventilation should be supported. Each patient should be considered individually and laboratory measurements

Table 21—3 Guidelines for Ventilatory Support in Adults with Acute Respiratory Failure

DATUM	NORMAL RANGE	TRACHEAL INTUBATION AND VENTILATION INDICATED
MECHANICS		
Respiratory rate	12–20	>35
Vital capacity (ml/kg body weight)	65–75	<15
FEV_1 (ml/kg body weight)	50–60	<10
Inspiratory force (cmH_2O)	75–100	<25
OXYGENATION		
PaO_2 (mmHg)	100–75 (air)	<70 (on mask)
$P(A-aDO_2)$ (mmHG)	25–65	>450
VENTILATION		
$PaCO_2$ (mmHg)	35–45	>55
V_D/V_T	0.25–0.40	>0.60

Table 21—4 Factors in Bedside Pulmonary Function Testing

Baseline "normal" values for the individual patient
Nature of the underlying disease process
Patient understanding of the test procedure
Patient cooperation and motivation
Knowledge and skill of the person administering the tests

used as adjunctive aids that precede any decision to employ mechanical ventilation.

TECHNIQUES OF MECHANICAL VENTILATION

ASSISTED VENTILATION

Assisted (patient-triggered) ventilation (AV) is used to (1) deliver humidified gases and aerosols to patients with acute or chronic airway and parenchymal disease by IPPB, (2) provide ventilatory support for both adults and infants (particularly infants) with acute respiratory failure, and (3) wean patients from controlled mechanical ventilation

(CMV) and initiate spontaneous respiratory activity (Fig. 21–8).

The arguments in support of this latter technique center primarily on the alleged normal physiologic aspects of such ventilation. Because the patient initiates the ventilator cycle, intrathoracic pressure decreases transiently before the mechanical respiratory phase, and venous return and cardiac output are enhanced. The patient sets his own ventilatory rate rather than being subjected to a superimposed, unsuitable pattern of ventilation. Theoretically, a more normal arterial pH and $PaCO_2$ result. Finally, periodic initiation of spontaneous effort reinforces normal ventilatory activity by preventing "disuse" of the respiratory muscles.

No convincing evidence exists that assisted ventilation provides the cited advantages to a clinically significant degree. If an assist mechanism operates properly, it will respond instantaneously. When the ventilator cycles, the events that follow are identical with those in the "control" mode, and it is doubtful whether the foregoing advantageous circulatory or respiratory effects ensue. Conversely, if the assist mechanism is not functioning properly, the patient expends considerable effort attempting to breathe, but cannot cycle the ventilator. He becomes agitated, hypoxic, hypercarbic, and "fights the ventilator." Controlled ventilation frequently is needed.

The effects of assisted ventilation on arterial pH and PCO_2 are not accurately ascertained without frequent arterial blood gas measurements. Underlying pulmonary abnormalities often increase a

Figure 21—8. Assisted (patient-triggered) ventilation (AV). An initial decrease in system pressure (P) results from the patient's spontaneous breathing effort. A sensing mechanism within the ventilator responds to the pressure decrement, and a mechanical cycle is initiated, producing gas flow and a positive pressure (T_I = inspiratory time; T_E = expiratory time). (Reproduced with permission from Eross B et al: Common ventilator modes: Terminology. In Kirby RR, Graybar GB (eds): Intermittent Mandatory Ventilation. Int Anesthesiol Clin 18(2):39, 1980)

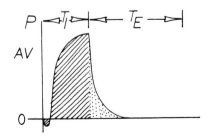

patient's minute ventilation to levels far above normal. Even though he is receiving assisted ventilation, his pH and $PaCO_2$ may be abnormal.

The greatest difficulty with assisted ventilation is improper adjustment of the ventilator, leading to unreliability of many assist mechanisms. One frequently experiences situations in which the assist mode is so sensitive that the ventilator autocycles. In other instances it is so insensitive that the ventilator does not respond to the patient's inspiratory effort, and controlled ventilation must be used.

CONTROLLED VENTILATION

Controlled mechanical ventilation (CMV) (Fig. 21–9) is used in several clinical settings:

1. When apnea is present, either because of primary CNS dysfunction (e.g., severe brain trauma, spinal cord injuries, poliomyelitis) or because of drug overdosage, intentional sedation, or neuromuscular paralysis by drugs, such as curare and pancuronium
2. As a backup (fail-safe) for assisted ventilation, should the patient fail to sustain spontaneous ventilatory activity
3. In conditions such as flail chest when spontaneous ventilatory effort is thought to be deleterious, and splinting of the chest wall is advocated
4. If therapy such as high-level PEEP makes the assist mode ineffective or of questionable reliability

Generally, physicians and respiratory therapists use controlled mechanical ventilation when a

certain level of ventilation must be "guaranteed" and when failure to supply this level of ventilation could be fatal. Most patients with severe respiratory insufficiency are initially treated with CMV to eliminate uncertainty over the adequacy of support. However, certain aspects of ventilation peculiar to CMV must be understood by all persons who use it therapeutically.

When spontaneous ventilation is depressed by muscle paralysis or heavy sedation, accidental disconnection of the ventilator circuit may occur. The ventilator alarm systems serve to decrease the possibility that such a disconnection will go unnoticed; nevertheless, such incidents are reported each year.

Often, controlled ventilation is not facilitated by sedative or paralytic drugs, but rather by deliberately increased minute ventilation so that hyperventilation ensues and the $PaCO_2$ falls below normal levels of 35 to 45 torr. As long as most patients are not hypoxemic, they will respond by becoming apneic, and their ventilation can then be controlled readily. Recent studies, however, suggest that the respiratory alkalemia induced by such techniques may be deleterious to the patient's overall physiologic status (Table 21–5). Such therapy may exacerbate the primary condition, increasing the patient's need for mechanical ventilation.

Controlled ventilation does not guarantee that patients will not attempt to initiate spontaneous ventilation. In such instances, the ventilator will not respond if it is used in a strictly control mode, and the ventilatory pattern becomes asynchronous: the patient attempts to take more breaths than the ventilator will provide. Failure to obtain a breath on demand leads to patient apprehension and may result in carbon dioxide retention.

The effects of CMV on cardiopulmonary function cannot be overlooked. Rapid controlled venti-

Figure 21–9. Controlled ventilation (CMV). Ventilator cycling is automatic at a preselected rate. An initial pressure (P) decrement is not present. (Reproduced with permission from Eross B et al: Common ventilator modes: Terminology. In Kirby RR, Graybar GB (eds): Intermittent Mandatory Ventilation. Int Anesthesiol Clin 18(2):39, 1980)

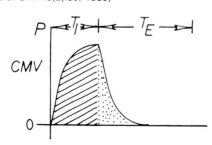

Table 21–5 Adverse Effects of Respiratory Alkalemia

Decreased
Cardiac output
Cerebral blood flow
Pulmonary compliance
Serum potassium concentration
Serum ionized calcium concentration
Increased
Oxygen consumption
Airway resistance
Oxyhemoglobin affinity (transient)

lation with large V_T increases mean intrathoracic pressure, particularly when combined with PEEP, and venous pressure return and cardiac output decrease. Consequently, cardiovascular function may be depressed both by respiratory alkalemia and by mechanical factors secondary to CMV.

INTERMITTENT MANDATORY VENTILATION

In 1971, IMV (Fig. 21–10) was introduced to wean infants from mechanical ventilation. Later, IMV was found to be similarly efficacious in adults. Additional work has established that certain benefits are derived when IMV is used as a primary form of ventilatory support, rather than solely as a weaning technique.

1. Conventional weaning techniques interpose periods in which the patient depends entirely on the ventilator with periods in which he must breathe on his own. Such alternating support may be physiologically as well as psychologically unsound. Abrupt disconnection of ventilation can produce anxiety and tachypnea, increase $\dot{V}O_2$ and ultimately result in failure to wean. IMV allows a smooth transition by gradually slowing the ventilator rate as the patient assumes an increasing percentage of the total work of breathing (WOB). No

other variables (e.g., V_T, FiO_2, PEEP) need be changed.

2. Throughout the entire period of ventilation, the $PaCO_2$ and pH are maintained relatively constant. Only enough ventilator support is given to maintain these arterial blood gas values within the range deemed appropriate for the individual patient. The patient is not forced to submit to a pattern of ventilation controlled by the ventilator; rather, the ventilator augments the patient's own ventilatory effort to the degree necessary. Respiratory alkalemia is avoided without resorting to depressant drugs or added mechanical dead space. This is particularly important in patients with COPD who suffer acutely superimposed respiratory failure and require mechanical ventilatory support. A very low IMV rate will return these patients' $PaCO_2$ and pH levels toward their own "normal" values. The patient with a baseline, steady-state $PaCO_2$ of 65 torr receives only enough IMV to achieve this level rather than being controlled at levels of 35 to 45 torr, as previously customary.

3. Very high levels of PEEP may be used with IMV, in contrast to the level that may be used successfully with CMV. Mean intrathoracic pressure is lower at any given level of expiratory positive pressure, and venous return is affected less deleteriously with IMV (Fig. 21–11). Patients who fail to respond to conventional therapy or who would otherwise have died or been consigned to extracorporeal membrane oxygenator support (ECMO) may be treated with PEEP as high as 30 to 40 torr because the nonmandated breaths reduce the cardiovascular effects of positive pressure.

4. Drugs such as morphine are required only for pain and not to induce respiratory depression. Neuromuscular-blocking drugs are seldom needed. Consequently, the dangers of profound hypoxemia are lessened, should the patient be disconnected from the ventilator accidentally.

Figure 21–10. Intermittent mandatory ventilation (IMV). A combination of both spontaneous and ventilator-controlled ventilation can be delivered at any ratio. Lower mean airway and intrapleural pressure result, compared with controlled ventilation.

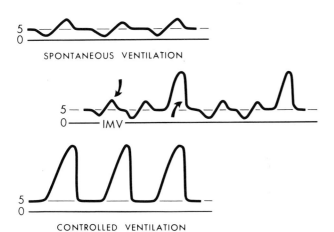

AIRWAY PRESSURES

SPONTANEOUS VENTILATION

IMV

CONTROLLED VENTILATION

As with any system of ventilator support, certain potential disadvantages may be noted:

1. Many IMV devices are "homemade." Improper assembly, such as unidirectional

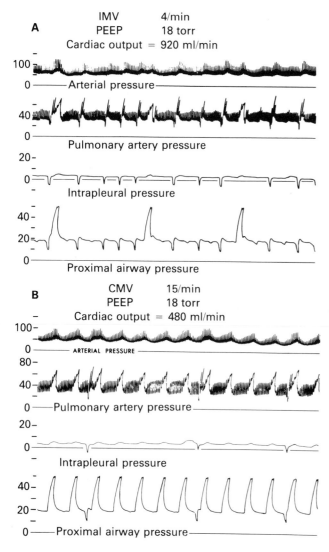

Figure 21—11. Hemodynamic effects of IMV compared with CMV at increased PEEP. (A) Fewer mechanical cycles and maintenance of spontaneous breathing result in decreased intrapleural pressure, augmentation of venous return, and maintenance of blood pressure, stroke volume, and cardiac output. (B) CMV (with the exception of three spontaneous breaths) significantly compromises cardiovascular function. (Reproduced with permission from Kirby RR: Mechanical ventilation in acute ventilatory failure: Facts, fiction and fallacies. In Brunner EA et al (eds): Current Problems in Anesthesia and Critical Care Medicine. Copyright 1977 by Year Book Medical Publishers, Chicago)

valves installed backward, may result in total malfunction and can be disastrous to the patient if not detected immediately. This problem is less frequent in manufactured units that incorporate IMV. Valves that

"stick" open during switchover to the non-mandated mode are also an occasional problem.

2. If a patient who has previously needed a low IMV rate becomes apneic, his ventilation will not be supported adequately. IMV should be used only in those patients in whom CNS function is intact enough to facilitate regular spontaneous ventilatory effort. The physician or respiratory therapist can be no less vigilant simply because the patient is receiving IMV!

3. The delivery of a mandated breath from the ventilator just as the patient finished spontaneous inspiration could lead to overdistention of the lung. Whether this concern is justified is debatable, particularly because a "sigh" mechanism has been used on many mechanical ventilators to achieve this very end: the delivery of a larger than normal V_T in the hope of preventing microatelectasis. However, newly designed IMV apparatuses are now available that deliver the mandated breath only at the beginning of the patient's spontaneous inspiration. The terminology applied to this modification of the basic IMV technique by the manufacturers of ventilators providing this option is synchronized intermittent mandatory ventilation (SIMV) or intermittent demand ventilation (IDV). Although this concept is attractive theoretically, published evidence shows that it offers no advantage over conventional IMV. Furthermore, the ventilator may fail to cycle appropriately, similar to the failure of certain assist mechanisms, a disturbing consideration.

PRESSURE-SUPPORT VENTILATION

The concept of pressure-support ventilation should be considered in three phases: initiation of inspiration, inspiratory flow generation, and cycling mechanism.

Initiation of Inspiration

Pressure support ventilation (PSV) is a form of assisted ventilation. The patient must initiate or trigger each breath by lowering airway pressure to a predetermined level set by the sensitivity control on the ventilator. Patients with an unstable respiratory drive should not be considered candidates for

PSV. Some, although not all, mechanical ventilators utilize backup modes of ventilation to avoid apneic episodes while on PSV or other ventilatory modes, dependent upon spontaneous ventilation.

Existing literature suggests that proper application of PSV may reduce patient WOB. In particular, PSV is useful in overcoming the added work of breathing imposed (WOB_{imp}) by artificial airways,[11] ventilator circuitry,[12] and demand valves.[13,14]

Two approaches have evolved for application of PSV. In the first, MacIntyre suggests the use of PSV_{max}, which is defined as the level of PSV that results in the slowest regular respiratory rate.[15] On the average, PSV_{max} produces tidal volumes (V_T) nearly identical with the preexisting V_T established while on SIMV or CMV. Patients appear to tolerate this ventilatory technique extremely well, when compared with SIMV or CMV. Evidence of this is provided by a reduction in respiratory frequency and arterial blood pressure. Patient comfort is also improved because patients determine their own respiratory rate, V_T, and inspiratory time. As patients improve clinically, weaning is accomplished by reducing the PSV level incrementally, gradually increasing the WOB_{imp}. When the PSV level approaches zero, the patient is considered to be a candidate for extubation.

A more conservative approach to the use of PSV is to select an assisting pressure level that will neutralize WOB_{imp}. Fiastro et al have quantitated the level of PSV required to overcome WOB_{imp} by various diameter artificial airways.[11] Despite this information, the workloads imposed by humidifiers, ventilator circuits, and demand valves prevent the easy quantification of appropriate levels of PSV to administer under all conditions. Several ventilator manufacturers incorporate a small amount of PSV (approximately 2 to 3 cmH_2O) with each spontaneous breath. This small boost occurs with or without activation of the PS mechanism and presumably overcomes the work required to move physiologic inspiratory flow rates across the inspiratory limb of the ventilator circuit (not including artificial airways). In addition, if the WOB_{imp} can be effectively neutralized, patients are more likely to tolerate weaning and their potential to maintain adequate, spontaneous alveolar ventilation upon extubation can more adequately be assessed.

Inspiratory Flow Generation

Pressure support transforms a conventional ventilator into an operator-adjusted, constant-pressure generator. The operator selects a pressure greater than the end-expiratory level; during mechanical inspiration, the ventilator will generate and maintain the selected pressure. Inspiratory flow generated by the ventilator will depend upon the selected pressure level, the flow-generating algorithm or drive pressure of the ventilator in use, and the lung–thorax compliance and airways resistance of the patient. The characteristic decelerating inspiratory flow pattern closely resembles a decaying, zero-approaching exponential curve and is the direct result of a reduced-pressure gradient across the ventilator circuit, which occurs concomitantly with filling of the lungs and the subsequent equilibration of pressure between the ventilator circuit and the pulmonary structures.

Cycling Mechanism

As a PS breath begins, an initial high flow of gas is directed into the ventilator circuit, establishing the selected PS level. As the lung fills, airway pressure rises and the pressure gradient across the ventilator circuit is reduced; concomitantly, inspiratory flow decelerates. When inspiratory flow reaches approximately 25% of the initial flow, the PS breath is terminated. Although flow is the primary cycling mechanism in PSV, most ventilators incorporate several added backup or safety-cycling mechanisms, such as time or pressure, or both. For example, if a patient on PSV developed an extensive leak around an artificial airway, it is possible that the ventilator might fail to cycle if the leak exceeded the critical value of 25% of the initial flow. A properly designed ventilator would terminate the PS breath after an appropriate time interval, generally 1 to 5 seconds.

PRESSURE-CONTROL VENTILATION

The concept of pressure-control ventilation (PCV) should be considered in three distinct phases: initiation of inspiration, inspiratory flow generation and pattern, and cycling mechanism.

Initiation of Inspiration

Until recently, ventilators offering PCV have provided the modality for use within the assist-control or control mode only. The Hamilton Medical ventilator, however, allows the operator to provide pressure-controlled, time-cycled breaths within the SIMV mode, in addition to the more traditional assist-control and control modes.

Existing literature implies that PCV is most beneficial when applied to patients in severe RDS (neonatal or adult) and should be implemented in conjunction with low control pressures, high ventilator rates, and inverse I/E ratios.[6,7,16–19] The technique permits the clinician to utilize reduced inflation pressures and PEEP settings (generally below 40 and 10 cmH$_2$O, respectively) while simultaneously increasing the mean airway pressure (Paw). The most significant benefits provided by PCV include reduced barotrauma and improved oxygenation.

The operating hypothesis for PCV suggests that low control pressures function to stabilize and recruit alveoli, while ventilation occurs during the exhalation phase as the lung deflates to the PEEP level.[7] This concept is contrary to conventional ventilatory methods that rely on positive-pressure V$_T$ delivery to provide ventilation and PEEP to prevent alveolar collapse.[6,7,18,19]

The appropriate adjustment of PCV, in general, requires the use of sophisticated monitoring equipment. The ability to measure expiratory flow is of particular importance. By utilizing such equipment, it is possible to begin each inspiratory phase immediately before the termination of expiratory flow. This allows sufficient time for complete exhalation, yet reduces the magnitude of airway collapse.

The preliminary studies, although provocative, will require a substantial amount of follow-up and additional study to elucidate the physiologic principles applicable to the technique. The prospect of dramatically lowering the levels of positive pressure required to ventilate patients with RDS, thereby reducing barotrauma, certainly warrants our attention.

Inspiratory Flow Generation

Pressure control, when selected, transforms a conventional ventilator into an operator-adjusted, constant-pressure generator. The operator selects a pressure above the end-expiratory level; then, during mechanical inspiration, the ventilator will generate and maintain the selected pressure. The inspiratory flow generated by the ventilator depends upon several factors, including the selected pressure level, because the higher the selected pressure level, the greater the pressure gradient across the ventilator circuit and subsequently higher flow rates that result; the flow-generating algorithm or drive pressure of the ventilator in use; and the lung–thorax compliance (CLT) and airways resistance of the patient. The characteristic decelerating inspiratory flow pattern closely resembles a zero-approaching, exponential curve. This pattern is the result of a reduced pressure gradient across the ventilator circuit, which occurs concomitantly with filling of the lungs and equilibration of pressure between the ventilator circuit and the pulmonary structures.

Cycling Mechanism

The principal cycling mechanism for PCV is time. If the lung fills and flow terminates before the completion of the allotted inspiratory interval, an inspiratory pause will result. As a safety feature, premature cycling will occur in the event airway pressures in excess of 2 cmH$_2$O above the selected PC level are sensed.

AIRWAY PRESSURE-RELEASE VENTILATION

The acronym APRV (airway pressure-release ventilation) was coined by John B. Downs in 1987.[20] In applying this technique, patients with acute lung injury are placed on a level of CPAP sufficient to restore the FRC to a more physiologic level. Spontaneous ventilation is allowed at all times. However, should additional ventilation be required, airway pressure is periodically reduced to ambient or a lower level of CPAP. Removal of the airway pressure reduces the FRC, with a resultant patient exhalation and ventilation. At the moment exhalation is complete, the CPAP level is restored. As a general rule, the exhalation phase is passive and dependent upon the expiratory time constant of the lung and the ventilator system in use. Exhalation can be considered to be complete after 2.5 time-constant intervals. Time constants can be difficult to estimate at the bedside, and a flow-monitoring device might be useful in determining the appropriate expiratory interval. In the absence of such equipment, an expiratory interval of 1.5 to 2 seconds is recommended.[21,22]

This ventilatory mode is similar to pressure-control ventilation (PCV). The only substantial difference is that spontaneous breathing is permitted by the APRV system. Advocates of the system claim that by allowing spontaneous breathing, patient comfort and acceptance of the mode is enhanced.[22] In addition, paralysis or sedation of the patient, or both, can be avoided.[23] On the other hand, the WOB imposed by 20 cmH$_2$O or more of CPAP is more than substantial. Without patient spontaneous contribution, the mode becomes essentially identical with PCV.

Although APRV may be similar to PCV, it is indistinguishable from constant flow, time-cycled, pressure-limited, inverse I/E ratio ventilation—a standard form of neonatal ventilation in many institutions. This statement was reinforced by Sechrist Industries Inc. when they modified an IV-100B infant ventilator to provide APRV by simply renaming the front panel controls. No internal modifications were necessary (personal communication).

Early reports[22,24,25,26] indicate APRV can significantly reduce peak inflation pressures and may reduce the frequency of barotrauma. In addition, the technique has been shown to maintain minute ventilation, PaO_2, $PaCO_2$, and cardiac output while concomitantly reducing mean airway pressure.

Interestingly, because ventilation occurs by the removal of airway pressure, the more the ventilator rate is increased, the lower the mean airway pressure becomes. This becomes a distinct advantage when unstable cardiovascular patients require significant levels of mechanical ventilation.

At present, this modality is experimental and is not available on commercial ventilators. Ongoing research into APRV should help to verify its application and to determine how it compares with PCV and other more conventional forms of therapy.

HIGH-FREQUENCY VENTILATION

High-frequency ventilation (HFV) represents a significant departure from conventional mechanical ventilation. It is an oversimplification to consider the various mechanisms employed as though they were only slight modifications of a basic principle. As originally described, HFPPV did not differ greatly from IPPV, as is now supposed. Frequencies ranged from 60 to 100 cycles per minute (cpm; 1 to 1.7 Hz), and V_T, although reduced, still exceeded calculated dead space. Of major significance was the reduction in peak and mean airway pressure to the intrapleural space.

Subsequent development has increased the frequencies used up to 3000 cpm (50 Hz) in clinical use and up to 7200 cpm (120 Hz) in experimental animals. To achieve the higher frequencies, drive mechanisms incorporate rotary fixed orifices and amplifier–speaker assemblies. Tidal volume delivery is often considerably less than predicted dead space, and the mechanism by which alveolar ventilation is achieved is highly controversial.

The present and future roles of HFV are difficult to define. Experimental protocols have been hampered because only a few existing high-frequency ventilators are available, and these are almost entirely in prototype form. Hence, the characteristics of one system often have little resemblance to those of another, and large-scale studies are difficult at best. Because of this limited availability, investigators cannot corroborate or refute the reported experimental and clinical findings of others. These same limitations have made it virtually impossible to define optimal frequencies, V_T, and pressure.

Many experimental studies have appeared in the published literature since 1978. However, clinical information has mostly been limited to case reports or series in which the small number of patients studied makes interpretation difficult. Nevertheless, most people involved in HFV research are optimistic that its proper role will eventually be defined and that the technique, in its many forms, will contribute significantly to reduced ventilator-related morbidity. In the meantime, if the studies of HFV do nothing more than elucidate mechanisms by which ventilation is possible under operant conditions, the gain in knowledge will be substantial.

COMPLICATIONS OF MECHANICAL VENTILATION

PULMONARY BAROTRAUMA

Among the most significant complications of mechanical ventilation are various forms of barotrauma, including

- Pulmonary interstitial emphysema
- Pneumomediastinum
- Pneumopericardium
- Pneumoperitoneum and pneumoretroperitoneum
- Tension pneumothorax
- Venous and arterial air embolism.

Current thought holds that the initiating event in "barotrauma" is overdistention of alveoli by either excessive pressure, volume, or both, with a resultant tearing of the alveolar wall and dissection into the interstitial space. There, it may tear into the mediastinum or through the pleural reflections of the great vessels to the pericardium. Additional dissection along the fascial planes into the subcutaneous tissues of the neck, head, thorax, and the rest of the body (subcutaneous emphysema) also occurs (see Fig. 12-21).

Except for vascular air embolism, which is often fatal (in massive cases it is instantaneously fatal), the most dangerous conditions are tension pneumothorax and pneumopericardium. In each condition the venous return is reduced substantially, producing a fall in arterial blood pressure and in cardiac output. With tension pneumothorax, decreased ventilation is also present.

The incidence of barotrauma (primarily pneumothorax) with mechanical ventilation has been cited at 10% to 20%, although in infants an incidence as high as 30% has been reported. Even though PEEP would seem to increase the risk, this possibility has not been proved. Lowering the number of mechanical ventilations per minute with IMV decreases mean intrathoracic pressure, compared with techniques by which ventilation is controlled, and may also lower the incidence of barotrauma.

Control of inspiratory flow rates to achieve more uniform distribution of gas flow appears warranted to prevent gross overdistention of areas of high $\dot{V}/\dot{Q}$. It also seems prudent to use exhalation systems that produce a minimal amount of retardation to flow (unless more is specifically desired for a given patient) to further decrease the mean intrathoracic pressure.

The presence of subcutaneous emphysema, although not necessarily dangerous in itself, indicates the presence of barotrauma. For early detection of complications of ventilator therapy, frequent physical examination to determine the adequacy of breath sounds bilaterally, constant monitoring of vital signs, and serial roentgenogram are all needed. Personnel should be familiar with simple techniques to decompress a tension pneumothorax in emergencies. Prophylactic bilateral chest tube thoracostomies should not be performed in patients undergoing mechanical ventilation with PEEP. No published evidence has demonstrated the efficacy of such treatment.

CARDIOVASCULAR COMPLICATIONS

Any mechanism that increases intrathoracic pressure tends to reduce venous return and cardiac output. This observation was documented by Cournand and his associates in studies on intermittent positive-pressure breathing.[27] Cournand's studies, however, were performed on animals and humans with normal pulmonary structure and function. More recent studies suggest that in pa-

tients who have acute respiratory failure and whose lungs have decreased compliance, the depressant cardiovascular effects of mechanical ventilation and PEEP may be minimal unless the patient is hypovolemic. Much of the high airway pressure dissipates within the noncompliant lung before it can be transmitted to the great vessels within the intrapleural space.

The effects of PEEP can be minimized by infusing judicious amounts of blood, plasma expanders, and balanced electrolyte solutions to maintain or expand the blood volume above normal. The depression of blood pressure and cardiac output by mechanical ventilation and PEEP can also be reduced markedly by IMV (see Fig. 21–11). Again, a low mean intrathoracic pressure resulting from fewer mechanical breaths and the patient's spontaneous breathing appears to be of paramount importance.

A major advantage of HFV may be reduced cardiovascular depressant effects, compared with conventional ventilation. The V_T approaches and, in some instances, is less than the calculated dead space; also, peak and mean airway pressures are very low (at least in normal experimental subjects). Unfortunately, these advantages may not be as great in patients with ARDS. Recent studies suggest that to improve PaO_2, a mean airway pressure equal to that achieved with conventional ventilatory techniques is needed. The technique should be particularly useful in certain specific forms of respiratory insufficiency that at present are poorly managed by conventional methods, including bronchopleural–cutaneous fistula, malignant pulmonary interstitial emphysema, diaphragmatic hernia in the newborn, and acute exacerbations of COPD that require mechanical ventilatory support.

MISCELLANEOUS COMPLICATIONS

Many other complications are associated with mechanical ventilation, including pulmonary infection, airway obstruction, and tracheal damage from improper occlusive cuffs. Most of these problems can be minimized, if not eliminated, through careful attention by the physician, nurse, and respiratory therapist.

CHOICE OF A MECHANICAL VENTILATOR

Several factors should be considered before a mechanical ventilator is purchased, including the purpose for which it will be used, the experience of the people who will be using it, the ease of maintenance or repair, the initial cost, and its reliability and versatility (see Table 21–2).

In the past decade the number of sophisticated ventilators (and their cost) has increased substantially. Volume-cycled ventilators that can be used in an ICU that cost less than 6000 dollars are rare. In some instances, the factors responsible for such high costs do not appear to offer sufficient improvement in care to justify the capital outlay.

Part of the difficulty in ventilator design has been that some manufacturers fail to heed the needs of patients, physicians, or respiratory therapists. Engineering masterpieces have been produced that were of little clinical usefulness. Performance characteristics in a laboratory frequently have little resemblance to those of the clinical setting. Recently, increasing cooperation has developed among manufacturers, their engineering staffs, and the physician/therapist consumer. Ventilators now more adequately meet the exacting physiologic requirements of patients with acute and chronic respiratory disease than those of the past.

The characteristics of an "ideal" ventilator are summarized in Table 21–6. Currently, no available device meets all suggested specifications, nor is it necessary that all ventilators should. A respiratory therapist primarily involved with IPPB therapy and routine postoperative ventilation has no need for the machine that can provide PEEP, IMV, high inspiratory pressures, and so forth. To spend money for such features is extravagant. On the other hand, a ventilator that will be used in an ICU to treat severely ill patients with acute respiratory failure should have most, if not all, of these features. No ventilator or ventilator technique can provide optimal ventilation to all patients.

Before purchase, one should use the ventilator for a trial period in the clinical setting. Reputable manufacturers confident of their products will comply with such a request. The purchase price of these intricate devices is too great to depend on advertising in brochures or journals or on exhibits using lung analogues at professional meetings.

The durability and the reliability of the ventilator are of paramount importance. Ease or availability of repair should be ascertained before purchase. Increased sophistication often is accompanied by increased fragility and "down time." Few consequences are more serious than those incidental to ventilator malfunction during the support of a critically ill patient.

The respiratory therapist should decide

Table 21–6   Ideal Mechanical Ventilator

OPERATIONAL CHARACTERISTICS

Volume or time-cycled

V_T = 10–200 mL (infants)
 = 50–500 mL (children)
 = 200–2000 mL (adult)

Variable inspiratory flow rate (up to 150 L/min for adult)
Variable I/E ratio
Peak inspiratory pressure limit
  60 torr (infants)
  100 torr (children, adults)
Control, assist, and IMV modes available
PEEP or CPAP up to at least 50 cmH$_2$O
  (ideal upper limit unknown at this time)
  (Threshold rather than flow resistor)
Frequency: 0–60 breaths/min (more for HFV)
Inspiratory plateau up to 2 sec
Expiratory retard

ALARMS

Minimum and maximum pressure in airway
Oxygen concentration
Inspiratory gas temperature
Humidifier/nebulizer water level
Electrical or pneumatic power failure

SERVOMECHANISMS (AUTOMATIC FEEDBACK CONTROL)

F$_\text{I}$O$_2$ (flow and pressure independent)
Inspiratory gas temperature
Humidifier/nebulizer water level

MONITORS

Airway pressure
Frequency
Tidal volume (patient)
Inspiratory gas temperature (at patient airway)

whether the features of the ventilator under consideration are necessary or, at the least, desirable. For example, many ventilators provide a "sigh" mode to increase the delivered V_T at periodic intervals. At one time, periodic sighing was considered essential in prolonged ventilatory support. Now, however, many clinicians believe that sighs are not indicated when PEEP is used. Accordingly, this mechanism may well add a needless cost.

Finally, there is indeed a difference in mechanical ventilators. In recent years, a rather trite observation has become popular to the effect that it is not the ventilator that is important, but rather the operator of the ventilator. Certainly, nobody will dispute that it is essential to have a knowledgeable and skilled person determining how the ventilator is to be used. However, it is patently untrue to assert that any one mechanical ventilator is as good as another. If such were true, those who espouse this philosophy would use the least complex ventilator available.

The problem facing the respiratory therapist is to catalogue those features that he or she considers most important to provide a continuing high level of respiratory care, and then to see which currently available model meets those requirements.

BEAR MEDICAL SYSTEMS
BEAR 1 VOLUME VENTILATOR

Classification

The Bear 1 (Fig. 21–12) adult volume ventilator is electrically and pneumatically powered, electronically operated, and may function as a constant or decelerating flow generator. Mechanical inspiration is terminated when a preselected V_T has been delivered and may be extended by a time-cycled plateau. End-expiratory pressure may be applied

SPECIFICATIONS

Inspiration	Norm 5–60
Rate (BPM)	10.5–10%
Volume (mL)	100–2000
Flow rate (L/min)	20–120
Pressure (cmH$_2$O)	0–100
Time (sec)	NC
Effort (cmH$_2$O)	(0.5)–(10)
Hold (sec)	0–2
Demand flow (L/min)	0–100
Safety pressure (cmH$_2$O)	110
Pressure support (cmH$_2$O)	NC
MMV (L/min)	NC
Expiration	
Time (sec)	NC
PEEP/CPAP (cmH$_2$O)	0–30
Retard (L/min)	NC
I/E ratio	NC

MODES

Assist	MMV
*Control	PS
*Assist/Control	APRV
IMV	PC
*SIMV	CPAP

* Asterisk refers to modes of ventilation available on this ventilator and in others throughout the text. Other modes are not available.

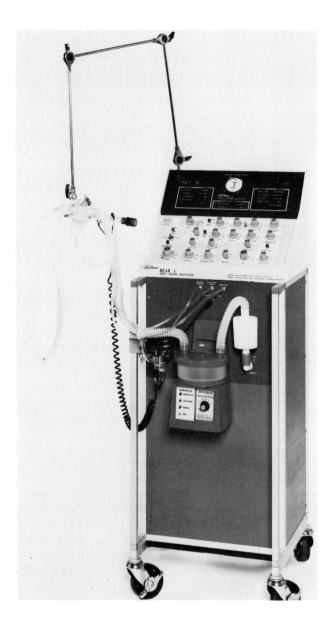

Figure 21–12. Bear 1 adult volume ventilator. (Courtesy of Bear Medical Systems)

during mechanical (PEEP) or spontaneous (CPAP) breathing. Initiation of mechanical inspiration is either control- or patient-triggered.

Operation

The ventilator is connected to a 50-psi oxygen source and a 115-V, 60-Hz electrical power source. If a 50-psi air source is available, the ventilator compressor system is bypassed. The type of ventilation desired is programmed by the mode selector knob (A, Fig. 21–13). In the assist-control mode, a

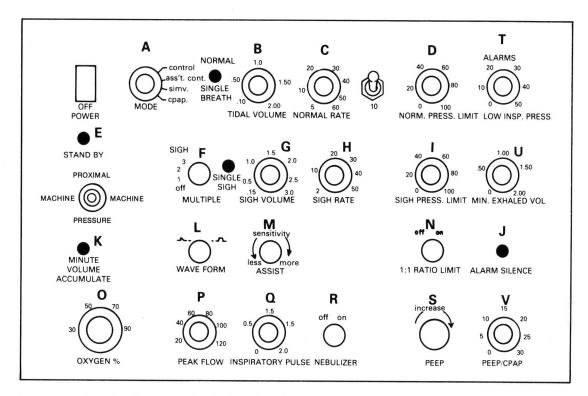

Figure 21—13. Control panel of the Bear 1 ventilator.

built-in safety feature does not allow the patient to initiate a breath until at least 100 milliseconds after termination of the previous exhalation. If the patient becomes apneic, the ventilator will revert to a control mode at the frequency set on the normal rate control.

In the SIMV mode, gas flow increases as necessary to meet the patient's spontaneous ventilatory demand. When the appropriate time interval has elapsed, the IMV breath is delivered in response (and synchronous with) the spontaneous effort.

The mechanical V_T is adjusted with control B, and the rate control C has a normal range of 5 to 60 breaths per minute; however, a "divisible by 10" toggle switch extends the range from 0.5 to 60 breaths per minute. The lower rates are used for SIMV. The pressure control, D, adjusts the pressure limit and the ventilator may be placed on "standby" by depressing button E. In this mode, the patient may breathe spontaneously. A standby light remains illuminated until 60 seconds have elapsed, at which time an audible alarm sounds.

Single or multiple sigh breaths F, may be programmed. A separate sigh volume, G, is selected from 150 to 3000 mL and may be delivered from 2 to 60 times per hour, H. The sigh breath has a sepa-

rate pressure limit, I, identical in operation with the normal pressure limit control.

A minute volume accumulator, K, measures both ventilator and spontaneous breaths and displays them as exhaled minute volume. After 1 minute of display the indicator automatically reverts back to V_T display. The inspiratory flow pattern is altered by waveform control L, which modifies the normal square wave by decelerating or tapering the flow as inspiration continues and as pressure in the circuit increases. Inspiratory flow deceleration from 120 down to 40 L/min is available.

The assist control knob M adjusts the degree of patient effort required to trigger the machine to the inspiratory phase. A ratio limit control N provides an audible alarm if the I/E ratio is 1:1.

The oxygen percentage control O is adjustable from 21% to 100%. The inspiratory flow control P is adjustable from 20 to 120 L/min. Spontaneous ventilation is not affected by this control. An inspiratory pause control Q delays the opening of the exhalation valve from 0 to 2 seconds. This delay is part of the inspiratory time and, therefore, is included in the I/E calculation. If this control is used to generate inverse I/E ratios, the I/E ratio limit control must be turned off.

A nebulizer control R activates the medication nebulizer. The PEEP control S adjusts PEEP and is self-adjusting to compensate for minor leaks within the system.

Monitoring and Alarms

The alarm systems have three controls on the main control panel. A low inspiratory pressure alarm, T, sets the lower limit of inspiratory positive pressure that must be generated by ventilator cycling. The minimum exhaled volume control U is adjustable from zero to 2000 mL. If the exhaled volume is less than the volume indicated for three consecutive breaths, the alarm is activated. All alarms can be silenced for 60 seconds by depressing alarm silence button J. The PEEP/CPAP alarm, V, is adjustable from zero to 30 cmH$_2$O. A visual and audible alarm is activated when the PEEP or CPAP level falls below the control setting. Multiple indicator and alarm lights are displayed on the upright ventilator panel, including pressure, exhaled volume, rate, and I/E ratio displays, as well as indicator lights for power-on, standby, alarm silence, nebulizer-on, control mode, assist–control mode, SIMV mode, CPAP mode, rate "divisible by 10", spontaneous breath, control breath, sigh breath, low oxygen pressure, low air pressure, pressure limit, inverse I/E ratio, low pressure, low PEEP/CPAP, low exhaled volume, apnea, and ventilator inoperative.

Mechanism

The ventilator is powered by 30- to 100-psi sources of air and oxygen. If a malfunction causes reduced pressure in either of the gases, a crossover solenoid, A, is activated so that the remaining functional gas continues ventilator operation (Fig. 21–14). If air pressure fails, a switch-over valve, B, activates a compressor, C. This compressor also functions if the high-pressure line is not connected to an external source of compressed air. Both air and oxygen pressure are matched in the system and delivered to a gas-blending device, D. This mixed gas then passes to a solenoid valve, E, which functions as the main on–off switch. Some gas also bypasses the main solenoid valve to perform other functions described in the following. From the main solenoid valve, the gas is adjusted through a set of two controls. The first, F, modifies the waveform delivered to the patient; the second, G, determines the peak flow rate. A vortex flow sensor, H, measures the volume of gas delivered to the patient. If the main solenoid-controlled time interval is not adequate to provide the preselected V$_T$, the flow transducer senses the discrepancy and signals the solenoid to remain open for an extended period until the volume has been delivered. An adjustable safety pop-off valve, I, limits the peak inspiratory pressure, and a subambient-pressure valve, J, allows the patient to inspire room air if a ventilator malfunction occurs. Humidification is provided by a cascade heated humidifier, K.

A secondary system bypasses the main patient supply flow. This system provides gas for spontaneous breathing in the synchronized IMV (SIMV) mode of ventilation. A patient-sensing pressure line, L, controls gas flow from a demand valve, M. With SIMV, the demand valve supplies gas flow to the patient distal to the main solenoid and wave-

Figure 21–14. Schematic diagram of the Bear 1 ventilator.

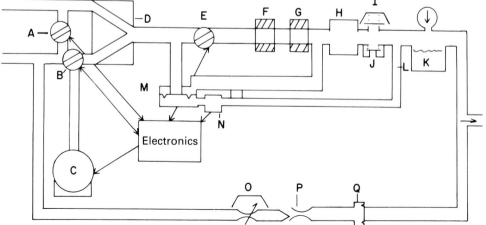

form control valves. If the assist sensor *N* is activated, the IMV is synchronized with the patient's inspiratory effort, and V_T is delivered through the main solenoid and flow modification valves. PEEP is adjusted by a PEEP control valve, *O*, and a Venturi, *P*, which pressurizes the exhalation valve, *Q*, during the expiratory phase.

Figure 21—15. Bear 2/3 adult volume ventilator. (Courtesy of Bear Medical Systems)

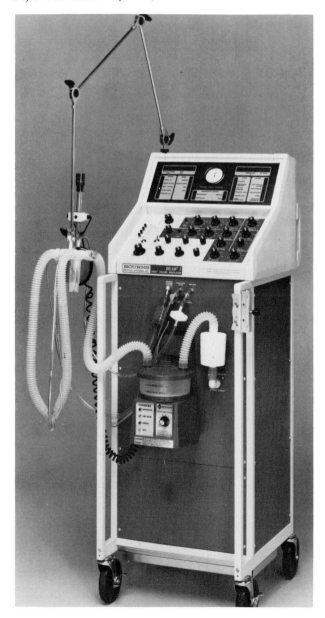

Troubleshooting

Troubleshooting is simplified by the 28 lights and monitors that indicate problems as they develop.

BEAR MEDICAL SYSTEMS, BEAR 2/3 ADULT VOLUME VENTILATOR

Classification

The Bear 2/3 (Fig. 21—15) adult volume ventilator is electrically and pneumatically powered, electronically operated, and may function as a constant, or decelerating, flow generator. Mechanical inspiration is terminated when a preselected V_T has been delivered and may be extended by a time-cycled plateau. End-expiratory pressure may be applied during mechanical (PEEP) or spontaneous (CPAP) breathing. Initiation of mechanical inspiration is either controlled or patient triggered. Pressure supported ventilation is standard on the Bear 3; however, any Bear 2 can be updated to provide this modality.

SPECIFICATIONS

Inspiration	Norm 5–60
Rate (BPM)	10.5–6%
Volume (mL)	100–2000
Flow rate (L/min)	
Pressure (cmH$_2$O)	0–120
Time (sec)	NC
Effort (cmH$_2$O)	1–5
Hold (sec)	0–2
Demand flow (L/min)	0–120
Safety pressure (cmH$_2$O)	130
Pressure support (cmH$_2$O)	4–72
MMV (L/min)	NC
Expiration	
Time (sec)	NC
PEEP/CPAP (cmH$_2$O)	0–50
Retard (L/min)	NC
I/E ratio	NC

MODES

Assist	MMV
*Control	*PS (Bear 3)
*Assist/Control	APRV
IMV	PC
*SIMV	CPAP

Operation

The ventilator is connected to a 50-psi oxygen source and a 115-V, 60-Hz electrical power source. If a 50-psi air source is available, the ventilator compressor system is bypassed. The type of ventilation desired is programmed by the mode selector knob A; Fig. 21–16). In the assist-control mode, a built-in safety feature does not allow a patient to initiate a breath for at least 350 milliseconds after termination of the previous exhalation. If the patient becomes apneic, the ventilator reverts to a control mode at the frequency set on the normal rate control, C.

In the SIMV and CPAP mode the patient breathes spontaneously, setting his rate, V_T, and peak flow up to 120 L/min. When a mandatory breath is delivered, all machine settings are met for V_T, peak flow, and so forth. The SIMV is triggered by activating the assist-control sensitivity after the designated spontaneous breathing period has elapsed. Should the patient not trigger a breath, one cycling period elapses, then the ventilator switches to control mode. The detection delay, U, may alarm during this period if the expiratory time exceeds the delay time and the patient is apneic.

The mechanical V_T is adjusted with control B,

mandatory (normal) rate with control C, and the high pressure limit with control D.

Single or multiple sigh breaths, E, may be programmed. A separate sigh volume is selected, F, from 150 to 3000 mL and may be delivered 2 to 60 times per hour, G. The sigh breath has a separate pressure limit, H, from zero to 120 cmH$_2$O.

The pressure can be measured from either a machine or a proximal tap. The pressure-sensing selector, I, can be directed to sample either source. There will be some difference between the two pressures because of system and humidifier resistance. A constant 1-L/min bleed in the proximal pressure measuring line prevents humidification buildup. A ¼- in. tubing should be used to connect the proximal tap. The waveform selector J may be used to deliver a square wave flow pattern in which the flow will decrease only 15% as the V_T is attained or a tapered flow pattern that reduces the flow by 50%. The flow taper cannot be used when the peak flow is set below 20 L/min because the minimum flow is 10 L/min. The nebulizer control K diverts a portion of the tidal volume through the nebulizer so that oxygen concentration and V_T are not altered during medication delivery. This nebulizer cannot be used if the peak flow, O, is set below 30 L/min. The assist control L adjusts the degree of

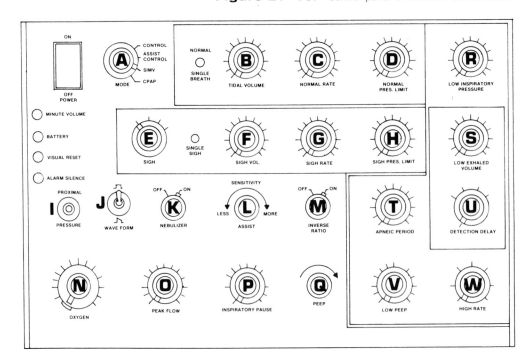

Figure 21–16. Control panel of the Bear 2/3 ventilator.

patient effort required to trigger the machine. Turning the control toward the "more" makes the system more sensitive both in the assist-control mode and the spontaneous-breathing mode. The volume of gas added to the system by the patient's inspiratory efforts will be added to the V_T as measured by the V_T flow tube. A ratio-limit control, M, provides an audible alarm if the I/E ratio exceeds 1 : 1 and inspiration is terminated. If this control is turned to OFF, inverse I/E ratios may be attained. This control is inactivated in the assist-control and SIMV modes.

The oxygen percentage control N is adjustable from 21% to 100%. The peak flow control O does not affect the spontaneous inspiratory flow but will affect the flow taper if it is set below 30 L/min. An inspiratory pause control P, delays the opening of the exhalation valve once the V_T has been delivered from zero to 2 seconds. Only in this configuration is the ventilator considered a time-cycled ventilator. This pause period is included in the inspiratory time and, therefore, should be considered when setting appropriate I/E ratios. The PEEP control, Q, can maintain its calibrated pressure with leaks up to 25 L/min for 7 to 9 seconds. In the CPAP mode, the patient breathes from the demand valve with flows up to 100 L/min.

Monitoring and Alarms

The alarm and monitoring systems have six adjustable controls on the face of the ventilator and multiple displays on the monitoring console. A low inspiratory pressure alarm, R, sets the lower limit of the inspiratory positive pressure that must be generated by ventilator cycling. The minimum exhaled volume control, S, is adjustable from zero to 2000 mL. If the exhaled volume is less than the volume indicated on the detection delay control U, the alarm is activated. Once the alarm has been activated, it can be deactivated within one breath with the appropriate V_T. The apneic period alarm, T, is adjustable from 2 to 20 seconds; if the breath interval exceeds the alarm setting, the alarm will activate. The low PEEP/CPAP alarm, V, is adjustable from zero to 50 cmH$_2$O; should the PEEP level fall below the level set, the alarm will activate. The high-rate alarm W, adjustable from 10 to 80 breaths per minute, is activated when respirations exceed the limit set. All alarms have corresponding lights that are activated on the display console to alert the therapist when an alarm has been activated. Besides these indicator lights, there are LED displays for V_T, minute volume, rate, temperature, and I/E

ratio. Should a "ventilator inoperative" display appear, the ventilator must be turned off to correct this alarm. If turning the ventilator off and then on again does not remedy the ventilator inoperative condition, the unit should be repaired by appropriately trained service personnel.

Signal outputs provided on the back of the ventilator allow for remote nurse call, 9-V DC outlet for accessories, pressure signal output, and flow signal output.

Mechanism

The ventilator is powered by 30- to 100-psi sources of air and oxygen. If a malfunction causes reduced pressure of either gas, a crossover solenoid, A, is activated so that the remaining functional gas continues ventilator operation (Fig. 21–17). If external air pressure fails or if internal air pressure falls below 9.5 psi, a switchover valve, B, activates a compressor, C. This compressor also functions if the high-pressure line is not connected to an external source of compressed air. Both air and oxygen pressures are reduced to about 11 psi and mixed at calibrated rates as selected by the blender control, D. The mixed gas passes to a solenoid valve, E, which functions as the main on–off switch. Some gas also bypasses the main solenoid valve to perform other functions, as controlled by the bypass solenoid, R.

A constant or decelerating (tapered) inspiratory flow pattern waveform may be selected by a toggle switch, F, which regulates driving pressure to the peak flow control, G. In the square-wave position, driving pressure is 3.0 psi, and the ventilator outflow is equal to the peak flow adjustment. When flow taper is activated, driving pressure is reduced to 1.8 psi, and inspiratory flow decelerates as circuit pressure increases. Flow will decelerate at 50% of the peak flow at 120 cmH$_2$O back-pressure to a minimum of 10 L/min.

When peak flow control, G, meters gas flow to the patient with the flow taper control set for square wave, there will be only a 15% drop in pressure shortly before termination of inspiration. Once the appropriate volume has passed through the flow transducer, H, a signal is sent through the electronic system to the main solenoid valve, E, to terminate inspiration, unless the pressure limit control, I, has already cycled the ventilator to exhalation. Should an inspiratory pause be desired, the patient exhalation valve, Q, will remain closed for the extended pause period once the V_T has been delivered. It is during this phase that the ventilator

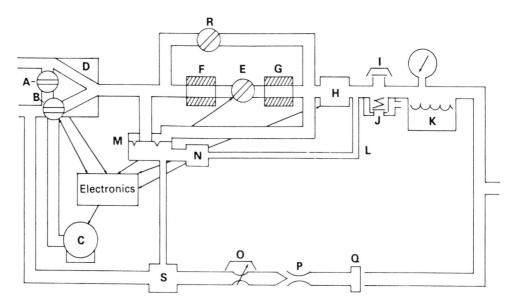

Figure 21—17. Schematic diagram of the Bear 2/3 ventilator.

is considered time-cycled. If all pneumatic and electronic systems fail, there is an antiasphyxiation valve, J, through which a spontaneously breathing patient may inspire. Humidification is provided by an adjustable heated humidifier, K.

A secondary system bypasses the main patient supply flow. This system supplies gas for spontaneous breathing in synchronized IMV (SIMV) and CPAP modes. A sensing line, L, controls gas from the demand valve, M, which is activated in the assist–control, SIMV, and CPAP modes. The demand valve system provides gas flow up to 120 L/min distal to the main solenoid valve, E, and waveform toggle, F. If the assist sensor, N, is activated, the IMV is synchronized with the patient's inspiratory efforts, and the tidal volume is delivered through the main solenoid, E, and flow waveform toggle F. PEEP is adjusted by the PEEP control valve, O, and a venturi, P, which pressurizes the exhalation valve, Q, during the expiratory phase. The compensation chamber, S, adjusts pressure on the exhalation valve during peak expiratory flow periods.

Troubleshooting

Troubleshooting is simplified by the 24 indicator lights and four LED displays on the monitoring console. This is coupled with a rather complete troubleshooting guide in the instruction manual available when purchasing this ventilator.

BEAR MEDICAL SYSTEMS, BEAR 5 ADULT VOLUME VENTILATOR

Classification

The Bear 5 adult volume ventilator (Fig. 21–18) is electrically and pneumatically powered, microprocessor operated, and may function as a constant, nonconstant, or decelerating flow generator and, in the pressure support mode, also as a constant-pressure generator (see Table 21–2). Mechanical inspiration is volume-, time-, or flow-cycled, may be extended by a time-cycled plateau, and is either control- or patient-triggered. End-expiratory pressure may be applied during mechanical (PEEP) or spontaneous (CPAP) breathing.

SPECIFICATIONS

Inspiration

Rate (BPM)	0–150
Volume (mL)	50–2000
Flow rate (L/min)	5–150
Pressure (cmH$_2$O)	0–140
Time (sec)	0.1–3*
Effort (cmH$_2$O)	0.5–0
Hold (sec)	0–2
Demand flow (L/min)	0–170
Safety pressure (cmH$_2$O)	220
Pressure support (cmH$_2$O)	0–72
MMV (L/min)	0.5–40

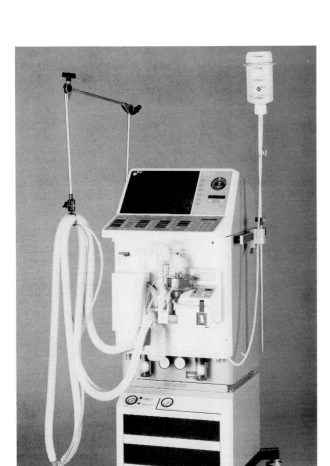

Figure 21—18. Bear 5 adult volume ventilator. (Courtesy of Bear Medical Systems)

The Bear 5 recalls all the settings from the previous use. They remain stored in memory by the microprocessor for at least 30 hours after power has been interrupted; otherwise, all controls must be reset. Ventilator controls are set by depressing specific keys, which cause the preexisting value (if any) to be displayed in the display window. Values are changed by pressing the requisite numeric keys or using the increment (up arrow key) or decrement (down arrow key) control and set stored in random access memory (RAM) by ⟨ENTER⟩, depressing as long as the magnitude of the setting is compatible with the ventilator specifications. When incompatible settings are entered, the letter E will appear in the display. Values may be reentered after clearing the display (⟨CLR⟩ key). Controls that do not require numeric values (e.g., ventilatory mode) have specific keys adjacent to the LEDs. If a selection is compatible with specifications, the setting is stored and the LED remains illuminated.

Ventilatory modes that can be selected (Fig. 21–19) include CMV, A; ASSIST/CMV, B; SIMV/IMV, C; CPAP, D; augmented minute ventilation (AMV), E, which is identical with SIMV except ventilator rate can be increased or decreased to maintain a minimum minute ventilation based on the patient's spontaneous contribution to the total minute volume; and TIME CYCLE, F, a pediatric mode allowing time-cycled termination of mechanical breaths at a desired peak inflation pressure

Figure 21—19. Control panel of the Bear 5 ventilator.

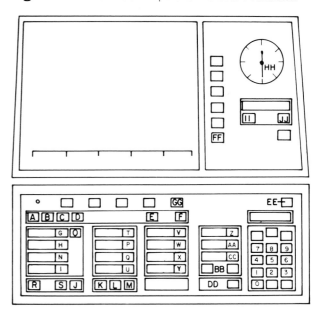

Expiration

Time (sec)	NC
PEEP/CPAP (cmH$_2$O)	0–50
Retard (L/min)	NC
I/E ratio	NC

* Available in time-cycle mode only.

MODES

*Assist	*MMV
*Control	*PS
*Assist–Control	APRV
*IMV	PC
*SIMV	CPAP

Operation

Before ventilation is applied, a series of self-checks, which take 12 seconds to complete, verifies the operational readiness of the ventilator.

(PIP). Mechanical V_T, G, must be programmed for volume delivery during CMV, ASSIST/CMV, SIMV/IMV, and AMV. Mechanical ventilator rates, H, can range from zero to 150 breaths per minute and FIO_2, I, from 21% to 100%. The flow pattern during mechanical V_T delivery may be constant, J; accelerating, K; decelerating, L; or sinusoidal, M. Constant flow, J, provides a set inspiratory flow rate, N, throughout V_T delivery. An accelerating contour, K, begins V_T delivery at 50% of the set flow rate; it increases incrementally to 100% at end inspiration. With decelerating flow, L, V_T delivery begins at the set flow rate; it then progressively decreases to 50% at end inspiration. With sinusoidal flow, M, it begins at zero and increases rapidly; the programmed peak coincides with midinspiration and flow rate decreases to zero at end inspiration. The programmed V_T will be automatically adjusted for compressional gas losses when the COMPLIANCE COMPENSATION function, O, is engaged; this compression factor must be known, or preferably should be measured, before it is set. For each volume-cycled breath, a volume equal to the product of the compression factor and the peak airway pressure of the previous breath is added to V_T. The added volume is also subtracted from the measured V_T sensed at the exhalation valve.

An inspiratory pause, P, can prolong the normal cycling interval. During ASSIST/CMV, SIMV/IMV, AMV, and CPAP, a patient may initiate machine breaths (selected V_T or demand flow) when inspiratory effort exceeds the sensitivity threshold, which is adjustable, Q. With SIMV/IMV or CPAP, a patient may breathe spontaneously from a demand system that can generate up to 170 L/min.

A manual breath, R, variable and magnitude are (programmed) administered; also, 100% oxygen can replace FIO_2 for 3 minutes, S. Both of these controls are manual options available at any time. End-expiratory pressure, T and pressure support, U may be engaged in any spontaneous breathing mode. During pressure-supported ventilation, a rapid flow of gas is directed into the breathing circuit to generate a level of pressure, up to 72 cmH_2O, including the CPAP level. The initial flow rate of the gas is allowed to decelerate as the lungs fill, and the pressure-supported breath terminates when the flow has decelerated to 25% of initial and the baseline circuit pressure is restored.

Minimum minute ventilation (MMV), adjustable to 40 L/min, is selected during the AMV mode, which functions nearly identically with SIMV. During AMV, however, the clinician sets an MMV level, a mechanical V_T, and a normal rate. When the total minute ventilation (spontaneous plus mechanical) exceeds the set MMV by 1.0 L or 10% the mechanical frequency is determined by the set rate. If the total minute ventilation falls below the set MMV by the same 1.0 L or 10%, the mechanical rate increases automatically and thereby restores MMV to its set level. If the normal rate is set to zero, the patient is automatically weaned from mechanical augmentation as long as spontaneous MV exceeds the MMV threshold.

With TIME CYCLE, inspiratory time, W, can range from 0.1 to 3.0 seconds; also, this requires a continuous flow, X, a normal rate, H, and a pressure-relief value, Y. In this mode, physiologic V_T is chiefly determined by the programmed flow (continuous) and the inspiratory time. Furthermore, the inspiratory phase is not terminated upon reaching the pressure-relief threshold; the exhalation valve opens enough to vent additional pressure to the ambient air and, thus, prevents further increase in pressure. This feature allows a timed, pressure plateau during which fresh gas is available for spontaneous breathing or operation that mimics most popular infant/pediatric ventilators.

Sigh volumes, Z, are possible at 2 to 60 machine-cycled breaths per hour, AA, in lieu of normally scheduled or patient-triggered breaths. The automatic sigh mechanism, BB, may be activated to administer one, two, or three consecutive breaths per sigh function, CC. Once the sigh function has been actuated, a manual sigh, DD, can be delivered during mechanical exhalation in any mode.

After the ventilatory controls are programmed, they can be rendered inoperative (panel lock key, EE), which makes the manual breath and the transient 100% oxygen functions inoperative as well.

Monitoring and Alarms

An extensive variety of ventilator and physiologic variables can be displayed. Data are derived from signals provided by the inspiratory flow transducer, expiratory flow transducer, and the two parallel airway pressure transducers. Monitored variables are exhaled V_T, exhaled minute volume, total breath rate, mechanical inspiratory time, peak airway pressure, mean airway pressure, PEEP/CPAP level, I/E ratio (mechanical breaths only), static compliance during volume-cycled breaths, resistance during volume-cycled breaths, volume added by compliance compensation, and the inspiratory source (i.e., ventilatory mode for a given breath). A calibrated aneroid manometer, *HH*, provides a continuous indication of the proximal airway pressure.

There are adjustable alarm thresholds for low exhaled V_T for spontaneous and mechanical breaths; low exhaled minute volume; high exhaled minute volume; low breath rate; high breath rate; low inspiratory time (TIME CYCLE only); high inspiratory time (TIME CYCLE only); high peak airway pressure (volume-cycled breaths only); pressure limit (TIME CYCLE only); high peak pressure (SIGH); low inspiratory pressure; high and low mean airway pressure; high and low PEEP/CPAP; inverse I/E ratio (mandatory breaths only); and low oxygen and air pressure (factory set at 27 psig). Programmed thresholds are displayed with the alarm page program (CRT) and may be reset, *JJ*, at any time. Alarm threshold ranges may also be set automatically by the central processing unit for variables specific to the set ventilatory mode. Audible alarms, with the exception of the ventilator-inoperative alarm, may be silenced, *II*, for 60 seconds.

With normal operation, the CRT screen primarily displays real-time graphics for flow, pressure, and volume. These waveforms can be helpful in diagnosing problems such as circuit leaks, air trapping, and disconnections. The graphics screen can be seen from across the room to provide visual confirmation of continued ventilator operation.

This screen can also display a mechanics menu that lists the current settings for mode, exhaled mandatory tidal volume, average exhaled minute volume, breath rate, inspiratory time, I/E ratio, peak normal pressure, compliance compensation volume, static compliance, and airways resistance.

Mechanism

The Bear 5 requires high-pressure, medical-grade air, oxygen (30 to 100 psig), and 115-V AC (receptacles on rear panel). An optional air compressor can provide air when the source pressure decreases below 28.5 psig or in areas for which compressed air is unavailable (Fig. 21–20). The gases are filtered, and then they flow to pressure regulators, *A* and *C*, set to 18.2 psig. Because of a pneumatic connection, *B*, the output of the air regulator, *A*, controls the output of the oxygen regulator, *C*, which ensures that both regulators have identical output pressure and that oxygen blending is accurate. In the event that either air or oxygen pressure is lost, a crossover valve, *D*, maintains ventilation with the remaining gas.

The FIO_2 is obtained with a stepper motor-controlled dual orifice, gas-blending valve, *E*. Stepper motors are small electric motors that rotate a shaft in a series of discrete steps defined by a precise change in voltage. The stepper motor and valve are linked mechanically, such that each step opens or closes the valve slightly according to a microprocessor program. This particular valve consists of 125 steps that can be changed at a rate of 83 steps per second; each step represents 0.6% oxygen and the FIO_2 can be adjusted from 21% to 100% in 1.5 seconds. Blended gas is routed into a 3.6-L reservoir, *F*, a rigid tank that stores a large volume of gas, which allows the ventilator to generate peak inspiratory flow rates that exceed the mixing capacity of the blender. A second advantage is a minimal response time and reduced work of breathing during

Figure 21–20. Schematic diagram of the Bear 5 ventilator.

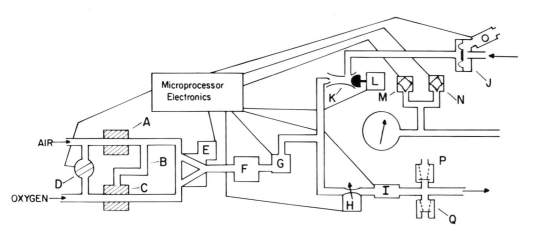

spontaneous ventilation. Gas flows from the reservoir through the shut-off valve, G, which terminates all gas flow when electric power is lost or during the ventilator inoperative mode.

The flow-control valve, H, comprises another stepper motor and valve complex; all gas delivered to the patient flows through this valve. This valve functions in conjunction with the internal flow transducer, I, as a closed-loop servosystem. To deliver the set V_T, the central processing unit (CPU) consults the ventilatory settings stored in RAM and adjusts the valve accordingly. As gas flows to the patient, the internal flow transducer measures the actual flow; the flow-control valve is automatically modulated until actual flow equals set flow throughout the inspiratory phase to produce the V_T, peak inspiratory flow rate, and flow pattern at the set values.

During spontaneous breathing, when inspiratory effort breaches the programmed sensitivity, the flow-control valve opens and functions like a constant-pressure generator. Thus, the flow-control valve is modulated according to airway pressure. As the spontaneous breath progresses, inspiratory flow decelerates and the breath is terminated when zero flow is reached, which will also maintain the PEEP/CPAP level.

To actuate the exhalation valve, I, the Bear 5 employs a Venturi, J, and a third valve and stepper motor complex, K. The stepper motor varies the position of a poppet at the outlet of the Venturi to control the output pressure of the Venturi. During any mechanical inspiration, the microprocessor manipulates the position of the poppet to maintain a pressure in the exhalation valve at approximately 20-cmH$_2$O above the proximal airway pressure. Upon completion of the breath, pressure in the breathing circuit is returned to the PEEP/CPAP level. Two pressure transducers, L, M, mounted in parallel, measure airway pressure and, for safety, must agree within ± 6 cmH$_2$O. An exhalation flow sensor, O, distal to the exhalation valve measures expired gas. To provide additional safety, breathing gases pass an overpressure relief valve, P, and an antisuffocation valve, Q.

Troubleshooting

The Bear 5 is extremely easy to troubleshoot because the patient-breathing circuit is simple in design and leaks are the only common problem. Mechanical or electronic problems can be diagnosed by an intricate, computer-operated, troubleshoot-

ing program contained within the software of the ventilator. It is recommended that only factory-trained technicians or service personnel attempt to repair this complex electropneumatic ventilator.

BEAR MEDICAL SYSTEMS BP-200 INFANT VENTILATOR

Classification

The Bear Medical Systems BP-200 infant ventilator (Fig. 21–21) is electrically and pneumatically powered, electronically operated, and functions as a constant-flow generator. Termination of mechanical inspiration is time-cycled and end-expiratory pressure may be applied during mechanical (PEEP) or spontaneous (CPAP) breathing. Initiation of mechanical inspiration is machine-cycled.

SPECIFICATIONS

Inspiration

Rate (BPM)	1–150
Volume (mL)	NC
Flow rate (L/min)	0–20
Pressure (cmH$_2$O)	12–80
Time (sec)	NC
Effort (cmH$_2$O)	NC
Hold (sec)	NC
Demand flow (L/min)	NC
Safety pressure (cmH$_2$O)	80
Pressure support (cmH$_2$O)	NC
MMV (L/min)	NC

Expiration

Time (sec)	NC
PEEP/CPAP (cmH$_2$O)	0–20
Retard (L/min)	NC
I/E ratio	1 : 10–4 : 1

MODES

Assist	MMV
Control	PS
Assist–Control	APRV
*IMV	PC
SIMV	CPAP

Operation

Ventilator function and settings are adjusted on a compact control panel (Fig. 21–22). A four-position control knob, A, serves as an electric power switch, alarm test, and ventilatory mode selector (IPPB/IMV or CPAP). In the alarm test position, an audible alarm buzzer should sound. When CPAP is selected, the pneumatic and electrical alarm circuit is activated. If air or oxygen inlet pressure decreases below 15 or 30 psi, respectively, or an electrical power interruption occurs, an audible battery alarm is activated. If IPPB/IMV is selected, the ventilator will time cycle in addition to engaging the electronic and pneumatic power loss surveillance alarm system. When the mode selection is in any position but off, the amber-colored power light, B, is illuminated. Mechanical V_T is the result of an adjusted breathing rate control, C, I/E ratio control, D, and continuous flow control, E. The continuous flow is indicated by means of a calibrated Thorpe tube, F. A manual breath, J, may be administered only in the CPAP mode and is determined by the ventilator settings similar to IMV/IPPB V_T. The FIO_2 is adjustable, N, from 0.21 to 1.0.

Monitoring and Alarms

Monitored and alarm settings are mixed in with the patient controls. At low IMV rates the maximum inspiratory time control, G, may be used to override I/E control, obviating prolonged inspiratory time. When maximum inspiratory time has been reached, a red indicator light, H, illuminates. If the electronic timer allows adjusted mechanical expiratory times less than 0.22 to 0.28 seconds, a red insufficient expiratory timer light, I, illuminates.

Peak inspiratory, K, and threshold expiratory, L, pressure may be regulated from 12 cmH_2O at 2 L/min to greater than 80 cmH_2O at 20 L/min, and zero to 20 cmH_2O at >45 psi oxygen inlet pressure, respectively. Each is adjusted by an uncalibrated control; consequently, the pressure limit must be observed on an aneroid manometer, M, while the proximal airway connection is occluded.

Mechanism

Air and oxygen, at 15 to 75 psi and 30 to 75 psi, respectively, are pressure-equilibrated and mixed to the desired FIO_2, A (Fig. 21–23). A continuous flow of blended gas is metered, B, into a calibrated Thorpe tube (not illustrated) and directed past a spring-tension pressure-relief valve, C. The gas is warmed and humidified, D, before it enters the breathing circuit. During mechanical inspiration a solenoid valve, E, closes, interrupting the continuous flow vent, thus diverting gas into the infant's

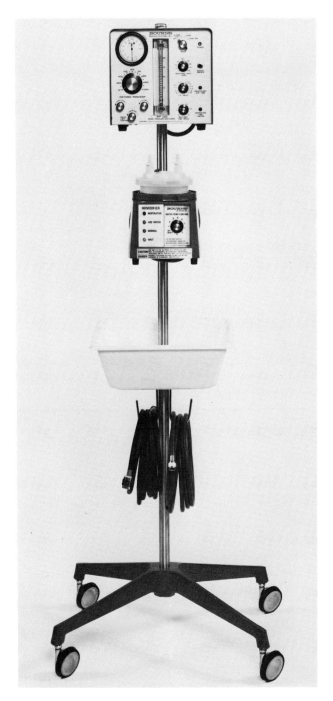

Figure 21—21. Bear Medical Systems BP-200 infant ventilator. (Courtesy of Bear Medical Systems)

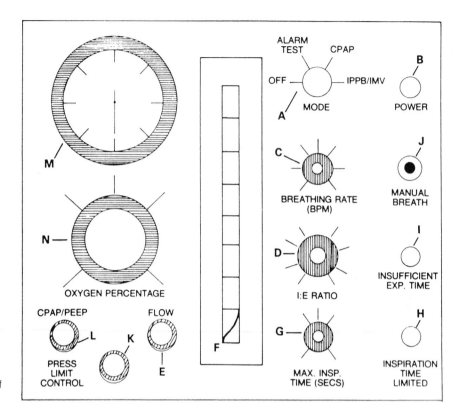

Figure 21–22. Control panel of the BP-200 ventilator.

airway. During mechanical expiration or CPAP, the patient breathes spontaneously from the continuous flow of gas. Gas flow may be opposed by a pressurized expiratory check-leaf valve, F. The amount of threshold expiratory generated depends on jet Venturi flow, G, metered by the PEEP/CPAP control, H.

Troubleshooting

The simplicity of this ventilator facilitates rapid recognition of problems. An audible alarm indicates either pneumatic or electrical power loss; if this occurs, gas inlet pressure gauges on the rear panel, the electrical connection, or the circuit

Figure 21–23. Schematic diagram of the BP-200 ventilator.

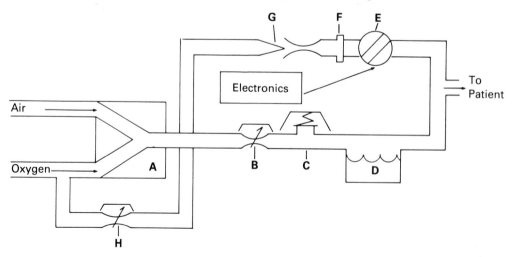

breaker should be checked. Failure to develop circuit pressure during IPPB/IMV is usually caused by circuit leaks or a low-pressure limit adjustment.

THE BEAR CUB INFANT VENTILATOR

Classification

The Bear Cub infant ventilator (Fig. 21–24), which is electrically and pneumatically powered and electronically operated, functions as a constant-flow generator (see Table 21–1). Initiation of mechanical inspiration is machine-generated and time-cycled. End-expiratory pressure may be applied during mechanical (PEEP) or spontaneous (CPAP) breathing.

SPECIFICATIONS

Inspiration	
Rate (BPM)	High 75–150
	Low 1–75
Volume (mL)	
Flow rate (L/min)	3–30
Pressure (cmH$_2$O)	0–72
Time (sec)	0.1–3
Effort (cmH$_2$O)	NC
Hold (sec)	NC
Demand flow (L/min)	NC
Safety pressure (cmH$_2$O)	87
Pressure support (cmH$_2$O)	NC
MMV (L/min)	NC
Expiration	
Time (sec)	NC
PEEP/CPAP (cmH$_2$O)	2–20
Retard (L/min)	NC
I/E ratio	NC

MODES

Assist	MMV
Control	PS
Assist–Control	APRV
*IMV	PC
SIMV	CPAP

Operation

The Bear Cub functions in a manner identical with that of the BABYbird and other popular infant ventilators. Gas flows continuously through the ventilator circuit and is periodically diverted to the patient by closure of the exhalation valve.

Ventilator function and variables are adjusted on a compact control panel (Fig. 21–25). A four-

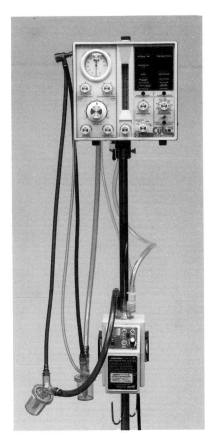

Figure 21—24. Bear Cub infant ventilator. (Courtesy Bear Medical Systems)

position selector switch, *A*, permits the operator to turn the ventilator off, test the battery and lamps, or select from the two available modes: CPAP or CMV/IMV. Next, the flowmeter, *B*, is adjusted, *C*, initially to a value approximately twice the patient's predicted maximal inspiratory flow rate. In the CMV/IMV mode, ventilator rate is adjusted with the control knob *D*, and range switching with the toggle *E* (1 to 75 or 76 to 170 breaths per minute); inspiratory time, *F*, PEEP/CPAP, *G*, and pressure limit, *H*, must also each be adjusted. In the CPAP mode, only the flow rate and the PEEP/CPAP setting need to be adjusted. The F$_{I}$O$_2$ is infinitely adjustable between 21% and 100%, *I*. A single manual breath button can be delivered, as defined by the setting on the control panel, *J*, in the CPAP mode only.

Monitors and Alarms

An array of five digital display windows provides a continuous display of monitored settings (see Fig.

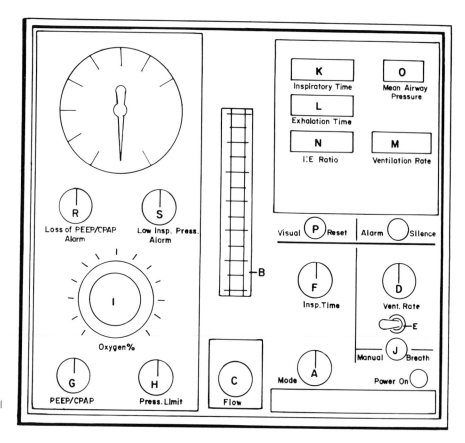

Figure 21—25. Control panel of the Bear Cub ventilator.

21–25): inspiratory time, K; expiratory time, L; ventilator rate, M; I/E ratio, N; and mean airway pressure, O. There are two operator-controlled alarms and five factory-adjusted alarms. To assist the operator in rapidly recognizing alarm conditions, each alarm consists of an audible alarm and a visual LED indicator and is listed in the display area. In the event that an alarm condition remits, the visual indicator remains lighted until the operator is able to determine which alarm limit was exceeded and resets the display, P. Audible alarms, with the exception of that indicating that the ventilator is inoperative, may be silenced for a period of 30 seconds, Q.

Adjustable alarms consist of low PEEP/CPAP, R, by which low-pressure limit is set and audible and visual alarms activated the instant proximal airway pressure exceeds the limit; and low inspiratory pressure, S, which provides a second pressure threshold that must be exceeded with each mechanical breath or audible and visual alarms are activated. If subsequent breaths return the airway pressure to proper limits, the audible alarms cease.

An additional alarm condition associated with the low PEEP/CPAP setting is referred to as pro-

longed inspiratory pressure. This audible and visual alarm activates if the airway pressure remains above the set low PEEP/CPAP setting plus 10 cmH$_2$O for 3.5 seconds or more. Therefore, the low PEEP/CPAP setting must be appropriately adjusted, particularly when elevated levels of PEEP or CPAP are required. Factory-adjusted alarms consists of I/E ratio alarm, which alerts the operator to inverse ratios in excess of 3 : 1 (expressed as 1 : 0.3); rate/time incompatibility, which warns that the rate and inspiratory time settings are such that the mandatory 0.25-second expiratory time has been violated; and the low air and oxygen pressure alarms, which sound when the inlet pressure of either gas falls below 22.5 psi.

The ventilator-inoperative alarm can be actuated for several reasons: failure of the ventilator to cycle, loss of electric power, disconnection, control panel problems, timing-circuit failure, prolonged on expiratory cycle, or excessive inspiratory time (±24% of programmed). This alarm interrupts all electronic functions and cannot be silenced until the problem is corrected. Gas flow and end-expiratory pressure are maintained during the alarm.

Mechanism

The Bear Cub is primarily pneumatic in design, with a three-way electronic solenoid responsible for changing ventilatory phases (Fig. 21–26). High-pressure (50 to 100 psi) medical-grade air, oxygen and 115-V, 60-Hz AC are required. Each gas is filtered before being reduced to 17 psi by precision regulators, A and B. To ensure gas is blended accurately, output pressures of the air and oxygen regulator must be within ±2 cmH_2O of each other; the gases are delivered to the dual orifice blender, C; and at the operator-selected FIO_2, flow through the flow control D and the flowmeter E. Gases entering the breathing circuit are regulated by an overpressure relief valve F, factory-adjusted to crack at approximately 87 cmH_2O, and an antisuffocation valve, G, which opens at −2 cmH_2O. The oxygen regulator, B, also powers two Venturi devices: the peak inspiratory pressure (PIP) venturi, H, and the PEEP Venturi, I, both of which are operator controlled, J or K. The air regulator, A, also includes a nonadjustable, expiratory Venturi, L, that reduces inadvertent CPAP generated by the movement of gas across the breathing circuit. The three-way solenoid, M, delivers pressure from the PEEP Venturi to the exhalation valve N and diaphragm during the expiratory phase. Mechanical inspiration begins with an electronic signal that actuates the three-way solenoid, which terminates flow from the PEEP Venturi, and delivers pressure from the PIP Venturi to the diaphragm of the exhalation valve, and diverts gas at a set flow rate to the patient's lungs. Airway pressure is monitored simultaneously with a pressure transducer, O, and mechanical, aneroid manometer, P.

Figure 21–26. Schematic diagram of the Bear Cub ventilator.

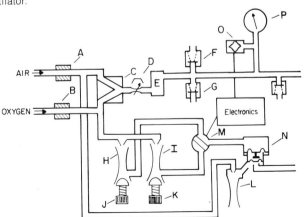

Troubleshooting

The Bear Cub has proved to be extremely reliable. The most frequently encountered problems are breathing circuit leaks and problems associated with the exhalation valve. In earlier models, the plunger within the exhalation valve sometimes would stick, which prevented cycling and resulted in a ventilator-inoperative alarm; these valves have been redesigned. The administration of nebulized medications to patients being ventilated on a Bear Cub, may also lead to problems related to the exhalation valve. The saline mixture used to dilute pharmaceutic solutions can leave a salt crust around the exhalation valve that may occlude the expiratory Venturi and, thereby, prevent the ventilator from cycling. A warm, damp rag can remove the crust, unless it is extremely thick and totally occluding the Venturi orifice. For this, the Venturi will need to be cleaned with a tool, which requires extreme care not to dilate or damage the orifice.

BENNETT 7200a SERIES MICROPROCESSOR VENTILATOR

Classification

The Bennett 7200a ventilator (Fig. 21–27), which is electrically and pneumatically powered and microprocessor operated, may function as a constant-,

Figure 21–27. Bennett 7200a Series microprocessor ventilator. (Courtesy of Puritan Bennett Corp.)

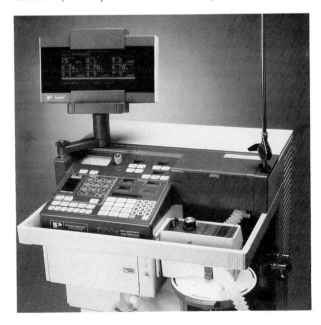

nonconstant-, or decelerating-flow generator (see Table 21–1). Mechanical inspiration ends once a preselected tidal volume has been delivered, but may be extended by a time-cycled plateau. End-expiratory pressure may be applied during mechanical (PEEP) or spontaneous (CPAP) breathing. Mechanical inspiration is either controlled or patient-triggered. Pressure-supported ventilation and numerous special functions are optional and may be purchased separately and installed at any time.

SPECIFICATIONS

Inspiration

Rate (BPM)	0.5–70
Volume (mL)	100–2500
Flow rate (L/min)	10–120
Pressure (cmH_2O)	10–120
Time (sec)	NC
Effort (cmH_2O)	0.5–20
Hold (sec)	0–2
Demand flow (L/min)	0–180
Safety pressure (cmH_2O)	140
Pressure support (cmH_2O)	0–20
MMV (L/min)	NC

Expiration

Time (sec)	NC
PEEP/CPAP (cmH_2O)	0–45
Retard (L/min)	NC
I/E ratio	NC

MODES

*Assist	MMV
*Control	*PS
*Assist–Control	APRV
*IMV	PC
*SIMV	CPAP

Operation

Upon receiving electrical power, the microprocessor of the 7200a ventilator initiates a series of tests known by the acronym POST (power on self-test) designed to verify the proper function of the microprocessor and associated circuitry, which requires approximately 15 seconds; all ventilator functions are disabled during this interval. After the POST, all previous ventilatory settings are recalled from memory and reset. This random access memory (RAM) receives power from an internal set of batteries, which prevent loss of data in the event of a power disruption. If batteries are absent or fail, the

7200a uses a set of default settings stored in a read-only memory (ROM). Failure to complete POST requires the attention of appropriately trained service personnel.

The ventilator is operated from the front panel (Fig. 21–28), partitioned into three sections: ventilator settings, physiologic data, and ventilator status. To change any settings except CPAP, there is a function key within the ventilator settings section that causes the preexisting value for that setting to be displayed in one of two windows, A. This preexisting value is replaced by pressing the numeric touchpad keys; the new setting is stored in RAM by touching the ENTER key, B, which is confirmed by two beeps. If the setting exceeds its specified range, the microprocessor rejects entry with four beeps and the message INVALID ENTRY is displayed. Pressing CLEAR, C redisplays the function to facilitate entry of an acceptable value. If the operator neglects to touch the ENTER key for 10 seconds, the display reverts to the previously selected value. CPAP is adjusted by a knob, D, that controls the output pressure of a small regulator that powers the PEEP venturi.

The ventilatory mode, selected by a mode key, includes CMV, E; SIMV, F: CPAP, G, and ++, H. The ++ key is reserved for special functions and optional modes, such as pressure support. Mechanical V_T, I; respiratory rate, J; peak inspiratory flow rate, K; oxygen percentage L, from 21% to 100%, and the desired waveform (constant, M; decelerating, N; or sinusoidal, O) key are sequentially entered into RAM. Peak inspiratory pressure, P, (PIP) during mechanical V_T delivery may be limited up to 120 cmH_2O. If the PIP threshold is exceeded, the inspiratory phase is terminated. Sensitivity, Q, for patient-initiated breaths, whether mechanical or spontaneous, is adjustable from 0.5 to 20 cmH_2O below the baseline pressure in the breathing circuit. A plateau, R, of up to 2.0 seconds extends inspiration. Other submodes and keys include: 100% O_2; suction, S; manual inspiration, T; manual sigh, U; automatic sigh, V; and nebulizer, W. A small LED on the touchpad indicates when the function is active.

During CMV all breaths are machine initiated, whereas assist breaths are triggered by the patient when inspiratory effort exceeds the sensitivity threshold. During the SIMV or CPAP mode, the patient is allowed to breathe spontaneously by a demand-flow system that can provide peak inspiratory flow rates of up to 180 L/min. With SIMV, the respiratory rate is divided into 60 seconds to create a timing window. The first patient-initiated breath

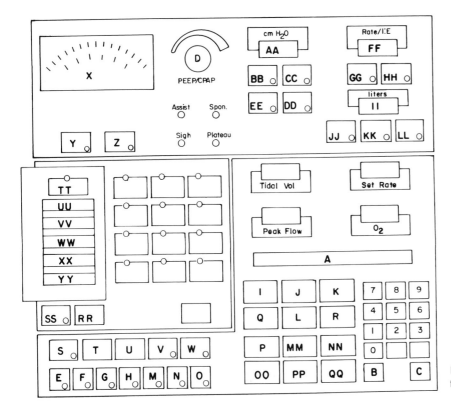

Figure 21–28. Control panel of the 7200a ventilator.

during a time window triggers a synchronized mechanical breath at the selected VT. For the remainder of the timing window, the patient may breathe spontaneously from the demand system. If the patient becomes apneic, the mechanical breath is delivered at the end of each window. Nebulization may be activated during each mechanical breath, but cannot function when peak flow is set at less than 20 L/min; nebulizer function automatically terminates after 30 minutes. Sigh volume, which is adjustable from 0.1 to 2.5 L, may not exceed twice the value of the VT. The automatic sigh mechanism is active only with CMV and allows 1 to 15 sighs per hour in lieu of normally scheduled mechanical or patient-triggered breaths. One, two, or three consecutive breaths or sighs can be delivered and the PIP for each sigh can be adjusted up to 120 cmH₂O. End-expiratory pressure (PEEP/CPAP) is continuously adjustable up to 50 cmH₂O with an uncalibrated rotary control.

With the ++ key, a series of messages and prompts are presented to the operator through the alphanumeric window and settings are keyed, as with ventilation settings. Pressure support may be set with any spontaneous-breathing mode. During pressure-supported ventilation, the 7200a becomes a constant-pressure generator. A rapid flow of gas directed into the breathing circuit generates the pressure level. As the physiologic airway pressure rises, flow decelerates until airway pressure and the pressure-support level are nearly equivalent. When flow has decelerated to 5 L/min, pressure support is terminated and baseline circuit pressure is restored. If the breathing circuit has a leak, inspiratory flow may not decelerate to 5 L/min, which will prolong inspiratory intervals. Pressure support would then terminate after 5 seconds.

Monitoring and Alarms

The physiologic data section comprises an analog meter, X, and three LED display windows (see Fig. 21–28). Under each data display is a series of touch pads by which the operator can select to view a variable. The analog meter indicates either airway pressure, Y, or exhaled minute volume, Z. Specific components of airway pressure, which are displayed in the cmH₂O window, AA, are mean airway pressure, BB; PIP, CC; plateau pressure, DD; and PEEP/CPAP level EE. Values in the digital display window and the analog meter may not agree on PEEP/CPAP level or plateau pressure. The digital PEEP/CPAP value is based on the output of the PEEP Venturi, the surface/area ratio of the exhalation valve, and the compressibility of the breathing circuit; surface/area ratio and circuit compressibility, in turn, are based on an extended self-test (EST). If the type of exhalation valve or compressibility of the breathing circuit have been changed, the digitally displayed value for PEEP/CPAP will be in error. Here, the operator must depend upon the analog meter or must disconnect the patient from the ventilator and rerun the EST.

Plateau pressure is calculated as the average of the previous four breaths and may not agree with the analog meter for any particular breath. The rate–I/E window, *FF*, displays ventilator rate, (*GG*, mechanical and/or spontaneous) or inspiratory/expiratory time (I/E ratio; *HH*) for mechanical breaths. In the liters window, *II*, the clinician may opt to view V$_T$, *JJ*; total (mechanical and spontaneous) minute volume (MV; *KK*); or spontaneous MV, *LL*. These data are averaged over ten breaths and mechanical and spontaneous breaths are not distinguished by the display for V$_T$ or MV. With SIMV, however, the difference between MV and spontaneous MV would be the mechanical contribution. A series of four LEDs below the PEEP/CPAP control representing assist, spontaneous, sigh, and plateau, each light after each breath to identify it.

There are limits or alarms for high pressure, *P*; low inspiratory pressure, *MM*, which detects ventilator–patient circuit leaks during mechanical inspiration; low PEEP/CPAP, *NN*, which facilitates detection of breathing circuit leaks, disconnection, or insufficient gas flow to meet spontaneous inspiratory requirements; low exhaled V$_T$, *OO*; low exhaled MV, *PP*; and high respiratory rate, *QQ*. Alarms are programmed in a manner identical with the procedure for programming ventilator settings. When limits are violated, an audible alarm and a visual indicator is illuminated, *Q*, and an associated message describing the conditions is presented in the message window *A*. The audible alarm automatically cancels if the alarm condition does not occur on the next breath. The LED indicator remains on, however, until the alarm has been reset, *RR*; thus, if the clinician is away from the patient, data from the event is retained for later reference. An alarm silencer, *SS*, gives a 2-minute period without audible alarms to permit undisturbed bedside procedures.

Factory-adjusted alarms consist of low oxygen and air source pressure, low battery power, exhalation valve leak, and I/E ratio. The apnea alarm is operator programmable. The apnea alarm settings are part of the special functions (++) key; the default setting is 20 seconds. When an exhaled volume is not detected within the assigned interval, audible and visual indicators are actuated, and the current ventilatory mode converts to apnea ventilation (AV). (AV ventilation settings are accessible beneath the ++ key.) Default values for apnea settings are a constant flow pattern, rate of 12 breaths per minute, V$_T$ of 500 mL, inspiratory flow rate of 45 L/min, O$_2$% of 100%, unless unavailable; sensitivity, PIP and PEEP/CPAP remain at current settings. A message in the alphanumeric display window indicates that AVL has been instituted. AV is cancelled when the alarm is reset, *R*.

The alarm summary display, *T*, includes: VENTILATOR INOPERATIVE, *TT*; ALARM, *UU*; CAUTION, *VV*; BACKUP VENTILATOR, *WW*; SAFETY VALVE OPEN, *XX*; and NORMAL, *YY*. The red VENTILATOR INOPERATIVE light will illuminate coincidentally with red SAFETY VALVE OPEN light, when the microprocessor has determined that the ventilator is not functional owing to an internal failure. The red ALARM light signals when an alarm has occurred and has not been reset. An indicator LED identifies which alarm is activated. When an alarm autoresets a yellow CAUTION light is illuminated. The red BACKUP VENTILATOR (BUV) lights up when the ventilator is in the emergency ventilatory mode; this mode, which is completely separate from the microprocessor, provides emergency ventilation in the event of computer problems or failure. Ventilatory settings during BUV are factory preset, constant flow, rate of 12 breaths per minute, V$_T$ of 0.5 L, PIP of PEEP/CPAP + 20 cmH$_2$O, and O$_2$% of 100%, if available, otherwise 21%. To restore normal operation, the 7200a must be repaired or, at the very least, must successfully pass EST. The red SAFETY VALVE OPEN is illuminated during emergency mode and the patient cannot be ventilated safely, so an internal valve is opened to allow room breathing when all inlet gas supply pressure is lost or when the microprocessor suspends normal ventilation to run POST. If POST fails, BUV is initiated. When the ventilator is operating normally and all limits and alarms are within acceptable ranges, a blue NORMAL light remains on.

Mechanism

The Bennett 7200a series ventilator features microprocessor control of electrical and electropneumatic subsystems (Fig. 21–29). The electropneumatic subsystem requires oxygen and air

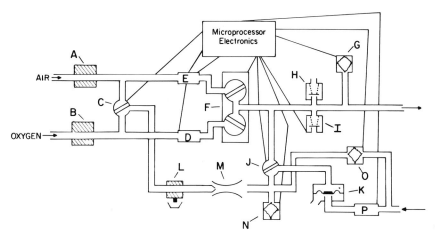

Figure 21–29. Schematic diagram of the 7200a ventilator.

compressed to between 35 to 100 psig. Air and oxygen flow through filters into regulators, A and B, which reduce pressure to a nominal 10 psig and deliver both gases to the crossover solenoid valve C, which can use oxygen for pneumatic power if necessary, through temperature-corrected, hot-film flow transducers Q1, D, and Q2, E, which measure oxygen and air, respectively; and, finally, into the proportional solenoid valve F, which, in conjunction with the flow transducers, form a closed servoloop. The microprocessor, using the operator-programmed physiologic settings, opens the solenoids within the valve, which provides the selected waveform and the proper amounts of air and oxygen to provide the set level of FiO_2, peak flow rate, and V_T. As gas flows to the patient, the microprocessor output signals from the flow transducers during each breath and makes adjustments accordingly; if, for example, flow is not sufficient, the processor opens the solenoids to increase flow. Accuracy is guaranteed. As it is delivered to the breathing circuit, gas passes a pressure transducer, G, that functions as an internal barometer and through a safety/check valve that functions as both an overpressure relief valve, H, and an antisuffocation valve, I. The overpressure valve, which is mechanical, vents circuit pressures in excess of 140 cmH_2O. The electronic antisuffocation valve opens in the event of gas or electric power loss and during POST.

Gas pressure to the exhalation valve is controlled by a three-way solenoid, J. During mechanical inspiration, the solenoid opens and allows pressure from the proportional solenoid to close the exhalation valve K. At the onset of exhalation, the solenoid closes and directs flow from the PEEP reg-

ulator, L, and PEEP Venturi, M, onto the diaphragm of the exhalation valve, which produces the set level of end-expiratory pressure (PEEP/CPAP). A pressure transducer, N, measures the output pressure of the PEEP Venturi and a differential pressure transducer, O, is used to measure airway pressure, as referenced to the output pressure of the PEEP Venturi. Once each hour the microprocessor opens a solenoid attached to each pressure transducer (not illustrated) to ambient and reestablishes the zero point. This ensures accuracy, because only the zero point is subject to drift. It also serves as a critical operational verification. Failure of a transducer to zero will necessitate the termination of normal ventilation and require that the ventilator be serviced before further use. Exhaled patient gas is directed through the temperature-compensated expiratory flow transducer, P, referred to as Q3. Signals from this flow transducer are integrated and displayed, providing the data for V_T and MV measurements. The measurements of V_T made at the expiratory flow transducer are constantly referenced against those made by the air and oxygen flow transducers coupled to the proportional solenoid. In the event that these two measurements disagree by more than 25%, normal operation is immediately discontinued and appropriate servicing is recommended.

Troubleshooting

Troubleshooting potential internal problems or failures with the 7200a is facilitated by the extended self-test (EST) procedure. This extensive battery of tests, performed in sequence, verifies the functional readiness of virtually every subsection of the ventilator, including microprocessor and associated electronics (POST), each pressure transducer and flow transducer, the exhalation valve and the patient-breathing circuit, the PEEP regulator, BUV, and the safety valve with associated overpressure relief. The test takes approximately 5 minutes to complete and must not be performed while the ventilator is on a patient. Each test sequence is given a code number, and if the test does not meet specifications, the code number is displayed in the alphanumeric message window. The Bennett Corporation suggests that the EST procedure be used to troubleshoot ventilator malfunctions and that a shortened version—quick extended self test (QUEST)—be used to verify day-to-day readiness for use.

Problems during routine use are minimized by a simple circuit and by ease of operation. One problem that is frequently encountered and not well understood is "autocycling." This will most likely occur in the SIMV mode when a spontaneously breathing patient becomes apneic. If the sensitivity is set too low, the exhalation phase of a mechanical breath may simulate the first patient-initiated breath in the next SIMV timing window. This produces two SIMV breaths in a row (one at the end of one timing window and the other at the beginning of the next window), followed by two SIMV intervals without a breath, and then the cycle repeats itself. In addition, if the apnea interval is less than two SIMV intervals, the ventilator will repeatedly convert to apnea ventilation and initiate alarms. The problem can be remedied by decreasing the sensitivity until SIMV breaths no longer trigger each other. Care should be taken that sensitivity is not decreased to the point that it inhibits spontaneous ventilation when the patient resumes spontaneous breathing.

BENNETT MA-1 VENTILATOR

Classification

The Bennett MA-1 ventilator (Fig. 21–30) is electrically and pneumatically powered, electronically controlled, and functions as a constant-flow generator that is volume-cycled (see Table 21–1). Because of low driving pressure, if compliance is low, constant flow may become constant pressure. There is an expiratory retard, and mechanical inspiration may be either machine cycled or patient triggered. The MA-1 may be modified to provide IMV, PEEP, or spontaneous CPAP.

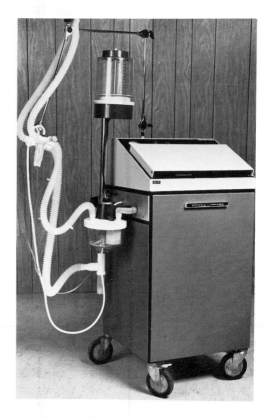

Figure 21–30. Bennett MA-1 ventilator. (Courtesy Puritan Bennett Corp.)

SPECIFICATIONS

Inspiration

Rate (BPM)	6–60
Volume (mL)	100–2200
Flow rate (L/min)	15–100
Pressure (cmH$_2$O)	10–80
Time (sec)	NC
Effort (cmH$_2$O)	0.5–10
Hold (sec)	NC
Demand flow (L/min)	NC
Safety pressure (cmH$_2$O)	85
Pressure support (cmH$_2$O)	NC
MMV (L/min)	NC

Expiration

Time (sec)	NC
PEEP/CPAP (cmH$_2$O)	Optional
Retard (L/min)	26–200
I/E ratio	NC

MODES

Assist	MMV
*Control	PS
*Assist–Control	APRV
*IMV (Optional)	PC
SIMV	CPAP

Operation

The Bennett MA-1 ventilator requires an electrical power source of 115 V, 60 Hz, and the power switch, *A*, is turned to ON (Fig. 21–31). To access oxygen, a hose is plugged into a 50-psi oxygen outlet. The humidifier should be filled and adjusted to the proper temperature at least 20 minutes before use so it will preheat while the ventilator is on standby. The ventilator sensitivity, *B*, must be adjusted for assisted ventilation. Peak flow, *C*, and mechanical ventilatory breathing rates, *D*, V⊤ up to 2200 mL, *E*; and normal high-pressure limit, *F* must be set. Pressure-cycled ventilation can be used, but, at the termination of each inspiration, the pressure-limit alarm, *P*, will sound unless it is silenced (switch just below front panel, inside cabinet). For sighs, the pressure limit, *G*, and the volume limit, *H*, function exactly as the normal pressure, volume limits, and rate, but at greater intervals; the sigh has its own volume and pressure that are independent of the ventilator breath. Up to three sighs may be administered, *I*. Manual breaths may be selected (normal or sigh) with button *J*.

The control for oxygen concentration is adjustable from 21% to 100%, *K*, and accurate to within ±2.5%. This is pneumatically powered with any high-pressure gas source. Thus, careful attention to the oxygen connection is essential. The amount of expiratory retard is controlled by the expiratory resistance control, *L*. Medication is nebulized by filling a nebulizer cup and activating the switch, *M*. PEEP is adjusted by an optional control on the side of the ventilator, and the level is registered on the ventilator system pressure gauge, *N*.

Monitoring and Alarms

The monitoring and alarm systems consist of lights on the front of the ventilator; the bulb function can

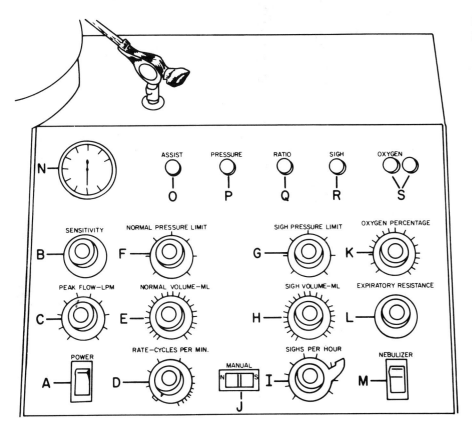

Figure 21–31. Control panel of the MA-1 ventilator.

be tested by depressing the light. These lights include an amber assist light, O, that indicates when the patient has initiated a breath; a pressure light, P, which turns red, is accompanied by an audible alarm when the pressure limit is exceeded; a ratio light, Q, is activated during controlled respiration when the I/E ratio becomes less than 1 : 1, thus, the inspiratory flow rate or ventilator frequency needs to be adjusted; and a sigh light, R, illuminates each time a sigh is administered.

An oxygen light system, S, functions when the ventilator is connected to a high-pressure gas source; a green light indicates when the oxygen concentration is greater than 21%, and a red light activates an audible alarm whenever a high-pressure gas source has not been connected to the ventilator and when the oxygen control knob, K, is turned to some value other than 21%. Use of the exhaled gas-collecting spirometer can assist the operator to ensure the delivery of adequate VT and that the patient is connected to the ventilator. Optional modes that require constant flow for spontaneous breathing, however, interfere with the spirometer and will require the clinician to provide additional monitoring to prevent accidental patient disconnection.

Mechanism

Air is drawn into the MA-1 (Fig. 21–32) through an air filter A to an oxygen blender C by the descending bellows. From a compressor, B, air is pumped into the power drive system, which causes the bellows to ascend. A solenoid valve, D, cycles the ventilator according to the logic of the electronic circuit and produces inspiratory and expiratory phases. The compressed gas passes through a Venturi, E, which boosts the flow, but can stall at a high peak inflation pressure. This is the mechanism by which the MA-1 is converted to a constant-pressure generator during ventilation of a patient with a noncompliant lung. Distal to the Venturi booster is a peak-flow control knob, F, which regulates the inspiratory flow rate by the rate of compression of the bellows. After passing the flow rate control, the major portion of gas flows into the bellows compression canister, G, through a one-way valve, and the remainder flows to a mushroom valve and compresses it, H. It then is exhausted from the bellows compression chamber; once inspiration has been complete.

On the front panel, the VT control (a potentiometer) provides a reference signal for the electronics. The bellows is attached to a pulley assembly that rotates a second potentiometer as the bellows ascends. When the VT signal from the front panel corresponds to the signal generated by the bellows pulley and potentiometer, VT has been delivered and mechanical inspiration is terminated.

In the patient intake circuit, air is drawn in through bacterial filter A, delivered to a blending chamber C, and mixed with oxygen according to the proportion set on the oxygen-control knob I.

Figure 21–32. Schematic diagram of the MA-1 ventilator.

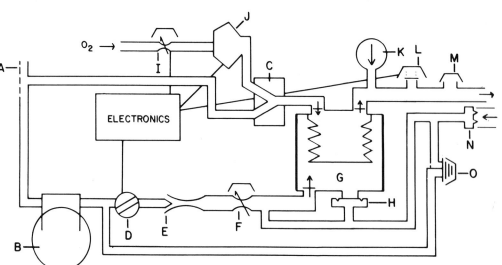

Oxygen flow to the blending chamber is controlled electronically and proportioned by an oxygen delivery bellows *J*. The oxygen–air mixture then enters the bellows through a one-way valve as it begins to descend (expiration). When the bellows begins to ascend, a second one-way valve opens, and the bellows gas is discharged into the patient circuit. Pressure is monitored by the ventilator system pressure gauge *K*, and is regulated by a pressure-relief control *L*. When the assist mode is used, sensitivity can be adjusted, *M*. The patient system bifurcates to seal the system during inspiration. Gas to this mushroom valve can also be controlled independently to obtain PEEP.

Troubleshooting

Because electronic components form a major part of this ventilator, most major malfunctions should be repaired by a manufacturer's representative.

If the ventilator will not develop pressure and there are no leaks, the exhalation mushroom valve may be incompetent or torn. Also, a thermometer should be placed in the orifice provided for this purpose or the orifice will leak. Similarly, if the ventilator is operated without the spirometer, the spirometer outlet must be plugged. If the humidifier does not heat satisfactorily, the water level may be inadequate, the heating element may be burned out, or the safety switch may not be making contact with the humidifier cover. One of the most difficult leaks to find is that from a loose screw in the heating element housed in the humidifier cover. Another leak that is difficult to find is a disconnection of the bacterial filter inside the ventilator door.

THE BIRD 6400ST VOLUME VENTILATOR

Classification

The Bird 6400ST volume ventilator (Fig. 21–33) is electrically and pneumatically powered, microprocessor operated, and may function as a constant- or decelerating-flow generator. It will also function as a constant-pressure generator when utilized in the pressure-support mode. Termination of mechanical inspiration is time-cycled; however, inspiratory flow becomes the cycling mechanism in pressure support. End-expiratory pressure may be applied during mechanical (PEEP) or spontaneous (CPAP) breathing. Initiation of mechanical inspiration is either machine-cycled or patient-triggered.

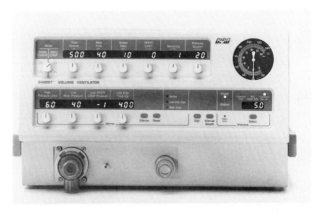

Figure 21–33. Bird 6400ST volume ventilator. (Courtesy of Bird Products Corp.)

SPECIFICATIONS

Inspiration

Rate (BPM)	0–80
Volume (mL)	50–2000
Flow rate (L/min)	10–120
Pressure (cmH$_2$O)	1–140
Time (sec)	NC
Effort (cmH$_2$O)	1–20
Hold (sec)	NC
Demand flow (L/min)	0–110
Safety pressure (cmH$_2$O)	NC
Pressure support (cmH$_2$O)	0–50
MMV (L/min)	NC

Expiration

Time (sec)	NC
PEEP/CPAP (cmH$_2$O)	0–30
Retard (L/min)	NC
I/E ratio	NC

MODES

*Assist	MMV
*Control	*PS
*Assist–Control	APRV
*IMV	PC
*SIMV	CPAP

Operation

Operation of the 6400ST is facilitated by a compact, easily understood control panel (Fig. 21–34). The top half of the panel is utilized for ventilatory settings, and the bottom is reserved for alarms and monitors.

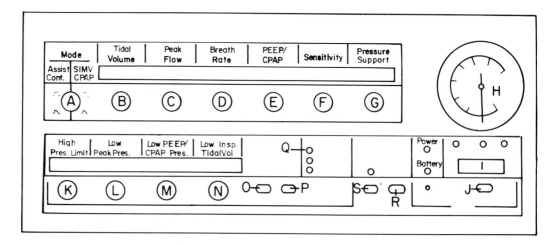

Figure 21–34. Control panel of the 6400ST ventilator.

The operator must first select a mode and flow pattern by placing the four-position mode selector switch, *A*, to the desired combination. Selections include assist–control (A/C) with square flow pattern, A/C with decelerating flow pattern, SIMV/CPAP with square flow pattern, and SIMV/CPAP with decelerating flow pattern. Selection of patient ventilator setting is monitored by a window, positioned above each control, that displays each selected value and changes as they are made. Ventilator settings with associated display window include mechanical tidal volume, *B*; peak flow rate, *C*; breath rate, *D*; PEEP/CPAP, *E*; sensitivity, *F*; and pressure support, *G*. Pressure support is available in the SIMV/CPAP mode only and cannot be adjusted in A/C.

Monitoring and Alarms

The 6400ST provides monitoring with an airway pressure manometer, *H*, and a message window, *I*, located on the front control panel (see Fig. 21–34). The message window is used to alert the operator to potential problems, or it can be used to select, *J*, one of the following for display: inspiratory time (seconds), total breath rate (breaths per minute), which includes both spontaneous and mechanical breaths; and calculated minute volume (L/min), which is simply the product of the V_T and rate settings. LEDs adjacent to the message window indicate use of battery power (not internal), or AC power, and any patient effort that surpasses the sensitivity setting. The 6400ST does not measure exhaled V_T; however, an external, optional monitor may be purchased to accompany the ventilator.

There are four primary patient alarms, each with a control knob and window to display the established value. The high-pressure limit control, *K*, establishes a pressure threshold that, when violated, terminates inspiration and activates an audible and visual alarm. If the airway pressure returns to the PEEP level within 3 seconds, normal ventilation resumes, and the audible alarm is cancelled. Should the airway pressure remain above the pressure limit setting or not return to the PEEP level, the internal safety solenoid will open. Airway pressure will then bleed to the PEEP level through an orifice in the main flow isolation valve. Upon reaching the PEEP level, the system will reset and attempt to deliver another breath. If the problem is not resolved, the scenario will repeat itself, and operator intervention will be necessary to rectify the situation. The pressure limit threshold is automatically increased to 150% immediately before each sigh breath, and returned to normal after the sigh has been delivered. However, the pressure limit cannot exceed 140 cmH$_2$O. The low peak pressure control, *L*, activates an alarm if the airway pressure fails to exceed the selected value during the inspiratory phase of any mechanical V_T. The low PEEP/CPAP control, *M*, is activated if the proximal airway pressure falls below the selected value for longer than 0.5 seconds. The low inspiratory tidal volume control, *N*, establishes a volume threshold that must be exceeded by both spontaneous and mechanical breaths. If four consecutive breaths fall below this setting, an alarm is activated. The alarm silence button, *N* will disable the audible alarm for 60 seconds, and the alarm reset, *P*, functions to reset the visual indicator for any alarm conditions that no longer exist. The ventilator-inoperative alarm cannot be silenced or reset.

Additional alarm conditions are listed with adjacent LED, Q. An apnea alarm occurs any time 20 seconds elapse without a mechanical or spontaneous breath. The low inlet alarm alerts the operator that the internal gas pressure has fallen below 17 psi and may be the result of low inlet pressure, internal regulator malfunction, or transducer error or malfunction. The ventilator-inoperative alarm terminates all ventilator functions; opens the safety solenoid, providing the patient access to room air; and activates audible and visual alarms. Conditions that will precipitate a ventilator-inoperative alarm include loss of electrical power, extended high or low system pressure, electrical or mechanical failure detected by the microprocessor, and improper installation of the exhalation valve housing. A manual breath, R, may be administered during any mode, provided that the patient is neither actively inhaling (mechanical or spontaneous) or exhaling. The sigh button, S, activates the automatic sigh function in all available modes and delivers a controlled sigh breath after each 100 breaths. The V_T of sigh breaths is 150% of the programmed mechanical V_T.

Mechanism

High-pressure (50 psi) blended gas and 115V AC electricity should be provided through the appropriate receptacles on the rear panel of the 6400ST ventilator (Fig. 21—35). The 6400ST requires an external blender capable of mixing 120 L/min at 50 psi. It is possible to substitute blenders, if they are capable of blending sufficient quantities of gas at 50 psig. Blended gas at the selected FiO_2 is filtered and delivered to a high-pressure 1.1L reservoir, A, and, subsequently, regulated, B, to 20 psi. The output

pressure of B is monitored by transducer C, which alerts the operator of potential regulator problems or low blended gas inlet pressure. The flow-control valve D receives blended gas from B and is responsible for the delivery of all breathing gases to the patient. The flow-control valve is defined as an *electromechanical* stepper valve. Such valves convert rotary motion into linear motion. Precise electrical signals from the microprocessor cause a motor to rotate a shaft. Rotation of the shaft occurs as a series of steps, each step opening or closing a poppet-type orifice located within the inspiratory flow valve. Resolution of flow through the orifice is claimed to be approximately 1 L per rotational step. The relationship between valve position and inspiratory flow rate is programmed into memory. This information allows the microprocessor to move the flow control valve in a sequence that will deliver the tidal volume, peak flow, and flow waveform selected by the operator. The exhalation valve E is also under microprocessor control and functions in a manner nearly identical with the flow control valve, except the rotating shaft applies pressure to the exhalation diaphragm rather than modulating an orifice.

To provide for spontaneous breathing, the microprocessor refers to information it receives from the proximal airway transducer F. As the airway pressure falls during a spontaneous breath, the microprocessor opens the flow-control valve in an effort to maintain the CPAP level. The microprocessor then regulates flow to simultaneously meet patient demand and hold the CPAP at the selected level. As the flow required to meet these demands approaches zero, the breath ends, and the exhalation valve opens.

Pressure-support breaths are delivered in a fashion similar to a spontaneous breath. The only difference is that the microprocessor attempts to

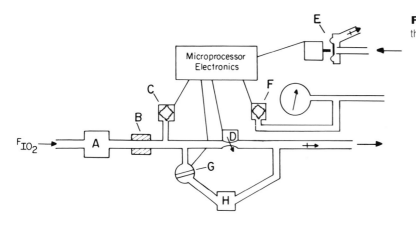

Figure 21—35. Schematic diagram of the 6400ST ventilator.

maintain the selected pressure-support level instead of the CPAP level.

The safety solenoid *G* can be opened during emergency alarm conditions, allowing the patient access to room air through ambient valve *H*, until appropriate action can be undertaken.

Troubleshooting

Troubleshooting is made easy through the judicious use of alarms and display windows. Potential patient circuit problems result in an audible alarm and the message "CIRC." The following conditions should be investigated as possible causes of the condition: disconnected proximal airway line, occluded or kinked proximal airway line, occluded or kinked inspiratory or expiratory limb of the breathing circuit, and transducer failure (either proximal or machine pressure transducer). Several problems can be avoided by ensuring that the exhalation valve diaphragm is properly engaged on the shaft of the valve-actuating motor and that the valve housing is securely latched. This is a complex pneumatic and electronic ventilator, and attempts to repair this ventilator should not be undertaken unless the operator is properly trained or qualified to make the repairs.

THE BABYBIRD VENTILATOR

Classification

The BABYbird ventilator (Fig. 21–36) is pneumatically powered, pneumatically controlled, and functions as a constant-flow generator that is time cycled. It may provide end-expiratory pressure during mechanical (PEEP) and spontaneous (CPAP) breathing. Mechanical inspiration is machine-cycled and may not be patient-initiated.

SPECIFICATIONS

Inspiration

Rate (BPM)	5.7–100
Volume (mL)	NC†
Flow rate (L/min)	0–30
Pressure (cmH$_2$O)	14–82
Time (sec)	0.4–2.5
Effort (cmH$_2$O)	NC
Hold (sec)	NC
Demand flow (L/min)	NC
Safety pressure (cmH$_2$O)	88

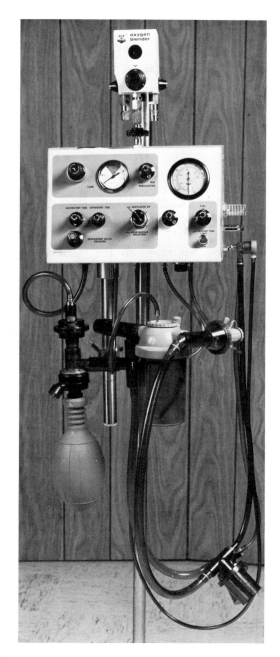

Figure 21–36. BABYbird ventilator, equipped with an oxygen blender. (Courtesy of Bird Products Corp.)

Pressure support (cmH$_2$O)	NC
MMV (L/min)	NC

Expiration

Time (sec)	0.4–10
PEEP/CPAP (cmH$_2$O)‡	0–20
Retard (L/min)	NC

I/E ratio   NC*

* Adjusted as a function of inspiratory and expiratory time
† A function of flow rate × inspiratory time
‡ At 10-L/min flow-rate

MODES

Assist	MMV
Control	PS
Assist–Control	APRV
*IMV	PC
SIMV	CPAP

Operation

The BABYbird operates easily, but it is occasionally misunderstood because IMV is the primary mode of ventilation (Fig. 21–37). In simplest terms, gas that flows continuously through the ventilator circuit is periodically diverted to the patient by closure of the exhalation valve.

The operator connects the air and oxygen lines to a 50-psi gas source and selects the desired FiO₂. Next, the flowmeter A is adjusted at B, according to the patient's needs. An arbitrary value, approximately twice the patient's predicted maximal inspiratory flow rate, is used initially. All flow from the ventilator is directed through the nebulizer; however, only part of the gas goes through the jet of the Venturi to produce particulate water. When the nebulization knob C is turned fully clockwise, a maximum of 12 L/min may be delivered through the venturi. As the nebulizer control is turned counterclockwise, less and less flow is directed through the nebulizer Venturi jet, and more is directed into the supplemental gas port of the nebulizer, the auxiliary flow input receiver. This auxiliary flow line should not be occluded or inadvertently connected to the nebulizer Venturi.

If the patient is to breathe spontaneously, these are the only controls that need to be adjusted. If the IMV mode is desired, the selector knob D is turned to IMV to activate the ventilator portion of the BABYbird. A suitable inspiratory time is set with the inspiratory time knob E. The duration of inspiration and the rate of flow is determined by the VT delivered by the ventilator. Selection of expiratory time with the expiratory time control F allows frequencies of 4 to 100 breaths per minute.

The inspiratory relief pressure control, G, determines the pressure limit of the system. Occlusion of the expiratory limb of the breathing circuit

Figure 21–37. Control panel of the BABYbird ventilator.

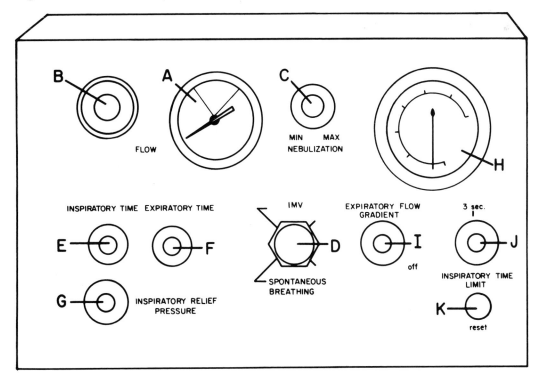

or kinking of the exhalation valve charging line will disable the inspiratory relief pressure control, allowing excessive and dangerous airway pressure to develop. To prevent this, an adjustable mechanical peak inspiratory pressure relief valve, factory set at 88 cmH₂O, is present. However, the operator must carefully adjust the relief pressure of this valve to suit the requirements of the individual patient and provide appropriate airway protection. The expiratory-flow gradient knob I reduces expiratory-flow resistance by decreasing resistance to flow through the breathing circuit. This is accomplished by a Venturi proximal to the outflow valve. The operator can stop inspiration manually, K, or by a time-cycled mechanism, J.

PEEP or CPAP can be adjusted between zero and 20 cmH₂O by a lever on the outflow valve. A test lung on the side of the BABYbird ventilator allows adjustment of these controls before the patient is connected to the breathing circuit. An additional safety device is the manual resuscitation bag attached to the lower part of the BABYbird ventilator. It can be used at any time to ventilate the patient.

Monitoring

The BABYbird contains an internal low-pressure alarm that will notify the operator that the supply pressure of blended gas has fallen to 40 psi. It is possible for the ventilator to fail in the inspiratory phase, when supply pressures fall below 35 psi, and appropriate action should be taken. As an additional safety feature, the operator may program an infinitely adjustable inspiratory timer control, J, with a calibrated mark at 3 seconds. If mechanical inspiration exceeds the programmed time period, inspiration will be terminated, and an audible alarm will be sounded. The audible alarm continues, and mechanical inspirations will not resume until the operator resets the alarm with the provided button, K. An aneroid manometer H, calibrated in cmH₂O, permits the operator to observe airway pressures. The clinician should be aware of the existence of a tiny orifice (0.013 in. diameter) located just before the manometer, within the proximal airway pressure line. This orifice functions to reduce oscillations in manometer readings, which may occur at high ventilatory rates when proximal airway pressures change rapidly. The orifice produces a "dampening" effect and, sometimes, will cause the manometer reading to lag behind the actual airway pressure. Under such conditions, an aneroid manometer cannot be relied upon to accu-

rately reflect proximal airway pressure and should not be utilized when making critical adjustments to ventilator settings. The BABYbird provides no additional monitoring capabilities, and an auxiliary monitoring device should be purchased to accompany this ventilator when in use.

Mechanism

The BABYbird is pneumatically operated by high-pressure air and oxygen mixed in the blender A to provide the desired FIO_2 (Fig. 21–38). This gas mixture is delivered into a source manifold where a low-pressure alarm, B, warns of any decreased pressure (less than 40 psig) within the ventilator system. A flowmeter, D, delivers the flow, C, to the patient with the appropriate jet nebulization. The inspiratory-breathing system also houses an adjustable pressure-relief valve, E, which vents pressure when it exceeds the adjusted limit in the breathing

Figure 21–38. Schematic diagram of the BABYbird ventilator.

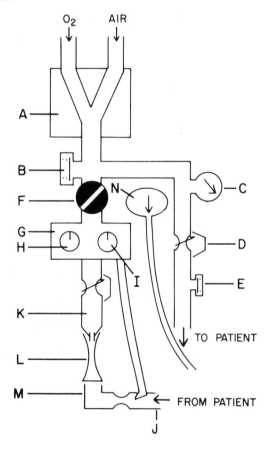

circuit. This is the entire inspiratory circuit when the patient is breathing spontaneously. However, during IMV, *F*, a second circuit is activated. Gas pressure is delivered to the cycling mechanism, *G*, which has inspiratory, *H*, and expiratory, *I*, timers to control intermittent flow. During the expiratory phase, pressure may be delivered to a Venturi system, *J*, which provides an expiratory flow gradient; during the inspiratory phase, pressure is delivered through a restricting valve, *K*, which controls the downstream pressure to a second Venturi system, *L*. This system occludes the outflow system, *M*, so that gas flow, rather than passing freely from the outflow valve, is delivered into the patient's lungs. A pressure gauge, *N*, measures the proximal airway pressure.

Troubleshooting

The most common problem is leakage. Leaks may occur because of a faulty gas supply system, because of loose connections in the breathing circuit, or because a part has been forgotten in reassembling the ventilator after it has been cleaned and sterilized. A decrease in line pressure activates an oxygen blender alarm if the pressure differential between oxygen and air exceeds 20 psi. An alarm at the bottom of the ventilator activates when the internal pressure of the ventilator has become less than 40 psi or the inspiratory time is prolonged excessively. If the patient is not receiving adequate nebulization, the auxiliary and nebulizer lines may be crossed or inserted into the wrong ports.

If residual positive-baseline pressure remains on the pressure gauge, the flow to the patient probably is too great for the breathing circuit. This baseline pressure can be eliminated by increasing the size of the breathing tubes, reducing the flow, or adjusting the expiratory-flow gradient control counterclockwise.

THE IMVBIRD VENTILATOR

Classification

The IMVbird (Fig. 21–39) is pneumatically powered, pneumatically controlled, and functions as a decelerating-flow generator. Termination of mechanical inspiration is time-cycled. End-expiratory pressure may be applied during mechanical (PEEP) and spontaneous (CPAP) breathing. Initiation of mechanical inspiration is machine-cycled and is not to be triggered by patient effort.

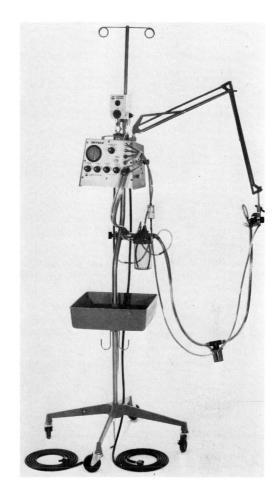

Figure 21–39. IMVbird ventilator. (Courtesy of Bird Products Corp.)

SPECIFICATIONS

Inspiration

Rate (BPM)	0.3–30
Volume (mL)	NC†
Flow rate (L/min)	10–72
Pressure (cmH$_2$O)	NC
Time (sec)	0.5–4
Effort (cmH$_2$O)	(1)
Hold (sec)	NC
Demand flow (L/min)	0–150
Safety pressure (cmH$_2$O)	110
Pressure support (cmH$_2$O)	NC
MMV (L/min)	NC

Expiration

Time (sec)	1.5–infinity
PEEP/CPAP (cmH$_2$O)	0–35
Retard (L/min)	NC

I/E ratio   NC*

* Adjusted as a function of inspiratory and expiratory time
† A function of flow rate × inspiratory time

MODES

Assist	MMV
Control	PS
Assist–Control	APRV
*IMV	PC
SIMV	CPAP

Operation

The oxygen blender is connected to 50-psi air and oxygen sources. As shown in Fig. 21–40, the inspiratory flow rate control knob *A* meters flow to the inspiratory-breathing circuit which, in conjunction with the adjustable inspiratory time control *B*, sets a wide range of V$_T$. The inspiratory timer increases the inspiratory time as the control is rotated clockwise. A lockout circuit is provided to depressurize the exhalation valve automatically should the ventilator fail to cycle during mechanical inspiration.

This internally adjustable mechanism is preset to terminate the mechanical inspiratory phase after approximately 5 seconds.

The mechanical expiratory time interval is adjusted with control *C*. Clockwise rotation will increase the expiratory phase from 1.5 seconds to more than 3 minutes. This interval allows the patient to breath spontaneously, and a wide range of IMV rates is possible. During the expiratory phase, the manual inspiration button *D* can be depressed to initiate a mandatory inspiration. If the button remains engaged, the ventilator will continue to deliver mechanical volume until the 5-second lockout mechanism terminates inspiration and dumps the V$_T$ to ambient. Proximal airway pressure is monitored on the pressure gauge, *E*, which is calibrated in both cmH$_2$O and mmHg. The end-expiratory pressure control, *F*, adjusts the amount of positive distending pressure desired during the expiratory phase. It should be pointed out, however, that the demand valve will not provide sufficient inspiratory flow unless some PEEP/CPAP has been adjusted. The manufacturer's recommendations suggest a minimum setting of 2 to 4 cmH$_2$O to pro-

Figure 21–40. Control panel of the IMVbird.

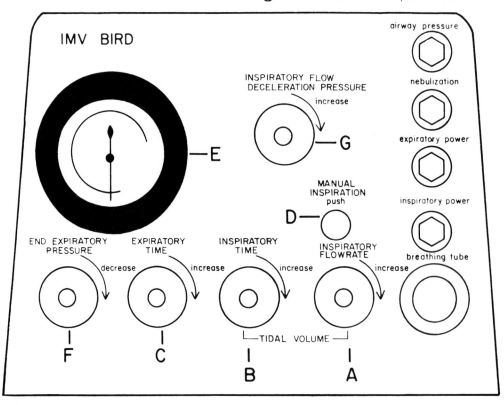

vide sufficient flow and minimize the inspiratory WOB.

The mechanical inspiratory flow pattern may be manipulated by adjusting the inspiratory flow deceleration pressure control, G, thus decreasing the flow rate at any preselected pressure between 20 and 75 cmH_2O. An internal overpressure governor provides a maximum pressure limit of 100 cmH_2O. Hose connections on the front panel are color-coded and indexed for the proper circuit connections.

Monitoring

The IMVbird provides no monitoring capabilities, and an auxiliary monitoring device should be purchased and used with this ventilator.

Mechanism

The IMVbird (Fig. 21-41) is pneumatically powered by a high-flow oxygen blender, A, which combines 50-psi sources of air and oxygen and delivers the 50-psi mixture to a manually operated on–off master switch B. This on–off switch must not be confused with the IMV on–off switch on the BABY-bird. In the OFF position, the IMVbird receives no gas power and all ventilatory functions are disabled, including spontaneous CPAP. In the ON position, blended gas is routed to a demand flow accelerator servo, C. As spontaneous inspiratory effort is initiated, the valve opens and provides accelerated gas flow to meet the patient's spontane-

ous inspiratory demand. Gas flow from B to the master cartridge D is metered to the timing circuit, which cycles the ventilator to inspiration or exhalation. The metering of gas from the master cartridge is regulated by the expiratory time E and the inspiratory time F control knobs. When gas is bled away, E, the master cartridge opens, initiating mechanical inspiration. The inspiratory phase is terminated when sufficient gas has metered through control F, closing the master cartridge and sequencing the ventilator into the exhalation phase.

During mechanical inspiration, a portion of the gas is diverted to pressurize the exhalation valve, G, facilitating the delivery of a mandatory breath. The inspiratory flow rate-metering valve, H, mediates flow during the controlled breath. The flow is directed into an injector, I, which entrains gas from a reservoir of equal oxygen concentration that is delivered into the inspiratory breathing circuit. The positive end-expiratory distending pressure is adjusted with control J delivering gas to a Venturi system, K, and simultaneously pressurizes the exhalation valve to the PEEP/CPAP level during the mechanical expiratory phase.

Troubleshooting

Leaks are a problem because of numerous hose connections. The small high-pressure tubing connections are vital to the function of this ventilator, but leaks are readily found because of the high flow of escaping gas through a small orifice that makes an audible hiss. Internal leaks are uncommon.

Figure 21—41. Schematic diagram of the IMVbird.

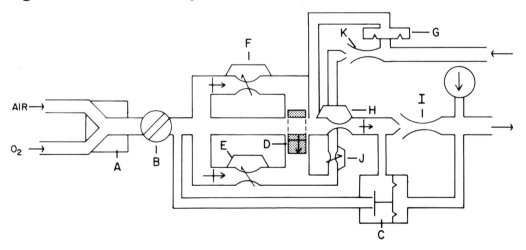

EMERSON IMVENTILATOR-3MV

Classification

The Emerson 3MV (Fig. 21–42) is electrically powered, electronically controlled, and functions as a nonconstant-flow generator that is time-cycled. It may provide end-expiratory pressure during mechanical (PEEP) and spontaneous (CPAP) breathing. The mechanical inspiration is machine-cycled and may not be patient initiated.

SPECIFICATIONS

Inspiration

Rate (BPM)	0.2–22
Volume (mL)	100–2200
Flow rate (L/min)	NC
Pressure (cmH$_2$O)	40–100
Time (sec)	1–5
Effort (cmH$_2$O)	NC
Hold (sec)	NC
Demand flow (L/min)	NC
Safety pressure (cmH$_2$O)	NC
Pressure support (cmH$_2$O)	NC
MMV (L/min)	NC

Expiration

Time (sec)	1.5–300
PEEP/CPAP (cmH$_2$O)	0–25
Retard (L/min)	NC

I/E ratio	NC

MODES

Assist	MMV
*Control	PS
Assist–Control	APRV
*IMV	PC
SIMV	CPAP

Operation

A modular control panel (Fig. 21–43) is provided to isolate functions, allow installation of various options, and facilitate repair service. The main power switch *A* activates all electronic functions, except the piston motor. Humidifier heat is regulated by the humidifier output control *B*. The FiO$_2$ is adjusted by an air–oxygen-blending device and is measured by an optional oxygen analyzer *C*.

Mechanical ventilation frequency is determined by adjusting the total cycle time (TCT) thumbwheel *D*. Inspiratory duration is selected

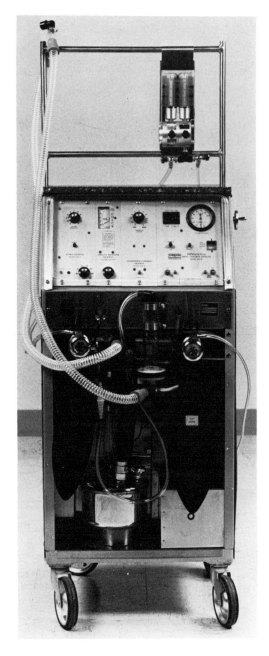

Figure 21–42. Emerson IMVentilator-3MV. (Courtesy of J.H. Emerson Co.)

with the inspiratory time (T$_I$) control *E*. The operator must remember, however, that expiratory time (T$_E$) is equal to the selected T$_I$ + 1 second, regardless of the total cycle time setting. This is important because random ventilator cycling will occur if T$_I$ + T$_E$ + 1 > TCT. In addition, this design prevents the use of inverse I/E ratio ventilation. Emer-

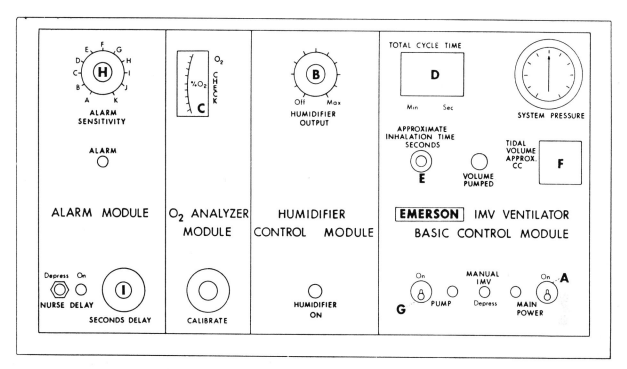

Figure 21—43. Control panel of the Emerson IMVentilator.

son offers an optional timing module that allows the use of inverse I/E ratios.

Mechanical V_T is adjusted with a hand crank on the right side of the ventilator chassis and is displayed on the panel in 100–mL intervals, *F*. The DC motor is activated by pump switch *G*. A mechanical inspiration may be administered (when the pump is on) by depressing an IMV manual button.

Monitoring and Alarms

An optional alarm module provides sensitivity control, *H*, to allow adjustment to sense the pressure. An audible alarm is activated when circuit pressure falls below the desired level (e.g., loss of CPAP or patient disconnect). A time delay allows tracheal suctioning or other procedures that require transient disconnection without an audible alarm. If purchased without the optional alarm, an auxiliary monitoring device should be purchased or available to accompany this ventilator when in use.

Mechanism

Air and oxygen are mixed at *A* to provide a desired FIO_2 for filling two 5-L anesthesia bags (Fig. 21–44).

One bag, *B*, serves as gas source for the mechanical V_T. The other, *C*, provides a reservoir of gas for spontaneous ventilation. Two pressure-relief valves, *D* and *E*, prevent overdistention of the anesthesia bags. An optional demand valve is available to replace the spontaneous reservoir bag. For proper operation, the demand valve option also requires the use of a high-flow oxygen blender in place of the standard oxygen–air mixing flowmeter.

During mechanical exhalation, gas from reservoir *B* is drawn into the cylinder, *F*, by the downward piston stroke. The cylinder displacement is regulated by a crank handle, *J*, connected to the piston rod linkage, *K*. As the piston terminates its downward motion, a microswitch, *I*, is closed by a rotating cam, *H*, initiating an electronic signal for mechanical inspiration. Power to the DC motor, *G*, is regulated by the inspiratory time control. An increased current flow accelerates motor speed, thus simultaneously shortening the inspiratory and expiratory duration.

Mechanical inspiration is initiated when positive displacement of the piston occurs, which forces most cylinder gas through a pass-over heated humidifier, *L*, into the patient circuit. A small amount of gas is shunted to pressurize and close the exhalation valve, *M*, which also may be loaded

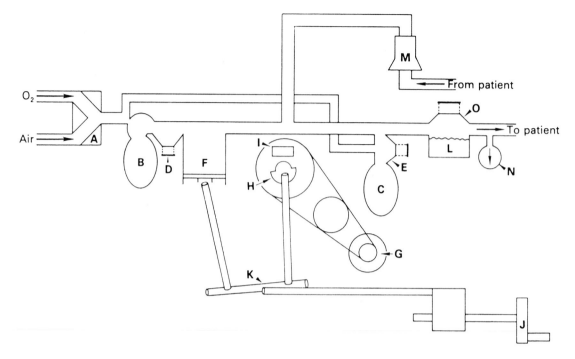

Figure 21—44. Schematic diagram of the Emerson IMVentilator.

with water to produce threshold expiratory pressure. System pressure increases simultaneously on each side of the exhalation valve and is indicated by an aneroid manometer, N. Maximum system pressure is adjustable by means of a relief valve, O, on the humidifier.

Troubleshooting

All connections must be tight and high back-pressure leak-proof. On occasion, an unexpectedly high level of CPAP may be observed. This problem is frequently traced to an excessive gas flow being used to fill anesthesia bag B. This problem is likely to occur when the filling flow exceeds the relieving ability of relief valve D. The rising pressure within the anesthesia bag is subsequently transmitted across the piston, which charges the exhalation valve M and elevates the CPAP level. Because of the practical design, few other problems are encountered.

EMERSON POSTOPERATIVE VENTILATOR-3PV

Classification:

The Emerson 3PV (Fig. 21-45) is electrically powered, electronically controlled, and functions as a nonconstant-pressure generator that is time-cycled. Mechanical inspiration is controlled and may not be patient initiated; it may provide end-expiratory pressure during mechanical ventilation (PEEP). The 3PV may be modified with optional accessories to provide the currently requisite modalities: IMV and spontaneous CPAP.

SPECIFICATIONS

Inspiration

Rate (BPM)	5–99
Volume (mL)	100–2200
Flow rate (L/min)	NC
Pressure (cmH$_2$O)	10–100
Time (sec)	0.3–6
Effort (cmH$_2$O)	NC
Hold (sec)	NC
Demand flow (L/min)	NC
Safety pressure (cmH$_2$O)	NC
Pressure support (cmH$_2$O)	NC
MMV (L/min)	NC

Expiration

Time (sec)	0.3–6
PEEP/CPAP (cmH$_2$O)	0–25
Retard (L/min)	NC
I/E ratio	NC

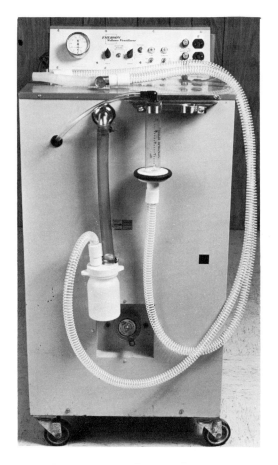

Figure 21—45. Emerson Postoperative 3PV ventilator. (Courtesy of J.H. Emerson Co.)

MODES

Assist	MMV
*Control	PS
Assist–Control	APRV
*IMV (Optional)	PC
SIMV	CPAP

Operation

The ventilator is connected to a 115-V, 60-Hz electrical outlet (Fig. 21–46). Sterile water is added to the humidifier and the filling port cap secured with the wrench provided. The humidifier heater is controlled by the three-position toggle switch B: HI, OFF, and LO. Generally, the HI (high) heating position is required to provide adequate humidification, especially when the continuous-flow modification for IMV is used. Mechanical V_T is set by turning the hand crank and the value read on the volume indicator (low center and center of chassis). A two-position toggle switch, A, turns the piston drive motor on or off. In the ON position, inspiratory, C, and expiratory, D, time adjustments determine the ventilator cycling frequency and because they are independent, inverse I/E ratios are possible. System pressure is indicated on an aneroid manometer, E.

Mechanism

The 3PV is operated and powered electronically (Fig. 21–47). Ambient air, drawn into a reservoir "trombone," A, may be enriched with oxygen by means of an inlet nipple, B, to provide the desired FIO_2. As the piston, C, moves downward (negative

Figure 21—46. Control panel of the Emerson 3PV ventilator.

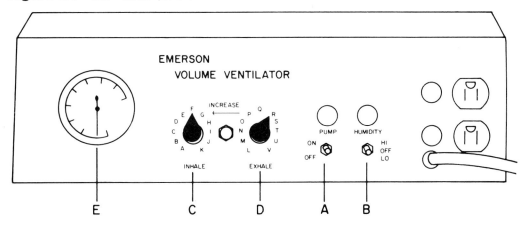

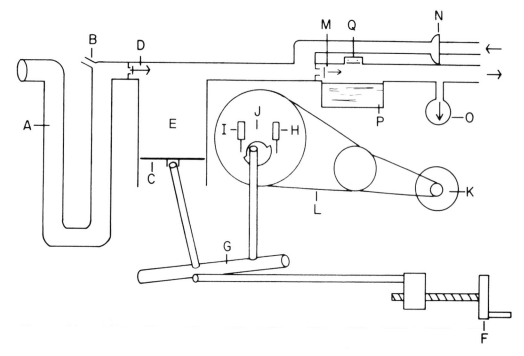

Figure 21—47. Schematic diagram of the Emerson 3PV ventilator.

displacement) reservoir gas is drawn into the chamber *E* through a unidirectional valve *D*. Chamber displacement is determined by turning a crank handle *F*, which regulates piston rod linkage *G*. A cam *J*, mounted on a pulley wheel, it designed such that microswitch *H* is closed when the piston is at its downward terminus and open at its maximum upward position. Inspiratory and expiratory time (I/E ratio) controls regulate a DC motor, *K*, and, thereby, piston speed by means of a pulley *L* when the microswitch is closed and open, respectively. A second microswitch, *H*, phases the optional sigh mechanism.

During positive-pressure displacement, the piston *C* compresses chamber gas, creating sufficient pressure to close intake valve *D*, open outflow valve *M*, and close exhalation valve *N*. System pressure equalizes on both sides of the exhalation valve and is indicated on an aneroid manometer, *O*. Gas flow to the patient is warmed and moistened by a pass-over humidifier, *P*. Peak pressure is limited by an adjustable relief valve, *Q*.

Monitoring and Alarms

The Emerson 3PV provides no monitoring capabilities, and an auxiliary monitoring device should be purchased to accompany this ventilator when in use.

Troubleshooting

Because of its functional design, the 3PV is a veritable workhorse. Potential system leaks may occur at welded seams (humidifier especially), exhalation valve, water trap, and, occasionally, the piston ring.

The electronic components of newer models have caused few problems, with the possible exception of the turn-screw on the panel between the inspiratory and expiratory timing knobs. This control adjusts the ventilator to hospital voltage. It should be adjusted for the lowest projected voltage drop. Indiscriminate tampering with the turn-screw may result in a malfunction.

THE HAMILTON AMADEUS VENTILATOR

Classification

The Hamilton Amadeus ventilator (Fig. 21—48) is electrically and pneumatically powered, is microprocessor operated, and may function as a constant- or decelerating-flow generator, or as a constant-pressure generator with pressure support (PS)

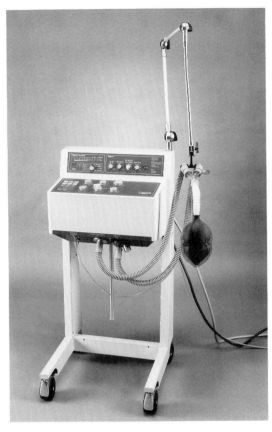

Figure 21—48. Hamilton Amadeus ventilator. (Courtesy of Hamilton Medical Corp.)

(see Table 21–1). Termination of mechanical inspiration is time-cycled and may be extended by a plateau. Inspiratory flow becomes the cycling mechanism in pressure support. End-expiratory pressure may be applied during mechanical (PEEP) or spontaneous (CPAP) breathing. Initiation of mechanical inspiration is either machine- or patient-cycled.

SPECIFICATIONS

Inspiration

Rate (BPM)	0.5–120
Volume (mL)	20–2000
Flow rate (L/min)	Up to 180*
Pressure (cmH$_2$O)	10–110
Time (sec)	NC†
Effort (cmH$_2$O)	(1)–(10)
Hold (sec)	NC†
Demand flow (L/min)	0–180
Safety pressure (cmH$_2$O)	120

Pressure support (cmH$_2$O)	0–100
MMV (L/min)	NC

Expiration

Time (sec)	NC†
PEEP/CPAP (cmH$_2$O)	0–50
Retard (L/min)	NC

I/E ratio	1 : 9–4 : 1

* Indirectly adjusted.
† Adjusted as function of TCT with I/E controls.

MODES

Assist	MMV
*Control	*PS
*Assist–Control	APRV
IMV	PC
*SIMV	CPAP

Operation

The front panel of the Amadeus ventilator (Fig. 21–49) is subdivided into three distinct sections: monitoring, alarm, and control subsections. All ventilator settings, except the pressure limit, are located in the control subsection.

To begin operation, the operator must select a mode by depressing the desired touchpad. To prevent accidental selection of settings, touchpads must be depressed for a minimum of 3 seconds before changes occur. The settings include ASSIST/CONTROL, A, which is either machine-cycled or may be patient triggered; SIMV, B, which provides access to fresh gas for spontaneous ventilation and periodic SIMV timing windows during which a mechanical breath may be patient triggered in lieu of a mandatory breath at the end of the window; and spontaneous breathing, C, with or without CPAP. When a mode is selected, only the controls requisite to that mode are activated. Green LEDs beside each control are used to indicate when a control is active (LED on) or not (LED off). Control knob D is used to determine ventilator frequency; however, for the purpose of determining inspiratory and expiratory time, the total cycle time (TCT) remains at 4 seconds at ventilator rates lower than 15 breaths per minute. In the SIMV mode, the maximum frequency is limited to 60 breaths per minute. The mechanical V$_T$ is active in both SIMV and CMV modes, and is regulated by a single control, E. The operator may select from either a constant or a decelerating flow pattern. Inline (DIP) switches (found on back) are used to access optional ventila-

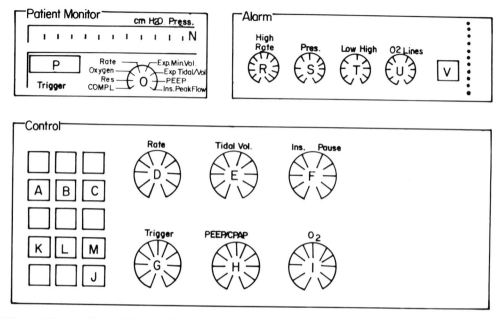

Figure 21—49. Control panel of the Amadeus ventilator.

tor routines. Option switch number 3 controls the waveform: *off* will yield a constant flow pattern and *on* a decelerating pattern. The microprocessor "consults" the position of the DIP switches only once during the first second after the ventilator is turned on. After this time, changing the position of the switch will have no effect upon ventilator operation.

The inspiratory and expiratory time controls are contained together in dual control knob *F*. The frequency control predetermines the TCT and the inspiratory and expiratory time controls divide this time up on a percentage basis. The expiratory time is set by a small, lighter-colored control and inspiratory time by the larger, darker-colored control. If the two controls are separated, an inspiratory plateau or pause will result. Pause time is considered part of the inspiratory time; therefore, the sum of the pause and the inspiratory time may not exceed 80% of the TCT. The trigger or sensitivity control *G* is active in all modes and is used to determine the reduction in breathing circuit pressure required to initiate the inspiratory phase cycling mechanism. The magnitude of pressure deflections is continuously adjustable and is referenced to the baseline circuit pressure (i.e., end-expiratory pressure). At the maximum counterclockwise position, the mechanism is off and will not permit patient initiation of breaths.

A second dual-function control, *H*, regulates the level of CPAP and inspiratory pressure support (range: zero to 100 cmH$_2$O). Pressure support may be utilized in any spontaneous-breathing mode. During PS ventilation, a rapid gas flow is directed into the breathing circuit and produces the desired pressure level. As the lungs fill and inspiratory demand decreases, flow decelerates, but the inspiratory pressure is maintained.

When flow decelerates to approximately 25% of the initial flow rate, PS is terminated and baseline circuit pressure is restored. The small, lighter-colored inner knob adjusts the CPAP and the outer, darker-colored knob adjusts the inspiratory PS level above the CPAP. It should be pointed out that when using PS and CPAP, any adjustments made to the CPAP level will require concomitant readjustment of the inspiratory PS level to maintain the equivalent level above CPAP.

Oxygen concentration, *I*, is infinitely adjustable between 21% and 100%.

The operator may depress one of four touchpads to facilitate calibration, testing, and temporary 100% oxygen delivery. The O$_2$ FLUSH key pad, *J*, allows the operator to provide 100% oxygen for 5 minutes, with an automatic return to the selected FIO$_2$. Depression of the CAL O$_2$ touchpad, *K*, results in an automatic calibration of the oxygen sensor. The CAL FLOW, *L*, and TEST TIGHTNESS,

M, touchpads permit the operator to calibrate the flow sensor and test the breathing circuit for leaks.

Monitoring and Alarms

The patient monitor subsection of the control panel (see Fig. 21–49) of the Amadeus contains a dynamic bar graph N, which provides a visual indication of airway pressure; an eight-position selector switch O, with accompanying display window P; and the trigger LED, which is illuminated to indicate patient-initiated breaths.

The Amadeus monitors in "real time" and each setting available for display has been measured. Information for display is gathered primarily from a miniature pneumotachograph located at the patient airway and pressure transducers within the ventilator. Location of the flow-sensing pneumotachograph at the airway, allows the measurement of exhaled V_T, without being affected by compressed gas trapped in the ventilator circuit. This location also prevents the erroneously high V_T readings that can result when the pneumotachograph is positioned distal to the exhalation valve.

Selector O may be rotated and situated to display PEEP/CPAP (cmH$_2$O), Rate (breaths per minute, total: spontaneous + machine-cycled), Exp Tidal Vol (mL), Exp Min Vol (L/min), Compliance* (static; mL/cmH$_2$O), Insp Resistance* cmH$_2$O/L/sec, Insp. Peak Flow (L/min), and oxygen concentration (%).

The dynamic bar graph N illuminates one segment for each 2 cmH$_2$O airway pressure, and the highest pressure segment remains lighted, providing the peak inflation pressure, until the next successive mechanical inspiration. The alarm section includes 5 operator adjustable alarms; 11 indicator LEDs with adjoining alarm description; and an alarm-silence touchpad. The operator must appropriately position each alarm control: high rate, R; the high pressure S; the high/low minute volume dual control knobs, T; and the oxygen limit, U; range: ±5% of selected F$_I$O$_2$ or off.

Alarm indicator LEDs provide nearby clinicians with immediate visual information to indicate which alarm or alarms have been violated. In addition to the adjustable alarm conditions, the Amadeus also monitors for APNEA, which is defined as no patient exhalation measured at the flow sensor for 15 consecutive seconds; POWER, which alerts the operator to a loss of electric power; DISCONNECTION, which indicates the patient has become detached from the ventilator; GAS SUPPLY, which signals a high-pressure gas (air or oxygen) source failure; FLOW SENSOR/USER, which alerts the operator that the flow sensor has been inserted backward or that there has been operator error in setting patient controls; and VENTILATOR INOPERATIVE, which signals that the internal diagnostics carried out by the microprocessors have detected a dysfunction. The ventilator-inoperative condition also terminates all ventilator function, opens the exhalation valve, and allows the patient to breath spontaneously through the internal safety (antisuffocation) valve. All alarm conditions provoke both audible and visual alarms. The audible portion of all alarms with the exception of the ventilator-inoperative may be silenced for 2 minutes by depressing the alarm silence touchpad V.

Mechanism

Mechanical operation (Fig. 21–50) is accomplished by three separate, but interconnected, microprocessor-controlled subsystems: the front panel, valve control, and the oxygen-mixing system. The front panel processor is responsible for interpreting the input of all physiologic data and controlling alarms and displays. The valve control processor integrates signals from the front panel into the appropriate mechanical function of the servovalve. The oxygen-mixing microprocessor is responsible for mixing air and oxygen in the proper quantities, providing gas flow to the servovalve during ventilatory maneuvers, and maintaining the reservoir in a full state. Each of the three microprocessors continuously monitors the operation of the other two, ensuring proper operation at all times, as well as facilitating the rapid diagnosis and subsequent termination of any unpredictable or errant behavior.

The Amadeus should be supplied with sources of medical-grade air and oxygen (29 to 86 psig) and 115-V AC through the provided receptacles on the rear panel. The gases are filtered and then delivered to separate electronic solenoids, A and B. Upon demand or depletion of the reservoir, the oxygen processor opens and closes the solenoids as required to produce the operator selected F$_I$O$_2$. A differential pressure transducer, C, monitors the flow generated by the mixer and terminates blender operation when the flow required to maintain the operational reservoir pressure approaches zero. The mixer is capable of blending approximately 90 L/min at an accuracy of ±3%. After being blended, the gas mix-

---

* The Amadeus requires that the operator provide an inspiratory pause, before the measurements of compliance and resistance can be made. $C_{static} = V_{T(exp)}/P_{plateau} - PEEP$; and $R_{insp} = P_{end-insp} - P_{plateau}/FLOW_{end-insp}$.

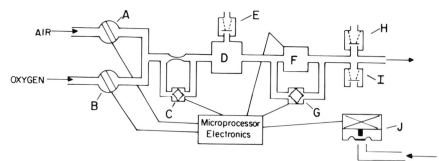

Figure 21—50. Schematic diagram of the Amadeus ventilator.

ture either flows directly to the patient or fills the large, cast aluminum reservoir, *D*, which, when pressurized to 350 cmH$_2$O, holds nearly 8 L of blended gas. An overpressure relief valve, *E*, ensures that the tank pressure does not exceed 350 cmH$_2$O, in the event of failure of the gas-mixing system. The large volume of compressed gas in this reservoir permits the Amadeus to achieve momentary peak inspiratory flow rates of nearly double the maximal mixing rate of the flow system.

The delivery of gas from the reservoir into the breathing circuit is accomplished by the servocontrolled flow valve, *F*, which separates the reservoir from the patient-breathing circuit. The entire process is under the coordination of the control microprocessor; however, the actual electronic servocontrol circuitry is analog. The flow valve comprises an electromagnetically actuated plunger (not illustrated), position sensor (not illustrated), and differential pressure transducer, *G*, coupled into a single unit. At the base of the plunger is an orifice configured as an isosceles triangle. During the delivery of a mechanical V$_T$, electric signals from the front panel and front panel processor are used to predict the flow required to meet requirements of the programmed settings. The control processor then raises the plunger in the flow valve to the desired height, creating an orifice of sufficient size to produce the requisite flow. The desired height and consequent orifice size are accurately verified by the position sensor.

Gas begins to flow from the reservoir into the breathing circuit. Transducer *G* measures the flow and compares the actual flow signal against the desired flow signal. If the actual flow signal is more or less than desired, the analog circuitry closes or opens the servovalve appropriately until the measured flow and desired flow signals are equivalent. This flow adjustment loop may be repeated as many as ten times per second, if necessary, and ensures extreme accuracy in the delivery of the selected flow and V$_T$. After leaving the flow valve, the

gas passes a mechanical overpressure relief valve, *H*, which is factory set to relieve at 120 cmH$_2$O; the oxygen-sensing fuel cell (not illustrated); and the ambient (antisuffocation) valve *I*, which allows the patient access to room air in the event of ventilator failure.

The exhalation valve *J* comprises a large silicon diaphragm, stabilized in the center with a metal plate. The diaphragm is seated during mechanical inspiration by an electromagnetic plunger. The same electronmagnetic plunger produces an extremely predictable threshold resistance and is responsible for generating CPAP.

Troubleshooting

Internal, electronic, or pneumatic problems are quickly diagnosed by the three microprocessors, which watch each other constantly and abort operation as soon as any errant behavior is diagnosed. A series of tests, stored in the software, can be accessed with the aid of a service manual and will help an interested operator or service technician quickly troubleshoot virtually any problem.

External or breathing circuit-related problems include tears or small holes in the silicon exhalation valve diaphragm and problems with the miniature pneumotachograph. Inability to calibrate the Amadeus is most frequently remedied by replacing the pneumotachograph.

THE HAMILTON VEOLAR VENTILATOR

Classification

The Hamilton Veolar ventilator (Fig. 21–51) is electrically and pneumatically powered, microprocessor operated, and may function as a constant-, nonconstant-, or decelerating-flow generator or as a constant-pressure generator, with either pressure support or pressure control (see Table 21–1). Termination of mechanical inspiration is time-cycled

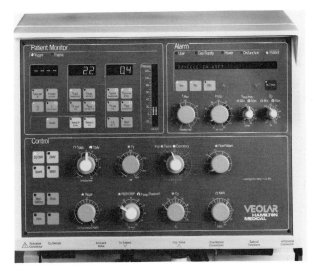

Figure 21–51. Hamilton Veolar ventilator. (Courtesy of Hamilton Medical Corp.)

and may be extended by a plateau. Inspiratory flow becomes the cycling mechanism in pressure support. End-expiratory pressure may be applied during mechanical (PEEP) or spontaneous (CPAP) breathing. Initiation of mechanical inspiration is machine- or patient-cycled.

SPECIFICATIONS

Inspiration		
	CMV	5–120
Rate (BPM)	SIMV	0.5–60
Volume (mL)		20–2000
Flow rate (L/min)	Up to 180†	
Pressure (cmH₂O)		10–110
Time (sec)		NC*
Effort (cmH₂O)		0–(15)
Hold (sec)		NC*
Demand flow (L/min)		0–180
Safety pressure (cmH₂O)		‡
Pressure support (cmH₂O)		0–100
MMV (L/min)		0–25
Expiration		
Time (sec)		NC†
PEEP/CPAP (cmH₂O)		0–50
Retard (L/min)		NC
I/E ratio		1:9–4:1

* Adjusted as function of TCT with I/E controls.

† Indirectly adjusted.

‡ Pressure-tracking relief valve (pressure limit + 10 cmH₂O) maximum relief 120 cmH₂O.

MODES

Assist	*MMV
*Control	*PS
*Assist–Control	APRV
IMV	*PC
*SIMV	CPAP

Operation

The front panel of the Veolar ventilator (Fig. 21–52) is subdivided into three distinct sections: monitoring, alarm, and control subsections. All ventilatory settings, except the pressure limit, are located in the control subsection.

When the Veolar is turned on (push button on the rear panel) a 31-character alphanumeric display, *A*, prompts the operator to select a mode: CMV, *B*, which is either controlled or may be patient initiated; SIMV, *C*, which provides access to fresh gas for spontaneous ventilation and periodic SIMV timing windows during which a mechanical breath may be patient triggered in lieu of a mandatory breath at the end of the window; spontaneous breathing, *D*, with or without CPAP; and MMV, *E*, which provides microprocessor-titrated pressure support of spontaneous inspiration to ensure delivery of the selected minute ventilation. When a mode is selected, only the controls requisite to that mode are activated. Green LEDs beside each control are used to indicate when a control is active (LED on) or not (LED off).

Ventilator frequency can be set for SIMV (small dark knob) or CMV (larger, light-colored knob; *F*). In addition, the CMV control serves as the primary control to determine the total cycle time (TCT) of mandatory breaths in either the SIMV or CMV modes. The expiratory time is set as a percentage of the TCT (small, dark knob). If the inspiratory (larger, light-colored knob) and expiratory controls, *G*, are separated, an inspiratory plateau or pause will result. Pause time is considered part of the inspiratory phase and, therefore, the sum of the pause and the inspiratory time may not exceed 80% of the total cycle time.

Mechanical V_T is active during both SIMV and CMV and is regulated by a single control, *H*. Mechanical V_T may be delivered with any of four possible flow waveforms, *I*: accelerating, decelerating, sinusoidal, or constant. Inspiratory time is not altered when flow pattern is changed; consequently, the microprocessor must adjust peak flow for the appropriate V_T to be delivered. As a point of reference, at any given V_T and inspiratory time, peak

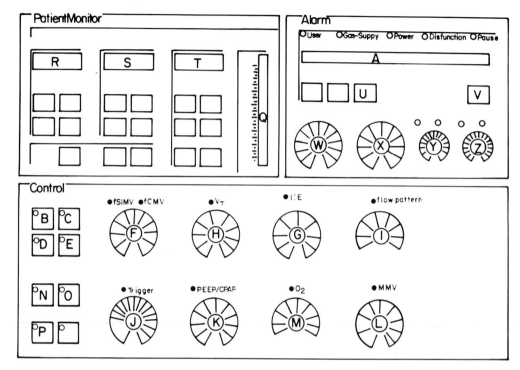

Figure 21—52. Control panel of the Veolar ventilator.

flow of the sinusoidal waveform is 57% higher than the constant-flow pattern, whereas the accelerating or decelerating patterns are 100% higher than constant flow. The trigger or sensitivity control, J, is active in all modes and is used to determine the reduction in breathing circuit pressure required to initiate the inspiratory–phase–cycling mechanism. The magnitude of pressure deflection is continuously adjustable and is referenced to the baseline circuit pressure (i.e., end-expiratory pressure; maximum counterclockwise position is off and will not permit patient initiation of breaths).

In regulating the level of CPAP and inspiratory pressure support (range: zero to 50 cmH₂O; K), the combined pressure levels cannot exceed 50 cmH₂O. During pressure support, which may be used in any spontaneous-breathing mode, a rapid gas flow is directed into the breathing circuit to produce the set pressure level. As the lungs fill and inspiratory demand decreases, flow decelerates, but inspiratory pressure is maintained. When flow decelerates to approximately 25% of the initial flow rate, PS is terminated and baseline circuit pressure is restored. When CPAP (small, dark inner knob) and PS (outer knob) are used together, adjusting CPAP requires concomitant adjustment of PS to

keep it at the same level above CPAP. Minimum minute ventilation, L, may be selected from 1 to 25 L/min. In the MMV mode, a minute volume and baseline level of PS are selected. The baseline PS will be automatically titrated upward in increments of 2 to 3 cmH₂O if the MV estimated from eight breaths is less than the selected MMV. If MV equals MMV, PS remains constant; when MV exceeds MMV, PS is progressively reduced toward the set baseline.

Oxygen concentration is continuously adjustable, M; from 21% to 100%). Manual breaths at set Vᴛ may be administered during mechanical exhalation, N. The reservoir tank and breathing circuit can be flushed with 60 L/min of fresh gas, O; this allows rapid changes in FᵢO₂ but flushing should be used judiciously because it reduces CPAP to approximately 5 cmH₂O as long as the flush is occurring. Bronchodilator and other pharmaceutic solutions may be administered, P, by a nebulizer placed into the inspiratory limb of the breathing circuit; mechanical Vᴛ is reduced by the volume of gas required to power the nebulizer. A hinged panel, located just below the control panel on the right side of the Veolar, contains several additional controls: an audible alarm volume control; a calibration button, which initiates calibration; a lamp test; a hold, which stops the ventilator and keeps the exhalation valve closed as long as the button is depressed; and option switches (a series of eight, on or off, dual inline package [DIP] switches). On all ventilators, all but switch 1 are reserved for options or future ventilatory enhancements. When switch number 1 is on, backup ventilation is activated, which provides mechanical ventilation in the event of patient apnea. The apnea alarm is not adjustable and is triggered when no exhaled gas passes the expiratory flow sensor for 15 seconds. The backup ventilation mode also requires switching to CMV; therefore, CMV settings should be adjusted when activating backup ventilation. The microprocessor detects the position of this switch only once during the first second after the ventilator is turned on; after that time, changing the position of the switch has no effect on ventilator operation.

Monitoring and Alarms

The monitoring section comprises a vertical airway pressure bar graph, Q, and three small alphanumeric display windows, R, S, T. A miniature pneumotachograph, located at the patient airway, and pressure transducers within the ventilator gather information for display. With the flow-sensing pneumotachograph at the airway, exhaled V_T can be measured without being affected by compressed gas trapped in the ventilator circuit, which prevents the erroneously high V_T readings that can result when the pneumotachograph is positioned distal to the exhalation valve.

Three of 14 possible variables may be displayed: peak inspiratory flow rate during mechanical V_T delivery (V_{peak}; L/min), mean airway pressure (P_{mean}; cmH_2O), oxygen percentage (O_2), effective compliance (C; L/cmH_2O), inspiratory or expiratory resistance (R_{insp}, R_{exp}; cmH_2O/L/sec), total respiratory frequency (f_{total}; breaths/minute),

peak inflation pressure (P_{max}; cmH_2O), spontaneous breathing frequency (f_{spont}; breaths per minute), I/E ratio (I/E), machine-delivered and exhaled V_T (V_{Tvent}, V_{Texp}; mL), exhaled minute volume ($V_{exp/min}$), and PEEP (cmH_2O). Trends can be obtained for the following variables: C, R_{insp}, R_{exp}, f_{spont}, and $V_{exp/min}$. Normally, these variables are displayed on a breath-by-breath basis; however, the measurements are stored in RAM. To display trends, a 15-minute or 2-hour time frame must be selected; the trend is displayed for 10 seconds and then the display returns to breath-by-breath monitoring. The 15-minute trend represents the most recent 15-consecutive minutes, and the 2-hour trend is the mean of the previous eight 15-minute trends. Alarms are conveniently grouped together in the control panel; a series of LEDs at the top identify the source of the problem: user, gas supply; power; dysfunction; and patient. Self-limited alarm conditions are stored in RAM, but may be recalled, U, and displayed, A. Alarms may be silenced for 2 minutes, V.

Adjustable alarms consist of maximum respiratory frequency, W; maximum airway pressure, X; maximum and minimum minute exhaled volume, Y; and maximum and minimum oxygen percentage, Z.

Mechanism

Operation of the Hamilton Veolar (Fig. 21–53) is accomplished by two separate but interconnected subsystems: the pneumatic gas-blending and flow system and the electronic control system. The pneumatic system employs two precision regulators, A and B, which accept medical-grade air and oxygen between 29 and 110 psig and reduce their pressure to 22 psig. These gases then enter the mechanical gas mixer C, where they are blended to a set FiO_2; maximal blending approaches 90 L/min. The blended gases are routed into a large, cast alu-

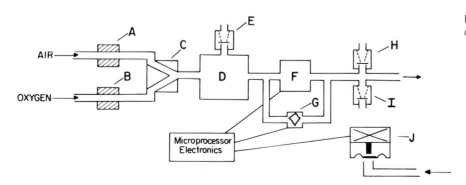

Figure 21–53. Schematic diagram of the Veolar ventilator.

minum reservoir, or surge tank *D*, compressed to 350 cmH₂O that holds nearly 8 L of blended gas. An overpressure relief valve *E* ensures that the tank pressure does not exceed 350 cmH₂O. The large volume of compressed gas in this reservoir permits the Veolar to achieve momentary peak inspiratory flow rates of nearly double the maximal mixing rate of the flow system. The delivery of gas from the reservoir into the breathing circuit is accomplished by a servocontrolled flow valve *F* under the coordination of a microprocessor; however, the actual electronic servocontrol circuitry is analog. The flow valve comprises an electromagnetically actuated plunger (not illustrated), position sensor (not illustrated), and differential pressure transducer, *G*, coupled into a single unit. At the base of the plunger is an orifice shaped like an isosceles triangle. During the delivery of a mechanical V_T, electric signals from the front panel and front panel processor are used to predict the flow required to meet requirements of the programmed physiologic variables. The control processor then raises the plunger within the flow valve to a set height, which opens the orifice to a size sufficient to produce the requisite flow; the height and size of the orifice are verified by the position sensor. Subsequently, gas begins to flow into the breathing circuit. The transducer *G* measures the flow and compares the actual flow signal with the flow-setting signal. If the actual flow signal is more or less than the setting, the analog circuitry closes or opens the servovalve as needed. This flow adjustment loop may be repeated as many as ten times per second, if necessary, and ensures extreme accuracy in the delivered flow and volume. After leaving the flow valve, the gases pass a mechanical overpressure relief valve, *H*, which is directly linked to the maximum pressure (P_max) control. A set P_max simultaneously sets the mechanical overpressure valve to approximately 10 cmH₂O higher than the P_max setting. The gas also passes the oxygen-sensing fuel cell (not illustrated) and the ambient valve *I*, which gives access to room air in the event of ventilator failure. The exhalation valve *J*, comprising a large silicon diaphragm, is stabilized in the center with a metal plate. The diaphragm is seated during mechanical inspiration by an electromagnetic plunger. The same electromagnetic plunger produces an extremely predictable threshold resistance force and generates CPAP.

Troubleshooting

Internal, electronic, or pneumatic problems are quickly diagnosed by the two microprocessors that sense each other constantly and abort ventilation as soon as any problem is detected. A series of tests stored in the software help troubleshoot virtually any problem. External or breathing circuit-related problems include tears or small holes in the silicon exhalation valve diaphragm and problems with the miniature pneumotachograph. Inability to calibrate the Hamilton is most frequently remedied by replacing the pneumotachograph. Initial reports on the Veolar indicate it is an extremely reliable and trouble-free ventilator.

THE INFRASONICS INFANT STAR VENTILATOR

Classification

The Infant Star ventilator (Fig. 21–54) is electrically and pneumatically powered, microprocessor operated, and may function as a constant- or nonconstant-flow generator. Termination of mechanical inspiration is time cycled, and end-expiratory pressure may be applied during mechanical (PEEP) or spontaneous (CPAP) breathing. Initiation of mechanical inspiration is machine-cycled.

SPECIFICATIONS

Inspiration

Rate (BPM)	1–150
Volume (mL)	NC

Figure 21–54. Infrasonics Infant Star ventilator. (Courtesy of Infrasonics Corp.)

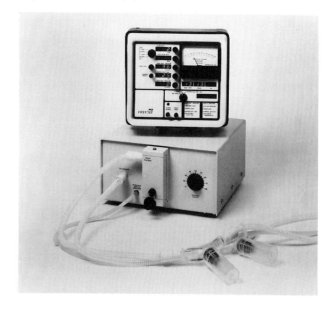

Flow rate (L/min)	4–40
Pressure (cmH_2O)	8–90
Time (sec)	0.1–3
Effort (cmH_2O)	NC
Hold (sec)	NC
Demand flow (L/min)	6–40
Safety pressure (cmH_2O)	80
Pressure support (cmH_2O)	NC
MMV (L/min)	NC
Expiration	
Time (sec)	NC
PEEP/CPAP (cmH_2O)	0–24
Retard (L/min)	NC
I/E ratio	NC

MODES

Assist	MMV
Control	PS
Assist–Control	APRV
*IMV	PC
SIMV	CPAP

Operation

The Infant Star comprises two separate, but interconnected, modules: the pneumatics unit and the electronics–display unit (Fig. 21–55). Ventilator operation is initiated by turning on the power switch, located on the back panel of the electronics–display module. The ventilator mode is selected with control knob A, and the selections include CPAP (continuous flow), CPAP (demand flow), IMV (continuous flow), and IMV (demand flow). The continuous-flow mode allows the Star to function similarly to other infant ventilators and establishes a set flow rate of gas that provides fresh gas for spontaneous breathing and mechanical breaths. However, should a patient's spontaneous inspiratory flow rate exceed the established continuous flow rate, the demand system will respond with an additional flow, a feature not found on other infant ventilators. The demand-flow mode provides a continuous flow of 4 L/min and spontaneous flow upon demand, up to a maximum of 40 L/min.

Ventilator controls are in a vertical row on the display panel, with the exception of PEEP/CPAP, B, which is located below switch A. The operator-selected value for each setting is displayed in an adjacent window that accompanies each control. As a safety feature, the control knobs must be depressed while they are rotated to effect a change,

preventing accidental movement. The flow rate control C, allows adjustment of the available flow for spontaneous breathing and mandatory breaths, Ventilator rate D is adjustable in one-breath increments between 1 and 60 BPM, two-breath increments between 60 and 130 BPM, and five-breath increments between 130 and 150 BPM. The peak inspiratory pressure (PIP; E) may be adjusted in 1-cmH_2O increments and inspiratory time F is adjustable in 0.01-second increments from 0.1 to 0.6 seconds, and in 0.1-second steps from 0.6 to 3.0 seconds. The manual breath button G may be utilized in any ventilatory mode. Each manual breath has the settings selected for mandatory breaths and the PIP and inspiratory time; care should be taken to appropriately adjust these controls before engaging the manual button when in the CPAP mode. The oxygen control H is located on the pneumatics module and is infinitely adjustable from 21% to 100%.

Monitoring and Alarms

The Infant Star measures and displays pertinent pressure data, while simultaneously monitoring the patient for numerous potentially dangerous conditions (see Fig. 21–55). Information utilized in the patient monitoring process is gathered by two airway pressure transducers: one located just before the patient gas flow outlet; the second monitors proximal airway pressure. The Infant Star also carries on numerous electronic checks and verifications to ensure proper operation at all times.

Only the operator-adjusted alarm, I, low inspiratory pressure (range: zero to 60 cmH_2O) will alert the clinician to the development of leaks or improper ventilator settings. Below the airway pressure manometer J are three patient-pressure display windows: peak inflation pressure (PIP; K), mean airway pressure (MEAN; L), and PEEP/CPAP, M. Each pressure setting is displayed in cmH_2O on a breath-by-breath basis, with the exception of the MEAN, which is an average based on a 30-second interval. A fourth display window, N, will exhibit the PEEP/CPAP setting (cmH_2O), I/E ratio, or the expiratory time (seconds) as determined by the position of selector switch O.

There are nine factory-specified alarm conditions, in addition to low inspiratory pressure, and they are each listed in the lower-right corner of the display panel, with an adjacent LED associated with each alarm. As alarm conditions occur, an audible alarm sounds and the associated LED lights up to inform the operator. The LED remains

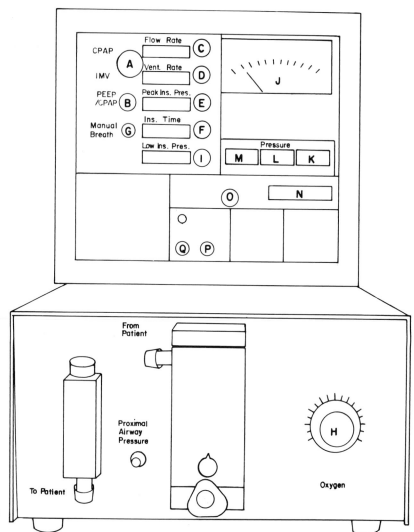

Figure 21–55. Control panel of the Infant Star ventilator.

lighted, even if the audible alarm stops, until the operator depresses the visual reset button, *P.* Alarms, with the exception of "vent inop," and "power loss," may be silenced with button *Q* for up to 60 seconds. Several alarm conditions may be precipitated by more than one problem, and operators should thoroughly familiarize themselves with all the possible problems.

Alarm conditions include low PEEP/CPAP, which is automatically adjusted by the microprocessor; airway leak, which signals the development of leaks by alarming when the continuous flow or background flow increases by 8 L/min for at least 4 seconds; insufficient expiratory time, which remains off when the expiratory time exceeds 0.3 seconds for rates under 100 breaths per minute and 0.2

seconds for rates over 100 breaths per minute; low oxygen–air pressure, which alerts the operator that the respective source gas pressure has fallen to 40 psi or less; internal battery and power loss, which alerts the operator that electric power is lost and the ventilator is being operated on internal batteries; and the obstructed tube, which utilizes the PIP display window to provide the operator with an error code message describing the type of violation that has occurred.

The operator should become thoroughly familiar with these error codes to prevent unnecessary delays in correcting potentially dangerous problems. The final alarm is the ventilator-inoperative condition. This alarm notifies the operator that the electronics have detected a problem that may render the ventilator unsafe to operate. The condition activates both audible and visual alarms, terminates gas flow, stops all ventilator functions, and opens the internal safety-vent valve, which reduces the airway pressure to ambient, and allows the patient access to fresh air. The ventilator-inoperative alarm will trigger if the exhalation valve remains closed for longer than 3.5 seconds; the exhalation valve does not close in a 66-second period during IMV; the airway pressure transducer does not zero during the autozero procedure; either or both microprocessors stop functioning; communications errors are detected; the internal battery fully discharges; or another electronics failure renders the ventilator unsafe. This alarm condition cannot be silenced.

Mechanism

The ventilator is connected to a 115-V, 60-Hz electrical outlet and 50-psi sources of medical-grade air and oxygen (Fig. 21–56). A precision regulator, A, reduces the air-source pressure to approximately 38 psi. A pneumatic connection, B, allows the regulated output from the air regulator to control the output of the oxygen regulator, C. This pneumatic "relay" system ensures that both regulators have identical pressure output. Any variation of the air regulator is immediately matched by the oxygen regulator. Accuracy of the oxygen-blending system is maintained with this design.

Regulated gases are mixed to the selected FIO_2 in the dual-needle valve blender, D, and subsequently flow through the blender control valve, E, and into a accumulator, F. As the pressure in the accumulator approaches 38 psi, the differential-

pressure transducer, G, will close the blender control valve. As ventilator function utilizes gas and reduces pressure in the accumulator, the blender control valve remains closed, until reservoir pressure reaches 29 psi. At this point, a signal from transducer G opens the control valve and gas flow rapidly fills the tank. This patented system ensures that when gas flows from the blender, it does so at high flow rates that are well within the calibrated range of the blender.

After the blending system and accumulator, a regulator, H, further reduces pressure to 18 psi and supplies each of six solenoids in the proportional flow manifold, I. When individually opened, each solenoid will deliver a precise flow rate: 2, 4, 8, 16, 16, 16 L/min. By opening selected solenoids, the ventilator can produce any flow rate between zero and 40 L/min in 2-L/min increments. For example, to produce 14 L/min, the microprocessor would open the 2-, 4-, and 8-L/min solenoids (14 = 2 + 4 + 8). During mechanical inspiration, the requisite solenoids are opened and the programmed flow is delivered. As the airway pressure approaches the selected peak airway pressure, the microprocessor reduces the selected flow rate in 2-L/min increments, resulting in a flow rate of zero at the point that airway pressure reaches the operator-selected PIP. If the selected inspiratory time has not elapsed or inverse I/E ratios are desired, the microprocessor turns the 2-L/min solenoid on and off, which maintains the airway pressure at the selected PIP until inspiration terminates.

Two additional pneumatic branch lines originate at the output of the air regulator A. The first passes through a solenoid, referred to as the Venturi valve, J, and subsequently, powers the expi-

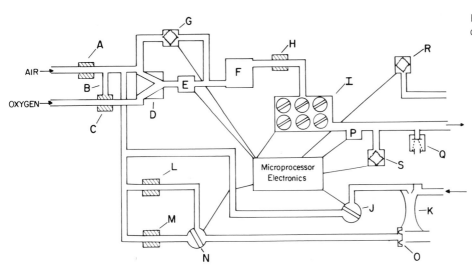

Figure 21–56. Schematic diagram of the Infant Star ventilator.

ratory Venturi, K. If inadvertent PEEP/CPAP develops, the microprocessor will increase the on cycle of the Venturi valve. The longer the Venturi valve remains on, the lower the baseline airway pressure will become. This system allows the Infant Star to automatically maintain the operator-programmed PEEP/CPAP under a wide variety of different conditions. The second pneumatic branch delivers gas to the PEEP regulator L and the PIP, M, regulator. The regulated pressure outputs of these regulators are connected to a three-way solenoid, N. During the mechanical inspiratory phase, N delivers the regulated PIP pressure to the exhalation valve diaphragm O. Termination of inspiration changes the configuration of N, and the regulated PEEP pressure is subsequently delivered to the exhalation valve diaphragm.

Located in the inspiratory limb is a safety valve P that functions as an antisuffocation valve during ventilator inoperative alarms. As an additional safety feature, an adjustable, mechanical overpressure-relief valve Q (range: 12 to 90 cmH$_2$O) is found just above the patient flow connection. This valve should be appropriately adjusted each time the ventilator is used.

Airway pressure is monitored by two separate transducers located in the proximal airway line, R, and in the patient flow delivery limb, S. This permits a cross-referencing of pressures, and facilitates the detection of a large variety of potentially dangerous circuit-related problems (e.g., expiratory limb occlusion and obstructed endotracheal tubes).

Troubleshooting

Nuisance alarms can be a problem unless operators are thoroughly familiar with the operation of this complex infant ventilator. However, troubleshooting is simplified by the ten indicator LEDs and the error codes displayed in the PIP display window. A complete troubleshooting guide can be found in the operator's manual and should help with most common and correctable problems.

This is a complex pneumatic and electronic ventilator and attempts to repair it should not be undertaken unless the operator is properly trained or qualified.

MONAGHAN 225/SIMV

Classification

The Monaghan 225/SIMV (Fig. 21–57) is pneumatically powered, fluidically controlled, and func-

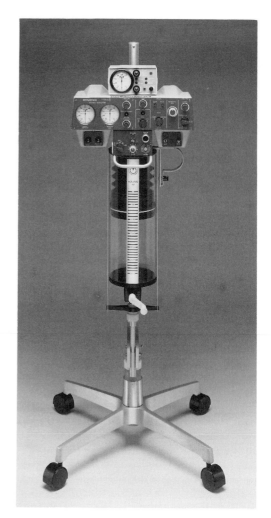

Figure 21—57. Monaghan 225/SIMV. (Courtesy of Monaghan Medical Corp.)

tions as a constant-flow generator. Termination of mechanical inspiration is pressure-, volume-, or time-cycled. End-expiratory pressure may be applied during mechanical (PEEP) and spontaneous (CPAP) breathing. Initiation of mechanical inspiration is machine-cycled or patient-triggered.

SPECIFICATIONS

Inspiration

Rate (BPM)	SIMV	0.3–5
Volume (mL)	SIMV	4–16
Flow rate (L/min)	CMV	6–60
Pressure (cmH$_2$O)		100–3000
Time (sec)		5–100
Effort (cmH$_2$O)		10–105

Hold (sec)	NC
Demand flow (L/min)	(0.5)–(10)
Safety pressure (cmH$_2$O)	NC
Pressure support (cmH$_2$O)	100
MMV (L/min)	120

Expiration

Time (sec)	NC
PEEP/CPAP (cmH$_2$O)	0–25
Retard (L/min)	NC
I/E ratio	NC

MODES

Assist	MMV
*Control	PS
*Assist–Control	APRV
IMV	PC
*SIMV	CPAP

Operation

The Monaghan 225/SIMV is connected to a 50-psi oxygen source and the humidifier plugged into an electrical outlet at least 20 minutes before use (Fig. 21–58). The desired mode is selected with switch A; options include assist, assist/control, and control. To access the SIMV function, the selector is placed in the assist/control mode and then the BPM (breaths per minute; B) control must be positioned to either 4 to 16 or 0.3 to 5 breaths per minute selections. If BPM switch is left in the off position, the mode will remain assist/control. Respiration rate control C may then be appropriately adjusted. The volume to be delivered is determined by a hand crank located at the bottom of the bellows (not illustrated). Any attempt to deliver volumes below 100 mL may result in erratic volume delivery. The ventilator also can be pressure-limited by adjustment of the pressure-limit control D. The maximal pressure attainable is 105 cmH$_2$O, and the selected limit may be observed on manometer E. The flow control F adjusts the rate of bellows compression. Peak flow of 100 L/min against zero back-pressure is possible. In the assist, assist/control, and control modes, mechanical inspiration is volume-cycled if the bellows is completely compressed; otherwise, it is time-cycled. Pneumatic "lights" indicate whether the tidal volume has been terminated by time-, G, or pressure-cycling, H. If neither of these lights flash, volume-cycling has occurred. If the ventilator time cycles, and the operator desires volume cycling, the flow rate control should be increased until volume cycling occurs. In the SIMV mode, the time-cycling mechanism is disabled, and the operator should appropriately adjust the flow rate to produce a desirable I/E ratio.

If the mode selector has been turned either to the assist or to the assist/control mode, assisted ventilation is possible. The trigger sensitivity control H adjusts the amount of subambient pressure the patient must generate. This control is also functional in the SIMV mode. When the patient has

Figure 21–58. Control panel of the Monaghan 225/SIMV.

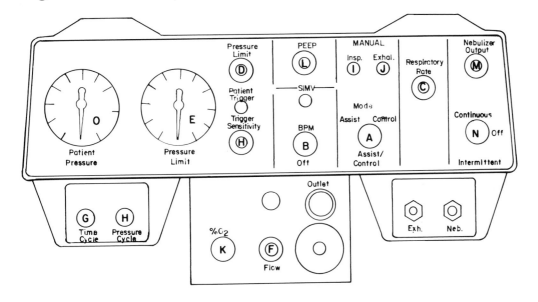

initiated an assisted breath, an indicator light will so inform the operator. A manual inspiratory start and hold button, I, is also present. Manual depression of button J will abort V_T delivery or indefinitely prolong the expiratory phase until it is released.

Oxygen concentration is selected by the percentage of oxygen control, K. This gas mixture requires no high-pressure air source to deliver oxygen concentrations from 21% to 100%. PEEP up to 20 cmH$_2$O can be dialed in by the PEEP control, L. Nebulization of medication can be provided by adjustment of switch M after being engaged by switch N.

Monitoring and Alarms

The Monaghan 225/SIMV provides no monitoring capabilities other than the airway pressure gauge, O; an auxiliary-monitoring device should be purchased to accompany this ventilator when in use.

Mechanism

The Monaghan 225/SIMV is pneumatically operated with fluid logic and is powered by a 50-psi oxygen source (Fig. 21–59). Oxygen is delivered to the main valve A, which is programmed by the logic system to align the valve system properly. The fluidic control is adjusted by controls on the front panel of the ventilator to determine the respiratory phasing of the ventilator. The inspiratory time, pressure limit, patient trigger, and the volume limit all have inputs and outputs from this programming center, B. Flow rate to the bellows chamber is controlled by the flow rate control C, which determines the rate at which the bellows is compressed.

Pressurization is developed in chamber D by this gas source when fluidic OR/NOR gate E closes the mushroom valve F. Simultaneous closure of the patient exhalation valve G is also accomplished by the fluidic OR/NOT gate. A mushroom valve F also serves as a safety pressure limit at 120 cmH$_2$O. Once inspiration has been completed, the oxygen that has compressed the bellows is exhausted through a control valve, H. This control delivers the amount of oxygen to be mixed with air brought in through a filter, I, to the prescribed oxygen concentration, as determined by control H. After the bellows volume has been delivered to the patient, it is humidified and the pressure monitored. The system can be pressure-limited by an inspiratory pres-

Figure 21–59. Schematic diagram of the Monaghan 225/SIMV.

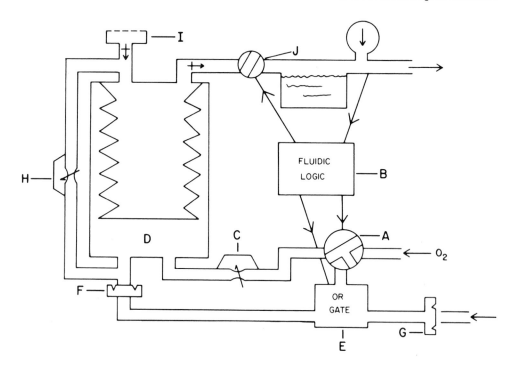

sure-relief control, J. The pressure-relief system, or gate, and main valve functions are controlled by the fluid logic system. Inspiratory effort can also be programmed into the logic system and adjusted to allow for assisted breaths.

In the SIMV mode, fresh gas for spontaneous breathing is supplied when inspiratory effort triggers a breath. The bellows is subsequently compressed, but the patient exhalation valve is not pressurized. This provides a volume of gas equivalent to the preselected V_T at the operator-adjusted flow rate. Spontaneous breaths that exceed the mechanical V_T or the inspiratory flow rate setting are not possible.

A special nonmagnetic version of the Monaghan 225–SIMV has been recently released and is compatible for use with magnetic resonance imaging (MRI) devices.

Troubleshooting

Fluid logic ventilators incorporate few moving parts; therefore, relatively trouble-free service should be expected. If the ventilator autocycles, the sensitivity may be too great or the PEEP control may be on. The PEEP control will autocycle the ventilator unless it is connected to a patient or test lung.

Improper oxygen delivery may result from the medication nebulizer being turned on, plugging of the air intake, or a hole in the bellows or bellows check-valve assembly. Erratic cycling and oxygen concentration delivery are expected if the V_T is set below 100 mL V_T; such attempts to obtain a low V_T should be avoided.

OHMEDA ADVENT VENTILATOR

Classification

The Ohmeda Advent ventilator (Fig. 21–60) is electrically and pneumatically powered, microprocessor and pneumatically operated, and functions as a constant- or decelerating-flow generator or a constant-pressure generator when spontaneous breathing occurs during pressure support. Mechanical inspiration can be either time- or pressure-cycled, can be extended by a time-cycled plateau, and is machine-cycled or patient-triggered. Inspiratory flow becomes the cycling mechanism in pressure support. End-expiratory pressure may be applied during mechanical (PEEP) and spontaneous (CPAP) breathing.

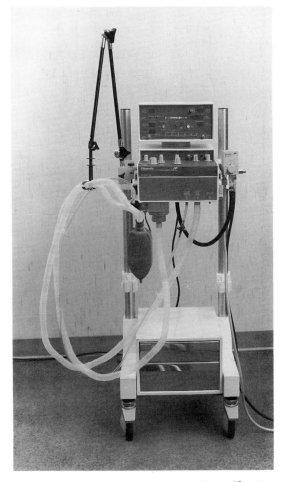

Figure 21—60. Ohmeda Advent ventilator. (Courtesy of Ohmeda Corp.)

SPECIFICATIONS

Inspiration

Rate (BPM)	0.5–85
Volume (mL)	70–2000
Flow rate (L/min)	10–120
Pressure (cmH$_2$O)	2–120
Time (sec)	0.3–4
Effort (cmH$_2$O)	(0.5)–(10)
Hold (sec)	0–1
Demand flow (L/min)	0–180
Safety pressure (cmH$_2$O)	0–130
Pressure support (cmH$_2$O)	0–30
MMV (L/min)	0.5–45

Expiration

Time (sec)	NC

PEEP/CPAP (cmH$_2$O)	0–30
Retard (L/min)	NC
I/E ratio	NC

MODES

*Assist	*MMV
*Control	*PS
*Assist–Control	APRV
IMV	*PC
*SIMV	CPAP

Operation

The Ohmeda Advent ventilator is composed of a display module and a control module. The front control panel (Fig. 21–61) comprises nine ventilatory controls, a mode selector switch, two alarm control knobs, and a power on–off button. Indica-tor lamps accompany each control knob and illuminate only when the controls are active and require adjustment.

The eight-position selector switch, *A*, allows the following settings: calibration, to calibrate the flow sensor; standby, a power on, but nonventilator mode; assist–control, SIMV, MMV, CPAP, and pressure control with assist. The eighth position is nonfunctional and is reserved for a future option. After selecting a mode, each of the ventilatory controls that are active within the mode must be adjusted. Ventilatory controls consist of frequency, *B*; V$_T$, *C*; sensitivity, *D*; flow, *E*; PEEP, *F*; T$_I$, *G*; inspiratory pause, *H*; and pressure support, *I*. Sigh, a mechanical sigh breath of 150% of the programmed V$_T$ each 100th mechanical cycle; nebulization, which does not alter the set V$_T$; and sigh–nebulizer, a combination, are set with a second switch, *J*. An options panel between the control panel and the

Figure 21–61. Control panel of the Advent ventilator.

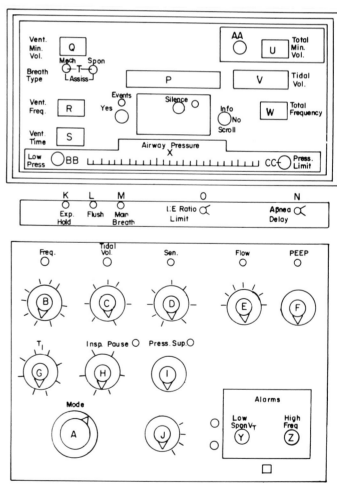

display module enables several options. An expiratory hold button, K, closes the exhalation valve during the next expiratory phase, which extends the expiratory phase and makes PEEP in the circuit comparable with the PEEP Venturi. When PEEP is elevated in the breathing circuit, "auto-PEEP" is displayed. This feature is useful in determining if enough time has been provided for exhalation. A "flush" button, L, enables the accumulator canister to be purged and facilitates rapid changes in FiO_2. The manual breath button M allows a programmed mechanical breath at the operator's discretion in any ventilatory mode. The apnea delay switch N interposes either a 30- or 45-second delay before the initiation of apnea alarms or apnea ventilation sequences. The ratio limit switch, O, either prevents (on) or allows inverse I/E ratios.

Pressure support is engaged in all spontaneous-breathing modes. Each spontaneous inspiration is assisted by at least 2 cmH_2O of pressure support, because the pressure-support function cannot be completely turned off. This feature, which is found on most ventilators that provide pressure support, reduces the work of spontaneous breathing for a patient receiving PEEP or CPAP. For patients who require additional assistance, pressure support, up to 30 cmH_2O, may be provided. Mandatory minute volume functions in a fashion similar to SIMV, except for mechanical frequency, which is calculated and adjusted (if required) every 24 seconds. All controls are adjusted the same as for the SIMV mode but, in addition, a minimal minute ventilation is selected. If minute ventilation ($\dot{V}E$) increases or decreases as a result of changes in spontaneous ventilatory activity, mechanical frequency is increased or decreased to maintain $\dot{V}E$ at the set value. A safety feature with MMV is that frequency cannot increase to the point that an inverse I/E ratio results. A disconnection freezes all variables and allows procedures, such as suctioning, to be performed.

Monitoring and Alarms

All monitored physiologic variables are displayed on a panel (see Fig. 21–61) that also includes several controls and alarms. Prompts and messages appear in a message window P, and monitoring data are displayed in two columns: ventilator function and physiologic variables. The ventilator function display, which provides a digital readout of ventilator minute volume, Q, is provided by mechanical ventilator breaths only; the total number of mechanical ventilator breaths each minute, R; and

ventilator %I time, S, which is the I/E ratio expressed as the percentage inspiratory time. Respective LEDs, T, illuminate to indicate a spontaneous or a machine-cycled breath. Both LEDs are lighted when a mechanical breath is patient-triggered. Physiologic data consists of total minute volume, U, which includes all spontaneous and mechanical contributions to the $\dot{V}E$; exhaled tidal volume, V; the total (mechanical and spontaneous) frequency, W; and an airway-pressure bar graph, X. The LED segments remain lighted during the expiratory phase to indicate the setting for PEEP, low-pressure threshold, and the pressure limit.

Safety is provided by five primary alarms, each requiring appropriate adjustments. The low spontaneous VT, Y, may be used with PS, SIMV, MMV, CPAP, or pressure control as a warning of insufficient tidal volumes. The high-frequency alarm, Z, can be used as a warning of tachypnea or autocycling; the latter may occur when sensitivity settings permit the ventilator to initiate breaths, without an inspiratory effort. The low minute volume alarm, AA, serves as the reference point during MMV and as a warning of reduced spontaneous contribution. The low-pressure threshold, BB, establishes a pressure threshold that must be surpassed with each mechanical VT. The pressure limit control, CC, determines the pressure at which volume delivery is terminated and airway pressure reduced to baseline. Pressure-limit violations produce a visual alarm only; however, three consecutive pressure-limit violations result in simultaneous audible and visual alarms. All alarms will self-cancel when violations cease. Data from self-cancelled alarms are stored and may be displayed one alarm at a time (review/cancel button). If more than one alarm occurs, the alarm with the highest priority is displayed first; lower priority alarms are displayed manually (info scroll button).

Mechanism

Pneumatic power is supplied to the Advent by an external and optional oxygen-mixing device (Fig. 21–62). Alternative, separately purchased mixers can be substituted provided they can blend 110 L/min at 50 psig. Otherwise, the performance characteristics of the Advent may be compromised. Before entering the control module, blended gas passes through a metallic, high-pressure reservoir A that has been filled with approximately 1 L of compressed gas and pressurized to 50 psig. The blended gas is regulated, B, to approximately 29 psig. A second regulator C, referred to as the low-

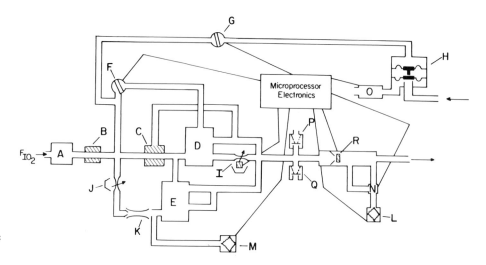

Figure 21–62. Schematic diagram of the Advent ventilator.

pressure regulator, provides an internal working pressure of 2.9 psig. Working pressure is subsequently supplied to the main flow-generating components: the inspiratory flow generator *D* and the demand valve *E*. Mechanical inspiration commences with actuation of two electropneumatic solenoids: the control solenoid *F*, which activates the inspiratory-flow generator, and the exhalation solenoid *G*, which closes the exhalation valve *H* pneumatically. The inspiratory flow generator provides a constant-drive pressure against the calibrated orifices of the inspiratory flow control *I*, which produces the constant-flow pattern characteristic of the Advent.

To provide V_T, the microprocessor determines the inspiratory time required to deliver the set V_T with the value set for inspiratory flow rate. To prevent decreases in inspiratory flow rate as airway pressure increases, the airway pressure is transmitted back to reference chambers located in both the inspiratory flow generator and the low-pressure regulator. This feedback system automatically increases pressure output of these components to maintain the set inspiratory flow rate, regardless of airway compliance or resistance. Mechanical inspiration is terminated when the programmed inspiratory time has elapsed. A pneumatic demand valve provides fresh gas for spontaneous breathing. A spontaneous inspiratory effort that exceeds 2 L/min triggers the valve, which can supply peak inspiratory flow rates of up to 180 L/min. When appropriately pressurized, the demand valve becomes a flow generator and, at high flow rates provides the constant pressure required for pressure support. During the expiratory phase, an operator-adjusted

needle valve *J* supplies gas to the PEEP Venturi *K*, which produces end-expiratory pressure (PEEP/CPAP).

To reduce the work of breathing required to initiate mechanical or pressure-support (PS) breaths, the Advent compares the output signals of two pressure transducers: a proximal airway pressure transducer *L*, used to generate the airway-pressure bar graph, and a reference transducer *M*, which measures the output pressure of the PEEP Venturi. When the pressure signals differ by a set amount, a breath is triggered.

The proximal airway pressure line is kept free of moisture and secretions by a purge flow of 100 mL/min. If the airway line becomes occluded, the purge flow will increase pressure at the proximal pressure transducer. A safety switch *N* located in a parallel, airway-sensing line will terminate inspiration and sound an alarm when back-pressure exceeds 25.4 cmH$_2$O.

Volume monitoring is provided by a hot-wire flow sensor *O*, distal to the exhalation valve. Several factors combine to make this a poor location for a flow sensor, especially for measurement of compressional gases and exhaled V_T. As the peak inflation pressure or the compression factor of the breathing circuit rises, compressional losses increase proportionally, as does the discrepancy between measured V_T and exhaled V_T.

Safety features include a mechanical over pressure relief valve *P*, which limits airway pressure to 122 cmH$_2$O, in the event that the primary, pressure-limiting apparatus fails, and an antisuffocation valve *Q*, which allows access to room air in the event of electric or pneumatic power loss. The antisuffocation valve opens at approximately −4 cmH$_2$O; an electromagnetic switch R isolates the patient from valve Q and permits the use of sensitivity settings in excess of −4 cmH$_2$O. A safety latch disables the switch during any emergency condition and, thereby, permits free access to fresh air for spontaneous breathing.

Troubleshooting

Troubleshooting the Advent is facilitated by a simple breathing circuit and by the microprocessor design. Microprocessor circuits ensure proper function and serve to alert the operator, with alarms and error codes in the display window, in the event of mechanical or electronic failure.

OHMEDA CPU-1 VENTILATOR

Classification

The CPU-1 ventilator (Fig. 21–63) is electrically and pneumatically powered, microprocessor and pneumatically controlled, and may function as a constant- or decelerating-flow generator or as a constant-pressure generator during spontaneous breathing in the pressure-support mode (see Table 21–1). Mechanical inspiration is initiated by machine or patient, terminated by either time or pressure cycling, and extended by a time-cycled plateau. Inspiratory flow becomes the cycling mechanism in the pressure-support mode. End-expiratory pressure may be applied during mechanical (PEEP) and spontaneous (CPAP) breathing.

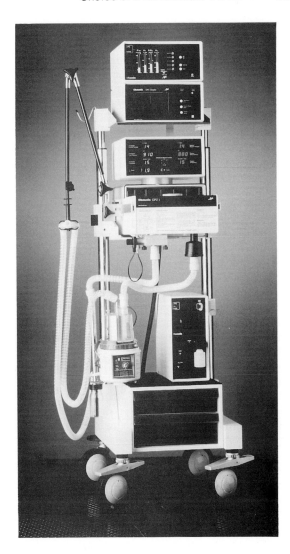

Figure 21–63. Ohmeda CPU-1 ventilator. (Courtesy of Ohmeda Corp.)

SPECIFICATIONS

Inspiration

Rate (BPM)	NC* 2–67
Volume (mL)	NC†
Flow rate (L/min)	5–120
Pressure (cmH$_2$O)	5–100
Time (sec)	0.3–3
Effort (cmH$_2$O)	NC
Hold (sec)	0–1
Demand flow (L/min)	0–100
Safety pressure (cmH$_2$O)	0–130
Pressure support (cmH$_2$O)	0–30
MMV (L/min)	0–30

Expiration

Time (sec)	0.6–30
PEEP/CPAP (cmH$_2$O)	0–30
Retard (L/min)	NC
I/E ratio	NC

* Adjusted as a function of inspiratory and expiratory time.
† A function of flow rate × inspiratory time.

MODES

*Assist	*MMV
*Control	*PS
*Assist–Control	APRV
*IMV	PC
*SIMV	CPAP

Operation

The CPU-1 is composed of a display and a control module that are interconnected (Fig. 21–64). Electric power supplied to the rear panel of the control module must be turned on or off with a switch on the back of the display module. The front control panel comprises seven ventilatory controls, a mode selector switch, and a pressure gauge. Indicator lamps accompany each control knob and illuminate to indicate that the control is operational within the selected mode.

Mode selector switch A allows the operator the option of choosing between CPAP, control IMV, SIMV, assist–control, or pressure-cycled ventilation mode. Mandatory minute volume (MMV) is possible by first placing the selector in the SIMV mode and then depressing the MMV button B. There is also a position that turns the ventilator off. Patient ventilatory controls include inspiratory time (T_I), C; inspiratory pause (T_P), D; expiratory time (T_E), E; pressure support (PS), F; inspiratory flow rate ($\dot{V}_{rate}$), G; PEEP, H; and sigh, I (on–off). The sigh mode offers the operator a series of options that are accessible by the appropriate positioning of a series of dual inline package (DIP) switches found on the rear panel of the control module. Placing the first option switch in the on

Figure 21–64. Control panel of the CPU-1 ventilator.

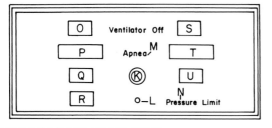

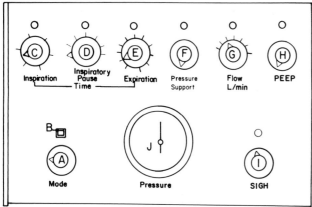

position results in a sigh breath that will be limited only by the maximum pressure setting of the ventilator. If the switch is in the off position, the microprocessor consults the position of the second switch. When on, the second option switch signals for a sigh volume of 200% of the programmed mechanical V_T; off results in a sigh volume of 150% of the programmed mechanical V_T. Sigh breaths will occur at a frequency of one sigh for each 100 machine cycles, in a series of three sighs, dependent upon the position of the sixth option switch (on = 3, off = 1). It should be noted, however, that regardless of the programmed sigh volume, airway pressure cannot exceed the maximum pressure setting.

Airway pressure is displayed on an aneroid pressure manometer, J. A rotating bezel, with a photoelectric reference cell, permits the selection of a maximum airway pressure (P_{max}) by aligning the photoelectric cell with the desired P_{max}. If the P_{max} threshold is violated, the inspiratory phase is immediately terminated, and the pressure limit display will light up. If the limit is exceeded for three consecutive breaths, an audible alarm activates to accompany the visual display.

The CPU-1 does not offer direct manipulation of mechanical V_T or ventilator rate. To achieve the desired V_T, the operator must select an appropriate inspiratory time and flow rate ($V_T = T_I \times \dot{V}_{rate}$). The ventilator rate may vary slightly in the SIMV, assist–control, and pressure-cycled modes, but can be determined by the formula: $f = 60/(T_I + T_P + T_E)$ when utilizing control–IMV. In the SIMV mode, the patient may breathe spontaneously from a demand valve during the expiratory phase. Near the end of the expiratory phase the CPU-1 establishes a variable waiting period (T_w), during which time the ventilator determines when the preceding spontaneous exhalation is complete. Subsequently, a 1-second triggering or synchronization window (T_f) is added to the end of the expiratory time. If a spontaneous effort is sensed during T_f, an SIMV breath is provided, otherwise a mechanical IMV breath is delivered at the termination of T_f. To prevent the possibility of breath stacking in patients with COPD, the waiting period of T_w may be extended up to 3 seconds and, as a result, the SIMV rate may not remain constant. If it is not necessary for the CPU-1 to provide extended T_w, the ventilator rate may be calculated by the formula: $f = 60/(T_i + T_p + T_e + 1)$. Ventilator rate will also vary in the assist–control and the pressure-cycled modes. In assist–control, the patient may assist at any time after a mandatory 0.6-second expiratory interval, and the inspiratory time in the pressure-cycled mode will be determined by the amount of time required to reach the cycling pressure (up to 3 seconds maximum) and can vary from breath to breath.

Pressure support is active in the CPAP, SIMV, and MMV modes. When employing these modes, each spontaneous inspiration is assisted by at least 2 cmH$_2$O of PS because it is not possible to completely turn off the PS function. This feature reduces the work of spontaneous breathing for patients on PEEP or CPAP and can be found on most ventilators that provide PS. During a PS breath, the airway pressure gauge will display a pressure that is the sum of the selected PS level and the CPAP level. Mandatory minute volume may be utilized by placing the selector switch in the SIMV mode, turning on option switch 7, turning the MMV reference level control to a value greater than zero, and depressing the MMV button. The current SIMV settings of T_I, T_P, and V_{rate} are retained; however, T_E is updated every 24 seconds, which requires an increase or decrease in the ventilator rate to maintain total patient minute ventilation at or above the selected MMV level. Changes to T_E occur when total patient minute ventilation exceeds ±12.5% of the selected MMV level.

Monitoring and Alarms

Patient monitoring is the sole function of the display module (see Fig. 21–64). The display is composed of seven display windows, the MMV control, K; the alarm silence button, L; the apnea alarm, M; and the pressure-limit alarm, N. The display windows are separated into two groups: ventilator status measurements that are calculated from the patient parameter settings taken from the control panel; and patient status measurements that are the result of measurements taken by a hot-wire flow sensor located distal to the exhalation valve. To clearly distinguish between ventilator and patient status displays, the four displays, on the left side of the display panel, monitor ventilator status and are displayed in yellow. Three displays on the right monitor patient status and are shown in red. Ventilator status displays include ventilator minute volume, O; ventilator tidal volume, P; ventilator frequency, Q; and I/E ratio, R. Patient status displays include patient minute volume, S, which is inclusive for all mechanical and spontaneous breaths over the last 60 seconds; patient tidal volume, T, which displays the most recently exhaled V_T, whether spontaneous or mechanical; and patient frequency, U, which represents the average total patient frequency for the previous five cycles, including mechanical, spontaneous, and patient-triggered breaths. The apnea alarm, M, illuminates with an audible alarm any time an apnea is noted. *Apnea* is defined as no detectable expiratory flow in a 15-second interval. If a spontaneous breath is detected in the next 15-second period, the "apnea" indicator switches off and the audible alarm stops. If the apnea continues, the display flashes, the audible alarm continues, and the ventilator begins one of the three emergency ventilation routines based on the operator-selected mode of operation.

The "pressure limit," N, indicator illuminates any time airway pressure exceeds the established limit. If three consecutive breaths violate the limit, the indicator flashes and the audible alarm sounds. When the airway pressure no longer breaches the limit, the alarm stops. Alarms may be silenced, L, for 1 minute to allow procedures, such as suctioning, to be performed.

Mechanism

Pneumatic power is supplied into the CPU-1 by an external and optional oxygen-mixing device (Fig. 21–65). It is possible to substitute any mixer, provided that it is capable of blending 110 L/min at 50 psig. Otherwise, the performance characteristics of the CPU-1 may be compromised. Inside the control module, blended gas is regulated to approximately 29 psig by the high-pressure regulator, A. A second regulator, B, referred to as the low-pressure regulator, regulates pressure further, to provide the working pressure of 2.9 psig. Working pressure is then supplied to the two main flow-generating components: the inspiratory flow generator, C, and the demand valve, D. Mechanical inspiration commences with actuation of two electropneumatic solenoids: the control solenoid E, which turns on the inspiratory flow generator; and the exhalation solenoid F, which provides pneumatic power to pressurize the exhalation valve, G. The inspiratory flow generator provides a constant-drive pressure against the calibrated orifices of the inspiratory flow control, H, producing the constant flow pattern that is characteristic of the CPU-1. To prevent reduced mechanical inspiratory flow rates as airway pressures rise, airway pressure is fed back into reference chambers located in both the inspiratory flow generator and low-pressure regulator. This feedback system provides an automatically increased pressure output from these components, which maintains the selected inspiratory flow rate, regardless of patient compliance or resistance. Mechanical inspiration is terminated by closure of

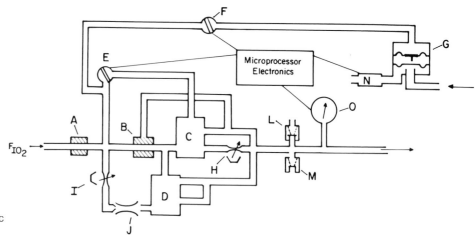

Figure 21—65. Schematic diagram of the CPU-1 ventilator.

the control and exhalation solenoids at the completion of the programmed inspiratory time.

A pneumatic demand valve provides fresh gas to the spontaneously breathing patient. Spontaneous inspiratory efforts that exceed a bias flow of 2 L/min, will trigger the valve, which is capable of supplying peak inspiratory flow rates of up to 110 L/min. In addition, when appropriately pressurized, the demand valve becomes a flow generator and provides the constant pressure and high flow rates required during PS. During the expiratory phase, an operator-adjusted needle valve *I* supplies gas to the PEEP Venturi *J*, producing the selected end-expiratory pressure (PEEP/CPAP).

A photoelectric cell and light beam (not illustrated) are used to permit patient initiation and synchronization. The same 2-L/min bias flow that charges the demand valve suspends an extremely lightweight ball, which occludes the optical path to the photoelectric cell. When patient effort removes the bias flow, the ball falls, which restores the optical path and triggers mechanical inspiration. Safety features within the CPU-1 include a mechanical overpressure relief valve, *L*, which will limit airway pressure to 122 cmH$_2$O, if the primary pressure limiting apparatus fails; and an antisuffocation valve, *M*, which allows the patient access to room air, in the event of electric or pneumatic power loss.

Volume monitoring is provided by a hot-wire flow sensor, *N*, located distal to the exhalation valve. Several factors combine to make this an undesirable location for a flow sensor. The measurement of compression volume along with the patient's exhaled V$_T$ is the most important factor. As the peak inflation pressure or the compression fac-

tor of the breathing circuit rises, compressional losses and the discrepancy between the measured V$_T$ and the actual exhaled V$_T$ will increase proportionally.

Airway pressure is displayed on an aneroid pressure manometer, *O*, and a rotating bezel with a photoelectric reference cell permits the selection of a maximum airway pressure (P$_{max}$) by aligning the photoelectric cell with the desired P$_{max}$. If the P$_{max}$ threshold is violated, the inspiratory phase is immediately terminated and appropriate alarms are triggered.

Troubleshooting

Troubleshooting the CPU-1 is facilitated by a simple breathing circuit and by the microprocessor design. Microprocessor watchdog circuits ensure proper function and serve to alert the operator, with alarms and error codes in the patient volume display window, in the event of mechanical or electronic failure.

SECHRIST IV 100B INFANT VENTILATOR

Classification

The Sechrist IV 100B ventilator (Fig. 21–66) is an electrically and pneumatically powered, fluidic and electronically operated, modifiable constant-flow generator that is time-cycled. It may provide end-expiratory pressure during mechanical (PEEP) and spontaneous (CPAP) breathing. Mechanical inspiration is machine-cycled and may not be patient-initiated.

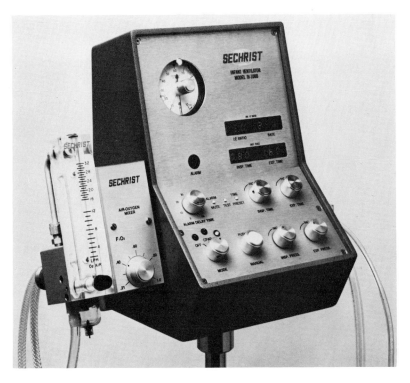

Figure 21—66. Sechrist IV-100B infant ventilator. (Courtesy of Sechrist Industries Corp.)

SPECIFICATIONS

Inspiration

Rate (BPM)	1–150
Volume (mL)	NC
Flow rate (L/min)	0–32
Pressure (cmH$_2$O)	7–70
Time (sec)	0.1–2.9
Effort (cmH$_2$O)	NC
Hold (sec)	NC
Demand flow (L/min)	NC
Safety pressure (cmH$_2$O)	85
Pressure support (cmH$_2$O)	NC
MMV (L/min)	NC

Expiration

Time (sec)	NC
PEEP/CPAP (cmH$_2$O)	(2)–15
Retard (L/min)	NC
I/E ratio	NC

MODES

Assist	MMV
Control	PS
Assist–Control	APRV
*IMV	PC
SIMV	CPAP

Operation

The Sechrist IV 100B ventilator (Fig. 21–67) is a compact neonatal ventilator that can easily be used for transport or long-term ventilation. Flow from the flow indicator, *A*, is blended in the air–oxygen mixer, *B*, to the desired concentration. The inspiratory time, *C*, is adjustable from 0.10 to 2.90 seconds. The time selected is indicated on the LED display for inspiratory time *D*. This real-time display will form the basis for the microprocessor's determination of "inspiratory time." Once the time-based generator has indicated the time dialed on the inspiratory time control *C*, the microprocessor terminates the inspiratory phase. The expiratory time control, *E*, and the expiratory time display, *F*, are similar to the inspiratory functions. Once the inspiratory time, *C*, and expiratory time, *E*, have been programmed into the unit, the microprocessor can calculate the I/E ratio, *G*, and rate, *H*, which may be adjusted up to 150 breaths per minute.

The inspiratory pressure limit, *I*, is adjustable from 7 to 70 cmH$_2$O, and the expiratory pressure (PEEP/CPAP), *J*, is adjustable up to 15 cmH$_2$O. A manual button, *K*, allows a single breath at any time. This breath will be limited to the inspiratory pressure limit, *I*, as set, but it will continue as long

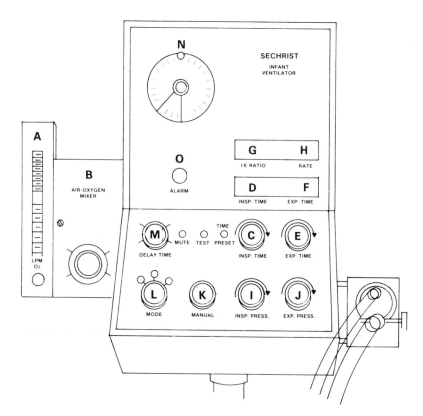

Figure 21–67. Control panel of the IV-100B ventilator.

as the button is held down. The mode selector switch L provides the choice of IMV or CPAP.

This light (16-lb) unit can be battery operated for use in transport.

Monitoring

The alarm systems provided are delay time, M, which is adjustable from 3 to 60 seconds, and a low-pressure alarm, N. The low-pressure alarm functions by passing the airway-pressure monitor needle through a photoelectric-sensing device that must be interrupted at frequent intervals. Should this light source not be interrupted for the period designated as the delay time, M, for reasons such as low airway pressure, leak, patient disconnection, failure to cycle, source gas failure, or power failure, the audible and visual alarms, O, will function. These alarms may be silenced for 25 seconds but then will sound again.

Mechanism

The Sechrist IV 100B ventilator (Fig. 21–68) is basically a gas-blending device, A, with a humidifier B that can occlude an exhalation valve C, by means of

an elaborate fluidic and microprocessor system. When an inspiration is desired, the microprocessor signals the solenoid valve D to close; this develops back-pressure through the fluidic unit E, which, in turn, sends pressure to fluidic unit F. Fluidic unit F provides 12-psi pressure through only one of its legs to the inspiratory pressure control G; gas continues to flow through various one-way valves and restricting orifices to the exhalation valve C. The main flow of gas to the exhalation valve may be supplemented by additional gas from the waveform modifier H. The waveform modifier, if fully open, opens and closes the exhalation valve abruptly, providing a square waveform pattern. Should the waveform modifier decrease the gas flow to the exhalation valve, the flow pattern will tend toward a sine flow pattern. During the expiratory phase the solenoid valve D is opened, and the normal route of gas flow is switched to the other leg of fluidic unit E; this provides gas flow to the proximal airway tap as a purge to remove humidity, the negative-pressure jet, I, and the expiratory pressure control, J. The expiratory pressure control J also provides gas flow to the exhalation valve to provide PEEP/CPAP when needed. A bleed, K, is necessary to allow the exhalation valve to cycle.

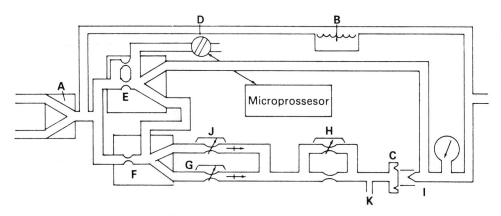

Figure 21—68. Schematic diagram of the IV-100B ventilator.

Troubleshooting

A comprehensive troubleshooting chart is included in the operator's manual to further simplify this simple and durable machine.

SIEMENS—ELEMA SERVO VENTILATOR 900C

Classification

The Servo 900C (Fig. 21—69) is electrically and pneumatically powered, electronically operated, and may function as a constant-, nonconstant-, or decelerating-flow generator. It will also function as a constant-pressure generator by appropriate adjustment of the working pressure regulator or when operated in the pressure-support or pressure-control modalities. The termination of mechanical inspiration is time-cycled and may be extended by a plateau. End-expiratory pressure may be applied during mechanical (PEEP) or spontaneous (CPAP) breathing. Initiation of mechanical inspiration is either machine- or patient-cycled.

Figure 21—69. Siemens—Elema Servo Ventilator 900C. (Courtesy of Siemens-Elema Corp.)

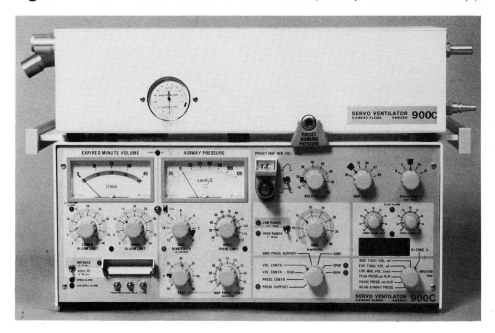

SPECIFICATIONS

Inspiration

Rate (BPM)	Low	4–10
Volume (mL)	High	0.4–4
Flow rate (L/min)		NC*
Pressure (cmH$_2$O)		NC
Time (sec)		15–120
Effort (cmH$_2$O)		20%–80%
Hold (sec)		0–(20)
Demand flow (L/min)		0–30%
Safety pressure (cmH$_2$O)		0–220 peak
Pressure support (cmH$_2$O)		0–100
MMV (L/min)		NC

Expiration

Time (sec)	NC
PEEP/CPAP (cmH$_2$O)	0–50
Retard (L/min)	NC

I/E ratio	1 : 4–4 : 1

MODES

Assist	MMV
*Control	*PS
*Assist–Control	APRV
*IMV	*PC
*SIMV	CPAP

Operation

Ventilator function and variables are adjusted and displayed on a compact control panel (Fig. 21–70). Mechanical V$_T$ is the result of an adjusted minute volume, *A*, and rate, *B*. The inspiratory time, *C* and pause time, *D*, are regulated as a percentage of the total ventilator cycle and are cumulative. If the inspiratory time exceeds 80% of the total ventilatory cycle, the pause time is automatically reduced. Inspiratory time is adjustable at 20%, 25%, 33%, 50%, 67%, and 80% of the ventilatory cycle. There are five pause times: zero, 5%, 10%, 20%, and 30%.

An accelerating or constant-flow inspiratory pattern may be selected, *E*. A decelerating inspiratory flow pattern can be used by adjusting *F*, the ventilator working pressure *G*, to a level equal to, or slightly higher than, peak airway pressure.

The desired ventilator mode is selected by an eight-position rotary knob *H*. Ventilatory modes include PS, pressure control, volume controlled with periodic sigh, volume controlled, SIMV with pressure support, SIMV, CPAP, and manual.

Pressure-supported ventilation (PRESS SUPPORT) provides an adjustable constant airway pressure during spontaneous breathing. If pressurized inspiration exceeds 80% of the breathing cycle, as determined by the existing control settings,

Figure 21–70. Control panel of the 900C ventilator.

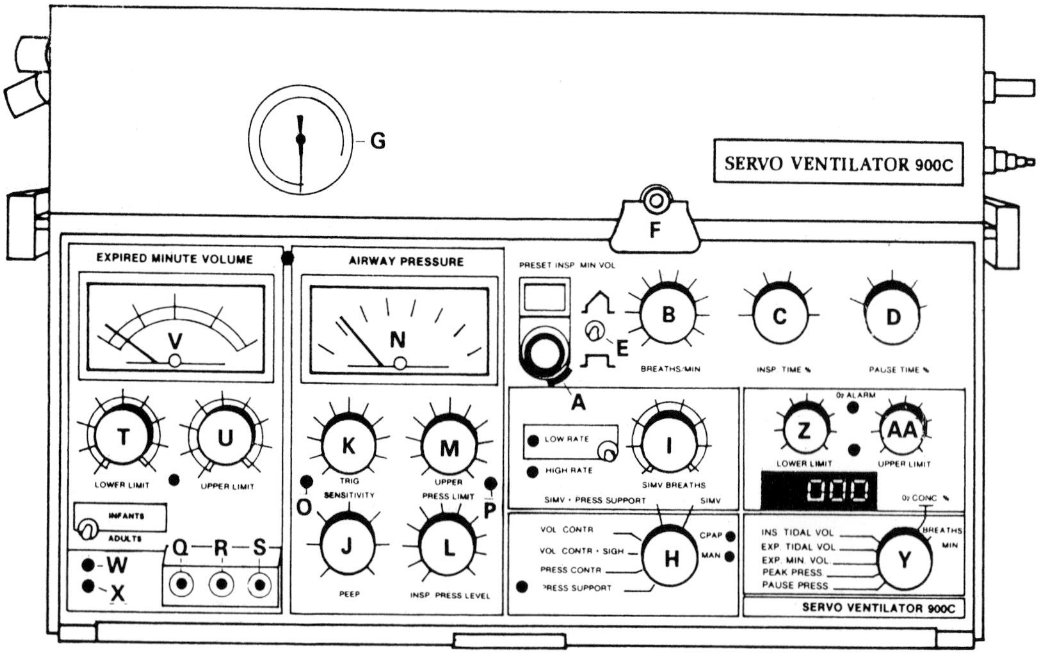

the inspiratory valve closes, and the exhalation valve vents pressure to a preset end-expiratory pressure level. The inspiratory pressure support is normally terminated when the inspiratory flow rate, as measured by the inspiratory flow transducer, has decelerated to approximately 25% of the initial flow. As a safety feature, PS will terminate if the expiratory pressure transducer senses an airway pressure in excess of the selected PS level.

Pressure-controlled (PRESS CONTR) ventilation provides a constant airway pressure during selected mechanical inspiratory time. This can be patient-triggered or controlled. The constant pressure is maintained by the inspiratory servo-feedback system (similar to INSP PRESS SUPPORT mode). Pressure-controlled breaths are normally time-cycled, but will also be terminated if the airway pressure exceeds the selected pressure level. Delivered mechanical V_T depends on inspiratory pressure, ventilatory rate, and inspiratory time and patient compliance.

Volume-controlled and sigh (VOL CONTR + SIGH) mode provides consistent V_T delivery to the circuit, with every 100th breath being doubled in volume. The volume-controlled (VOL CONTR) mode provides tidal ventilation without a sigh.

In the SIMV and PS (SIMV + PRESS SUPPORT) mode, the patient breathes spontaneously at a selected constant airway pressure and intermittently triggers a mechanical V_T. The SIMV rate is adjustable, I, in two ranges: low-rate, 0.4 to 4/min, and high-rate, 4 to 40/min. While in the SIMV mode, spontaneous ventilation occurs at baseline (i.e., ambient or end-expiratory) pressure. In the CPAP position, spontaneous ventilation at end-expiratory pressure is not augmented with any mechanical breaths.

The manual (MAN) mode is used in conjunction with an anesthesia bag and manual ventilation valve (accessory equipment) attached to the ventilator outflow port and connected to the inspiratory line of the breathing circuit (e.g., anesthesia system). During manual inflation (bag compression), circuit pressure rises; when it reaches 4 cmH_2O the ventilator exhalation valve closes, diverting the compressed volume to the patient. During exhalation, as the circuit pressure decreases to less than 4 cmH_2O, the ventilator exhalation valve opens. When circuit pressure is <2 cmH_2O, demand flow from the ventilator refills the bag. The apnea alarm is deactivated while in the manual mode.

Airway pressure during mechanical or spontaneous breathing modes is manipulated by the following control knobs: PEEP, J; TRIG SENSITIVITY

BELOW PEEP, K; INSP PRESS LEVEL ABOVE PEEP, L; and UPPER PRESS LIMIT, M. The airway pressure (range: -20 to 120 cmH_2O) is indicated on an analog meter, N.

PEEP is adjustable, up to 50 cmH_2O, with a safety catch at 20 cmH_2O. Inspiratory effort (below PEEP) necessary for patient-triggered breaths is adjustable from zero to 20 cmH_2O subatmospheric. Each patient-triggered breath activates an indicator light, O. During PRESS SUPPORT, PRESS CONTR, and SIMV and PRESS SUPPORT modes, the constant airway pressure above PEEP is adjustable from zero to 100 cmH_2O, with a safety catch at 30 cmH_2O.

Peak airway pressure may be limited from 20 to 120 cmH_2O. When the upper pressure limit is exceeded, the ventilator cycles to exhalation.

A small hood located beneath the UPPER ALARM LIMIT encloses push buttons for the following functions: inspiratory pause hold (INSP PAUSE HOLD), Q; expiratory pause hold (EXP PAUSE HOLD), R; and GAS EXCHANGE, S. Each function is activated for as long as the push button is depressed. The INSP PAUSE HOLD may be used to enhance alveolar gas mixing to provide an accurate mean expired carbon dioxide analysis. Stable end-expiratory pressure measurements may be affected by extending exhalation via EXP PAUSE HOLD. To quickly change the patient's inspiratory gas mixture, the GAS CHANGE button is depressed, which rapidly "washes" the internal and external circuits with the "new" gas mixture.

Monitoring and Alarms

The Siemens 900C provides extensive display, monitoring, and alarm capabilities. Electronic signals are collected from two flow transducers and two pressure transducers, one of each being located in the inspiratory and expiratory limbs of the breathing circuit. After appropriate electronic conditioning, these signals provide information that is displayed or used to trigger alarm conditions. A digital display window, capable of presenting one measured variable at a time, is controlled by an eight-position rotary knob, Y. Selections include mean airway pressure (MEAN AIRWAY PRESS; cmH_2O), pause or inspiratory plateau pressure (PAUSE PRESS; cmH_2O), peak airway pressure (PEAK PRESS; cmH_2O), expired minute volume (EXP MIN VOL; mL), inspired V_T (INSP TIDAL VOL; mL), expired V_T (EXP TIDAL VOL), oxygen concentration (O_2 CONC; %), and breaths per minute.

The primary patient monitors include expired minute volume and apnea. The lower, T, and upper, U, limit for exhaled minute volume is adjustable in two ranges: infants, 0 to 4 L/min and adults, 0 to 40 L/min. When either the lower or upper limit has been reached, an audible and visual alarm is activated. The exhaled minute volume is displayed on an analog meter, V, in addition to the display of exhaled minute volume, if selected.

If the expiratory flow sensor does not detect any flow for 15 seconds, the apnea alarm, W, which is both audible and visual is activated. A visual and audible alarm occurs if the gas supply, X, fails to maintain adequate pressure in the concertina bag.

The lower, Z, and upper, AA, limits for FIO_2 are adjustable from 0.20 to 1.0. If either has been reached, an audible and visual alarm is activated.

Violation of the peak pressure threshold results in the ventilator immediately cycling to the exhalation phase and the initiation of audible and visual, P, alarms.

Mechanism

The Servo 900C is electronically operated and pneumatically powered (Fig. 21–71). An air–oxygen mixer A provides gas at the prescribed FIO_2. Metered gas may be added by means of an auxiliary inlet B. On demand, a valve C opens, allowing mixed gas to flow by an oxygen sensor and through a bacterial filter (not illustrated) into a pressurized concertina bag D. The pressure is indicated on manometer E and is generated by adjustable spring tension F. During mechanical inspiration, gas from the concertina bag is directed into the patient circuit by means of an inspiratory flow valve, controlled by a "closed feedback loop" or servosystem. The servo system is composed of an inspiratory flow transducer, electronic comparator circuitry, and an inspiratory flow valve, which comprises a stepper motor that actuates a lever arm and a silicone rubber tube. The function of the lever is to open and close the rubber tubing by pinching it against a fixed part of the valve, thereby allowing or terminating flow through the silicone tube.

This pinching or scissorslike effect occurs in a series of 48 discrete steps. From the closed position, each additional step will increase the opening within the tube. Each step open will increase the flow through the silicone tubing by approximately 10%. The valve can be opened from the closed position in as little as 0.1 second, or at a rate of 480 steps per second. As inspiration begins, the inspiratory valve opens a predetermined number of steps, creating an appropriate aperture that permits the desired inspiratory flow as calculated by the front panel control settings. Flow passes the inspiratory flow transducer, where it is measured. If the measured and desired flows do not agree, the electronic comparator circuitry modulates the valve aperture to produce the specific flow required to guarantee volume delivery in the allotted inspiratory time. In the pressure-support mode, the inspiratory pressure transducer signal is processed electronically and referenced to the set valve. The inspiratory flow valve is subsequently modulated, allowing only sufficient flow to maintain the selected pressure. The exhalation valve is also a lever arm and silicone tube assembly. The expiratory lever arm, however, is actuated by a two-position (opened/closed) electromagnetic solenoid or pull-magnet. During mechanical inspiration, the solenoid closes, pinching the silicone tube and permitting the delivery of the mechanical VT. Termination of inspiration releases the lever arm and the patient exhales freely.

PEEP/CPAP is regulated by a second servoloop. Exhaled gas enters the expiratory servocircuit, comprising a flow transducer, K, pressure transducer, L, and expiratory valve, M, interfaced in a

Figure 21–71. Schematic diagram of the 900C ventilator.

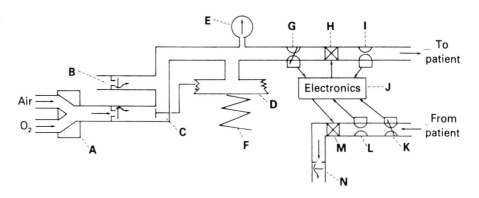

feedback loop with the electronics. PEEP/CPAP is regulated as a function of flow resistance by altering the exhalation orifice. During exhalation, the pressure transducer signal to the electronics is compared with the selected PEEP level. The expiratory valve is then opened or closed by a process referred to as "pulse width modulation," which is various sequences of rapid open–close signals to the solenoid that will create a series of discrete apertures within the expiratory valve. The size of the exhalation orifice is thereby altered until the desired PEEP and the measured PEEP coincide. Exhaled gas is ultimately vented through a unidirectional valve N.

Troubleshooting

Performance failures may be caused by internal system leaks in valve assemblies or the concertina bag. Valve system leaks are correctable but may be difficult to detect. When the rubber valves are inserted, twisting must be avoided to prevent unnecessary flow resistance. If the meter reads erroneously elevated minute volume, the flow transducer screen may have accumulated moisture.

Despite its sophisticated electronics, the Siemens 900C has no electronic troubleshooting software and troubleshooting may be difficult, often requiring a trip to the factory for proper diagnosis and repair.

APPENDIX

Ventilator compressible volume is that volume of a total ventilator system subject to increased pressure during inspiration. Determining the volume contained in the ventilator system from the piston or bellows to the exhalation valve by water displacement allows calculation of a compressibility factor for any particular ventilator. Once the total ventilator system volume has been determined, Boyle's law can be used to determine the particular compressibility factor. Manipulation of the formula is as follows:

Compliance formula:

$$C^* = \frac{V_1 - V_2}{P_2 - P_1}$$

$$= \frac{V_1 - V_2}{\dfrac{P_1 V_1}{V_2} - P_1}$$

*In a rigid container.

$$= \frac{V_1 - V_2}{\dfrac{P_1 V_1}{V_2} - \dfrac{P_1 V_2}{V_2}}$$

$$= \frac{V_1 - V_2}{\dfrac{P_1(V_1 - V_2)}{V_2}}$$

$$= \frac{V_2(V_1 - V_2)}{P_1(V_1 - V_2)}$$

$$C_F = \frac{V_2}{P_1}$$

where P_1 = ambient pressure and V_2 = ventilator system volume.

Example: A ventilator has a system volume of 4200 mL. You are using a tidal volume that attains a peak inspiratory pressure of 20 cmH$_2$O. What is the compressibility factor?

$$C_F = \frac{V_2}{P_1}$$

$$= \frac{4200}{1033}$$

$$= 4.07 \text{ mL/cmH}_2\text{O}$$

Therefore, this ventilator would deliver a true tidal volume of

$$600 - (4.07 \times 20) = 518.6 \text{ mL}.$$

REFERENCES

1. Herholdt JD, Rafn CG: An Attempt at an Historical Survey of Life-Saving Measures for Drowning Persons and Information on the Best Means by Which They Can Be Brought Back to Life. Stiftsbogtrykkeriet, Aarhus, Denmark, 1960
2. Emerson H: Artificial respiration in the treatment of edema of the lungs. Arch Intern Med 3:368, 1909
3. Gregory GA et al: Treatment of the idiopathic respiratory distress syndrome with continuous positive airway pressure. N Engl J Med 284:1333, 1971
4. Herman S, Reynolds EOR: Methods for improving oxygenation in infants mechanically ventilated for severe hyaline membrane disease: Arch Dis Child 48:612–617, 1973
5. Manginello FP, Grassi AE, Schechner S et al: Evaluation of methods of assisted ventilation in hyaline membrane disease. Arch Dis Child 53:878–881, 1978
6. Lachmann B, Grossmann G, Freyse J et al: Lung-thorax compliance in the artificially ventilated premature rabbit neonate in relation to variations in inspiration : expiration ratio. Pediatr Res 15:833–838, 1981
7. Lachmann B, Jonson B, Lindroth M, Robertson B: Modes of artificial ventilation in severe respiratory distress syndrome. Crit Care Med 10:724–732, 1982

8. Mapleson WW: The effect of changes of lung characteristics on the functioning of automatic ventilators. Anaesthesia 17:300, 1962

9. Elam JO, Kerr JH, Janney CD: Performance of ventilators. Effect of changes in lung-thorax compliance. Anesthesiology 19:56, 1958

10. Pontoppidan H, Geffin B, Lowenstein E: Acute respiratory failure in the adult. N Engl J Med 287:743, 1972

11. Fiastro JF, Habib MP, Quan SF: Pressure support compensation for inspiratory work due to endotracheal tubes and demand continuous positive airway pressure. Chest 93:499–505, 1988

12. Forrette TL, Cook EW, Jones LE: Determining the efficacy of inspiration assist during mechanical ventilation [Abstract]. Respir Care 30:864, 1985

13. Nagy RS, MacIntyre NR: Patient work during pressure support ventilation [Abstract]. Respir Care 30:860–861, 1985

14. Linn CR, Gish GB, Mathewson HS: The effect of pressure support on work of breathing [Abstract]. Respir Care 30:861–862, 1985

15. MacIntyre NR: Respiratory function during pressure support ventilation. Chest 89:677–683, 1986

16. Herman S, Reynolds EOR: Methods for improving oxygenation in infants mechanically ventilated for severe hyaline membrane disease. Arch Dis Child 48:612–617, 1973

17. Manginello FP, Grassi AE, Schechner S et al: Evaluation of methods of assisted ventilation in hyaline membrane disease. Arch Dis Child 53:878–881, 1978

18. Gurevitch MJ, Van Dyke J, Young ES, Jackson K: Improved oxygenation and lower peak airway pressure in severe adult respiratory distress syndrome. Chest 89:211–213, 1986

19. Lain DC, DiBenedetto R, Morris SL et al: Pressure control inverse ratio ventilation as a method to reduce peak inspiratory pressure and provide adequate ventilation and oxygenation. Chest 95:1081–1086, 1989

20. Downs JB: Airway pressure release ventilation: A new concept in ventilatory support [Editorial]. Crit Care Med 15:459–461, 1987

21. Stock MC, Downs JB: Airway pressure release ventilation: A new approach to ventilatory support. Respir Care 32:517–524, 1987

22. Garner W, Downs JB, Stock CM, Rasanen J: Airway pressure release ventilation: A Human Trial. Chest 94:779–781, 1988

23. Stock MC, Downs JB: Airway pressure release ventilation: A new approach to ventilatory support. [Editorial] Crit Care Med 15:459, 1987

24. Stock MC, Downs JB, Frolicher DA: Airway pressure release ventilation. Crit Care Med 15:462–466, 1987

25. Banner MJ, Kirby RR, Banner T et al: Airway pressure release ventilation in patients with acute respiratory failure [Abstract]. Crit Care Med 17:S32, 1989

26. Cane RD, Stock MC, Lefebvre DL et al: Airway pressure release ventilation in severe acute respiratory failure. [Abstract] Crit Care Med 17:S32, 1989

27. Cournand A et al: Physiologic studies of the effects of intermittent positive pressure breathing on cardiac output in man. Am J Physiol 152:162, 1948

BIBLIOGRAPHY

General Texts

Avery ME, Fletcher BD, Williams R: The Lung and Its Disorders in the Newborn Infant, 4th ed. Philadelphia, WB Saunders, 1981

Bendixon HH et al: Respiratory Care. St Louis, CV Mosby, 1965

Dobkin AB: Ventilators and Inhalation Therapy. Boston, Little, Brown & Co, 1972

Goldsmith JP, Karotkin EH: Assisted Ventilation in the Neonate. Philadelphia, WB Saunders, 1981

Grenard S: Introduction to Respiratory Therapy, Monsey, NY, Glenn Educational Medical Services, 1971

Grenard S et al: Advanced Study in Respiratory Therapy. Monsey, NY, Glenn Educational Medical Services, 1971

Heironomous T, Bageant RA: Mechanical Artificial Ventilation, 3rd ed. Springfield, Ill, Charles C Thomas, 1977

Hunsinger DL et al: Respiratory Technology. Reston, Va, Prentice-Hall, 1973

Kirby RR: Design of mechanical ventilators. In Thebault DW, Gregory GA (eds): Neonatal Pulmonary Care, pp 154–167. Menlo Park, Calif, Addison-Wesley, 1979

Kirby RR: Intermittent mandatory ventilation. In Refresher Courses in Anesthesiology, pp 169–188. Philadelphia, JB Lippincott, 1979

Kirby RR, Graybar GB (eds): Intermittent mandatory ventilation. In International Anesthesiology Clinics, Boston, Little, Brown & Co, 1980

Mushin WW, Rendell-Baker L, Thompson PW et al: Automatic Ventilation of the Lungs. Oxford, Blackwell Scientific, 1980

Petty TL: Intensive and Rehabilitative Respiratory Care, 2nd ed. Philadelphia, Lea & Febiger, 1974

Safar P, Kunkel HG: Respiratory Therapy. Philadelphia. FA Davis, 1965

Scanlan C: Egan's Fundamentals of Respiratory Therapy, 3rd ed. St Louis, CV Mosby, 1989

Shapiro BA: Clinical Applications of Respiratory Care, pp 319–392; 439–459. Chicago, Year Book Medical Publishers, 1979

Smith RA: Respiratory care. In Miller RD (ed): Anesthesia, pp 1379–1434. New York, Churchill Livingstone, 1981

Swyer PR: An assessment of artificial respiration in the newborn. In Lucey JF (ed): Problems of Neonatal Intensive Care Units, p 25. Columbus, Ohio, Ross Laboratories, 1969

Young J, Crocker D: Principles and Practice of Respiratory Therapy, 2nd ed. Chicago, Year Book Medical Publishers, 1976

Journals

Ashbaugh DG, Petty TL, Bigelow DB et al: Continuous positive pressure breathing (CPPB) in adult respiratory distress syndrome. J Thorac Cardiovasc Surg 57:31, 1969

Avery AE, Morch ET, Benson DW: Critically crushed chests: A new method of treatment with continuous hyperventilation to produce alkalotic apnea and internal pneumatic stabilization. J Thorac Surg 32:291, 1956

Banner MJ, Lampotang S, Boysen PG: Flow resistance of expiratory positive pressure valve systems. Chest 90:212, 1986

Barach AL: Recent advances in inhalation treatment of cardiac and respiratory disease: Principles and methods. NY State J Med 37:1095, 1937

Barach AL, Bickerman HA, Petty TL: Perspectives in pressure breathing. Respir Care 20:627, 1975

Barach AL, Marin S, Eckman M: Positive pressure respiration and its application to the treatment of acute pulmonary edema. Ann Intern Med 12:754, 1938

Beach T, Miller E, Grenivik A: Hemodynamic response to discontinuance of mechanical ventilation. Crit Care Med 1:85, 1973

Bendixon HH, Bullwinkel B, Hedley-Whyte J et al: Atelectasis and shunting during spontaneous ventilation in anesthetized patients. Anesthesiology 25:297, 1964

Benjaminsson E, Klain M: Intraoperative dual-mode independent lung ventilation of a patient with bronchopleural fistula. Anesth Analg 60:118, 1981

Bjork VO, Engstrom CE: The treatment of ventilatory insufficiency after pulmonary resection with tracheostomy and prolonged artificial ventilation. J Thorac Surg 30:356, 1955

Bland RD, Kim MH, Light MJ et al: High frequency mechanical ventilation in severe hyaline membrane disease: An alternative treatment? Crit Care Med 2:275, 1980

Boysen PG: Respiratory muscle function and weaning from mechanical ventilation. Respir Care 32:572, 1987

Bunnell S: The use of nitrous oxide and oxygen to maintain anesthesia and positive pressure for thoracic surgery. JAMA 58:835, 1912

Burgess WA, Anderson DE: Performance of respiratory expiratory valves. Am Hyg Assoc J 28:216, 1966

Carlon GC, Howland WS, Turnbull AD et al: Pulmonary venous admixture during mechanical ventilation and varying FIO_2 and PEEP. Crit Care Med 8:616, 1980

Carlon GC, Kahn RC, Howland WS et al: Clinical experience with high frequency jet ventilation. Crit Care Med 9:1, 1981

Cheney FW: The need for standards of performance. Anesthesiology 34:307, 1971

Civetta JM, Bron R, Gabel JC: A simple and effective method of employing spontaneous positive-pressure ventilation. J Thorac Cardiovasc Surg 63:312, 1972

Cullen P, Modell JH, Kirby RR et al: Treatment of flail chest—use of intermittent mandatory ventilation and positive end expiratory pressure. Arch Surg 110:1099, 1975

de Lemos RA et al: Continuous positive airway pressure as an adjunct to mechanical ventilation in the newborn with respiratory distress syndrome. Anesth Analg 52:328, 1973

Downs JB, Klein EF, Desautels D et al: Intermittent mandatory ventilation: A new approach to weaning patients from mechanical ventilators. Chest 64:331, 1973

Elder JD et al: An evaluation of mechanical ventilating devices. Anesthesiology 24:95, 1963

Elsbert CA: Clinical experiences with intratracheal insufflation (Metzler), with remarks upon the value of the method for thoracic surgery. JAMA 54:23, 1910

Engstrom C: Treatment of severe cases of respiratory paralysis by the Engstrom universal respirator. Br Med J 2:666, 1954

Epstein RA: The sensitivities and response times of ventilatory assistors. Anesthesiology 34:321, 1971

Fairley HB, Hunter DD: The performance of respirators used in the treatment of respiratory insufficiency. Can Med Assoc J 90:1397, 1964

Fleming WH, Bowen JC: A comparative evaluation of pressure-limited and volume-limited respirators for prolonged postoperative ventilatory support in combat casualties. Ann Surg 176:49, 1972

Froese AB, Bryan AC: Effects of anesthesia and paralysis on diaphragmatic mechanics in man. Anesthesiology 41:242, 1974

Froese AB, Bryan AC: Editorial: High frequency ventilation. Am Rev Respir Dis 123:249, 1981

Garg GP, Hunter JW, Adair DL: A simple modification of an adult volume ventilator for use with infants. Respir Care 19:199, 1974

Green NW, Janeway HH: Artificial respiration and intrathoracic esophageal surgery. JAMA 52:58, 1909

Greenbaum DM, Millen EJ, Eross B et al: Continuous positive airway pressure without tracheal intubation in spontaneously breathing patients. Chest 69:615, 1976

Greer JR, Donald I: A volume controlled patient-cycled respirator for adults. Br J Anaesth 30:32, 1958

Grogono AW, Sinopoli LM: A new classification system for intermittent positive pressure ventilators. Respir Care 19:199, 1974

Han HY, Lowe HJ: Humidification of inspired air. JAMA 205:303, 1968

Hillman KM, Barber JD: Asynchronous independent lung ventilation (AILV). Crit Care Med 8:390, 1980

Holaday DA, Rattenborg CC: Automatic lung ventilators. Anesthesiology 23:493, 1962

Hunter AR: The classification of respirators. Anaesthesia 16:231, 1961

Inkster JS, Pearson DT: Some infant ventilator systems. Br J Anaesth 39:667, 1967

James OF: The place of mechanical ventilation in management of thoracic injury. Semin Respir Med 3:240, 1982

Katz JA, Marks JD: Inspiratory work of breathing during assisted mechanical ventilation. Anesthesiology 63:598, 1985

Keats AS: A simple and versatile mechanical ventilator for infants. Anesthesiology 29:591, 1968

Kirby RR: A new pediatric volume ventilator. Anesth Analg 50:533, 1971

Kirby RR: Intermittent mandatory ventilation in the neonate. Crit Care Med 5:18, 1977

Kirby RR: Mechanical ventilation of the newborn: Pitfalls and practice. Perinatol Neonatol 5:47, 1981

Kirby RR, Downs JB, Civetta JM et al: High level positive end-expiratory pressure (PEEP) in acute respiratory insufficiency. Chest 67:156, 1975

Kirby RR, Perry JC, Calderwood HW et al: Cardiorespiratory effects of high positive end-expiratory pressure. Anesthesiology 43:533, 1975

Kirby RR, Robinsin EJ, Schultz J et al: Continuous flow ventilation as an alternative to assisted or controlled ventilation in infants. Anesth Analg 51:871, 1972

Kumar A, Pontoppidan H, Falke KJ: Pulmonary barotrauma during mechanical ventilation. Crit Care Med 1:181, 1973

Kumar A et al: Continuous positive pressure ventilation in acute respiratory failure. N Engl J Med 283:1430, 1970

Lassen HCA: A preliminary report on the 1952 epidemic of poliomyelitis in Copenhagen with special reference to the treatment of acute respiratory insufficiency. Lancet 1:37, 1953

Lewinsohn GE et al: Control of inspired oxygen concentration in pressure cycled ventilators. JAMA 211:301, 1970

Lewis FR, Blaisdell FW, Schlobohm RM: Incidence and outcome of post-traumatic respiratory failure. Arch Surg 112:436, 1977

Llewellyn MA, Swyer PR: Assisted and controlled ventilation in the newborn period: Effect on oxygenation. Br J Anaesth 43:926, 1971

Lohand L, Charabarti MK: The internal compliance of ventilators. Anaesthesia 26:414, 1971

Lutch JS, Murray JF: Continuous positive pressure ventilation: Effects on systemic oxygen transport and tissue oxygenation. Ann Intern Med 76:193, 1972

MacIntyre NR: Pressure support ventilation: Effects on ventilation reflexes and ventilatory–muscle workloads. Respir Care 32:447, 1987

McPherson SP et al: A circuit that combines ventilator weaning methods using continuous flow ventilation (CFV). Respir Care 20:261, 1975

Maloney JV, Derrick WS, Whittenberger JL: A device producing regulated assisted respiration. II. The prevention of hypoventilation and mediastinal motion during intrathoracic surgery. Anesthesiology 13:23, 1952

Maloney JV et al: Importance of negative pressure phase in mechanical respirators. JAMA 152:21, 1953

Marini JJ, Capps JS, Culver BH: The inspiratory work of breathing during assisted mechanical ventilation. Chest 87:612, 1985

Marini JJ, Culver BH, Kirk W: Flow resistance of exhalation valves and positive end-expiratory pressure devices used in mechanical ventilation. Am Rev Respir Dis 131:850, 1985

Marini JJ, Rodriquez RM: Bedside estimation of the inspiratory work of breathing during mechanical ventilation. Chest 89:56, 1986

Marini JJ, Rodriquez RM, Lamb V: The inspiratory workload of patient initiated mechanical ventilation. Am Rev Respir Dis 134:902, 1986

Matas R: Artificial respiration by direct intralaryngeal intubation with a modified O'Dwyer tube and a new graduated air pump, in its applications to medical and surgical practice. Am Med 3:97, 1902

Modell JH: Ventilation/perfusion changes during mechanical ventilation. Dis Chest 55:447, 1969

Morganroth ML, Morganroth JL, Nett LM, Petty TL: Criteria for weaning from prolonged mechanical ventilation. Arch Intern Med 144;1012, 1984

Musgrove AH: Controlled respiration in thoracic surgery: A new mechanical respirator. Anaesthesia 7:77, 1952

Nash G, Blennerhasserr JB, Pontoppidan H: Pulmonary lesions associated with oxygen therapy and artificial ventilation. N Engl J Med 276:309, 1967

Norlander OP et al: Controlled ventilation in medical practice. Anaesthesia 16:285, 1961

Peslin RL: The physical properties of ventilators in the inspiratory phase. Anesthesiology 30:315, 1969

Petty TL: IMV vs IMC. [Editorial] Chest 67:630, 1975

Petty TL, Ashbaugh DG: The adult respiratory distress syndrome. Chest 60:233, 1971

Piergeorge AR: Modification of the Bennett MA-1 ventilator for intermittent mandatory ventilation. Respir Care 20:255, 1975

Pollack MM, Fields AI, Holbrook PR: Cardiopulmonary parameters during high PEEP in children. Crit Care Med 8:372, 1980

Pontoppidan H, Berry PR: Regulation of the inspired oxygen concentration during artificial ventilation. JAMA 201:290, 1967

Pontoppidan H, Geffin B, Lowenstein E: Acute respiratory failure in the adult. N Engl J Med 287:690, 1972

Popovitch J, O'Neal A, Deepak VIJ et al: Differential lung ventilation with a modified ventilator. Crit Care Med 9:490, 1981

Powers SR, Manual R, Neclerio M et al: Physiologic consequences of positive end-expiratory pressure (PEEP) ventilation. Ann Surg 178:265, 1973

Prakash O, Meij S: Cardiopulmonary response to inspiratory pressure support during spontaneous ventilation vs conventional ventilation. Chest 88:403, 1985

Qvist J et al: Hemodynamic response to mechanical ventilation with PEEP: The effect of hypervolemia. Anesthesiology 42:45, 1975

Reynolds EOR: Effect of alterations in mechanical ventilator settings on pulmonary gas exchange in hyaline membrane disease. Arch Dis Child 46:152, 1971

Reynolds RN: A pulmonary ventilator for infants. Anesthesiology 25:712, 1965

Robbins L, Crocker D, Smith RM: Tidal volume losses of volume-limited ventilators. Anesth Analg 46:294, 1967

Rochford J, Welch RF, Winks DP: An electronic time-cycled respirator. Br J Anaesth 30:23, 1958

Rose DM, Downs JB, Heenan TJ: Temporal responses of functional residual capacity and oxygen tension changes in PEEP. Crit Care Med 7:79, 1981

Sahn SA, Lakshminarayan S, Petty TL: Weaning from mechanical ventilation. JAMA 235:2208, 1976

Schlobohm RM, Falltrick RT, Quan SF, Katrz JA: Lung volumes, mechanics and oxygenation during spontaneous positive-pressure ventilation: The advantage of CPAP over EPAP. Anesthesiology 55:416, 1981

Simbrunner G, Gregory GA: Performance of neonatal ventilators: The effects of changes in resistance and compliance. Crit Care Med 9:509, 1981

Sjostrand U: High frequency positive pressure ventilation (HFPPV): A review. Crit Care Med 8:345, 1980

Sjostrand U, Eriksson IA: High rates and low tidal volumes in mechanical ventilation—not just a matter of ventilatory frequency. Anesth Analg 59:567, 1980

Smith RA, Kirby RR, Civetta JM et al: Continuous positive airway pressure (CPAP) by face mask. Crit Care Med 8:483, 1980

Snider GL: Thirty years of mechanical ventilation. Arch Intern Med 143:745, 1983

Steir M, Ching N, Roberts ER: Pneumothorax complicating continuous ventilator support. J Thorac Cardiovasc Surg 67:17, 1974

Sugarman HJ, Rogers RM, Miller LD: Positive end-expiratory pressure (PEEP): Indications and physiologic considerations. Chest 62:86, 1972

Suter PM, Fairley HB, Isenberg MD: Optimum end-expiratory pressure in patients with acute pulmonary failure. N Engl J Med 292:284, 1975

Swartz MA, Marino PL: Diaphragmatic strength during weaning from mechanical ventilation. Chest 88:736, 1985

Trimble C et al: Pathophysiologic role of hypocarbia in post traumatic respiratory insufficiency. Am J Surg 122:633, 1971

Urban BJ, Weitzner SW: The Amsterdam infant ventilator and the Ayre T-piece in mechanical ventilation. Anesthesiology 40:423, 1974

Vidyasager D, Pildes RS, Salem MR: Use of Amsterdam infant ventilator for continuous positive pressure breathing. Crit Care Med 2:89, 1974

Webb P, Troutman SJ, Annis JF: Comparison of three IPPB respirators on a mechanical lung analog. Inhalation Ther 15:112, 1970

Weigl J: Gas trapping in the respiratory system: An analytical study. Third International Conference on Neonatal Intensive Care. Alberta, Canada, August 30, 1973

Weill H, Williams TB, Burk RH: Laboratory and clinical evaluation of a new volume ventilator. Chest 67:14, 1975

Weisman IM, Rinaldo JE, Rogers RM, Sanders MH: Intermittent mandatory ventilation. Am Rev Respir Dis 127:641, 1983

TWENTY-TWO

Mechanical Ventilation: Initiation, Management, and Weaning

Dean Hess
John E. Hodgkin
George G. Burton

INDICATIONS FOR MECHANICAL VENTILATION

There are numerous indications for mechanical ventilation (Table 22–1).[1,2] These include gas exchange as well as mechanical indicators of acute respiratory failure. Although these criteria are useful in establishing the need for mechanical ventilation, clinical judgment may be as important as strict adherence to absolute guidelines. If acute respiratory failure appears imminent, it may be prudent to electively intubate the patient and initiate mechanical ventilation, thereby avoiding overt respiratory failure and respiratory arrest.

Hyperventilation therapy and major surgery are indications for mechanical ventilation that may not involve primary respiratory failure. Although hyperventilation therapy is specifically used in the treatment of acute head injury, these patients often have associated respiratory failure. Short-term mechanical ventilation is also commonly used after major surgery, such as open-heart surgery or major abdominal surgery.

COMPLICATIONS OF MECHANICAL VENTILATION

Although mechanical ventilation can be life-saving, it is not a benign treatment, and it can have major effects on the homeostasis of the patient.

Complications of mechanical ventilation are listed in Table 22–2.

Mechanical ventilation for acute respiratory failure includes placement of an artificial airway such as an endotracheal tube or tracheostomy. Thus, mechanically ventilated patients are at risk for all of the complications associated with the use of artificial airways. These include laryngeal trauma, tracheal mucosal trauma, contamination of the lower respiratory tract, and loss of the normal humidifying function of the upper respiratory tract.

Numerous mechanical complications of ventilators are associated with the use of continuous ventilation. The most serious of these is accidental disconnection, which can result in the death of an apneic patient. It is critically important that the ventilator disconnect alarm is functional on all mechanically ventilated patients. Another common mechanical complication is leaks within the ventilator circuit. These must be detected and corrected promptly to prevent hypoventilation of the patient. Internal or external electrical and pneumatic failures can also occur, which can result in failure to ventilate the patient. A self-inflating bag-valve resuscitator should be at the bedside of all patients receiving continuous ventilation so that the patient can be manually ventilated in the event of a mechanical failure.

Ironically, mechanical ventilation can harm the lungs. Pulmonary barotrauma (pneumothorax, pneumomediastinum, subcutaneous emphysema) can result from excessive ventilation pressures.

Table 22–1   Indications for Mechanical Ventilation

Mechanical	
Respiratory rate	> 35/min
Minute ventilation	> 10 L/min
Maximal inspiratory pressure	< −20 cmH$_2$O
Vital capacity	< 10–15 mL/kg
Respiratory muscle paradox	
Gas Exchange	
P($_A$ − a) O$_2$	> 300 torr on 100% O$_2$
PaO$_2$/PAO$_2$	< 0.15
PaO$_2$	< 60 torr on FiO$_2$ > 0.60
PaO$_2$/FiO$_2$	< 100–150
V$_D$/V$_T$	> 0.60
PaCO$_2$	> 50 torr (acutely)
Hyperventilation Therapy	
Major Surgery	

Pulmonary barotrauma is also a problem when the expiratory time is too short, so that gas is trapped in the lungs at end-exhalation. Oxygen toxicity can occur if a high FiO$_2$ is used. Bronchopulmonary dysplasia can occur in the lungs of premature infants who are ventilated with high pressures and a high FiO$_2$.

Because mechanical ventilation increases intrathoracic pressure, it can decrease venous return, which may result in decreased cardiac output and decreased arterial blood pressure. Fluid challenge and drug therapy may be necessary to maintain cardiac output, blood pressure, and urine output.

Patients who are ventilated mechanically are at risk for gastrointestinal bleeding. Many ventilated patients are treated with antacids or histamine H$_2$ blockers (e.g., cimetidine) to avoid this complication. However, raising the gastric pH with these medications leads to an increased risk of nosocomial pneumonia. The use of oral sucralfate reduces the risk of gastric mucosal bleeding, without altering gastric pH.

It is also important to be aware of the nutritional needs of the mechanically ventilated patient. Undernourished patients are at risk for respiratory muscle weakness and pneumonia. On the other hand, excessive caloric intake can result in an increase in carbon dioxide production, which can markedly increase the patient's ventilatory requirements.

Mechanical ventilation can affect the patient's renal function and fluid balance. Elevations in plasma antidiuretic hormone (ADH) and reductions in atrial natriuretic peptide (ANP) can occur as a result of mechanical ventilation. The result of these alterations in ADH and ANP is a decrease in urine output and fluid retention. Urine output may also decrease during mechanical ventilation as a result of decreased renal perfusion, which occurs because of a decrease in cardiac output and blood pressure, attributable to mechanical ventilation.

The increase in intrathoracic pressure from mechanical ventilation can result in an increase in intracranial pressure. This may be a particular problem when mechanical ventilation is used with positive end-expiratory pressure (PEEP) in head-injured patients. In patients with head injury, it is prudent to keep the mean airway pressure as low as possible during mechanical ventilation.

An acid–base disturbance frequently observed during mechanical ventilation is respiratory alkalosis. This may be desirable in the treatment of head-injured patients. Otherwise, respiratory alkalosis should be avoided because of its effects on the oxyhemoglobin dissociation curve, electrolyte imbalance, and cardiac function.

Table 22–2   Complications of Mechanical Ventilation

Airway: laryngeal edema, tracheal mucosal trauma, contamination of lower respiratory tract, loss of humidifying function of the upper airway
Mechanical: accidental disconnection, leaks in the ventilator circuit, loss of electrical power, loss of gas pressure
Pulmonary: barotrauma, oxygen toxicity, atelectasis, nosocomial pneumonia
Cardiovascular: decreased venous return, decreased cardiac output, hypotension
Gastrointestinal/nutritional: gastrointestinal bleeding, malnutrition
Renal: decreased urine output, changes in antidiuretic hormone and atrial natriuretic peptide
Neurologic: increased intracranial pressure
Acid–base: respiratory alkalosis

INITIAL VENTILATOR SETTINGS

MODE OF VENTILATION

Assist–control (A/C) ventilation delivers a clinician-preset tidal volume (V_T) at a clinician-preset minimum rate. The patient can trigger additional breaths above the minimal rate, but the V_T is constant at the preset level. Intermittent mandatory ventilation (IMV), on the other hand, allows the patient to breathe spontaneously between ventilator-delivered breaths. With IMV, the clinician sets a ventilator V_T and rate, but the patient determines the V_T and rate of the spontaneous breaths between the ventilator breaths. During IMV, the ventilator breaths may be delivered at regular intervals, or the ventilator may be synchronized with the patient's spontaneous breaths (SIMV). In practice, if the rate set on the ventilator is high enough to satisfy the patient's ventilatory need, IMV and A/C ventilation are similar. Figure 22–1 illustrates the breath patterns for A/C, IMV, and SIMV. Controlled ventilation can also be used, but this mode is not desirable because the patient is unable to increase ventilation above that set on the ventilator. If control mode is used, the patient must often be hyperventilated, sedated, or paralyzed to suppress the respiratory drive.

Since its introduction in the early 1970s, IMV has become a popular mode of ventilation. Although it was initially regarded as a weaning mode, it is now commonly used as an alternative to A/C, even though weaning per se is not occurring. Al-

Table 22–3 Theoretical Advantages and Disadvantages of IMV

ADVANTAGES

  Avoids respiratory alkalosis
  Improves ventilator synchrony
  Lowers mean airway pressure
  Prevents respiratory muscle atrophy
  Facilitates safe weaning

DISADVANTAGES

  Respiratory muscle fatigue if IMV rate too low
  CO_2 retention if IMV rate too low
  Increased work of breathing
  Prolonged weaning, if IMV rate lowered too slowly

---

though IMV originally required a homemade add-on circuit to the existing ventilator circuit (with potentially disastrous mistakes in valve placement or alarm disconnections), most currently available ventilators feature built-in IMV, using either a demand valve or a continuous-flow system. Although there are several theoretical advantages of IMV, there are also potential disadvantages of its use (Table 22–3).

With A/C ventilation, the patient may trigger an inappropriate number of breaths, resulting in respiratory alkalosis. Because a patient's spontaneous V_T will usually be lower than the ventilator-delivered V_T, IMV should theoretically produce less risk of hyperventilation. However, switching to IMV from A/C does not necessarily correct acute respiratory alkalosis because patients who hyperventilate during mechanical ventilation usually do so for pathophysiologic reasons.[3] There may be some patients in whom respiratory alkalosis will be ameliorated with IMV, and a trial of IMV may be reasonable for patients who hyperventilate with A/C.

Some clinicians believe that IMV may produce improved synchrony between the patient and the ventilator, thereby decreasing the need for sedatives, narcotics, and muscle relaxants; however, there is no scientific support for this. For patients with high ventilation requirements (increased V_D or increased V_{CO_2}), use of IMV might actually result in less synchrony and carbon dioxide retention. During A/C, ventilator synchrony can usually be accomplished by appropriate adjustments in trigger sensitivity and inspiratory flow.

Figure 22–1. Assist–control ventilation (A), IMV (B), and SIMV (C). For the assist–control pattern (A), the second and third breaths are assisted, and the first and last breaths are ventilator controlled.

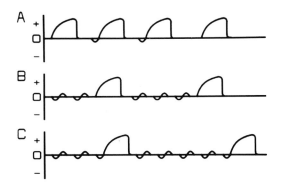

Because IMV reduces the number of ventilator breaths and increases the number of spontaneous breaths, it may result in a lower mean airway pressure. It is theoretically reasonable to assume that cardiac output will be improved and the frequency of barotrauma will be reduced with IMV. A few studies with patients and animals have suggested that IMV with high-level PEEP may produce a better cardiac output and less risk of barotrauma than A/C (or controlled ventilation) with PEEP. In contrast, other studies have been unable to show a beneficial effect of IMV with PEEP on cardiac output, when compared with the A/C–PEEP combination. It remains unclear whether IMV has any clinical advantage over A/C relative to cardiac output or barotrauma.

Respiratory muscle inactivity can result in disuse atrophy. By maintaining spontaneous breathing, it has been suggested that IMV may prevent respiratory muscle atrophy. However, it is also known that excessive respiratory muscle exertion may result in fatigue. If respiratory muscles are fatigued, they must be rested if they are to recover. Because IMV does not rest the respiratory muscles, its use during periods of fatigue is contraindicated. It may either provide training or produce fatigue. Unfortunately, it is currently unknown whether IMV trains respiratory muscles or fatigues them.

Most commercially available ventilators have a built-in IMV mode, and many of them deliver spontaneous breaths from a demand valve. Several studies have shown that the work imposed by a demand valve exceeds that of a continuous-flow system. Although this additional work is well tolerated by many patients, it may fatigue some. If fatigue occurs during demand-valve IMV, the patient should be switched to A/C or continuous-flow IMV. If continuous-flow IMV is used, the flow should be high (perhaps as much as 70–90 L/min). It should also be noted that A/C ventilation may not result in complete respiratory muscle rest. During A/C ventilation, the ventilator settings must be adjusted to minimize triggering effort, and to provide an inspiratory flow that exceeds patient effort. With either IMV or A/C, it is important to minimize the resistance imposed by the external circuitry of the ventilator and the endotracheal tube.

Many patients can be ventilated equally well with either A/C or IMV. The choice of the ventilation mode is one of institutional policy or individual bias; there is no clear superiority of A/C or of IMV. When mechanical ventilation is initiated, it is often best to use either A/C or high-rate IMV to produce nearly complete respiratory muscle rest.

MINUTE VENTILATION, TIDAL VOLUMES, AND RATES

During mechanical ventilation, $\dot{V}_E$ is set by the respiratory rate (f) and the tidal volume (V_T):

$$\dot{V}_E = (f \times V_T)$$

Commonly recommended settings for mechanical ventilation of patients with relatively normal lungs include a V_T of 10–12 mL/kg ideal body weight and a rate of 8–12/min. Patients are often mechanically ventilated at a V_T greater than their spontaneous V_T, and a rate less than their spontaneous rate. High-V_T ventilation may result in improved oxygenation, lower V_D/V_T, increased surfactant production, and less dyspnea. However, high-V_T ventilation may also decrease cardiac output and increase the risk of barotrauma. The low rate associated with high-V_T ventilation may also be useful because this is associated with longer expiratory times, which decreases the risk of air-trapping. Air-trapping has been shown to be a frequent occurrence in mechanically ventilated patients, particularly those with chronic obstructive pulmonary disease (COPD). Slow-rate ventilation may also allow inspiratory time to be increased, with a resultant improvement in distribution of ventilation.

During spontaneous ventilation, the respiratory rate associated with the lowest work of breathing (WOB) depends upon the patient's pulmonary mechanics (Fig. 22–2). Patients with a high elastic work (i.e., low lung compliance) have the lowest WOB with high-rate/low-V_T ventilation, whereas patients with high resistive work (high airway resistance) have the lowest WOB with low-rate/high-V_T ventilation. Thus, a patient with COPD (or other disease with airway obstruction) will breathe most efficiently at a high V_T and low rate, whereas a patient with pulmonary fibrosis (or other disease with pulmonary restriction) will breathe most efficiently at a low V_T and high rate. Although the physiology of mechanical ventilation is different from spontaneous breathing, patients with COPD should usually be mechanically ventilated with high V_T and low rate, but patients with chronic pulmonary restriction should be ventilated with smaller V_T and higher rate. Although tidal volumes of 12 to 15 mL are recommended, patients with acute lung injury (such as adult respiratory distress syndrome; [ARDS]) may need to be ventilated at lower V_T and higher rates to avoid dangerously high ventilating pressure; this is particularly important if the patient is being ventilated with PEEP.

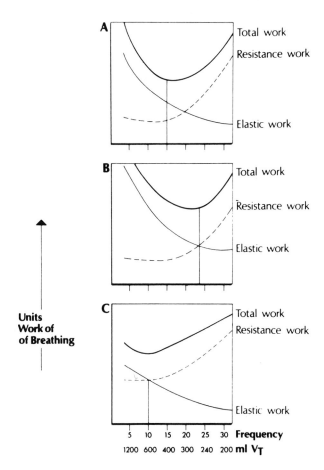

Figure 22—2. The effect of elastic and resistive work on the respiratory rate and tidal volume. (*A*) Normal lungs; (*B*) an increase in elastic work; and (*C*) an increase in resistive work (Kacmarek RN, Venegas J: Mechanical ventilatory rates and tidal volumes. Respir Care 32:466–478, 1987, with permission)

Table 22—4 Recommended Settings for Tidal Volume and Rate

PATIENT TYPE	TIDAL VOLUME*	RATE
Normal lungs	10–15 mL/kg	8–12/min
COPD	10–15 mL/kg	≤ 8–10/min
Chronic restrictive disease	< 10 mL/kg	12–20/min
Severe acute lung injury	< 12–15 mL/kg	12–20/min

* Based on ideal body weight.

for use of sighs is that the hyperinflation will decrease the risk of atelectasis. The use of sighs is controversial and may not be necessary if large VTs are used. Sighs should be avoided if they are associated with high ventilating pressures, particularly if the patient is being ventilated with PEEP.

INSPIRATORY FLOW PATTERNS

Numerous flow patterns are available on many modern ventilators. These include sine waves, square waves, accelerating flows, and decelerating flows. Although a sine-wave or decelerating-flow pattern theoretically should be better than a square wave, none of these flow patterns has been shown to be superior to the others during mechanical ventilation. An end-inspiratory pause can also be used, which may improve distribution of ventilation. However, an inspiratory pause may have a deleterious effect on hemodynamics if it significantly prolongs inspiratory time.

The inspiratory flow is the principle determinant of inspiratory time and the inspiratory/expiratory (I/E) ratio. A slow inspiratory flow may improve distribution of ventilation, but it will also prolong inspiratory time and adversely affect hemodynamics. A higher inspiratory flow will shorten the inspiratory time, allowing a longer expiratory time and better hemodynamics.

If the patient is assisting the ventilator, the flow set on the ventilator must exceed the patient's inspiratory demand. Otherwise, the patient's WOB will be increased, and the patient may not breathe in synchrony with the ventilator.

If the ventilator rate is less then 12/min and the patient is not assisting, a flow of 40 L/min may be appropriate. Higher flows must be used at faster rates, particularly if the patient is assisting. Here, flows of 60 L/min or greater may be required.

Recommended settings for VT and rate are listed in Table 22–4.

It has been suggested that static and dynamic compliance measurements can be used to determine an appropriate VT in mechanically ventilated patients.[4] With this approach, VT is increased until compliance drops. If VT increases and compliance drops, it implies that the elastic limits of the lung–thorax have been exceeded, and the patient is at increased risk for barotrauma. This method for determining VT is not commonly used, and its clinical usefulness has not been clearly established.

Some ventilators are capable of providing periodic sigh volumes. When sighs are used, they are usually set at a volume of 1.5 to 2.0 times the VT and delivered every 4 to 6 minutes. The rationale

INSPIRED OXYGEN CONCENTRATION

When instituting mechanical ventilation, it is usually best to begin with a high inspired oxygen concentration (FIO_2). Hypoxia is more deleterious than hyperoxia. Some practitioners prefer to use 100% oxygen until the PaO_2 is known. After the first arterial blood gas measurement, the FIO_2 can be decreased to produce the desired PaO_2. The FIO_2 required for a desired PaO_2 can then be estimated using the formula:[5]

FIO_2 needed

$$= \frac{(PaO_2 \text{ desired})/(PaO_2/P_AO_2) + PaCO_2}{\text{Effective barometric pressure}}$$

This estimation of FIO_2 may be clinically useful, but it should be considered an underestimate of the FIO_2 needed to prevent a PaO_2 lower than desired. Pulse oximetry is a useful guide to assist in lowering the FIO_2 while maintaining an adequate blood oxygen level. Although it has been common practice to wait 20 to 30 minutes before obtaining arterial blood gas measurements after an FIO_2 or other ventilator change, 10 minutes may be an adequate wait time, unless the patient has obstructive lung disease.[6]

SETTING APPROPRIATE POSITIVE END-EXPIRATORY PRESSURE LEVELS

Positive end-expiratory pressure is commonly used in the care of patients with acute respiratory failure. It has even been suggested that low-level PEEP (3 to 5 cmH$_2$O) should be used with all intubated patients, although there is little evidence that this is useful or important. PEEP is used to increase functional residual capacity, decrease intrapulmonary shunting ($\dot{Q}s/\dot{Q}t$), and improve PaO_2. The PEEP level is often determined by personal bias or institutional policy. There are two more quantitative approaches to the choice of PEEP level, re-ferred to as "optimal PEEP" and "least PEEP" (Table 22–5).

The primary goal of the optimal PEEP approach is to lower the shunt ($\dot{Q}s/\dot{Q}t$) to a target level, which is usually less than 15%, and to obtain the highest mixed venous PO_2 ($P\bar{v}O_2$), ideally greater than 34 torr. This may result in PEEP levels higher than 15 cmH$_2$O. Use of optimal PEEP requires insertion of a pulmonary artery catheter, which is used for sampling mixed venous blood and hemodynamic monitoring. Because of the high PEEP levels often produced with this approach, hemodynamics may need to be supported by increasing blood volume and administration of inotropes. Although high levels of PEEP may increase the PaO_2, it might actually worsen tissue hypoxia because of its adverse effects on cardiac output. There is currently little scientific evidence that the optimal PEEP approach is superior to other approaches for the treatment of ARDS. This approach is also labor-intensive and expensive because of the amount of monitoring required.

With the least-PEEP approach, PEEP is used at a level that provides an acceptable PaO_2 at a safe FIO_2. An acceptable PaO_2 is usually 60 torr or higher, which produces a hemoglobin oxygen saturation greater than 90%. Most clinicians consider an $FIO_2 < 0.60$ safe. The least-PEEP approach requires less monitoring, is less labor-intensive, and is probably less expensive.

The prophylactic use of PEEP in patients at risk for ARDS is controversial. Although some studies have suggested that PEEP may affect the natural course of ARDS, others have found no prophylactic benefit of PEEP. The question is: Does PEEP affect the functional abnormality in ARDS, or does PEEP treat the hypoxemia associated with ARDS? How one answers this question affects whether the optimal-PEEP or least-PEEP approach is used.

Not only is it important to determine an appropriate level of PEEP when this therapy is initiated,

Table 22–5 Optimal PEEP Compared with Least PEEP

OPTIMAL PEEP	LEAST PEEP
Goal is decreased shunt	Goal is decreased FIO_2
Pulmonary artery catheter required	Pulmonary artery catheter not needed
Belief that PEEP affects disease course	Belief that PEEP has little effect on disease course
Extensive labor-intensive monitoring	Ordinary ICU monitoring
Hemodynamic support needed	Often no hemodynamic compromise
PEEP > 15 cmH$_2$O may be required	PEEP < 15 cmH$_2$O usually required
High cost	Low cost

Table 22—6 Criteria to Discontinue PEEP

Stable, nonseptic patient
$FiO_2 \leq 0.40$
$PaO_2 \geq 80$ torr and stable or rising
Compliance ≥ 25 mL/cmH$_2$O
3-min PEEP reduction trial

but it is also important to correctly determine when PEEP can be lowered. Although prolonged PEEP therapy may increase the risks of barotrauma and hemodynamic derangements, premature lowering of PEEP can also be deleterious. Objective criteria to predict successful lowering of PEEP have been identified (Table 22–6).[7–10] A useful component of these criteria is the 3-minute PEEP reduction trial (Fig. 22–3);[8–10] if the 3-minute PEEP PaO$_2$ falls less than 20% of the baseline PEEP PaO$_2$, a prolonged PEEP reduction is attempted. By use of pulse oximetry, the 3-minute PEEP trial may be performed noninvasively. The PEEP should not be decreased by more than 5 cmH$_2$O, and generally 4 to 6 hours should elapse between PEEP reductions.

ALARMS

It is particularly important that all alarms are correctly set on the ventilator. The most important alarm is the disconnect alarm, which can be a low-pressure alarm or a low–exhaled-volume alarm. A sensitive alarm should detect not only disconnection of the ventilator from the patient but also leaks

Figure 22—3. The 3-minute PEEP reduction trial. Blood gas samples are drawn at the times indicated by the asterisks. A fall in PaO$_2$ of 20% or more indicates that PEEP is still indicated. (Craig KC, Pierson DJ, Carrico CJ: The clinical application of positive end-expiratory pressure (PEEP) in the adult respiratory distress syndrome (ARDS). Respir Care 30:184–201, 1984, with permission)

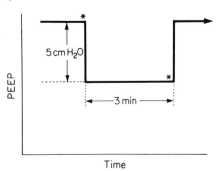

in the system. Failure to properly set the disconnect alarm on the ventilator could result in serious harm to the patient should a disconnection or leak occur. Other alarms set on the ventilator include high-pressure alarms, I/E ratio alarms, loss of PEEP alarms, and overtemperature alarms.

CIRCUIT AND HUMIDIFIER

A technical consideration in the determination of an adequate V$_T$ for a mechanically ventilated patient is the effect of compressible volume loss. Because of the volume compressed within the ventilator circuit, and the compliance (elasticity) of the ventilator circuit tubing, as much as 3–5 mL/cmH$_2$O can be "lost" in the ventilator circuitry. In other words, at a peak airway pressure of 40 cmH$_2$O, 120 to 200 mL of the gas delivered from the ventilator will not be delivered to the patient. Thus, if the ventilator is set to deliver an 800 mL V$_T$, only 600 to 680 mL will be delivered to the patient. For patients who are being ventilated with small tidal V$_T$, compressible gas volume can greatly affect alveolar ventilation.

Not only should the volume loss in the circuit be considered, but mechanical dead space should be considered as well. Mechanical dead space is that part of the ventilator circuit through which the patient rebreathes and, as such, becomes an extension of the patient's anatomic dead space. Theoretically, if the sum of the volume loss in the circuit and the V$_D$ is greater than the V$_T$ set on the ventilator, then V$_A$ will be zero. Although in the past it was popular to use mechanical dead space to produce changes in PaCO$_2$, this therapy is now seldom used.

Because mechanically ventilated patients usually have their upper airway bypassed with an artificial airway, it is important that a humidifier is part of the ventilator circuit. This is usually a heated humidifier. A hygroscopic humidifier (artificial nose or heat-moisture exchanger) can be used, but is usually not recommended for continuous ventilation; the most appropriate use for these devices is during transport ventilation.

MONITORING OF THE PATIENT ON A VENTILATOR

Critically ill patients on ventilators require the constant surveillance of the health care team. Frequent monitoring of physical findings, oxygenation, ventilation, compliance, hemodynamics, and renal and neurologic functions are essential to good patient care. It is also important to frequently monitor the function of the mechanical ventilator, including checks of the correct ventilator settings, the ventilator alarm systems, the humidifier and circuitry, and the patient's airway. Flowsheet charting is often used at 2- to 4-hour intervals to document the monitoring of patients on ventilators (Fig. 22–4).

PHYSICAL ASSESSMENT

Much important information can be obtained by simply observing the patient. Cyanosis may be seen in very hypoxemic patients. Asymmetric chest motion may indicate main stem intubation, pneumothorax, or atelectasis. Paradoxic chest motion may be seen with flail chest or respiratory muscle fatigue. Retractions may be seen if the inspiratory flow and sensitivity are inappropriately set on the ventilator, or if the airway is obstructed. If the patient does not appear to be breathing in synchrony with the ventilator (i.e., "bucking the ventilator"), this may indicate that the settings on the ventilator are not appropriate or that the patient may need sedation.

Palpation of the chest in conjunction with inspection can be used to assess symmetry of chest movement. Palpation of the trachea can be useful; pneumothorax causes the trachea to be deviated away from the affected side, and atelectasis causes it to be deviated toward the affected side. Palpation of fremitus in a ventilated patient indicates the presence of secretions in the airway. Palpation of crepitation in the subcutaneous tissues is indicative of subcutaneous emphysema, resulting from an air leak from the lungs.

Percussion can also be useful in the assessment of patients on ventilators. Unilateral hyperresonance or tympany may indicate the presence of a pneumothorax. Dullness may indicate consolidation, atelectasis, or pleural effusion.

The chest of a patient on a ventilator should be auscultated frequently. Unilateral decreased breath sounds may indicate main stem intubation, pneumothorax, atelectasis, or pleural effusion. Decreased breath sounds and crackles at the lung bases usually indicates basilar atelectasis, which may be corrected with a higher V_T, PEEP, or chest physiotherapy. Bibasilar rales are heard with congestive heart failure, fluid overload, or basilar atelectasis. Coarse rales are heard with retained secretions, and wheezing usually indicates bronchospasm. An end-inspiratory squeak over the trachea usually indicates that there is insufficient air in the cuff in the airway.

EVALUATION OF OXYGENATION

The earliest indicators of hypoxemia are often changes in the clinical status of the patient, which include restlessness and confusion, changes in level of consciousness, tachycardia or bradycardia, changes in blood pressure, tachypnea, bucking the ventilator, and cyanosis.

The most commonly used indicator of oxygenation is the PaO_2 value. A low PaO_2 value indicates hypoxemia and a dysfunction in the ability of the lungs to oxygenate arterial blood. The PaO_2 must always be interpreted in relation to the FIO_2. This can be done by calculation of $P(A-a)O_2$, PaO_2/PAO_2, or PaO_2/FIO_2. A high $P(A-a)O_2$, low PaO_2/PAO_2, or low PaO_2/FIO_2 indicates lung dysfunction.

The PaO_2 is not necessarily a good indicator of tissue oxygenation (hypoxia). Mixed venous oxygenation ($P\overline{v}O_2$) is a better indicator of overall tissue oxygenation. A $P\overline{v}O_2$ less than 35 torr (or an $S\overline{v}O_2$ less than 70%) indicates tissue hypoxia. The $P\overline{v}O_2$ may be decreased as the result of arterial hypoxemia, anemia, decreased cardiac output, or increased oxygen consumption. It is important to recognize that the PaO_2 value may be normal, or even increased, but the patient may be hypoxic with a decreased $P\overline{v}O_2$ value. Unfortunately, a pulmonary artery catheter (Swan–Ganz) must be placed in the patient to obtain blood to measure $P\overline{v}O_2$.

In critically ill mechanically ventilated patients, it may be useful to calculate shunt ($\dot{Q}s/\dot{Q}t$). The $\dot{Q}s/\dot{Q}t$ is calculated from the equation

$$\dot{Q}s/\dot{Q}t = (Cc'O_2 - CaO_2)/(Cc'O_2 - C\overline{v}O_2)$$

where $Cc'O_2$ is pulmonary end-capillary oxygen content, CaO_2 is the arterial oxygen content, and $C\overline{v}O_2$ is the mixed venous oxygen content. To correctly calculate $\dot{Q}s/\dot{Q}t$, it is important to account for the small amounts of endogenous carboxyhemoglobin and methemoglobin in the blood. Unless the patient is breathing 100% oxygen, the $\dot{Q}s/\dot{Q}t$ is referred to as physiologic shunt and results from low $\dot{V}/\dot{Q}$ regions in the lung as well as zero $\dot{V}/\dot{Q}$ regions (true shunt). Although administration of 100% oxygen can be used to assess the degree of true shunt, this is usually not recommended because 100% oxygen can result in an increase in $\dot{Q}s/\dot{Q}t$ caused by absorption atelectasis. PEEP may be useful in patients with high $\dot{Q}s/\dot{Q}t$. However, if $\dot{Q}s/\dot{Q}t$ is elevated because of a low but finite $\dot{V}/\dot{Q}$ (such as occurs with chronic airway disease), PEEP will have little effect on the $\dot{Q}s/\dot{Q}t$.

Pulse oximetry, transcutaneous PO_2 ($PtcO_2$), and conjunctival PO_2 monitors are available to continuously and noninvasively monitor oxygenation.

RUSH-PRESBYTERIAN-ST. LUKE'S MEDICAL CENTER
CHICAGO, ILLINOIS

RESPIRATORY THERAPY DEPARTMENT
VENTILATOR CHECK SHEET

Date _____   Page _____

				Circuit Change			Working Pressure				Cal			
Time														
Mode														
VT Preset (L)														
Rate														
FIO2														
Pmax / Pressure Support														
Peep														
Preset Insp. MV. (L)														
Control Breaths														
Inspiratory Time (Secs)														
Expiratory Time (Secs)														
Inspiratory Time %														
Pause Time %														
VT Spontaneous (L)														
VT Exhaled (L)														
VT Exp ÷ Wt. KG. _____														
Total Rate														
Minute Volume (Exp)														
Peak Pressure														
Pause (Plateau) Press														
Mean Pressure														
Flow														
Sensitivity														
Gas Temp (°C)														
Pressure Limit														
Pressure (Hi – Lo)														
FIO2 (Hi – Lo)														
Therapist Initials														
Blood Gas Time														
Site														
pH														
PCO2														
PO2														
HCO3 / BE														
SaO2														

M/R FORM NO. 2505 – REV. 12/84

Figure 22—4. An example of a ventilator monitoring flowsheet.

PNP — Peak Neg. Pressure
V$_T$ — Tidal Volume
MV — Minute Volume

WEANING PARAMETERS

Time	VT	MV	Time	VT	MV	Time	VT	MV
Rate	VC	PNP	Rate	VC	PNP	Rate	VC	PNP

RESPIRATORY TREATMENTS

Time	Therapy	TX Freq	Med	TX #	Pulse			Sputum	General Information	Initials

PATIENT ASSESSMENT

					Heart Rate				Temp		
Time					Airway Type				Airway Size		
Color					**OXYGEN EQUIPMENT**						
Activity					Bag + Mask						
Anterior Apical	L	R	L	R	L	R					
Anterior Basal											
Posterior Apical											
Posterior Basal					**ANALYZER CALIBRATION**						
Respirations					Comments:						
Retractions											
Sputum: Color											
Consistency											
Amount											
Initials											

Initials	Signature Plus Credential

BREATH SOUNDS		**RESPIRATIONS**		**ACTIVITY**	
G — Good Air Entry	R — Rales	Diaphragmatic — D		Active — A	
↓ — Decreased Air	A — Apices	Sternal		Active With	
Entry	B — Bases	Retractions — SR		Stimulation — AS	
RH — Rhonchi		Intercostal		Quiet — Q	
		Retractions — IR		Lethargic — L	
		Periodic — P		Irritable — I	
		Shallow — SH			
		Labored — LA			

Figure 22—4 (continued)

Pulse oximetry is useful in infant, pediatric, and adult patients. Transcutaneous PO_2 monitoring is used primarily in infants. Conjunctival PO_2 monitoring has not gained widespread clinical acceptance.

Pulse oximetry uses the principles of spectrophotometry and plethysmography to measure SaO_2, pulse rate, and pulse amplitude. Pulse oximetry is useful to continuously assess the oxygenation of unstable mechanically ventilated patients requiring high FIO_2s and PEEP. When using pulse oximetry, one must appreciate the relationship between PaO_2 and SaO_2. For example, if the patient's PaO_2 is on the flat part of the oxyhemoglobin dissociation curve, large changes in PaO_2 may result in little or no change in the SaO_2 measured by the pulse oximeter. Also, if there is a change in pH (with a resultant change in the position of the oxyhemoglobin dissociation curve) concurrent with a change in PaO_2, there can be a change in PaO_2 with no associated change in SaO_2.

Transcutaneous PO_2 ($PtcO_2$) monitoring uses a miniaturized Clark electrode to measure skin PO_2. The $PtcO_2$ is a function of tissue oxygen delivery (i.e., PaO_2 and cardiac output). The $PtcO_2$ correlates well with PaO_2, provided that cardiac output is adequate. If cardiac output is low, $PtcO_2$ may correlate better with cardiac output than with PaO_2. Because the skin of the newborn is more permeable to oxygen than that of the adult, $PtcO_2$ more closely approximates PaO_2 in infants than in adults.

The use of noninvasive monitors of oxygenation generally reduces the need for arterial blood gas analysis of PaO_2. Noninvasive monitoring allows the assessment of arterial oxygenation between PaO_2 measurements. Changes in oxygenation detected by noninvasive monitors signal the need to measure the PaO_2. In mechanically ventilated patients, pulse oximetry and $PtcO_2$ monitoring should not be used without periodic PaO_2 determinations.

In mechanically ventilated patients, a number of factors affect the PaO_2 (Table 22–7). A change in PaO_2 can be affected by changing the patients lung function, FIO_2, and PEEP level. During mechanical ventilation, attempts should be made to improve the patient's lung function, while using appropriate levels of FIO_2 and PEEP to avoid hypoxemia and hypoxia.

EVALUATION OF VENTILATION

Minute ventilation ($\dot{V}E$) is the sum of alveolar ventilation ($\dot{V}A$) and dead space ventilation ($\dot{V}D$):

$$\dot{V}E = \dot{V}A + \dot{V}D$$

For a given $\dot{V}A$, an increase in $\dot{V}D$ will require a greater $\dot{V}E$. Dead space volume is normally limited to the volume of the conducting airways, which is about one-third of the total V_T. Several clinical conditions will increase V_D (Table 22–8). The ratio of dead space volume to total V_T(V_D/V_T) can be calculated by the Bohr equation:

$$V_D/V_T = ([PaCO_2 - P\overline{E}CO_2]/PaCO_2)$$

where $P\overline{E}CO_2$ is the PCO_2 of mixed exhaled gas.

An increase in $\dot{V}A$ will also require a greater $\dot{V}E$. The $\dot{V}A$ is determined by $\dot{V}CO_2$ and $PaCO_2$:

$$\dot{V}A \propto (\dot{V}CO_2/PaCO_2)$$

where $\dot{V}CO_2$ is tissue CO_2 production. Thus, an increased $\dot{V}CO_2$ or a decreased $PaCO_2$ (hyperventilation) will require a higher $\dot{V}A$. Clinical conditions that will increase $\dot{V}CO_2$ are also listed in Table 22–8. The $\dot{V}CO_2$ can be calculated by the equation:

$$\dot{V}CO_2 = (\dot{V}E \times F\overline{E}CO_2)$$

where $F\overline{E}CO_2$ is the fraction (concentration) of carbon dioxide in exhaled gas.

Table 22–7 Factors Affecting PaO_2 in Mechanically Ventilated Patients

Lung disease	Mean airway pressure
Secretions	Tidal volume
Infection	PEEP
Bronchospasm	I/E ratio
Atelectasis	Sighs
ARDS	FIO_2
Congestive heart failure	
Fluid overload	

Table 22–8 Causes of Increased $\dot{V}D$ and Increased $\dot{V}CO_2$

INCREASED $\dot{V}D$	INCREASED $\dot{V}CO_2$
Pulmonary embolism	Fever
High-rate/low-V_T ventilation	Sepsis
Pulmonary hypoperfusion	Exercise
Positive airway pressure	Excessive caloric intake (especially glucose)
	Hyperthyroidism

The $PaCO_2$ is determined by $\dot{V}CO_2$ and $\dot{V}A$. If $\dot{V}CO_2$ is constant, $PaCO_2$ varies inversely with $\dot{V}A$. The $\dot{V}E$ affects the $PaCO_2$ indirectly because of the relationship between $\dot{V}E$ and $\dot{V}A$. An increase in $\dot{V}E$ will decrease $PaCO_2$, and a decrease in $\dot{V}E$ will increase $PaCO_2$.

The transcutaneous PCO_2 ($PtcCO_2$) electrode and end-tidal PCO_2 are used to noninvasively monitor carbon dioxide levels. Many transcutaneous electrode systems use a combination PO_2–PCO_2 electrode to simultaneously monitor $PtcO_2$ and $PtcCO_2$. Although the $PtcCO_2$ tends to correlate with $PaCO_2$ (particularly in newborns), it should not be assumed that the $PtcCO_2$ and $PaCO_2$ are identical. In patients with normal lungs, the end-tidal PCO_2 will closely approximate $PaCO_2$. However, in patients with an elevated V_D/V_T, such as those commonly seen in the critical care unit, there can be a large and inconsistent gradient between the $PaCO_2$ and end-tidal PCO_2.

MONITORING VENTILATION PRESSURES

The pressure required to ventilate a patient at a given tidal volume and inspiratory flow is determined by airway resistance and lung-thorax compliance. Static and dynamic compliance can be calculated and used to evaluate the resistance and compliance of mechanically ventilated patients.

Static compliance is calculated by dividing tidal volume by plateau pressure. Plateau pressure is measured by instituting a period of no-flow for about 0.5 seconds at the end of inhalation. To accurately measure static compliance, tidal volume must be corrected for ventilator tubing compression and compliance, and PEEP pressure must be subtracted from the plateau pressure. In critically ill patients, an acceptable static compliance is about 50–100 mL/cmH$_2$O. Factors that can decrease static compliance are listed in Table 22–9.

Dynamic compliance is calculated by dividing tidal volume by peak airway pressure. Tidal volume must be corrected for tubing compression and compliance, PEEP pressure must be subtracted from peak airway pressure, and peak airway pressure should be measured at the proximal airway. A decrease in dynamic compliance without a change in static compliance indicates an increase in airway resistance. Causes of decreased dynamic compliance are also listed in Table 22–9.

Peak airway pressure, therefore, is affected by airway resistance and respiratory system compliance, plateau pressure is affected by static compliance, and the difference between peak airway pressure and plateau pressure is affected by airway resistance. Airway pressure ideally should be monitored at the proximal airway.

Airway pressure monitoring may also be useful to evaluate mean airway pressure, which can be calculated from the airway pressure curve or be measured electronically. Many of the beneficial and adverse effects of positive-pressure ventilation may be the result of mean airway pressure. Factors affecting mean airway pressure are listed in Table 22–10.

It is also useful to check for the presence of auto-PEEP, which is positive alveolar pressure that remains at end-exhalation because of an insufficient exhalation time.[11,12] Auto-PEEP can result in hypotension and barotrauma, as well as increased WOB and miscalculation of static and dynamic compliance. Auto-PEEP can be measured by occluding the expiratory port of the ventilator at end-exhalation. Occlusion should occur just before the next ventilator-delivered breath. Measurement of auto-PEEP is facilitated in ventilators that have a manual exhalation-hold function (such as Servo

Table 22–9 Causes of Low Static and Dynamic Compliance

DECREASED STATIC COMPLIANCE

Pneumothorax
Atelectasis
Pneumonia
Main stem intubation
Congestive heart failure
ARDS
Pleural effusion
Chest wall restriction
Pneumonectomy
Fibrotic lung disease

DECREASED DYNAMIC COMPLIANCE

Low static compliance
Bronchospasm
Airway secretions

Table 22–10 Factors Affecting Mean Airway Pressure

Peak airway pressure	Respiratory rate
PEEP pressure	Inspiratory hold
I/E ratio	Inspiratory flow pattern

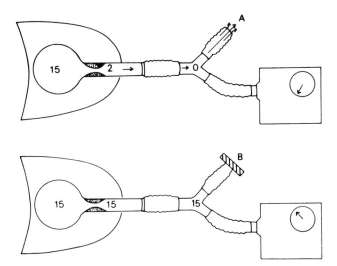

Figure 22–5. Measurement of auto-PEEP. If flow is stopped at end-exhalation, pressure equilibrates throughout the system and is indicated on the ventilator's manometer. (Marini JJ: The role of the inspiratory circuit in the work of breathing during mechanical ventilation. Respir Care 32:419–430, 1987, with permission).

900C or Hamilton Veolar). Measurement of auto-PEEP is illustrated in Figure 22–5.

EVALUATION OF POSITIVE END-EXPIRATORY PRESSURE

The beneficial and hazardous effects of PEEP should be monitored frequently. Arterial oxygenation should be evaluated. It may also be useful to evaluate $\dot{Q}s/\dot{Q}t$. The effects of PEEP on blood pressure, cardiac output, and urine output should also be evaluated. If the patient has head injury, the effects of PEEP on neurologic function should be monitored.

Several noninvasive techniques have been described to determine appropriate PEEP levels. One of these uses bedside measurement of static compliance.[13] By utilizing this method, PEEP is increased to the level that produces the best static compliance. In spite of the simplicity and noninvasiveness of this method, it has not been particularly useful in many critically ill patients. Another noninvasive method to determine appropriate PEEP uses the arterial minus end-tidal CO_2 gradient ($PaCO_2 - PetCO_2$).[14] With this method, appropriate PEEP corresponds to the lowest ($PaCO_2 - PetCO_2$). Although this method has been shown to be useful in experimental dogs,[14] its usefulness in critically ill patients has not yet been determined.[15]

VENTILATOR WEANING

The weaning of a patient from continuous ventilation can be a difficult, frustrating task. The weaning period is critical for the patient both physiologically and psychologically. Many such patients have marginal respiratory reserve, and determining whether or not the patient can maintain adequate alveolar ventilation with spontaneous breathing may be challenging to the respiratory care team. The weaning process ranges from simple (as with the patient recovering from acute drug overdose) to complex (as with the patient recovering from ARDS). If proper guidelines are followed, weaning need not be a risky experience for the patient.

FACTORS TO BE IMPROVED BEFORE WEANING

The patient's general condition must be evaluated and any problems that are identified must be resolved or improved. As a general rule, patients who are homeostatically unstable are not good candidates for weaning from the ventilator. General factors to be improved before weaning are listed in Table 22–11. The time to begin thinking about weaning is at the onset of continuous ventilation. The respiratory care team should keep a daily record of variables that indicate when weaning is feasible (Fig. 22–6).

Acid–base abnormalities are commonly associated with continuous mechanical ventilation. Alkalemia of both respiratory and metabolic origin is

Table 22–11 General Factors to Improve Before Ventilator Weaning Is Initiated

Acid–base abnormalities (particularly metabolic alkalosis)
Anemia
Arrhythmias
Caloric depletion or excess
Electrolyte abnormalities
Fever
Fluid balance
Hyperglycemia
Infection
Protein loss
Reduced cardiac output (hemodynamic instability)
Renal failure
Sepsis
Shock
Sleep deprivation
State of consciousness

Pt Name_____ Age: _____ Height: _____ Sex: _____

Diagnosis: _____

	Date/Time	Date/Time	Date/Time
Correctable Parameters			
Hb-g.%			
Temp. F.			
Blood Pressure			
Electrolytes			
Chest X-ray			
Secretions			
Cardiac Output			
Arterial Blood Gases	pH____PaCO₂____ HCO₃____BE____ PaO₂____SaO₂____ Vt____Rate____ F₁O₂____	pH____PaCO₂____ HCO₃____BE____ PaO₂____SaO₂____ Vt____Rate____ F₁O₂____	pH____PaCO₂____ HCO₃____BE____ PaO₂____SaO₂____ Vt____Rate____ F₁O₂____
Tests			
$\dot{V}/\dot{Q}$ Matchup:			
V_D/V_T			
$P(A-a)O_2$ on 100% O_2			
Shunt			
Mechanical Ability:			
Maximal Inspiratory Pressure			
Vital Capacity			
Minute Ventilation and MVV			
FEV₁			

Figure 22–6. Daily record of indices that indicate when weaning is feasible.

common and physiologically troublesome. The normal compensatory mechanism for metabolic alkalemia is alveolar hypoventilation, which can produce hypoxemia and atelectasis. Alkalemia also causes a leftward shift of the oxyhemoglobin dissociation curve, resulting in an increased hemoglobin affinity for oxygen and, thereby, impaired release of oxygen to tissues. Metabolic acidemia may also interfere with weaning because it increases the ventilation requirement to compensate for the acidemia.

Hyperventilation, with resultant hypocapnia, often occurs during continuous ventilation. Hypocapnia itself may produce ventilation–perfusion imbalance with the lung. Respiratory alkalemia, if prolonged, may be compensated by renal mechanisms, with a decreased plasma bicarbonate concentration. After spontaneous ventilation has been resumed, the $PaCO_2$ may increase, resulting, with the decreased bicarbonate level, in acidosis. This

is particularly a problem in patients who have chronic hypercapnia. It is useful to review the patient's past medical records to ascertain the prerespiratory failure blood gas values, since the ultimate goal is achievement of these values. The "relative" hypocapnia, whether or not alkalemia is present, must be corrected before weaning is initiated because the patient may not be able to maintain a $PaCO_2$ lower than the premechanical ventilation value once weaning is initiated. Unfortunately, the patient's $PaCO_2$ value before the onset of mechanical ventilation is not always known.

Although frequently only the PaO_2 is considered, there are multiple determinants of systemic oxygen transport. Anemia results in a decreased oxygen-carrying capacity. Generally, a hemoglobin of at least 10 g/dL is preferable for weaning. Cardiac output and blood pressure should be optimized to ensure adequate oxygen delivery to tissues. Cardiac arrhythmias should be controlled because they may decrease the cardiac output, as well as being potentially life-threatening. Because of the life-threatening potential of arrhythmias, a cardiac monitor should be used on all patients during weaning. Arrhythmias may be aggravated by the hypoxemia, acidosis, and stress that may accompany weaning.

Hypokalemia may cause myocardial irritability and, therefore, must be corrected; it may also lead to metabolic alkalemia. The combination of hypoxemia, alkalemia, and hypokalemia strongly predisposes to arrhythmias. Hyponatremia, hyperglycemia, and renal failure should all be treated and restored to normal if possible before weaning is begun. Hypophosphatemia should also be corrected, because this can result in respiratory muscle weakness. Hypocalcemia, hypomagnesemia, or hypermagnesemia should also be corrected.

Caloric and protein depletion may occur over a period of mechanical ventilation in the patient being sustained solely by intravenous fluids. Respiratory muscles may atrophy from inactivity and may also be weakened by catabolism as a result of malnutrition. Therefore, proper nutrition and an exercise program should be started in advance of weaning in the patient who has spent a prolonged period on the ventilator. Excessive caloric intake with intravenous or enteral nutrition should be avoided when weaning is initiated, because this can increase O_2 consumption and CO_2 production; it has also been associated with failure to wean from mechanical ventilation.

Fever should be controlled because it increases O_2 consumption and CO_2 production. Its presence often signifies infection, which also increases O_2 demand. Thus, both fever and infection should be controlled, if possible, before weaning patients with minimal respiratory reserve. Septic patients usually cannot be successfully weaned.

Fluid balance can be critical, especially if borderline pulmonary edema is present. Continuous ventilation can promote fluid retention, which could further compromise the patient's respiratory reserve. This is particularly likely in malnourished patients with low colloidal osmotic pressure secondary to hypoalbuminemia. Patients receiving inadequate fluids or diuretics may develop hypovolemia, which in turn can reduce the cardiac output and blood pressure. Body weight and fluid intake and output should be monitored carefully to prevent further compromise of the patient's reserve.

Sleep deprivation and pain are common in critically ill patients and interfere with the patient's ability to resume spontaneous ventilation. Narcotics and sedatives should be reduced or discontinued, if possible, to ensure alertness and to avoid respiratory center depression. However, a minimal analgesic dose is often useful in weaning the postoperative patient, since it dulls pain sufficiently to enable the patient to take deep breaths, optimizing alveolar ventilation and preventing atelectasis. Adequate rest enhances the patient's ability to cooperate. Therefore, sedatives should not be totally abandoned but should be used judiciously. Ideally, patients should be alert, conscious, and cooperative at the start of weaning, but this is not always possible. In patients with severe head injury or cerebral vascular accident, consciousness may be slow in returning and may follow successful weaning by weeks or months.

As a general rule, patients who are homeostatically unstable cannot be weaned. Patients with multisystem failure usually require mechanical ventilation.

RESPIRATORY MUSCLES AND WEANING

In recent years, there has been increasing interest in the role of respiratory muscles during acute respiratory failure, mechanical ventilation, and weaning from mechanical ventilation. Respiratory muscle fatigue occurs if the load placed on the muscles is excessive, if the muscles are weak, or if the duty cycle is too long (duty cycle is the inspiratory time relative to total cycle time). A fatiguing load can result from a high airway resistance, a low lung compliance, or a high WOB imposed by the ventilator breathing circuit. Respiratory muscles may be weakened by disease, disuse, malnutrition, hypoxia, or electrolyte imbalance. A long duty cycle may result from tachypnea. Respiratory muscle fatigue is clinically recognized by tachypnea, abnormal respiratory movements (respiratory alternans and abdominal paradox), and finally an increase in $PaCO_2$. Because maximal inspiratory pressure (MIP) is a good indicator of overall respiratory muscle strength, a low MIP may indicate respiratory muscle fatigue.

To avoid respiratory muscle weakness, appropriate amounts of oxygen and other nutrients must be supplied to these muscles. This requires an adequate tissue perfusion (cardiac output) and arterial oxygen content. Nutritional status is also important because inadequate caloric intake can result in catabolism of respiratory muscle protein.

Respiratory muscles must be rested if fatigue occurs. Respiratory muscle rest is usually provided by a period of A/C ventilation or an IMV rate fast

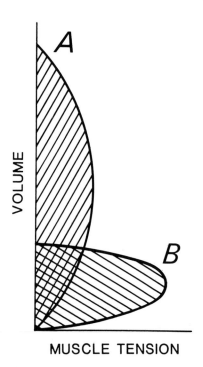

Figure 22—7. Low-tension/high-volume work (*A*) and high-tension/low-volume work (*B*).

enough to eliminate spontaneous breathing. However, A/C ventilation does not necessarily result in complete muscle rest. To maximize rest during A/C ventilation, the ventilator settings must be adjusted to minimize triggering effort and to provide an inspiratory flow that exceeds patient effort.

If respiratory muscle fatigue is the result of an excessive load, then that load should be reduced

before attempts are made to wean the patient from the ventilator. This is done by increasing lung compliance and decreasing airway resistance. Xanthines, such as aminophylline, may be useful because they decrease airway resistance and increase diaphragmatic contractility. Patients with low compliance or high airway resistance are usually not good candidates for weaning, since this high respiratory load may result in muscle fatigue.

Respiratory muscle performance, like that of other skeletal muscles, can be improved by training. Respiratory muscles can be trained for strength or endurance. High-tension/low-volume work tends to stimulate strength conditioning through the development of increased sarcomeres (Fig. 22—7). Low-tension/high-volume work tends to stimulate endurance training through development of increased mitochondrial density. Spontaneous breathing during T-piece trials or IMV may tend to promote respiratory muscle strengthening, whereas pressure-support ventilation (PSV) may tend to promote respiratory muscle endurance. Inspiratory muscle training using isocapnic hyperpnea or a resistive training device has been useful in a few cases of difficult weaning.[16] A commercially available resistive-training device can be incorporated into the ventilator circuit for such training (Fig. 22—8).

DETERMINATION OF ADEQUATE PULMONARY FUNCTION

It must be determined whether a patient has the ventilatory capacity to maintain adequate spontaneous ventilation and oxygenation off the ventila-

Figure 22—8. An adjustable inspiratory resistor can be added to the inspiratory limb of the ventilator circuit by a one-way valve to produce inspiratory resistive training (Reprinted, with permission, from Aldrich TK, Uhrlass RM: Weaning from mechanical ventilation: Successful use of modified inspiratory resistive training in muscular dystrophy. Crit Care Med 15:247–249, © by Williams & Wilkins, 1987)

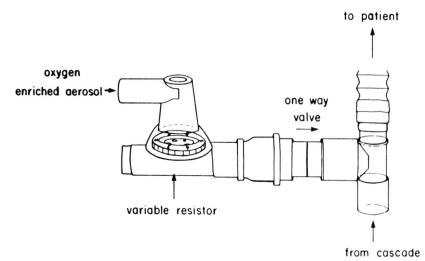

Table 22–12 Physiologic Parameters That Suggest Weaning Is Possible

TESTS OF MECHANICAL CAPABILITY

Maximal inspiratory pressure	> -20 cmH$_2$O
Vital capacity	$> 10–15$ mL/kg
FEV$_1$	> 10 mL/kg
Spontaneous resting minute ventilation (can be doubled with MVV maneuver)	< 10 L/min
Spontaneous tidal volume	> 5 mL/kg
Spontaneous respiratory rate	< 30/min and > 6/min
Compliance on ventilator	> 30 mL/cmH$_2$O

TESTS OF OXYGENATION CAPABILITY

P(a − a)O$_2$ on 100% O$_2$	$< 300–350$ torr
PaO$_2$ on 100% O$_2$	> 300 torr
PaO$_2$ on $\leq 40\%$ O$_2$	≥ 60 torr
PaO$_2$/P$_A$O$_2$	> 0.15
PaO$_2$/F$_I$O$_2$	> 100
$\dot{Q}$s/$\dot{Q}$t	$< 15\%$
V$_D$/V$_T$	$< 0.55–0.6$

tor. This evaluation can be divided into two categories: the patient's mechanical or neuromuscular ability to breathe, and the lungs' ability to adequately oxygenate the arterial blood (e.g., ventilation–perfusion inequality, diffusion defect, or shunt). The variables listed in Table 22–12 give the minimal values considered necessary to institute weaning. Although these values are a useful guide to weaning potential, they are less valuable in predicting weaning success or failure in patients who have been on long-term ventilatory support than in those who have required mechanical ventilation for a shorter period.[17]

If the patient must be disconnected from the ventilator to perform the weaning test, a standard procedure should be followed. First, while the patient is still connected to the ventilator, one should carefully explain the testing procedure and familiarize the patient with the equipment that will be used. Next, the patient should be allowed to practice the test to be performed. The test should then be repeated several times, with the best effort being recorded. After each test, the patient should be placed back on the ventilator for a short time to prevent dyspnea. The vital capacity and MIP can be tested without providing supplemental oxygen. The maximal voluntary ventilation (MVV) and $\dot{V}$E, however, may require supplemental oxygen during testing.

The MIP is measured by attaching an aneroid manometer to the endotracheal or tracheostomy tube. The patient then forcibly inhales after maximal exhalation. When MIP is measured, it is recommended that a undirectional valve be used, and that the airway is completely obstructed for 20 to 25 seconds (Fig. 22–9). An MIP greater than −20 cmH$_2$O suggests adequate inspiratory muscle strength for sighs, as well as for the deep inhalations necessary for an effective cough. However, if the patient has a high WOB, an MIP of −20 cmH$_2$O may not be large enough to prevent fatigue. Serial MIP measurements may be useful during weaning to evaluate fatigue; a drop in MIP indicates fatigue.

The vital capacity (VC) can be measured easily with any instrument that measures exhaled volume

Figure 22–9. The one-way valve system used to measure inspiratory force: The patient is connected at *A*, the manometer (*D*) is connected at *C*, and the patient exhales through *B*. In this way, maximal inspiratory pressure will be measured at FRC.

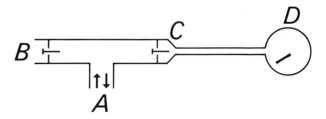

(e.g., a Wright Respirometer or portable electronic spirometer). The patient is instructed to take a maximal inspiration and then exhale maximally. Serial vital capacity measurements are better indicators of respiratory reserve than is tidal volume or respiratory rate, and are particularly useful in following the status of patients with neuromuscular weakness (e.g., Guillain-Barré syndrome or myasthenia gravis). The (VC) should be more than 15 mL/kg body weight to be able to sigh deeply enough to avoid atelectasis.

The FEV_1 is considered by some practitioners to be a useful indicator of weaning ability in COPD patients. The vital capacity may be nearly normal if the patient slowly exhales. However, airway collapse may occur with forced exhalation. An FEV_1 of at least 10 mL/kg makes successful weaning more likely. The FEV_1 may be difficult to measure in intubated patients and may be affected by the resistance of the endotracheal tube.

Although a patient may be able to produce an acceptable vital capacity when removed from the ventilator, the ability to sustain the muscular effort necessary for normal gas exchange is crucial. The MVV, although criticized because of its dependence on patient effort, is a test of this ability. The patient is a candidate for weaning if the spontaneous resting ventilation is less than 10 L/min and the resting ventilation can be doubled with an MVV maneuver.

A spontaneous tidal volume of at least 5 mL/kg with a respiratory rate less than 30/min is considered acceptable for weaning. Tachypnea is often associated with failure to wean. A patient who requires more than 10 L/min of ventilation while on the ventilator is not a good candidate for weaning because it is unlikely that he or she will be able to maintain this level of ventilation spontaneously without fatigue.

The alveolar–arterial difference of oxygen [$(P(A-a)O_2$] is an index of the lungs' ability to transfer oxygen from the inspired gas to the blood. A $P(A-a)O_2$ of less than 300 to 350 torr or a PaO_2 greater than 300 torr on 100% oxygen indicates adequate pulmonary oxygenation ability to allow weaning. However, since 100% oxygen predisposes to atelectasis, the use of 100% oxygen for the sole purpose of measuring $P(A-a)O_2$ should be avoided. If the PaO_2 is at least 60 torr on an FIO_2 of 0.4 or less, the patient's ventilation–perfusion relationship, diffusing capacity, and shunt are acceptable to allow satisfactory weaning. Some practitioners prefer to use PaO_2/PAO_2 or PaO_2/FIO_2, rather than $P(A-a)O_2$.[18]

The presence of significant shunting interferes with the ability to adequately oxygenate arterial blood. Frequent causes of intrapulmonary shunting in ventilator-dependent patients include retained secretions, bronchospasm, atelectasis, pulmonary edema, and pneumonia. These conditions can usually be corrected by use of suctioning, bronchodilators, chest physiotherapy, diuretics, and antibiotics. Infrequently, more invasive procedures such as bronchoscopy may be required. Shunts greater than 20% make weaning difficult, with a shunt less than 15% being preferable.

The V_D/V_T should be less than 0.55 to 0.60 before weaning is begun. Sometimes it is also useful to measure $\dot{V}CO_2$ and $\dot{V}O_2$ to assess weaning ability. An increase in $\dot{V}CO_2$ and $\dot{V}O_2$ implies hypermetabolism, which results in an increased ventilatory requirement.

Some of these tests of weaning ability should be performed daily, with both the absolute value and trend being observed (see Fig. 22–6). Some patients may never achieve an acceptable score on many of these tests. The patient, nonetheless, may be successfully weaned if there is a trend toward improvement in these values. An overall evaluation of the patient is more important than rigid conformance to specific weaning criteria.

TECHNIQUES OF WEANING

Weaning a ventilator patient may involve one or a combination of several methods: T-piece trials of spontaneous breathing; IMV, which allows the patient to breathe spontaneously while receiving a specified, decreasing number of ventilator-delivered breaths per minute; and PSV, in which the patient's spontaneous breaths are augmented by a clinician-determined level of pressure support.

Psychological preparation is very important and must begin before the patient has been disconnected from the ventilator. The respiratory therapists and nurses in whom the patient has shown the most confidence should be used during the weaning process. Before each weaning trial or weaning evaluation, the respiratory therapist or nurse should explain every detail of the procedure to the patient. The patient should be assured that there will be continuous monitoring during the weaning trial and mechanical ventilation will be reinitiated when necessary. Early in the weaning process, someone should always be with the patient for reassurance, to monitor the patient's tolerance of the weaning trial, and to check the equipment for malfunction. Frequent encouragement is needed because the success of weaning depends largely on the attitude of, and effort exerted by, the patient. The need for psychological preparation appears to be directly proportional to the length of continuous ventilation. During the weaning period setbacks are common; the patient and staff must be prepared to accept this.

T-PIECE WARNING

The goal of the T-piece method is to allow spontaneous ventilation while providing supplemental oxygen as needed. The tubing from the gas source attaches to the T-piece, which in turn is connected to the endotracheal tube. While the patient is receiving humidified oxygen by a T-piece, care must be taken to prevent significant entrainment of room air. The application of a reservoir tubing distal to the patient's T-piece can prevent room air entrainment (Fig. 22–10). With an adequate flow and a reservoir, an FIO_2 of at least 0.5 can be delivered if necessary. Patients with high inspiratory flows may require significantly higher gas flows, sometimes as high as 70–90 L/min.

The design of the T-piece system should be as simple as possible. One-way valves, reservoir bags, and elaborate systems can be hazardous. Valves can be inadvertently placed in the system in the wrong direction, and reservoir bags can fill with water. A nebulizer is usually used for humidity, but a heated humidifier should be used if the patient has reactive airways and is at risk for bronchospasm. A

Figure 22–10. Diagram of T-piece setup. (Gray LS, Hodgkin JE: Ventilator Weaning. New York, Parke–Davis, 1981)

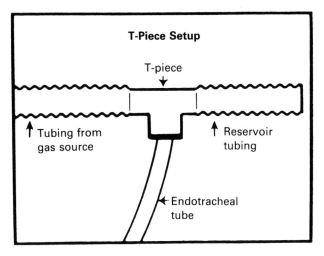

heated humidifier may also be needed in high flows and high FIO_2s are required.

During periods of spontaneous breathing on the T-piece system, the cuff on the airway can often be deflated, removing pressure from the tracheal mucosa and allowing gas to pass around as well as through the tube. The cuff should not be deflated if there is a significant risk of aspirating upper airway secretions or gastric contents. The cuff must be inflated whenever ventilator-initiated breaths are being delivered.

Suctioning the patient before and during a T-piece weaning trial may help clear the airway, resulting in a reduced WOB and improved gas exchange. It is useful to hyperoxygenate the patient before and after suctioning to prevent hypoxemia and subsequent deterioration. Hyperinflation should also be used after suctioning to reverse suctioning-related atelectasis.

Initially, spontaneous breathing may result in a decreased PaO_2. Hypoventilation, with smaller tidal volumes, and atelectasis, with resultant physiologic shunting, may occur. Therefore, the patient will initially need a higher FIO_2 off the ventilator. Increasing the FIO_2 by 0.1 above the ventilator setting is an acceptable rule of thumb to prevent hypoxemia. However, one should remember that the patient with chronic CO_2 retention may need a hypoxic drive to breathe; thus, routinely raising the FIO_2 in these patients may be hazardous.

A sitting or semirecumbent position is usually best tolerated during the weaning trial. The patient should be as comfortable as possible before disconnecting him or her from the ventilator. An ECG monitor should be attached during weaning, since both early detection and early treatment of arrhythmias are essential. Stress and blood gas changes during weaning may induce arrhythmias.

A flowsheet (Fig. 22–11) may be useful to chart a patient's progress during weaning. The initial values of pulse, blood pressure, and ECG are taken just before the patient is disconnected from the ventilator. The initial values for tidal volume and respiratory rate are taken during the first 2 minutes of the weaning trial. Volume measurements are more accurate if one measures a cumulative volume and divides it by the respiratory rate to produce an average tidal volume. During the time the patient is disconnected, the ventilator tubing should be protected from contamination.

The patient should be monitored closely during the T-piece trial. Factors indicating that the patient should be returned to the ventilator are listed in Table 22–13. These values are guidelines and

Date/ Time	Pulse	Blood Pressure	Tidal Volume	Resp. Rate	EKG Rhythm	Exhaled CO_2	Total Time Off	F_iO_2	pH	PaO_2	$PaCO_2$	Tech. Comments

Figure 22—11. Weaning flowsheet.

may not be applicable to all patients. For example, one may accept a lower PaO_2 or pH with a higher $PaCO_2$ in patients with chronic carbon dioxide retention. When the patient can tolerate being off the ventilator for about 15 to 20 minutes, it is useful to evaluate arterial blood gas values on the T-piece. The ability to monitor end-tidal PCO_2 may allow detection of hyperventilation or hypoventilation, and pulse oximetry allows continuous monitoring of arterial oxygenation.

During weaning trials, the patient should be monitored for signs of respiratory muscle fatigue. Early signs of fatigue include tachypnea and respiratory muscle paradox. A decrease in MIP during weaning also implies respiratory muscle fatigue. If fatigue occurs, the patient should be returned to the ventilator.

After each T-piece trial, the patient is returned to the ventilator for a period of rest. Ventilation during the rest periods is best provided by A/C mode or high IMV rates. Intermittent mandatory ventilation with low rates, which requires significant spontaneous breathing, may not allow sufficient rest for the respiratory muscles. With T-piece

Table 22—13 Factors Indicating That Patient Should Be Returned to Ventilatory Support During Weaning

Blood pressure	Change of 20 mmHg systolic or 10 mmHg diastolic
Pulse	Increase of 20/min or rate > 110/min
Respiratory rate	Increase of 10/min or rate > 30/min
Tidal volume	< 250–300 mL or < 5 mL/kg
MIP	A drop indicates respiratory muscle fatigue
Breathing pattern	Discoordinate breathing indicates respiratory muscle fatigue
PaO_2	< 60 torr
$PaCO_2$	> 55 torr
pH	< 7.35
Significant ECG change	

weaning, the periods of spontaneous breathing become longer relative to the periods of ventilation until the patient is eventually completely weaned from the ventilator.

A T-piece trial is not the same as a trial of spontaneous breathing with the patient attached to a ventilator in continuous positive airway pressure (CPAP) mode. In CPAP mode, most currently available ventilators supply spontaneous breaths from a demand valve. It has been shown that spontaneous breathing from a demand valve increases the inspiratory workload imposed on the patient. In some patients this increased workload may promote fatigue.

Weaning may begin while the patient is still being ventilated with low levels of PEEP. In these patients, breathing by T-piece may result in a drop in functional residual capacity, with deleterious effects on ventilatory mechanics, $\dot{Q}s/\dot{Q}t$, and PaO_2. In such cases, spontaneous breathing trials should be performed using a high-flow CPAP system rather than an ambient pressure T-piece.

Advantages of T-piece weaning include low cost and simplicity. The equipment is usually easy to assemble, with little risk of problems related to the equipment. The major disadvantage of T-piece weaning is that it requires the patient to abruptly resume complete spontaneous ventilatory support, thus requiring close monitoring of the patient during T-piece weaning trials.

WEANING BY INTERMITTENT MANDATORY VENTILATION

The use of IMV involves gradually reducing the number of ventilator-delivered breaths, thereby allowing the patient to increase the amount of spontaneous breathing between the mandatory ventilator breaths (Fig. 22–12). Thus, ventilatory support is gradually withdrawn, allowing the patient to slowly resume spontaneous ventilation.

As with T-piece weaning, the patient should be closely monitored when IMV weaning is begun (see Table 22–13). If the patient shows signs of fatigue during IMV weaning, an increase in the ventilator IMV rate is necessary, or the patient may need to be switched to A/C mode. Initially, during IMV weaning, the patient may still need rest periods of full ventilatory support.

A major advantage of IMV weaning is convenience. Simply changing the ventilator rate alters the patient's weaning progress. The patient's safety may be more readily ensured, since ventilator-delivered breaths continue at the IMV rate. By gradu-

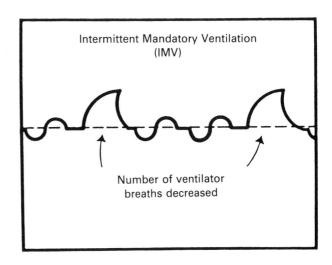

Figure 22–12. Diagram of IMV. (Gray LS, Hodgkin JE: Ventilator Weaning. New York, Parke–Davis, 1981)

ally decreasing the IMV rate, the best $PaCO_2$ can be safely determined in those patients in whom the $PaCO_2$ before mechanical ventilation is unknown. This method may also be less stressful to the patient psychologically because of the gradual withdrawal of ventilatory support.

Although most currently available ventilators have a built-in IMV mode, older ventilators require add-on circuitry to achieve IMV. This setup may be relatively complex, with the risk of incorrectly placed valves and disconnection of ventilator alarms. If add-on IMV circuits are used, extreme care must be taken to guarantee their correct assembly and function.

Virtually all commercially available ventilators deliver the spontaneous breaths during IMV from a demand valve. Although the additional work imposed by the demand valve may be well tolerated by many patients, there may be a substantial number of patients in whom this additional work results in fatigue. If fatigue occurs during demand-valve IMV weaning, weaning may be successful if a continuous-flow IMV system is used, or if T-piece weaning is used.

Although IMV may be a convenient weaning technique, it does not necessarily reduce weaning time. It may actually prolong the weaning process. With a graded reduction in ventilator rate on IMV, patients may remain intubated significantly longer than with T-piece weaning. The use of very low IMV rates (i.e., fewer than 4/min) can result in respiratory muscle fatigue and should be avoided.

WEANING BY PRESSURE-SUPPORT VENTILATION

Pressure-support ventilation (PSV), the newest weaning technique, appears to be a promising alternative to T-piece weaning and IMV. With PSV, patient effort is augmented by a clinician-determined level of pressure during inspiration (Fig. 22–13). Although the clinician sets the level of pressure support, the patient sets the respiratory rate, inspiratory flow, and inspiratory time. The V_T is determined by the level of pressure support, the amount of patient effort, and the resistance and compliance of the patient's lungs. At high levels of pressure support (>20 cmH₂O), PSV is similar to pressure-limited assisted ventilation. Several approaches can be used when weaning with PSV. One of these involves choosing a level of PSV that provides a targeted V_T and respiratory rate, then decreasing the pressure-support level in a stepwise fashion (provided that V_T and rate remain adequate). The second approach involves a combination of IMV and PSV, in which the patient's spontaneous breaths are supported by a low level of pressure.

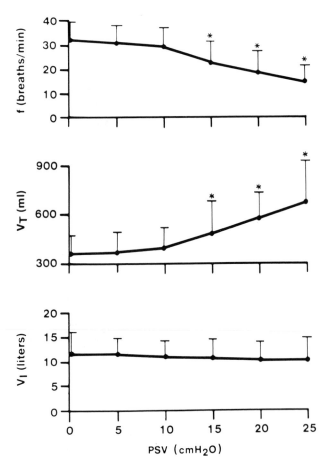

Figure 22–14. Effect of PSV on breathing pattern. Note the increase in tidal volume and decrease in respiratory rate with increasing levels of PSV. (Reprinted with permission from Ershowsky P, Krieger B: Changes in breathing pattern during pressure support ventilation. Respir Care 32:1011–1016, © Williams & Wilkins, 1987)

Figure 22–13. Airway pressures, flows, and volumes with PSV (*dashed lines*) and spontaneous breathing (*solid line*). (Reprinted with permission from MacIntyre NR: Pressure support ventilation: Effects on ventilatory reflexes and ventilatory muscle workloads. Respir Car 32:447–457, 1987)

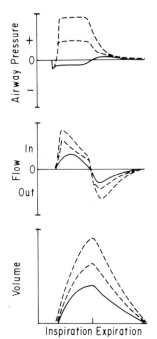

With this approach, the patient is weaned by decreasing the number of ventilator breaths (as in standard IMV weaning). Low-level PSV may be beneficial because it eliminates the inspiratory work imposed by ventilator demand-valves during spontaneous breathing, because it may be a more comfortable mode of ventilation than IMV for some patients, and because it promotes endurance training of respiratory muscles. Pressure-support ventilation may also be useful in overcoming the work of breathing through artificial airways. It has been shown that PSV may improve the efficiency of breathing patterns in some difficult-to-wean patients (Fig. 22–14). The precise role of PSV in weaning still needs clarification.

WHICH WEANING TECHNIQUE IS BEST?

Specific weaning protocols are usually based upon institutional policy or individual bias. A single rigid approach to weaning will not be appropriate for all patients. Most patients can be weaned easily with any of the foregoing techniques. It is the occasional difficult-to-wean patient who presents a clinical dilemma. If a weaning attempt is not successful for a specific patient, it seems prudent to try another approach. With T-piece trials, IMV, PSV, and variations and combinations, a successful weaning plan can be tailored to the needs of most patients.

WEANING FROM THE AIRWAY

Although weaning and extubation are often closely related in clinical practice, they are technically separate events. For a patient to be extubated, not only does the patient need to be able to breathe spontaneously, but the patient also needs to be able to protect the airway and be able to adequately clear secretions. Prolonged spontaneous breathing before extubation is usually not desirable because of the high WOB imposed by the artificial airway (Fig. 22–15), and prolonged low-rate IMV may not be desirable because of the additional work imposed by the ventilator demand valve. Consequently, some patients can be successfully extubated without a successful trial of spontaneous breathing. However, it is usually best to evaluate the patient's ability to breathe spontaneously without any ventilatory support before extubation.

When weaning from a tracheostomy, a fenestrated tube may be useful (Fig. 22–16). With the cuff deflated and the inner cannula removed from this tube, the patient can breathe through the normal tube channel, through the fenestration in the posterior (superior) portion of the tube, and around the tube. This results in an increased inspired volume for the same amount of effort by reducing the resistance to airflow. This tube can also be plugged to evaluate the patient's ability to breathe through the upper airway. However, this tube should *never* be plugged unless the fenestration is open and the cuff is deflated; otherwise, the patient's airway may be totally obstructed! If the patient needs to be reconnected to the ventilator, the inner cannula must be inserted and the cuff inflated. Unfortunately, the fenestration in the tracheostomy tube is often not located in the lumen of the airway, but is occluded by tissue anterior to the trachea or by the posterior

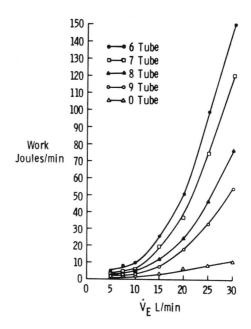

Figure 22–15. Effect of endotracheal tube size on work of breathing. (Reprinted with permission from Shapiro M, Wilson RK, Casar G et al: Work of breathing through different sized endotracheal tubes. Crit Care Med 14:1028–1031, © Williams & Wilkins, 1986)

Figure 22–16. Fenestrated tracheostomy tube.

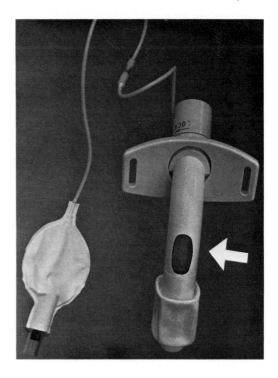

tracheal wall. Unless the fenestration is properly located in the trachea, these fenestrated tubes should not be used.

REFERENCES

1. Grum CM, Chauncey JB: Conventional mechanical ventilation. Clin Chest Med 9:37–46, 1988
2. Pierson DJ: Indications for mechanical ventilation in acute respiratory failure. Respir Care 28:570–578, 1983
3. Hudson LD, Hurlow RS, Craig KC, Pierson DJ: Does intermittent mandatory ventilation correct respiratory alkalosis in patients receiving assisted mechanical ventilation? Am Rev Respir Dis 132:1071–1074, 1985
4. Suter PM, Fairley HB, Isenberg MD: Effect of tidal volume and positive end-expiratory pressure on compliance during mechanical ventilation. Chest 73:158–162, 1978
5. Maxwell C, Hess D, Shefet D: Use of the arterial/alveolar oxygen tension ratio to predict the FiO_2 needed for a desired PaO_2. Respir Care 29:1135–1139, 1984
6. Hess D, Good C, Didyoung R et al: The validity of assessing arterial blood gases 10 minutes after an FiO_2 change in mechanically ventilated patients without chronic pulmonary disease. Respir Care 30:1037–1041, 1985
7. Luterman A, Horovitz JH, Carrico CJ et al: Withdrawal from positive end-expiratory pressure. Surgery 83:328–332, 1978
8. Weaver LJ, Haisch CE, Hudson LD, Carrico CJ: Prospective analysis of PEEP reduction [abstract]. Am Rev Respir Dis 119:182, 1979
9. Weaver LJ, Hudson LD, Carrico CJ: Prospective analysis of PEEP reduction [abstract]. Chest 78:544, 1980
10. Craig KC, Pierson DJ, Carrico CJ: The clinical application of positive end-expiratory pressure (PEEP) in the adult respiratory distress syndrome (ARDS). Respir Care 30:184–201, 1985
11. Brown DG, Pierson DJ: Auto-PEEP is common in mechanically ventilated patients: A study of incidence, severity, and detection. Respir Care 31:1069–1074, 1986
12. Pepe PE, Marini JJ: Occult positive end-expiratory pressure in mechanically ventilated patient with airflow obstruction. The auto-PEEP effect. Am Rev Respir Dis 126:166–170, 1982
13. Suter PM, Fairley HB, Isenberg MD: Optimum end-expiratory pressure in patients with acute pulmonary failure. N Engl J Med 292:284–289, 1975
14. Murray IP, Modell JH, Gallagher TJ, Banner MJ: Titration of PEEP by the arterial minus end-tidal carbon dioxide gradient. Chest 85:100–104, 1984
15. Jardin F, Genevry B, Pazin M et al: Inability to titrate PEEP in patients with acute respiratory failure using end-tidal carbon dioxide measurements. Anesthesiology 62:530–533, 1985
16. Aldrich TK, Uhrlass RM: Weaning from mechanical ventilation: Successful use of modified inspiratory resistive training in muscular dystrophy. Crit Care Med 15:247–249, 1987
17. Fiastro JF et al: Comparison of standard weaning parameters and the mechanical work of breathing in mechanically ventilated patients. Chest 94:232–238, 1988
18. Hess D, Maxwell C: Which is the best index of oxygenation: $P(A-a)O_2$, PaO_2/PAO_2, or PaO_2/FiO_2? [editorial]. Respir Care 30:961–963, 1985

BIBLIOGRAPHY

Complications of Mechanical Ventilation

Strieter RM, Lynch JP: Complications in the ventilated patient. Clin Chest Med 9:127–139, 1988

Zwillich CW, Pierson DJ, Creagh CE et al: Complications of assisted ventilation: A prospective study of 356 consecutive cases. Am J Med 57:161–170, 1974

Initial Ventilator Settings

Banner MJ, Downs JB, Kirby RR et al: Effects of expiratory flow resistance on inspiratory work of breathing. Chest 93:795–799, 1988

Banner MJ, Lampotang S, Boysen PG et al: Flow resistance of expiratory positive-pressure valve system. Chest 90:212–217, 1986

Christopher KL, Neff RA, Bowman JL et al: Demand and continuous flow intermittent mandatory ventilation systems. Chest 87:625–630, 1985

Downs JB, Klein EF, Desautels D et al: Intermittent mandatory ventilation: A new approach to weaning patients from mechanical ventilation. Chest 64:331–334, 1973

Gibney RTN, Wilson RD, Pontoppidan H: Comparison of work of breathing on high gas flow and demand valve continuous positive airway pressure systems. Chest 82:692–695, 1982

Henry WC, West GA, Wilson RS: A comparison of the oxygen cost of breathing between a continuous-flow CPAP system and a demand-flow CPAP system. Respir Care 28:1273–1281, 1983

Hess D: Controversies in respiratory critical care. Crit Care Nurs Q 11(3):62–78, 1988

Hudson LD, Weaver J, Haisch CE, Carrico CJ: Positive end-expiratory pressure: Reduction and withdrawal. Respir Care 33:613–619, 1988

Kacmarek RM, Vemegas J: Mechanical ventilatory rates and tidal volumes. Respir Care 32:466–478, 1987

Katz JA, Kraemer RW, Gjerde GE: Inspiratory work and airway pressure with continuous positive airway pressure delivery system. Chest 88:519–526, 1985

Luce JM, Pierson DJ, Hudson LD: Intermittent mandatory ventilation. Chest 79:678–685, 1981

Marini JJ: Mechanical ventilation: Taking the work out of breathing? Respir Care 31:695–702, 1987

Marini JJ, Capps JS, Culver BH: The inspiratory work of breathing during assisted mechanical ventilation. Chest 5:612–618, 1985

Marini JJ, Culver BH, Kirk W: Flow resistance of exhalation valves and positive end-expiratory pressure devices used in mechanical ventilation. Am Rev Respir Dis 131:850–854, 1985

Marini JJ, Rodriguiz M, Lamb V: The inspiratory workload of patient-initiated mechanical ventilation. Am Rev Respir Dis 134:902–909, 1986

Marini JJ, Smith TC, Lamb VJ: External work output and force generation during synchronized intermittent mechanical ventilation. Am Rev Respir Dis 138:1169–1179, 1988

Nelson LD, Civetta JM, Hudson-Civetta J: Titrating positive end-expiratory pressure in patients with early, moderate arterial hypoxemia. Crit Care Med 15:14–19, 1987

Opt't Holt TB, Hall MW, Bass JB, Allison RC: Comparison of changes in airway pressure during continuous positive airway pressure (CPAP) between demand valve and continuous flow devices. Respir Care 27:1200–1209, 1982

Shapiro BA, Cane RD, Harrison RA: Positive end-expiratory pressure in adults with special reference to acute lung injury: A review of the literature and suggested clinical correlations. Crit Care Med 12:127–141, 1984

Shelly MP, Lloyd GM, Park GR: A review of the mechanisms and methods of humidification of inspired gases. Intensive Care Med 14:1-9, 1988

Smith RA: Physiologic PEEP. Respir Care 33:620–629, 1988

Van Hook CJ, Carilli AD, Haponik EF: Hemodynamic effects of positive end-expiratory pressure. Historical perspective. Am J Med 81:307–310, 1986

Venus B, Copiozo GB, Jacobs HK: Continuous positive airway pressure. The use of low levels in adult patients with artificial airways. Arch Surg 115:824–828, 1980

Weisman IM, Rinaldo JE, Rogers RM, Sanders MH: Intermittent mandatory ventilation. Am Rev Respir Dis 127:641–647, 1983

Monitoring of the Patient on a Ventilator

Benson MS, Pierson DJ: Auto-PEEP during mechanical ventilation of adults. Respir Care 33:557–568, 1988

Bone RC: Thoracic pressure–volume curves in respiratory failure. Crit Care Med 4:148–150, 1976

Demers RR, Pratter MR, Irwin RS: Use of the concept of ventilator compliance in the determination of static total compliance. Respir Care 26:644–648, 1981

Fallat RJ: Respiratory monitoring. Clin Chest Med 3:181–194, 1982

Fernandez R, Benito S, Blanch L, Net A: Intrinsic PEEP: A cause of inspiratory muscle ineffectivity. Intensive Care Med 15:51–52, 1988

Forbat AF, Her C: Correction for gas compression in mechanical ventilators. Anesth Analg 59:488–493, 1980

Hess D: Bedside monitoring of the patient on a ventilator. Crit Care Q (4):23–32, 1983

Hess D, Evans C, Thomas K et al: The relationship between conjunctival PO_2 and arterial PO_2 in 16 normal persons. Respir Care 31:191–198, 1986

Hess D, Maxwell D, Shefet D: Determination of intrapulmonary shunt: Comparison of an estimated shunt equation and a modified shunt equation with the classic shunt equation. Respir Care 32:268–273, 1987

Kirby RR: Best PEEP: Issues and choices in the selection and monitoring of PEEP levels. Respir Care 33:569–580, 1988

Marini JJ: Monitoring during mechanical ventilation. Clin Chest Med 9:73–100, 1988

Ventilator Weaning

Agusti AGN, Torres A, Estopa R, Agusti-Vidal A: Hypophosphatemia as a cause of failed weaning: The importance of metabolic factors. Crit Care Med 12:142–143, 1984

Aldrich TK, Karpel JP, Uhrlass RM et al: Weaning from mechanical ventilation: Adjunctive use of inspiratory muscle resistive training. Crit Care Med 17:143–147, 1989

Annest SJ, Gottlieb M, Paloski WH et al: Detrimental effects of removing end-expiratory pressure prior to endotracheal extubation. Ann Surg 191:539–545, 1980

Aubier M, Murciano D, Lecocguic Y et al: Effect of hypophosphatemia on diaphragmatic contractility in patients with acute respiratory failure. N Engl J Med 313:420–424, 1985

Benotti PN, Bistrian B: Metabolic and nutritional aspects of weaning from mechanical ventilation. Crit Care Med 17:181–185, 1989

Boysen PG: Respiratory muscle function and weaning from mechanical ventilation. Respir Care 32:572–583, 1987

Brochard L, Harf A, Lorino H, Lemaire F: Inspiratory pressure support prevents diaphragmatic fatigue during weaning from mechanical ventilation. Am Rev Respir Dis 139:513–521, 1989

Brochard L, Pluskwa F, Lemaire F: Improved efficiency of spontaneous breathing with inspiratory pressure support. Am Rev Respir Dis 136:411–415, 1987

Cohen CA, Zagelbaum G, Gross D et al: Clinical manifestations of inspiratory muscle fatigue. Am J Med 73:308–316, 1982

Ershowsky P, Krieger B: Changes in breathing pattern during pressure support ventilation. Respir Care 32:1011–1016, 1987

Feeley TW, Saumarex R, Klick JM et al: Positive end-expiratory pressure in weaning patients from controlled ventilation. Lancet 2:725–728, 1975

Hall JB, Wood LDH: Liberation of the patient from mechanical ventilation. JAMA 257:1621–1628, 1987

Hess D: Perspectives on weaning from mechanical ventilation—with a note on extubation. Respir Care 32:167–171, 1987

Hodgkin JE, Bowser MA, Burton GG: Respiratory weaning. Crit Care Med 2:96–102, 1974

Kacmarek RM: The role of pressure support ventilation in reducing work of breathing. Respir Care 33:99–120, 1988

MacIntyre NR: Respiratory support during pressure support ventilation. Chest 89:677–683, 1986

MacIntyre NR: Weaning from mechanical ventilatory support: Volume-assisting intermittent breaths versus pressure-assisting every breath. Respir Care 33:121–125, 1988

Marini JJ, Smith TC, Lamb V: Estimation of inspiratory muscle strength in mechanically ventilated patients: The measurement of maximal inspiratory pressure. J Crit Care 1:32–38, 1986

Menzies R, Gibbons W, Goldberg P: Determinants of weaning and survival among patients with COPD who require mechanical ventilation for acute respiratory failure. Chest 95:398–405, 1989

Morganroth ML, Morganroth JL, Nett LM, Petty TL: Criteria for weaning from prolonged mechanical ventilation. Arch Intern Med 144:1012–1016, 1984

Pierson DJ: Weaning from mechanical ventilation in acute respiratory failure: Concepts, indications, and techniques. Respir Care 28:646–662, 1983

Pingleton SK: Nutritional support in the mechanically ventilated patient. Clin Chest Med 9:101–112, 1988

Quan SF, Falltrick RT, Schlobohm RM: Extubation from ambient or expiratory positive airway pressure in adults. Anesthesiology 55:53–56, 1981

Roussos C, Macklem PT: The respiratory muscles. N Engl J Med 307:786–797, 1982

Sahn SA, Lakshminarayan S: Bedside criteria for discontinuation of mechanical ventilation. Chest 63:1002–1005, 1973

Sahn SA, Lakshminarayan S, Petty TL: Weaning from mechanical ventilation. JAMA 235:2208–2212, 1976

Schachter EN, Tucker D, Beck GJ: Does intermittent mandatory ventilation accelerate weaning? JAMA 246:1210–1214, 1981

Sporn PHS, Morganroth ML: Discontinuation of mechanical ventilation. Clin Chest Med 9:113–126, 1988

Tobin MJ, Perez W, Guenther SM et al: The pattern of breathing during successful and unsuccessful trials of weaning from mechanical ventilation. Am Rev Respir Dis 134:1111–1118, 1986

Weaning from the Airway

DeHaven CB, Hurst JM, Branson RD: Evaluation of two different extubation criteria: Attributes contributing to success. Crit Care Med 14:92–94, 1986

Gorbach MS, Kantor K: Extubation without a trial of spontaneous ventilation in the general surgical population. Respir Care 32:178–182, 1987

Shapiro M, Wilson K, Casar G et al: Work of breathing through different sized endotracheal tubes. Crit Care Med 14:1028–1031, 1986

TWENTY-THREE

Chest Physical Therapy

L. Jack Faling

Many of the techniques of chest physical therapy were first described in the late 1800s and early 1900s, and these methods have remained remarkably unchanged since then. On the other hand, newer investigational approaches, such as the study of respiratory mechanics and lung radioaerosol clearance, are now providing physiologic understanding of how chest physical therapy modalities work, which of the physical therapy methods are most helpful to patients, and which types of lung diseases are benefited from their use. The first portion of this chapter discusses the controlled breathing techniques of pursed-lip breathing, the bending-forward posture, and diaphragmatic-breathing exercises, which are employed to diminish dyspnea and increase the efficiency of the respiratory muscles as part of the long-term care of patients with severe chronic obstructive lung disorders. The second half deals with chest physical therapy techniques that enhance airway secretion clearance, including postural drainage, chest percussion, vibration, directed cough, and the forced expiratory technique. Although some chest physical therapy methods are of proven usefulness in managing neonates and young children with a variety of lung disorders, this chapter focuses mainly on the application of these techniques to adult patients.

CONTROLLED-BREATHING TECHNIQUES (BREATHING TRAINING)

Controlled-breathing techniques or "breathing training" are employed primarily in the long-term ambulatory management of patients with severe chronic obstructive lung disorders, although they may also prove helpful to patients during an acute exacerbation of their disease. Although most such patients have conventional chronic obstructive pulmonary disease (COPD) with emphysema and chronic bronchitis, breathing training is also of benefit in patients with significant airways obstruction caused by bronchiectasis, cystic fibrosis, and chronic asthma.

Breathing training was first promoted in the United States over 30 years ago by Alvan Barach and William F. Miller who recognized that patients with obstructive lung disease could improve their dyspnea by consciously altering their breathing pattern.[1,2] These physicians, along with their medical coworkers, described and employed the three major breathing-training techniques we use today: pursed-lip breathing, the bending-forward posture, and controlled abdominal breathing. It was some time later before we began to understand the physiologic perturbations in obstructive lung disorders and how these breathing techniques relieve dyspnea and improve respiratory function.

The chronic obstructive pulmonary disorders cause numerous physiologic abnormalities that interact to increase the work of breathing and reduce the efficiency of the respiratory muscles. Loss of pulmonary elastic recoil in emphysema, along with obstruction of small airways in obstructive bronchitis, bronchiectasis, and cystic fibrosis increases airways resistance and hyperinflates the lungs, producing elevations in total lung capacity (TLC), function residual capacity (FRC), and residual volume (RV). As hyperinflation progresses, the diaphragm becomes increasingly flattened, with loss of apposition of its costal components to the lower ribs so that its insertions on the ribs become oriented transversely inward rather than caudally. In addition, the diaphragm's muscle fibers shorten and its radius of curvature increases. As a result, the diaphragm contracts less effectively, losing its ability to pull up and inflate the lower rib cage (instead the rib cage may be pulled inward during inspiration, clinically manifested as lower costal retractions or Hoover's sign). The diaphragm is thus made to function on a less advantageous portion of its length–tension curve. According to Laplace's law,* the diaphragm would now generate a reduced transdiaphragmatic pressure for a given tension, and when completely flattened with an infinite radius of curvature, it becomes incapable of generating any useful inspiratory pressure.[3]

Hyperinflation also adversely influences the geometry of the ribs, shifting them from their normal oblique (downward) orientation to a more horizontal position. As a result, the inspiratory intercostal muscles function less effectively in lifting the ribs and expanding the thoracic rib cage. In addition, in disorders of airways obstruction, demands on the respiratory muscles are greater owing to the increased work of breathing. This stems from an elevated airway resistance, as well as from an increased minute ventilation brought about by the enlarged physiologic dead space. As a result, respiratory muscle fatigue will occur when the transdiaphragmatic pressures generated by a patient's respiratory muscles consistently exceed a critical fraction of his maximum transdiaphragmatic pressure.[4] Clinically, this is manifested by an increased respiratory rate, respiratory alternans (a cyclic alternation between the diaphragm and other inspiratory muscles), and a paradoxic inward motion of the abdomen during inspiration because of ineffective diaphragmatic contraction. These findings are usually noted in severe airways obstruction and often herald the onset of respiratory failure. A rapid respiratory rate also promotes further air-trapping, because of incomplete exhalation, and this accelerates inspiratory muscle dysfunction, weakness, and fatigue.

The intent of breathing training is to (1) restore the diaphragm to a more normal position and function, (2) control the respiratory rate and breathing pattern to diminish air-trapping, (3) decrease the work of breathing, and (4) allay patient dyspnea and anxiety.

* Laplace's law: $Pdi = Tdi/R$, where Pdi is the transdiaphragmatic pressure, Tdi is the trangential tension developed by the diaphragm and R is the radius of curvature of the diaphragm.

PURSED-LIP BREATHING

Pursed-lip breathing (PLB) is usually the easiest breathing technique to learn for patients with chronic airflow obstruction and is often employed instinctively by those who benefit from its use. Patients inhale through the nose over several seconds with their mouth closed, and then exhale slowly over 4 to 6 seconds through pursed lips held in a whistling or kissing position. This is done with or without contraction of the abdominal muscles during expiration. During this maneuver, no expiratory airflow occurs through the nose, because of involuntary elevation of the soft palate with total occlusion of the entrance to the nasopharynx.[5] Pursed-lip breathing should be employed during and following exercise and with any activity that makes the patient tachypneic or dyspneic. It is also useful in controlling panic attacks. Dyspnea is relieved almost immediately after PLB is begun.[6]

Only a few studies have investigated the physiologic responses to PLB, and as yet there is no full explanation of why dyspnea improves. Mueller and coworkers have noted a substantially increased tidal volume, (V_T) along with a reduced respiratory rate (RR) and minute ventilation. ($\dot{V}_E$), both at rest and during exercise following PLB training.[7] Those COPD patients with the greatest relief of dyspnea while employing PLB demonstrated the largest increases in V_T, together with the most marked falls in resting and exercise respiratory rate. Patients with and without symptomatic relief from PLB had a modest but significant improvement in PaO_2 during rest, but no arterial gas changes occurred in either group during exercise. Also noted was that the ventilatory equivalent for oxygen ($\dot{V}_E$)/$\dot{V}O_2$) fell with PLB during rest and exercise in all patients, solely because of a reduction in $\dot{V}_E$. The investigators concluded that inability of PLB to decrease the oxygen uptake ($\dot{V}O_2$) meant that this breathing method failed to improve the work of breathing. The anticipated fall in respiratory muscle oxygen consumption resulting from a decrease in $\dot{V}_E$ must have been offset by an increased work per breath consequent to the greater V_T and the added expiratory resistance of pursed lips.

Thoman and coworkers obtained similar results, with PLB increasing V_T while decreasing the respiratory rate.[8] Importantly, these workers also demonstrated that FRC fell insignificantly following PLB. This failure to reduce end-expiratory lung volume makes it unlikely that the improved dyspnea with PLB is related to restoration of the diaphragm to a higher position in the thorax or to a reduction in rib cage volume, with improved positioning of the intercostal muscles. Currently, there are no studies that have examined the specific effects of PLB on diaphragm or other respiratory muscle function.

Another recognized benefit of PLB is its inhibition of dynamic airway collapse during exhalation. Expiratory airway collapse often occurs in patients with chronic airways obstruction because of the loss of lung elastic recoil forces (as in emphysema) and diffuse airways narrowing. Such patients must actively employ their expiratory muscles during the expiratory phase of breathing. The positive pleural pressure created by a forced exhalation is transmitted to the collapsible intrathoracic airways, causing premature airway closure and expiratory flow limitation.

Ingram and Schilder devised an ingenious model of the interaction of PLB with lung mechanics, employing a rubber stopper with a 4-mm orifice to mimic the pursed-lips technique[9] (Fig. 23–1). A two-way valve always permitted a low inspiratory resistance and a low expiratory resistance, except when the obstructing stopper was inserted. Inspiratory and expiratory nonelastic resistance was measured with the stopper inserted or not inserted in 15 older men with COPD; eight of them experienced relief of dyspnea using true self-generated PLB and seven did not. The difference in expiratory nonelastic resistance across the lung, with and without the stopper in place, was the decrease in pulmonary resistance owing to the simulated pursed-lip technique. The effectiveness of this stopper system in diminishing nonelastic expiratory resistance was significantly greater in the eight men who gained relieve of dyspnea by true PLB, compared with those who claimed no benefit. The investigators concluded that those patients with dynamic airway collapse had improved symptoms of dyspnea with PLB, whereas those without dynamic airway collapse did not. Exactly how this maneuver relieves dyspnea remains uncertain.

Like Mueller and associates,[7] these workers calculated that, overall, the pursed-lip technique required more pressure for flow and volume change, so that expiratory and total respiratory work were actually increased. Like Thoman and coworkers, they found no reduction in lung volume at end-expiration to improve respiratory muscle position. Also, no present theory on the mechanism of dyspnea considers dynamic airway collapse as a possible cause. Higenbottam and Payne recently observed that there is reflex narrowing of the glottic chink in COPD patients, particularly during exhalation, which becomes more marked as 1-second forced expiratory volume (FEV_1) falls, further suggesting that expiratory narrowing of the upper respiratory tract favorably influences respiratory function as well as the sensation of dyspnea.[10] Although COPD patients who do not intuitively employ PLB can significantly increase their arterial oxygen saturation following properly taught but imposed PLB, such patients do not take to pursed-lip training naturally and appear to work harder while employing this technique, making it only transiently helpful.[11] For unclear reasons, PLB also

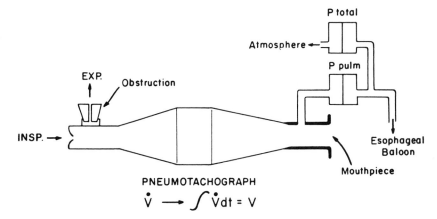

Figure 23–1. Diagram of the experimental apparatus. Volume (V) was obtained by electronic integration of flow ($\dot{V}$). The intraesophageal balloon catheter, used to estimate intrapleural pressure, connects to two separate pressure transducers. The other side of one transducer connects to a lateral oral pressure tap to give transpulmonary pressure to the airway opening (P pulm). The other side of the second transducer opens to atmospheric pressure to give total transpulmonary pressure (P total). P pulm was used to calculate nonelastic inspiratory and expiratory resistance across the lung (R pulm). (Ingram RH Jr, Schilder DP: Effect of pursed-lips expiration on the pulmonary pressure–flow relationship in obstructive lung disease. Am Rev Respir Dis 96:381–387, 1967, with permission)

reduces hyperventilation-induced bronchoconstriction in susceptible asthmatics and may play a role in attenuating exercise-induced asthma.[12]

HEAD-DOWN AND BENDING-FORWARD POSTURE

Respiratory physiologists have long known that the supine position, and even more so the head-down (Trendelenburg) and leaning-forward postures, often relieve dyspnea in COPD patients. These techniques could be used alone but were frequently combined with abdominal-breathing exercises and pursed-lips breathing to improve patients' dyspnea. Barach, over 30 years ago, noted that these positions appeared to alleviate dyspnea by reducing respiratory effort, and they were accompanied by a prompt decline in accessory respiratory muscle use.[1] He postulated that elevation of a depressed, flattened diaphragm by the upward (cephalad) shift in weight of the abdominal contents was responsible for these improvements. As an adjunct to these positions, physicians frequently utilized abdominal weights and binders, and even pneumoperitoneum to further elevate the diaphragm.[13] Fluoroscopy has confirmed that these positional changes will displace the diaphragm headward, and greater than 3-cm shifts have been observed in COPD patients[14] along with 6-cm shifts in normal persons.[15]

On the other hand, these positional changes have produced less dramatic effects on total diaphragmatic excursions. Barach and Beck recorded about a 2-cm increase in diaphragmatic excursion in COPD subjects during quiet respiration with a downward head tilt of 12° to 18°,[1] whereas Gayrard and associates, also using the head-down position both with and without abdominal weights, observed only negligible changes in diaphragmatic excursions, compared with excursions in the supine position during tidal breathing or with forced respiratory maneuvers.[14]

The head-down position, used infrequently, is achieved using a slant board (identical with that employed for postural drainage) or an equivalent device, such as foot blocks, to elevate the foot of the bed or a cot. Patients seem most comfortable when a 10° to 20° Trendelenburg position is employed. During the more commonly employed leaning-forward position, patients assume a posture with the trunk bent forward 20° to 45° from the vertical position. This posture can be used when seated or during walking. While seated, patients can support themselves by bracing their elbows or hands on

their knees or on a table. During walking, this posture can be taught or assisted by employing a walker or using a cane in both hands.

Improved mechanical efficiency of the diaphragm is probably responsible for the relief of dyspnea and physiologic benefit of the head-down and leaning-forward positions. Other physiologic gains have been minimal, except for a 20% reduction in $\dot{V}_E$ without deteriorating arterial blood gases recorded in two studies employing the head-down position.[1,16] Sharp and coworkers have identified those COPD patients who are most likely to benefit from these postures, and have also unraveled the physiologic basis of why the diaphragm functions more effectively and why dyspnea is reduced.[17] They recognized that the subgroup of COPD patients with paradoxic (inward) inspiratory motion of their anterior abdominal wall caused by passive ascent of the diaphragm in the standing and upright seated positions, experienced major relief of their dyspnea while in the leaning-forward position. About half of these patients also had relief of dyspnea while supine. Many times, simple observation of these patients' breathing patterns permitted detection of this inspiratory paradox.

In contrast with COPD subjects without paradoxic abdominal motion and with no postural relief of dyspnea, this subgroup had overinflated lungs with much higher TLC, FRC, and RV, causing greater depression of their diaphragms. Recordings of respiratory muscle electromyograms (EMGs), transdiaphragmatic pressures (p esophagus − p gastric), and thoracoabdominal diameters using magnetometers, showed that these COPD patients, when supine or when leaning forward while seated, switched to a normal outward abdominal motion during inspiration. Their inspiratory transdiaphragmatic pressures were higher during these positions, compared with when they were standing or sitting erect, because their inspiratory gastric pressures became more positive or less negative, indicating a partial restoration of diaphragmatic function. At the same time, EMG activity of their sternocleidomastoid and scalene muscles diminished significantly, signifying less accessory inspiratory muscular work. The COPD patients who had no decrease in their dyspnea with these postural changes did not manifest these physiologic benefits or demonstrated them to a smaller extent.

Subsequently, Druz and Sharp further elucidated the effects of various postures on respiratory muscle function with studies of electrical and mechanical activity of the diaphragm in eight normal persons and six COPD patients with markedly hyperinflated lungs.[18] In contrast with the normal subjects, the four COPD subjects who achieved postural relief of dyspnea in the supine and leaning-forward positions had a substantial fall in their ΔP_{di} (the inspiratory phasic range in transdiaphragmatic pressure) while standing or seated erect, indicating reduced diaphragmatic function. Like the normal subjects, they displayed a marked increase in their ΔE_{di} (the phasic inspiratory amplitude of their diaphragmatic EMG and an index of phrenic nerve activity), while in these positions. Therefore, the diminished mechanical output of their diaphragm in the standing and seated-erect postures resulted from a further unfavorable change in diaphragmatic configuration and muscle fiber length and was not due to reduced phrenic nerve activity. However, while supine or leaning forward, these four COPD postural responders displayed both a substantial decrease in their ΔE_{di} and an increase in their ΔP_{di} (Fig. 23–2). As a result, their neuromuscular efficiency index ($\Delta P_{di}/\Delta E_{di}$) increased significantly because of improved diaphragmatic contraction strength. The improved length–tension status of their diaphragm while supine or leaning forward permitted it to generate more pressure for a reduced neurogenic input. These changes, along with previously recognized declines in accessory respiratory muscle activity, probably account for the improved dyspnea these patients experienced. The two COPD patients who noted no postural relief of dyspnea had little improvement of their $\Delta P_{di}/\Delta E_{di}$ when supine or bent forward. In these patients, there was a slight increase of their Edi and Pdi in these positions. For unclear reasons, the reflex that attempts to stabilize the reciprocal relationship between transdiaphragmatic pressure change (ΔP_{di}) and change in diaphragmatic EMG (ΔE_{di}) was inoperative in this COPD subgroup. It should also be noted that all six COPD patients studied had a marked degree of hyperinflation, with low flat diaphragms seen on their chest radiographs. Similar studies in patients with chronic airflow obstruction but with less hyperinflation remain to be done.

An advantage of the leaning-forward posture during exercise is supported by the recent observations by Delgado and associates that dyspnea diminished and exercise tolerance improved during walking in the leaning-forward posture (at a 45° angle) in COPD patients who developed paradoxic diaphragmatic motion with upright exercise.[19] This improvement was accompanied by a return of normal chest wall–abdominal motion during breathing in one patient, and a shift to only partial inspiratory paradox in the second. Therefore, the

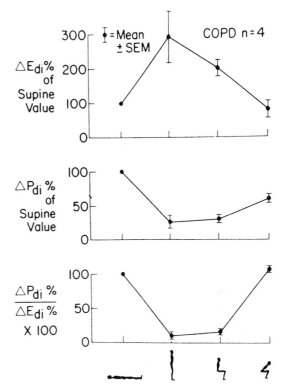

Figure 23—2. Data on four COPD patients in supine, standing, erect-sitting, and forward-leaning positions. (ΔE_{di} = inspiratory phasic change in the moving average integral of the diaphragmatic EMG; ΔP_{di} = inspiratory phasic change in the transdiaphragmatic pressure.) The $\Delta P_{di}\%/\Delta E_{di}\%$ ratio is an index of the efficiency of the diaphragm. (Druz WS, Sharp JT: Electrical and mechanical activity of the diaphragm accompanying body position in severe chronic obstructive pulmonary disease. Am Rev Respir Dis 125:275–288, 1982, with permission)

leaning-forward posture merits a trial during exercise as well as during inactivity, especially in patients with paradoxic breathing.

CONTROLLED SLOW, DEEP BREATHING

Patients with COPD often breathe shallowly and rapidly, and this pattern usually accelerates as they develop respiratory failure.[20] For several reasons, it would be physiologically beneficial for these patients to breathe slowly and deeply; resistive work and dead space ventilation would be less, and ventilation–perfusion relationships might improve through more equal distribution of inspired air during lengthier inhalations. Opening of previously closed basilar airways by deeper breaths should also be of benefit. As discussed earlier, tachypnea in COPD patients can also lead to progressive air-trapping with hyperinflation caused by inadequate expiratory time.

Two studies have examined the effects of slow, deep breathing on ventilation and gas exchange in patients with severe COPD, using an electronic respiration simulator to help reduce respiratory rate.[21,22] Both showed a significantly increased $\dot{V}_T$, but one demonstrated a significant decrease in $\dot{V}_E$[22] and the other a slight increase.[21] Both noted no major change in the work of breathing, with oxygen consumption slightly increased in one[21] and minimally reduced in the other.[22] Alveolar ventilation and ventilation–perfusion relationships were also relatively unaffected, with $PaCO_2$ and either PaO_2 or SaO_2 only modestly improved. In the study of Paul and coworkers, some patients actually complained that slow, deep breathing was tiring and uncomfortable, and all patients quickly returned to their normal breathing frequency after removing the breathing stimulus.[22] It seems unlikely, therefore, that voluntary-breathing control can initiate a permanent change in the normal automatic pattern of breathing.

Grassino and coworkers have recently formulated an explanation of why COPD patients do not spontaneously breathe more slowly and deeply.[23] They monitored several indices of muscle fatigue in five COPD patients during normal resting breathing and during an imposed breathing pattern with an increased V_T, a slow respiratory rate, a prolonged inspiratory phase, and a brisk exhalation. They watched for changes in transdiaphragmatic pressure (P_{di}) with time,* the ratio of high-frequency/low-frequency diaphragmatic EMG components (H/L),† and the diaphragmatic tension–time index (TT_{di}).‡ The $\dot{V}_E$ was always maintained at the resting level. After only a 6- to 10- minute trial, the slow deep-breathing pattern caused clear-cut diaphragmatic fatigue, characterized by a progressive fall in mean P_{di} from about 25 cmH_2O to about 16 cmH_2O (solely from a decrease in gastric- or dia-

---

* P_{di} = P esophagus − P gastric

† EMG recordings of diaphragmatic activity are passed through two band-pass filters to isolate the high-frequency (about 100 to 600 Hz) and low-frequency (approximately 10 to 40 Hz) components. As diaphragmatic fatigue develops, a characteristic change occurs in the frequency spectrum of the EMG, with a decrease in the higher-frequency components and an increase in its low-frequency components. As a result, the high-frequency/low-frequency ratio (H/L) falls as an early indicator of diaphragmatic fatigue.

‡ The TT_{di} is calculated as the product of two ratios, the mean transdiaphragmatic pressure per breath/maximum static transdiaphragmatic pressure (P_{di}/P_{dimax}) and the inspiratory time/total respiratory cycle time (T_i/T_t). It represents the time integral of the transdiaphragmatic pressure swing.

phragmatic-induced pressure), a fall in H/L to 70% of control EMG levels, and an increased TT_{di} to an average of 0.17 (fatigue occurs when TT_{di} approaches or exceeds 0.15 to 0.18).

It appears obvious that this breathing pattern is unsatisfactory because it fatigues the diaphragm. It is apparent that slow, deep breathing will help COPD patients only when it is a by-product of another breathing technique, such as pursed-lip breathing or diaphragmatic-breathing training. On the other hand, patients should be taught to avoid the tendency to breathe rapidly, with its propensity for air-trapping during anxious times or when they become frightened, often by dyspnea.

DIAPHRAGMATIC-BREATHING EXERCISES AND ALLIED MANEUVERS

Early investigators emphasized the importance of diaphragmatic-breathing exercises in the management of patients with obstructive lung disorders. Many echoed Barach's belief that a "change from an upper thoracic to a predominantly diaphragmatic respiration is the single most valuable contribution of the various physiologic methods employed to improve the mechanics of breathing."[24] In contrast, although patients often claim clinical improvement and reduced dyspnea with this method, physiologic studies have shown inconclusive and conflicting results of its effectiveness. Therefore, the prescription of this technique should not be an arbitrary or fixed decision, but requires close clinical monitoring to assess its efficacy. If a patient fails to experience clinical improvement, with less dyspnea or an increased work tolerance, after a reasonable trial of properly performed diaphragmatic breathing, this treatment approach should be discontinued.

Although any patient with obstructive lung disease can be taught breathing exercises, they appear most helpful to patients with hyperinflated lungs and depressed, flattened diaphragms who have pulmonary emphysema as a major component of their lung disease. Such persons often respond poorly to other treatment modalities.

Inspection of a patient's breathing pattern, along with palpation of the lower thorax and upper abdomen, is usually adequate to assess if he or she is using the respiratory muscles correctly and effectively. Accessory neck muscle use, predominantly upper chest wall expansion, together with inward movement of the lower ribs, and failure of the abdomen to distend on inspiration (or paradoxically move inward), all signify diaphragmatic dysfunc-

Table 23—1   Instructions for Diaphragmatic Breathing

1. Diaphragmatic exercises should be preceded by an inhaled bronchodilator, if a patient has reversible airway obstruction, and by postural drainage or controlled cough, or both, if airway secretions are a major problem. Patients should employ O_2 if on home O_2 therapy.
2. Patient lies supine or tilted 15° to 25° in head-down position.
3. Patient places dominant hand on upper midabdomen and the nondominant hand on the upper anterior chest. This permits monitoring of an inspiratory outward motion of the abdomen while minimizing chest excursions. The patient relaxes the chest wall and accessory respiratory muscles.
4. Patient breathes more slowly and deeply, inspiring through the nose and expiring slowly with pursed lips. A conscious effort is made to employ only the diaphragm during inspiration and to maximize abdominal protrusion. The anterior abdominal wall muscles are consciously contracted during inspiration to facilitate diaphragmatic movement and to improve lower rib cage expansion.
5. Patient can employ abdominal wall muscle contraction during expiration to displace the diaphragm more cephalad. An 8 to 10 lb abdominal weight placed on or strapped to the lower abdomen can also be used to assist this activity.
6. Once mastered lying down, the same exercises should be repeated sitting and, later, standing in a forward-leaning posture.

(Faling LJ: Pulmonary rehabilitation—physical modalities. Clin Chest Med 7:599–618, 1986 with permission)

tion. Such findings help identify patients who might benefit the most from diaphragmatic breathing instruction. This breathing technique requires conscious patient effort, and it has never been documented to become an automatic function.

Breathing training should be initiated by a specialist in this technique. The appropriate maneuvers are easily taught to most patients, but the technique can be difficult for some, especially those with the most depressed and poorly functioning diaphragms. Specific instructions for diaphragmatic breathing are recorded in Table 23–1. Once they have learned diaphragmatic breathing, patients should practice these exercises for at least 30 minutes, two to three times daily, and after mastering it in the supine or Trendelenburg (head-down) position, they should learn it while sitting, and finally while standing, walking, and during daily-living activities. Diaphragmatic breathing is frequently combined with pursed-lip exhalation and the leaning-forward position to attain maximum symptomatic benefit. Bimanual compression of lower ribs and the upper subcostal abdomen beginning in midexhalation can also be performed by patients to maximize expiratory ascent of the diaphragm. However, this practice, like the use of a mechanical chest compressor,[25] is impractical and rarely used today.

The results of six studies that assessed the extended benefits of breathing exercises in obstruc-

tive lung disease patients are shown in Table 23–2.[2,26–30] Supervised breathing instruction was provided to all patients, although the prescribed exercises varied somewhat among patient groups. Patients performed their breathing exercises several times daily in most studies, although Miller's patients exercised four to six times daily.[31] Clinical or physiologic assessment was performed before and after a variable period of training; reassessment varied from about 2 weeks to 1 year after beginning the exercise program, with most programs having a duration of 1 to 3 months. Assessment consisted of clinical evaluation alone in one study,[26] physiologic testing only in three,[2,28,30] and both clinical and physiologic studies in two.[27,29] A wide range of physiologic studies were employed.

Although substantial clinical benefit was observed in most patients in the three studies that employed clinical evaluation, betterment of pulmonary function indices was inconsistent, with Miller alone showing statistically significant changes in multiple tests.[2] He recorded significant improvement in forced expiratory flow, lung volumes, ventilatory parameters, and arterial blood gases. All the other investigators who assessed pulmonary function changes[27–30] concluded that diaphragmatic breathing failed to provide significant long-term benefit to pulmonary function. As a result, Becklake commented that ". . . benefit claimed by the subject was more likely to be the result of his men-

Table 23–2 Benefits of Breathing Exercises in Patients with Obstructive Lung Disease

REF.	PATIENT POPULATION	NO. OF PATIENTS	BREATHING TECHNIQUE	TIME TECHNIQUE EMPLOYED	MEASUREMENT MADE	IMPROVEMENT
Livingstone et al[26]	Asthma	75	Asthma Research Council[156] Emphasize lung expiration to elevate diaphragm For 10 minutes 2–3x/day	1 year	Clinical assessment	52/75 had excellent, very good, or much improved status.
Becklake et al[27]	Emphysema (± bronchitis, asthma)	10	Prolong expiration; improve diaphragmatic movement; general relaxation 2x/day	mean 24 days, range 13–46 days	Subjective improvement, VC, TLC, FRC, RV, MBC, SaO_2	8/10 moderate to marked subjective improvement. Only 1 patient showed improvement of multiple physiologic tests. Average % change of all tests considered insignificant
Miller[2]	Obstructive bronchitis; asthmatic bronchitis; bronchiectasis	24	Diaphragmatic training as per Asthma Research Council[156] and Miller[31] 4–6x/day	6 weeks to 2 months	(Rest only) maxiumum diaphragmatic excursion, RR, V_T, $\dot{V}_E$, FVC, FEV_3, MBC, IC, ERV, MEP, SaO_2, $PaCO_2$, pHa, Hct	(Rest only) Significant ↑ max. diaphragmatic excursion, V_T, IC, FVC, FEV_3, MBC, MEP, SaO_2, and pHa. Significant ↓ RR, $PaCO_2$, and Hct
McNeill et al[28]	Asthma Bronchitis	33 (17 completed exercises)	Asthma Research Council[156] 2x/day	1–3 months	EFR 40 ($FEV_{0.25} \times 40$)	Improvement in 11 patients, worsening in 6; mean improvement for group was 4% (not significant)

Study	Disease	N	Method	Duration	Tests	Results
Sinclair[29]	Emphysema (± asthma, bronchitis)	22	Reed[157] (emphasize abdominal–diaphragmatic breathing) Taught daily to weekly	3 to 14 weeks (mean 8.1 weeks)	Clinical assessment. Maximum diaphragmatic excursion, VC, TLC, FRC, RV, MBC, $\dot{V}_E$, Alveolar $N_2\%$, SaO_2 (all tests not made in all subjects)	Slight increases in VC, MBC, $\dot{V}_E$, SaO_2, and max. diaphragmatic excursion (none significant for entire group). Slight decreases in RV, TLC, Alv $N_2\%$ (none significant for entire group); 5 patients had appreciable improvement of PFTs; 7 claimed marked clinical improvement; 7 moderate improvement; and 8 unchanged
Campbell et al[30]	Emphysema	12	Reed[157] Taught 3x/week for 4–6 weeks	Immediate effects after instruction; long-term effects after 3 months	*Acute Effects* V_T, RR, $\dot{V}_E$, He mixing efficiency, $\dot{V}_{O_2}$, slow space/FRC *Long-term effects* Lung volumes, MBC; He mixing efficiency	*Acute* ↑V_T, ↓RR, ↓$\dot{V}_E$; $\dot{V}_{O_2}$, He mixing efficiency and slow space/FRC were unchanged. *Long-term* No change in lung volumes, He mixing efficiency, or MBC

VC, vital capacity; TLC, total lung capacity; FRC, functional residual capacity; RV, residual volume; MBC, maximum breathing capacity; SaO_2, oxygen saturation; RR, respiratory rate; V_T, tidal volume; $\dot{V}_E$, minute ventilation; FVC, forced vital capacity; FEV_3, forced expired volume in 3 seconds; IC, inspiratory capacity; ERV, expiratory reserve volume; MEP, maximum expiratory pressure; $PaCO_2$, arterial partial pressure of carbon dioxide; pHa, arterial pH; EFR_{40}, forced expiratory flow at 0.25 seconds of a forced vital capacity × 40; alveolar $N_2\%$, intrapulmonary gas-mixing efficiency as percentage alveolar nitrogen after 7 minutes of O_2 breathing; He, helium; $\dot{V}_{O_2}$, oxygen consumption; slow space/FRC, poorly ventilated space/functional residual capacity (%) (determined from helium breathing). (Faling LJ: Pulmonary rehabilitation—physical modalities. Clin Chest Med 7:599–618, 1986, with permission)

tal attitude than of true physical improvement."[27] The explanation of why Miller's patients achieved significant pulmonary function improvement is not certain, but may be due to his more comprehensive training regimen and his requirement that patients "practice prodigiously" (at least four to six times a day).[31] Although overall improvement in lung function was not significant in the other studies, most noted that a few of their subjects improved considerably. Sinclair had five such patients,[29] McNeill and McKenzie three,[28] and Becklake and coworkers one.[27] It is apparent that some patients will be helped by breathing training; however, no common factor that will permit early recognition of responders has been identified. Only Miller studied the long-term effects of breathing training on a number of physiologic indices following exercise; however, the amount of exercise was limited to 1 minute of one-step climbing.[2] When compared with postexercise studies before training, he noted a significant rise in SaO_2 values and oxygen removal per liter of ventilation, together with a significant decline in $PaCO_2$ values, indicating improved alveolar ventilation and alveolar gas exchange. Those patients with a maximum breathing capacity (MBC) > 40% of predicted (indicating less severe disease) also had a reduced ventilatory requirement, with a decrease in their exercise minute ventilation. On the other hand, patients with more severe disease (MBC < 40% of predicted) had an unfavorable response, with an increase in their postexercise minute ventilation needs.

The immediate consequences of diaphragmatic training have been assessed for its influence on ventilatory indices, on inspiratory gas distribution, and on chest wall mechanics. Campbell and Friend (see Table 23–2) observed that the early effects of diaphragmatic-type breathing included a major decline in respiratory rate and $\dot{V}_E$, along with an increased V_T and "an increasedly expiratory position" (reduced FRC).[30] Willeput and coworkers made similar observations.[32] These changes were precisely the same as those observed with slow, deep-breathing and pursed-lip respiration. Several other groups have also recorded falls in respiratory rate and increases in V_T; however, $\dot{V}_E$ and FRC were unchanged.[33,34]

Theoretically, diaphragmatic breathing should locally alter the configuration of the chest wall and create a greater pleural pressure swing at the base of the lung than at its apex. This shift from a constant pleural pressure gradient down the lung should cause a further preferential delivery of inspired gas to the more compliant lung bases and, thereby, improve ventilation–perfusion relationships. Nevertheless, in COPD patients, three studies that evaluated this possibility, with use of nitrogen washout curves or inhaled or intravenous ^{133}Xe, were unable to confirm any alteration in the distribution of ventilation when comparing diaphragmatic with conventional breathing.[33–35] This was true even though Sackner and associates, using strain gauges, recorded larger abdominal excursions with diaphragmatic breathing,[34] and Grimby and coworkers, employing magnetometers, demonstrated that the contribution of the abdomen to ventilation increased from 40% to 67% with this breathing technique.[33] All patients had received professional instruction in diaphragmatic breathing and were judged to be highly skilled in this modality. Patients performed while seated and breathed from either residual volume (RV)[34] or FRC.[33,35]

With one important exception, studies of diaphragmatic breathing in *normal* humans have also produced disappointing results. Several studies, in 38 normal persons, that examined nitrogen washout curves,[36] the distribution of an inhaled bolus of ^{133}Xe[34,37], or ^{133}Xe washout curves,[35] found that diaphragmatic breathing only infrequently increased ventilation to the lung bases. Subjects were evaluated in both the erect seated[34–36] and supine positions[37] and inhaled from RV[34,36] or FRC.[34,35,37] Of Shearer and coworkers' 15 normal young subjects, only two expert physical therapists were able to preferentially direct an inspired nitrogen bolus to their lower lung zones when they breathed in from RV.[36] On the other hand, Roussos and associates have convincingly demonstrated that abdominal (diaphragmatic) inspiration in nine normal persons could enhance distribution of inspired gas to dependent lung zones.[38] When inhaling either ^{133}Xe or helium at FRC, these normal subjects could preferentially "steer" the inspired gas to their lung bases in the upright, supine, and lateral decubitus positions after inhaling either small boluses or a larger tidal volume of the tracer at a constant low inspiratory flow (<0.5 L/sec). In a similar fashion, they could redirect inspired gas to upper lung zones when they selectively employed intercostal breathing. Why the results of this study are at such variance with other published reports in normal subjects is not readily apparent. Unfortunately, Roussos and his coworkers have not repeated these studies in COPD patients; thus, it remains uncertain if diaphragmatic-breathing testing in their laboratory might enhance basilar lung ventilation in this group (Roussos, personal communication).

Sackner and associates[39] and Willeput and

coworkers[32] studied the effects of diaphragmatic breathing on thoracoabdominal motion in COPD patients. Sackner et al. monitored separate rib cage and abdominal movement in the supine and upright positions with use of respiratory inductive plethysmography, whereas Willeput et al. examined these movements in seated subjects with magnetometers. Both groups discovered that diaphragmatic breathing gave rise to increased asynchronous* and paradoxic† motion between the rib cage and abdomen. Willeput et al. found these changes almost exclusively for the rib cage, with a paradoxic expiratory outward movement in 9 to 11 patients. Sackner et al., calculating inspiratory and expiratory asynchrony indices to quantitatively assess discoordination between the rib cage and abdomen, noted that both were increased in supine COPD subjects during abdominal (diaphragmatic), compared with normal breathing. Paradoxic rib cage motion during inspiration and expiration was also increased, but resolved when patients were returned to an upright posture. Both Willeput et al. and Sackner et al. concluded that these chest wall effects of diaphragmatic breathing would cause distortion of the rib cage and abdominal compartments away from their relaxation characteristics, thereby increasing patients' work of breathing. In this sense, diaphragmatic breathing in COPD patients is probably less mechanically efficient than natural breathing.

In conclusion, the long- and short-term benefits of diaphragmatic-breathing exercises remain uncertain. Although clinical benefit is sometimes apparent, this could represent a placebo effect, and only a few investigators have recorded physiologic alterations that appear beneficial. Further investigation is needed to fully justify the use of this technique as an effective modality in the management of COPD patients and to explain why some COPD patients appear to benefit clinically from its use.

CHEST PHYSICAL THERAPY

NORMAL RESPIRATORY MUCUS AND CLEARANCE OF MUCUS

The mucociliary system of the lung is responsible for normal airway mucous transport and comprises ciliated epithelial cells covered by a thin layer of mucus. This system protects the airways by trapping and eliminating a wide range of inhaled materials, including dusts, chemical vapors, and microorganisms. On the other hand, abnormalities of ciliary function or conditions that markedly increase the production of mucus can disable this system, causing mucous impaction of airways and impairing essential gas exchange. Obstructive atelectasis and bronchopulmonary suppuration often occur in this setting.

The ciliary apparatus consists of ciliated epithelial cells that extend from the nose to the respiratory bronchioles. These cells progressively increase in proportion to other airway surface cells at higher levels of the bronchial tree, with a ciliated cell/goblet cell ratio in the trachea of about 4:1 to 5:1. Each ciliated cell projects 200 to 250 cilia, with each cilia in the trachea having a 5 to 7-mm length, which becomes shorter toward the lung periphery. The ciliary beat frequency is also faster in the larger airways (between 8 and 15 Hz).[40] The airway cilia beat in one plane with a fast power stroke directed toward the upper respiratory tract, and a slower recovery stroke.[41] Groups or fields of cilia normally beat in the same upward direction in coordinated waves, and, although many groups of cilia may display slightly different directions of beat and wave movement, the net result is the steady flow of mucus toward the pharynx.[41] To prevent a "log-jamming" effect from mucus converging from the many smaller airways, mucous transport velocity progressively increases from the small to the large airways, with a speed of 4–10 mm/min in the trachea of normal nonsmokers.[42]

The volume of tracheobronchial secretions in normal persons has been estimated to range from 10 to 100 mL/day.[43] This material is the product of numerous cells lining the airways, including Clara cells, goblet cells, plasma cells (producing immunoglobulins), and the serous and mucous cells of the submucosal glands. Although goblet cells extend throughout the bronchial tree to the level of the alveolar ducts, submucosal glands are present only in cartilaginous airways, whereas Clara cells reside in the bronchioles and terminal conducting units.[40,41,43] However, normal submucosal gland cells outnumber goblet cells by about 40:1 and, overall, produce considerably more mucus.[43] The function of the Clara cell is less certain, but it appears to contribute to the bronchiolar periciliary fluid.[41]

The airway mucus is 2- to 5-mm thick,[43] and lines the airways in a continuous fashion from alveoli to the tracheolaryngeal juncture. It consists of a

---

* *Asynchronous:* a difference in rate of change of rib cage and abdominal compartmental excursions during tidal breathing.

† *Paradoxic:* opposite movement of one compartment (rib cage or abdomen) during tidal breathing.

basilar, nonviscous serous layer (the *sol*) that surrounds the airway cilia, as well as a discontinuous upper mucous layer, with viscoelastic properties (the *gel*), with which the tips of cilia interact. It is the gel layer that is propelled mouthward by the cilia. The viscosity and elasticity of mucus are mainly attributed to mucoglycoproteins, a heterogeneous family of extremely large acidic macromolecules, the basic structure of which is a highly glycosylated protein core.[43] It is the disulfide crosslinkages between these glycoprotein subunits, along with physical entanglements of these molecules, that give the gel its rheologic properties.[44] A change in these viscoelastic properties that is outside an optimal range can impair ciliary function and, therefore, mucociliary clearance.[40]

In normal persons, cough is a reserve clearance mechanism only and is employed during emergency situations, such as following the accidental aspiration of liquids or solids, or during lower respiratory tract infections, when the capacity of the normal mucociliary apparatus to clear mucus is temporarily exceeded.

ABNORMAL MUCOCILIARY CLEARANCE AND COUGH

Many factors and conditions adversely affect mucociliary transport and may cause retention and stasis of airway secretions (Table 23–3). They do this by increasing the production of mucus, altering its physical properties, impairing ciliary function, destroying ciliated epithelial cells, and by various combinations of these disturbances. It is quite apparent that many of these situations, either alone or in combination, are present in hospitalized and ambulatory patients with a variety of pulmonary disorders.

Although bronchiectasis has become an infrequent pulmonary disease, chronic obstructive lung disease caused by chronic bronchitis and emphysema is by far the most common chronic lung condition in adults. Many of these patients continue to smoke. They have increased sensitivity to air pollutants as well as to common respiratory tract viruses and other airway pathogens. Status asthmaticus continues to be a potentially lethal complication of asthma in both adults and children, and diffuse airway plugging by mucus is characteristic in this setting. Other than asthma, cystic fibrosis (CF) is the most frequently seen chronic lung disorder in pediatric patients, and many of these children are now living to young adulthood. The severity of their lung disease necessitates frequent hospitalization

Table 23–3 Factors That Can Adversely Affect Mucociliary Function

Airway disorders
  Asthma
  Chronic bronchitis
  Bronchiectasis
  Allergic bronchopulmonary aspergillosis (ABPA)
Congenital defects
  Cystic fibrosis
  Primary ciliary dyskinesia syndrome
  Young's syndrome
  Hypogammaglobulinemia
Medications
  Narcotics
  Ethyl alcohol
  Atropine
  Acetylsalicylic acid (aspirin)
  β-Adrenergic antagonists
Inhaled and intravenous anesthetics
Acute respiratory tract infections
  Mycoplasma pneumoniae
  Influenza virus
  Other airway viruses
  Acute bacterial bronchitis
Physical mechanisms
  Hyperoxia
  Dehydration
  Low humidity
  Hypercapnia
  Tracheal intubation
  Tracheal suctioning
Cigarette smoke
Air pollutants
  Sulfur dioxide
  Nitrogen dioxide
  Ozone
Other gases and aerosols
  Ammonia, chlorine
  Hydrochloric acid, sulfuric acid
  Formaldehyde, hydrogen sulfide
  Cyanide, smoke inhalation
Lung transplantation
Increasing age
Sleep
Blood and tissue factors
  Serum
  Complement factors (C3a, C5a)
  Neutrophil elastase
  Monocyte-derived mucus secretagogue
  Mast cell products (histamine, prostaglandins [A_2, D_2, E_1, F_2a] and leukotrienes [C_4, D_4])

as well as intensive outpatient care. Persons with acute smoke inhalation are exposed to multiple noxious gases and particulates that damage the airway mucosa and stimulate production of mucus. Protracted bronchorrhea may occur, and some patients go on to develop irreversible bronchiectasis.[45]

In surgical patients, mucociliary function is jeopardized by intubation, general anesthesia, and the narcotics used for postoperative pain control. In cardiothoracic surgery, lobectomy or pneumonectomy can lead to secretion stasis and temporary dysfunction of unresected lung, and cardiac surgery may impair left phrenic nerve activity, with resultant left lower lobe atelectasis.[46] In addition, unilateral lung transplantation for pulmonary fibrosis and combined lung–heart transplantation are rapidly becoming accepted procedures, and transection of a major airway with an end-to-end anastomosis can decrease mucociliary clearance for periods of up to a month or longer.[47] Denervation of the lungs following transplantation may be permanent, and the resulting anesthesia of the bronchi prevents patients from sensing secretions in their airways.[48]

Many patients within intensive care units require prolonged tracheal intubation and high concentrations of inhaled oxygen, often with suboptimal airway humidification. Such persons may also need frequent tracheal suctioning, which damages the airway mucosal surface, and are given multiple medications potentially harmful to mucociliary function, including narcotics, salicylates, and β-adrenergic blockers.[40,47] The airways of patients with the adult respiratory distress syndrome (ARDS) are exposed to serum exudates, complement factors, neutrophil elastases, and various prostaglandin and leukotriene products of arachidonic acid metabolism; these substances all have been demonstrated to stimulate airway mucous secretion.[42,43] During sleep, mucociliary clearance is significantly less than during the awake state,[49] and many patients with acute and chronic lung disorders require greater assistance to clear their respiratory tract secretions immediately after awakening.

Patients may have impaired cough for a number of reasons. Those with muscle weakness or paralysis may not be able to generate the high intrapleural pressures required for effective cough, and persons with pain on breathing, as a result of surgery or trauma, are often unwilling to cough. Following upper abdominal surgery, cough is also impaired by a period of diaphragmatic dysfunction.[50] Individuals with disorders of airflow limitation have impaired cough because maximum expiratory flow rates are often substantially reduced. Dynamic airways collapse may occur farther upstream (closer to alveoli) in airways with a greater cross-sectional area, reducing exhaled air velocity and shear forces. Increased airways collapse may totally occlude airways impeding mucous clearance, and abnormal mucus with altered viscoelastic properties is more difficult to expel.[51]

GOAL OF CHEST PHYSICAL THERAPY

The goal of chest physical therapy (PT) is to facilitate removal of excess or retained airway secretions and thereby reduce resistance to airflow, improve pulmonary gas exchange, and decrease the frequency of bronchial infection. In addition, atelectasis may be prevented or, if already present, corrected. Techniques used in chest PT include postural drainage, chest percussion, vibration, directed cough, and the forced expiration technique (FET). Chest PT is employed in hospitalized patients with a variety of pulmonary disorders and to reduce postoperative complications, as well as in ambulatory patients with chronic airways disorders characterized by mucous hypersecretion such as cystic fibrosis, bronchiectasis, and chronic bronchitis.

DEFINITION OF TECHNIQUES

Postural drainage (PD) uses gravity to help drain the airways of individual lung lobes and segments. The specific positions used for PD are shown in Figure 23–3. The Trendelenburg (head-down) position with varying degrees of rotation is generally employed, with a drainage angle between 10° and 45°, except for the upper lobes, which are drained with the patient upright or flat. Whereas large angles are often poorly tolerated by many patients with severe airways obstruction, patients with COPD were shown to have negligible alterations in lung volumes and had no decline in arterial oxygen saturation when evaluated in as much as a 25° head-down tilt.[52] In patients with a predominantly unilateral lung disorder, positioning the "good" lung in the down position will improve oxygenation, but caution must be taken to make certain that drainage from the uppermost diseased lung does not gravitate to the dependent "normal" lung and jeopardize it.

To create the various PD positions, patients can employ a tilt board (such as an ironing board) or tilt a bed or cot. Patients can also successfully and

(text continues on p. 640)

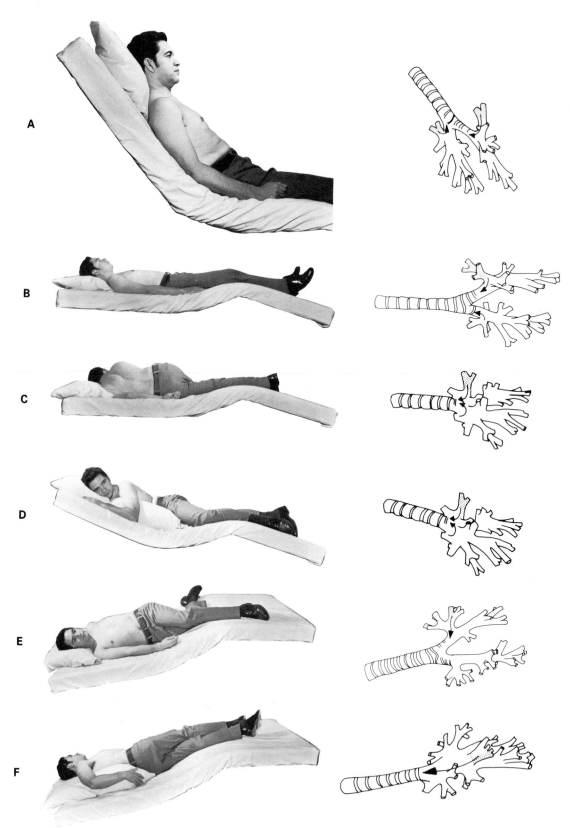

Figure 23–3. Postural drainage positions for specific pulmonary segments. (A) Left and right upper lobes (apical segment); (B) left and right upper lobes (anterior segments); (C) right upper lobe (posterior segment); (D) left upper lobe (posterior segment); (E) left upper lobe (lingular segment); (F) middle lobe of right lung;

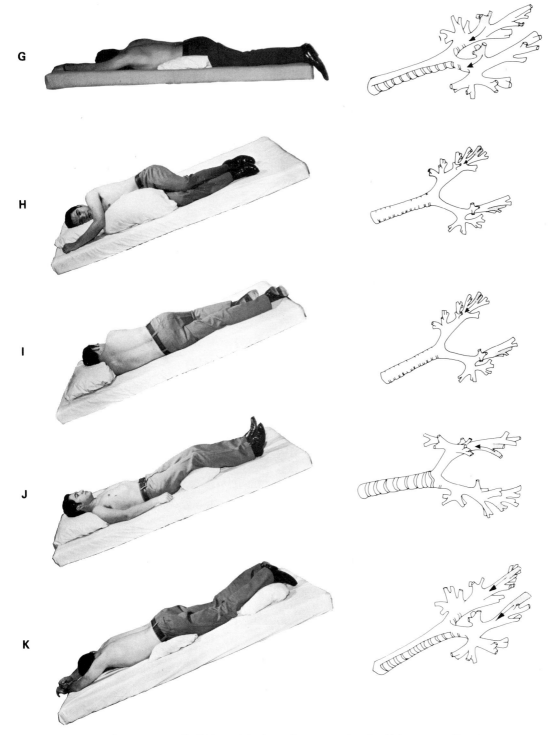

Figure 23–3 (continued) (*G*) lower lobe (superior segment), patient lying prone with one pillow under abdomen; (*H*) left lower lobe (lateral basal segment); (*I*) left and right lower lobes (anterior basal segments); (*J*) left and right lower lobes (anterior basal segments); (*K*) left and right lower lobes (posterior basal segments).

comfortably employ pillows on a bed, couch, or on the floor to create the various PD positions. An inhaled bronchodilator can be given 10 to 20 minutes before beginning PD. A generous fluid intake (1–2 L/day) appears desirable, considering the adverse effects of dehydration on tracheal clearance in dogs, and its reversal by rehydration.[53] However, the beneficial effects of hydration on the viscoelastic properties of bronchial mucus, as well as on ease of expectoration, are more controversial.[54] Inhaled moisture from a nebulizer or humidifier is of value mostly in patients with a tracheostomy who have lost the "air-conditioning" function of their upper respiratory tract.

Postural drainage should be performed two to three times daily, with each total treatment lasting 30 to 45 minutes. Each position can be maintained for 5 to 10 minutes or even longer if secretion clearance is incomplete. Because airway secretions are retained during sleep, the technique is most helpful after awakening in the morning, and it can be increased in frequency during periods of increased sputum production. To prevent gastroesophageal reflux, nausea, or emesis, it seems prudent to delay head-dependent drainage for 1 to 2 hours after eating; this may be of even greater importance in patients receiving nasogastric tube feedings, because such tubes encourage reflux by impairing lower esophageal sphincter function. Controlled cough or the forced expiratory technique (FET) after a period of PD is considered essential to help clear bronchial secretions that have been directed to the large airways by PD.[55]

Lung sites requiring drainage are selected by a knowledge of the patient's underlying lung disorder, as determined from medical records and interviewing the patient's physician; by carefully auscultating the patient's thorax for coarse rales, wheezes, and diminished breath sounds caused by airway plugging; and by examining chest roentgenographs for evidence of focal or diffuse disease. Ambulatory patients quickly learn to use the drainage positions that benefit them the most.

Percussion, vibration, and shaking have been frequently employed during PD to loosen airway secretions. Percussion is administered by striking the rib cage throughout inspiration and expiration with cupped hands or by employing a mechanical percussor. A frequency of about 5 Hz is employed, and the technique is thought to transmit energy from the chest wall to the airways, loosening airway secretions from bronchial walls. Percussion is given by trained personnel or family members and is administered for 1 to 5 minutes over the portion of the chest that is draining. However, optimal force and duration of percussion remain unclear, and periods of percussion longer than 5 minutes appear justified if there is evidence of persistent secretions in the percussed lung zone. A thin towel or other suitable protection is draped over the percussed area in patients with sensitive skin and should probably be employed routinely in elderly persons whose skin is fragile. Caution is required in patients with severe osteoporosis or other bone disorders, and percussion should not be applied to the spine, sternum, or soft tissue overlying the kidneys or other vital organs.

Vibration is applied by exerting a downward pressure over a draining zone, using crossed hands (similar to that used in cardiopulmonary resuscitation) at a frequency of 10 to 15 Hz. When administered manually, it is most effective during exhalation. Mechanical vibrators can also be used, and they should be applied continuously during breathing at an ideal frequency of about 13 Hz.[56] Shaking (2 Hz) has also been applied to help loosen secretions, but these low-frequency movements are unlikely to provide additional benefit.[56]

Cough, either voluntarily or as a reflex, is an effective technique to remove excess mucus from the larger airways. By creating rapid expiratory flow rates at high lung volumes and by compressing and narrowing airways through the generation of large intrapleural pressures, high but transient air velocities approaching 200 to 250 m/sec can be attained in normal persons.[57] These high linear air flows generate large shear forces through a coupling of expired air with mucus that is adherent to airway walls; such shearing causes airway secretions to be expelled.

Whereas only large airways up to the sixth or seventh generation of branching are cleared by cough at high lung volumes, airways collapse extends upstream to smaller airways with cough at lower lung volumes, raising the possibility that cough under these circumstances might also propel mucus from small to larger central bronchi.[55] In a mechanical tracheal model, the clearance of mucus stimulants by artificial cough was increased linearly with the increasing depth of mucus.[51] This supports the clinical observation that cough is an ineffective method for clearing mucus from the airways of normal persons or persons with lung disease who do not have an excess of mucus production;[58] it seems that a critical depth of airway mucus is required before cough becomes beneficial. Cough is most effective in the upright or seated positions because higher cough pressures and flow rates can be generated in these positions, compared with other body positions.[59]

Because the "cleansing" action of cough in large airways occurs mostly during the first one or two coughs in a cough sequence,[60] and because frequent uncontrolled cough may induce fatigue, chest wall pain, and dyspnea, as well as worsen bronchospasm, controlled cough and the forced expiration technique (FET or huffing) have been advocated as constructive alternatives.[61] During controlled cough, patients are taught to inspire deeply, hold their breath for several seconds and then cough two or three times with their mouths open, without taking another breath. Manual self-compression of the upper abdomen may assist such coughing. Patients can then take another slow deep inhalation, preferably by breathing through their nose, and repeat the cough procedure. After performing this two or three times, patients should rest and breath normally for several minutes before repeating their controlled coughing.

The FET consists of one or two forced exhalations (but without glottic closure, as in cough) starting at midlung volume and continuing to low lung volume. This is followed by expectoration or a controlled cough at high lung volume to clear mucus from the central airways, and then a period of relaxed (preferably diaphragmatic) breathing. Patients can supplement FET by compressing the sides of their chest wall with a brisk adduction of their upper arms. The rationale for FET is that it causes less fatigue, is less likely to provoke bronchospasm, and produces less dynamic airways collapse than does a cough, because lower transpulmonary pressures are produced. It is also possible that this technique decreases cough-induced damage with focal ciliary impairment in flow-limiting airway segments.[62] Although most of the published studies on FET have dealt with patients with cystic fibrosis and bronchiectasis, this approach should also prove useful for the many COPD patients with mucous hypersecretion, and perhaps for other patients with conditions associated with abnormal mucociliary transport.

Another adjunct to cough is *positive expiratory pressure (PEP) physiotherapy*.[63] Theoretically, this represents another method for preventing dynamic expiratory closure of airways, while also increasing lung volume and perhaps directing air downstream to or behind airway secretions so that they can be more readily expelled. The technique is performed in the sitting position and can be carried out without assistance. The PEP setup employs either a face mask or a mouthpiece with nose clips, along with a one-way valve to which variable expiratory resistance is attached.[63] The system, including a pressure manometer, is commercially available. (Astromeditec, Denmark). A resistance is selected that provides a PEP level of 10 to 15 cmH_2O in midexhalation. The technique is employed for 5 to 15 breaths and is followed by the FET, with spontaneous cough as needed. The entire procedure can be repeated over 10 to 30 minutes.

ASSESSMENT OF THE VARIOUS COMPONENTS OF CHEST PHYSICAL THERAPY

There has been considerable recent interest in attempting to better understand how the various components of chest PT facilitate the clearance of mucus from the lung, and which of these components, alone or in combination, is the most important element of chest PT. However, the methods used to assess the efficacy of chest PT vary considerably and often have limitations. Improvement of patients' symptoms is important, but a major placebo effect limits the objectivity and reliability of this approach.

Determination of sputum volume is often inaccurate, because patients are known to frequently swallow sputum, and sputum volume often correlates poorly with physiologic disturbances in the obstructive airway disorders. A wide range of physiologic measurements, including tests of large and small airways function as well as arterial blood gas levels, have been recorded following chest PT, but specific tests vary considerably between studies, making comparisons difficult.

A reduction in the frequency of lower respiratory tract infections is one goal of chest PT, but there are no long-term studies assessing this possibility. The best technique to determine if chest PT improves bronchial clearance is the use of radioaerosol clearance studies. This method employs particles that are insoluble in lung fluids and are permanently tagged with a γ-emitting radionuclide, such as technetium-99m. After a controlled inhalation of the aerosol, frequent radiation monitoring of the chest permits measurements of initial deposition of the radioaerosol, as well as its progressive clearance out of the lungs. Ideally, clearance rates from both peripheral and central lung zones should be determined. However, peripheral distribution of inhaled particles is often impaired in patients with airways obstruction or with excess bronchial secretions, making clearance measurements in this zone difficult. Other variables that may confound the results include differences in particle size; the use of mono- or heterodispersed particles; the type, number, and location of scintillation detectors; and the degree of control of spontaneous cough during a study.[47] Cough itself is a highly effective means for clearing the larger airways. Thus, it is important to construct coughed-up sputum-corrected tracheobronchial clearance curves to quantitate the maximum contribution of mucociliary clearance or adjuvantive techniques, such as postural drainage, to the removal of deposited radioaerosol.[64] Another limitation of radioaerosol studies is that present methods have restricted their use to short-term trials in patients with stable respiratory disorders.

BENEFITS OF CHEST PHYSICAL THERAPY AND ITS VARIOUS COMPONENTS

The benefits of chest PT and its various components for sputum production and radioaerosol clearance from the lungs are shown in Table 23–4.[65] Comprehensive chest PT, including PD, cough, percussion, and vibration, has substantially increased sputum volume and radioaerosol clearance from both central and peripheral lung zones in stable patients with COPD[66,67] and in young adults with cystic fibrosis.[68] Of importance, these individuals, with rare exception, all produced large daily sputum volumes exceeding 30 mL/day and often greater than 100 mL/day. On the other hand, chest PT is thought to be much less useful in patients who expectorate little or no sputum.[69] Since comprehensive chest PT is time-consuming, burdensome to the patient, and requires the help of an assistant, a critical assessment of its components has been the subject of a number of recent investigations and reviews.[55,65,69]

With one exception,[70] radioaerosol studies of PD alone have shown enhanced lung mucous clearance. This was the case in 11 of 13 stable CF patients placed in a 25° head-down tilt,[71] as well as in eight heterogeneous patients with copious sputum production who either had bronchiectasis, CF, or chronic bronchitis.[72] Chopra and associates also showed that PD increased tracheal mucous velocity by 40% in normal dogs.[53] A study by Oldenburg and coworkers, with negative results in bronchitic patients, has been criticized because natural cough during PD was prohibited, and the patients were placed at a tilt angle of only 15°.[70]

The contribution of percussion and vibration to chest PT has become much less certain. In a study by Sutton and associates, percussion failed to improve central or peripheral bronchial clearance over PD alone.[72] This modality also failed to supplement the benefit of PD and cough in radioaerosol clearance studies of COPD patients by Wollmer and coworkers[73] and by Van der Schans and associates.[74] In addition, percussion failed to enhance re-

Table 23—4 Benefits of Chest PT and Its Components on Sputum Production and Lung Radioaerosol Clearance

TECHNIQUE	SPUTUM CLEARANCE	RADIOAEROSOL CLEARANCE	REF.
Complete chest PT	+	+	66, 67, 68
PD	−	+	53, 71, 72
PD	−	0	70
PC	+	0	72
PC	−	0	68, 73, 74
V	+	0	72
V	0	0	77
Cough	−	+	68, 70
Cough	+	+*	67
FET	+	+	61
FET and PD	+	+	61
FET and PD	+	−	85

* Increased central clearance only.

+, Increased clearance; 0, no benefit; −, not assessed.

Abbreviations: PD, postural drainage; PC, percussion; V, vibration; FET, forced expiration technique.

(Modified from Sutton PP: Chest physiotherapy: Time for reappraisal. Br J Dis Chest 82:127–137, 1988)

moval of lung radioactivity over PD alone in six young adults with CF.[68] Nevertheless, two of Wollmer's patients with the greatest sputum production did have substantially higher clearance rates when percussion was added to their treatment regimen.[73] Manual percussion may still be useful in this setting, as well as for the occasional patient who cannot cough or tolerate PD. Although mechanical percussors have been developed that allow many patients to do their own chest percussion, such devices are no more effective than manual percussion in generating sputum[75] and actually may worsen pulmonary function in some patients.[76]

Conventional chest vibration has not been as extensively evaluated as percussion, but Sutton et al., who used manual vibration and shaking together with PD,[72] and Pavia and coworkers, who used an electrically driven vibration pad with PD at a 45° tilt angle,[77] were unable to document a significant clearance advantage for chest vibration over PD alone in a mixed group of patients with bronchiectasis, chronic bronchitis, and CF, or in COPD patients who had difficulty raising sputum. However, the high vibrational frequency Pavia et al. used (41 ± 5.4 Hz) considerably exceeded the compression frequency that is thought to maximize tracheobronchial clearance of mucus.[56] On the other hand, Gross and coworkers have clearly demonstrated that high-frequency chest wall oscillation in dogs can substantially increase peripheral and central airway clearance of mucus with peak clearance at 13 Hz.[78] This frequency is in resonance with natural ciliary beat frequency, and it should augment ciliary beat amplitude. Oral high-frequency oscillation, in the same frequency range, failed to improve clearance in dogs,[79] but modestly enhanced it in normal persons[80] and in adults with CF.[81] This comfortable, simple technique can be self-administered and warrants further clinical trials.

Cough, especially controlled cough, and FET are now recognized as key elements in chest physical therapy and are easier to perform than the other PT maneuvers. Radioaerosol studies in patients with chronic bronchitis[70] and in those with CF[68] showed that controlled[70] or directed vigorous cough[68] accelerates both central and, to a lesser extent, peripheral lung clearance, and it does this as effectively as a comprehensive PT regimen.[68] Two nonradioaerosol studies that measured changes in sputum production and pulmonary function indicators also concluded that vigorous or directed cough was as beneficial as complete chest PT.[82,83] These findings are somewhat surprising, since

cough is thought to expel mucus primarily from central airways, but not from the lung periphery. This premise is supported by the radiotracer study by Bateman and coworkers that showed that comprehensive chest PT, but not cough, enhanced peripheral lung clearance in stable COPD patients, whereas both methods were equally effective in accelerating central clearance.[67] Sputum yield was also greater during chest PT than following cough,[67] and Lorin and Denning recorded the same finding while comparing cough with PD in a nonradioaerosol study in CF patients.[84] Although further investigation seems appropriate, controlled cough is clearly beneficial in removing excessive large airway secretions and, as discussed earlier, may also cleanse smaller airways when performed at low lung volume.

Sutton and coworkers have championed FET (or huffing) as preferable to directed coughing in clearing airway secretions. They showed that FET (plus natural cough) significantly enhanced whole-lung radioaerosol clearance in resting, upright patients with CF or bronchiectasis, whereas directed coughing did not.[61] However, FET *plus* postural drainage further enhanced pulmonary clearance and produced significantly more sputum than either FET or directed cough alone, in this group of patients. Sutton's belief that FET plus PD provides close to optimal chest PT is supported by the findings of Pryor and associates, who showed that FET plus self-administered PD cleared more sputum in less time than conventional PT that requires a therapist for assistance.[85] Controlled cough can be substituted for FET if patients dislike or are unable to perform this technique, whereas percussion or vibration may be added if patients produce copious sputum or if significant secretion retention persists. Because many patients find PD uncomfortable,[61,86] those with only mild to modest secretion excess can attempt a trial of FET with natural cough alone; however, they should be closely monitored to make certain their pulmonary status does not deteriorate on this regimen. A nebulized β-adrenergic bronchodilator just before chest PT will further significantly improve central and peripheral clearance of lung mucus, as well as enhance sputum expectoration in patients with obstructive lung disease and mucous hypersecretion, although the precise mechanism for this is not yet known.[87]

The use of a PEP mask or mouthpiece for chest PT has been studied only in patients with CF. Published treatment results up to now have been variable, with patients doing better,[88] worse,[63] or the same,[89] compared with standard chest PT. Because the PEP system is well accepted and allows independent treatment, it warrants a trial in older CF patients.

CHEST PHYSICAL THERAPY IN SPECIFIC LUNG DISORDERS

The various components of chest PT have been critically assessed in a number of lung disorders (such as bronchiectasis and CF), permitting a logical treatment approach. However, this has not been done for all lung diseases benefited by chest PT. In these conditions, chest PT is described in more general terms, including PD, percussion, and vibration, without a clear understanding of *which* chest PT components are most effective in a specific setting.

Chest Physical Therapy in Patients with Chronic Obstructive Lung Disease

Stable Disease. Chest PT in stable COPD patients promotes an immediate increase in sputum expectoration volume, greatest in patients who produce the largest amount of daily sputum before treatment. All five studies that have recorded changes in sputum volume or weight[66,67,90-92] observed an increased sputum production during, or immediately following, chest PT, except Mohsenifar and coworkers who noted no sputum increase (all but one patient produced less than 5 mL of sputum during chest PT).[92] Similarly, chest PT in stable COPD patients enhanced clearance of mucus from central and, to a lesser extent, peripheral lung zones, based on radiotracer studies.[66,67] It appeared that PD and cough were both required to maximize this effect.

Chest PT in stable COPD patients has had much less benefit on pulmonary function indicators. Of the five studies that measured pulmonary function changes,[70,90-93] only Feldman and coworkers noted significant improvement following a regimen of PD, percussion, vibration, and cough;[93] however, this benefit was limited to flows at low lung volume, that is, after 75% of the FVC has been exhaled ($\dot{V}max_{25\%}$; usually called $\dot{V}max_{75\%}$), indicating some improvement of small airways function, with no improvement of FEV_1, and a transient fall in peak expiratory flow rate (PEFR). The other studies noted no significant change in a range of functions, including arterial blood gases, spirometric indices (FVC, FEV_1), and flows at high (PEFR, $FEF_{200-1200}$), and low ($FEF_{50\%}$, $FEF_{75\%}$, $FEF_{25\%-75\%}$) lung volumes. This lack of improvement may be due to a poor correlation of airway function (especially

large airway) with the quantity of sputum produced[70,90-93] and a need for longer-term PT, since pulmonary function improvement may lag considerably behind changes in sputum expectoration and bronchial clearance, perhaps because of difficulty in clearing small-airway secretions.

Acute Disease. The value of chest PT in acute COPD exacerbations is even more uncertain. In six studies,[73,94-98] chest PT produced little, if any, improvement of the indicators that were monitored. Except for a few cases of pneumonia,[97] these episodes were all an acute bronchitis. Both Anthonisen and coworkers[94] and Newton and associates[97] compared the course of acutely ill COPD patients managed either with conventional therapy alone (O_2, antibiotics, bronchodilators, diuretics) or by conventional treatment plus chest PT (Newton et al. also employed IPPB[97]). The duration of hospitalization[97] and temperature curves[94] were unaltered when compared with the control population who did not receive chest PT. There were also no significant differences in the course of arterial blood gas values,[94,97] spirometric indices,[97] and daily sputum volume,[94,97] except for a subgroup of men with initial mild hypoxemia ($PaO_2 > 60$ mmHg), who produced more sputum when treatment included chest PT and IPPB.[97] Both groups of investigators concluded that chest PT failed to improve conventional management of their acutely ill patients.

Three studies have evaluated the immediate effects of chest PT on either lung mechanics[95,96] or arterial gases[96,98] in COPD patients with an acute exacerbation. Whereas Newton et al. noted no improvement in FEV_1, vital capacity (VC), specific conductance (SGaw), or arterial blood gas values following a regimen of postural drainage, vibration, and chest percussion,[97] and Buscaglia and associates recorded a stable oxygen saturation with vigorous chest PT,[98] Campbell and coworkers actually observed a fall in FEV_1 in patients treated similarly.[95] This did not occur if chest percussion and vibration were omitted from their chest PT regimen.

Is chest PT ever beneficial in COPD patients with an acute bronchitic exacerbation? This remains uncertain, but patients who are producing large quantities of sputum may have an immediate benefit, given Campbell and coworkers' observation of an increased FEV_1 in one such patient[95] and Wollmer and coworkers discovery of greater radioaerosol clearance in two patients with very high sputum yield when percussion and PD were both administered.[73]

Bronchiectasis

Bronchiectasis is characterized by abnormal dilatation of airways associated with varying degrees of airway inflammation or infection, or both. This disorder may be focal in one segment or lobe or be bilateral and multilobar. Patients often expectorate large quantities of sputum, sometimes as much as a cup or more per day, and those with the diffuse form of the disorder often manifest substantial airways obstruction on pulmonary function testing. Tracheobronchial mucociliary clearance, as assessed by radioaerosol studies, is often markedly impaired,[99] and may be totally absent in patients with primary ciliary dyskinesia (the immotile cilia syndrome). Accordingly, chest PT has long been the cornerstone of therapy for bronchiectasis. Ideal treatment consists of self-administered PD and FET.[61] The addition of percussion or vibration further increases sputum production but does not improve tracheobronchial clearance.[72] On the other hand, an aerosolized β-agonist immediately before PD and FET substantially increases both sputum expectoration and lung clearance in bronchiectasis.[87] Family members can usually be taught to assist with chest PT if this becomes necessary, especially during acute exacerbations. Such therapy has achieved an immediate improvement in airflow obstruction in one study,[100] but not in another.[101] There was also no short-term improvement in oxygen saturation.[101] Although the long-term effects of chest PT on pulmonary function in bronchiectasis remain to be studied, clinical experience attests to its value in maintaining patients' functional capacity and limiting infectious exacerbations.

Cystic Fibrosis

Chest PT is an essential modality in the management of CF and should be administered throughout the lifetime of CF patients. Such treatment is responsible, in part, for the increased life expectancy of these children and young adults and may retard the development of severe airways obstruction, progressive bronchiectasis, and destructive respiratory tract infections caused by *Staphylococcus aureus*, *Pseudomonas aeruginosa*, and other bacterial pathogens. In addition to increasing airway clearance of mucus, short-term benefits of chest PT in CF include improvement in large[93,102] and small-airways function.[93]

Failure to administer chest PT for several weeks leads to deteriorating pulmonary function, which is reversible once PT is renewed.[103]

Although conventional chest PT, with an emphasis on PD, is the mainstay for managing infants and young children with CF, alternative methods, which may be self-administered, warrant a trial in older children and adults. Vigorous self-directed cough[68,82] and the FET[61] are both effective for removing pulmonary secretions in stable patients and are as efficacious as therapist-administered chest PT. Sleeping in the head-down position (20° tilt) further improves sputum expectoration in patients with copius secretions and may obviate the need for daytime PD if combined with FET.[104]

The frequency of treatments must be individualized, depending on the severity of CF, but, at a minimum, should be conducted at least on awakening in the morning and before sleep at night, even if the subject is well, with minimal or no sputum production. Supervised directed coughing, together with FET, has also been as beneficial as conventional PT for managing acute exacerbations of CF,[83] but it seems prudent to include traditional chest PT in this circumstance, since PD can augment the clearance benefit of FET in CF.[61]

Mechanical chest percussors have also been employed in CF patients,[75,105] but probably add nothing to the benefits of FET plus PD.[76] Mask positive expiratory pressure (PEP) can also enhance clearance of mucus in CF;[88,89] however, this technique can reduce the effectiveness of PD plus FET when combined with them.[63] Because these PT adjuncts are easy to apply, may shorten treatment sessions, and allow independent therapy, their value in CF warrants further study. All but the most disabled patients should be encouraged to engage in daily physical exercise, especially running and swimming; these techniques can be as effective as chest PT in clearing airway secretions.[106]

Asthma

There is no evidence supporting the use of chest PT in the management of asthma.[69] Even in acute asthma and status asthmaticus, pharmacologic treatment with bronchodilators and corticosteroids is the keystone of therapy. Nevertheless, occlusion of large and especially small airways by thick, tenacious mucus is probably universally present in status asthmaticus, and patients have serious difficulty coughing up these mucous plugs. Gentle chest PT can be attempted in such cases, although there is no consensus on which PT techniques are most effective in this setting (and least likely to worsen bronchospasm). Treatment sessions with PD, percussion, and vibration should be short, and their impact judged by alterations in dyspnea, arterial blood gas concentrations, and the quantity of sputum expectorated. An anecdotal report indicates that vigorous chest PT in mechanically ventilated patients with status asthmaticus can mobilize large amounts of sputum (30 to 40 mL per treatment), significantly decrease peak inspiratory ventilator pressures, and reduce chest radiographic findings of hyperinflation caused by air-trapping behind obstructed airways.[107]

CHEST PHYSICAL THERAPY IN TRAUMATIC QUADRIPLEGIA AND OTHER NEUROMUSCULAR DISEASES

Secretion retention, atelectasis, and bronchopneumonia occur frequently in patients with traumatic quadriplegia and in those with a number of advanced neuromuscular disorders affecting the muscles of respiration. Mucous plugging of major bronchi may even occasionally simulate acute pulmonary embolism in such patients, with sudden onset of shortness of breath, chest pain, worsening hypoxemia, a normal or near-normal chest film, and a perfusion defect on perfusion lung scan.[108] Clinical awareness of this problem, along with poor ventilation on ventilation scintiscan in the hypoperfused lung zones, should lead to a correct diagnosis and appropriate secretion management. Excessive airway secretions and atelectasis in this patient group are due to reduced respiratory muscle strength, with impaired cough and deep breathing, along with generalized immobility stemming from paralyzed extremity and trunk muscles. Cough is especially impaired in cervical spinal cord injury because such an injury causes paralysis of all the expiratory muscles.[109]

Early institution of a regimen to prevent secretion retention has decreased pulmonary complications, the need for mechanical ventilation, and mortality in patients with traumatic quadriplegia.[110] Such a program should include frequent changes in a patient's position in bed, deep-breathing exercises (including incentive spirometry), assisted coughing, and chest PT with PD and percussion. The Trendelenburg (head-down) position favors airway secretion clearance and probably improves patients' vital capacity through a reduction in residual volume and improved inspiratory function of the diaphragm.[110] A turning bed such as a Stryker frame is ideal for positioning because it permits the prone position as well as the other postures. Intermittent positive-pressure breathing (IPPB) does not appear to provide any additional benefit to these patients.[111] A modified version of this program should also be instituted in quadriplegic patients who require mechanical ventilation at the outset, and in other neurologically impaired patients with significant respiratory muscle dysfunction. Because of impaired sympathetic nervous system function in traumatic quadriplegia, especially in the period immediately after the cervical injury, rapid or major change in body position can lead to hemodynamic compromise; cardiovascular efficacy should be monitored.

Secretion retention often eventually becomes less of a problem in quadriplegics because of a substantial improvement in their vital capacity between the third and fifth week after injury, with the V_C doubling by 3 months.[112] Inspiratory muscle training can also be employed to increase the strength and endurance of the diaphragm in these patients in the interval and, indeed, indefinitely.[113]

Pneumonia

There is no evidence that chest PT (including PD, percussion, and vibration) hastens the clinical or roentgenographic resolution of primary pneumonia in otherwise well patients without an endobronchial lesion, underlying chronic obstructive lung disease, respiratory muscle weakness, or the need for mechanical ventilatory support.[114,115] To the contrary, younger patients (< 47 years) with mainly interstitial infiltrates on chest radiographs, suggesting a nonbacterial pneumonia, actually had a longer duration of fever and required a lengthier hospital stay if they received chest PT.[115] Similarly, chest PT does not appear to benefit children with an uncomplicated pneumonia.[116] Clearly, chest PT in pneumonia should be limited to patients who cannot clear their own airway secretions or whose pneumonia is complicated by mucoid impaction of airways with atelectasis. In addition, there is a single case report documenting the efficacy of long-term scheduled coughing (seven times daily for 10 minutes each) in normalizing restrictive pulmonary function in pneumonia resulting from the long-term aspiration of mineral oil. This was accompanied by the expectoration of large amounts of this material over a 17-month period.[117]

Lung Abscess

As for any localized collection of pus, proper drainage and appropriate antimicrobial therapy are considered essential in the management of lung abscess.[118] Endobronchial evacuation of infected material is the preferred drainage method, and this is facilitated through PD (using chest film localization of the abscess to select positioning), cough, and careful chest percussion. This therapy should be performed for 15 to 20 minutes three or four times daily. If major hemoptysis develops during such treatment, PD and percussion should be withheld, and the patient should be placed with the abscess in a dependent position until the hemoptysis has resolved. The same steps should be taken if an abscess suddenly discharges a large quantity of pus into the airways, threatening asphyxiation and massive aspiration pneumonia. Occasionally, conservative management fails to drain a lung abscess. In this situation, other drainage techniques, such as bronchoscopy, transbronchial catheterization,[119] and percutaneous tube drainage[120] can be employed; only rarely is surgical resection of an abscess necessary.

CHEST PHYSICAL THERAPY IN PREOPERATIVE AND POSTOPERATIVE RESPIRATORY CARE

Atelectasis is the most common postoperative pulmonary complication and occurs most often after upper abdominal and cardiothoracic surgery. Additional risk factors include older age (> 60 years), obesity, cigarette use, and underlying lung disease, especially COPD. The cause of postoperative atelectasis is multifactorial and includes reduced tracheobronchial mucociliary clearance following general anesthesia,[121] poorly understood diaphragmatic dysfunction,[50] pain, impairment of cough and sigh maneuvers, excessive analgesia, and immobility. Intraoperative lung contusion and phrenic nerve injury by cold cardioplegia are additional mechanisms unique to cardiothoracic surgery.[46]

Preventive measures are the cornerstone to appropriate pre- and postoperative respiratory care. The most important of these are deep-breathing techniques that generate maximum inspiratory volumes. Their ability to significantly decrease postoperative pulmonary complications is well documented. Such methods include IPPB, incentive spirometry, and deep-breathing exercises.[122] Mask continuous positive airway pressure (CPAP), with a pressure of 7.5 to 15 cmH$_2$O can also prevent postsurgical atelectasis and quickly restores FRC to near preoperative levels.[123,124] Because IPPB is expensive and causes more side effects,[122] we prefer the use of other expansion modalities, especially *incentive spirometry*.

Patients should receive instruction in these techniques before surgery, and undergo treatment postoperatively for 15 minutes every 2 to 3 hours while awake during the first 3 to 5 days after operation. These methods should be prescribed primarily for patients undergoing upper abdominal and cardiothoracic surgery, including those with a normal pulmonary status [122,125] as well as for those who have underlying lung disease. The routine addition of chest PT to lung expansion maneuvers is unnecessary and has even been reported to be detrimental, with more frequent atelectasis[126] as well as increased patient discomfort[127] resulting.

The addition of chest PT to deep-breathing techniques should be reserved for patients who are major sputum producers (> 30 mL/day). This approach, plus general prophylactic measures, including smoking cessation before elective operations, late morning surgery for patients with excess morning secretions, frequent side-to-side turning postoperatively, judicious use of analgesics, and early ambulation can substantially reduce the incidence of postsurgical pulmonary complications from as high as 60% to about 20%.[125] Furthermore, the *severity* of lung complications (should they occur) is reduced.[125]

OBSTRUCTIVE ATELECTASIS CAUSED BY RETAINED AIRWAY SECRETIONS

In contrast with its lesser role in atelectasis prevention, chest PT should be routinely provided to patients who develop obstructive atelectasis caused by mucous plugging of airways. This problem is often encountered in postoperative patients who have undergone abdominal or thoracic surgery, as well as in other seriously ill patients, often in an intensive care setting, with a wide range of disorders including drug overdose, trauma, paralysis, and obstructive lung diseases. In addition to bronchodilator therapy, intensified breathing exercises, and directed cough, such persons should receive ample chest PT with PD and percussion directed to the involved lung lobes or segments. This strategy is usually effective in quickly resolving atelectasis resulting from large-airway plugging; one report noted complete resolution of atelectasis in three of eight patients following a single treatment, with 50% restoration of lung volume in three others.[128] Most of the volume loss in this group was restored by 24 hours.

On the other hand, atelectasis caused by retained secretions within small airways resolved more slowly with restoration of only about 60% of normal lung volume after 48 hours of aggressive therapy. Atelectasis of this type is recognized by the presence of an air bronchogram within the atelectatic lung on plain chest roentgenograms, signifying patency of the large central bronchi.

Fiberoptic bronchoscopy with lavage and suctioning of obstructed airways is no better than conventional chest PT in managing atelectasis caused by either large- or small-airway obstruction[128] and should be reserved for patients whose atelectasis is unresponsive to chest PT. This conservative approach is also justified before instituting other techniques to treat atelectasis, such as maximum volume IPPB[129] and lung reexpansion employing a fiberoptic bronchoscope with a balloon cuff.[130] On the other hand, continuous positive-pressure breathing (CPPB) with expiratory pressures between 5 and 15 cmH$_2$O, administered as PEEP on a ventilator[131] or as CPAP by nasal[132] or facial mask,[133] may provide more rapid resolution of atelectasis not associated with large-airway obstruction. Further studies are needed to compare the efficacy of chest PT and CPPB in resolving atelectasis of this type.

CHEST PHYSICAL THERAPY IN CRITICALLY ILL PATIENTS

Chest PT is a routine procedure in most intensive care units, and its use is predicted to increase or remain at the same level at most hospitals during the next 5 years.[134] Its main indication is to facilitate the clearance of airway secretions in both intubated and nonintubated patients by conventional techniques of PD, percussion, vibration, and directed cough. Also, nasotracheal or endotracheal suctioning must often be employed to complete secretion removal.

Although a controlled, carefully conducted study documenting the efficacy of chest PT in this patient population remains to be done, its value is generally accepted on the basis of widespread clinical experience. The largest study is reported in the monograph by Mackenzie and coworkers, documenting the results of more than 11,000 chest PT treatments in over 3,000 critically ill trauma patients.[135] These investigators stressed the need to direct PT to lung zones that were abnormal on recent chest radiographs or on chest physical examination, and to continue treatment until auscultation revealed improved air entry and reduced adventitious (abnormal) breath sounds.

An ingenious array of supportive rolls, slings, pulleys, and body frames can be employed in even the sickest and most severely injured patients to help hospital personnel position them to carry out the appropriate chest PT maneuvers.[135] Following treatments lasting from 30 minutes to 1 hour, Mackenzie reported increases in total lung–thorax compliance (perhaps owing to recruitment of alveoli through the clearance of secretions from small airways),[136,137] along with a reduced intrapulmonary shunt, in most patients, and a modest improvement in arterial PaO$_2$.[137] This approach also obviated the need for bronchoscopy to remove retained airway secretions in all but a small number of patients. Percussion and vibration can be employed even in trauma patients with rib fractures or with a flail chest, as long as such treatment is not given directly over the trauma site and monitoring for accidental rib displacement during treatment is performed.[138]

Although physiologic indicators, such as arterial blood gas concentrations, only rarely deteriorated following chest PT in Mackenzie's patients[137] other investigators have not uniformly reported favorable results (see following section). In addition, chest PT can substantially increase a patient's metabolic rate, with increases in oxygen consumption and carbon dioxide production averaging close to 40% above levels found during sleep.[139] These values may remain above the resting ones for up to 45 minutes after chest PT is completed. Since major increases in heart rate and the heart rate–systolic blood pressure product (an indicator of myocardial oxygen demand) also occur, chest PT is felt to constitute a major metabolic and hemodynamic stress, which might be hazardous to patients with underlying cardiovascular disorders.[139] Neither therapeutic doses of bolus or continuous intravenous morphine[140] nor small (1.5 μg/kg) intravenous doses of fentanyl, a short-acting narcotic analgesic,[141] reduced the hypermetabolic response to chest PT. However, higher doses of fentanyl (3μg/kg) appeared to attenuate the hemodynamic responses, with suppression of the blood pressure and heart rate increases.[141] It seems prudent to institute close electrocardiographic and hemodynamic monitoring in patients with serious underlying cardiovascular disorders who undergo chest PT, and higher concentrations of inspired oxygen should probably be employed during and, for 30 minutes to 1 hour, after chest PT is completed. The routine use of analgesics and sedatives during chest PT requires further study.

Alterations in body position can promote major changes in oxygenation and may significantly benefit patients with ARDS[142] and unilateral parenchymal lung disease, such as pneumonia.[143] The prone position has improved the arterial PaO_2 in ARDS by a mean of 47 to 69 mmHg in two separate studies.[142,144] With unilateral lung disease, the PaO_2 often improves significantly when the good lung is in the decubitus (down) position, through directing blood flow to the better aerated lung.[143] This benefit is present in both spontaneously breathing patients and in those undergoing mechanical ventilation, with or without PEEP.[145] The effects of the sitting position on oxygenation is less certain, but this posture is unlikely to be employed in seriously ill patients except for those with acute cardiogenic pulmonary edema, in whom it is known to be beneficial.

COMPLICATIONS OF CHEST PHYSICAL THERAPY

Serious complications are infrequent during chest PT. Only a few deaths have been reported,[146] usually owing to massive pulmonary hemorrhage from a lung abscess or bronchopulmonary fistula. In these patients a small amount of bleeding had been noted during routine care or with chest PT before the terminal hemorrhage. Therefore, chest PT should be administered cautiously to any patient with a necrotizing lung process that has recently bled, and percussion and vibration are probably contraindicated in this setting because they may loosen a clot. Modest blood streaking of sputum, however, should not be considered a harbinger of major hemorrhage; chest PT should be continued, although carefully, in this circumstance.

Other adverse side effects of chest PT, such as those due to the mechanical effects of changes in body position (displacement of intravascular lines, endotracheal tubes, fractures, dislocations, and such) are more common,[135] but can often be anticipated and minimized. The most important adverse occurrence is hypoxemia, with an average fall of PaO_2 of 19 mmHg in one group of 17 patients after postural drainage and chest percussion,[147] with significant falls in SaO_2 from above 90% to 85% or below in five of nine patients in another group.[148] However, hypoxemia with chest PT has not been reported in all studies that monitored its occurrence,[149] and PaO_2 may also improve in some.[150] Hypoxemia with chest PT has been observed in postcardiac surgery patients,[151] acutely ill medical patients with a variety of lung disorders,[152] and in adolescents and young adults with CF.[148] It occurs in patients with minimal or no airway secretions[152] as well as in patients who produce copious sputum.[148] Importantly, the PaO_2 value appears to decrease less as baseline hypoxemia becomes more pronounced, so that chest PT need not be withheld from patients with low baseline PaO_2 values.[153] Chest PT-related hypoxemia may be worsened by chest percussion,[152] especially when the diseased lung is placed in the dependent position,[147] and by endotracheal suctioning.[151]

Supplemental oxygen (at 3 L/min nasal cannula) did not prevent chest PT-related hypoxemia in CF patients, but did promote a quicker return of SaO_2 to baseline levels after completed PT.[148] On the other hand, 100% oxygen in two acutely ill, mechanically ventilated patients completely averted the fall in PaO_2 after PD and chest percussion in a study by Connor and associates, eliminating an increased shunt fraction as the cause of the hypoxemia.[152]

Although the mechanism of hypoxemia after chest PT is not certain, it may be due to a shifting of mucus from the peripheral to the central airways, causing blockage at this level with ventilation–perfusion mismatch. The widespread availability of ear oximetry now permits continuous monitoring of SaO_2 during chest PT, and if needed, supplemental oxygen can be easily adjusted to maintain the SaO_2 at a safe level of 90% or higher. Cardiac output has also been observed to fall during chest PT,[154,155] and this can significantly diminish tissue oxygen delivery, especially if the blood oxygen content is reduced by chest PT as well. However, only a few such studies have been carried out, and the patients were either seriously ill on mechanical ventilators[154] or had just undergone cardiac surgery.[155] These patients, therefore, do not accurately reflect the wide range of patients undergoing chest PT, and cardiac output is likely to remain unchanged or may even increase in many of these.[154]

Chest PT does not appear to have a major adverse effect on lung mechanics. One study, however, noted a modest but transient fall in FEV_1 immediately after chest percussion in 40% of patients treated during an acute exacerbation of chronic bronchitis, most of whom had evidence of hyperreactive airways disease.[95] Chest percussion should probably be preceded by an aerosolized bronchodilator in such patients, and special caution is warranted when this technique is administered to asthmatics with an acute asthma attack or in status asthmaticus. Neither postural drainage alone nor directed cough seems to cause a similar decline in FEV_1.

Because coughing or the head-down position can raise intracranial pressure, such techniques pose some risk to patients with intracranial hypertension resulting from trauma, craniotomy, or other causes.[146] When an intracranial pressure-measuring device has been inserted, the pressure effects of chest PT can be directly monitored and chest PT modified if unsafe pressures are recorded. Without such monitoring, chest PT should be administered very cautiously in patients with intracranial hypertension. Elevation of the head with a rolled towel may limit increases in central nervous system pressure during Trendelenburg posturing.[138]

REFERENCES

1. Barach AL, Beck GJ: The ventilatory effects of the head-down position in pulmonary emphysema. Am J Med 16:55–60, 1954
2. Miller WF: A physiologic evaluation of the effects of diaphragmatic breathing training in patients with chronic pulmonary emphysema. Am J Med 17:471–477, 1954
3. Celli BR: Respiratory muscle function. Clin Chest Med 7:567–584, 1986
4. Macklem PT: The diaphragm in health and disease. J Lab Clin Med 99:601–610, 1982
5. Rodenstein DO, Stanescu DC: Absence of nasal air flow during pursed lips breathing. Am Rev Respir Dis 128:716–718, 1983
6. Barach AL: Physiologic advantages of grunting, groaning and pursed-lip breathing: Adaptive symptoms related to the development of continuous positive pressure breathing. Bull NY Acad Med 49:666–673, 1973
7. Mueller RE, Petty TL, Filley GF: Ventilation and arterial blood gas changes induced by pursed lips breathing. J Appl Physiol 28:784–789, 1970
8. Thoman RL, Stoker GL, Ross JC: The efficacy of pursed-lips breathing in patients with chronic obstructive pulmonary disease. Am Rev Respir Dis 93:100–105, 1966
9. Ingram RH Jr, Schilder DP: Effect of pursed lips expiration on the pulmonary pressure–flow relationship in obstructive lung disease. Am Rev Respir Dis 96:381–387, 1967
10. Higenbottam T, Payne J: Glottis narrowing in lung disease. Am Rev Respir Dis 125:746–750, 1982
11. Tiep BL, Burns M, Kao D et al: Pursed lips breathing training using ear oximetry. Chest 90:218–221, 1986
12. Wardlaw JM, Fergusson RJ, Tweeddale PM, McHardy G Jr: Pursed-lip breathing reduces hyperventilation-induced bronchoconstriction. Lancet 1:1483–1484, 1987
13. Callaway JJ, McKusick VA: Carbon-dioxide intoxication in emphysema: Emergency treatment by artificial pneumoperitoneum. N Engl J Med 245:9–13, 1951
14. Gayrard P, Becker M, Bergofsky EH: The effects of abdominal weights on diaphragmatic position and excursion in man. Clin Sci 35:589–601, 1968
15. Wade OL, Gilson JC: The effect of posture on diaphragmatic movement and vital capacity in normal subjects with a note on spirometry as an aid in determining radiological chest volumes. Thorax 6:103–124, 1951
16. Erwin WS, Zolov D, Bickerman HA: The effect of posture on respiratory function in patients with obstructive pulmonary emphysema. Am Rev Respir Dis 94:865–872, 1966
17. Sharp JT, Drutz WS, Moisan T et al: Postural relief of dyspnea in severe chronic obstructive pulmonary disease. Am Rev Respir Dis 122:201–211, 1980
18. Druz WS, Sharp JT: Electrical and mechanical activity of the diaphragm accompanying body position in severe chronic obstructive pulmonary disease. Am Rev Respir Dis 125:275–280, 1982
19. Delgado HR, Braun SR, Skatrud JB et al: Chest wall and abdominal motion during exercise in patients with chronic obstructive pulmonary disease. Am Rev Respir Dis 126:200–205, 1982
20. Milic-Emili J, Aubier M: Some recent advances in the study of the control of breathing in patients with chronic obstructive lung disease. Anesth Analg 59:865–873, 1980
21. Motley HL: The effects of slow deep breathing on the blood gas exchange in emphysema. Am Rev Respir Dis 88:485–492, 1963
22. Paul G, Eldridge F, Mitchell J, Fiene T: Some effects of slowing respiration rate in chronic emphysema and bronchitis. J Appl Physiol 21:877–882, 1966
23. Grassino A, Bellemare F, Laporta D: Diaphragm fatigue and the strategy of breathing in COPD. Chest 85(suppl):51S–54S, 1984
24. Barach AL: Breathing exercises in pulmonary emphysema and allied chronic respiratory disease. Arch Phys Med Rehabil 36:379–390, 1955
25. Petty TL, Guthrie A: The effects of augmented breathing maneuvers on ventilation in severe chronic airway obstruction. Respir Care 16:104–111, 1971
26. Livingstone JL, Gillespie M: The value of breathing exercises in asthma. Lancet 2:705–708, 1935
27. Becklake MR, McGregor M, Goldman HI, Braudo JL: A study of the effects of physiotherapy in chronic hypertrophic emphysema using lung function tests. Dis Chest 26:180–191, 1954
28. McNeill RS, McKenzie JM: An assessment of the value of breathing exercises in chronic bronchitis and asthma. Thorax 10:250–252, 1955
29. Sinclair JD: The effect of breathing exercises in pulmonary emphysema. Thorax 10:246–249, 1955
30. Campbell EJM, Friend J: Action of breathing exercises in pulmonary emphysema. Lancet 1:325–329, 1955
31. Miller WF: Physical therapeutic measures in the treatment of chronic bronchopulmonary disorders. Methods for breathing training. Am J Med 24:929–940, 1958
32. Willeput R, Vachaudez JP, Lenders D et al: Thoracoabdominal motion during chest physiotherapy in patients affected by chronic obstructive lung disease. Respiration 44:204–214, 1983
33. Grimby, G, Oxhoj H, Bake B: Effects of abdominal breathing on distribution of ventilation in obstructive lung disease. Clin Sci Mol Med 48:193–199, 1975
34. Sackner MA, Silva G, Banks JM et al: Distribution of ventilation during diaphragmatic breathing in ob-

structive lung disease. Am Rev Respir Dis 109:331–337, 1974

35. Brach BB, Chao RP, Sgroi VL et al: Xenon washout patterns during diaphragmatic breathing. Studies in normal persons and patients with chronic obstructive pulmonary disease. Chest 71:735–739, 1977

36. Shearer, MO, Banks JM, Silva G, Sackner MA: Lung ventilation during diaphragmatic breathing. Phys Ther 52:139–147, 1972

37. Bake B, Dempsey J, Grimby G: Effects of change of the chest wall on distribution of inspired gas. Am Rev Respir Dis 114:1113–1120, 1976

38. Roussos CS, Fixley M, Genest J et al: Voluntary factors influencing the distribution of inspired gas. Am Rev Respir Dis 116:457–466, 1977

39. Sackner MA, Gonzalez HF, Jenouri G, Rodriguez M: Effects of abdominal and thoracic breathing on breathing pattern components in normal subjects and in patients with chronic obstructive pulmonary disease. Am Rev Respir Dis 130:584–587, 1984

40. Pavia D, Agnew JE, Lopez-Vidriero MT, Clarke SW: General review of tracheobronchial clearance. Eur J Respir Dis 71(suppl 153):123–129, 1987

41. Gail DB, Lenfant CJM: State of the art. Cells of the lung: Biology and clinical implications. Am Rev Respir Dis 127:366–387, 1983

42. Konietzko N: Mucus transport and inflammation. Eur J Respir Dis 69(suppl 147):72–79, 1986

43. Kaliner M, Shelhamer JH, Borson B, Nadel J: Human respiratory mucus. Am Rev Respir Dis 134:612–621, 1986

44. Lopez-Vidriero MT: Biochemical basis of physical properties of respiratory tract secretions. Eur J Respir Dis 71(suppl 153):130–135, 1987

45. Loke J, Matthay MA, Putman CE: Pulmonary complications of acute smoke inhalation [Abstract]. Am Rev Respir Dis 117:146, 1978

46. Pearce W, Baile EM, Hards J et al: Phrenic nerve function and its relationship to atelectasis after coronary artery bypass surgery. Chest 93:693–698, 1988

47. Wanner A: State of the art. Clinical aspects of mucociliary transport. Am Rev Respir Dis 116:73–125, 1977

48. Estenne M, Ketelbant P, Primo G, Yernault JC: Human heart–lung transplantation: Physiologic aspects of the denervated lung and post-transplant obliterative bronchiolitis. Am Rev Respir Dis 135:976–978, 1987

49. Bateman JRM, Pavia D, Clarke SW: The retention of lung secretions during the night in normal subjects. Clin Sci Mol Med 55:523–527, 1978

50. Dureuil B, Vires N, Cantineau J-P et al: Diaphragmatic contractility after upper abdominal surgery. J Appl Physiol 61:1775–1780, 1986

51. King M, Brock G, Lundell C: Clearance of mucus by simulated cough. J Appl Physiol 58:1776–1782, 1985

52. Marini JJ, Tyler ML, Hudson LD et al: Influence of head-dependent positions on lung volume and oxygen saturation in chronic air-flow obstruction. Am Rev Respir Dis 129:101–105, 1984

53. Chopra SK, Taplin GV, Simmons DH et al: Effects of hydration and physical therapy on tracheal transport velocity. Am Rev Respir Dis 115:1009–1014, 1977.

54. Shim C, King M, Williams MH Jr: Lack of effect of hydration on sputum production in chronic bronchitis. Chest 92:679–682, 1987

55. Sutton PP, Pavia D, Bateman M Jr, Clarke SW: Chest physiotherapy: A review. Eur J Respir Dis 63:188–201, 1982

56. King M, Phillips DM, Gross D et al: Enhanced tracheal mucus clearance with high frequency chest wall compression. Am Rev Respir Dis 128:511–515, 1983

57. Evans JN, Jaeger MJ: Mechanical aspects of coughing. Pneumonologie 152:253–257, 1975

58. Camner P, Mossberg B, Philipson K, Strandberg K: Elimination of test particles from the human tracheobronchial tract by voluntary coughing. Scand J Respir Dis 60:56–62, 1979

59. Burford JG, George RB: Respiratory physical therapy in the treatment of chronic bronchitis. Semin Respir Infect 3:55–60, 1988

60. Harris RS, Lawson TV: The relative mechanical effectiveness and efficiency of successive voluntary coughs in healthy young adults. Clin Sci 34:569–577, 1968

61. Sutton PP, Parker RA, Webber BA et al: Assessment of the forced expiration technique, postural drainage and directed coughing in chest physiotherapy. Eur J Respir Dis 64:62–68, 1983

62. Smaldone GC, Itoh H, Swift DL, Wagner HN Jr: Effect of flow-limiting segments and cough on particle deposition and mucociliary clearance in the lung. Am Rev Respir Dis 120:747–758, 1979

63. Hofmeyr JL, Webber BA, Hodson ME: Evaluation of positive expiratory pressure as an adjunct to chest physiotherapy in the treatment of cystic fibrosis. Thorax 41:951–954, 1986

64. Pavia D, Agnew JE, Clarke SW: Cough and mucociliary clearance. Bull Eur Physiopathol Respir 23(suppl 10):41S–45S, 1987

65. Sutton PP: Chest physiotherapy: Time for reappraisal. Br J Dis Chest 82:127–137, 1988

66. Bateman JRM, Newman SP, Daunt KM et al: Regional lung clearance of excessive bronchial secretions during chest physiotherapy in patients with stable chronic airways obstruction. Lancet 1:294–297, 1979

67. Bateman JRM, Newman SP, Daunt KM et al: Is cough as effective as chest physiotherapy in the removal of excessive tracheobronchial secretions? Thorax 36:683–687, 1981

68. Rossman CM, Waldes R, Sampson D, Newhouse MT: Effect of chest physiotherapy on the removal of mucus in patients with cystic fibrosis. Am Rev Respir Dis 126:131–135, 1982

69. Kirilloff LH, Owens GR, Rogers RM, Mazzocco MC: Does chest physical therapy work? Chest 88:436–444, 1985

70. Oldenburg FA Jr, Dolovich MB, Montgomery JM, Newhouse MT: Effects of postural drainage, exercise, and cough on mucus clearance in chronic bronchitis. Am Rev Respir Dis 120:739–745, 1979

71. Wong JW, Keens TG, Wannamaker EM et al: Effects of gravity on tracheal mucus transport rates in normal subjects and in patients with cystic fibrosis. Pediatrics 60:146–152, 1977

72. Sutton PP, Lopez-Vidriero MT, Pavia D et al: Assessment of percussion, vibratory-shaking and breathing exercises in chest physiotherapy. Eur J Respir Dis 66:147–152, 1985

73. Wollmer P, Ursing K, Midgren B, Eriksson L: Inefficiency of chest percussion in the physical therapy of

chronic bronchitis. Eur J Respir Dis 66:233–239, 1985

74. Van Der Schans CP, Piers DA, Postma DS: Effect of manual percussion on tracheobronchial clearance in patients with chronic airflow obstruction and excessive tracheobronchial secretion. Thorax 41:448–452, 1986

75. Maxwell M, Redmond A: Comparative trial of manual and mechanical percussion technique with gravity-assisted bronchial drainage in patients with cystic fibrosis. Arch Dis Child 54:542–544, 1979

76. Murphy MB, Concannon D, Fitzgerald MX: Chest percussion: Help or hindrance to postural drainage? Ir Med J 76:189–190, 1983

77. Pavia D, Thomson ML, Phillipakos D: A preliminary study of the effect of a vibrating pad on bronchial clearance. Am Rev Respir Dis 113:92–96, 1976

78. Gross D, Zidulka A, O'Brien C et al: Peripheral mucociliary clearance with high-frequency chest wall compression. J Appl Physiol 58:1157–1163, 1985

79. King M, Phillips DM, Zidulka A, Chang HK: Tracheal mucus clearance in high-frequency oscillation. II: Chest wall versus mouth oscillation. Am Rev Respir Dis 130:703–706, 1984

80. George RJD, Johnson MA, Pavia D et al: Increase in mucociliary clearance in normal man induced by oral high frequency oscillation. Thorax 40:433–437, 1985

81. George RJD, Pavia D, Woodman G et al: Oral high frequency oscillation (OHFO) as an adjunct to physiotherapy (Physio) in cystic fibrosis (CF) [Abstract]. Thorax 41:235–236, 1986

82. deBoeck C, Zinman R: Cough versus chest physiotherapy. A comparison of the acute effects on pulmonary function in patients with cystic fibrosis. Am Rev Respir Dis 129:182–184, 1984

83. Bain J, Bishop J, Olinsky A: Evaluation of directed coughing in cystic fibrosis. Br J Dis Chest 82:138–148, 1988

84. Lorin MI, Denning CR: Evaluation of postural drainage by measurement of sputum volume and consistency. Am J Phys Med 50:215–219, 1971

85. Pryor JA, Webber BA, Hodson ME, Batten JC: Evaluation of the forced expiration technique as an adjunct to postural drainage in treatment of cystic fibrosis. Br Med J 2:417–418, 1979

86. Currie DC, Munuro C, Gaskell D, Cole PJ: Practice, problems and compliance with postural drainage: A survey of chronic sputum producers. Br J Dis Chest 80:249–253, 1986

87. Sutton PP, Gemmell HG, Innes N et al: Use of nebulised saline and nebulised terbutaline as an adjunct to chest physiotherapy. Thorax 43:57–60, 1988

88. Falk M, Kelstrup M, Anderson JB et al: Improving the ketchup bottle method with positive expiratory pressure, PEP, in cystic fibrosis. Eur J Respir Dis 65:423–432, 1984

89. Van Asperen PP, Jackson L, Hennessy P, Brown J: Comparison of a positive expiratory pressure (PEP) mask with postural drainage in patients with cystic fibrosis. Aust Paediatr J 23:283–284, 1987

90. March H: Appraisal of postural drainage for chronic obstructive pulmonary disease. Arch Phys Med Rehabil 52:528–530, 1971

91. May DB, Munt PW: Physiologic effects of chest percussion and postural drainage in patients with stable chronic bronchitis. Chest 75:29–32, 1979

92. Mohsenifar Z, Rosenberg N, Goldberg HS, Koerner SK: Mechanical vibration and conventional chest physiotherapy in outpatients with stable chronic obstructive lung disease. Chest 87:483–485, 1985

93. Feldman J, Traver GA, Taussig LM: Maximal expiratory flows after postural drainage. Am Rev Respir Dis 119:239–245, 1979

94. Anthonisen P, Riis P, Sogaard-Anderson T: The value of lung physiotherapy in the treatment of acute exacerbations in chronic bronchitis. Acta Med Scand 175:715–719, 1964

95. Campbell AH, O'Connell JM, Wilson F: The effect of chest physiotherapy upon the FEV_1 in chronic bronchitis. Med J Aust 1:33–35, 1975

96. Newton DAG, Stephenson A: Effect of physiotherapy on pulmonary function. Lancet 2:228–229, 1978

97. Newton DAG, Bevans HG: Physiotherapy and intermittent positive-pressure ventilation of chronic bronchitis. Br Med J 2:1525–1528, 1978

98. Buscaglia AJ, St Marie MS: Oxygen saturation during chest physiotherapy for acute exacerbation of severe chronic obstructive pulmonary disease. Respir Care 28:1009–1013, 1983

99. Currie DC, Pavia D, Agnew JE et al: Impaired tracheobronchial clearance in bronchiectasis. Thorax 42:126–130, 1987

100. Cochrane GM, Webber BA, Clarke SW: Effects of sputum on pulmonary function. Br Med J 2:1181–1183, 1977

101. Mazzocco MC, Owens GR, Kirilloff LH, Rogers RM: Chest percussion and postural drainage in patients with bronchiectasis. Chest 88:360–363, 1985

102. Tecklin JS, Holsclaw DS: Evaluation of bronchial drainage in patients with cystic fibrosis. Phys Ther 55:1081–1984, 1975

103. Desmond KJ, Schwenk WF, Thomas E et al: Immediate and long-term effects of chest physiotherapy in patients with cystic fibrosis. J Pediatr 103:538–542, 1983

104. Verboon JML, Bakker W, Sterk PJ: The value of the forced expiration technique with and without postural drainage in adults with cystic fibrosis. Eur J Respir Dis 69:169–174, 1986

105. Flower KA, Eden RI, Lomax L et al: New mechanical aid to physiotherapy in cystic fibrosis. Br Med J 2:630–631, 1979

106. Zack M, Oberwaldner B, Hansler F: Cystic fibrosis: Physical exercise versus chest physiotherapy. Arch Dis Child 57:587–589, 1982

107. Kigin CM: Breathing exercises in chest physical therapy. Chest 92:190, 1987

108. Dee PM, Suratt PM, Bray ST, Rose CE Jr: Mucous plugging simulating pulmonary embolism in patients with quadriplegia. Chest 85:363–366, 1984

109. Estenne M, De Troyer A: Mechanism of the postural dependence of vital capacity in tetraplegic subjects. Am Rev Respir Dis 135:367–371, 1987

110. McMichan JC, Michel L, Westbrook PR: Pulmonary dysfunction following traumatic quadriplegia. JAMA 243:528–531, 1980

111. McCool FD, Mayewski RF, Shayne DS, et al: Intermittent positive pressure breathing in patients with respiratory muscle weakness. Alterations in total re-

spiratory system compliance. Chest 90:546–552, 1986

112. Ledsome JR, Sharp JM: Pulmonary function in acute cervical cord injury. Am Rev Respir Dis 124:41–44, 1981

113. Gross D, Ladd HW, Riley EJ et al: The effect of training on strength and endurance of the diaphragm in quadriplegia. Am J Med 68:27–35, 1980

114. Graham WGB, Bradley DA: Efficacy of chest physiotherapy and intermittent positive-pressure breathing in the resolution of pneumonia. N Engl J Med 299:624–627, 1985

115. Britton S, Bejstedt M, Vedin L: Chest physiotherapy in primary pneumonia. Br Med J 290:1703–1704, 1985

116. Stapleton T: Chest physiotherapy in primary pneumonia. Br Med J 291:143, 1985

117. Heckers H, Melcher FW, Dittmar K et al: Long-term course of mineral oil pneumonia. Lung 155:101–109, 1978

118. Delarue NC, Pearson FG, Nelems JM, Cooper JD: Lung abscess: Surgical implications. Can J Surg 23:297–302, 1980

119. Schmitt GS, Ohar JM, Kanter KR, Naunheim KS: Indwelling transbronchial catheter drainage of pulmonary abscess. Ann Thorac Surg 45:43–47, 1988

120. Yellin A, Yellin EO, Lieberman Y: Percutaneous tube drainage: The treatment of choice for refractory lung abscess. Ann Thorac Surg 39:266–270, 1985

121. Gamsu G, Singer MM, Vincent HH et al: Postoperative impairment of mucous transport in the lung. Am Rev Respir Dis 114:673–679, 1976

122. Celli BR, Rodriguez KS, Snider GL: A controlled trial of intermittent positive pressure breathing, incentive spirometry, and deep breathing exercises in preventing pulmonary complications after abdominal surgery. Am Rev Respir Dis 130:12–15, 1984

123. Stock MC, Downs JB, Gauer PK et al: Prevention of postoperative pulmonary complications with CPAP, incentive spirometry, and conservative therapy. Chest 87:151–157, 1985

124. Paul WL, Downs JB: Postoperative atelectasis: Intermittent positive pressure breathing, incentive spirometry, and facemask positive end-expiratory pressure. Arch Surg 116:861–863, 1981

125. Roukema JA, Carol EJ, Prins JG: The prevention of pulmonary complications after upper abdominal surgery in patients with noncompromised pulmonary status. Arch Surg 123:30–34, 1988

126. Reines HD, Sade RM, Bradford BF, Marshall J: Chest physiotherapy fails to prevent postoperative atelectasis in children after cardiac surgery. Ann Surg 195:451–455, 1982

127. Torrington KG, Sorenson DE, Sherwood LM: Postoperative chest percussion with postural drainage in obese patients following gastric stapling. Chest 86:891–895, 1984

128. Marini JJ, Pierson DJ, Hudson LD: Acute lobar atelectasis: A prospective comparison of fiberoptic bronchoscopy and respiratory therapy. Am Rev Respir Dis 119:971–978, 1979

129. O'Donohue WJ Jr: Maximum volume IPPB for the management of pulmonary atelectasis. Chest 76:683–687, 1979

130. Harada K, Mutsuda T, Saoyama N et al: Reexpansion of refractory atelectasis using a bronchofiberscope with a balloon cuff. Chest 84:725–728, 1983

131. Fowler AA, Scoggins WG, O'Donohue WJ Jr: Positive end-expiratory pressure in the management of lobar atelectasis. Chest 74:497–500, 1978

132. Duncan SR, Negrin RS, Mihm FG et al: Nasal continuous positive airway pressure in atelectasis. Chest 92:621–624, 1987

133. Williamson DC III, Modell JH: Intermittent continuous positive airway pressure by mask. Arch Surg 117:970–972, 1982

134. Luce JM, Breeling JL: Critical care practice of chest physicians. Chest 93:163–165, 1988

135. Mackenzie CF, Ciesla N, Imle PC, Klemic N: Chest Physiotherapy in the Intensive Care Unit. Baltimore, Williams & Wilkins, 1981

136. Mackenzie CF, Shin B, Hadi F, Imle PC: Changes in total lung/thorax compliance following chest physiotherapy. Anesth Analg 59:207–210, 1980

137. Mackenzie CF, Shin B: Cardiorespiratory function before and after chest physiotherapy in mechanically ventilated patients with post-traumatic respiratory failure. Crit Care Med 13:483–486, 1985

138. Kigin CM: Advances in chest physical therapy. In O'Donohue WJ Jr (ed): Current Advances in Respiratory Care, pp 37–71. Park Ridge, Ill, American College of Chest Physicians, 1984

139. Weissman C, Kemper M, Damask MC et al: Effect of routine intensive care interactions on metabolic rate. Chest 86:815–818, 1984

140. Swinamer DL, Phang PT, Jones RL et al: Effect of routine administration of analgesia on energy expenditure in critically ill patients. Chest 92:4–10, 1988

141. Klein P, Kemper M, Weissman C et al: Attenuation of the hemodynamic responses to chest physical therapy. Chest 93:38–42, 1988

142. Piehl MA, Brown MS: Use of extreme position changes in acute respiratory failure. Crit Care Med 4:13, 1976

143. Zach MB, Pontoppidan H, Kazemi H: The effect of the lateral positions on gas exchange in pulmonary disease. Am Rev Respir Dis 110:49–55, 1974

144. Douglas WW, Rehder K, Beynen FM et al: Improved oxygenation in patients with acute respiratory failure—the prone position. Am Rev Respir Dis 115:559–566, 1977

145. Norton LC, Conforti CG: The effects of body position on oxygenation. Heart Lung 14:45–51, 1985

146. Tyler ML: Complications of positioning and chest physiotherapy. Respir Care 27:458–466, 1982

147. Huseby J, Hudson L, Stark K, Tyler M: Oxygenation during chest physiotherapy [Abstract]. Chest 70:430, 1976

148. McDonnell T, McNicholas WT, FitzGerald MX: Hypoxaemia during chest physiotherapy in patients with cystic fibrosis. Ir J Med Sci 155:345–348, 1986

149. Mackenzie CF, Shin B, McAslan TC: Chest physiotherapy: The effect on arterial oxygenation. Anesth Analg 57:28–30, 1978

150. Holody B, Goldberg HS: The effect of mechanical vibration physiotherapy on arterial oxygenation in acutely ill patients with atelectasis or pneumonia. Am Rev Respir Dis 124:372–375, 1981

151. Gormezano J, Branthwaite MA: Effects of physiotherapy during intermittent positive pressure ventilation. Anaesthesia 27:258–264, 1972

152. Connors AF Jr, Hammon WE, Martin RJ, Rogers RM: Chest physical therapy. The immediate effect on oxygenation in acutely ill patients. Chest 78:559–564, 1980

153. Tyler ML, Hudson LD, Grose BL, Huseby JS: Prediction of oxygenation during chest physiotherapy in critically ill patients. Am Rev Respir Dis 121(part2):218, 1980

154. Laws AK, McIntyre RW: Chest physiotherapy: A physiological assessment during intermittent positive pressure ventilation in respiratory failure. Can Anaesth Soc J 16:487–493, 1969

155. Barrell SE, Abbas HM: Monitoring during physiotherapy after open heart surgery. Physiotherapy 64:272–273, 1976

156. Asthma Research Council: Physical Exercises for Asthma, 8th ed. Londom, Asthma Research Council, 1949

157. Reed JMW: Chapter 32 in Marshall G, Perry KMA (eds): Diseases of the Chest. London, Butterworths, 1952

TWENTY-FOUR

Pulmonary Rehabilitation

Gerilynn A. Connors
John E. Hodgkin

The term *pulmonary rehabilitation* is becoming a "household name" to those caring for patients with lung impairment. At one time, pulmonary rehabilitation (PR) was considered only for patients with chronic obstructive pulmonary disease (COPD), such as chronic bronchitis and emphysema. Now it is better recognized that patients with asthma, cystic fibrosis, and some restrictive lung diseases may also benefit from PR. Therefore, PR should no longer be viewed as a treatment (the last treatment) for the patient with end-stage lung disease but, rather, as an integral component of good care for individuals with pulmonary disease.[1] Care of the pulmonary patient is often medically challenging and, at times, frustrating. These patients have specialized needs that can best be met by members of the medical community who are uniquely trained in the art of pulmonary rehabilitation. The intent of this chapter is to provide a broad understanding of PR for the respiratory care practitioner.

It is important to remember that PR is *not* only therapeutic but *preventative!* A clear understanding of this simple yet important concept will assist health care providers to utilize the information presented in this chapter to optimize their care of patients with lung disease.

ECONOMIC IMPACT OF LUNG DISEASE

The cost of lung disease in terms of dollars spent and lives affected is immense, and it continues to grow each year. Impairment and disability from lung disease is now a critical economic concern in the United States. In 1987, the National Health Interview Survey estimated that 9.6 million Americans have asthma, 12.7 million have chronic bronchitis, and 2 million have emphysema.[2] One in five people in the United States reports some form of chronic respiratory problem, according to the National Institutes of Health (NIH) Taskforce Report of July 1979. Chronic obstructive pulmonary disease shows the most rapid increase among the leading causes of death in the United States.[3] In fact, COPD and allied conditions are the fifth leading cause of death in the U.S. with an estimated 78,000 deaths in 1987 (Table 24–1).[4]

The actual death rate from COPD is thought to be underestimated owing to inconsistent reporting of respiratory diagnoses in the past. It is believed that 10% of all disability benefits paid by the Social Security Administration are to persons with COPD and that as many as 250 million work hours each year are lost because of the condition. In 1984, the total cost of health care related to respiratory diseases was estimated at 30 billion dollars.[3] In 1985, the cost of care including deceased productivity due to morbidity and mortality, for COPD and asthma, was estimated at 14.1 billion dollars.[5]

Although one can look at statistics for the economic impact of COPD, the *total* cost of COPD to patients themselves cannot be measured. The emotional, physical, social, and spiritual losses that these individuals endure must also be considered. Loss of self-respect, self-confidence, and ego strength, and the patient's increased dependency on others, can often lead to depression, emotional

Table 24–1 Deaths from the Leading Causes, U.S., 1987

TOTAL	2,123,000
1 Heart disease*	760,000
2 Cancer	477,000
3 Cerebrovascular disease (stroke)	150,000
4 Accidents	95,000
5 COPD and allied conditions	78,000
6 Pneumonia and influenza	69,000
7 Diabetes	39,000
8 Suicide	31,000
9 Chronic liver disease	26,000
10 Atherosclerosis	22,000
All other causes of death	376,000

* Includes 512,000 deaths from coronary heart disease.

disorders, and possible suicide. The effect that lung disease has on a person, his family, and his friends can be much more significant than the actual economic impact.

DEFINITION

The concept of rehabilitation is not new. In 1942 the Council on Rehabilitation defined *rehabilitation* as "the restoration of the individual to the fullest medical, mental, emotional, social, and vocational potential of which he/she is capable."

Pulmonary rehabilitation is not only concerned with control of symptoms and disease but also with *promotion and maintenance of health*. Rehabilitation is a process whereby it is hoped that a change in the patient reflects a movement toward health and an increased level of wellness.

Patients must understand their rehabilitative potential so that they have the information needed for decision-making. Rehabilitation helps the person to identify his or her "assets and liabilities," as well as the available avenues for change. The patient must have a goal or purpose to appropriately enter into a PR program.

The American College of Chest Physicians adopted the following definition of pulmonary rehabilitation:

> An art of medical practice wherein an individually tailored multidisciplinary program is formulated, which, through accurate diagnosis, therapy, emotional support, and education, stabilizes or reverses both the physio- and psychopathology of pulmonary diseases and attempts

to return the individual to the highest possible functional capacity allowed by his pulmonary handicap and overall life situation.[6]

As pointed out in the official American Thoracic Society Statement on Pulmonary Rehabilitation,[7] ". . . in the broadest sense, pulmonary rehabilitation means providing good, comprehensive respiratory care for patients with pulmonary disease."

RESOURCES FOR DELIVERY OF A REHABILITATION PROGRAM

The number and type of personnel needed for a PR program vary from one facility to another. To provide good rehabilitation, one does not have to be in a university setting or a large tertiary hospital. None of the resources discussed in this chapter are beyond that available to most physicians in private practice.

The key member of any rehabilitation team is, of course, the *patient*; the patient should be the focus of the rehabilitation program. It is the patient's understanding of his disease and individual goals that will determine the success of the program. The rehabilitation program must be individualized for each patient; consideration is given to such factors as type and severity of lung disease, the presence of other medical problems, background, family situation, vocation, and level of education.

The *rehabilitation team* most simply comprises a physician and a nurse or respiratory therapist. Other programs utilize the skills and services of a multidisciplinary team, including a physician, nurse, respiratory care practitioner, cardiopulmonary technologist, physical therapist or exercise physiologist, psychiatrist or psychologist, social worker, occupational therapist, vocational rehabilitation specialist, recreational therapist, dietitian, and chaplain. Not all of the members of a multidisciplinary team will be needed for each patient, although their services should be available. In smaller programs, the services of one allied health specialist may be provided by another member of the team if the person is knowledgeable in that area.[8]

Table 24–2 lists the services that should be available for patients during a PR program, even though not all patients with COPD will need all these services. Multidisciplinary teams are particularly appropriate for teaching or research purposes and if large numbers of patients are seen.

Table 24–2 Pulmonary Rehabilitation Services

ESSENTIAL SERVICES

Initial medical evaluation and care plan
Patient education, evaluation, and program coordination
Respiratory therapy techniques
Chest physical therapy techniques
Exercise conditioning
Daily performance evaluation
Social service evaluation
Nutritional evaluation

ADDITIONAL SERVICES

Psychological evaluation
Psychiatric evaluation
Vocational evaluation
Spiritual evaluation

Table 24–3 Sequence of a Pulmonary Rehabilitation Program

1. Select patient
2. Perform initial assessment
3. Determine goals
4. Outline components of care
5. Assess patient's progress
6. Arrange for long-term follow-up

Pulmonary rehabilitation programs are now largely carried out in the outpatient setting, since third-party payers are unwilling to pay for hospital care for nonacute patients.[9] However, those facilities that have designated rehabilitation units often care for the respiratory patient on an inpatient basis. The PR team certainly may become involved with a patient during his or her acute hospitalization and outline a program that will continue on an outpatient basis.

Outpatient programs generally vary from 4 to 6 weeks in length and may be arranged around a patient's employment responsibilities. Some programs provide home care services for the respiratory patient, which can help assist with the patient's follow-up care. These services may be provided directly by the rehabilitation program itself or in cooperation with a local visiting nurses' association.

SEQUENCE OF CARE

An appropriate sequence of care should be followed for patients in a PR program (Table 24–3).[7,10]

The following factors may affect the ultimate success, or lack thereof, of a patient in a PR program. Because the usual course of COPD is 30 years or more and because symptoms of early disease are often mild, the condition frequently is not diagnosed until it has reached an advanced stage.[11] This often means a patient will first be seen by a pulmonary specialist after the age of 60. The presence of other coexisting diseases, such as heart disease, hypertension, rhinitis–sinusitis, and gastrointestinal

disease, needs to be determined because these conditions may adversely affect the patient's rehabilitation potential.[12] Cancer, organic brain syndrome, cerebrovascular accident, severe heart failure, respiratory failure, chemical dependency, or severe arthritis may make it difficult for a patient to obtain much benefit from a rehabilitation program. Such conditions should be assessed before the start of rehabilitation.[13] Some of the other factors that may affect the success of the rehabilitation program are the age of the patient, intelligence, and occupation.[14] Those patients with good family support and strong personal motivation probably have greater potential for success than those who do not.

INITIAL EVALUATION

The initial evaluation of a patient should include a thorough history and physical examination, chest x-ray, pulmonary function tests, an electrocardiogram, and, when indicated, arterial blood gas analysis, sputum examination, blood theophylline levels, electrolyte and complete blood count (CBC) analyses (Table 24–4).[7,14] This initial assessment helps to establish a baseline for determining a patient's response to treatment and to outline his or her individual program.

This careful initial evaluation should include an examination by the medical director of pulmonary rehabilitation or by another pulmonary specialist to determine the proper pulmonary diagnosis and to detect the presence of other important

Table 24–4 Initial Medical Tests

Spirometry	Arterial blood gas
Diffusion capacity	Chest roentgenogram
Lung volume study	Complete blood count
Electocardiogram	Blood chemistry profile*
Exercise test*	

* The precise exercise protocol and blood chemistries ordered are determined by the pulmonologist after the initial evaluation of the patient.

medical problems that can affect the patient's rehabilitative potential.[13]

A psychosocial evaluation can assist health professionals in determining the patient's and family's attitudes about the disease. The psychosocial assessment should include assessment of the patient's family and other personal relationships, financial status, and life-style. Psychological tests that assess the impact of the illness on the patient, his moods, attitudes, and stress, as measured by recent life changes, may also be utilized to help us understand the patient and his or her needs.

It is critical that a psychosocial assessment be included in every examination of the patient with chronic lung disease, since the disease is often characterized by anxiety, social withdrawal, and low self-esteem. Patients often need immediate attention to these problems, with the same amount of concern as is directed to shortness of breath and bronchospasm.

DETERMINATION OF GOALS

Short- and long-term goals should be established after the initial evaluation. The goals established must be attainable and tailored to the level of impairment, extent of disease, patient's personality, physical ability, and life-style. The patient must be able to express his or her own expectations and, along with the PR team, establish reasonable goals.

The immediate goal of any program is to alleviate and to control any acute symptoms. This may be accomplished primarily by medication. For the setting of long-range goals, the patient should be intimately involved. These goals should include improvement of the patient's capacity to carry out activities of daily living, as well as his understanding of the pathophysiology of dyspnea so that exacerbations may be avoided or minimized. By understanding his disease process, the patient can lessen the frequency of exacerbations. The purpose of rehabilitation is to decrease reliance on others, promote independence in the patient, and prevent or delay worsening of the lung disease.

COMPONENTS OF A PULMONARY REHABILITATION PROGRAM

PATIENT EDUCATION

The goals of patient education include patient control of symptoms, promotion of health and wellness, and reduced anxiety.[15,16] A proper understanding of how a patient and his or her family relate to the disease and its limitations is helpful in educating the patient.

Behavior that demonstrates a step toward improving or maintaining health should be rewarded. This positive reinforcement should encourage more desired behavior. Attainable goals should be the focus of the educational program. By successfully completing minimal skills initially, the patient will also gain more confidence to attempt more complicated behaviors later.

Some basic principles of learning that should be considered when implementing an educational program for patients include the following:[16]

- The capacity of the person being educated (for example, the educational background) must be established to help define the learner.
- The intrinsically motivated person may learn better.
- Learning is facilitated by reward.
- People need practice in setting up goals for themselves. Without practice, their goal-setting may be too low or unrealistically high.
- Active participation, rather than passive reception, encourages learning.
- Material presented should be meaningful.
- Individual learners need to have opportunity to practice skills.
- The learner must understand what constitutes "good results" as well as what constitutes a "mistake."
- Experience should be provided for the learner to apply his learning.
- The learner should be able to discover relationships between what is learned and himself.
- The individual learner should also have opportunities to test his recall of pertinent information.
- Healthier patients are able to gain greater knowledge and retain it longer than severely impaired patients.

The environment provided for the individual's learning should be an "open" one that encourages asking questions, enhances self-confidence, and fosters independence. Health education should be designed to promote *patient compliance* as much as possible. The educational material must explain the need for, as well as the importance of, compliance.[17] Consideration should be given to misconceptions that the person already has learned, and efforts should be made to "unlearn" these misconceptions early in the educational process.

A problem common to the treatment of many chronic diseases is the failure of patients to adhere to regimens known to be beneficial. One reason for such "noncompliance" is the discouraging prospect of lifelong adherence to a regimen, or lifelong change in previously established behavior patterns or life-styles. Davis estimated in 1966 that about 30% to 35% of patients fail to follow medical recommendations.[18]

Researchers have explored reasons for noncompliant, as well as for compliant, behavior. Contradictory data have emerged, and as yet many questions have not been fully answered. Until a clearer picture develops concerning the factors that influence compliance, we should continue measuring compliance with the "tools" available—serum drug levels, pill counts, the keeping of appointments, and patient reports—and wait for information to emerge that will help us become more effective. Common sense suggests that continuity in care may help eliminate factors that contribute to noncompliance. Evaluation of the possible causes of the noncompliant act should be accomplished in an effort to remove as many distracting items as possible, so that the patient can be free to follow a path to optimal health and well-being.

Several components of the health belief model are thought to affect one's compliance:[19]

- The individual's belief in his or her susceptibility to the disease.
- His or her feelings about the severity of the disease.
- The person's understanding of benefits of the treatment program.
- The patient's understanding of certain "clues" to action that make the individual aware of his or her health beliefs and the need to act.
- His or her belief in the value of good health.

Patient education in the course of a PR program can help reduce the length of hospitalization, improve the quality of life, and increase the knowledge and skills of the pulmonary patient.

GENERAL MANAGEMENT

An important factor in the general management of a patient with COPD is the *avoidance of smoking*.[20,21] There has been some evidence that the course of COPD may be altered if the patient with very early airway obstruction stops smoking. Stopping smoking during any stage of COPD will likely slow down deterioration. Smoking cessation should be an integral part of any treatment program.[22] Many times it takes more than just an encouraging word from the physician to help a patient stop smoking; there are many different types of smokers, and the physician should work with the patient to help find the smoking cessation technique best suited for him or her.

Nicotine chewing gum can reduce withdrawal symptoms related to nicotine addiction,[23] and preliminary reports have suggested that clonidine can minimize adverse symptoms during acute withdrawal. Release of nicotine through the skin with a patch could simplify nicotine administration.

Patients should avoid *air pollution* and other inhaled irritants as much as possible. They should avoid contact with *individuals suffering from respiratory tract infections* and with large crowds when respiratory infections are prevalent.

Consideration should be given to such environmental factors as *temperature, humidity,* and *altitude.* Extremes of temperature and humidity can aggravate airway obstruction. The use of air conditioners, humidifiers, and filtering systems may be helpful. High altitude can cause significant lowering of the PaO_2. Commercial airliners are pressurized at the equivalent of 5000 to 8000 ft elevation. Air travel, thus, may lead to serious hypoxemia. *Adequate hydration* should be maintained in an attempt to liquefy airway secretions. An *influenza immunization* should be given yearly, and a pneumococcal vaccine should be administered once.

MEDICATIONS

Medications are an important component in the treatment program for patients with COPD, being not only therapeutic but also preventative. Medications are useful in achieving the short-range goal of relieving symptoms, but they should be combined with other therapeutic modalities as part of a comprehensive respiratory care program.[24,25] With the large amount of medications given to COPD patients, care must be taken to avoid adverse side effects and cross-reactions. One should also schedule medications and other treatments so that they do not disrupt the patient's life-style. It is important to coordinate activities of daily living, including exercise, with the patient's medication program. Inhaling a bronchodilator 15 to 20 minutes before activity may improve the patient's ability to be active by reversing or preventing bronchospasm.

Of the several categories of medications commonly used in respiratory patients, bronchodilators are those most commonly used. There are three major types: the methylxanthines, the sympathomimetic (β-agonist) preparations, and the anticholinergics. Long-acting anhydrous theophylline preparations maintain constant blood levels, with the additional advantage of less frequent administration.[26] The therapeutic theophylline blood level is 10–20 μg/mL. β-sympathomimetic agents are available for use by both the oral and aerosol routes, with the inhaled β_2-type agents being preferred. Parenteral sympathomimetic preparations and methylxanthines are usually reserved for hospitalized patients with an exacerbation of their lung disease. Ipratropium bromide (Atrovent), an inhaled anticholinergic bronchodilator, may be used in combination with a β-agonist and theophylline to provide more optimal bronchodilation than may occur with any one of these agents alone.

Broad-spectrum antibiotics (e.g., ampicillin, amoxicillin, tetracycline, doxycycline, trimethoprim–sulfamethoxazole) are used during episodes of acute bronchitis. Recently, some oral antimicrobials with a very broad spectrum (e.g., ciprofloxacin and cefuroxime) have become available. Corticosteroids can be given either orally or by inhalation and are indicated in patients with intermittent bronchospasm whose symptoms are not controlled by β_2 or anticholinergic bronchodilators. Other medications that are sometimes useful in patients with COPD or asthma include diuretics, expectorants, cromolyn sodium, psychopharmacologic agents, and digitalis. Almitrine has been reported to reduce the $PaCO_2$ and increase the PaO_2 in some hypoxemic patients with COPD. Theoretically, its use might delay the need for supplemental oxygen in patients with significant hypoxemia; however, whether it will be helpful still needs to be determined. Chapter 19 discusses the use of medications in patients with respiratory disease.

RESPIRATORY THERAPY MODALITIES

Respiratory therapy provides several modalities of benefit for the patient with lung disease, including aerosol therapy, oxygen therapy, breathing retraining, and bronchial hygiene.

Inhalation of bronchodilators is particularly effective because it results in a quick response with minimal systemic side effects, compared with the oral route. Aerosolization of bronchodilators may be accomplished by inexpensive cartridge inhalers (metered-dose inhalers), hand-bulb nebulizers, or

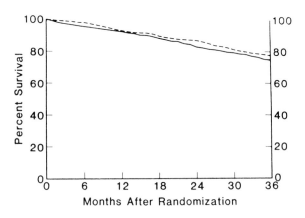

Figure 24–1. Survival of randomized COPD patients enrolled in the NIH/IPPB study. Survival differences between those receiving IPPB therapy (———) and those using compressor nebulizers (———) was insignificant. (Reproduced with permission from: The IPPB Trial Group: Intermittent positive pressure breathing therapy of chronic obstructive pulmonary disease: A clinical trial. Ann Intern Med 99:612–620, 1983)

compressor pump nebulizers. Various holding chambers (spacers) are available to aid in the proper use of metered-dose inhalers and to minimize topical and systemic side effects. Intermittent positive-pressure breathing (IPPB) is occasionally used for aerosolization of bronchodilators, although there are no data that it works more effectively than other methods available for aerosolization of bronchodilators. The NIH collaborative study comparing IPPB and compressor nebulizers in outpatients with COPD did not demonstrate any advantage for IPPB therapy, nor was any significant difference noted in the variables that were monitored, including survival (Fig. 24–1).[27]

Although aerosolization of bland mist or mucolytic agents is sometimes used in patients with thick secretions, there is little evidence of their efficacy in the liquefaction of lower airway secretions.

When low-flow oxygen is used in COPD patients who have significant hypoxemia, there is improvement in psychological testing, motor coordination, exercise tolerance, and sleep patterns.[28,29] One report suggests that supplemental oxygen for at least 15 hr/day will delay the onset of pulmonary hypertension and cor pulmonale in the hypoxemic COPD patient.[30] In the NIH cooperative Nocturnal Oxygen Therapy Trial, 203 patients with COPD, with either a PaO_2 of 55 mmHg or less or a PaO_2 of less than 60 mmHg plus either polycythemia or evidence of cor pulmonale, were randomly allocated to continuous oxygen therapy or 12-hour nocturnal oxygen therapy. The results show that mortality in the nocturnal oxygen therapy group after 12 months of follow-up was nearly twice that seen in the continuous oxygen therapy group.[31]

Although the use of low-flow oxygen is important in patients with COPD, increasing the PaO_2 above 60 to 65 mmHg in patients with hypercapnia may lead to worsening of the hypercapnia and respiratory acidosis.

The reader is referred to Chapter 15 for a thorough discussion of oxygen therapy and to Chapter 17 for a discussion of aerosol therapy.

CHEST PHYSIOTHERAPY AND EXERCISE RECONDITIONING

Chest physiotherapy techniques used in pulmonary rehabilitation programs may include relaxation techniques, breathing retraining, chest percussion, and bronchial drainage techniques[32,33] (see Chap. 23).

Relaxation techniques have been used to help the patient control anxiety, agitation, and fear. Stress can exacerbate and aggravate existing physical and psychological symptoms. For patients with COPD, the sensation of dyspnea can create tension and fear. Relaxation techniques may include biofeedback, imagery, or simply listening to soothing music in a quiet environment.

Breathing retraining has the following goals: to help control dyspnea through a relaxed pattern of slow breathing, and to increase alveolar ventilation in an attempt to improve or to maintain adequate gas exchange.

The use of pursed lips along with abdominal–diaphragmatic breathing is the breathing technique most commonly used to reduce the respiratory rate and improve respiratory muscle coordination. With this technique, the patient inhales deeply with the abdominal muscles relaxed and then exhales through pursed lips, augmented by abdominal muscle contraction. Although improved ventilation, a reduced respiratory rate and a decreased alveolar–arterial oxygen difference have been reported in patients who use this breathing pattern,[34,35] similar improvements in blood gas levels have occurred with slow deep breathing alone. For many patients, however, these breathing techniques help relieve dyspnea.

Respiratory muscle strength and endurance may be enhanced by voluntary normocapnic hyperpnea as well as by periodic breathing through a high-resistance device.[36,37] Patients with cystic fibrosis have achieved the same increase in ventila-

tory muscle function by participating in a 4-week physical activity training program at a summer camp that included intensive swimming and canoeing.[38]

Chest percussion and bronchial drainage techniques can improve clearance of secretions in those COPD patients who have excessive amounts of secretions and who are unable to clear their airways spontaneously because of an inability to take a deep breath or to cough effectively, or because of tenacious sputum.[39] This technique should be reserved for those COPD patients who expectorate more than 30 mL (2 tbsp) of sputum daily and who have difficulty eliminating the mucus with proper cough techniques.[40]

Patients with COPD generally lack activity and exercise endurance. Dyspnea and fatigue are the usual limiting factors in exercising COPD patients. Many patients reduce their physical activity dramatically to avoid this discomfort. This results in a worsening condition and leads to a cycle of increasing deconditioning. The physiologic effects of exercise and its benefits in this patient population have been described in many reports and include improved appetite, better sleep, enhanced tolerance of dyspnea, and ability to achieve a higher level of work.[41–46]

A 6- or 12-minute walk test or an incremental exercise (pulmonary or cardiac) stress test may be done to assess the patient's current exercise tolerance and to document an impaired ability to exercise. An exercise prescription has four parts: (1) the mode of exercise, (2) the intensity, (3) the duration, and (4) the frequency. Modes of exercise that could be selected include walking, swimming, and riding a stationary bicycle. The mode selected for the patient should be the one that the patient prefers.

There has been considerable controversy over how to determine the appropriate intensity level of exercise for the COPD patient. A target heart rate (THR) can be used by most patients with COPD. However, this may be a less reliable indicator of the intensity desired in those with very severe impairment. *Karvonen's formula*, using 0.6 as the factor in the equation, has been shown to select a THR that works well for most patients initiating an exercise training program:[47]

$$THR = (0.6 \times (PHR - RHR)) + RHR$$

where PHR is the peak heart rate during a maximal exercise stress test and RHR is the resting heart rate. Karvonen's formula is particularly helpful in that it takes both the PHR and the RHR into account when determining a THR. If, for example, we used the formula $THR = 0.7 \times PHR$, the calculated THR might, in fact, be lower than the patient's RHR!

In patients with very severe impairment, for whom a THR may be a less reliable indicator of the level of work and in those who have difficulty monitoring their heart rate, an acceptable alternative for determining the intensity of exercise is to teach the patient the level of dyspnea or "perceived exertion" that would be safe to achieve during exercise. Although this is less objective than using the THR, it has been successful in many programs for patients with pulmonary impairment.

It is important to increase the intensity of exercise gradually to achieve improved conditioning. The exercise session preferably should last at least 20 to 30 minutes, with the patient exercising at least three to four times a week.[48]

When exercise is performed regularly, the patient usually gains an increased tolerance for dyspnea, has an improved appetite, and demonstrates an increased physical capability, with resultant improvement in quality of life. The use of an ear oximeter to monitor oxygen saturation is a noninvasive, reliable way of evaluating blood oxygen levels during the exercise period. In patients with significant hypoxemia that limits exercise ability (i.e., $PaO_2 \leq 55$ mgHg or O_2 saturation $\leq 88\%$), supplemental oxygen may allow patients to participate in an exercise-conditioning program and thereby improve their level of activity.[49]

ACTIVITIES OF DAILY LIVING EVALUATION

Evaluation of activities of daily living can identify problem areas. Outlining various energy-saving maneuvers can assist the patient in carrying out desired activities. Adaptive devices can be prescribed for patients to help them avoid excessive exertion when picking up objects from the floor, dressing, or bathing. The goal is to modify activities to consume less oxygen and become energy efficient.[50]

NUTRITIONAL EVALUATION

A low-fat, complex carbohydrate diet is generally advised for COPD patients. For patients with hypercapnia, a lower-carbohydrate, higher-fat diet may be considered to help reduce the carbon dioxide production. A nutritional evaluation should be performed and dietary instructions given to meet the patient's needs.[51] Some general recommendations can be made about dietary patterns, such as

avoidance of an increased amount of fluids during a meal, which can cause bloating. Patients with decreased appetite related to dyspnea, abdominal fullness from air swallowing, or nausea from medications should use multiple small feedings throughout the day rather than two or three large meals. Nutritional supplements may be useful in patients with a poor appetite. The use of oxygen during meals may help hypoxemic patients to eat more comfortably.

Often these patients have concomitant disease—for example, cardiovascular problems that require other special dietary instructions. For the obese patient, losing weight reduces the work of breathing. For the patient who is progressively losing weight unintentionally as a result of his or her increased caloric expenditure owing to COPD and excess accessory respiratory muscle work, proper nutritional support is important. The patient must have adequate (normal) serum potassium, magnesium, and phosphorus levels to assure muscle strength and endurance. Deficiencies of these nutrients may result in respiratory failure and cardiac arrhythmias.

PSYCHOSOCIAL EVALUATION

Psychosocial assessment focuses on the patient's reaction to COPD, how to handle the illness, and its effects on daily life.[52,53] It deals with the patient's work, social, recreational, interpersonal, and family relationships, and sex. The COPD patient's sexual activity and how he feels about it are basic components of his identity and ego strength and affect how he relates to his spouse. Psychotherapy and psychopharmacologic agents should be considered for those patients not responding satisfactorily to usual attempts by the physician and team members to help with their emotional problems.

Although counseling and strong supportive care are important in dealing with patients with COPD, psychopharmacologic agents are sometimes used as adjuncts in controlling the emotional disorder. Agents to treat anxiety should be used only on a short-term basis, since long-term use can lead to significant habituation. Diazepam and hydroxyzine are relatively safe anxiolytic agents. They can, however, result in undesirable side effects such as drowsiness, dizziness, and confusion. A potential problem with the use of tranquilizers is sedation and potentiation of depression.

When anxiety and depression coexist, the symptoms of anxiety often mask the depression. If the anxiety alone is treated, the depression may worsen significantly. When selecting an antidepressant agent, one should ascertain the need for a sedating effect versus an activating effect.[52] Doxepin is an excellent medication for agitated, depressed patients because it can reduce or eliminate agitation, in addition to its antidepressant effect. Protriptyline is a good antidepressant for depressed patients with low drive and motivation. Imipramine falls between doxepin and protriptyline and would be particularly useful when neither sedation nor activation is needed. Doxepin should be administered near bedtime to assist with sleep, whereas morning administration of protriptyline promotes daytime energy.

VOCATIONAL REHABILITATION

The basic goal of rehabilitation is to return the patient with COPD to society as a self-sufficient, useful member. Once a patient's activity level has been optimized after a rehabilitation program, one should evaluate his or her potential for vocational restoration.[54,55] A patient may be able to return to his or her previous employment or to the same occupational field in a different job or location. Sometimes a patient may need to be retrained in another field.

Successful vocational rehabilitation is difficult to achieve in patients with COPD. Factors that can hinder successful vocational rehabilitation include a recent significant change in life-style, evidence of rapid clinical deterioration, major personality change, alcoholism, and inability to mobilize psychological and social assets.[56] The level of intelligence is also a factor in vocational options.[14] Other factors that lessen vocational rehabilitation potential include advanced age, the progressive nature of the disease, and limitations in the ability of the patient with respiratory impairment to retrain. A proper approach to disability and impairment evaluation is essential when attempting to determine a patient's ability to work.[57]

ASSESSMENT OF PATIENT'S PROGRESS

The patient's pulmonary rehabilitation goals should be continually assessed and reassessed while a patient is in the program. This allows for any necessary modifications to the program, as well as an evaluation of its overall effectiveness. The patient's program must change as he or she does.

LONG-TERM FOLLOW-UP

It is critical to send the patient back to his or her own primary care physician for follow-up, to help assure that the PR program will receive future referrals from these physicians! The medical director or program director of pulmonary rehabilitation should also send a complete summary of the patient's assessment and the team's recommendations to the patient's primary care physician.

Once the patient has completed the rehabilitation program, follow-up care is generally resumed by the primary care physician. The rehabilitation team may work with the primary care physician in continuing to assess the patient periodically and in helping to modify the patient's program as his or her condition changes.

BENEFITS OF PULMONARY REHABILITATION

Reported benefits of pulmonary rehabilitation include an improved quality of life and enhanced ability to carry out daily activities.[58,59] Patients have achieved a significant reduction in their symptoms, anxiety, depression, and somatic concerns, with an associated improvement in ego strength.[52,60,61] The number of hospital days required per patient per year has been significantly reduced,[62,63] and some patients have been able to continue or to return to gainful employment.[54,56,58] An improvement in exercise tolerance has already been discussed.

A study of patients with COPD undergoing PR at Loma Linda University Medical Center demonstrated a significant reduction in hospital days required following the rehabilitation program (Fig. 24–2). One might, at first glance, conclude that the reduction in hospital days noted simply reflects death of the sickest patients during the first several years of follow-up, leaving the healthier patients toward the end. However, the reduction in hospital days required for only those patients surviving for the full 8 years is virtually identical. Obviously, this marked reduction in hospitalization results in a significant cost saving.[63,64] In a comparison of COPD patient survival between the NIH/IPPB study and Burrows study, the survival in both groups was similar for patients with an FEV_1 higher than 42.5% of predicted. However, patients with more severe obstruction had a better survival in the NIH/IPPB group than in Burrows patients[65] (Fig. 24–3). It is

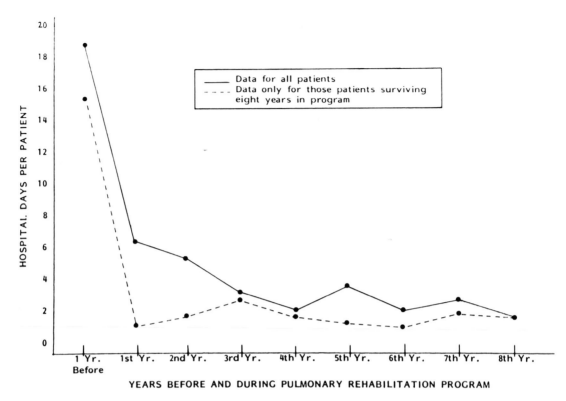

Figure 24—2. Analysis of hospital days before and during a pulmonary rehabilitation program. (Data from the Loma Linda University Medical Center Pulmonary Rehabilitation Program)

Figure 24—3. Survival curves from the NIH/IPPB trial were compared with those of the Burrows group according to patients' baseline FEV$_1$ and age at entry into the trial. Patients in both groups with baseline FEV$_1$ greater than 42.5% of predicted had similar survival rates. In the NIH/IPPB study, patients with more severe obstruction had improved survival rates, perhaps related to comprehensive long-term care. (Adapted from Anthonisen NR, Wright EC, Hodgkin JE et al: Prognosis in chronic obstructive pulmonary disease. Am Rev Respir Dis 133:14–20, 1986)

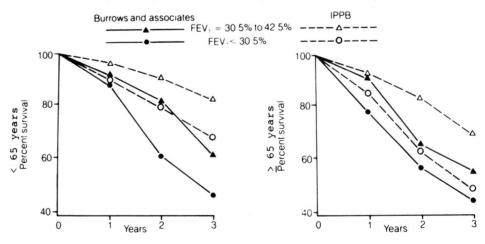

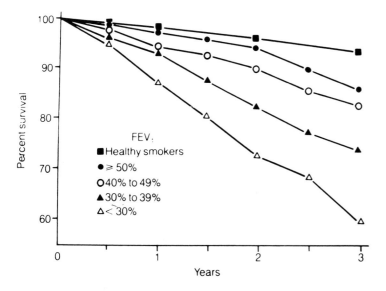

Figure 24—4. Baseline FEV$_1$ was clearly shown to be a predictor of survival when patients from the NIH/IPPB study were segregated according to baseline FEV$_1$ after administration of a bronchodilator. Patients whose baseline FEV$_1$ was 50% of predicted or greater had mortality only slightly different from that of a group of healthy smokers, whereas those with lower FEV$_1$ values had a higher probability of death. (Reproduced with permission from Anthonisen NR, Wright EC, Hodgkin JE et al: Prognosis in chronic obstructive pulmonary disease. Am Rev Respir Dis 133:14–20, 1986)

reasonable to believe that the improved survival in patients in the NIH/IPPB study is at least partly a result of the comprehensive respiratory care and PR that included close follow-up with home and clinic visits.

Although no improvement in survival or slowing of the deterioration of respiratory function has been documented in most reports, it is hoped that by implementing the components of care described in this chapter in patients with relatively mild obstructive airway disease, the course of the disease may be altered favorably. The lower the FEV$_1$, the worse the expected survival becomes[65] (Fig. 24–4).

Pulmonary rehabilitation is not something that happens *to* a patient but *with* a patient. It allows a patient to return to as normal a life as possible. Each program must be individualized to meet the patient's needs. The PR program that provides only education and exercise, without a comprehensive individual assessment, will fail to help the pulmonary patient achieve the highest level of function possible. It is logical that the course of lung disease is more likely to be altered favorably by instituting the principles of PR earlier than has generally been done in the past.

REFERENCES

1. Hodgkin JE, Petty TL: Definition and epidemiology of COPD. In Hodgkin JE, Petty TL (eds): Chronic Obstructive Pulmonary Disease: Current Concepts. Philadelphia, WB Saunders, 1987

2. Estimated prevalence and incidence of respiratory disease by Lung Association territory. American Lung Association, Sept. 1989
3. National Heart, Lung, and Blood Institute Fact Book. Fiscal Year 1986. U.S. Dept. of Health and Human Services, Oct. 1986
4. Morbidity and Mortality Chart book on Cardiovascular, Lung, and Blood Diseases. National Heart, Lung, and Blood Institute. U.S. Department of Health and Human Services, 1990
5. Hodgkin JE (ed): Chronic obstructive pulmonary disease. Clin Chest Med 11:9–10, 1990
6. Petty TL: Pulmonary Rehabilitation. Basics of RD, Vol 4, p 1. New York, American Thoracic Society, 1975
7. Pulmonary rehabilitation: Official statement of the American Thoracic Society. Am Rev Respir Dis 124:663–666, 1981
8. Hodgkin JE: Pulmonary rehabilitation: Structure, components, and benefits. J Cardiopulmonary Rehabil 11:423–434, 1988
9. Elkousy NM, Komorowski D, Foto M et al: Outpatient pulmonary rehabilitation: A Medicare fiscal intermediary's viewpoint. J Cardiopulmonary Rehabil 11:492–497, 1988
10. Hodge-Hilton T, Herrmann DW, Hills RL et al: Initial evaluation of the pulmonary rehabilitation candidate. In Hodgkin JE, Zorn EG, Connors GL (eds): Pulmonary Rehabilitation: Guidelines to Success. Boston, Butterworth Publishers, 1984
11. Hatch TF: Changing objectives in occupational health. Am Ind Hyg Assoc J 23:1, 1962
12. Connors GA, Hodgkin JE, Asmus RM: A careful assessment is crucial to successful pulmonary rehabilitation. J Cardiopulmonary Rehabil 11:435–438, 1988
13. Branscomb BV: Aggravating factors and coexisting disorders. In Hodgkin JE, Petty TL (eds): Chronic Obstructive Pulmonary Disease: Current Concepts. Philadelphia, WB Saunders, 1987
14. Connors GC: Evaluation and testing of the COPD patient prior to rehabilitation. In Hall LK, Meyer GC

(eds): Epidemiology, Behavior Change, and Intervention in Chronic Disease. Champaign, Life Enhancement Publications, 1988

15. Hopp JW, Maddox SE: Education of patients and their families. In Hodgkin JE. Zorn EG, Connors GL (eds): Pulmonary Rehabilitation: Guidelines to Success. Boston, Butterworth Publishers, 1984

16. Neish CM, Hopp JW: The role of education in pulmonary rehabilitation. J Cardiopulmonary Rehabil 11:439–441, 1988

17. Hills RL, Gerkin CM, Jezerinac L: Compliance and the patient with pulmonary disease. In Hodgkin JE, Zorn EG, Connors GL (eds): Pulmonary Rehabilitation: Guidelines to Success. Boston, Butterworth Publishers, 1984

18. Davis MD: Variations in patients' compliance with doctors' orders: Analysis of congruence between survey responses and results of empirical investigations. J Med Educ 41:1037, 1966

19. Respiratory Diseases Task Force Report on Prevention, Control, Education: US Department of Health, Education, and Welfare Publ No. (NIH) 77-1248, p 133. Bethesda, National Heart, Lung & Blood Institute, 1977

20. Buist AS, Sexton GJ, Nagy JM et al: The effect of smoking cessation and modification on lung function. Am Rev Respir Dis 114:115, 1976

21. Peters JA, Lim VJ: Smoking cessation techniques. In Hodgkin JE, Zorn EG, Connors GL (eds): Pulmonary Rehabilitation: Guidelines to Success. Boston, Butterworth Publishers, 1984

22. Campbell IA: Smoking cessation. In Hodgkin JE, Petty TL (eds): Chronic Obstructive Pulmonary Disease: Current Concepts. Philadelphia, WB Saunders, 1987

23. Jarvin MJ, Raw M, Russell MAH et al: Randomized controlled trial of nicotine chewing gum. Br Med J 285:537–540, 1982

24. Yee AR, Connors GL, Cress DB: Pharmacology and the respiratory patient. In Hodgkin JE, Zorn EG, Connors GL (eds): Pulmonary Rehabilitation: Guidelines to Success. Boston, Butterworth Publishers, 1984

25. Ziment I: Pharmacologic therapy of obstructive airway disease. In Hodgkin JE (ed): Chronic obstructive pulmonary disease. Clin Chest Med Sept. 1990

26. Muriciano D, Ambier M, Lecocguic Y et al: Effects of theophylline on diaphragmatic strength and fatigue in patients with chronic obstructive pulmonary disease. N Engl J Med 1311:349–353, 1984

27. The Intermittent Positive Pressure Breathing Trial Group: Intermittent positive pressure breathing therapy of chronic obstructive pulmonary disease. Ann Intern Med 99:612–620, 1983

28. Block AJ: Low-flow oxygen therapy, treatment of the ambulant outpatient. Am Rev Respir Dis 110(suppl):71, 1974

29. Block AJ, Castel JR, Keitt AS: Chronic oxygen therapy: Treatment of chronic obstructive pulmonary disease at sea level. Chest 65:279, 1974

30. Stark RD, Finnegan P, Bishop JM: Daily requirement of oxygen to reverse pulmonary hypertension in patients with chronic bronchitis. Br Med J 3:724, 1972

31. Continuous or nocturnal oxygen therapy in hypoxemic chronic obstructive lung disease: A clinical trial. Ann Intern Med 93:391, 1980

32. Cherniack RM: Physical therapy techniques. In

33. Hodgkin JE, Petty TL (eds): Chronic Obstructive Pulmonary Disease: Current Concepts. Philadelphia, WB Saunders, 1987

33. Sexton DL: Relaxation techniques and biofeedback. In Hodgkin JE, Petty TL (eds): Chronic Obstructive Pulmonary Disease: Current Concepts. Philadelphia, WB Saunders, 1987

34. Mueller RE, Petty TL, Filley GF: Ventilation and arterial blood gas changes induced by pursed lip breathing. J Appl Physiol 28:784, 1970

35. Thomas RL, Stoker GL, Ross JC: The efficacy of pursed-lip breathing in patients with chronic obstructive pulmonary disease. Am Rev Respir Dis 93:100, 1966

36. Belman MJ, Mittman C: Ventilatory muscle training improves exercise capacity in chronic obstructive pulmonary disease patients. Am Rev Respir Dis 121:273, 1980

37. Pardy RL, Rivington RN, Despas PJ et al: Inspiratory muscle training compared with physiotherapy in patients with chronic airflow limitation. Am Rev Respir Dis 123:421, 1981

38. Keens TG, Krastins IRB, Wannamaker EM et al: Ventilatory muscle endurance training in normal subjects and patients with cystic fibrosis. Am Rev Respir Dis 116:853, 1977

39. Jones NL: Physical therapy—present state of the art. Am Rev Respir Dis 110(suppl):132, 1974

40. Murray JF: The ketchup-bottle method. N Engl J Med 300:1155, 1979

41. Bass H, Whitcomb JF, Forman R: Exercise training: Therapy for patients with chronic obstructive pulmonary disease. Chest 57:116, 1970

42. Belman MJ, Wasserman K: Exercise training and testing in patients with chronic obstructive pulmonary disease. Basics of RD 10, No. 2, November 1981 (available from the American Thoracic Society)

43. Shephard RJ: Exercise and chronic obstructive lung disease. Exerc Sport Sci Rev 4:263, 1976

44. Wasserman K, Whipp BJ: Exercise physiology in health and disease. Am Rev Respir Dis 112:219, 1975

45. Woolf CR, Suero JT: Alterations in lung mechanics and gas exchange following training in chronic obstructive lung disease. Dis Chest 55:37, 1969

46. Hodgkin JE: Exercise testing and training. In Hodgkin JE, Petty TL (eds): Chronic Obstructive Pulmonary Disease: Current Concepts. Philadelphia, WB Saunders, 1987

47. Hodgkin JE, Litzau KL: Exercise training target heart rates in chronic obstructive pulmonary disease. Chest 94:30S, 1988

48. Adams WC, McHenry MM, Bernauer EM: Long-term physiologic adaptions to exercise with special reference to performance and cardiorespiratory function in health and disease. In Amsterdam EA, Wilmore JH, Demaria AN (eds): Exercise in Cardiovascular Health and Disease. New York, Yorke Medical Books, 1977

49. Stein DA, Bradley BL, Miller WC: Mechanisms of oxygen effects on exercise in patients with chronic obstructive pulmonary disease. Chest 81:6, 1982

50. Shanfield K, Hammond MA: Activities of daily living. In Hodgkin JE, Zorn EG, Connors GL (eds): Pulmonary Rehabilitation: Guidelines to Success. Boston, Butterworth Publishers, 1984

51. Peters JA, Burke K, White D: Nutrition and the pulmo-

nary patient. In Hodgkin JE, Zorn EG, Connors GL (eds): Pulmonary Rehabilitation: Guidelines to Success. Boston, Butterworth Publishers, 1984

52. Dudley DL, Glaser EM, Jorgenson B et al: Psychosocial concomitants to rehabilitation in chronic obstructive pulmonary disease. Chest 77:413, 544, 677, 1980

53. Glaser EM, Dudley DL: Psychosocial rehabilitation and psycho-pharmacology. In Hodgkin JE, Petty TL (eds): Chronic Obstructive Pulmonary Disease: Current Concepts. Philadelphia, WB Saunders, 1987

54. Kass I, Daughton DM, Fix AJ: Respiratory impairment disability and vocational rehabilitation. In Hodgkin JE, Zorn EG, Connors GL (eds): Pulmonary Rehabilitation: Guidelines to Success. Boston, Butterworth Publishers, 1984

55. Kawner RE: Impairment and disability evaluation and vocational rehabilitation. In Hodgkin JE, Petty TL (eds): Chronic Obstructive Pulmonary Disease: Current Concepts. Philadelphia, WB Saunders, 1987

56. Kass I, Dyksterhuis JE, Rubin H et al: Correlation of psychophysiological variables with vocational rehabilitation: Outcome in chronic obstructive pulmonary disease patients. Chest 67:433, 1975

57. Evaluation of impairment/disability secondary to respiratory disorders. Am Rev Respir Dis 133:1205–1209, 1986

58. Haas A, Cardon H: Rehabilitation in chronic obstructive pulmonary disease: A five-year study of 252 male patients. Med Clin North Am 53:593, 1969

59. Shapiro BA, Vostinak-Foley E, Hamilton BB et al: Rehabilitation in chronic obstructive pulmonary disease: A two-year prospective study. Respir Care 22:1045, 1977

60. Fishman DB, Petty TL: Physical, symptomatic, and psychological improvement in patients receiving comprehensive care for chronic airway obstruction. J Chronic Dis 24:775, 1971

61. Agle DP, Baum GL, Chest EH et al: Multidiscipline treatment of chronic pulmonary insufficiency: Psychologic aspects of rehabilitation. Psychosom Med 35:41, 1973

62. Hudson LD, Tyler ML, Petty TL: Hospitalization needs during an outpatient rehabilitation program for severe chronic airway obstruction. Chest 70:606, 1976

63. Burton GG, Gee G, Hodgkin JE et al: Cost effectiveness studies in respiratory care: An overview and some possible early solutions. Hospitals 49:61, 1975

64. Bebout DE, Hodgkin JE, Zorn EG et al: Clinical and physiological outcomes of a university-hospital pulmonary rehabilitation program. Respir Care 28:1468–1473, 1983

65. Anthonisen NR, Wright EC, Hodgkin JE et al: Prognosis in chronic obstructive pulmonary disease. Am Rev Respir Dis 133:14–20, 1986

SECTION THREE

Respiratory Care in Critical Illness

Care of Ventilator-Assisted Individuals in the Home and Alternative Community Sites

Barry J. Make
Mary E. Gilmartin

The concept of home care for individuals requiring mechanical assistance to ventilation was originally pioneered in the 1940s and 1950s in patients suffering from poliomyelitis.[1–6] Those patients used respiratory assist devices, such as the iron lung,[7,8] chest cuirass,[9] rocking bed,[10,11] and pneumobelt,[12] which were developed earlier in the 20th century but today are considered crude and ineffective by intensivists caring for critically ill patients in modern critical care units. Nevertheless, respiratory care practitioners in the late 1980s rediscovered both the concepts and the equipment of the polio era and applied them to the care of the rapidly increasing number of ventilator-assisted individuals managed outside the acute care hospital setting.[13–15] This chapter will address the management of ventilator-assisted persons cared for in the home and other locations in the community such as long-term care hospitals and skilled nursing facilities, where the goals are different from those for patients receiving mechanical ventilation in intensive care units (ICUs). The goals of home care for this population are the following:[15]

- Reduce mortality
- Decrease morbidity
- Improve the quality of life
- Improve physical and physiologic function
- Provide an environment that will enhance individual potential
- Be cost-effective

EXTENT OF THE PROBLEM

Three major factors have led to an increased interest in home care for ventilator-assisted persons: (1) an increase in the number of candidates for home ventilation; (2) improvements in respiratory care in the home; and (3) increased societal awareness of the potential of handicapped individuals. The rapid increase in knowledge about respiratory disorders over the last two decades has been followed by an expansion of the number of training programs for all types of respiratory care practitioners (respiratory therapists, nurses, and pulmonary physicians). As a result of the widespread implementation of improved respiratory care techniques by an increased number of skilled professionals, there has been increased survival not only of seriously ill hospitalized patients, but also of individuals with chronic progressive respiratory and neurologic disorders. This, in turn, has led to an increase in the number of candidates for mechanical assistance to ventilation in the home. Increasing emphasis on reducing hospital costs has also created a greater demand for home care.

Two studies have documented inequities in Medicare's Medical Diagnosis Related Group (DRG) prospective payment system for prolonged ventilator care.[16,17] Douglas et al. found that costs exceeded reimbursement by an average of 23,129 dollars per case in 95 nonsurgical Medicare patients receiving mechanical ventilation for 3 or more days in a Chicago teaching hospital.[16] The average cost for hospital care was 38,486 dollars per patient, and each day on a ventilator added 439 dollars for respiratory-related services. The magnitude of the problem appears to be similar in community hospitals.[17] These findings led to a change in the DRG classification of ventilator patients in 1987.

Although prospective payment systems have encouraged hospitals to discharge patients earlier, pressures placed upon respiratory practitioners by hospital administrators should not be the prime motivation for discharging ventilator-assisted individuals. Rather, medical professionals should act as patient advocates and place the interests of their patients foremost in determining the optimal location for continued care of ventilator-assisted individuals. Potential candidates for mechanical ventilation in the home or alternative site in the community should be carefully screened to assure that they are appropriate for such care and will thrive in the nonhospital environment. Moreover, patients should not be sent home until they and the personnel participating in their care are appropriately trained in the necessary respiratory care.

Several studies[18–20] have reported a substantial number of ventilator-assisted individuals in acute care hospitals, many of whom cannot be discharged because of lack of community resources, both in less acute institutions, such as skilled nursing facilities, and in the home. In 1983, a study in Massachusetts identified 143 individuals who had been ventilator-dependent for more than 3 weeks.[18] The majority (60%) were in acute care hospitals, and 60% of hospitalized patients were in intensive care units. Twenty-four percent of patients were in long-term care hospitals (a setting more readily available in southeastern Massachusetts than in many other areas of the United States), and two patients were in a skilled nursing facility. The most common diagnoses of these ventilator-assisted individuals were chronic obstructive pulmonary disease (20%), amyotrophic lateral sclerosis (13%), other neuromuscular disorders (13%), central nervous system diseases (8%), and spinal cord injury (5%). Given the prevalence of ventilator-assisted individuals ($3:100,000$ population) in this study, the authors estimated there were at least 6800 long-term ventilator-assisted individuals in the United States. The cost of caring for hospitalized long-term ventilator-assisted individuals was estimated at 1.7 billion dollars yearly, about 1.5% of the total hospital costs for the United States in 1983! The results of the Massachusetts study suggested that up to 40% of

acute care hospital patients were candidates for transfer to chronic care hospitals, and 15% were candidates for home care, with a potential cost reduction of 251 million dollars per year in medical costs. A follow-up study 6 months later showed that 35% of the patients had died; 81% of patients still alive remained ventilator-dependent.

A 1983 survey conducted by the American Association of Respiratory Care (AARC) identified 2272 ventilator-dependent individuals in 106 hospitals in 21 states, 13% of whom were "deemed medically able to go home," but remained in acute care hospitals, presumably because of lack of third-party payment for other types of care or because of fewer acute care community facilities capable of caring for ventilator-assisted patients.[19] The AARC estimated the mean cost of hospital care per patient was 270,830 dollars per year, but only 21,192 dollars for home care. Although the number of patients is small, the cost savings of home care compared with hospital care was estimated to be over 64 million dollars per year.

As documented by Bone,[20] there are inadequate resources in chronic care facilities to appropriately manage patients requiring prolonged ventilatory assistance. In the metropolitan Chicago area, there is a 50 to 80 patient waiting list for the 33 available beds in two chronic care facilities.[20] In the Boston area, there is a waiting list of 25 to 50 patients for the 25 available beds in chronic care hospitals.

BENEFICIAL EFFECTS OF PROLONGED MECHANICAL VENTILATION

The benefits of mechanical ventilation when employed over an extended period in the home include (1) reduction of $PaCO_2$ and often maintenance of eucapnia during periods off the ventilator; (2) improved oxygenation; (3) improved ability to perform activities; (4) decrease in hospitalizations; (5) decreased respiratory symptoms, dyspnea, and cor pulmonale; (6) increased respiratory muscle strength; and (7) decreased mortality.[21–25]

Garay et al. reported the course of eight patients with alveolar hypoventilation, without parenchymal lung disease, who were treated with "noninvasive" forms of ventilatory assistance not requiring a tracheostomy.[21] Ventilatory assistance was required because of muscular dystrophy, kyphoscoliosis, postpolio muscular weakness, postthoracic surgery and phrenic nerve crush, and primary alveolar hypoventilation. These patients were leading active lives but were unable to maintain normal alveolar ventilation outside the hospital; they were begun on home ventilatory assistance only after repeated hospital admissions for carbon dioxide narcosis, hypersomnolence, or coma. Patients successfully received ventilatory assistance in the home, using negative-pressure ventilators or positive-pressure ventilation by mouthpiece for 3 to 14 years, with sustained reversal of hypercapnia and a decrease in hospital admissions to 1.5 per patient during a mean follow-up of 10.6 years. Pulmonary function studies were stable or showed mild improvement in some cases, and pulmonary hypertension resolved in three patients who had repeat cardiac catheterization.

Similarly, Hoeppner et al. described four patients with symptomatic chronic respiratory failure with secondary kyphoscoliosis caused by polio who did not respond to supplementary oxygen, diuretics, intermittent positive-pressure breathing treatments, and tracheostomy.[22] Within 3 days of institution of positive-pressure ventilation for 12 hours at night through a tracheostomy, symptoms of dyspnea and restless sleep improved. Within 1 to 3 weeks, the $PaCO_2$ during the day while breathing spontaneously had decreased from 60 to 38 mmHg, and the PaO_2 increased from 38 to 68 mmHg. In addition, vital capacity, erythrocytosis, and right heart failure improved, allowing an almost normal pattern of daytime activity. Improvement was maintained over a mean follow-up of 3.4 years.

Studies of the effect of negative-pressure ventilation electively employed in patients with chronic obstructive pulmonary disease (COPD) have produced conflicting results. Braun and Marino tested the hypothesis that respiratory muscle rest could alleviate chronic respiratory failure by electively using external negative-pressure ventilators (the Pulmowrap, or poncho, from J. H. Emerson Co., Cambridge, Mass.) in 35 patients with a variety of thoracic and extrathoracic disorders.[23] After 5 months of 4 to 10 hours of daily ventilator use, the mean PCO_2 decreased from 54 to 43 mmHg, with improvement in vital capacity; inspiratory and expiratory muscle strength, measured by maximal mouth pressures; endurance, measured by maximal voluntary ventilation; and functional activity, with a subsequent reduction in hospitalizations. Cropp and associates showed similar results in a group of nine COPD patients after only 3 days of negative-pressure ventilator use for 4 to 8 hours daily,[24] and Gutierrez et al. reported improvement in five patients ventilated 8 hours, once a week.[25] On the other hand, Pluto et al.[26] and Zibrak et al.[27] could not demonstrate improvement in similar patients. In addition, Celli et al. failed to show an improvement in diaphragm strength or exercise tolerance with negative-pressure ventilation in COPD patients randomized to receive either negative-pressure ventilation plus rehabilitation or rehabilitation alone.[28] All patients received rehabilitation, including exercise training, which resulted in improved exercise endurance and clinical status, with decreased respiratory muscle work and improved efficiency. In general, COPD patients with hypercapnia seem to demonstrate improvement following use of negative-pressure ventilation, whereas eucapneic individuals experience no improvement.

Rochester et al. suggested that the beneficial effects of negative-pressure ventilation in patients with chronic hypercapnia secondary to obstructive lung disease and chest wall disorders were due to reduced activity of inspiratory muscles.[29] They demonstrated decreased diaphragmatic electrical activity and accessory muscle activity with consequent relief of dyspnea, with use of a tank ventilator. In contrast, body respirators were able to reduce diaphragmatic activity only when the subject's upper airway resistance was increased. It has been suggested that negative-pressure ventilation may be ineffective in some studies of patients with COPD because of failure to reduce respiratory muscle work. Rodenstein et al. have demonstrated that diaphragmatic electromyographic (EMG) activity is not initially reduced in untrained COPD subjects placed in a negative-pressure ventilator.[30] Only a 20% reduction in EMG activity was apparent after a 20- to 60-minute trial of ventilation in Rodenstein's patients. Further research is required to determine exactly which COPD patients are likely to benefit from elective use of negative-pressure ventilation.

Other respiratory-assist devices used in the home, including rocking beds and pneumobelts, may also be of benefit in patients with chronic respiratory failure.[31–37] Alexander and coworkers used these external respiratory-assist devices in ten patients with Duchenne muscular dystrophy, ranging in age from 10 to 20 years, for an average of 3.5 years at home.[35] Similarly, Curran used body respirators intermittently in nine patients with muscular dystrophy, for an average of 2 years, with reduction in $PaCO_2$.[31] Body respirators are also useful in patients with other chest wall disorders.[32,36,37]

INDICATIONS FOR HOME MECHANICAL VENTILATION

MEDICAL DIAGNOSIS

Mechanical ventilation is usually initiated in acute care settings for one of the following disorders: (1) the new onset of acute respiratory failure with severe hypoxia, such as in patients with adult respiratory distress syndrome (ARDS) following trauma or surgical procedures: (2) treatment of acute neurologic disorders; (3) management of progressive hypercapnia in patients with chronic, underlying neuromuscular or skeletal disorders; and (4) management of progressive hypercapnia in patients with COPD. In the first two situations, home mechanical ventilation is not appropriate. In the first situation, the expectation is that the application of ventilatory support is a temporary lifesaving measure and will be discontinued when the underlying pulmonary and systemic disorders are reversed. Owing to the inherent physiologic and clinical instability of these patients, home care is not appropriate. In the second situation, use of mechanical ventilation may be applied briefly in an emergency setting and may also be expected to be of only temporary duration in patients with reversible neurologic disorders of recent onset such as Guillain-Barré syndrome or an overdose of narcotic or sedative drugs.

As indicated in Table 25–1, home mechanical ventilation is appropriate for individuals with a variety of disorders.[15,38] In patients with chronic, irreversible neurologic or skeletal disorders such as amyotrophic lateral sclerosis, the use of mechanical ventilation to treat progressive hypercapnia or recurrent episodes of respiratory failure may be needed over a prolonged period as a life-supporting measure. In patients with COPD, mechanical ventilation has traditionally been reserved for patients who develop acute respiratory failure with respiratory acidosis unresponsive to intensive inpatient medical care. Although health professionals hope that the use of mechanical ventilation will be of only short duration, sometimes it is impossible to remove such patients from ventilatory assistance, despite advances in our understanding of the physiologic determinants of ventilator dependence.

ELECTIVE INITIATION OF VENTILATION

In many cases when respiratory failure can be anticipated in patients with chronic neuromuscular disorders and respiratory status is monitored se-

Table 25–1 Disorders That May Benefit From Home Mechanical Ventilation

---

NEUROMUSCULAR DISORDERS

Central nervous system
  Idiopathic (Ondine's curse)
  Acquired (Arnold-Chiari malformation)
Spinal cord
  Traumatic injury
  Syringomyelia
Anterior horn cell
  Amyotrophic lateral sclerosis
  Poliomyelitis
  Spinal muscle atrophy (Werdig-Hoffman)
Peripheral nerve
  Neuropathy (Charcot-Marie-Tooth, isolated phrenic neuropathy)
Muscle
  Muscular dystrophy
  Myopathy
Chest wall disorders
  Kyphoscoliosis
  Postsurgical (thoracoplasty)

CHRONIC OBSTRUCTIVE LUNG DISEASE

Adult (emphysema, chronic bronchitis, bronchiectasis)
Child (bronchopulmonary dysplasia)

---

quentially over time, the decision to institute ventilatory support may be made electively with the input of the patient and family. In these situations, effective application of mechanical assistance to ventilation may be "noninvasive" (i.e., not require a tracheostomy). Negative-pressure external ventilation, rocking bed, pneumobelt, or positive-pressure ventilation through a nasal mask may be effective in patients with chronic neuromuscular disorders. In such cases, respiratory care professionals should educate the patient and family so that they understand the progressive nature of the disease and the eventual outcomes, with and without ventilatory support. Patients and families should be given a realistic view of the future and encouraged to speak with other persons receiving long-term ventilatory support; speaking with other patients is of great educational value and may allay patient and family anxiety. The patient and family should play an integral role in the process of making a decision about whether to institute ventilatory support, and these decisions should be made well in advance of an acute episode of respiratory failure.[13] Elective initiation of mechanical ventilation in patients with neuromuscular disorders should be strongly considered on the basis of clinical and physiologic factors in patients who have

- Repeated hospital admissions for respiratory failure
- Unexplained development of pneumonia in the setting of reduced ventilatory function
- Marked reduction in exercise capacity and functional ability
- Dyspnea with minimal activity, tachypnea > 30/min, and thoracoabdominal inspiratory paradox
- Hypercapnia ($PaCO_2 > 45$ mmHg)
- Marked reduction in vital capacity (<25% predicted or <600 to 900 mL)
- Severely decreased respiratory muscle strength ($PI_{max} < 25$ cmH$_2$O)

FAILURE TO WEAN

Individuals who cannot be successfully weaned from mechanical ventilation should be considered chronically ventilator-dependent. There is no uniformly accepted definition of *ventilator dependence,* but the following are key elements that must be met before home ventilation is considered:

1. Multiple attempts to completely wean the patient from the mechanical ventilator for 24 hr/day have been unsuccessful over a period of at least 1 month.
2. Weaning attempts have been performed when the patient's medical condition is optimal and when the acute illnesses that led to initiation of ventilatory assistance have been reversed, if possible.
3. Weaning attempts have occurred when the patient is receiving an adequate bronchodilator regimen.
4. Weaning has been attempted in a meticulous manner by a skilled, respiratory care team.

It is unreasonable to consider long-term home mechanical ventilation unless the patient is truly ventilator-dependent, because of the intense effort on the part of many health professionals, and great expense necessary to discharge a ventilator-assisted individual. Although there are anecdotal stories of patients weaning from ventilatory assistance after discharge home, implying psychological im-

provement related to the home setting, there are no clear indications that these patients would not have weaned in the hospital with additional time and effort. Patients who are truly ventilator-dependent may then be considered as potential candidates for home care. Children with bronchopulmonary dysplasia (BPD) do have a greater potential to eventually wean from the ventilator than adults. Controversy exists over whether or not unweanable COPD patients should be considered for home mechanical ventilation.[15,38–40]

PATIENT SELECTION

The most important factor in assuring the success of mechanical ventilation in the home is selection of patients who are appropriate for such care. However, determining that a patient is a candidate for ventilatory assistance in the home or alternative site is not a simple task. The guidelines for long-term ventilatory support developed by the American College of Chest Physicians,[15] large published series on home ventilation,[3,5,13,39,41,42] and other reports,[20,43,44] give some indications of the types of patient who can be successfully managed outside the acute care hospital. These may assist the physician and respiratory care health professional in making a decision about the feasibility for home or alternative site care.

Factors other than the diagnosis that caused respiratory failure and the determination that, indeed, the patient is ventilator-dependent must be assessed before a decision is made to discharge a patient receiving ventilatory assistance (Table 25–2). The other important medical factors in selecting patients for home mechanical ventilation are clinical and physiologic stability (Tables 25–3, 25–4). Patients who are not clinically or physiologically stable have a high incidence of readmission and require intensive resources in the home. Patients should be considered for home care only if it is expected that they can spend most their time at home, rather than in the hospital, in the years following discharge. Coexisting diseases of other organ systems should be stable and not interfere with the patient's progress through the discharge-planning phase, nor with care in the home.

Frequent changes in ventilatory settings should not be required. Patients who have recurring deterioration in blood gas concentrations, despite optimal medical management, should be cared for in a hospital setting. Such unstable patients may need frequent medical, nursing, and respiratory therapy

Table 25—2 Factors Influencing the Decision for Home or Alternative Site Care

Medical diagnosis	Social support
Ventilator dependence	Psychological health
Clinical stability	Financial support
Physiologic stability	Home resources
Desires of the patient	Physical environment
Desires of the family	Health professional support
Patient and family ability	Technical support
to learn and perform	Community support
necessary care	

interventions that are unavailable in the home. Table 25—4 lists the criteria for physiologic stability of the respiratory system necessary for successful home ventilatory support. Nevertheless, many children with BPD are managed with positive end-expiratory pressure (PEEP) in the home. The ventilator characteristics listed are necessary because of the increased complexity and difficulty inherent in delivering high inspired oxygen concentrations and PEEP with the current generation of small, home ventilators.

Ventilators used in the home are generally less sophisticated than those used in the intensive care setting. The addition of complex devices to the basic ventilator to provide more sophisticated care

Table 25—3 Criteria for Clinical Stability

Absence of significant sustained dyspnea or severe dyspneic episodes and/or tachypnea
Absence of intercostal retractions (child)
Acceptable arterial blood gas levels, with $FiO_2 \leq 0.40$
Psychological stability
Progression on growth curve and developmental program (infants and children)
Absence of life-threatening cardiac dysfunction or arrhythmias
No major change in management requiring readmission to the hospital for 1 month
Ability to clear secretions
Evidence of gag/cough reflex or protected airway
Absence of significant aspiration
Presence of a tracheostomy (rather than an oral or nasal tracheal tube)

(O'Donohue WJ, Giovannoni RM, Goldberg AF et al: Long-term mechanical ventilation: Guidelines for management in the home and at alternate community sites. Chest 90(suppl):1S–37S, 1986, with permission)

reduces the safety so important to successful home care. At times a hospital-type ventilator may be required in the home because the patient's needs exceed the capabilities of portable home ventilators. However, such ventilators are relatively large and stationary; a second portable ventilator may be necessary for mobility.[15,45] An important principle of home care is to employ as simple a technology as possible in the home, rather than attempting to recreate the intensive care unit environment.

Nonmedical factors are important and must be assessed when considering the feasibility of home ventilation. These factors include the desires of the patient and family and the presence of family to assist with care (see Table 25–2). Many family members may be fearful about their ability to provide all the care required in the home. These fears may be overcome by allowing them to meet other families involved in home care, read educational materials, or view audiovisual materials that provide a detailed description of the process of discharge planning, and participate in an extensive hands-on educational program designed to help them feel at ease and confident with their ability to perform the required tasks. The amount of support that patients and families will receive in the home should also be discussed in a realistic fashion, since the type of insurance and financial resources often dictate the amount of support that can be provided. The caretaker's physical health and age is crucial when making a decision about the feasibility of home care. The elderly potential caretaker may also have multiple medical problems, poor eyesight, or reduced eye-hand coordination, limiting their ability to partake in the care even when he or she is willing. The psychological health of the patient and family should be assessed before mak-

Table 25—4 Criteria for Physiologic Stability

Other organ systems stable
Absence of acute infections
Optimal acid–base and metabolic status
Ventilator parameters
  FiO_2 stable and <0.40
  PEEP < 10 cmH$_2$O
  IMV not used
  Stable impedance
  Stable time on and off the ventilator

ing a final decision because the stress involved in home care of a ventilator-assisted individual can unravel the structure and function of the family and thereby impair the safety of home care. The patient's coping mechanisms (i.e., optimism, resourcefulness, flexibility, and adaptability) and motivation should be assessed.[46] Although the perfect patient is rare, it is important to have a model of the ideal home care candidate when assessing the patient and family.[46]

Payment sources available for home care should be determined for each individual; third-party payments are necessary for the vast majority of patients. It should be determined early in the hospital course whether the patient can qualify for additional funding from alternative sources such as a state Medicaid program. The amount of skilled health care professional services needed in the home is the major determinant of home care costs; in a patient who requires around-the-clock professional help, home care costs may exceed the cost of care in a hospital or chronic care facility.

EXPERIENCE WITH HOME MECHANICAL VENTILATION

Since 1980, there have been numerous reports of both adults and children successfully managed at home with mechanical ventilatory assistance.[3,5,18,22,23,35,39,41,42,44,47–60] Although many of these reports document the successful discharge of

patients to the home, few have addressed the issue of maximizing the functional ability of patients receiving home ventilation. Garay mentioned that most of his patients were leading active, productive lives using body respirators for only a portion of each day.[21] When positive-pressure ventilators are used, patient activity has been more limited. Fischer and Prentice commented on the activity status of 6 of their 14 COPD patients and 11 of 15 patients with restrictive respiratory disorders.[3] Of the COPD patients, one was confined to bed, two were homebound, one occasionally traveled outside the home, and two were "independent." Of patients with restrictive disorders, five were occasionally able to perform outside activities, one was homebound, and one was confined to bed. Many patients mentioned in other reports have been confined to home or bed or require extensive home-nursing services because of inability to care for themselves. On the other hand, many patients who were ventilated during the polio epidemic have led productive lives.

It is interesting to note the relative paucity of COPD patients in the large series reports of patients receiving home ventilation[3,5,41,44,55,56,61] (Table 25–5). The reasons for the lower number of COPD patients relate to their greater respiratory care requirements, such as suctioning, variability of airflow obstruction, and the progressive nature of the lung disease. Dull and Sadoul in France followed eight COPD patients for over 1.5 years and demonstrated reduction in $PaCO_2$, but no decrease in hospitaliza-

Table 25—5 Large Series of Ventilator-Assisted Patients in the Home

AUTHOR/YEAR	RESTRICTIVE LUNG DISEASE PATIENTS	COPD PATIENTS	POSITIVE-PRESSURE VENTILATORS	YEARS OF FOLLOW-UP
Make, 1988	39	33	29	1–6
Sivak, 1986[42]	33	2	25	0.2–17
Ontario, 1985[55]	33	4	37	2
Kopacz, 1984[56]	14	4	18	0.2–3.6
Indihar, 1984[44]	11	3	14	0.1–2.1
Robert, 1983[41]	162	60	222	1–25
Splaingard, 1983[5]	47	0	47	1 day–11 years
Fischer, 1982[3]	15	14	29	0.1–5.5
Dull, 1981[61]	1	7	8	1–7
Total	355	127		

tion, after institution of home ventilation. They therefore suggested that quality of life may not be improved.[61] Robert and coworkers have followed a large group of ventilator-assisted individuals in the home in France and reported the survival rates of COPD patients as 55% at 3 years, 30% at 5 years, and 18% at 8 years, with substantially better survival rates for patients with neuromuscular disorders.[41]

Czorniak et al. reported the clinical course of 14 patients with COPD and 21 with neuromuscular disorders followed at home for an average of 31 months (range, 5 to 66 months) after hospital discharge.[62] The COPD patients had an average of 2.7 hospital admissions per patient per year at home and averaged 54 days in the hospital each year, whereas patients with neuromuscular disorders had significantly fewer hospitalizations (0.7 admissions and 9.8 hospital days per patient for each year at home). Seven patients with neuromuscular diseases (33%) had no hospital admissions; these patients were generally younger and were receiving positive-pressure ventilation by tracheostomy, rather than noninvasive forms of ventilation. The reasons for hospitalization were similar in both COPD and neuromuscular patients. The most common reasons (54%) for admission were related to the lungs: 29% were for increased ventilatory requirements, 10% were related to pneumonia, and 9% were for bronchitis. Twenty-three percent of hospital admissions were for nonpulmonary problems unrelated to mechanical ventilation. Upper airway problems related to the tracheostomy (gran-

ulation tissue, stoma revision, cuff leak) led to 14% of the admissions. Hospitalization was uncommonly (9%) related to power failure or mechanical ventilation system malfunction. As shown in Figure 25–1, mortality in the COPD group was higher than in the neuromuscular group. Although the long-term survival of COPD patients is less than that of individuals with neuromuscular or skeletal disorders, our experience at Boston University suggests that physical capacity, independence, and possibly the quality of life may be greater in carefully selected COPD patients than in individuals with neurologic disorders.

BOSTON UNIVERSITY EXPERIENCE

Make and Gilmartin have shown that persons can be largely independent when a rehabilitation program is integrated into the to-home discharge of ventilator-assisted individuals, and have described the details of such a rehabilitation program.[39,60,63] From 1981 to 1988, 72 ventilator-assisted patients were admitted to the Respiratory Care Center at the University Hospital at the Boston University Medical Center. All patients were screened and thought to have a reasonable potential for discharge home. Characteristics of these patients are shown in Table 25–6. Of the patients with neuromuscular disorders, eight had muscular dystrophy, eight had sequelae of polio, five had spinal cord injury, four had amyotrophic lateral sclerosis, and four had kyphoscoliosis. All but one patient with COPD and 23 (59%) of the patients with neuromuscular disorders

Figure 25–1. Survival of adults receiving mechanical assistance to ventilation in the home. NM, patients with neuromuscular disorders; COPD, patients with chronic obstructive pulmonary disease.

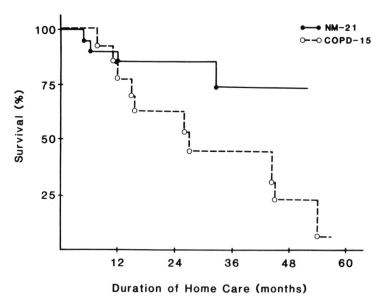

Table 25—6 Outcomes of 72 Ventilator-Assisted Patients Admitted to Boston University Hospital (1981—1988)

	COPD	NEUROMUSCULAR
ADMISSIONS AGE	33	39
Mean	61.3	50.1
Range	46–78	22–81
OUTCOME		
Home care	23	35
Chronic hospital	2	4
Died in hospital	8	0
INDEPENDENCE*		
Maximal	6	13
Moderate	11	7
Minimal	16	10
None	0	9

* Maximal, performs own care independently; moderate, performs most of own care except for showering and meal preparation; minimal, can wash, dress, and eat at bedside once materials are set up; none, needs complete assistance with almost all personal care.

Table 25—7 Ventilatory Requirements* of Ventilator-Assisted Individuals in Boston University Hospital Program

	COPD	NEUROMUSCULAR
Positive-pressure ventilator		
Tracheostomy	33	29
Nasal	0	4
Negative-pressure ventilator	0	6
Ventilator-free time		
<2 hr	13	8
2–7 hr	8	3
8–16 hr	13	26
16–24 hr	0	2

* At the time of discharge, transfer, or death.

were initially placed on mechanical ventilation as an acute life-saving procedure because of progressive hypercapnia, respiratory acidosis, and respiratory failure. The remaining patients were electively ventilated for gradually progressive hypercapnia, exercise intolerance, and dyspnea.

As shown in Table 25–6, all but four patients with neuromuscular disorders were successfully discharged home, but only 23 of 33 patients with COPD were discharged home. The COPD patients who did not go home included two who died in the hospital secondary to complications of abdominal surgery, three who died of cardiac disease, and five whose care was too complex to be managed independently or whose families were older and not physically capable of providing as much support as required. These results and those reported by others suggest that ventilator-assisted persons with neuromusculoskeletal disorders are strong candidates for discharge, whereas patients with COPD, even with careful screening and intensive rehabilitation efforts, may possibly not be successfully discharged home. We also found, as Table 25–6 shows, that many patients who are discharged can lead active, independent lives at home.

Complete "weaning" from mechanical ventilation was rarely possible in this patient population, but provision of as much "free time" off the ventilator as possible is an extremely useful goal. To attain this goal, weaning patients once or twice a day using a T-piece and gradually increasing the length of the wean is suggested. At the same time, increasing ventilator rate to minimize spontaneous respiratory efforts while receiving ventilatory assistance, and thereby decreasing ventilatory work, has been effective. During ventilator-free time, patients can more easily perform activities of daily living (ADL) at home or participate in community activities. The amount of ventilator-free time tolerated by our 72 patients is shown in Table 25–7. For those patients discharged home, the amount of ventilator-free time that was tolerated at the time of discharge grew shorter during exacerbations of their disease, during respiratory infections, and as the disease progressed.

VENTILATORS AND OTHER EQUIPMENT

Ventilatory support in the home has evolved from the polio era when patients were transferred home with simple equipment individualized for each patient. The patient and family became experts in the care and use of this equipment and generally were able to make modifications to suit their needs. They altered their equipment so they could travel, utilized batteries or generators in the event of power outages, and were well known to the ventilator companies. Negative-pressure ventilators were the main mode of ventilatory support, other forms of ventilatory assistance included rocking beds and pneumobelts. Many of these patients are still at home today and are using the equipment originally prescribed 30 years ago.

Because ventilator-assisted individuals discharged home today have a wider variety of medical disorders causing respiratory failure, different modes of therapy are often required. The three major types of mechanical ventilation used today are (1) positive-pressure ventilation provided through a tracheostomy or noninvasively through a nasal mask or mouthpiece, (2) negative-pressure ventilation provided by an iron lung or chest cuirass, and (3) other devices such as a pneumobelt or rocking bed. The type of device used will depend on the cause of respiratory failure, compliance of the lung and chest wall, and the presence of increased airway resistance. The ability of the patient to protect his or her airway and the presence of obstructive sleep apnea are also important determinants of the type of ventilatory support.

POSITIVE-PRESSURE VENTILATORS

Positive-pressure ventilation is the most commonly used approach to ventilatory assistance in the home today.[33] Until recently, if patients had intrinsic lung or airway disease a more sophisticated hospital-type ventilator had to be used in the home.[33,34] These ventilators were reliable for long-term use and inspiratory flow rate could be altered for patients with severe airway or lung disease. The ability to provide supplemental oxygen was fairly simple, and the delivered FIO_2 was usually constant. These ventilators usually had more than one alarm, important in the hospital but unnecessary in the home environment.[33] The problem with using sophisticated ICU-type ventilators is that they are not "user friendly" to caregivers who have either no medical education or no education at all, and who may not be mechanically oriented. The most typical of the ICU ventilators used in the home were the Emerson Post-Op and 3MV (J. H Emerson Co., Cambridge, Mass.), Bennett MA-1 and MA2 (Puritan-Bennett Co., Overland Park, Kan.), and Bear 1 and 2 (Bourne Medical Systems, Riverside, Calif.) ventilators.

Today there are more home-style ventilators available, although many of their features are similar.[33,34,64] In general, when selecting a ventilator for the home the following features should be considered: reliability, portability, size, ease of operation,

and ease of maintenance. The advantages of all of the home ventilators are their compact size and weight; they all weigh under 40 pounds. They can easily be placed on a cart or mounted on a motorized or manual wheelchair. They also can operate on normal household current, an internal DC battery, and an external DC battery. The internal battery is useful only as a very short-term power source in the event of power failure or for limited transportation. One major disadvantage of the small ventilators is that when operated in the intermittent mandatory ventilation (IMV) or synchronized IMV (SIMV) mode, the patient effort required for spontaneous breathing is very high.[65] Although work of breathing could be reduced by use of an external continuous-flow system for IMV, such systems add to the complexity of the ventilator. Simple methods to decrease the amount of patient effort are to (1) replace the filter at the air inlet on the back of the ventilator with a bacterial filter and add a bacterial filter at the outlet port, (2) remove the tower when using a cascade humidifier, (3) reduce patient spontaneous ventilatory effort by increasing the ventilator rate, and (4) use assist–control mode.

A potential drawback to small ventilators is the difficulty in delivering additional oxygen. Although a reservoir or accumulator may be added to the ventilator intake, oxygen may also be delivered through a small nipple adapter attached at the patient port proximal to the humidifier. With these latter methods, the oxygen flow will be constant, but the actual delivery to the patient may vary owing to changes in patient effort or respiratory rate. For most patients, this variability in the FIO_2 will not be of significance, since most home patients are receiving low oxygen concentrations. For those patients who require a precise FIO_2 or higher oxygen concentrations, a reservoir or accumulator might be appropriate. These systems add to the complexity of the ventilator and should be considered only when strict attention to oxygen delivery is mandatory. Table 25–8 lists some of the features of each of the currently available portable ventilators.

An increasingly popular and effective approach to home ventilation is the use of positive-pressure ventilation by a nasal mask, the origin of which can be traced to the use of nasal masks developed for continuous positive airway pressure (CPAP) in patients with obstructive sleep apnea. This form of ventilation is most appropriate for patients with neuromuscular disorders.[58,66,67] Positive-pressure ventilation with a mouthpiece has been used successfully for patients with polio.[57]

Table 25—8 Features of Positive-Pressure Home Care Ventilators

PRODUCT	MODE	TIDAL VOLUME	RATE	I/E RATIO	ALARMS	POWER SOURCES
Aequitron (Minn, MN) LP-6	C AC SIMV	100–2200 mL	1–38	Variable	Low-pressure, high-pressure, low-power, apnea, I/E ratio, power switchover, ventilator malfunction	AC DC Int.
Life Care (Lafeyette, Colo.) PVV	C	50–3000 mL	8–30	Fixed 1 : 1	Low-pressure, high-pressure, low-power, power failure	AC DC Int.
PLV-100	C AC SIMV Sigh	50–3000 mL	2–40	Variable	Low-pressure, high-pressure, low-power, power failure, apnea, I/E ratio, power switchover, inspiratory flow, ventilator malfunction, reverse battery cable connection	AC DC Int.
PLV-102	C AC SIMV	50–3000 mL	2–40	Variable	Low-pressure, high-pressure, low-power, apnea, I/E ratio, power switchover, inspiratory flow	AC DC Int.
Puritan-Bennett (Overland Park, Kan.) Companion 2800	C AC SIMV Sigh	50–2800 mL	1–69	Variable	Low-pressure, high-pressure, low-power, power failure, apnea, I/E ratio, power switchover, inspiratory flow, ventilator malfunction	AC DC Int.
Bear Medical Systems (Riverside, Calif.) Bear 33	C AC SIMV Sigh	100–2200 mL	2–40	Variable	Low-pressure, high-pressure, power failure, apnea, power switchover, inspiratory flow, I/E ratio, ventilator inoperable	AC DC Int.

Custom-made nasal masks and mouthpieces have been utilized at some centers to increase patient comfort.

NEGATIVE-PRESSURE VENTILATION

Recently there has been renewed interest in the use of negative-pressure ventilation for patients with neuromuscular disease faced with the need for ventilatory support; these patients would often rather use less invasive negative-pressure ventilation rather than tracheostomy and positive-pressure devices. There has also been significant interest in this form of ventilatory assistance for patients with severe COPD, to provide elective rest of fatigued respiratory muscles. Negative-pressure ventilation can be accomplished with the use of an iron lung, a self-contained device that is an effective pressure generator and that can be manually operated during a power failure. The major disadvantage is the bulk and lack of portability of these machines and the difficulty of gaining access to the patient.

A portable version of the iron lung is available (Porta-Lung, W. W. Weingarten, Denver, Colo.). The chest cuirass ("turtle shell") is a much less confining negative-pressure ventilator chamber placed over the chest and abdomen. Ready-made shells are available, but custom-made shells are often necessary for patients who have kyphoscoliosis, protuberant abdomens, or thoracic deformity. A negative-pressure generator is attached to the center of the shell by a flexible tubing. Even though these devices are well tolerated, as chest wall compliance worsens or skeletal deformity increases, adequate ventilation may not be possible, and other forms of ventilation may need to be considered. The Pulmowrap ("raincoat," pneumosuit) is made from nylon or other airtight material that surrounds the patient and requires the use of a negative-pressure generator. These are more cumbersome to get into for some patients, and the poncho type requires patience to reduce leaks around the arms and lower abdomen. A major complaint with some patients is back discomfort since a relatively hard surface is needed for the grid (which provides for maintenance of an air space inside the suit) to rest upon, thus requiring the patient to be in bed and limiting mobility.

A major contraindication to using negative-pressure ventilation is obstructive sleep apnea. If sleep-disordered breathing is a diagnostic consideration, a sleep study should be performed before instituting this form of ventilation. If there is objective or symptomatic deterioration without other explanation, a sleep study is indicated to evaluate the possibility of upper airway obstruction while the patient is using the negative-pressure device. A common complaint of patients using negative-pressure ventilators is that of being cold; this can be remedied by having the patient wear appropriate clothing.

PNEUMOBELT

The pneumobelt consists of a corset fitted around the abdomen and lower rib cage. Inflation of the "bladder" inside the corset by a positive-pressure ventilator compresses the abdominal contents, pushing the diaphragm cephalad and actively assisting expiration. When the "bladder" deflates, the diaphragm is allowed to descend, decreasing intrathoracic pressure and allowing gas to enter the lungs during inspiration.[12] The pneumobelt is most useful for patients who need some ventilatory support during the day and do not have significant airway or parenchymal disease. This assist device can be used during sleep, but the patient cannot lie flat. Patients with significant deformity of their thoracic or lumbar spine are unable to use this device, but patients with lower cervical spinal cord injury who do not require ventilatory support when lying flat may use this device to increase diaphragmatic motion when sitting upright.[68]

ROCKING BED

The rocking bed functions by alternately rotating the head of the bed down to shift the abdominal contents cephalad and assist expiration, and then rotating the foot of the bed down, to shift abdominal contents caudally and assist inspiration.[10,11] The rocking bed moves the diaphragm up and down, thereby assisting ventilation. The rate of the rocking motion and the pitch of the bed are adjustable. Generally, the tidal volume cannot be greatly enhanced, but it may be adequate for many patients with neuromuscular disease. The motion of the bed seems to mobilize secretions, which can be quite

bothersome to some patients and interfere with sleep. It also takes up much more space than a regular bed, which is an important factor to consider when choosing a ventilatory-assist device for the home. The bed does have an automatic stop as a safety device if something interferes with its motion.

ACCESSORY EQUIPMENT

The most important piece of accessory equipment needed in the home of a ventilator-assisted person is a self-inflating manual resuscitator and mask. This is necessary for several reasons. First, the resuscitator can provide ventilation, if there is a power failure or ventilator malfunction, as a short-term remedy until a battery or another ventilator is available. Second, the resuscitator can be used to assist ventilation when the patient is experiencing shortness of breath unrelieved by other modalities such as suctioning or bronchodilators. Third, during ventilator tubing changes the resuscitator is helpful in patients who do not have free time from the ventilator. Furthermore, the resuscitator can assist in mobilizing secretions before or during suctioning. Finally, it may provide ventilation to the patient by face mask if the tracheostomy tube inadvertently falls out or during failure of noninvasive ventilatory equipment.

A second ventilator is necessary for any patient who has limited free time off the ventilator or who lives in a very rural area. As a general rule, a second ventilator should be considered if the patient requires 20 or more hours of mechanical assistance each day or if he or she cannot wean for 4 or more consecutive hours.[45] A second ventilator may also be helpful to improve mobility by permanently mounting it on a wheelchair.[15,45] Other accessory equipment used in the home is listed in Table 25–9.

Adaptive equipment useful for improving the patient's performance of ADL includes devices that help the caregivers, such as the Hoyer lift or hydraulic shower chair. Team members need to collaborate to decide what equipment is necessary and what will be reimbursed by third-party payers. Some adaptive devices may be funded through nonprofit agencies, such as the Muscular Dystrophy Association. A list of equipment and supplies[14,34] necessary for home care of ventilator-assisted patients should be developed before discharge, and the equipment should be made available for use by the patients and caregivers during their training. The necessary equipment and

Table 25–9   Accessory Equipment Used
in the Home

Self-inflating manual resuscitation face mask
Ventilator—backup
Ventilator filters
Humidifier
Water trap
Suction machines—electrical/battery powered
Oxygen source
Compressors—for medication delivery or aerosols
Battery—12 V DC
Battery charger
Battery cable
Mobility devices
Bathing and toileting devices
Environmental control unit
Bed
Safety devices

---

supplies should then be placed in the home before
the patient is discharged.

AIRWAY MANAGEMENT

Maintenance of an adequate airway in the patient
using positive-pressure ventilation by tracheostomy should be a top priority to the team caring for
the patient. Potential problems to be anticipated by
the discharge or home care team are (1) complications already encountered with the airway owing to
a stormy and prolonged ICU course, (2) a poorly
placed tracheostomy stoma, (3) an ill-fitting tracheostomy tube, (4) granulation tissue formation interfering with the patency of the airway associated
with bleeding and increasing the difficulty of tube
changes, (5) stomal infection or inflammation related to poor healing and continuous drainage of
secretions around the stoma, and (6) peristomal fibrosis, making tube changes difficult.

The airway complications associated with a
prolonged ICU hospitalization include tracheomalacia, subglottic stenosis, tracheal stenosis, and
poorly healed tracheal stomas. These may be related to prolonged endotracheal intubation; repeated endotracheal intubations before tracheostomy; relatively high ventilatory pressures,
necessitating increasing amounts of air and pressure in the cuff to prevent a loss of ventilation; poor
perfusion to the tracheal mucosa, secondary to low
cardiac output or overinflation of the cuff; and poor
healing related to chronic infection and nutritional

deficits. At times, the tracheotomy stoma may be
placed either too high or too low in the neck, causing problems with tube positioning. If the stoma is
not placed centrally, the tip of the trachostomy tube
may place constant pressure on the tracheal wall,
causing erosion or scarring.

Many patients have tracheal tubes that are
much too large, in which the angle of tube insertion
is not appropriate for their anatomy. There is a tendency to place larger-diameter tubes when the cuff
requires increasing amounts of air for a seal because of tracheomalacia, with the result that the
patient ends up with a very large tube in place that
still requires a large volume of air to create a seal.
The patient with a thick neck often has tracheal
tube positional problems, with the cuff bulging upward in the airway and the distal tip of the tube
pressing on the posterior wall of the trachea, with
potential erosion into the esophagus.

Granulation tissue formation at the stomal site
may occur and is not always preventable. We have
encountered granulation tissue inside the tracheal
stoma of sufficient degree to impair spontaneous
patient ventilation through a fenestrated tracheostomy tube. The presence of a foreign body constantly irritating the mucosa and skin surface
causes formation of granulation tissue. If the patient is a candidate for long-term ventilation and
the tracheostomy is not an emergency, then a permanent stoma may be created with skin flaps
brought down to the level of the trachea; this may
facilitate tube changes and reduce the incidence of
problems with granulation tissue and bleeding. Inside the trachea, there may be granulation tissue at
the subglottic level, at the superior aspect of the
stoma, or at the tube tip site. If granulation tissue
causes significant airflow obstruction, causes
bleeding, or interferes with tube changes, it should
be surgically removed.

Stomal infection or inflammation may be associated with repeated tracheobronchial infection,
immunosuppression, and continuous drainage of
upper airway secretions and saliva around the
stoma. Loss of skin integrity secondary to maceration of the skin will also predispose to infection.
Repeated use of antibiotics and the use of an antimicrobial ointment may predispose to a fungal infection.

When a patient enters a rehabilitation program
or is being prepared for home, an assessment of the
airway and tracheal tube should be done. Visual
inspection of the stoma and tracheal tube should
consist of an examination for skin breakdown
around the stoma and under the tracheal tape or

ties, type and amount of drainage, presence of granulation tissue, redness or swelling, shape of the neck, protrusion of the tube out of the neck, and relationship of the neck plate or phalange of the tube to the neck, itself. If the patient has a fenestrated tracheostomy tube that is used for phonation and spontaneous ventilation during free time from the ventilator, proper position of the fenestration must be assured. A limited examination can be performed by removing the inner cannula and inspecting the fenestration with a flashlight to determine if the fenestration is patent and positioned well in the airway lumen. An anteroposterior film of the neck or a well-positioned chest roentgenogram will show whether the cuff is bulging out the tracheal wall and whether the tube is midline. The lateral chest or neck film will show if the tip of the tube or cuff is bulging into the posterior wall of the trachea and toward the esophagus, which may impair swallowing and esophageal motility and increase the risk of aspiration.[69] The lateral film will also aid in determining the position of the fenestration.

A limited bronchoscopy can assess the presence of vocal cord edema, paralysis, or stenosis and determine subglottic abnormalities such as granulation tissue or stenosis. Direct visualization of the tube in the trachea can aid in properly placing the fenestration. Collapse or loss of support of the tracheal wall, especially at the level of the cuff site, may necessitate a longer tracheostomy tube, which can be placed under direct visualization to prevent inadvertent location in the right main stem bronchus. The position of the cuff can also be noted, and one can assess bulging into the proximal airway, which can decrease the adequacy of the seal with changes in patient position or movement of the tracheal tube. Not all tracheostomy problems can be corrected, but by using these assessment measures, at least the state of the airway can be observed, and further problems can be prevented.

Care of the stoma should consist of cleaning the stoma and surrounding skin as well as the portion of the tube that is visible. This should be done at least twice daily if there is minimal drainage, and the area should be kept dry to prevent maceration of the skin. Diluted hydrogen peroxide is generally used for cleaning the stoma and the inner cannula. An antiseptic ointment may also be used. The stoma should be observed for redness, swelling, itchiness, blisters, and signs of fungal infection. If any of these occur, procedures should be reviewed to make sure patients are properly caring for the stoma. If lack of care is not the problem, then altering the care may be necessary; omitting the hydro-

gen peroxide or stopping the antiseptic ointment may decrease irritation. If there is a fungal infection, an antifungal ointment combined with hydrocortisone will alleviate the problem. The patient should be taught to keep the inner cannulas and buttons clean and dry to prevent infection.

Cuff inflation, assessment of leaks in the system, and troubleshooting similar problems are a major part of home care and probably some of the hardest concepts for the patient and caretakers to learn. If the volume of air in the cuff cannot be maintained because of a leak, and the patient cannot tolerate the loss of ventilator volume, the patient or caregiver needs to know temporary measures to maintain ventilation, how to change the tube, or how to obtain care in a local emergency room for a tube change.

RESOURCES IN THE HOME

The discharge of a patient to home on a ventilator may seem relatively simple. However, if the patient is a key part of the team approach and if the goal of home care is to allow maximal patient self-responsibility and independence, then a comprehensive inpatient program of rehabilitation must be individualized for each patient. The process of discharging a patient home on life-support equipment requires the expertise and cooperation of many different people from different disciplines (Fig. 25–2). When a large number of people are involved, communication may be enhanced and goals shared among personnel if they organize into a team.[15,45,63] The role of each team member should be defined, and the patient and family should be considered an integral part of the team and the discharge planning effort.

In the home, many patients can provide much or all of their own care if their potential is maximized through a program of rehabilitation and education. Even patients who cannot physically participate in their own care may be able to direct their care providers. In other cases, family members or parents will provide the care or direct others in the delivery of care. Children represent a special case, since they require care totally given by others; in addition, children and neonates have special needs that are very different from those of adults.[49,54,70–75] The roles of the patient, family, and other home care providers should be clearly and precisely identified well in advance of discharge. Home care agencies should be integrated into discharge plan-

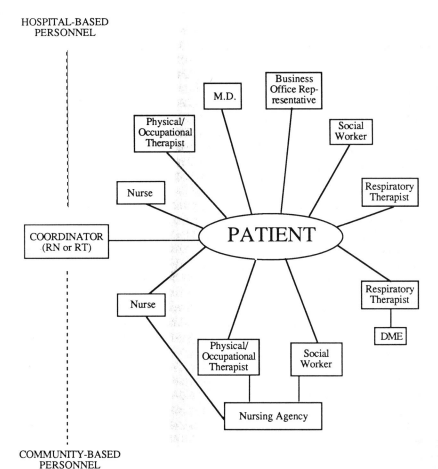

HOSPITAL-BASED
PERSONNEL

COMMUNITY-BASED
PERSONNEL

Figure 25—2. Members of the discharge-planning team for ventilator-assisted individuals.

ning early in the hospitalization. If the patient and family will be providing most of the care, a community nursing agency may be involved to assess the patient in the home setting and to coordinate the functions of other allied health professionals when needed, such as physical or occupational therapists and social workers. If assistance with personal care, such as bathing, feeding, or meal preparation, is necessary, a home health aide or nursing assistant provided by a community nursing agency may be utilized. Usually, these nonprofessionals cannot provide respiratory care, such as suctioning, bronchodilator treatments, or ventilator care, because of liability concerns of the home health care agencies. Some agencies allow their home health aides to administer chest physical therapy and assist with cleaning of ventilator circuits, but only after training and under supervision of a registered nurse. In the absence of a family member, chest physical therapy may be performed by nurses or physical therapists.

If the patient requires more comprehensive care in the home and is unable to physically provide his or her own care, then a personal care attendant (PCA) may be helpful. The PCAs are generally lay people without prior experience who can be trained by the patient or family to provide the necessary care. In many areas, they are hired by the patient and, therefore, there is no liability to the home care agency. A PCA may cost much less than a home health aide, professional nurse, or therapist, and the cost may be reimbursed by a state Medicaid program or rehabilitation commission. They can be hired for day or night hours, and their salary may be supplemented with room and board. Many patients with neuromuscular disorders, such as polio, spinal cord injury, or muscular dystrophy, have utilized such caregivers for years. An important point to remember about PCAs is that they are nonprofessional caregivers. Thus, the patient and family must be directive of the care, capable of providing the necessary education, and able to discipline the PCA if he or she is not providing the care as directed. State-funded "centers of independent living" can educate the patient and family in the methods of recruitment, reimbursement, and termination of a PCA.

Another option for short-term respite care or companionship is community volunteer organizations. If the patient needs continuous professional care, many factors may be considered, not the least of which is cost. Twenty-four-hour care by registered nurses may cost 500 to 800 dollars a day, which is unaffordable for most people. Some insurance plans cover this level of care, but the patient may have to pay the caregivers themselves and apply for reimbursement by the insurance carrier—a process that requires some financial resources. State and federal insurance programs may reimburse continuous skilled nursing care but at a lower rate, thereby excluding participation by many nursing agencies. Other problems that must be considered with round-the-clock care are lack of coverage because of paucity of health professionals, availability of backup help in the event of illness or transportation problems, and inadequate training and experience of the caregivers.

It is important to stress that one of the most important resources necessary in home care is the emotional health of the patient and family and their ability to cope with changes in their lives that are imposed by chronic disease. The patient can be physically stable, but if there is deterioration in the psychological health of the patient or caretakers, home care will fail. Many patients and families will require a great deal of psychological support, and this can be provided by the referring institution or the home care agency. If respite care is available or if the family can afford to pay privately for respite care, it should become a routine part of the home program. If the caregiver does not get adequate sleep or rest, he or she will not be able to continue to provide optimal care, and his or her physical and psychological health may deteriorate, thereby placing the patient at risk, since an unhealthy caregiver makes mistakes.

Other types of community support may be necessary, such as transportation for medical care, meal preparation, homemaking, and shopping. Many communities have an emergency telephone service that connects directly to the local hospital; this service is particularly helpful for the ventilatory-assisted individual who may be alone during part of the day. The local utility company, ambulance service, and fire department should be aware of the patient at home on life-support equipment so that they can respond to emergency situations such as a power failure or need for transport to the hospital.

A home assessment should be performed by representatives from both the hospital team and the home respiratory care company, to determine if the home physical environment is adequate for the patient's needs and to make necessary modifications before the patient's hospital discharge. If the patient requires extensive adaptation to the physical layout because of wheelchair dependence or because of severe functional impairments, a physical or occupational therapist should also be involved in the home assessment. The physical layout should be assessed for any barriers to mobility, such as narrow doorways, stairs, thick carpets, and thresholds. The patient's bedroom should not only be large enough to accommodate the required equipment, but also easily accessible to the rest of the house, so that the patient will not be isolated. If a hospital bed is required, the patient may not be able to remain in his or her own bedroom because of lack of space. There should be adequate ventilation and heat, and the electrical supply should be appropriate for the additional equipment. A separate electrical circuit for the ventilator and accessory equipment is preferable, but not mandatory, since all home care equipment will function with normal 110 V AC household current. Grounded outlets are preferable and should be available for such items as the ventilator, suction machine, humidifier, electric bed, and compressor. An evaluation by a licensed electrician is required for any patient that has a lot of electrical equipment and should be mandatory in older houses. Fortunately, the respiratory equipment does not draw much electrical power and will not usually exceed the capabilities of most homes. There should be a designated area to charge wheelchair and ventilator batteries; acid-filled batteries should not be charged in the patient's room because of potential danger from fumes emitted from the battery, sparks, and fire. Home modifications are not covered by third-party payment but funding may be available through community agencies, such as the Muscular Dystrophy Association.

There must be space in the home for the cleaning, drying, and storage of equipment. Many patients utilize their kitchen sink for cleaning and then use a basin for the sterilizing process. A clothes rack placed in the bathtub is very useful for drying ventilatory tubing.

RESPIRATORY HOME CARE COMPANIES

One of the most important resources in the home is the respiratory care or durable medical equipment company (DME). Mechanical ventilators, other equipment such as suction machines and wheelchairs, and disposable items are most often supplied to ventilator-assisted individuals in the home by respiratory home care companies. Many of these durable medical equipment vendors were founded in the 1970s to supply oxygen to patients at home. With the increased recognition of the importance of long-term oxygen therapy and subsequent reimbursement for this outpatient therapy, these local companies flourished and were merged with the several larger national concerns that currently dominate the marketplace. These larger vendors have the resources to provide any type of equipment or supply needed in the home and have expanded their personnel to satisfy the needs of the growing number of home ventilator patients. All the large national DMEs have developed written policies, procedures, and guidelines for home care of ventilator-assisted individuals and will gladly participate in the planning and education of caregivers before a patient's hospital discharge. However, the translation of such policies developed on a national level to care provided by local branches is not always optimal and depends heavily upon the expertise and experience of local branch personnel. There may be regional differences in home care techniques and equipment that are based upon common practice in the community. Competition among companies for a larger share of the home care market has traditionally been the motivating factor for development of a comprehensive, high-quality program by vendors.

The primary responsibility for planning and implementation of a comprehensive home care program for hospitalized ventilator-assisted persons should reside in the hands of a single, clearly designated, health care professional (usually either a respiratory therapist or clinical respiratory nurse specialist) who has the most knowledge and experience in respiratory home care. This discharge coordinator may be hospital- or community-based and should draw upon both hospital and community resources, as needed, to assure a smooth transition to the home.[45]

A reputable DME and community nursing agency should be involved early in the discharge process so that equipment needs can be determined and the necessary equipment provided for patient use and teaching before discharge. Backup equipment must be readily available in the event of equipment failure; consequently, a small company may not be the optimal choice for home care of ventilator-assisted individuals. Larger home care companies usually stock required home care equipment. The home care therapists may not be involved with the education of the patient and family in the hospital but will definitely be involved with continuing education in the home setting. They may also be involved with the education of other home care providers such as community nursing agencies or PCAs. The hospital team and the respiratory home care company need to coordinate their efforts to provide optimal initial and continuing education for patients and caregivers. All educators must teach identical home care procedures and methods to avoid confusing patients and families. A comprehensive home management plan (Table 25–10) and specific respiratory care plan (Table 25–11) must be individualized for each patient before his or her hospital discharge, and the personnel responsible for each component must be adequately trained. The responsibilities of each person, as well as what procedures will be taught to the patient and family, need to be delineated well in advance of discharge; this will prevent confusion of the caregivers and assure a smooth transition from hospital to home.

Table 25–10   Comprehensive Management Plan

The written comprehensive management plan for a home ventilator patient should:

- Identify primary and consulting physicians
- Identify local hospital emergency room
- Specify appropriate medical center for care reevaluation
- Designate roles of health care providers
- Designate roles of patients and others in daily care
- Provide a method to select and train future caregivers
- Guarantee comprehensive funding
- Determine necessary modifications of the care environment
- Assess community resources to meet health, social, educational, and vocational needs
- Itemize equipment and supplies needed
- Identify equipment dealers and services they provide (maintenance, surveillance, and such)
- Outline alternative emergency and contingency plans

(O'Donohue WJ, Giovannoni RM, Goldberg AF et al: Long-term mechanical ventilation: Guidelines for management in the home and at alternate community sites. Chest 90(suppl):1S–37S, 1986, with permission)

Table 25–11 Respiratory Care Plan

Mechanical ventilator
  Type and characteristics (including backup when indicated)
Manual resuscitator
Ventilator power source
  Electrical requirements
  Battery or generator powered
Ventilator circuit
  Detailed description of circuits
  Description of alarms
  Instructions for cleaning, assembly, and use
  Documentation of the education of caregivers
Use of ventilators
  Specific times on and off the ventilator
  FiO_2 and range of oxygen
  Mode of ventilation
  Desired change with exercise or sleep
  Acceptable limits of dialed/measured exhaled volume
  Desired pressure ranges
Appropriate alarms and monitors
  For ventilator dysfunction, power failure
  For high and low pressure, exhaled volume
  Others as needed
Name and type of artificial airway
  Size and type
  Cuffed, uncuffed, fenestrated
  Double or single cannula
Instructions for care of artificial airway
  Cuff inflation (conditions for inflation/deflation)
  Airway care plan (tube changes, cleaning, problem solving)
  Airway suctioning
  Speaking tube operation, if appropriate
Adjunctive techniques
  Medications
  Aerosol (bronchodilator)
  Chest physiotherapy
  Oxygen therapy
Communication systems
  Intercom
  Physical sound (bell/siren)
  Telephone/beeper system

(O'Donohue WJ, Giovannoni RM, Goldberg AF et al: Long-term mechanical ventilation: Guidelines for management in the home and at alternate community sites. Chest 90(suppl):1S–37S, 1986, with permission)

Once the patient is stabilized in the home, the respiratory home care company should make periodic routine visits, at least monthly, to monitor the overall function of the ventilator and other accessory equipment, provide preventive maintenance, assess the patient's response to therapy, and assure compliance with the prescribed respiratory care plan. They may also participate in noninvasive monitoring to assure adequate oxygenation during various activities in the home. They usually provide disposable supplies, such as suction catheters, tubings, medication nebulizers, and gloves. The DME may also provide medications, a service that may be very helpful for the patient who is not mobile or does not have ready access to a pharmacy. The home care company should not be responsible for medical problems that occur in the home, but if the therapist determines that a medical problem or psychological deterioration is interfering with patient progress at home, the company should communicate with the referring physician or institution. At times, the patient or family may not be able to differentiate between a medical or equipment problem, and an on-site assessment should be performed by the home care therapist. Often, a telephone conversation between therapist and patient will provide important insight concerning the nature of the problem, but unscheduled home calls will also be necessary. Communication between the home care company, nursing agency, and referring physician is extremely important to ensure optimal continuing care in the home. Often the home health aide, nurse, or therapist is the first to notice increasing emotional problems that interfere with optimal delivery of care in the home; these problems may not be detected by the physician during a brief office visit.

It is imperative that the hospital discharge planning team assure the presence of a comprehensive program for daily care in home. Because the respiratory home care vendor plays an important role in patient management, a company should be chosen on the basis of its ability to provide a continuous level of quality care—to deliver the necessary equipment and supplies to the patient in the home on a timely basis, provide experienced, qualified home care respiratory therapists, and to meet the Joint Commission on Accreditation of Health Care Organizations (JCAHO) standards.

COSTS OF HOME VENTILATOR CARE

Although improved and more humane patient care, and not cost reduction, should be the motivating factor for home care,[76] costs cannot be completely overlooked. The Boston University program has evaluated the home care costs for ventilator-assisted individuals with COPD and with neuromuscular disorders.[77] The average cost of home care in 1987 for these patients was 2974 dollars a month, with a wide variation between individual patient costs. Figure 25–3 shows the costs of various components of care in the home. Other investigators

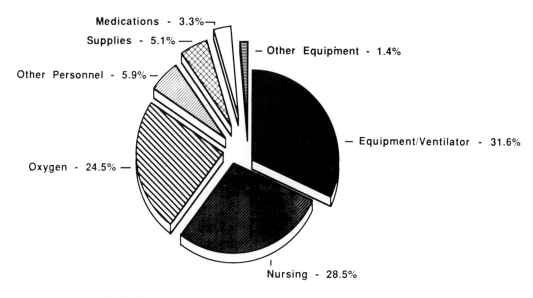

TOTAL MONTHLY COST - $2976

Figure 25–3. Average payments for home care for ventilator-assisted individuals in 1987 reported by the Boston University program.[77]

have reported that substantial savings can be achieved by home care. The American Association for Respiratory Care[19] conducted a 20-state hospital survey in 1984 and estimated the cost of home care to be 1766 dollars per person per month and hospital care to be 22,569 dollars per patient per month. Giovannoni[52] reported an average hospital cost of 32,800 dollars a month for five ventilator-assisted patients in the hospital, compared with an average cost of 20,000 dollars for the first month at home for three patients successfully discharged. However, many chronic ventilator-dependent patients do not require the ICU level of care used by Giovannoni in her hospital cost estimates. Sivak and coworkers[78] estimated the average monthly cost of hospital care for ventilator-dependent patients to be 15,600 dollars (about half the cost estimated by Giovannoni), whereas the range of monthly costs for ten home care patients was 30 to 5673 dollars not including equipment purchase. Unfortunately, home care equipment costs are often high, and equipment is often rented rather than purchased to ensure continued maintenance and home monitoring. In other reports, costs of home care have been reported to be as high as 16,000 dollars a month.[5,51]

It is clear that the single most expensive item in the home is the professional services of a nurse. If patients who are clinically stable are selected for home care, and if patients and families can become independent and self-sufficient through a comprehensive rehabilitation program, professional services required in the home may be lessened.

CARE IN ALTERNATIVE SITES

It is often difficult to determine the optimal site for continued care of ventilator-assisted individuals.[43,79] Unfortunately, all the options shown in Figure 25–4 are not available in all communities. Therefore, the decision to place a patient in a site outside the hospital is based upon the presence and availability of facilities and resources in the local community, as well as on the medical condition of the individual patient. All patients are managed in ICUs of acute care hospitals when positive-pressure mechanical ventilation is initiated on an emergency basis. Because many hospitals do not have other units with adequate skilled personnel and resources, ventilator-assisted patients often must remain in critical care units for the duration of their hospital stay. However, owing to the large number of ventilator patients, hospitals often develop step-down units or other specialized areas to manage their patients, often with "noninvasive" monitoring.[44,80–82] In some regions of the United States, a limited number of beds are available in long-term care hospitals for patients.[20] Selected skilled nurs-

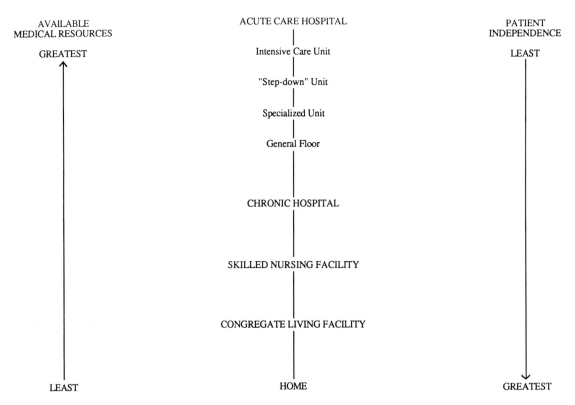

Figure 25—4. Sites for care of ventilator-assisted individuals. In general, facilities toward the bottom of the figure have fewer medical resources (physician, therapists, nurses, equipment), but allow greater patient independence.

ing facilities (SNF) may admit such patients who are very stable, but SNF do not usually have 24-hour in-house physicians or therapists. Congregate living facilities are rarely available in the United States. Care for ventilator-assisted people is often more available and organized in a variety of non-hospital sites in other countries.[83]

Health care professionals must carefully assess the options for care available within their community and make the best choice of location, with patient safety as their foremost concern. Just as in home care, adequate skilled personnel, equipment, and supplies, sufficient to meet the needs of a comprehensive patient management plan must be available in an alternative care site.

REFERENCES

1. Affeldt JE, Bower AG, Dail CW, Aratan N: Prognosis for recovery in severe poliomyelitis. Arch Phys Med Rehabil 38:290–295, 1957
2. Alcock AJW, Hildelin H, Rasanen O et al: Chronic respiratory paralysis. Acta Paediatr Scand 228:1–32, 1972
3. Fischer DA, Prentice WS: Feasibility of home care for certain respiratory-dependent restrictive or obstructive lung disease patients. Chest 82:739–743, 1982
4. Harrison GM, Mitchell MB: The medical and social outcome of 200 respirator and former respirator patients on home care. Arch Phys Med 42:590–598, 1961
5. Splaingard ML, Frates RC Jr, Harrison GM et al: Home positive pressure ventilation: Twenty year's experience. Chest 84:376–382, 1983
6. Christensen MS, Kristensen HS, Hansen EL: Artificial hyperventilation during 21 years in 3 cases of complete respiratory paralysis. Acta Med Scand 198:409–413, 1975
7. Drinker P, Shaw LA: An apparatus for the prolonged administration of artificial ventilation. J Clin Invest 7:229, 1929
8. Collier CR, Affeldt JE: Ventilatory efficiency of the cuirass respirator in totally paralyzed chronic poliomyelitis patients. J Appl Physiol 6:531–538, 1954
9. Flaum A: Experience in the use of a new respirator in the treatment of respiratory paralysis in poliomyelitis. Acta Med Scand Suppl 78:849–855, 1936
10. Eve FG: Activation of inert diaphragm by gravity method. Lancet 2:995–997, 1932
11. Plum F, Whedon GD: The rapid-rocking bed: Its effect on the ventilation of poliomyelitis patients with respiratory paralysis. N Engl J Med 245:235–241, 1951

12. Adamson JP, Stein JD: Application of abdominal pressure for artificial respiration. JAMA 169:1613–1617, 1959

13. Gilmartin ME, Make BJ (eds): Mechanical ventilation in the home—issues for health care providers. Probl Respir Care 1(2), 155–295 1988

14. Johnson DL, Giovannoni RM, Driscoll SA: Ventilator-Assisted Patient Care: Planning for Hospital Discharge and Home Care. Rockville, Md, Aspen, 1986

15. O'Donohue WJ, Giovannoni RM, Goldberg AF et al: Long-term mechanical ventilation: Guidelines for management in the home and at alternate community sites. Chest 90(suppl):1S–37S, 1986

16. Douglas PS, Rosen RH, Butler PW, Bone RC: DRG payment for long-term ventilator patients: Implications and recommendations. Chest 91:413–417, 1987

17. Gracey DR, Gillespie D, Nobrega F et al: Financial implications of prolonged ventilator care of Medicare patients under the prospective payment system. Chest 91:424–427, 1987

18. Make B, Dayno S, Gertman P: Prevalence of chronic ventilator-dependency. Am Rev Respir Dis 132(4, part 2):A167, 1986

19. Association holds press conferences on ventilator survey. AARTimes 8(Apr):28–31, 1984

20. Bone RC: Long-term ventilator care. A Chicago problem and a national problem. Chest 92:536–539, 1987

21. Garay SM, Turino GM, Goldring RM: Sustained reversal of chronic hypercapnia in patients with alveolar hypoventilation syndromes: Long-term maintenance with noninvasive nocturnal mechanical ventilation. Am J Med 70:269–274, 1981

22. Hoeppner VH, Cockcroft DW, Dosman JA et al: Nighttime ventilation improves respiratory failure in secondary kyphoscoliosis. Am Rev Respir Dis 129:240–243, 1984

23. Braun NMT, Marino WD: Effect of daily intermittent rest on respiratory muscles in patients with chronic airflow limitation. Chest 85:595–605, 1984

24. Cropp AJ, DiMarco AF, Altose MD: Effect of intermittent negative pressure on respiratory muscle function in patients with severe chronic obstructive pulmonary disease. Am Rev Respir Dis 135:1056–1061, 1987

25. Gutierrez M, Beroiza T, Contreras G et al: Weekly cuirass ventilation improves blood gases and inspiratory muscle strength in patients with chronic airflow limitation and hypercarbia. Am Rev Respir Dis 138:617–623, 1988

26. Pluto LA, Fahey PJ, Sorenson L, Chandrosekhar AJ: Effects of 8 weeks of INPV on exercise parameters in patients with severe chronic obstructive lung disease. Am Rev Respir Dis 131(4, part 2):64A, 1985

27. Zibrak JD, Hill NS, Federman EC, O'Donnell C: Evaluation of intermittent long-term negative pressure ventilation in patients with severe chronic obstructive pulmonary disease. Am Rev Rispir Dis 138:1515–1518, 1988

28. Celli B, Lee H, Criner G et al: Controlled trial of external negative pressure ventilation in patients with severe chronic airflow obstruction. Am Rev Respir Dis 140:1251–1256, 1989.

29. Rochester DF, Braun NMT, Laine S: Diaphragmatic energy expenditure in chronic respiratory failure. Am J Med 63:223–231, 1977

30. Rodenstein DO, Stanescu DC, Cuttita G et al: Ventilatory and diaphragmatic EMG responses to negative pressure ventilation in airflow obstruction. J Appl Physiol 65:1621–1626, 1988

31. Curran FJ: Night ventilation by body respirators for patients in chronic respiratory failure due to late-state Duchenne muscular dystrophy. Arch Phys Med Rehabil 62:270–274, 1981

32. Holtackers TR, Loosbrock LM, Gracey DR: The use of the chest cuirass in respiratory failure of neurologic origin. Respir Care 27:271–275, 1982

33. Kacmarek RM, Spearman CB: Equipment used for ventilatory support in the home. Respir Care 31:311–328, 1986

34. O'Donnell C, Gilmartin ME: Home mechanical ventilators and accessory equipment. Probl Respir Care 1(2):217–240, 1988

35. Alexander MA, Johnson EW, Petty J et al: Mechanical ventilation of patients with late stage Duchenne muscular dystrophy: Management in the home. Arch Phys Med Rehabil 60:289–292, 1979

36. Hill NS: Clinical application of body ventilators. Chest 90:897–905, 1986

37. Wiers PWJ, LeCoultre R, Dallingo OT et al: Cuirass respirator treatment of chronic respiratory failure in scoliotic patients. Thorax 32:221–228, 1977

38. O'Donohue WJ Jr: Patient selection and discharge criteria for home ventilator care. Probl Respir Care 1(2):167–174, 1988

39. Make BJ: Long-term management of ventilator-assisted individuals: The Boston University experience. Respir Care 31:303–313, 1986

40. Davis PB, di Sant'Agnese PA: Assisted ventilation for patients with cystic fibrosis. JAMA 239:1851–1854, 1978

41. Robert D, Gerard M, Leger P et al: Domiciliary mechanical ventilation by tracheostomy for chronic respiratory failure. Rev Fr Mal Resp 11:923–936, 1983

42. Sivak ED, Cordasco EM, Gipson WT et al: Home care ventilation: The Cleveland Clinic experience from 1977 to 1985. Respir Care 31:294–302, 1986

43. Prentice WS: Placement alternatives for long-term ventilator care. Respir Care 31:288–293, 1986

44. Indihar FJ, Walker NE: Experience with a prolonged respiratory care unit revisited. Chest 86:616–620, 1984

45. O'Donohue W, Petty TL, Plummer A et al: Consensus conference on problems in home mechanical ventilation. Am Rev Respir Dis 140:555–560, 1989

46. LaFond L, Horner J: Psychological issues related to long-term ventilatory support. Probl Respir Care 1(2):241–256, 1988

47. Alba A, Pilkington LA, Kaplan E et al: Long-term pulmonary care in amyotrophic lateral sclerosis. Respir Ther 16:49–105, 1986

48. Banaszak EF, Travers H, Fraizer M et al: Home ventilator care. Respir Care 26:1262–1268, 1981

49. Burr BH, Buyer B, Todres ID et al: Home care for children on respirators. N Engl J Med 309:1319–1323, 1983

50. Dunkin LJ: Home ventilatory assistance. Anaesthesia 38:644–649, 1983

51. Feldman J, Tuteur PG: Mechanical ventilation: From hospital intensive care to home. Heart Lung 11:162–165, 1982

52. Giovannoni R: Chronic ventilator care: From hospital to home. Respir Ther 14:29–33, 1984

53. Glover DW: Three years at home on an MA-1. Respir Ther 11:69–70, 1981

54. Goldberg AI, Kettrick R, Buzdygan D et al: Home ventilation program for infants and children. Crit Care Med 31:238–243, 1980

55. Home ventilation: Status in Ontario. Ont Med Rev (Jan):14–16, 1986

56. Kopacz MA, Moriarty-Wright R: Multidisciplinary approach for the patient on a home ventilator. Heart Lung 13:255–262, 1984

57. Bach JR, Alba AS, Bohatuik G: Mouth intermittent positive pressure ventilation in the management of post polio respiratory insufficiency. Chest 91:859–864, 1987

58. Bach JR, Alba A, Mosher R: Intermittent positive pressure ventilation via nasal access in the management of respiratory insufficiency. Chest 92:168–170, 1987

59. Splaingard ML, Frates RC, Jefferson LS et al: Home negative pressure ventilation: Report of 20 years experience in patients with neuromuscular disease. Arch Phys Med Rehabil 66:239, 1985

60. Make B, Gilmartin M, Brody JS et al: Rehabilitation of ventilator-dependent subjects with lung diseases: The concept and initial experience. Chest 86:358–365, 1984

61. Dull WL, Sadoul P: Home ventilators in patients with severe lung disease. Am Rev Respir Dis 123(suppl):74, 1981

62. Czorniak MA, Gilmartin ME, Make BJ: Home mechanical ventilation: Clinical course of patients with neuromuscular disease (NMD) and chronic obstructive pulmonary disease (COPD). Am Rev Respir Dis 135(4, part 2):194A, 1987

63. Gilmartin M, Make B: Home care of ventilator-dependent persons. Respir Care 28:1490–1497, 1983

64. McPherson SP: Respiratory Home Care Equipment. Dubuque, Kendall/Hunt, 1988

65. Kacmarek RM, Stanck KS, McMahon K et al: Improved work of breathing during synchronized intermittent mandatory ventilation (SIMV) via home care ventilators. Am Rev Respir Dis 137(4, part 2):64, 1988

66. Leger P, Jennequin J, Gerard M, Robert D: Home positive pressure ventilation via nasal mask for patients with neuromuscular weakness or restrictive lung or chest wall disease. Respir Care 34:73–77, 1989

67. Kerby GR, Mayer LS, Pingleton SK: Nocturnal positive pressure ventilation via nasal mask. Am Rev Respir Dis 137:738–740, 1987

68. Miller JH, Thomas E, Wilmont CB: Pneumobelt use among high quadriplegic population. Arch Phys Med Rehabil 69:369–372, 1988

69. Wilson DJ: Airway management of the ventilator-assisted individual. Probl Respir Care 1(2):192–203, 1988

70. Schreiner MS, Downes JJ, Kettrick RG et al: Chronic respiratory failure in infants with prolonged ventilator failure. JAMA 258:3398–3404, 1987

71. Lawrence PA: Home care for ventilator-dependent children: Providing a chance to live a normal life. Dimens Crit Care Nurs 3:42–52, 1984

72. Report of the Brook Lodge Symposium on the Ventilator-Dependent Child: La Rabida Children's Hospital and Research Center, 1984. (Copies may be obtained from Children's Home Health Network of Illinois. East 56th Street, Chicago, IL 60649)

73. Report of the Surgeon General's Workshop on Children with Handicaps and Their Families. Washington, DC, US Department of Health and Human Services, 1982

74. Kettrick RG, Donar ME: Ventilator-assisted infants and children. Probl Respir Care 1(2):269–278, 1988

75. Frates RC, Splaingard ML, Smith DO et al: Outcome of home mechanical ventilation in children. J Pediatr 106:850, 1985

76. Moser KM: Home mechanical ventilation and the cost of humane care. J Respir Dis 7(3):15, 1986

77. LaFond L, Make BJ, Gilmartin ME: Home care costs for ventilator-assisted individuals. Am Rev Respir Dis 137(4, part 2):62, 1988

78. Sivak ED, Cordasco EM, Gipson WT: Pulmonary mechanical ventilation at home: A reasonable and less expensive alternative. Respir Care 28:42–49, 1983

79. Prentice WC: Transition from hospital to home. Probl Respir Care 1(2):174–191, 1988

80. Krieger BP, Ershowsky P, Spivack D et al: Initial experience with a noninvasive respiratory monitoring unit as a cost-saving alternative to the intensive care unit for Medicare patients who require long-term ventilator support. Chest 93:395–397, 1988

81. Bone RC, Balk RA: The noninvasive respiratory care unit—a cost-effective solution for the future. Chest 93:390–394, 1988

82. O'Donohue WJ, Branson RD, Hoppough JM, Make BJ: Criteria for establishing units for chronic ventilator-dependent patients in hospitals. Respir Care 33:1044–1046, 1988

83. Goldberg AI: Home care for life-supported persons: Is a national approach the answer? Chest 90:744–748, 1986

TWENTY-SIX

Bronchoscopy

W. Mark Brutinel
Denis A. Cortese

Bronchoscopy is an established and useful tool in patient care and medical research. The ability to visualize the tracheobronchial tree has been available since the development of rigid bronchoscopy. However, until the introduction into clinical practice of the flexible fiberoptic bronchoscope in 1968, this procedure was limited to specialists, most often surgeons, and was performed in operating suites or dedicated bronchoscopy suites. The flexible fiberoptic bronchoscope has proved to be easy to use and highly portable. Once its efficacy was established, a wide range of medical specialists found it useful in their practice and have taken bronchoscopy out of the operating room into the intensive care units, and procedural rooms, and even into outpatient settings away from the hospital.

In this chapter, we will attempt to give an overview of the clinical indications and contraindications to the use of the flexible fiberoptic instrument. A more detailed discussion will be presented of necessary equipment; the procedure itself; how to set up for a bronchoscopy, assist the bronchoscopist, and collect specimens; and how to clean the bronchoscope after the procedure. Unless otherwise stated, the discussion will deal with the flexible fiberoptic bronchoscope.

INDICATIONS

The diagnostic and therapeutic indications for bronchoscopy are shown in Tables 26–1 and 26–2.[19,63,66] The decision to perform a bronchoscopy must be undertaken with a full knowledge of the patient's history, physical findings, and laboratory data. The appropriate timing and selection of the most effective diagnostic maneuvers cannot be done without detailed information about the patient. Care and attention must always be directed to the overall medical condition of the patient and, particularly, to the patient's respiratory reserve. The relative contraindications to bronchoscopy must be kept in mind and suitable decisions made for the patients to whom they apply (see Table 26–3).[66]

The most common indication for a bronchoscopic procedure is an abnormal roentgenographic study. Chest roentgenograms, tomograms, computed tomograms (CT scan), and magnetic resonance imaging (MRI) scans can all show abnormalities. The approach to these lesions depends on their location and the clinical situation. The procedure begins with a thorough visual inspection of the upper and lower respiratory tract. This should include the nasal passages, pharynx, hypopharynx, larynx, vocal cords, subglottic area, trachea, bronchi, lobar bronchi, and segmental bronchi down to the third or fourth divisions. If abnormalities are seen, diagnostic maneuvers are done,

Table 26–1 Diagnostic Indications for Bronchoscopy

Abnormal radiographic findings
  Localized lesion
    Mass lesion
    Recurring pulmonary infiltrates
    Unresolved pulmonary infiltrates
    Persistent atelectasis/collapse
      Segmental
      Lobar
      Lung
    Mediastinal and hilar abnormalities
    Malignant pleural effusions
    Abnormalities of the tracheobronchial air shadow
  Diffuse parenchymal lung disease
    Immunocompetent host
    Nonimmunocompetent host
Acute inhalation injury
Assessment of intubation damage
Assessment of rejection of transplanted lung
Bronchiectasis
Bronchopleural fistulas
Broncholithiasis
Diaphragmatic paralysis
Foreign body
Hemoptysis
Lung abscess
Major thoracic trauma
Positive sputum cytology for malignancy
Recurrent laryngeal nerve (vocal cord) paralysis
Stridor or localized wheezing
Unexplained cough
Upper esophageal lesions

Table 26–2 Therapeutic Indications for Bronchoscopy

Endotracheal intubation
Retained secretions or mucus plugs
  Postoperatively
  In mechanically ventilated patients
Foreign body aspiration
Management of life-threatening hemoptysis
Bronchopleural fistulas
Lung abscess
Bronchial strictures
  Dilatation (rigid bronchoscopy)
  Placement of stents (rigid bronchoscopy)
  Laser therapy (rigid and flexible bronchoscopy)
Endobronchial malignant obstruction
  Dilatation (rigid bronchoscopy)
  Placement of stents (rigid bronchoscopy)
  Laser therapy (rigid and flexible bronchoscopy)
    Photodynamic therapy
    Carbon dioxide laser
    Neodymium:YAG laser
Brachytherapy

which may include any or all of the following: brushings, biopsies, needle aspirations, and washings. If no abnormalities of the visible airways are seen, then fluoroscopy may be used to direct the brush, needle, and biopsy forceps to the area of interest.[63] With these maneuvers the diagnosis and extent of disease frequently can be determined for various disorders. These include cancer, sarcoidosis, infection, foreign bodies, and other more unusual disorders of the lung parenchyma and bronchial tree.

The bronchoscopist is commonly called to diagnose diffuse lung disease. In the immunocompetent host, the procedure is most effective in diagnosing neoplastic and infectious causes of diffuse disease.

In the immunocompromised host, the bronchoscope is highly efficacious in diagnosing infectious causes of new pulmonary infiltrates.[11,18,24,35,39,47,48,69]

Bronchoalveolar lavage (BAL) is now routinely used in an attempt to diagnose bacterial, fungal, mycobacterial, Pneumocystis, Legionella, and viral infections that can occur in these patients. If, in both immunocompetent and immunocompromised patients, after physical examination, initial laboratory testing, and analysis of the patient's sputum a diagnosis is not made,[35,46] bronchoscopy is performed and a segment of the lung containing the infiltrate is lavaged. Appropriate microbiologic tests are then performed on the aspirated fluid. If appropriate, brushing and biopsies can be performed. The yield on these procedures is excellent and helps avoid an open-lung biopsy. Because of the efficacy of bronchoscopy with BAL, the bronchoscopist is often asked to perform the procedure on patients who are very ill and with little respiratory reserve. This requires care on the part of the medical team to ensure the patient's comfort and safety.

Acute inhalation injury from toxic or heated gases can be a life-threatening situation. Initially, judgments need to be made about the degree of respiratory support that will be needed. A bronchoscopic examination of the upper and lower airways can be helpful in judging the extent of the damage and planning therapy. One of the most immediate dangers is laryngeal edema causing upper airway obstruction, usually at the level of the vocal cords. An experienced observer can judge the degree of laryngeal damage and proceed to elective intubation with the help of the bronchoscope before the edema can make intubation difficult or impossible to accomplish. Knowledge of the degree and extent of mucosal damage can help determine whether careful observation or early therapy with steroids and possibly antibiotics is indicated.[3,12,55,58]

Endotracheal intubation carries with it the risk of damage to the larynx, vocal cords, and trachea. The bronchoscope is an excellent tool to assess the possibility of damage to these areas. Hemoptysis from an endotracheal tube or postintubation shortness of breath, stridor, or wheezing are reasons to perform a bronchoscopy. The bronchoscope is also an excellent tool to assess the patency of the airway in an intubated patient. A quick examination can discover if the endotracheal tube is placed correctly and whether any mucus, blood, or foreign body is obstructing the endotracheal tube. Difficulty ventilating the patient without obvious cause and difficulty passing a suction catheter are reasons to examine the airway.[15,44,56]

Bronchiectasis is fortunately less common in this age of antibiotic therapy, but it still occurs. It is important to assess the bronchial anatomy in individuals with bronchiectasis to rule out an endobronchial cause and look for the extent of involvement. *Bronchopleural fistulas* with persistent leakage of air into the pleural space can be troublesome. The bronchoscope can be used to attempt to locate the fistula. Particularly after a lung resection, inspection of the bronchial suture line for dehiscence is important. *Broncholithiasis* presenting as hemoptysis, lithoptysis, or bronchial obstruction can be diagnosed with the bronchoscope in conjunction with appropriate roentgenographic studies.[31] Unfortunately, it is not as useful for removal of the broncholiths because of the dangers of massive hemorrhage.[54]

Diaphragmatic paralysis can be idiopathic or iatrogenic from surgical manipulation. However, it can also be caused by neoplasms of the airway, and some clinicians have recommended a bronchoscopic examination to look for endobronchial lesions. The advent of CT scanning has made this less necessary in our view. The likelihood of there being a visible endobronchial lesion causing a phrenic nerve paralysis in the face of a negative CT scan of the chest is quite small.

Foreign bodies in the airway can almost always be removed with bronchoscopy. The flexible fiberoptic bronchoscope is excellent for diagnosing the presence of a foreign body, and some authors feel that they can be removed with the flexible instrument.[31] However, when the foreign body cannot be easily withdrawn through an endotracheal tube, the rigid bronchoscope is the instrument of choice for removal of the foreign body.[37,68] In children, the rigid bronchoscope allows ventilation of the patient under general anesthesia; in both children and adults, the rigid bronchoscope facilitates safe delivery of large foreign bodies through the subglottic area and the larynx.[43]

Most patients with *hemoptysis* have benign bronchitis. Unfortunately, hemoptysis is also a sign of bronchiectasis, broncholithiasis, foreign body aspiration, endobronchial tumor, and bronchogenic carcinoma. In patients who are older, have a smoking history, have had hemoptysis longer than 1 week, or have an abnormal chest x-ray, the risk of a significant pathologic cause of the hemoptysis is increased. Bronchoscopy is indicated in selected patients with increased risk factors for cancer or in whom the clinical situation suggests a diagnosis that can be investigated by a visual inspection of the airway.[29,32,51]

A *lung abscess* is a strong indication for a bronchoscopic examination. The abscess may be a result of endobronchial obstruction, which may be due to a foreign body, tumor, extrinsic compression, or mucosal lesions. The bronchoscopist can also help therapeutically by attempting to establish drainage from the abscessed area of the lung.[57,64]

Major blunt thoracic trauma can result in a pulmonary contusion as well as a laceration or disruption of the tracheobronchial tree. The disruptions can range from small tears to complete transection and can occur in the trachea and major bronchi. They present as pneumothorax, pneumomediastinum, and subcutaneous emphysema. Airway obstruction and asphyxia can occur with transection of the trachea. The bronchoscope is invaluable in determining the integrity of the tracheobronchial tree.[22]

A patient who has *cancer cells* on cytologic examination of the sputum and a negative chest roentgenogram or CT scan presents a diagnostic dilemma. An ear, nose, and throat examination will rule out an upper airway cause; bronchoscopy will then be needed to search for a cancer of the tracheobronchial tree. If this is negative, a repeat examination is performed under general anesthesia with selective brushing of all 20 lobar segments. If malignancy is confirmed by biopsy, positive brush cytology on two separate occasions, or both, the cancer is considered localized and treatment begins. If the malignancy cannot be localized, careful observation with repeat roentgenographic and bronchoscopic studies is advised. Localization with hematoporphyrin fluorescence is another technique that can be used, but it is performed in only a few medical centers.[13]

Recurrent laryngeal nerve (vocal cord) paralysis suggests the possibility of a lesion along the distribution of the recurrent laryngeal nerve. Imaging of the chest with a CT scan is appropriate. If the CT scan is abnormal, bronchoscopy can be performed to look for an endobronchial lesion (most commonly malignant) to make the diagnosis for the cause of the nerve dysfunction. A transbronchial needle aspiration could be performed if the diagnosis cannot be made with inspection of the tracheobronchial tree and if a mediastinal mass is present on the CT scan.[62] Bronchoscopy performed when the CT scan is negative has less chance of finding the cause of the nerve paralysis, but it can be performed to be sure there is no occult extrabronchial lesion.

Stridor or localized wheezing suggests a functional or structural narrowing of the airway from various causes. Pulmonary function tests can be helpful, along with roentgenographic studies, in attempting to localize the point of narrowing. Asthma should be considered, but care must be taken not to confuse a localized obstruction with the more diffuse bronchial narrowing of asthma. Bronchoscopy is an excellent technique to look for vocal cord paralysis, laryngeal pathology, tumors (benign and malignant), and extrinsic compression of the tracheobronchial tree.[17,25,70]

Unexplained *cough* can be a diagnostic dilemma. Once common causes such as respiratory infections, chronic obstructive pulmonary disease, and asthma have been ruled out, bronchoscopy should be considered. Occult endobronchial lesions can cause chronic persistent coughing and are often small and treatable. A careful evaluation for treatable causes of cough should be undertaken and appropriate therapy should be instituted. If no cause for the cough is found and no significant improvement occurs in 2 to 3 months, bronchoscopy is advised.[50]

Cancer of the upper esophagus can invade the tracheobronchial tree. It is important for the thoracic surgeon attempting to resect this type of cancer to know the extent of the spread of the tumor. A bronchoscopic examination of the trachea and main bronchi can accomplish this.[7,8,27,33,67]

The bronchoscope is also an excellent therapeutic tool. It is extremely useful in placing endotracheal tubes by the oral or nasal route. It is the instrument of choice to assist with *difficult intubations*. Patients who cannot move their necks or who have unusual upper airway anatomy can be intubated safely while awake with this technique.[15,44,56]

Probably the most frequent therapeutic use of the bronchoscope is to *remove retained secretions*. In a hospitalized patient in whom new atelectasis or collapse of a lung or its segments develops and who has not responded to aggressive chest physiotherapy and suctioning, bronchoscopy is indicated to assess the airway for retained secretions and to remove them. If the patient is stable and has an adequate blood oxygen tension, increasing those measures that improve pulmonary toilet are as likely to resolve the atelectasis and collapse as bronchoscopy. These include instituting or increasing chest physical therapy, cough, deep inspiratory maneuvers, pain relief, and ambulation. If these measures are already in place, or if after 12 to 24 hours of intensive treatment there is no improvement, bronchoscopy is indicated. If the patient is hypoxemic despite oxygen supplementation and it is judged that relief of the presumed obstruction caused by secretion retention will improve the hypoxemia, then bronchoscopy should be done promptly while the oxygen saturation is monitored.[28,38]

Management of life-threatening *hemoptysis* is a difficult clinical problem.[9,20,26,42,45,52,54] The degree of danger to the patient is dependent on the amount of hemorrhage and the patient's pulmonary reserve. Therapy should be directed toward protecting what pulmonary function remains. The flexible instrument can be used to attempt to localize the site of bleeding, remove blood and clot from the airway, place single- and double-lumen endotracheal tubes,[61] and place balloon catheters to tamponade that portion of the lung that is bleeding. However, in massive hemoptysis, the flexible instrument is often not adequate. Its small fiberoptic bundle is quickly obscured, making vision difficult if not impossible, and the relatively small suction channel is easily clogged with fibrin clot. Rigid bronchoscopy has the advantage of being able to simultaneously ventilate the patient through the instrument and maintain a clear airway. Larger instruments can be passed through the scope. This permits the use of large suction catheters, and more than one suction catheter can be used at once.

In addition, the bronchus leading to the bleeding area of the lung can be packed with umbilical tape soaked in epinephrine.[45] The rigid bronchoscope cannot examine the upper lobes well, but if required the flexible bronchoscope can be passed through the rigid scope to examine these areas. The optimum management of massive hemoptysis is with a combination of flexible and rigid instruments.

Bronchial strictures, other than thin webs, are treated definitively with surgical resection. In patients in whom this is not possible, dilatation with a rigid bronchoscope can be a temporizing measure. Placement of Silastic bronchial stents can be tried,[10,65] and laser resection with the neodymium:YAG or carbon dioxide laser has been used.[60]

Endobronchial malignant obstruction is best treated with surgical resection, but when that is not possible, bronchoscopic techniques can help in palliation of respiratory symptoms and prolongation of life. Dilatations can be performed with the rigid bronchoscope. Laser therapy with either the neodymium:YAG or carbon dioxide laser has been helpful.[6] Endobronchial Silastic stents can be placed to maintain airway patency.[10,65] Photodynamic therapy with hematoporphyrin has been used by some clinicians to treat malignant airway obstruction.[1,2,30,41]

Photodynamic therapy is also used to treat small-airway carcinomas for cure in patients who are not candidates for surgical resection.[14] *Brachytherapy* performed with small plastic tubes temporarily placed in the airways with bronchoscopic guidance can help decrease malignant obstruction in patients who have received maximal external beam radiation therapy. The catheters are subsequently loaded with iridium-192 beads on a wire, and local radiation therapy is delivered to the airway obstruction.[59]

COMPLICATIONS

Fortunately, complications from a fiberoptic bronchoscopy examination are rare. Overall mortality should be less then 0.1%. All complications should be fewer than 8.1%. Other complications not leading to death have been reported, including fever (1.2%), pneumonia (0.6%), vasovagal reaction (2.4%), obstruction of the airways (0.9%), respiratory arrest (0.1%), cardiac arrhythmias (0.9%), pneumothorax (0.7%), nausea and vomiting (0.2%), psychotic reaction (0.1%), and aphonia (0.1%).[49] Bacteremias can occur after bronchoscopic examination, and antibiotics are recommended for subacute bacterial endocarditis prophylaxis. Laser bronchoscopy increases the risk of death to 2%.[6]

Complications can be minimized if thought is given to the clinical status of the patient. For exam-

ple, before the procedure the asthmatic should be treated for bronchospasm, the unstable cardiac patient stabilized medically, and the hypoxic chronic lung disease patient adequately oxygenated. With careful preparation and monitoring, bronchoscopy can be made safe.

CONTRAINDICATIONS

The contraindications to bronchoscopy are shown in Table 26–3.[19,63,66] They are all relative. If after careful evaluation it is thought that the possible benefit of bronchoscopy outweights the risks, then the procedure should be performed by an experienced bronchoscopist. Bronchoscopy frequently can cause a decrease in the arterial oxygen tension, both during and after the procedure. Oxygen supplementation should be provided, and a finger pulse oximeter to monitor the need for oxygen before, during, and after the procedure should be used.[4,5,23,34,36,40] If the patient is already significantly hypoxemic despite medical management, oxygen supplementation, and mechanical ventilation, bronchoscopy may worsen the hypoxemia and could be a serious risk to the patient. Patients who have borderline or low arterial oxygen tensions should continue to receive supplemental oxygen after the procedure until their oxygen saturation is at an acceptable level.

Acute hypercapnia with acidosis is a significant contraindication. Bronchoscopy will increase airway resistance and the work of breathing and can quickly worsen the situation. If it is thought that the procedure is necessary, mechanical venti-

Table 26–3 Contraindications to Bronchoscopy

Hypoxemia
Unresponsive to
Medical management
Oxygen supplementation
Hypercapnia
Unresponsive to
Medical management
Mechanical ventilation
Cardiovascular instability
Hypotension
Uncontrolled angina
Myocardial infarction
Malignant arrhythmias
Asthma
Patient unable to cooperate with the procedure

lation will be required. If the patient is hypercapnic and acidotic on a ventilator, the procedure should be performed if the potential benefit is judged to be high. In a patient with stable compensated respiratory acidosis, bronchoscopy can be performed, depending on the degree of hypercapnia, with careful attention to the use of premedication, sedation during the procedure, and the amount of oxygen supplementation.

Cardiac instability should be treated before the bronchoscopy. Elective bronchoscopy should not be performed until the situation is stabilized. However, if the cause of cardiac instability can be corrected by the bronchoscopy, then the risks of the procedure must be weighed against the benefits.

Asthma is a relative contraindication because bronchoscopy can stimulate or worsen bronchospasm. If the asthma is adequately treated and controlled, asthmatics can be examined safely.

Coagulopathies are contraindications only to brushings, needle aspirations, and biopsies. Patients can safely undergo a bronchoscopy while receiving full anticoagulation therapy as long as care is taken not to irritate the mucosa. Bronchoalveolar lavage can be performed with low platelet counts, and it is useful in the immunocompromised hematologic patient, who often has a coagulopathy. Uremia increases the risk of bleeding owing to platelet dysfunction, and the serum creatinine level should be routinely measured; if the creatinine level is increased, a blood urea nitrogen measurement is indicated before a bronchoscopy in which brushings, needle aspirations, or biopsies are planned.

If the patient is unable to cooperate with the procedure, then consideration can be given to performing the bronchoscopy under heavy sedation or general anesthesia. This is best done in an operating room, outpatient surgical area, or intensive care unit, with assistance from an anesthesiologist or nurse anesthetist.

PERSONNEL SAFETY

All members of the bronchoscopy team should wear masks, eye protection, and gloves. It is good practice to use nonsterile protective gowns to keep secretions and blood off clothes and bodies. The entire procedure should be done carefully to prevent contamination of the bronchoscopy team with secretions. In the past, the main concern was transmission of airborne disease organisms, such as *Mycobacterium tuberculosis*, to personnel. With the advent of the acquired immunodeficiency syndrome (AIDS), there has been concern that the virus could be transmitted by the patient's respiratory secretions. Fortunately, there is no documented case of human immunodeficiency virus (HIV) transmission to bronchoscopy personnel. Of more concern is contact with the patient's blood. Care with handling of blood products should be exercised at all times, but particularly when handling the needle catheters used for cytologic aspiration. They should be handled in the same manner as any contaminated sharp instrument. Because the needle is passed from the bronchoscopist to the assistant, special care must be taken not to puncture the person receiving the needle catheter.[21]

EQUIPMENT

The proper selection of equipment is important to ensure a safe and effective procedure. Table 26–4 lists suggested equipment that can be placed on a portable cart and moved to wherever the bronchoscopy is to be performed (Figs. 26–1, 26–2). If possible, a system should be devised to store the bronchoscopes on the side of the cart such that they hang straight and are protected from injury (Fig. 26–3). Particular attention should be paid to avoid catching the scope in the hinges of a door, drawer, or case. Oxygen, suction, and a cardiac monitor should be available where the procedure is to be performed. A regular program of inspection and stocking of the bronchoscopy cart should be instituted, especially in the situation in which more than one physician uses the equipment.

ASSISTING IN THE PROCEDURE

Before a bronchoscopy is performed, a certain amount of preparation is required to ensure a safe and smooth procedure. The patient's history should be carefully reviewed for possible contraindications to the procedure. Special attention should be directed to the patient's mental status, cardiovascular status, history of asthma, respiratory reserve, and arterial blood gas values. A recent hemoglobin value, platelet count, electrolyte values, and creatinine level should be available. If there is any concern about the patient's respiratory reserve, an arterial blood gas measurement and possibly pulmonary function testing should be done. If the history or laboratory results suggest a coagulopathy, then a prothrombin time, activated partial thromboplastin time, and, if indicated, a bleeding

Table 26—4 Bronchoscopy Equipment

Portable cart
Light source
Bronchoscopes
    Adult scope (5.0-mm OD)
    Adult lavage scope (6.0-mm OD)
    Pediatric scope (3.5-mm OD)
    Suction adapters, valves, and caps
Oxygen source
    Tubing, nasal cannulas, close-fitting mask
Assortment of endotracheal tubes
Swivel adapters with rubber diaphragms
Cardiac monitor
Pulse oximeter
Isotonic saline
Syringes (non–Luer-lock)
    10–12 mL
    30–50 mL
Sterile needles
Lidocaine
    Viscous 2%
    Injectable 2%
    Injectable 4%
Benzocaine 20% oral spray
Direct laryngoscopes
Laryngeal mirror
Laryngeal cannula
Heal lamp
Wall suction
Suction tubing and connectors
Specimens
    Secretion traps
    Glass slides
    Cytology jars
    Formalin jars
    Sterile containers
    Sterile capped plastic tubes with 1 mL of isotonic saline
Cytology brushes
Biopsy forceps
    Cup forceps
    Alligator forceps
Foreign body forceps
    Basket
    Grasping
Bronchoalveolar lavage kit
    Tubing
    Stopcock
    Connectors
    Specimen containers

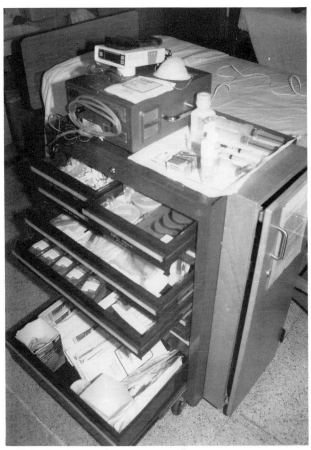

Figure 26—1. Portable bronchoscopy equipment cart at bedside.

time should be measured; these need to be performed only if brushings, aspirations, or biopsies are contemplated.

The bronchoscopist selects the appropriate instruments for the procedure planned. The bronchoscopy cart should be set up close to the patient so that the bronchoscope's light guide is not under tension. The patient should have a cardiac monitor and finger-pulse oximeter attached and supplemental oxygen given by nasal cannula or close-fitting mask. If a close-fitting mask is used, a small hole can be cut in the disposable mask to allow insertion of the bronchoscope. If the patient is intubated or is going to be intubated, a swivel adapter with a rubber diaphragm should be available. Also, if the patient is to be intubated, an appropriate-sized endotracheal tube, 7.5 or larger, should have its balloon tested, lubricated, and placed over the bronchoscope before intubation. A means to hand-ventilate the patient during the procedure should be ready, and a mechanical ventilator should be available.

On the top of the bronchoscopy cart spread a sterile towel and place the basic items required for the procedure (Fig. 26–4). These may vary some-

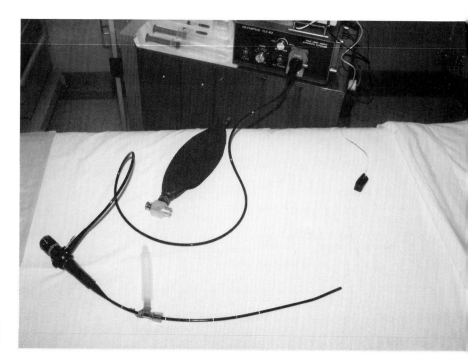

Figure 26—2. Flexible fiberoptic bronchoscope with swivel adaptor and anesthesia bag.

what with the individual requirements of each physician. A clear water-soluble lubricant is needed to lubricate the insertion tube of the scope. Four-by-four sponges are helpful to apply the lubricant and wipe off excess lubricant and secretions. Isotonic saline is used to clear the suction channel and to fill the lavage syringes. Two 50-mL non–Luer-lock syringes filled with 30 mL of isotonic saline and 10 mL of air are needed for lavage. For instilling local anesthetic, two 10-mL non–Luer-lock syringes filled with 1 mL of 2% lidocaine and 9 mL of air should be prepared. Wall suction should be available and, if secretions are to be collected, a secretion trap should be inserted in the suction line. The trap must be held upright or taped to an object to prevent tipping and losing secretions.

Depending on the diagnostic procedures planned (Table 26–5), the appropriate instruments should be readily available (see Table 26–4). Wire brushes are needed for cytologic specimens. Transbronchial needle catheters vary according to the type of aspiration planned. Flexible biopsy forceps should be tested to ensure that the jaws work smoothly. If BAL is planned, it is best to have a kit available (see Table 26–4).

Most bronchoscopists in this country will perform the procedure facing a sitting patient, who is receiving supplemental oxygen. The bronchoscope is inserted through an anesthetized naris, without

Table 26—5 Diagnostic Procedures Performed With Fiberoptic Bronchoscope

Inspection
Collection of secretions
  Fungal cultures
  Mycobacterial cultures
  Cytology
Brushings
  Bacterial culture
    Double-sheathed protected catheter brush
  Cytology
Needle aspirations
  Cytology
  Biopsy
  Culture
    Bacterial cultures
    Fungal cultures
    Mycobacterial cultures
  Aspiration of cystic structures
Biopsy
Bronchoalveolar lavage
  Research
  Cultures
    Bacterial
    Fungal
    Mycobacterial
    Legionella
    Pneumocystis carinii
    Viral

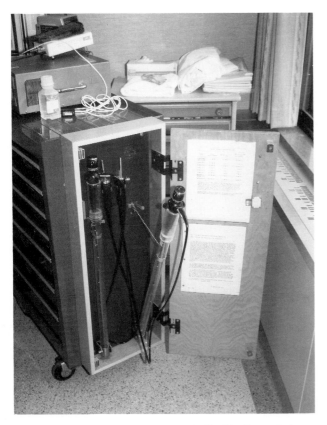

Figure 26–3. Storage cabinet for flexible fiberoptic bronchoscopes attached to a portable bronchoscopy equipment cart. This allows the scopes to be stored in a straight position and reduces the chance of damage to them.

an endotracheal tube, and 2% lidocaine is given through the suction channel of the scope to anesthetize the hypopharynx, larynx, vocal cords, and tracheobronchial tree, as needed. Other alternatives are use an endotracheal tube placed through the naris or through the mouth. When performing the bronchoscopic examination through the mouth, the use of an endotracheal tube is also optional. Endotracheal tubes may be used when the patient will need ventilatory support during the procedure, when thick tenacious secretions are expected, or when there is a risk of hemorrhage. A swivel adapter is used to allow assisted ventilation while bronchoscopy is performed (Fig. 26–5). If one elects to examine the patient through the mouth, local anesthetic can be instilled in the back of the throat and tongue with a spray, such as 20% benzocaine, and the hypopharynx, larynx, and vocal cords can be anesthetized with 2% lidocaine by us-

ing a laryngeal mirror and cannula. Other techniques include the use of 5 mL of 4% lidocaine delivered by nebulizer, superior laryngeal nerve block, and direct instillation of 2 mL of 2% lidocaine through the cricothyroid membrane into the trachea with a syringe and a small-gauge needle.

If secretions are being collected for culture, suction should not be attached to the bronchoscope until it is inside the trachea. This prevents aspiration of saliva and pharyngeal contents. The bronchoscopist asks for lidocaine and isotonic saline when needed, and the syringes should be handed to his or her free hand. Because of the small volume involved, when the bronchoscopist is going to inject lidocaine through the suction channel, the suction should be temporarily stopped.

The handling of specimens is dependent on the requirements of the microbiologist, pathologist, and cytopathologist who will interpret the results. What follows is a description of how specimens are handled in our institution.

If brushings are performed for cytologic examination, the brush is handed to the bronchoscopist such that it can be grasped just behind the bristles. The brush is inserted through the suction channel, and the area of interest is brushed. After this the brush will either be pulled back through the suction channel and handed to the assistant, or the scope will be removed from the patient and the brush removed by grasping the wire behind the bristles and pulling it out of the distal tip of the bronchoscope's suction channel. The brushings should be smeared on a series of slides and placed in the fixative. At some institutions the end of the brush is clipped off and also placed in the fixative.

A double-sheathed protected catheter brush is used to obtain specimens for sterile bacterial cultures. There are several available; instructions on how to use them are included in their packaging. In general, the procedure is performed before applying any suction to the suction channel. Consequently, this catheter brush is often used first, even before inspecting the airways. The tip of the catheter should be treated in a sterile manner. The catheter brush is advanced, as is, into the area of interest. Then the inner catheter is advanced out of the outer catheter sheath. The glycerol plug is advanced out of the outer catheter sheath and will be absorbed in the airway. The brush is advanced out of the inner catheter sheath. The brush is pulled back into the inner catheter sheath, and the whole catheter brush is removed from the bronchoscope channel. The inner catheter sheath is cleaned with alcohol and its tip is cut off with sterile scissors. The brush is

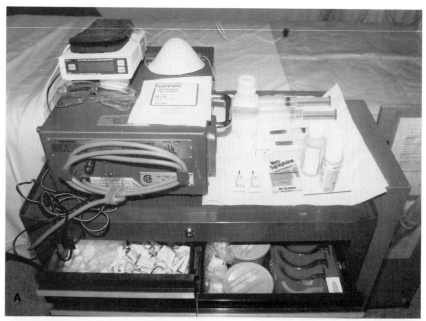

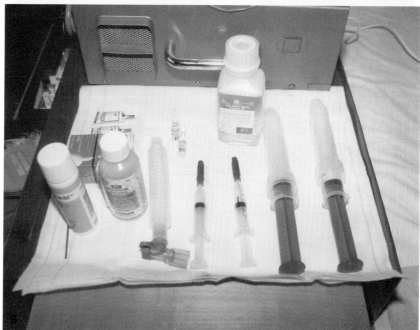

Figure 26—4. (*A* and *B*) Portable bronchoscopy equipment cart setup with equipment needed for a basic bronchoscopic examination.

advanced out of the inner catheter sheath and clipped into a small container with 1 mL of isotonic saline. This is tightly sealed and transported to the microbiology laboratory, where it can be quantitatively cultured for aerobic and anaerobic bacteria.

Transbronchial needle aspirations are performed with needle catheters, which come in various sizes and styles. The bronchoscopy assistant should be familiar with, and have practiced with, the needle catheters that are used. All needle catheters are inserted through the suction channel of the scope. The needle is prepared by either withdrawing the stylet or extending and locking the needle. The bronchoscopist punctures the bronchial wall

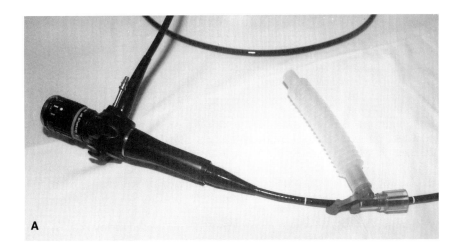

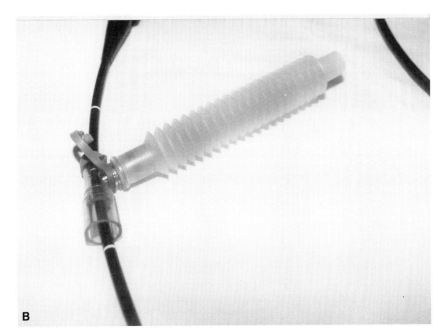

Figure 26—5. (*A* and *B*) Flexible fiberoptic bronchoscope with swivel adaptor. The swivel adaptor is used to ventilate an intubated patient during a bronchoscopic examination.

and asks for suction, which is created by using a syringe attached to the end of the needle catheter. A stylet will need to be withdrawn slightly from the proximal end of the catheter to allow the suction to reach the needle tip. The syringe should contain a small amount of isotonic saline. The needle is agitated in the bronchial wall and then withdrawn through the suction channel of the scope. The assistant flushes the needle catheter and needle with the saline in the syringe. If a small needle is used, the aspirations are placed on a cytologic slide and submitted in fixative. Excess fluid is separately sub-

mitted in a jar for cytologic examination. If a large biopsy needle was used, the core of tissue is flushed into a fixative jar to be submitted for histologic analysis. The catheter is then prepared for the next aspiration. Usually several aspiration/biopsies will be done in the area of interest.

The assistant should be familiar with the control and function of the biopsy forceps. The forceps jaws should work smoothly. The forceps is handed to the bronchoscopist in the closed position. It will be inserted in the suction channel and directed to the area of interest; then the assistant is asked to open and close the jaws as needed. Once the sample is acquired, either the forceps is removed from the suction channel or the entire bronchoscope, with the forceps still in place, is removed from the patient. The forceps jaws are then opened and the sample is removed. The sample is placed either on a glass slide with isotonic saline, if frozen sections are desired, or in formalin for histologic examination. If the forceps are shaken in formalin to remove the specimen, then that part of the forceps should be washed with isotonic saline before being inserted again into the suction channel.

If BAL is to be done, it should be performed before aspirating secretions through the suction channel. If we are also using a double-sheathed protected catheter brush, we perform the BAL after the brushings are done. The wall suction should be set at 80 mmHg for BAL. The bronchoscopist inserts the bronchoscope in the airway and, without suction, advances it until it is wedged into a segmental bronchus that has been selected. The suction tubing is attached with a three-way stopcock between the scope and the collection jar. The stopcock is initially turned off to suction. We use five 30-mL syringes filled with 20 mL of isotonic saline and 10 mL of air. The contents of one syringe are then injected slowly. The syringe points down so that at the end of the injection the line is flushed with air. The stopcock is then turned off to the syringe and opened to suction. A new syringe is inserted into the stopcock after the return of isotonic saline has stopped. The maneuver is repeated with each of the subsequent four syringes until 100 mL of saline is instilled. The actual amount of isotonic saline used may vary and will depend on the bronchoscopist's preference. The volume of lavage fluid aspirated by the end of the procedure should be 40 mL or more if a total of 100 mL of lavage fluid was injected. The BAL fluid is sent to laboratories where standard protocols are followed to be sure that all appropriate tests are performed on the specimen. The actual laboratory tests done will depend on the clinical situation and should be specified by the bronchoscopist.

CLEANING UP

At the end of the procedure the suction channel should be cleansed immediately by suctioning clean water or saline through it. The bronchoscopes should be cleaned carefully following the manufacturer's instructions. A protocol should be established for your institution and followed routinely

to protect both the patients and the bronchoscopes. Currently, we use a soaking time of 45 minutes in glutaraldehyde, and the scope can be ready for use in approximately 1 hour.[16] It is helpful to have a designated area for cleaning, with all necessary equipment and solutions available. In contaminated cases, if exposure to tuberculosis, hepatitis virus, or HIV is known or suspected, the bronchoscope should be gas sterilized. This requires 24 hours to complete; manufacturer's instructions should be followed to prevent damage to the bronchoscope. When planning more than one bronchoscopy in 24 hours, depending on the number of bronchoscopes available, consideration needs to be given to examining contaminated cases last. Biopsy forceps also need to be cleaned carefully to keep their mechanisms working smoothly. Gas sterilization of biopsy forceps will also be needed in contaminated cases.

CONCLUSION

Bronchoscopy is a safe and efficacious procedure that has become a routine part of respiratory care. Understanding the indications and contraindications for the procedure, how to set up and assist the bronchoscopist, and how to care for the equipment will increase the respiratory care practitioner's usefulness, patient comfort, and physician satisfaction with the procedure.

REFERENCES

1. Balchum OJ, Doiron DR, Huth GC: HpD photodynamic therapy for obstructive lung cancer. Prog Clin Biol Res 170:727–745, 1984
2. Balchum OJ, Doiron DR: Photoradiation therapy of endobronchial lung cancer. Large obstructing tumors, nonobstructing tumors and early-stage bronchial cancer lesions. Clin Chest Med 6:255–275, 1985
3. Bingham HG, Gallagher TJ, Powell MD: Early bronchoscopy as a predictor of ventilatory support for burned patients. J Trauma 27:1286–1288, 1987
4. Breuer HW, Charchut S, Worth H: Effects of diagnostic procedures during fiberoptic bronchoscopy on heart rate, blood pressure, and blood gases. Klin Wochenschr 67:524–529, 1989
5. Brutinel WM, McDougall JC, Cortese DA: Bronchoscopic therapy with neodymium–yttrium–aluminum–garnet laser during intravenous anesthesia. Effect on arterial blood gas levels, pH, hemoglobin saturation, and production of abnormal hemoglobin. Chest 84:518–521, 1983
6. Brutinel WM, Cortese DA, McDougall JC et al: A two-year experience with the neodymium-YAG laser in endobronchial obstruction. Chest 91:159–165, 1987

7. Choi TK, Siu KF, Lam KH, Wong J: Bronchoscopy and carcinoma of the esophagus II. Carcinoma of the esophagus with tracheobronchial involvement. Am J Surg 147:760–762, 1984

8. Choi TK, Siu KF, Lam KH, Wong J: Bronchoscopy and carcinoma of the esophagus I. Findings of bronchoscopy in carcinoma of the esophagus. Am J Surg 147:757–759, 1984

9. Conlan AA: Massive hemoptysis—diagnostic and therapeutic implications [Review]. Surg Annu 17:337–354, 1985

10. Cooper JD, Pearson FG, Patterson GA et al: Use of silicone stents in the management of airway problems. Ann Thorac Surg 47:371–378, 1989

11. de Blic J, Blanche S, Danel C et al: Bronchoalveolar lavage in HIV infected patients with interstitial pneumonitis. Arch Dis Child 64:1246–1250, 1989

12. Desai MH, Rutan RL, Herndon DN: Managing smoke inhalation injuries. Postgrad Med 86(8):69–70, 73–76, 1989

13. Edell ES, Cortese DA: Bronchoscopic localization and treatment of occult lung cancer [Review]. Chest 96:919–921, 1989

14. Edell ES, Cortese DA: Bronchoscopic phototherapy with hematoporphyrin derivative for treatment of localized bronchogenic carcinoma: A 5-year experience. Mayo Clin Proc 62:8–14, 1987

15. Edens ET, Sia RL: Flexible fiberoptic endoscopy in difficult intubations. Ann Otol Rhinol Laryngol 90(4 part 1):307–309, 1981

16. Elford B: Care and cleansing of the fiberoptic bronchoscope. Chest 73(5 suppl):761–763, 1978

17. Filston HC, Ferguson TB Jr, Oldham HN: Airway obstruction by vascular anomalies. Importance of telescopic bronchoscopy. Ann Surg 205:541–549, 1987

18. Frankel LR, Smith DW, Lewiston NJ: Bronchoalveolar lavage for diagnosis of pneumonia in the immunocompromised child. Pediatrics 81:785–788, 1988

19. Fulkerson WJ: Current concepts. Fiberoptic bronchoscopy. N Engl J Med 311:511–515, 1984

20. Garzon AA, Gourin A: Surgical management of massive hemoptysis. A ten-year experience. Ann Surg 187:267–271, 1978

21. Hanson PJ, Collins JV: AIDS and the lung. 1. AIDS, aprons, and elbow grease: Preventing the nosocomial spread of human immunodeficiency virus and associated organisms [Review]. Thorax 44:778–783, 1989

22. Hara KS, Prakash UB: Fiberoptic bronchoscopy in the evaluation of acute chest and upper airway trauma. Chest 96:627–630, 1989

23. Hendy MS, Bateman JR, Stableforth DE: The influence of transbronchial lung biopsy and bronchoalveolar lavage on arterial blood gas changes occurring in patients with diffuse interstitial lung disease. Br J Dis Chest 78:363–368, 1984

24. Heurlin N, Lonnqvist B, Tollemar J, Ehrnst A: Fiberoptic bronchoscopy for diagnosis of opportunistic pulmonary infections after bone marrow transplantation [Review]. Scand J Infect Dis 21:359–366, 1989

25. Hirschler-Schulte CJ, Postmus PE, van Overbeek JJ: Endoscopic treatment of a whistling middle-lobe bronchus. Chest 88:635–636, 1985

26. Imgrund SP, Goldberg SK, Walkenstein MD et al: Clinical diagnosis of massive hemoptysis using the fiberoptic bronchoscope. Crit Care Med 13:438–443, 1985

27. Inculet RI, Keller SM, Dwyer A, Roth JA: Evaluation of noninvasive tests for the preoperative staging of carcinoma of the esophagus: A prospective study. Ann Thorac Surg 40:561–565, 1985

28. Jaworski A, Goldberg SK, Walkenstein MD et al: Utility of immediate postlobectomy fiberoptic bronchoscopy in preventing atelectasis. Chest 94:38–43, 1988

29. Johnston H, Reisz G: Changing spectrum of hemoptysis. Underlying causes in 148 patients undergoing diagnostic flexible fiberoptic bronchoscopy. Arch Intern Med 149:1666–1668, 1989

30. Lam S, Muller NL, Miller RR et al: Predicting the response of obstructive endobronchial tumors to photodynamic therapy. Cancer 58:2298–2306, 1986

31. Lan RS, Lee CH, Chiang YC, Wang WJ: Use of fiberoptic bronchoscopy to retrieve bronchial foreign bodies in adults. Am Rev Respir Dis 140:1734–1737, 1989

32. Lederle FA, Nichol KL, Parenti CM: Bronchoscopy to evaluate hemoptysis in older men with nonsuspicious chest roentgenograms. Chest 95:1043–1047, 1989

33. Leipzig B, Zellmer JE, Klug D: The role of endoscopy in evaluating patients with head and neck cancer. A multi-institutional prospective study. Arch Otorhinolaryngol 111:589–594, 1985

34. Lennon RL, Hosking MP, Warner MA et al: Monitoring and analysis of oxygenation and ventilation during rigid bronchoscopic neodymium-YAG laser resection of airway tumors. Mayo Clin Proc 62:584–588, 1987

35. Luce JM, Clement MJ: Pulmonary diagnostic evaluation in patients suspected of having an HIV-related disease. Semin Respir Infect 4:93–101, 1989

36. Macgillivray RG, Zulu S: Oxygen saturation after bronchography under general anaesthesia. S Afr Med J 76:151–152, 1989

37. Mantor PC, Tuggle DW, Tunell WP: An appropriate negative bronchoscopy rate in suspected foreign body aspiration. Am J Surg 158:622–624, 1989

38. Marini JJ, Pierson DJ, Hudson LD: Acute lobar atelectasis: A prospective comparison of fiberoptic bronchoscopy and respiratory therapy. Am Rev Respir Dis 119:971–978, 1979

39. Martin WJ II, Smith TF, Sanderson DR et al: Role of bronchoalveolar lavage in the assessment of opportunistic pulmonary infections: Utility and complications. Mayo Clin Proc 62:549–557, 1987

40. Matsushima Y, Jones RL, King EG et al: Alterations in pulmonary mechanics and gas exchange during routine fiberoptic bronchoscopy. Chest 86:184–188, 1984

41. McCaughan JS Jr, Hawley PC, Bethel BH, Walker J: Photodynamic therapy of endobronchial malignancies. Cancer 62:691–701, 1988

42. McCollun WB, Mattox KL, Guinn GA, Beall AC Jr: Immediate operative treatment for massive hemoptysis. Chest 67:152–155, 1975

43. McGuirt WF, Holmes KD, Feehs R, Browne JD: Tracheobronchial foreign bodies. Laryngoscope 98(6 part 1):615–618, 1988

44. Messeter KH, Pettersson KI: Endotracheal intubation with the fibre-optic bronchoscope. Anaesthesia 35:294–298, 1980

45. Noseworthy TW, Anderson BJ: Massive hemoptysis [Review]. Can Med Assoc J 135:1097–1099, 1986

46. Obrien RF, Quinn JL, Miyahara BT et al: Diagnosis of *Pneumocystic carinii* pneumonia by induced sputum

in a city with moderate incidence of AIDS. Chest 95:136–138, 1989

47. Pattishall EN, Noyes BE, Orenstein DM: Use of bronchoalveolar lavage in immunocompromised children with pneumonia. Pediatr Pulmonol 5:1–5, 1988

48. Pedersen U, Hansen IM, Bottzauw J: The diagnostic role of fiberoptic bronchoscopy in AIDS patients with suspected *Pneumocystis carinii* pneumonia. Arch Otorhinolaryngol 246:362–364, 1989

49. Pereira W Jr, Kovnat DM, Snider GL: A prospective cooperative study of complications following flexible fiberoptic bronchoscopy. Chest 73:813, 1978

50. Poe RH, Israel RH, Utell MJ, Hall WJ: Chronic cough: Bronchoscopy or pulmonary function testing? Am Rev Respir Dis 126:160–162, 1982

51. Poe RH, Israel RH, Marin MG et al: Utility of fiberoptic bronchoscopy in patients with hemoptysis and a nonlocalizing chest roentgenogram. Chest 93:70–75, 1988

52. Porter DK, Van Every MJ, Anthracite RF, Mack JW Jr: Massive hemoptysis in cystic fibrosis. Arch Intern Med 143:287–290, 1983

53. Prakash UB: The use of the pediatric fiberoptic bronchoscope in adults. Am Rev Respir Dis 132:715–717, 1985

54. Rees JR: Massive hemoptysis associated with foreign body removal. Chest 88:475–476, 1985

55. Robinson L, Miller RH: Smoke inhalation injuries. Am J Otolaryngol 7:375–380, 1986

56. Rogers SN, Benumof JL: New and easy techniques for fiberoptic endoscopy-aided tracheal intubation. Anesthesiology 59:569–572, 1983

57. Schmitt GS, Ohar JM, Kanter KR, Naunheim KS: Indwelling transbronchial catheter drainage of pulmonary abscess. Ann Thorac Surg 45:43–47, 1988

58. Schneider W, Berger A, Mailander P, Tempka A: Diagnostic and therapeutic possibilities for fibreoptic bronchoscopy in inhalation injury. Burns Incl Therm Inj 14:53–57, 1988

59. Schray MF, McDougall JC, Martinez A et al: Management of malignant airway compromise with laser and low dose rate brachytherapy. The Mayo Clinic experience. Chest 93:264–269, 1988

60. Shapshay SM, Beamis JF Jr, Hybels RL, Bohigian RK: Endoscopic treatment of subglottic and tracheal stenosis by radial laser incision and dilation. Ann Otol Rhinol Laryngol 96:661–664, 1987

61. Shivaram U, Finch P, Nowak P: Plastic endobronchial tubes in the management of life-threatening hemoptysis. Chest 92:1108–1110, 1987

62. Shure D: Transbronchial biopsy and needle aspiration [Review]. Chest 95:1130–1138, 1989

63. Shure D: Fiberoptic bronchoscopy—diagnostic applications. Clin Chest Med 8:1–13, 1987 [published erratum appears in Clin Chest Med 8(2):following xii, 1987]

64. Sosenko A, Glassroth J: Fiberoptic bronchoscopy in the evaluation of lung abscesses. Chest 87:489–494, 1985

65. Tsang V, Goldstraw P: Endobronchial stenting for anastomotic stenosis after sleeve resection. Ann Thorac Surg 48:568–571, 1989

66. Van Gundy K, Boylen CT: Fiberoptic bronchoscopy. Indications, complications, contraindications [Review]. Postgrad Med 83:289–294, 1988

67. Weaver A, Fleming SM, Knechtges TC, Smith D: Triple endoscopy: A neglected essential in head and neck cancer. Surgery 86:493–496, 1979

68. Wood RE, Gauderer MW: Flexible fiberoptic bronchoscopy in the management of tracheobronchial foreign bodies in children: The value of a combined approach with open tube bronchoscopy. J Pediatr Surg 19:693–698, 1984

69. Xaubet A, Torres A, Marco F et al: Pulmonary infiltrates in immunocompromised patients. Diagnostic value of telescoping plugged catheter and bronchoalveolar lavage. Chest 95:130–135, 1989

70. Zalzal GH: Stridor and airway compromise. Pediatr Clin North Am 36:1389–1402, 1989

TWENTY-SEVEN

Patient Monitoring in the Intensive Care Unit

Robert A. Balk
Roger C. Bone

The use of specialized units for the care of the critically ill reportedly began in Scandinavia in 1952.[1] The first such unit was created in response to growing problems associated with the poliomyelitis epidemic; since then, the field of intensive care medicine has continued to grow rapidly. Tremendous advances in technologic support systems have fueled this growth pattern. It has been estimated that intensive care medicine now accounts for approximately 15% of hospital-associated health care costs.[2] Although it is usually assumed that a major role of the intensive care unit (ICU) is to provide the aggressive care needed to salvage critically ill patients, a recent study has demonstrated that 40% of medical intensive care unit (MICU) and 30% of surgical intensive care unit (SICU) patients were admitted strictly for monitoring purposes.[3] Obviously, all patients admitted to the ICU require intense monitoring to promptly detect potentially life-threatening changes in the underlying condition, the development of complications, and the response to therapeutic maneuvers.

This chapter will discuss a variety of patient-monitoring techniques as they involve the respiratory care practitioner. We will begin with the rationale behind the need for the intense monitoring and then discuss in some detail various noninvasive monitors of respiratory function; monitors of other organ systems will follow. The chapter will conclude with some speculations on future trends in patient monitoring and technology.

RATIONALE FOR INTENSIVE CARE MONITORING

The rationale for proper monitoring is obvious. Despite the vast array of technologic advances in medicine, adverse occurrences and complications continue. This problem is compounded by the fact that patients in ICUs constitute the most unstable group of patients in the hospital; they are the ones least able to tolerate such mishaps. A study of adverse occurrences in a combined medical–surgical ICU found that harm resulted more frequently if the adverse occurrence took place when the patient was unattended.[4] This emphasizes the importance of trained support staff, available at the bedside, who are able to respond to a given situation.

The use of mechanical ventilation is associated with frequent adverse occurrences and complications. In one prospective study, 400 real or potential complications of mechanical ventilation occurred in 354 separate episodes of acute respiratory failure in 304 consecutive patients.[5] Three of these complications—right main stem bronchus intubation, endotracheal tube malfunction, and alveolar hypoventilation—were all associated with an increased mortality.

Recent technologic advances have provided several types of monitors to assist in the care of the patient. It is reasonable to assume that these monitors will result in improved patient care. Be that as it may, there is no substitute for the presence of a properly trained health care provider. The respiratory practitioner needs to be able to use monitor technology as an aid in providing proper patient care. As such, monitors have a role in directing therapy and in demonstrating response to therapeutic maneuvers. The practitioner must learn how to properly discriminate the data that are provided by the monitors. There can be hazards when too little (or too much) data are available, especially if the staff is relatively inexperienced and unable to properly analyze the information provided.

BASIC CLINICAL MONITORS

The trained observer should rely on all of his or her clinical skills to assist with the monitoring of the critically ill patient. The importance of obtaining the pertinent patient history and of performing a detailed physical examination cannot be overemphasized. The patient's mental status, degree of comfort, and position in bed can give valuable clues for monitoring. The fluid status can be assessed by evaluating the patient's intake and output, weight, tissue turgor, and mucous membrane hydration. The peripheral perfusion can be assessed by evaluating the color and temperature of the skin.

The most commonly applied clinical monitors include indicators that have traditionally been referred to as the *vital signs*. The vital signs include the temperature, pulse rate and rhythm, blood pressure, and respiratory rate. These indices are easy to measure with use of simple bedside skills; they can be easily accomplished by lay persons. Measurements of vital signs can be repeated often and do not require sophisticated equipment.

A patient's *temperature*, when measured orally, in the axilla, or on an extremity, can be used to reflect skin temperature. Measurements of the rectal, esophageal, or pulmonary artery temperatures are used to reflect the core temperature of the patient. A variety of disturbances can lead to an alteration in temperature (Table 27–1). Recognition of a change in the temperature-regulating ability should prompt an evaluation into the cause of the disturbance and of the treatment of the underlying condition. The difference between the core and the big-toe temperature can reflect the peripheral blood flow. A large gradient is seen with decreased peripheral blood flow, and a narrow difference results with improved flow.[6]

The absolute or changing *pulse rate* is also a valuable diagnostic and monitored indicator. It is

Table 27–1 Abnormalities of Temperature

Hyperthermia
  Infection
  Tissue necrosis
  Late-stage carcinomatosis
  Hodgkin's disease
  Leukemia
  Hyperthyroidism and other metabolic states
Low-grade temperature elevation
  Accidental or surgical trauma
  Hematomas
  Foreign bodies
  Fistulae
  Urinary extravasation or retention
  Atelectasis
Hypothermia
  Metabolic diseases (hypothyroidism, diabetic ketacidosis, renal failure, hypoglycemia, hypopituitarism, hepatic encephalopathy)
  Central nervous system diseases (CVA, subdural hematoma, tumors, local trauma)
  Drugs (phenothiazines, tricyclic antidepressants, benzodiazepines)
  Substances and overdose (ethanol, ethylene glycol, organophosphates, heroin, carbon monoxide.)

usually recorded and interpreted in context with changes in the blood pressure. The regularity and rhythm of the pulse rate are noted in addition to the rate itself. Sinus tachycardia is a frequent type of rapid heart beat. This condition is a specific response to an underlying disturbance (e.g., fever and anemia) and should prompt a search for the responsible disorder. When there is a question about the exact type of rhythm disturbance, an electrocardiogram (ECG) should be obtained for better definition.

The patient's *systemic blood pressure* can be easily monitored with a cuff applied to a limb or with an indwelling catheter placed in an accessible artery. New noninvasive monitors of blood pressure can give trend analysis, alert the staff to changes in pressure, and reliably monitor the pressure at a set interval of time. More detailed information is included in the section on cardiovascular monitoring later in this chapter.

The *respiratory rate* is a frequently overlooked monitor of respiratory function in adults. Abnormalities may occur in both rate and rhythm (or pattern) of respiration. An elevation of the respiratory rate has been shown to be a sensitive and a reasonably specific indicator of respiratory dysfunction.[7]

Unfortunately, respiratory rate is not specific in identifying the etiology of the dysfunction, and it is still necessary to rely on additional clinical clues and diagnostic tests to uncover the underlying disorder.

The *synchrony of the respiratory muscles* can give valuable information on the likelihood of respiratory failure and the ability of the patient to maintain spontaneous ventilation. As the diaphragm descends for a normal inspiration, the chest wall expands and there is outward expansion of the abdomen. During expiration the chest wall and abdomen both return to their resting positions. However, with respiratory muscle dysfunction there may be paradoxic motion of the diaphragm, during which the abdominal wall may move inward during inspiration and outward during expiration. These findings can be easily seen by a trained individual and can be documented using *respiratory inductive plethysmography.*[8] Respiratory muscle synchronization, when observed in conjunction with respiratory rate, can serve as reliable indicators of inspiratory muscle fatigue. In a study of patients who encountered difficulty during the weaning trial, it was found that the initial abnormality was electromyographic evidence of muscle fatigue. This was accompanied or followed by an increase in the respiratory rate. Paradoxic respiratory motion was next seen, followed by a decrease in respiratory rate and minute ventilation and the production of hypercapnia and respiratory acidosis.[9]

RESPIRATORY MONITORS

A number of additional respiratory monitors are useful in assessing the critically ill patient. Included in this group are the standard weaning indices, compliance studies, airway resistance, and respiratory inductive plethysmography. In addition, any patient who is being treated with mechanical ventilatory support should be carefully monitored for proper ventilator function and adverse patient–ventilator interactions. Although mechanical failures are infrequent, they are encountered as the most common of the ventilator-associated complications. Regular ventilator checks should be a part of the respiratory therapist's responsibilities in the ICU (see Chaps. 20, 21, and 22).

The *standard ventilator weaning* measurements (Table 27–2) include the vital capacity (VC), tidal volume (V_T), respiratory rate, spontaneous minute ventilation ($\dot{V}_E$), negative inspiratory force

Table 27–2 Standard Weaning Indicators

Tests of mechanical ability
    Tidal volume >5 mL/kg
    Vital capacity >10–15 mL/kg
    Resting minute ventilation ($\dot{V}_E$) < 10 L
    Maximum voluntary ventilation (MVV) >2 × $\dot{V}_E$
    Respiratory rate <30
Tests of Oxygenation–Ventilation
    P(A–a)O$_2$ on 100% FiO$_2$ < 300–350 mmHg
    Shunt fraction on 100% FiO$_2$ < 10%–20%
    Dead space/tidal volume (V_D/V_T) < 0.55–0.60

(NIF), and the maximal voluntary ventilation (MVV).[10,11] Although these measurements serve as a guide to determine a patient's weanability, clinical acumen is probably of equal weight in deciding whether to wean a patient. In one study, patients with an NIF more negative than −30 cmH$_2$O pressure were able to be weaned.[10] In patients who required prolonged ventilatory assistance, the weaning indices had much less prognostic value, and an "adverse factor score" and a "ventilator score" were developed to assist the clinician in deciding the proper time for weaning the patient.[12]

The standard weaning measurements also include tests of oxygenation and ventilation. A favorable set of indicator values would include (and may be predicted by) alveolar–arterial oxygen difference (A–a gradient) on 100% oxygen of less than 300 to 350 mmHg, a shunt fraction on 100% oxygen less than 10% to 20%, and a dead space/tidal volume ratio (V_D/V_T) less than 0.55 to 0.60.[10,11]

Serial measurements of the weaning indicators can be useful in monitoring the clinical progress of the respiratory patient. The tests of mechanical function can be particularly useful in patients with neuromuscular dysfunction, serving as a gauge for changes in function in response to treatment. The tests of oxygenation and ventilation can be used to assess the clinical response of the pulmonary system to the specific treatment of the underlying disorder. When using the same FiO$_2$, a narrowing of the A–a gradient can be a signal of improved oxygenation. When comparisons are desired at different FiO$_2$s, the a/A ratio can be followed as a measure of improved lung function.[13]

A number of important physiologic measurements can be derived from formulas. The dead space/tidal volume ratio (V_D/V_T) can be calculated using the Enghoff modification of the Bohr equation:

$$\frac{V_D}{V_T} = \frac{PaCO_2 - P\bar{E}CO_2}{PaCO_2}$$

The shunt fraction can also be calculated according to the following formula:

$$\frac{\dot{Q}s}{\dot{Q}T} = \frac{CcO_2 - CaO_2}{CcO_2 - C\bar{v}O_2}$$

where CcO_2 is the ideal oxygen content of capillary blood, the CaO_2 is the oxygen content of arterial blood, and the $C\bar{v}O_2$ is the oxygen content of mixed venous blood.

Pulmonary compliance reflects the volume–pressure relationship of the lung and is the inverse of elasticity.[13,14] Compliance is computed as the change in volume divided by the change in pressure. The pulmonary system has both a dynamic (peak) characteristic and a static (plateau) compliance. The dynamic characteristic takes into account the compliance of the ventilator tubing, the pressures needed to overcome the resistance encountered in the endotracheal tube, the airways of the lung, and the compliance of the lung and chest wall. The static compliance is measured during an inspiratory pause or a time of no gas flow and reflects the compliance of the lung and chest wall. Compliance curves can be analyzed to determine the optimal ventilator tidal volume for a given patient. This volume is present just below the point at which a sudden increase in airway pressure occurs. Aside from this use, single compliance curves are not as useful as the trend of compliance over time.

The relative changes in the position of these curves can be used to assess the possible causes for hypoxemia.[14] A rightward shift of the dynamic characteristic curve, without a similar shift in the plateau curve, would suggest an airway process such as bronchospasm, retained secretions, or the insertion of an endotracheal tube with a smaller internal diameter. A shift of both the dynamic characteristic and the plateau curves to the right is seen in main stem bronchus intubation, increased fluid in the lung (pulmonary edema, pneumonia), collapse of the lung (atelectasis), tension pneumothorax, or large pleural effusion.

The *airway resistance* is an important measure of pulmonary mechanics.[15] Until recently, it was difficult to measure in patients requiring ventilator support. The resistance can be obtained by dividing the pressure difference by the flow. Some of the newer ventilators are equipped with a respiratory mechanics package that monitors both resistance and compliance. The greatest source of airway resistance in most ventilated patients is the endotracheal tube. The work of breathing and airway resistance rise exponentially as smaller-sized tubes are used.[15] The use of inappropriately small endotracheal tubes frequently results in the need to overinflate the endotracheal tube cuff to produce a proper seal. The excessive cuff pressure can lead to tracheal trauma (tracheal stenosis, tracheomalacia, infection of the cartilaginous rings) if the cuff pressure exceeds the capillary perfusion pressure.[16] Endotracheal tube cuff pressures must be monitored frequently (at least once each shift) to prevent such complications. Nonetheless, the initial approach should always be to use a proper-sized endotracheal tube, with a high-volume–low-pressure cuff.

Respiratory inductive plethysmography can be used to supplement the physical examination in monitoring the respiratory function of patients.[8] Some investigators have used the technique to aid in the weaning process and as an apnea monitor. It is relatively simple and is very well tolerated by patients. Paradoxic motion of the muscles of respiration can easily be seen on the visual display of rib cage and abdominal motion. Bands are placed around the thorax and the abdomen and connected to transducers that are interpreted with the aid of a computer. Data on the respiratory rate, qualitative or semiquantitative tidal volume, functional residual capacity, respiratory cycle times, and the synchrony or coordination of the respiratory pattern are obtained.

In taking care of a patient on a mechanical ventilator, it is important to ensure that the ventilator is functioning the way it is intended. Frequent checks are necessary and should be noted on a specialized ventilator monitor sheet (Fig. 27–1). In patients with an increased lung compliance or an increased resistance, the expiratory phase may not be sufficient to allow complete expiration before the next breath is administered. The result is a stacking of breaths or the creation of auto or occult positive end-expiratory pressure (PEEP).[17] When occult PEEP is noted, the ventilatory cycle should be modified to lengthen expiration and shorten inspiration in an attempt to avoid stacking breaths and to allow a sufficient time interval for complete expiration.

Mechanical problems are not frequent, but the trained respiratory therapist needs to be alert to their possibility as they monitor patients on mechanical ventilators. Approximately 40% of these

RUSH-PRESBYTERIAN-ST. LUKE'S MEDICAL CENTER

CHICAGO, ILLINOIS

RESPIRATORY THERAPY DEPARTMENT

VENTILATOR CHECK SHEET

Date _____   Page _____

			Circuit Change			Working Pressure				Cal			
Time													
Mode													
V_T Preset (L)													
Rate													
FIO_2													
Pmax / Pressure Support													
Peep													
Preset Insp. MV. (L)													
Control Breaths													
Inspiratory Time (Secs)													
Expiratory Time (Secs)													
Inspiratory Time %													
Pause Time %													
V_T Spontaneous (L)													
V_T Exhaled (L)													
V_T Exp ÷ Wt. KG. _____													
Total Rate													
Minute Volume (Exp)													
Peak Pressure													
Pause (Plateau) Press													
Mean Pressure													
Flow													
Sensitivity													
Gas Temp (°C)													
Pressure Limit													
Pressure (Hi – Lo)													
FIO_2 (Hi – Lo)													
Therapist Initials													
Blood Gas Time													
Site													
pH													
PCO_2													
PO_2													
HCO_3 / BE													
SaO_2													

M/R FORM NO. 2505 ▪ REV. 12/84

Figure 27—1. The Rush-Presbyterian–St. Luke's Hospital ventilator check sheet.

PNP — Peak Neg Pressure
VT — Tidal Volume
MV — Minute Volume

WEANING PARAMETERS

Time	VT	MV	Time	VT	MV	Time	VT	MV
Rate	VC	PNP	Rate	VC	PNP	Rate	VC	PNP

RESPIRATORY TREATMENTS

Time	Therapy	TX Freq	Med	TX #		Pulse		Sputum	General Information		Initials

PATIENT ASSESSMENT

				Heart Rate				Temp			
Time				Airway Type				Airway Size			
Color				**OXYGEN EQUIPMENT**							
Activity				Bag + Mask							
Anterior Apical	L	R	L	R	L	R					
Anterior Basal											
Posterior Apical											
Posterior Basal				**ANALYZER CALIBRATION**							
Respirations				Comments:							
Retractions											
Sputum: Color											
Consistency											
Amount											
Initials											

Initials	Signature Plus Credential

BREATH SOUNDS		**RESPIRATIONS**		**ACTIVITY**	
G — Good Air Entry	R — Rales	Diaphragmatic	— D	Active	— A
↓ — Decreased Air	A — Apices	Sternal		Active With	
Entry	B — Bases	Retractions	— SR	Stimulation	— AS
RH — Rhonchi		Intercostal		Quiet	— Q
		Retractions	— IR	Lethargic	— L
		Periodic	— P	Irritable	— I
		Shallow	— SH		
		Labored	— LA		

Figure 27–1 (continued)

problems comprise leaks and disconnections.[18] Other potential mechanical problems include failure of the electrical circuits, failure of the alarms, humidifier problems, and human engineering problems.[19]

ARTERIAL BLOOD GAS MONITORING

An indispensable test for the monitoring of a patient's respiratory status is the arterial blood gas (ABG) determination. The ABG has been considered to be the "gold standard" and gives information about the oxygenation, ventilation, and acid–base status of the patient. The test is usually easily obtained, and the cost of running the specimen is relatively inexpensive.

The disadvantages of an ABG determination is that it is an invasive procedure and does have some associated morbidity and discomfort.[20] Currently, ABG sampling is intermittent and not continuous. Work is currently underway to develop an indwelling arterial catheter that will give continuous data on the PaO_2, $PaCO_2$, and pH. Another potential disadvantage is the time lag between obtaining the specimen and reporting the results, which occurs in many institutions.

ADEQUACY OF OXYGENATION

Although the ABG determinations may be the "gold standard" by which other monitors of oxygenation are judged, several other oxygenation monitors currently exist, including pulse oximeters, tissue oxygen sensors, transcutaneous oxygenation monitors, conjunctival oxygen sensors, and monitors of the oxygen saturation in mixed venous blood.[21–28]

The practice of noninvasive oxygenation monitoring has been revolutionized with the advent of the new generation of *pulse oximeters*. These devices are much smaller and easier to use then the older bulkier models. They employ smaller probes that can be placed on the ear lobe, finger, toe, bridge of the nose, or the infant's foot. Pulse oximeters emit two different wavelengths of light—red and infrared. Deoxygenated blood has a greater optical absorption of red light than does oxygenated hemoglobin, whereas oxygenated hemoglobin has a greater optical absorption of infrared light than does deoxygenated blood. Many studies have shown good correlation between the measured SaO_2 of arterial blood and the SaO_2 determined by

the pulse oximeter.[29] Certain clinical settings have been associated with less than optimal function of pulse oximeters. These include the presence of carboxyhemoglobin or other abnormal hemoglobins, increased skin pigmentation, jaundice, or decreased perfusion of the probe site.[25]

The major advantages of pulse oximeters are their ability to perform continuous and real-time monitoring, portability, affordability, simplicity, and ease of use. In patients with normal or stable ventilation, the pulse oximeter is a very convenient way to titrate the FiO_2 to a desired level of oxygen saturation.

The Clark oxygen electrode has been incorporated into devices to monitor the *tissue, conjunctival,* and *transcutaneous oxygen tension.* The transcutaneous oxygen monitor has been predominantly utilized in the pediatric population.[27–29] Good correlation has been demonstrated between the transcutaneous oxygen tension ($PtcO_2$) and the PaO_2 in neonates and small children; however, in older children, adults, and in low-output states the correlation has decreased considerably.[27–30] A series of animal studies that used transcutaneous oxygen monitors to assess oxygenation during periods of hypoxia, low cardiac output, and hypovolemia, demonstrated that the $PtcO_2$ correlated best with tissue oxygen delivery[31] (Fig. 27–2).

The transcutaneous electrode requires the addition of heat for proper function. The skin site is heated to 44° to 45° C. There is a significant risk of skin burning if this electrode is left in place too long; it is recommended that the site be changed every 4 hours. Another drawback to the use of $PtcO_2$ is the need to frequently calibrate the monitor. The $PtcO_2$ does not correlate well if the skin is too thick; it seems to be most useful as a trend monitor, rather than an approximation of the PaO_2. Some authors point out that the $PtcO_2$ is actually reflective of the tissue oxygen level and not the PaO_2. A low level may indicate a decrease in tissue oxygenation or a decrease in tissue oxygen delivery.[30–31]

Tissue oxygen determinations involve placing the Clark oxygen electrode directly into the tissue or a mucous membrane, such as the conjunctiva. The conjunctiva is easily accessible and monitoring probes placed there can be relatively well tolerated.[24] Advocates of conjunctival oxygen tension ($PcjO_2$) stress that the conjunctival capillary bed derives its blood supply from the internal carotid artery, which also supplies the brain.

The mixed venous oxygen saturation ($P\bar{v}O_2$) can also be monitored to assess the adequacy of

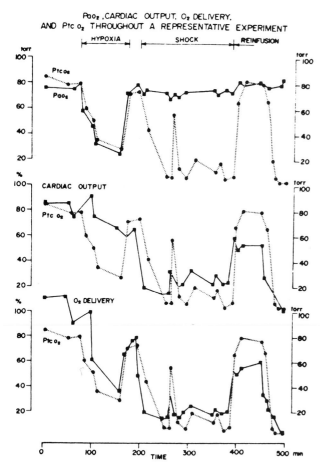

Figure 27—2. Serial PtcO₂ and PaO₂ values (*upper section*), PtcO₂, and cardiac output (*middle section*), and PtcO₂ and O₂ delivery values throughout a representative experiment. O₂ delivery and cardiac output are plotted as percentage of control. Note PtcO₂ values follow the PaO₂ values during hypoxia, but not during shock; PtcO₂ values follow cardiac output during shock, but not during hypoxia; however, PtcO₂ values most closely follow O₂ delivery throughout the entire experiment. (Tremper KK: The effects of hypoxemia in shock on transcutaneous PO₂ values in dogs. Crit Care Med 7(12):529, 1979 © Williams & Wilkins, with permission)

oxygenation. This technique has become popular in the past several years since the introduction of Swan–Ganz catheters equipped to continuously monitor mixed venous oxygen saturation. A more detailed description of this technique will be found in Chapter 35.

ADEQUACY OF VENTILATION

Ventilation is predominantly concerned with the elimination of carbon dioxide (CO_2) from the respiratory system. As with oxygenation, the gold standard for assessing the adequacy of ventilation is the ABG. Ventilation can also be monitored by evaluating the CO_2 content of expired air. The $PaCO_2$ is inversely proportional to the minute ventilation and is dependent on the pulmonary blood flow, cardiac output, CO_2 production, and the ventilation–perfusion relationships of the lung.[20,32] In patients with relatively normal lungs, the end-tidal CO_2 (PETCO₂) correlates with the $PaCO_2$.[20,32] In the presence of lung disease this correlation is less precise; however, changes detected over time may still give useful trend information.

The PETCO₂ can be monitored with rapid-response infrared *capnometers* or *mass spectrometers*.[32–34] Two types of capnometers are currently utilized. The direct-sampling method places the infrared monitor directly in the ventilator circuitry as close to the endotracheal tube as possible. This may result in an increased dead space; the weight of the apparatus may also present some problems for the patient. The sidestream-sampling method siphons off a portion of the expired gas, and there is an associated delay with this method. The sidestream method also is frequently hampered by the presence of water droplets in the sampling port that may interfere with the function of the monitor. The use of a mass spectrometer is a very expensive method of monitoring. Some of these systems are extremely complex and can monitor several patients at the same time.

Capnometry has a number of uses in clinical medicine (Table 27–3); It is noninvasive and relatively easy to perform. In the ICU, capnometers can

Table 27—3 Applications of Capnometry/Capnography

Monitoring the adequacy of mechanical ventilation
Monitoring airflow for polysomnography/apnea detection
Regulating hyperventilation in craniocerebral trauma
Monitoring cardiopulmonary resuscitation
Verifying a steady-state before respiratory calorimetry
Monitoring anesthesia (disconnects, proper tube position, hypoventilation)

assist with weaning from mechanical ventilation, assess changes in ventilation or cardiac output, and detect increased CO_2 elimination that may suggest increased CO_2 production. Capnometers can be used to detect apnea and disconnections from the mechanical ventilator.

The CO_2 tension of the skin capillaries ($PtcCO_2$) can also monitor ventilation. A Severinghaus electrode is heated to 44° to 45° C in a fashion similar to the transcutaneous oxygen electrode and placed on the skin. Like $PtcO_2$, $PtcCO_2$ is predominantly utilized in neonates and small children.[27,35] Newer monitors have incorporated the Clark and Severinghaus electrodes into one probe to make application easier. However, the site needs to be changed every 4 hours to avoid burns, and the electrodes require frequent calibration, which is time-consuming. The reliability of the information will vary depending on skin thickness and blood flow, in a manner similar to the $PtcO_2$ monitors.

CHEST ROENTGENOGRAPHY

Chest x-ray examinations are frequently performed in the ICU. They give useful information concerning tube and line placement and position, the presence of infiltrates, atelectasis, fluid, changes in heart size, the development of barotrauma, and the response to therapy. A daily chest x-ray film is particularly important when an endotracheal tube is in place. The tip of an endotracheal tube can move 2 cm down or up with flexion or extension of the head, respectively.[36] This potential for a 4-cm change in endotracheal tube position makes it extremely important to know the daily location of the tube, to avoid accidental extubation or intubation of a main stem bronchus.

Pulmonary barotrauma includes pneumothorax, pneumomediastinum, pneumocardium, pneumoperitoneum, and subcutaneous emphysema. The prevalence of barotrauma in mechanically ventilated medical ICU patients has been estimated to be 15%.[37] Nosocomial infections and sepsis complicating multiple organ system failure are common complications in critically ill patients.[38] The chest x-ray film is a valuable test to monitor the ICU patient for these potential complications.

A study of routine daily chest x-ray films of intubated patients in the MICU found that 64% of the useful films revealed an unexpected new finding or progressive improvement.[39] Forty-three percent of the useful films demonstrated an unex-pected finding and brought about a change in therapy or management. This high yield would support the use of a routine daily chest x-ray examination for intubated patients in the MICU as a cost-effective form of management. For more details on this topic of chest roentgenography, see Chapter 12.

CARDIOVASCULAR MONITORING

Cardiovascular monitors are an integral component of patient monitoring in the ICU.[21,22,40] The importance of evaluating the patient's heart rate and blood pressure have already been emphasized in the section dealing with vital signs. The ECG or rhythm strip is continuously monitored in almost every patient in the ICU. The changes in cardiac rate or rhythm can be an early marker for, or a result of, changes in other organ systems. Detection of such a change should prompt an evaluation into the cause.

Commonly, more in-depth information concerning cardiovascular function is needed, and invasive monitors of arterial blood pressure and right-sided cardiac and pulmonary artery pressures are placed.[21,22,40] The pulmonary artery catheters allow the measurement of cardiac output, mixed venous oxygen tension and saturation, and pulmonary artery occlusion pressure. An in-depth discussion of these more invasive monitors is included in Chapter 35.

NEUROLOGIC MONITORING

Neurologic disorders are frequently encountered in the ICU. The importance of serial and frequent neurologic monitoring in patients with neurologic disorders is obvious; however, we are just beginning to appreciate some of the more subtle forms of neurologic dysfunction. In patients with sepsis and multiple organ system failure, a form of neuropathy termed *critical illness polyneuropathy* has been described.[41] The clinical manifestations include changes in the deep tendon reflexes (DTRs), and this disorder has been associated with difficulty weaning from mechanical ventilatory support and with a prolonged convalescence.

Neurologic monitoring includes the assessment of mental status and the ability to follow commands and answer questions appropriately. The Glasgow coma scale has been used to assist with this evaluation (Table 27–4). The mental status ex-

Table 27—4 Glasgow Coma Scale

TEST	RESPONSE	RATING
Eyes	Open spontaneously	4
	Open to verbal command	3
	Open to pain	2
	No response	1
Best motor response	Obeys verbal command	6
	Localizes painful stimulus	5
	Flexion/withdrawal to pain	4
	Decorticate response to pain	3
	Decerebrate response to pain	2
	No response to pain	1
Best verbal response	Oriented and converses	5
	Disoriented and converses	4
	Inappropriate words	3
	Incomprehensible sounds	2
	No response	1

amination includes the level of consciousness and the patient's ability to react to the environment (respond to pain, and so forth).

Patients may require electroencephalographic (EEG) monitoring to help diagnose central nervous system (CNS) lesions, coma, define brain death, or monitor seizure activity. The EEG can be followed on a continuous or intermittent basis.

The brain is enclosed in a rigid structure, and increased intracranial pressure can lead to brain stem herniation and death.[42] Increased intracranial pressure has been associated with closed head trauma, intracranial operations, subarachnoid hemorrhage, cerebrovascular accidents (CVA), Reye's syndrome, brain tumors, meningitis, and encephalitis. Intracranial pressure changes frequently precede changes in clinical neurologic function. The changes in intracranial pressure may be hard to distinguish from those caused by medications, shock, sepsis, hypoxia, and electrolyte or CNS abnormalities. *Intracranial pressure* can be monitored with a subarachnoid bolt, a Richmond subdural screw, or a Scott cannula placed in the lateral ventricle. The Scott cannula is the more accurate system and is the least likely to become dampened. It allows easy access to cerebrospinal fluid (CSF) for culture or chemical analysis or to relieve elevated CSF pressures.

Certain patients who are in the ICU may develop an acute psychotic reaction, termed ICU psychosis.[43] This usually affects elderly people who have difficulty perceiving their environment and may be related to sleep deprivation. Phenothiazines and continued attempts at reality orientation frequently help this situation.

MONITORING OF GASTROINTESTINAL FUNCTION

Stress ulceration is a common occurrence in patients who are critically ill.[44,45] The patient's stool and nasogastric tube (NG) aspirate should be tested for occult blood loss to determine clinically inapparent bleeding. Past studies have used large doses of antacids or histamine type 2 (H$_2$) blockers to elevate the gastric pH above 4, as a means of preventing stress ulceration.[46–48] Enteral alimentation has also been useful as a form of prophylaxis for gastrointestinal bleeding. However, recent studies have shown that raising the gastric pH may predispose the patient to nosocomial infections (particularly pneumonia). The cytoprotective agent sucralfate has been suggested as a more beneficial agent for stress ulcer prophylaxis.[49]

An ileus or decreased intestinal function is also a common occurrence in seriously ill patients in the ICU. Careful auscultation of the abdomen and radiographic examinations will help determine the nature of the problem and differentiate this disorder from bowel obstruction. Metabolic derangements may also be responsible for the alterations in intestinal function.

MONITORING OF RENAL FUNCTION

Oliguria is defined as a urine output of less than 400 mL/day or less than 20 mL/hr.[50,51] *Polyuria* is a daily urine output of more than 2400 mL or 100 mL/hr. The sudden appearance of oliguria should lead the clinician to determine if the cause is prerenal, postrenal, or renal. Prerenal failure is functional renal insufficiency resulting from a decreased plasma volume, deficient cardiac output, or decreased renal perfusion. Postrenal insufficiency may result from obstruction or the extravasation of urinary outflow from the urethra, bladder, ureters, or pelvis. A plugged Foley catheter is the most common cause of an abrupt decrease in urine flow and can be quickly treated by irrigating the catheter. The laboratory evaluation of acute renal insufficiency should include a determination of BUN, serum creatinine, BUN/serum creatinine ratio, serum and urine electrolytes, urine creatinine, and glomerular filtration rate.[51] A careful microscopic examination of the urine and its sediment is also an important part of this evaluation. A renal ultrasound should be obtained to evaluate renal size and to assess for signs of obstruction.

NUTRITIONAL AND METABOLIC MONITORS

Adequate nutritional replacement has been emphasized in critically ill patients.[52–57] Malnutrition may have a variety of adverse effects on the respiratory and host defense systems. Poor nutritional status has been associated with a diminished response to hypoxia.[52] Hypoxic and hypercapnic drives have improved with the addition of nutritional therapy.[52] Malnutrition has been associated with decreased diaphragmatic muscle mass, area, and thickness, decreased respiratory muscle strength, and decreased contractile properties of the diaphragm.[52] There may be diminished cell-mediated immunity, altered immunoglobulin turnover, and possibly altered alveolar macrophage function in severely malnourished patients.

The response to nutritional therapy should be monitored to assess the adequacy of the replacement and to detect complications that may result from its administration.[58] Some measure of nutritional assessment should be performed before initiating replacement therapy. The Harris–Benedict equation or anthropometric studies can be performed to help determine the proper constituents and amount of nutritional replacement.[58] Anthropometric studies include the patient's height, weight, triceps skinfold thickness, and midarm circumference.[58] Other measurements that can reflect nutritional status include indirect calorimetry, T-cell function, lymphocyte count, serum albumin, serum transferrin, vitamin levels, and trace metal levels.[58] As nutritional therapy progresses, these indices can be followed at intervals to determine the adequacy of the nutritional replacement.[58] Determination of nitrogen balance is also useful to assess the replacement therapy.[58] Careful attention should be given to the serum electrolyte, magnesium, calcium, phosphorus, and glucose concentrations to ensure that they are being properly maintained. In patients with respiratory limitation of either the obstructive or restrictive type, it is important to monitor the $PaCO_2$ since acute respiratory acidosis can result from diets high in carbohydrates in patients who are unable to meet the increased ventilatory requirements.[59–61] Carbohydrates have been partic-ularly implicated in this phenomenon because they have a high respiratory quotient ($R = 1.0$). Fat-containing energy sources can be substituted for carbohydrates because they have a lower respiratory quotient ($R = 0.7$).[62]

SUMMARY

This review has emphasized the importance of proper monitoring in the care of the critically ill patient. The trained observer at the bedside is the most important component in the proper care of the patient and detection of adverse consequences. The development of new monitors and other technologic advances have aided clinicians in their ability to provide quality patient care. In the future, as more attention is focused on patient monitoring, we can anticipate an even greater role for advanced technology, working in concert with the highly trained clinical staff. The proper marriage of these two ingredients is particularly important, as there is currently no machine that can adequately fill the role of the well-trained health care professional.

REFERENCES

1. Lawin P: Reflections on the development of intensive care medicine. In Vincent JL (ed): Update in Intensive Care and Emergency Medicine, pp 547–551. New York, Springer-Verlag, 1986
2. Birnbaum ML: Cost-containment in critical care. Crit Care Med 14:1068–1077, 1986
3. Henning RJ, McClish D, Daly B et al: Clinical characteristics and resources utilization of ICU patients: Implications for organization of intensive care. Crit Care Med 15:264–269, 1987
4. Abramson NS, Wald KS, Grenvik ANA et al: Adverse occurrences in intensive care units. JAMA 244:1582–1584, 1980
5. Zwillich CW, Pierson DJ, Creagh CE et al: Complications of assisted ventilation: Prospective study of 354 consecutive episodes. Am J Med 57:161–170, 1974
6. Shoemaker WC: Monitoring of the critically ill patient. In Shoemaker WC, Thompson WL, Holbrook PR (eds): Textbook of Critical Care Medicine, pp 105–121. Philadelphia, WB Saunders, 1984
7. Gravelyn TR, Weg JG: Respiratory rate as an indicator of acute respiratory dysfunction. JAMA 244:1123–1125, 1980
8. Tobin MJ: Noninvasive evaluation of respiratory movement. In Nochomovitz ML, Cherniak NS (eds): Noninvasive Respiratory Monitoring, pp 29–57. New York, Churchill Livingstone, 1986
9. Cohen CA, Zagelbaum G, Gross D et al: Clinical manifestations of inspiratory muscle fatigue. Am J Med 73:308–316, 1982
10. Sahn SA, Lakshminarayan S, Petty TL: Weaning from mechanical ventilation. JAMA 235:2208–2212, 1976

11. Sahn SA, Lakshminarayan S: Bedside criteria for discontinuation of mechanical ventilation. Chest 63:1002–1005, 1973

12. Morganroth ML, Morganroth JL, Nett CM, Petty TL: Criteria for weaning from prolonged mechanical ventilation. Arch Intern Med 144:1012–1016, 1984

13. Bone RC: Monitoring ventilatory mechanics in acute respiratory failure. Respir Care 28:597–604, 1983

14. Bone RC: Diagnosis of causes for acute respiratory distress by pressure–volume curves. Chest 70:740–746, 1976

15. Marini JJ: Monitoring during mechanical ventilation. Clin Chest Med 9:73–100, 1988

16. Lewis RF, Schlobohm RM, Thomas AN: Prevention of complications from prolonged tracheal intubation. Am J Surg 135:452–457, 1978

17. Pepe PE, Marini JJ: Occult positive end-expiratory pressure in mechanically ventilated patients with airflow obstruction: The auto-PEEP effect. Am Rev Respir Dis 126:166–170, 1982

18. Feeley TW, Bancroft ML: Problems with mechanical ventilators. Int Anesthesiol Clin 20:83–93, 1982

19. Bone RC, Balk R: Mechanical ventilation. In Simmons DH (ed): Current Pulmonology, Vol 5, pp 201–228. New York, John Wiley & Sons, 1989

20. Balk RA, Bone RC: Noninvasive monitors of respiratory function. Hosp Physician 23:72–77, 1987

21. Goldenheim PD, Kazemi H: Current concepts: Cardiopulmonary monitoring of critically ill patients. N Engl J Med 311:717–720, 1984

22. Wiedemann HP, Matthay MA, Matthay RA: Cardiovascular–pulmonary monitoring in the intensive care unit (Part II). Chest 85:656–667, 1984

23. Saunders NA, Powles ACP, Rebuck AS: Ear oximetry: Accuracy and practicability in the assessment of arterial oxygenation. Am Rev Respir Dis 113:745–749, 1976

24. Kram HB: Noninvasive tissue oxygen monitoring in surgical and critical care medicine. Surg Clin North Am 65:1005–1024, 1985

25. Chapman KR, Rebuck AS: Oximetry. In Nochomovitz ML, Cherniak NS (eds): Noninvasive Respiratory Monitoring, pp 203–221. New York, Churchill Livingstone, 1986

26. Anderson WM, George RB: Techniques for bedside pulmonary assessment in the ICU. J Crit Ill 2:57–64, 1987

27. Monaco F, Nickerson BG, McQuitty JC: Continuous transcutaneous oxygen and carbon dioxide monitoring in the pediatric ICU. Crit Care Med 10:765–766, 1982

28. Tremper KK, Shoemaker WC: Transcutaneous oxygen monitoring of critically ill adults, with and without low flow shock. Crit Care Med 9:706–709, 1981

29. Rebuck AS, Chapman KR, D'Urzo A: The accuracy and response characteristics of a simplified ear oximeter. Chest 83:860–864, 1983

30. Eberhard P, Mindt W, Schafer R: Cutaneous blood gas monitoring in the adult. Crit Care Med 9:702–705, 1981

31. Tremper KK, Waxman K, Shoemaker WC: Effects of hypoxia and shock on transcutaneous P_{O_2} values in dogs. Crit Care Med 7:526–531, 1979

32. Rebuck AS, Chapman KR: Measurement and monitoring of exhaled carbon dioxide. In Nochomovitz ML,

33. Cherniak NS (eds): Noninvasive Respiratory Monitoring, pp 189–201. New York, Churchill Livingstone, 1986

33. Linnarsson D, Lindborg B: Breath-by-breath measurement of respiratory gas exchange using on-line analogue computation. Scand J Clin Lab Invest 34:219–224, 1974

34. Harris K: Noninvasive monitoring of gas exchange. Respir Care 32:544–557, 1987

35. Monaco F, McQuitty JL: Transcutaneous measurements of carbon dioxide partial pressures in sick neonates. Crit Care Med 9:756–758, 1981

36. Conrardy PA, Goodman LR, Lainge F, Singer MM: Alteration of endotracheal tube position. Crit Care Med 4:8–12, 1976

37. Peterson GW, Baier H: Incidence of pulmonary barotrauma in a medical ICU. Crit Care Med 11:67–69, 1983

38. Bell RC, Coalson JJ, Smith JD, Johanson WG: Multiple organ system failure and infection in adult respiratory distress syndrome. Ann Intern Med 99:293–298, 1983

39. Greenbaum D, Marschall KE: The value of routine daily chest x-rays in intubated patients in the medical intensive care unit. Crit Care Med 10:29–30, 1982

40. Weidemann HP, Matthay MA, Matthay RA: Cardiovascular pulmonary monitoring in the intensive care unit (Part I). Chest 85:537–548, 1984

41. Zochodne DW, Bolton CF, Wells GA et al: Critical illness polyneuropathy. A complication of sepsis and multiple organ failure. Brain 110:819–841, 1987

42. Ward JD, Becker DP: Intracranial pressure monitoring. In Shoemaker WC, Thompson WL, Holbrook PR (eds): Textbook of Critical Care Medicine, pp 955–959. Philadelphia, WB Saunders, 1984

43. Cassem NH: Critical care psychiatry. In Shoemaker WC, Thompson WL, Holbrook PR (eds): Textbook of Critical Care Medicine, pp 981–989. Philadelphia, WB Saunders, 1984

44. Harris (Pingleton) SK, Bone RC, Ruth WE: Gastrointestinal hemorrhage in a respiratory intensive care unit. Chest 72:301–304, 1977

45. Schuster DP, Rowley H, Feinstein S et al: Prospective evaluation of the risk of upper gastrointestinal bleeding after admission to a medical intensive care unit. Am J Med 76:623–630, 1984

46. Priebe HJ, Skillman JJ, Bushnell LS et al: Antacid versus cimetidine in preventing acute gastrointestinal bleeding. N Engl J Med 302:426–430, 1980

47. Peura DA, Johnson LF: Cimetidine for prevention and treatment of gastroduodenal mucosal lesions in patients in an intensive care unit. Ann Intern Med 103:173–177, 1985

48. Zinner MJ, Zuidema GD, Smith PL, Mignosa M: The prevention of upper gastrointestinal tract bleeding in patients in an intensive care unit. Surg Gynecol Obstet 153:214–220, 1981

49. Dirks MR, Craven DE, Celli BR et al: Noscomial pneumonia in intubated patients given sucralfate as compared with antacids or histamine type 2 blockers. N Engl J Med 317:1376–1382, 1987

50. Kramer S, Khan F, Patel S et al: Renal failure in the respiratory intensive care unit. Crit Care Med 7:263–266, 1979

51. Danielson RA, McDougal WS: Renal dysfunction. In Berk JL, Sampliner JE, Artz JS, Vinocur B (eds): Hand-

book of Critical Care, pp 389–417. Boston, Little, Brown & Co, 1976

52. Pingleton SK: Nutritional support in the mechanically ventilated patient. Clin Chest Med 9:101–111, 1988

53. Barrocas A, Tretola R, Alonso A Jr: Nutrition and the critically ill pulmonary patient. Respir Care 28:50–61, 1983

54. Brown RO, Heizer WD: Nutrition and respiratory disease. Clin Pharm 3:152–161, 1984

55. Benotli P, Blackburn GL: Protein and caloric or macronutrient metabolic management of the critically ill patient. Crit Care Med 7:520–525, 1979

56. Larca L, Greenbaum DM: Effectiveness of intensive nutritional regimens in patients who fail to wean from mechanical ventilation. Crit Care Med 10:297–300, 1982

57. Heymsfield SB, Bethel RA, Ansely JD et al: Enteral hyperalimentation: An alternative to central venous hyperalimentation. Ann Intern Med 90:63–71, 1979

58. Mann S, Westenskow DR, Houtchens BA: Measured and predicted caloric expenditure in the acutely ill. Crit Care Med 13:173–177, 1985

59. Sheldon GF, Baker C: Complications of nutritional support. Crit Care Med 8:35–37, 1980

60. Askanazi J, Rosenbaum SH, Hyman AI et al: Respiratory changes induced by the large glucose loads of total parenteral nutrition. JAMA 243:1444–1447, 1980

61. Covelli HD, Black JW, Olsen MS, Beckman JF: Respiratory failure precipitated by high carbohydrate loads. Ann Intern Med 95:579–581, 1981

62. Skeie B, Askanasi J, Rothkopf MM et al: The beneficial effects of fat on ventilation and pulmonary function. Nutrition 3:149–154, 1987

TWENTY-EIGHT

Neonatal Lung Disease and Respiratory Care

John M. Fiascone
Patricia N. Vreeland
Ivan D. Frantz III

Since early in this century the *infant mortality rate*, defined as the number of deaths in the first year of life per 1000 live births, has been falling steadily. Initially this decline was due to a reduction in deaths from infections, malnutrition, and diarrheal diseases. More recently, however, the decline in infant mortality has been due to a reduction in *neonatal mortality rate*, the number of deaths in the first 28 days of life per 1000 live births. Currently, in developed countries neonatal mortality is the major determinant of infant mortality. Most deaths in the first year of life happen in the first 28 days of life. Fatal disease in newborns most often involves the respiratory system. These facts underscore the importance of fetal lung development and neonatal pulmonary disease within the field of respiratory care.

FETAL LUNG DEVELOPMENT

STRUCTURAL DEVELOPMENT

Development of the human lung can be conveniently divided into five phases, each with distinct morphologic alterations that mark its beginning and end. The *embryonic period* begins between the fourth and fifth week of gestation. Its most prominent feature is the formation of the proximal conducting airways. This period begins when the embryonic foregut, an endodermal derivative, gives rise to a single lung bud as an outpouching structure at the caudal end of the laryngotracheal groove (Fig. 28–1). Shortly after its appearance, the single lung bud divides to give rise to two bronchial buds. Subsequent divisions and growth form the segmental bronchi. Formation of the segmental bronchi establishes the future bronchopulmonary segments, occurs by the end of the sixth postconceptional week, and marks the end of the embryonic period.

The *pseudoglandular period* of lung development extends from the 7th through the 16th week. During this time all of the conducting airways are formed. Study of this period gives rise to Reid's first law of lung development: the entire bronchial tree is developed by the 16th week of intrauterine life, and this development with its subsequent deposition of cartilage proceeds from lung hilum to periphery (centrifugal development). Reid's second law of lung development also applies to the pseudoglandular period and states that preacinar blood vessels (i.e., arteries and arterioles leading to alveoli or to structure that will be alveoli) develop in parallel with the conducting airways (Table 28–1). However, the intra-acinar arteries and veins (i.e., those vessels closest to the future gas-exchanging units) develop in parallel with alveoli and, thus, will make their appearance and begin to develop in the next period of lung development. The pseudoglandular stage takes its name from the microscopic appearance of the lung (Fig. 28–2), which resembles that of an exocrine gland, with

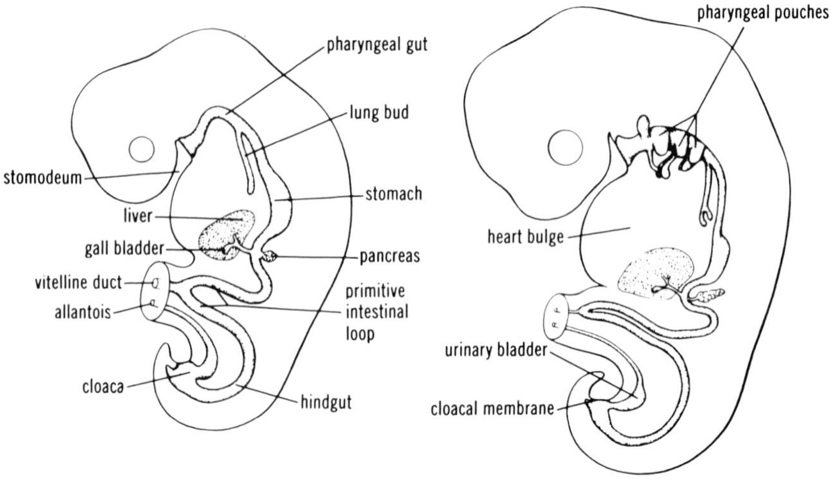

Figure 28—1. Diagrammatic embryos at different stages of development between 4 and 8 weeks illustrating the endodermal origin of the lungs. The single lung bud shown in the figure on the *left* is a derivative of the gastrointestinal tract. The figure on the *right* illustrates the subsequent appearance of the bronchial buds. (Reproduced with permission from Langman J: Medical Embryology, 3rd ed. © 1975, Williams & Wilkins Co, Baltimore)

columnar epithelial cells surrounding lumena that are approximately circular.

The *canalicular period* is characterized by the beginning of formation of the pulmonary gas-exchanging unit—the acinus. This period lasts from the 17th through the 28th week of gestation. The acinus may be thought of as the functional gas-exchanging unit of the mature lung and, ultimately, consists of a respiratory bronchiole, with its subsequent six to ten additional generations of airways, and their blood supply. During the canalicular period, the basic structure of the acinus is formed and the vascularization process is begun as intra-acinar vessels develop within the mesenchyme adjacent to the forming acini (Reid's second law). Histologically, the fetal lung shows potential airspaces that are lined with cuboidal epithelium; a thick, cellular interstitium is present; and the lung as a whole contains more tissue space than potential airspace (Fig. 28–3).

During the *saccular period*, 29 through 36 weeks after conception, formation of the gas-exchanging units continues in association with a dramatic change in the microscopic appearance of the

Figure 28—2. Microscopic appearance of the lung during the pseudoglandular stage. This stage is named for the resemblance of the lung to an exocrine gland.

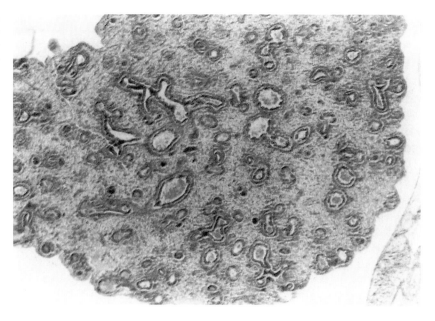

Table 28—1   Reid's Laws of Lung Development

1. All the conducting airways of the tracheobronchial tree are formed by the end of the 16th week of gestation. Deposition of cartilage proceeds from hilum to periphery.
2. The preacinar blood vessels follow the development of the conducting airways and the intra-acinar vessels develop along with the alveoli. The canalicular phase is characterized by capillary invasion of the acini.
3. Alveolar development takes place predominantly during postnatal life. Alveoli increase in number during the first 8 years and in size until adulthood. Alveolar development proceeds from the periphery to the hilum; alveoli first appear on saccules and later in life on terminal bronchioles.

lung (Fig. 28–4). There is reversal of the tissue–airspace relationship that was present in the previous period, and the lung comes to contain much more potential airspace than tissue space. The interstitium is thin, and the walls between airspaces become very compact. Capillary networks are present and are easily visible within the lung interstitium.

The final period of lung development is the *alveolar period*, which begins at 37 weeks after conception but continues into postnatal life to the eighth year. However, primitive alveoli can first be seen at 29 weeks, and by full-term the infant lung should be extensively alveolarized (Fig. 28–5). The absolute number of alveoli varies linearly with body weight. There is an average of 150 million alveoli present at term, although the range of normal appears to be quite wide. At term there are 50% as many alveoli present as in the adult lung, but the infant lung weighs only 5% as much as the adult lung. New alveoli continue to form until 8 years of age and increase in size until adulthood (Table 28–2).

CYTODIFFERENTIATION

The human lung contains more than 40 cell types. The two cell types of greatest interest are the type 1 alveolar epithelial cells, which line alveoli and across which gas exchange occurs, and the type 2 alveolar epithelial cells, which synthesize, store, and secrete pulmonary surfactant. Neither of these two cell types is recognizable before the canalicular stage of development. After 20 weeks' gestational age the respiratory epithelial cells accumulate large quantities of glycogen, probably in preparation for differentiation and surfactant synthesis. Distinct type 2 cells appear between 22 and 26 weeks of gestation, but become more prominent after 34 weeks. These cells are distinguished by easily identified subcellular organelles involved in surfactant metabolism: polyribosomes, endoplasmic reticu-

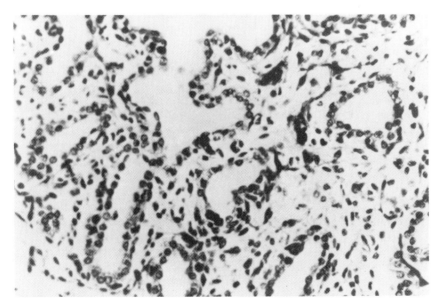

Figure 28–3. Microscopic appearance of the lung during the canalicular stage. Potential air spaces are present but are lined with cuboidal epithelium, the interstitial tissue is thick, and there is more tissue space than air space. (Thibeault DW, Gregory GA (eds): Neonatal Pulmonary Care, 2nd ed. Norwalk, Conn, Appleton & Lange, 1987, with permission)

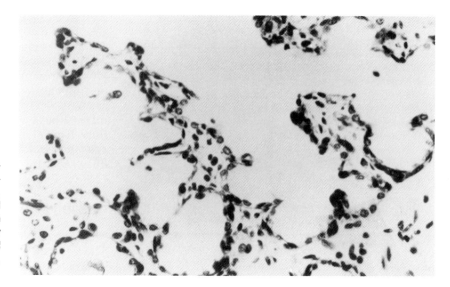

Figure 28—4. Saccular stage microscopic appearance of the lung: Potential airspace now exceeds tissue space, the interstitial area is much thinner, and epithelial lining cells are flatter than in previous stages. (Thibeault DW, Gregory GA (eds): Neonatal Pulmonary Care, 2nd ed. Norwalk, Conn, Appleton & Lange, with permission)

Table 28—2   Stages of Lung Development

PERIOD	TIME	MAJOR DEVELOPMENTS
Embryonic	4–6 wk	Formation of proximal conducting airways to level of segmental bronchi; establish bronchopulmonary segments.
Pseudoglandular	7–16 wk	Formation of all conducting airways, preacinar blood vessels, columnar epithelial cells surround future airspaces
Canalicular	17–28 wk	Formation of acini and intra-acinar vessels, cuboidal cells line future airspaces, type 2 cells distinguishable from type 2 cells, lamellar bodies present in type 2 cells
Saccular	29–36 wk	Decrease in tissue space, increase in airspace, extensive capillary network
Alveolar	37 wk–on	Progressive increase in number and size of alveoli

Figure 28—5. Early, histologic structure of the alveolar period lung: Microscopic appearance is now very similar to that of a mature lung. (Thibeault DW, Gregory GA (eds): Neonatal Pulmonary Care, 2nd ed. Norwalk, Conn, Appleton & Lange, 1987, with permission)

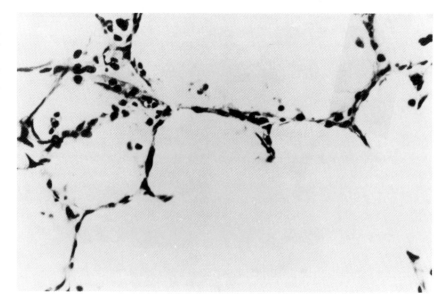

lum, Golgi apparatus, multivesicular bodies, and lamellar bodies.

The lamellar bodies contain surfactant and are eventually excreted by the type 2 cell. Type 2 cells constitute less than 15% of the lung parenchyma but have great functional importance. At the same time that type 2 cells are first identified, other alveolar cells are differentiating into type 1 cells. These cells are flat, with long extensions of thin cytoplasm, a large surface area, and few subcellular organelles. Most gas exchange takes place across these cells because they cover the major portion of the alveolar surface. Junctions between type 1 cells constitute the alveolar epithelial barrier to fluids and molecules. This barrier, in the normal lung, is virtually impermeable to protein.

Connective Tissue Development

Relatively little is known about the developmental aspects of lung connective tissue. Pulmonary fibroblasts, located in the interstitium, synthesize and secrete both collagen and elastin. Collagen synthesis is required for branching of airways and, as such, has a major influence in airway development. Elastin, in contrast, is more intimately involved with the structure of the lung parenchyma distal to the conducting airways. Whereas collagen is present in lung primordia from very early in gestation, elastin does not appear earlier than 20 weeks. Elastin, subsequent to its appearance, is closely involved in the structure of the acinus. Elastin has both immature and mature forms. In human development, immature forms appear first and then are replaced with more mature elastin as gestation progresses.

The human fetal lung parenchyma contains only small quantities of collagen and elastin. Postnatally there is a rapid deposition of these proteins and, at approximately 6 months of age, adult levels (12% of dry lung weight) are reached.

BIOCHEMICAL DEVELOPMENT AND SURFACE TENSION IN THE LUNG

Surface tension can conveniently be thought of as the attractive force between molecules in a liquid at an air–liquid interface. The alveolar surface is lined by a thin liquid layer; hence, any expansion of alveoli, as during inspiration, not only requires the force necessary to expand the lung tissue itself (referred to as frictional resistance) but also that force necessary to overcome surface tension. *Pulmonary surfactant* is a complex phospholipid and

Table 28–3 Composition of Pulmonary Surfactant

Protein		7%
Lipid		93%
Neutral lipid	9%	
Phospholipid	91%	
Phosphatidylcholine	92%	
Other phospholipids	8%	

(Adapted from Sanders RL: The composition of pulmonary surfactant. In Lung Development: Clinical and Biological Perspectives. New York, Academic Press, 1982)

protein mixture secreted into the alveolus by type 2 cells (Table 28–3). The function of pulmonary surfactant seems to be to reduce surface tension within the alveolus at the air–liquid interface and thereby greatly decrease the force or pressure required for alveolar expansion. In the absence of adequate quantities of surfactant, as a result of surface tension, the alveolus has a force directed toward collapse that becomes strongest at end-expiration when the alveoli are smallest. The presence of adequate quantities of surfactant reduces surface tension at end-expiration to nearly zero and, in this manner, stabilizes alveoli. An inadequate quantity of surfactant, leading to end-expiratory alveolar collapse and to a requirement for greater pressure to produce lung expansion (i.e., decreased lung compliance) is the central feature of surfactant deficiency disease (SDD), also known as the respiratory distress syndrome (RDS) or hyaline membrane disease (HMD). Recognition of the critical role of surfactant in RDS has led to the term *surfactant deficiency disease* to replace both of the preceding names, as this new term is more specific in its description.

The term *lung maturity* is generally used to describe the fetal or newborn lung when it comes to contain adequate quantities of surfactant in the airspaces to support alveolar stability and gas exchange. In uncomplicated pregnancies, type 2 cells are first discernible shortly after 20 weeks' gestation, during the canalicular period. As these cells increase in number the subcellular synthetic organelles involved in surfactant synthesis become more prominent and surfactant synthesis increases. *Lamellar bodies*, the intracellular storage sites of surfactant, can first be found between 20 and 24 weeks. Limited quantities of surfactant release can be shown between 25 and 30 weeks; secretion becomes more extensive after 35 weeks. There is wide

Table 28—4 Maternal Conditions Influencing Fetal Lung Maturation

Accelerated Maturation
  Chronic hypertension
  Placental insufficiency
  Prolonged rupture of the membranes
  Black race
Delayed Maturation
  Maternal diabetes mellitus
  Rh isoimmunization with fetal hydrops
  Male sex
  Second-born twin

variation in the timing of normal development relative to the quantity of surfactant synthesized, stored, and available for secretion should birth occur earlier than 37 weeks (full-term). There is an approximate 10-week window, from 25 to 35 weeks, when early lung maturity may be present. Several conditions of pregnancy, and specific pharmacologic interventions, are capable of accelerating or delaying fetal lung maturity (Tables 28–4, 28–5).

Large amounts of information from both laboratory and clinical studies indicate that corticosteroid exposure results in increased synthesis of surfactant and in precocious maturation of the fetal lung. Similar, although not as extensive, data indicate that the thyroid hormones triiodothyronine (T3), thyroxine (T4), and thyrotropin-releasing hormone (TRH), as well as aminophylline have similar effects. The precise mechanism of action of corticosteroids is as yet unclear. They may act directly on the type 2 cell or, more likely, may induce the production of small polypeptides such as fibroblast pneumonocyte factor in surrounding lung fibroblasts. This peptide, in turn, may accelerate surfactant production by alveolar type 2 cells. On the other hand, chronic hyperglycemia, as found in infants of diabetic mothers, leads to fetal hyperinsulinemia, which, in turn, delays fetal lung maturation. Male fetal lung development is generally delayed in comparison with that of females.

Although maturity of the pulmonary surfactant system is paramount in determining lung function after birth, there are other biochemical systems within the lung, the development of which is important to the neonate. The system of enzymes that function to prevent lung tissue damage by oxygen radicals is one example. Molecular oxygen in tissue is capable of undergoing several reactions that may lead to the formation of unstable molecular species such as hydrogen peroxide (H_2O_2), the hydroxyl radical ($OH\cdot$), and the superoxide anion (O_2^-). These species may interact with membrane lipids in a reaction called *peroxidation*, which results in cellular and tissue damage. Iron may accelerate and exacerbate this process. The enzymes of the pulmonary antioxidant system are catalase, glutathione peroxidase, and superoxide desmutase. Their activity in fetal lung tissue, as gestation progresses, parallels the increasing activity of the pulmonary surfactant system. In addition to the antioxidant enzymes, there are nonenzymatic antioxidant compounds, such as vitamin E and ascorbic acid, that can interfere with lipid peroxidation. Tissue stores of these compounds also accumulate as pregnancy progresses. Exposure of the fetus to corticosteroids accelerates the development of at least the enzymatic portion of the antioxidant system.

At birth, the degree of maturation of lung structure and the surfactant system are the most important determinants of lung function. When oxygen therapy is required in high concentrations and for prolonged periods of time there will be formation within the newborn lung of oxygen radicals, and the potential for lung damage from these species exists. Additionally, during neonatal lung diseases, polymorphonuclear leukocytes migrate into the lung and release toxic products that can lead to lipid peroxidation reactions. The degree of maturity of the antioxidant system may determine in part if, and how much, secondary lung damage will occur when oxygen therapy is required for treatment of severe neonatal lung disease.

Table 28—5 Drugs Accelerating Fetal Lung Maturation

Corticosteroids
Thyroid hormones
Methylxanthines: theophylline, caffeine
Estrogens

FETAL PULMONARY FLUID

In fetal life, the pulmonary epithelial cells secrete fluid into the alveoli. This fluid fills the potential airspaces during development, is very rich in chloride, has almost no protein, and exhibits a net flux up the conducting airways and outward into the amniotic fluid. As term approaches mammalian lungs contain a volume of fetal pulmonary fluid that exceeds their functional residual capacity, approximately 20–30 mL/kg body weight of fluid. This pulmonary fluid is essential for normal lung development. In animal experiments in which this fluid is removed, abnormal lung growth and pulmonary hypoplasia develop.

Although fetal pulmonary fluid is essential for normal lung development, this liquid must be removed from the airspaces before or very soon after birth for gas exchange to occur. Evidence indicates that the process of removal of lung fluid begins prior to delivery. As part of preparation for the onset of labor, the pulmonary epithelium decreases its secretion of fluid. When labor commences, further reductions in lung fluid are initiated. The processes that determine fetal lung fluid content are incompletely understood, but regulation by several hormones is involved. The stress of labor for the fetus and the accompanying high levels of circulating epinephrine and perhaps arginine vasopressin (AVP) seem to be responsible, in large part, for the reduction in fluid content. There is some evidence that prostaglandin E_2 (PGE_2) may also be involved. Animal and human infants delivered by cesarean section without prior labor have increased volumes of pulmonary fluid in comparison with the amount found after vaginal delivery following labor. Premature birth is associated with a higher lung fluid content than is found after term birth, regardless of the manner of delivery.

Removal of fluid from airspaces continues in the several hours that follow birth. The onset of respiration creates a transpulmonary pressure gradient. Conducting airways pressure is equal to atmospheric pressure, whereas intrapleural pressure is -5 to -8 cmH_2O. This pressure gradient favors shifting of the remaining fluid in the airspaces into the perivascular spaces around large blood vessels and conducting airways (the pulmonary interstitium) where lymphatic vessels and small blood vessels take the fluid up and remove it. In addition to this fluid shift, caused by a pressure gradient, there is reason to believe that active transport of sodium and fluid across the pulmonary epithelium contributes to removal of fluid from the airspaces. At present the site of this active transport seems to be the type 2 cell. Following the displacement of fluid from airspaces to perivascular and peribronchial spaces, most fluid is removed by small vessels in the lung microcirculation, with a small amount (11% in lambs) being removed through the lymphatics. On the basis of animal experiments, the final clearance of this pulmonary fluid occurs within 6 hours after delivery.

FETAL CIRCULATION

Most of the information on fetal circulation has been obtained from the study of fetal lambs; it is generally believed that the human fetal circulation is similar. Recent studies of the fetal circulation in humans, which used pulsed Doppler ultrasound and Doppler color-flow mapping technology, indicate that this is true. Several features of the circulation that are present before birth are very different from the circulation that exists shortly after birth (Fig. 28–6). These features are (1) the presence of the placenta, which functions as the organ of gas exchange and as a very low resistance circuit for blood flow; (2) a very high pulmonary vascular resistance owing to constriction of the pulmonary arterioles, resulting in very little flow of blood through the fetal lungs; and (3) two channels for shunting of blood from the pulmonary system to the systemic circulation, the patent ductus arteriosus, and the foramen ovale.

Blood returning from the placenta is carried in the umbilical vein, which has a PaO_2 close to 35 mmHg and an SaO_2 in the range of 85% to 90%. Some 50% of umbilical venous blood is shunted through the liver by the ductus venosus to the inferior vena cava, with no change in oxygen content. The remainder is divided between the hepatic venous system, supplying the major circulation to the left lobe of the liver, and the portal venous system, supplying blood to the right lobe of the liver. Blood distributed through the liver in this manner delivers oxygen to those tissues; as a consequence, there is a decrease in blood oxygen content.

The distal vena cava, the ductus venosus, and the right and left hepatic veins all contribute blood flow to the thoracic inferior vena cava (IVC). Blood entering the thoracic IVC from each of these sources has a different oxygen content. Blood from the ductus venosus has the highest oxygen content because it has not participated in tissue oxygen delivery.

Recent information indicates that within the thoracic IVC there is selective streaming of blood. Blood from the ductus venosus is directed into the right atrium and across the patent foramen ovale (in the atrial septum) into the left atrium. From the left atrium this blood, with its relatively high oxygen content, is pumped into the left ventricle and then out into the proximal aorta from which the coronary arteries and the cerebral vessels arise. In this manner, the heart and brain tissues are selectively supplied with the fetal blood that has the highest oxygen content. In contrast, blood in the thoracic

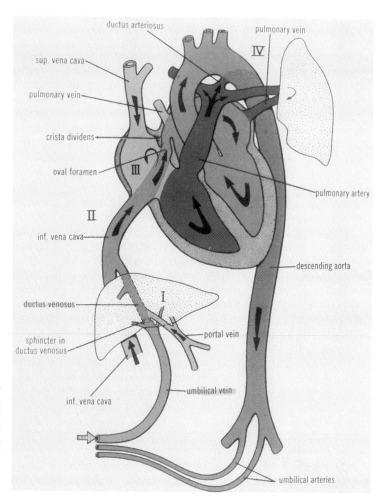

Figure 28—6. The fetal circulation. Note selective streaming of blood returning from the placenta, with the highest P_{O_2} across the foramen ovale. This blood supplies the coronary arteries and brain selectively, as these vessels leave the aorta proximal to the entry of the ductus arteriosus. (Reproduced with permission from Langman J: Medical Embryology, 3rd ed. © Baltimore, Williams & Wilkins, 1975)

IVC returning to the heart from the liver or lower body, upon reaching the heart, is selectively directed to the right atrium where atrial contractions then force it, along with blood returning to the right atrium from the superior vena cava, into the right ventricle, with subsequent ventricular contractions ejecting this more desaturated blood into the main pulmonary artery. Once in the main pulmonary artery, approximately 90% of blood crosses the patent ductus arteriosus, with only 10% entering the pulmonary circulation because of the high pulmonary vascular resistance. Blood that crosses the patent ductus arteriosus enters the descending thoracic aorta, where it mixes with blood ejected from the left ventricle, which has a higher oxygen content. This arrangement places the ventricles in series, rather than in parallel as they will be in extrauterine life. Of the combined ventricular output into the aorta, approximately 60% will enter the placenta and 35% will be distributed to supply other organs.

FETAL HEMOGLOBIN

The hemoglobin molecule synthesized by fetal red blood cells is structurally different from that synthesized after several months of age. All hemoglobin molecules consist of four peptide chains. Both fetal and adult hemoglobin contain two α-chains, but these hemoglobins differ in that whereas adult hemoglobin also contains two β-chains, fetal hemoglobin instead has two δ-chains. The β- and δ-chains differ in their amino acid sequence, and this structural difference confers functional differences that are of consequence for the fetus. The β-chains of adult hemoglobin will bind small phosphate-containing compounds involved in energy metabolism, and such binding will result in a diminished binding affinity for oxygen. The most important of these compounds is 2,3-diphosphoglycerate (2,3-DPG) because it is present in significant amounts in red blood cells. Binding of 2,3-DPG results in a rightward shift of the oxyhemoglobin dissociation curve; adult hemoglobin will bind less oxygen at any given P_{O_2} within the physiologic range (Fig. 28–7). In contrast, the δ-chains of fetal hemoglobin do not bind 2,3-DPG and, as a result, have an oxyhemoglobin dissociation curve that lies to the left of that for adult hemoglobin (see Fig. 28–7). Thus, at any given P_{O_2} fetal hemoglobin has a greater affinity for oxygen and will have a higher percentage saturation than adult hemoglobin. The increased binding of oxygen by fetal hemoglobin, in comparison with adult hemoglobin, is responsible for the transplacental passage of oxygen from mother to fetus. However, the high affinity of fetal hemoglobin for oxygen may be a disadvantage in the setting of neonatal anemia, during which the total oxygen content of blood is reduced because of a reduced amount of hemoglobin, and the high affinity of fetal hemoglobin for oxygen results in less release of oxygen to tissues.

Figure 28–7. Fetal and adult oxyhemoglobin dissociation curves. Note that the neonate, with a high proportion of fetal hemoglobin, will have a low PaO_2 (33 to 42 mmHg) before cyanosis will be observed. (Reproduced by permission from Lee MH, King DH: Cyanosis in the newborn. Pediatr Review 9:36–42, 1987)

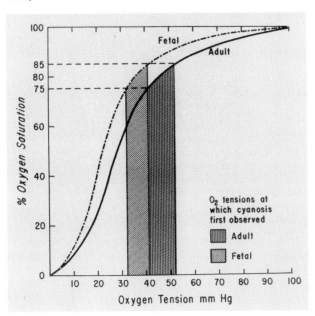

ADAPTATION TO EXTRAUTERINE LIFE

The first few minutes after delivery of an infant are a critical time when marked pulmonary and cardiovascular changes in function must occur smoothly if the newborn is to survive. At the moment of delivery, the infant has no functional residual capacity (FRC) and hence is unable to perform gas exchange. As a result of stimulation from touch and the abrupt change in temperature, newborns in good condition initiate a series of deep inspiratory efforts. These initial inspirations or cries are very forceful and can generate pressures in excess of 60 cmH_2O. Their purpose is to rapidly establish the newborn's FRC, which forms the basis for effective gas exchange. At the end of several minutes of crying, a normal infant will have a well-established FRC. This initial inflation of the lungs leads to the secretion of large amounts of surfactant from type 2 cells into the airways, which in turn assists in stabilizing the neonate's FRC and leads to normal lung mechanics. Premature infants who have severe surfactant deficiency, the basis for SDD, often have difficulty initiating effective respirations because of their inability to expand the lungs repeatedly and achieve a stable FRC.

Sustained inflation of the lungs, along with removal of the placenta from the circulation, lead to transition from the fetal to the neonatal pattern of circulation. As a direct consequence of lung expansion and an increase in alveolar P_{O_2}, the pulmonary arteriolar vasconstriction, which maintained a high pulmonary vascular resistance in fetal life, remits and pulmonary vascular resistance falls. Removal of the placenta from the circulation causes a marked increase in systemic vascular resistance. With the expansion of the lungs, arterial P_{O_2} rises and the ductus arteriosus constricts. As a result of these changes, blood in the right ventricle is pumped into the main pulmonary artery and flows into the lungs, with their newly decreased resistance to blood flow. Blood that has perfused the lungs returns to the left atrium, where a high left atrial pressure, the result of increased blood flow and increased systemic vascular resistance, results in functional closure of the foramen ovale.

With functional closure of the foramen ovale and ductus arteriosus and with a reversal of the relationship between pulmonary and systemic vascular resistances, the transition to the normal neonatal circulation is complete. It is, however, important to realize that early on in neonatal life the transition is tenuous. Hypoxia, acidosis, cold stress, and unstable pulmonary function may be associated with a partial return of the fetal pattern of circulation. In the absence of a placenta, this leads to shunting of blood from the right side of the circulation (pulmonary) to the left side of the circulation (systemic), resulting in arterial desaturation.

NEONATAL RESUSCITATION AND STABILIZATION

ANTICIPATION AND PLANNING

As previously stated, the first moments of life are critical because of the need for rapid establishment of a new system for gas exchange and a new pattern of circulation. Approximately 80% of full-term neonates will have a smooth transition and require no help beyond avoidance of cold stress, suctioning of the airway, and gentle tactile stimulation. Approximately 6% of all newborns will require more extensive resuscitative care in the delivery room. However, among those infants whose birth weight is less than 1500 g, nearly 80% will require resuscitation. Some infants will require supplemental oxygen, others will require positive-pressure ventilation with bag and mask for a time, and a smaller group will require a combination of endotracheal intubation, chest compressions, and therapy with drugs.

An important aspect of stabilization of those neonates who require more than minimal help at delivery is anticipation. Although it is not possible to foresee all situations in which resuscitation will be required, there are warning signs that should

Table 28–6 Conditions with Increased Risk of Need for Neonatal Resuscitation

Prematurity (less than 37-wk gestation)
Intrauterine growth retardation
Fetal heart monitor pattern indicating fetal distress
Acidosis in fetal scalp pH assessment
Birth by emergency cesarean section
Umbilical cord prolapse
Abnormal presentation with difficult extraction
Meconium staining of amniotic fluid
Multiple gestation
Maternal drug therapy
  General anesthesia
  Magnesium sulfate
  Narcotics
Placental abruption
Maternal cardiorespiratory compromise

Table 28–7 Resuscitation Equipment That Should Always Be Available for Neonatal Resuscitation

Radiant warmer
Bulb syringe
Warm towels
Stethoscope
Wall oxygen with flowmeter
Suction with manometer
Suction catheters, sizes 5 or 6, 8 and 10 French
Neonatal resuscitation bag (vol. 250–500 mL) with manometer
Facemasks (full-term and preterm sizes)
Laryngoscope with blades, Miller 0 and Miller 1
Endotracheal tubes, sizes 2.5, 3.0, 3.5, and 4.0
Endotracheal tube stylets

alert the responsible personnel to the increased risk of need for resuscitation at birth (Table 28–6).

The preparation for resuscitation of a newborn involves having both the appropriate people and the proper equipment in place in advance of the actual delivery. At least two people are required, and a third is highly desirable. Tables 28–7 and 28–8 list the equipment required. Two types of resuscitation bags are available: self-inflating bags and anesthesia bags. Self-inflating bags are easier to use and, hence, require less training and experience, whereas anesthesia bags provide more control over pressure delivery. Self-inflating bags are preferred, unless the operators are experienced in the use of anesthesia bags.

Several companies have begun to market adapters that will allow direct connection between

Table 28–8 Equipment That Should Be Readily Available for Neonatal Resuscitation

ECG with oscilloscope
Umbilical catheters, 3.5 and 5.0
Three-way stopcocks
Sterile umbilical artery catheterization tray
Needles, syringes
Drugs in these forms
  Epinephrine 1 : 10,000 dilution
  Albumin 5%
  Sodium bicarbonate, 0.5 mEq/mL
  Neonatal naloxone (Narcan) 0.02 mg/mL
10% dextrose in water IV solution
IV therapy equipment

wall suction and the endotracheal tube. These devices obviate the need for mouth-to-endotracheal tube suctioning for removal of meconium or blood from the airways and should be immediately available in the delivery room.

In addition to having the appropriate number of people and equipment available for deliveries, when the need for resuscitation is anticipated, each person on the team should have a clear understanding of his or her role and tasks before the infant is delivered. In general, it is wise to have one person assigned to manage the airway; a second person given the task of assessing the heart rate, respiratory effort, and breath sounds; and a third person available to perform other tasks.

One way of assessing newborns, which is currently in widespread use, is the Apgar scoring system. In this method an infant is assessed by hands-on examination and scored on the basis of specific findings at age 1 minute and again at age 5 minutes. For distressed infants, scoring is repeated at 10 minutes of age and again every 5 minutes until stabilization. On the basis of the score given at 1 minute of age the type of intervention required is determined. Subsequent scores at 5-minute intervals reflect the response to preceding interventions and again determine what further interventions are necessary. Table 28–9 summarizes the Apgar scoring system.

When the infant is delivered, he or she should be placed under the radiant warmer and dried off with warm towels. The head should be placed in the slightly extended "sniffing" position while the mouth and hypopharynx are gently suctioned with a bulb syringe by the person assigned the responsibility of airway management. During this same time, the person responsible for heart rate and breath sounds should be assessing these findings. As this is being done, other characteristics of the infant that should also be noted are muscle tone and whether the child is crying and turning pink or making less than desirable respiratory effort and remaining cyanotic. Very rapid and accurate assessment of the condition of a newborn at delivery is possible by determining the heart rate, respiratory effort, and rapidity of color change.

Infants whose score is 7 or higher at 1 minute require only protection from hypothermia by warming and drying and continued maintenance of an airway free of secretions. Continuous observation is also required. Babies whose Apgar score at 1 minute is between 4 and 6 are those babies who at delivery have a heart rate of approximately 100 or faster and have some muscle tone; however, they may have inadequate respiratory effort or apnea. In general, they require blow-by oxygen, continued tactile stimulation and warming with repositioning of the head, and bulb suctioning to ensure airway patency. Those infants with scores in this range who exhibit no or ineffective respirations will require a brief period of positive-pressure ventilation with the resuscitation bag and face mask. Infants in this group generally do not require extended positive-pressure ventilation.

Newborns whose Apgar scores are 3 or less as 1 minute approaches are in definite need of intervention. Although continued warming is important, continued tactile stimulation of babies exhibiting this degree of depression is unlikely to be productive and generally wastes time. These babies should have their airway repositioned and positive-pressure ventilation with bag and mask should com-

Table 28—9   Apgar Scoring*

SIGN	0	1	2
Heart rate	Absent	<100	>100
Respirations	Absent	Slow, gasps	Good, crying
Muscle tone	Limp	Some flexion	Active motion
Irritability	None	Grimace	Cough, sneeze
Color	Blue	Pink body, dusky extremities	Completely pink

(Adapted from Apgar V: Proposal for a new method of evaluation of the newborn infant. Anesth Analg 32:260, 1953; Apgar V et al: Evaluation of the newborn infant—second report. JAMA 168:1985, 1958)
* The condition of the newborn infant is expressed as a score that is the sum of five numbers obtained from the above variables. The numbers should be determined at 1 and 5 min after birth and thereafter until the baby is stable. Possible scores range from 0 to 10. The predictive value of this scoring system as an indicator of neonatal outcome is excellent.

mence without delay. For ventilation to be effective, the chest must be seen to rise and fall, and breath sounds must be audible. Often, surprisingly high amounts of pressure (40 to 60 cmH$_2$O) are required for the first few breaths for this to occur. This relates to the need to expand atelactatic alveoli, remove lung liquid, and establish an FRC. Infants in this group not infrequently will require extended periods of positive-pressure ventilation. Effectively performed bag-and-mask ventilation with 100% oxygen results in a rapid increase in heart rate to values faster than 100 beats/min (BPM) in less than 1 minute in almost all children. Failure to obtain this response or the need for positive-pressure ventilation beyond 2 minutes' duration is an indication for endotracheal intubation.

Once effective ventilation is established, either by bag and mask or bag and endotracheal tube, 15 to 30 seconds should be allowed to ascertain the response of the heart rate to ventilation. Ventilation is the foundation of good neonatal resuscitation and, as stated, almost all babies will respond to ventilation, with a prompt increase in heart rate and change in color to pink. The most frequent cause of failure to respond to ventilation is failure of the resuscitator to ventilate the infant appropriately. Reasons for inadequate ventilation include equipment failure, use of inadequate pressure to expand the lungs, improper positioning of the head, inadequate seal between infant and mask, obstructed airway, and malpositioning of the endotracheal tube. If at the end of 15 to 30 seconds of effective ventilation the heart rate is fewer than 60 BPM or is 60 to 80 BPM, but not increasing rapidly, external cardiac compressions are indicated. This infrequent circumstance is also the one in which placement of an umbilical venous catheter, vascular volume expansion, and cardiotropic drugs are indicated. Standards for neonatal advanced life-support have recently been developed and adopted under the combined auspices of the American Heart Association and the American Academy of Pediatrics.

Delivery of an infant with *meconium staining of the amniotic fluid* requires modification of the foregoing principles. Infants with meconium-stained amniotic fluid are at risk for aspiration of this highly irritating material and for the subsequent development of the meconium aspiration syndrome. This is a severe disease with a significant mortality rate; the prevention of this disease deserves high priority. When an infant with meconium-stained amniotic fluid is delivered, the oro-pharynx and hypopharynx should be thoroughly suctioned while the infant's head is still on the mother's perineum. Following delivery of the baby, no attempt should be made to stimulate the infant to initiate respiration. Instead, the baby should be rapidly given to the resuscitation team. Many infants will cry spontaneously at delivery and this imposes an unavoidable risk of meconium aspiration that can be minimized by predelivery suctioning as described. However, under no circumstances should positive-pressure ventilation be administered until the trachea has been suctioned.

The individual responsible for airway management should clear the hypopharynx of secretions and meconium, perform direct laryngoscopy and endotracheal intubation, and suction the trachea with wall suction at approximately 80 mmHg, while slowly withdrawing the endotracheal tube. This procedure should be repeated until the tracheal secretions seen in the tube are free of meconium and may require two or three intubations, although most commonly one will suffice. At the time of laryngoscopy, endotracheal intubation should be performed even if no meconium is seen "on the cords" because it is still possible that there will be substantial quantities of meconium in the trachea below the level of the vocal cords. Once the pharynx and trachea are free of meconium, the management of the infants should proceed, as described previously, and Apgar scores should be assigned.

CLINICAL ASSESSMENT OF RESPIRATORY STATUS

In the immediate hours that follow delivery there are ongoing adaptations to extrauterine life. Fluid continues to be removed from alveoli, recruitment of new lung units is ongoing, central control of respiratory effort stabilizes, and the infant, for the first time, participates in its own thermoregulation. The usual signs of respiratory difficulty in newborn infants are an elevated respiratory rate (the normal range being 40 to 60 BPM), intercostal or sternal retractions, grunting, nasal flaring, and central cyanosis or a requirement for supplemental oxygen to avoid cyanosis. Although these are signs of respiratory difficulty, it is not unusual for normal infants to have these findings in a mild form for the first 4 to 6 hours of life as part of transition to ex utero life. Arterial blood gas values obtained during this period may show mild hypercarbia and the need for small amounts of supplemental oxygen in babies who, at 6 or 8 hours of age, will be completely well and no longer have an oxygen requirement. It is often difficult to distinguish the infant who will be well after a several-hour transition period from the infant who is in the initial stages of surfactant deficiency disease, transient tachypnea of the newborn, pneumonia, or meconium aspiration syndrome. The exact point at which diagnostic and therapeutic interventions are indicated in infants such as these is a matter of judgment that is based on the constellation of various risk factors present in the maternal history, the exact findings on physical examinations and the clinical sense of whether the child is improving or worsening during a period of observation.

MANAGEMENT OF NEONATAL RESPIRATORY PROBLEMS

SURFACTANT DEFICIENCY DISEASE

General Considerations

Surfactant deficiency disease, also known as respiratory distress syndrome (RDS) or hyaline membrane disease (HMD), remains a major cause of illness and death for newborns. It is involved in 30% of all neonatal deaths and 70% of deaths among preterm newborns. The greatest risk factor for SDD is preterm birth, and the more premature the baby, the greater the risk. Other factors that increase the risk at any gestational age are maternal diabetes, maternal bleeding, perinatal asphyxia, second-born twin status, and birth by cesarean section. The size and maturity of infants with SDD have been decreasing progressively for the past several years, a finding that is consistent with an increasing birth weight–specific survival rate during the same period.

Pathophysiology

In recent years the understanding of the functional abnormalities of SDD has expanded and may be conveniently described as consisting of four basic elements: (1) a quantitative deficiency of pulmonary surfactant, (2) immaturity of the lung structure, (3) pulmonary capillary leak, and (4) patency of the ductus arteriosus. These elements in varying combinations lead to progressive alveolar atelectasis, pulmonary edema, right-to-left shunting of blood through atelectatic alveoli, poor lung compliance, and a markedly increased work of breathing. The result is hypoxemia, hypercarbia, and metabolic acidosis. The abnormalities of lung mechanics and gas exchange bring about the clinical picture that is associated with SDD.

Pulmonary surfactant has been recognized for several decades as a complex of phospholipids (90%) and proteins (10%) that is synthesized, stored, and secreted by alveolar type 2 cells. It is widely believed that the essential action of surfactant is to lower surface tension at an air-liquid interface, such as occurs within the aveolus. Such lowering of surface tension is believed to result in stable lung volumes at end-expiration and to be required for normal lung compliance. As noted previously, there is a window of time during gestation within which the pulmonary surfactant system matures; this window is between 25 and 35 weeks. Birth earlier than this maturation is associated with a deficiency of surfactant and SDD.

In addition to a deficiency of surfactant, premature babies have lungs the structure of which corresponds to their gestational age. Accordingly a 28-week-old infant will have lungs in the canalicular stage, and there will be a paucity of alveoli. Even in more mature babies at, for example, 34 weeks, there may be an insufficient number of alveoli for normal lung function in gas exchange.

In the absence of surfactant and with the presence of an immature lung structure, there is a leak of serum proteins into the alveolar space from the vascular space. One of these proteins has the unique ability to inhibit the function of surfactant in lowering surface tension and, thus, has the potential to further aggravate the alveolar deficiency of surfactant, which leads to abnormal respiratory function. This protein is known as the *surfactant inhibitor*.

Although in full-term, healthy infants, functional closure of the ductus arteriosus occurs within several hours of birth, this is not necessarily true for premature infants with SDD. In these infants continued patency of the ductus arteriosus (PDA) is common. The smaller and less mature the baby, the more common is a PDA. In the presence of a PDA there will be shunting of blood from the aorta to the main pulmonary artery and subsequent overcirculation through the pulmonary vascular bed. This leads to pulmonary edema. Pulmonary edema in turn worsens lung compliance and thereby exacerbates the consequences of surfactant deficiency.

Fetal Lung Maturity Testing

In pregnancies complicated by maternal or fetal illness and when labor begins before 37 weeks of completed gestation, it is desirable to know whether or not the fetal lungs contain an adequate quantity of surfactant to prevent the deficiency disease. Several laboratory studies currently in use are able to predict fetal lung maturity accurately, by quantifying the amount of surfactant present in the amniotic fluid. One such test is the lecithin/sphingomyelin (L/S) ratio, which has been in use for several years. Lecithin is phosphatidylcholine, and its concentration in amniotic fluid increases with increasing duration of gestation, as the components of lung surfactant move from within the type 2 cell to the alveoli to amniotic fluid as part of the outward flux of fetal pulmonary fluid. Sphingomyelin is a phospholipid derived primarily from nonsurfactant sources, and its concentration in amniotic fluid is relatively constant as gestation progresses. The L/S ratio value that predicts fetal lung maturity varies somewhat among laboratories, depending on the exact methodology used, but it is usually close to a value of 2 : 1. In pregnancies that are not complicated by diabetes, a mature L/S ratio will correctly predict the absence of SDD in 98% of fetuses. The L/S ratio is less reliable in pregnancies complicated by diabetes, and it cannot be performed on amniotic fluid samples contaminated by meconium or blood. Another shortcoming of the L/S ratio test is its technical difficulty, which creates the need for great attention to detail and leads to a 3- to 4-hour time required to perform the test. A further limitation of the test is its inability to accurately predict lung immaturity. Approximately 50% of fetuses with an immature L/S ratio, if delivered, will not develop SDD. An immature L/S ratio at term, a time in gestation when SDD does not occur, is not uncommon.

Phosphatidylglycerol (PG) is a surfactant phospholipid, the appearance of which in amniotic fluid is coincident with lung maturity. The presence of detectable PG in the amniotic fluid correctly predicts lung maturity virtually 100% of the time. However, the absence of PG does not predict lung immaturity with any degree of accuracy. Approximately 50% of full-term pregnancies with mature L/S ratios still will not have detectable quantities of PG present in the amniotic fluid. Determination of PG is most helpful in diabetic pregnancies, for which the L/S ratio may be falsely mature, and on occasions when the amniotic fluid is contaminated with blood or meconium. This test is now commercially available as a slide agglutination test (AmnioStat-FLM).

Several other tests for fetal lung maturity exist and are used by specific medical center laboratories with experience in using their own results to predict fetal lung maturity in their population. Examples include saturated phosphatidylcholine concentration, fluorescence polarimetry, and the delta optical density 650 test. Each of these methods has specific advantages and disadvantages. None has found acceptance beyond that of the L/S ratio and the presence or absence of PG.

Clinical Features

The delivery of an infant at risk for SDD can be anticipated on the basis of gestational age and the presence or absence of risk factors in the pregnancy history. At the time of delivery, larger, more mature infants who will develop SDD may initially be vigorous and have good Apgar scores. It may be only later in the newborn nursery that the typical symptoms of tachypnea, grunting, flaring, retracting, and cyanosis in room air, or a requirement for supplemental oxygen to avoid cyanosis, become manifest. The chest radiograph in SDD shows hypoinflation and a unique pattern of reticulogranularity and air bronchograms that are diagnostic of SDD (Fig. 28–8). Infants such as these will usually be symptomatic by several hours of age at the latest. In contrast, smaller less mature infants (under 30 weeks' gestation or under 1500 g) destined to develop SDD may not be strong enough to initiate respirations and establish an FRC at the time of delivery. They may be apneic or have only ineffective gasping. Such infants require resuscitation and positive-pressure ventilation in the delivery room if they are to survive.

Newborns with SDD typically exhibit an increasing degree of illness for some 3 to 5 days after birth. The smaller and more immature the infant, the greater the duration of illness. Many infants with SDD will exhibit respiratory failure, despite supplemental oxygen, and will require mechanical ventilation. The smaller the infant, the greater the duration of mechanical ventilation that can be anticipated. Ultimate survival from SDD is birth weight- and gestational age-specific, with the larger, more mature infants having distinctly better survival. Most neonatal units report a greater than 90% survival in infants with birth weight heavier than 1250 g, in contrast to the less than 10% survival seen when birth weight is between 500 and

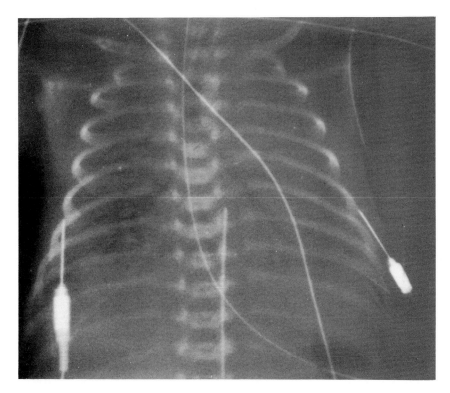

Figure 28—8. Chest radiograph of an infant with surfactant deficiency disease. Note the reticulogranularity and gray background with superimposed air bronchograms.

600 g. An unintended consequence of successful mechanical ventilation of smaller infants with lung disease has been a chronic pulmonary illness, referred to as *bronchopulmonary dysplasia* (BPD) or chronic lung disease of infancy.

Although successful mechanical ventilation of the newborn has been the single largest contributor to the increased survival of preterm infants, there are other aspects of their care that deserve mention. Obstetric management in relation to the avoidance of perinatal asphyxia and the readiness to provide respiratory support in the delivery room have produced babies in better condition to undergo the mechanical ventilation that supports them during SDD. Cautious administration of glucose, fluids, and electrolytes, with frequent monitoring of body weights, has been helpful, in that overhydration exacerbates a PDA and increases the risk of bronchopulmonary dysplasia, whereas underhydration leads to metabolic acidosis. Availability of total parenteral nutrition has improved the survival and the developmental outcome of the smallest infants whose duration of lung disease precludes adequate caloric intake by the gastrointestinal tract.

There are several therapies that are expected to undergo trials to determine if they will improve the results of treatment of preterm infants with SDD. Early closure of the PDA with indomethacin on the first day of life is one such therapy. Several preparations of surfactant from animal sources are undergoing field trials to determine what their effect will be on the course and outcome of SDD. Early results from *surfactant replacement therapy* trials indicate that there is a dramatic, but temporary, improvement in lung function following a single dose; further data will determine if the ultimate outcome is improved when serial doses are used. Mechanical ventilators that have unconventional mechanisms of gas exchange and operate at very high rates—high frequency ventilators—are undergoing trials to determine whether survival, occurrence of chronic lung disease, or other outcome measures will improve.

MECHANICAL VENTILATION OF THE NEWBORN

Continuous Positive Airway Pressure

The application of continuous positive airway pressure (CPAP) to the airways of newborns with respiratory difficulty has been thought to be beneficial in a number of circumstances. The pulmonary effects of CPAP are (1) to prevent end-expiratory collapse of alveoli in the setting of surfactant deficiency and thereby help to increase and stabilize an infant's FRC; and (2) to cause a redistribution of alveolar fluid into the lung interstitium, which will result in improved lung function, but no alteration in total lung water content. These effects result in an increase in PaO_2 after the application of CPAP that can be very dramatic and occurs in two stages. The early increase is related to an improvement in FRC, which leads to superior gas exchange; the later increase is related to the redistribution of pulmonary water.

Consistent with its mode of action, the use of CPAP seems to be most effective in the setting of SDD and in diseases, such as transient tachypnea of the newborn (TTNB), in which the alveoli are filled with retained fetal lung fluid. Continuous positive airway pressure has also been used to treat infants with apnea of prematurity when the basis for the apnea is hypotonia and incoordination of the muscles of the upper airway. In these infants, the airway pressure is believed to maintain patency of the upper airway and prevent obstruction. Infants with lung disease respond to the application of CPAP with a decrease in respiratory rate, a decrease in retractions, an increase in PaO_2 values and, usually, with no change in the $PaCO_2$ value. The decrease in respiratory rate in the setting of a stable $PaCO_2$ implies an improvement in matching of ventilation to perfusion within the lung.

The use of CPAP may actually result in a decrease in dynamic lung compliance, whereas it increases static lung compliance. The effect of CPAP on airways resistance is inconsistent. The application of excessive levels of CPAP will result in a worsening of arterial blood gas values. During CPAP therapy of SDD, there is a very rapid loss of FRC when CPAP is interrupted, as for suctioning or with inadvertent disconnection. In infants and experimental animals with normal lungs, application of CPAP results in prompt transmission of approximately 60% of applied pressure to the thoracic vasculature. This has the potential to decrease venous return to the heart and thereby compromise cardiac output. However, in the setting of lung disease, reduced transmission of airway pressures to thoracic vessels occurs, perhaps as little as 25%, and cardiac output is usually unimpaired. As an infant's lung condition improves, transmission of pressures increases, and compromise of cardiac output may supervene during the recovery phase of an illness such as SDD.

There are several methods for application of CPAP. Nasal prongs are perhaps the most frequently used at present (Fig. 28–9). A major difficulty with this approach is frequent inadvertent dislodgment with subsequent rapid loss of FRC and clinical deterioration. Also, secretions may plug the prongs and result in failure to deliver pressure and supplemental oxygen. This is easily determined when the sounds of gas flow are no longer audible over the infant's lung fields. Gastric distention is not infrequent with this technique, and decompression with a nasogastric tube should be accomplished during the application of nasal CPAP. Prongs may also cause local irritation and ischemia, and infants must be examined for these inadvertent effects. In the past, masks that cover the nose and mouth have been used. This technique has been largely abandoned because of the complications of posterior fossa intracranial hemorrhage, carbon dioxide retention, and gastric perforation.

An endotracheal tube may also be used to apply CPAP. Appropriately sized endotracheal tubes must be used (Table 28–10). Advantages are the increased stability of the delivery system, compared with nasal prongs, and the ability to deliver a more constant FIO_2 and CPAP level. The disadvantage of this delivery method relates to the increased resistance to airflow through the endotracheal tube, which is narrower and longer than the trachea. This increased resistance increases the newborn's work of breathing and may result in carbon dioxide retention or frank respiratory failure.

Therapy with CPAP should be considered for any newborn who exhibits clinical signs of respiratory difficulty, such as tachypnea, grunting, flaring, and retracting, and who requires substantial amounts of supplemental oxygen. It is especially easy to begin nasal CPAP in this circumstance, and 5 cmH_2O is a reasonable starting point. Opinions differ on how high CPAP should be raised if the response to lower levels is not satisfactory. Levels as low as 7 cmH_2O, and as high as 15 cmH_2O have been recommended by various authors. In general, if the required FIO_2 exceeds 0.8, the CPAP is 10 cmH_2O, and the PaO_2 is not consistently greater than 50 mmHg, then mechanical ventilation will be required.

Mechanical Ventilation

Indications for mechanical ventilation in neonates are (1) respiratory failure, which is defined by arterial blood gas criteria; (2) apnea, which is common in neonates; (3) impending cardiovascular collapse,

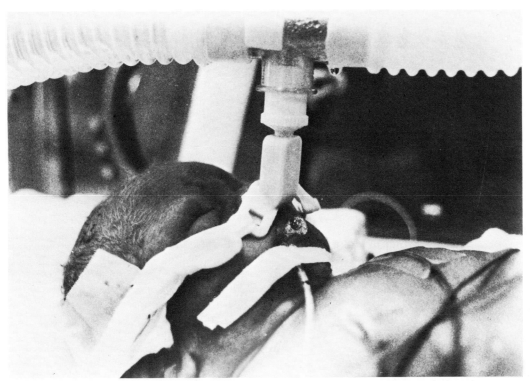

Figure 28—9. Use of the nasal CPAP cannula (see text). (Reproduced by permission of Sherwood Medical Industries)

Table 28—10 Selection of Endotracheal Tubes in Infants

| WEIGHT OF INFANT (g) | ID* (mm) | LENGTH WITHOUT CONNECTOR | |
		Nasotracheal Tube (cm)	Orotracheal Tube (cm)
500–1000	2.5	8.0	6–7.0
1001–1400	3.0	8.5	
1401–1900		9.0	
1901–2200		9.5	7–8.0
2201–2600		10.0	
2601–3000	3.5	10.5	8–9.0
3001–3400		11.0	
3401–3700		11.5	
3701–4100		12.0	9–10.0
4101–4500	4.0	12.5	
>4500		13.0	

* ID = internal diameter.

as in severe sepsis or shock; and (4) clinical evidence of respiratory difficulty in premature infants with birth weight less than 1500 g, such as tachypnea, inspiratory retractions, and poor air entry on auscultation of the chest. Arterial blood gas criteria for respiratory failure vary somewhat from one author to another. A PaO_2 of less than 50 mmHg with an FIO_2 in excess of 0.60, or a $PaCO_2$ more than 50 mmHg is in the range constituting respiratory failure given by most authors.

Ventilators for use on newborns generally function in a time-cycled, pressure-limited manner. A high flow of fresh gas is circulated by the endotracheal tube at a rate rapid enough to preclude rebreathing of exhaled carbon dioxide; flow rates are usually 5–15 L/min. This permits the infant to breath spontaneously at whatever respiratory rate is desired. Mechanical inspiration occurs by periodic obstruction of the expiratory limb of the gas flow, which results in an increase in pressure proximal to the endotracheal tube. This pressure is conducted down the tube and applied to the infant's lungs. When a preset pressure limit is reached, the expiratory obstruction is released.

The frequency of these ventilator breaths, the duration of expiratory limb obstruction, and the preset pressure limit are chosen by the operator of the ventilator. The frequency of periodic obstructions is the ventilator rate or intermittent mandatory ventilation (IMV) rate, the duration of obstruction of the expiratory limb is the inspiratory time, and the pressure limit chosen becomes the peak inspiratory pressure. By manipulating the degree of resistance in the expiratory circuit, the positive end-expiratory pressure (PEEP) can also be chosen by the operator of the ventilator.

Choosing the initial ventilator settings can be done well by careful observation of the child during ventilation with a resuscitation bag and in-line manometer, immediately following endotracheal intubation and stabilization of heart rate and color. Chest excursions with inflation should be approximately 0.25 to 0.50 cm in the anteroposterior plane. On auscultation of the chest, air entry should be clearly audible. If the infant has SDD, then faint end-inspiratory crackles, corresponding to opening of the terminal air sacs, should be audible. The peak inspiratory pressure that produces these findings is the one with which ventilation should be initiated. Ventilation at a rate of between 30 and 50 BPM is a common starting point. The FIO_2 chosen should be that which produces a pink infant and generally will be similar to that required before beginning mechanical ventilation. During initiation of mechanical ventilation following endotracheal intubation, noninvasive monitoring of oxygenation (pulse oximetry or transcutaneous PO_2 monitoring) can be very helpful. Recommended inspiratory times during mechanical ventilation differ greatly among authors and are dependent upon the type of ventilatory strategy to be employed. This will be discussed in detail later.

The concept of mean airway pressure, Paw, is one that is of considerable importance in newborn ventilation. The Paw can be thought of as the average airway pressure over the course of a respiratory cycle, and its importance lies in the linear relationship between Paw and PaO_2 in infants with SDD (Fig. 28–10). That is, for any given FIO_2 an infant's PaO_2 rises or falls in direct proportion to the Paw applied. Thus, there are two ways to improve oxygenation during mechanical ventilation: increase the FIO_2 or increase the Paw. However, mechanical ventilators do not allow the operator to directly select the Paw to be applied. The determinants of Paw that are selectable during mechanical ventilation are peak inspiratory pressure, end-expiratory pressure, and inspiratory time. Increases in any of these variables will increase the Paw and result in improved oxygenation. Of these variables, the most powerful in determining Paw is the inspiratory time; hence, this variable is particularly important. Longer inspiratory times (equal to or beyond 0.6

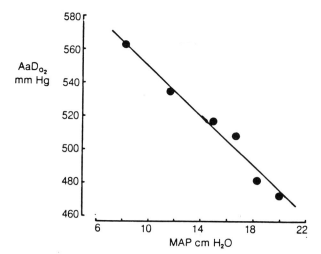

Figure 28–10. A linear relationship exists between the alveolar–arterial O_2 gradient and mean airway pressure (MAP) in infants with surfactant deficiency disease undergoing mechanical ventilation. (Herman S, Reynolds ER: Methods for improving oxygenation in infants mechanically ventilated for hyaline membrane disease. Arch Dis Child 48:612–617, 1973, with permission)

Table 28–11   Ventilatory Management Considerations

VARIABLE	PHYSIOLOGIC AND CLINICAL EFFECTS
F_IO_2	P_AO_2 and PaO_2 will change in the same direction as F_IO_2 administered
PIP	Increases/decreases in PIP produce changes that are in the same direction for both Paw and in tidal volume. PaO_2 will vary directly with Paw, and $PaCO_2$ will change in the opposite direction in which tidal volume (and thus minute ventilation) is changed.
PEEP	Changes in PEEP produce changes in Paw that are in the same direction. Paw and PaO_2 will change in the same direction. Application of PEEP reduces ventilation–perfusion mismatch leading to an increase in PaO_2
Rate	Changes in ventilator rate will change minute ventilation and $PaCO_2$ in the opposite direction leading to alteration of $PaCO_2$.
T_I	Lengthening T_I (inspiratory time) will increase Paw leading to an increase in PaO_2; shortening T_I will have the opposite effect.
Flow Rate	Changes in flow rate will alter the respiratory waveform and may change Paw. Effects of manipulating flow rate may be complicated.

seconds) are associated with an ability to use lower peak inspiratory pressures and low end-expiratory pressures, because of the impact of inspiratory time on Paw (which is the principal determinant of PaO_2 at any given F_IO_2). However, this ventilatory strategy is associated with a higher frequency of pneumothorax. Conversely, use of a shorter inspiratory time (between 0.3 and 0.6 seconds) requires the use of a higher peak inspiratory pressure, a faster rate, and higher end-expiratory pressure to achieve comparable oxygenation. These shorter inspiratory times are associated with fewer air leak phenomena, such as pneumothorax, and some have reported a decreased prevalence of chronic lung disease with this approach to treatment. Except at very high ventilator rates (e.g., a rate greater than 60 BPM) the rate chosen has only a small influence on the Paw.

When rapid ventilator rates are used, as with rates faster than 60 BPM, there may not be adequate time for complete exhalation. This is especially probable if the ventilator rate is increased by a large amount, without a compensatory shortening of the inspiratory time. When inadequate expiratory time is allowed, there is "stacking" of breaths wherein inspiration begins before the previous expiration is complete. This leads to increasing positive end-expiratory pressure in the alveoli and alveolar overdistention, with a progressive increase in lung volume over time. Because of this, arterial blood gases may deteriorate. This situation also predisposes to alveolar rupture and pneumothorax.

Even among infants requiring mechanical ventilation, spontaneous respiratory efforts may contribute substantially to total alveolar ventilation. For breaths given by the mechanical ventilator, tidal volume will be determined by the difference between the peak inspiratory pressure and the end-expiratory pressure. Therefore, the determinants of minute ventilation that involve the mechanical ventilator are: the rate and the difference between peak inspiratory pressure and end-expiratory pressure. The influence of mechanical ventilation on arterial pH is mainly through changes in arterial carbon dioxide levels. Table 28–11 is helpful in assessing the most likely effects of various parameter changes in ventilator management.

Alterations in flow rate through the mechanical ventilator will alter the inspiratory waveform delivered to the baby, which may increase the Paw. The physiologic effects of altering the waveform are complicated, and only rarely is manipulation of this variable required. Delivered flows should always be twice a baby's minute ventilation; rates of 5–15 L/min are usually chosen.

TRANSIENT TACHYPNEA OF THE NEWBORN

Transient tachypnea of the newborn (TTNB) is a common entity, which has several names in common use: wet lung syndrome, retained fetal lung fluid, and RDS type 2. Incidence data are not widely available, but TTNB is a quite common illness and is probably the most common reason for respiratory symptoms in larger babies who are nearly full-term or full-term. Among unselected deliveries this disorder may be as common as 2:100 births; among infants admitted to a neonatal intensive care nursery with symptoms of respiratory difficulty, the final diagnosis will be TTNB as often as 40% of the time.

The functional disorder of TTNB is a delay in removing fetal pulmonary fluid from the alveoli. Retention of this fluid results in partial airway obstruction, which has two effects. First, there is obstruction to air entry, which results in lung units with low ventilation/perfusion ratios. Lung units that function with low ventilation/perfusion ratios result in arterial hypoxemia. Second, there is inadequate emptying of these units during expiration, resulting in air-trapping and lung hyperinflation. As a result of hyperinflation, the lung compliance is lower than normal; the infant's work of breathing increases, and excessive respiratory effort is required to maintain normal gas exchange.

There is evidence from echocardiographic studies of children with TTNB that sometimes the high pulmonary artery pressure that characterizes fetal life does not completely remit. These infants seem to have a more severe form of the disease. The cause for the high pulmonary artery pressures may be hyperinflation of groups of alveoli, leading to mechanical compression of the pulmonary capillary bed and, thereby, resistance to blood flow. Resistance to blood flow would then lead to an increased pulmonary artery pressure. In babies with this additional feature to their illness, the persistently high pulmonary artery pressure may lead to shunting of blood from the pulmonary circulation to the systemic circulation, with subsequent arterial desaturation.

Another recent development in the understanding of TTNB relates to the role of pulmonary surfactant. Several authors have offered preliminary data that indicate that some babies with TTNB may have a mild deficiency of pulmonary surfactant quantity or function. Whether this deficiency represents a quantitative or a qualitative deficiency, or whether it really exists at all, is not completely clear at present.

Risk factors for TTNB are considered to be a borderline prematurity with gestational age 34 to 37 weeks, delivery by cesarean section without preceding labor, absent phosphatidylglycerol from the amniotic fluid, and low Apgar scores. Clinically, these infants usually come to attention because of persistent tachypnea, retractions, nasal flaring, grunting, and a requirement for supplemental oxygen to prevent cyanosis. The chest radiograph shows hyperinflation to varying degrees, fluid in one or both lung fissures, perihilar haziness, and a normal to slightly large heart size (Fig. 28–11).

The course of this illness is usually uncomplicated, with infants remaining tachypneic in the range of 80 to 90 BPM for 2 to 5 days, with gradual improvement noted toward the end of this time.

Some infants may require an FiO_2 of 0.30 to 0.40, although some authors believe that infants with TTNB should have no requirement for supplemental oxygen. It is important to note, however, that there are a few infants who will have a much more severe illness. These infants will be discernible by their extreme elevation in respiratory rate to faster than 90 to 100 BPM, and the need for high FiO_2 in the 0.60 to 0.80 range. Some of these infants will benefit from a constant distending pressure (such as with nasal CPAP), whereas others will experience frank respiratory failure and require mechanical ventilation. Echocardiographic data indicate that these latter infants are those with persistence of a high pulmonary artery pressure.

The diagnosis of TTNB is best thought of as one of exclusion. Other diagnoses that must be considered are pneumonia, SDD, and aspiration syndromes. The prognosis for infants with TTNB is quite good, with most recovering rapidly and completely.

PNEUMONIA AND SEPSIS IN THE NEONATAL PERIOD

Infections in newborn infants (sepsis) most often take the form of pneumonia and, generally, have a bacterial origin. The most common etiologic agents are group B *Streptococcus*, *Escherichia coli*, *Klebsiella pneumoniae*, and *Listeria monocytogenes*, although other bacteria can produce illness as well. Less typically, a newborn will be infected by cytomegalovirus or herpesvirus, and the infection will manifest as pneumonia. In the last few years, it has become clear that approximately two-thirds of cases of neonatal sepsis and pneumonia are acquired during labor. Thus, affected children are most often ill at the time of birth or within several hours immediately following birth. These children have acquired infection with an organism that ascended from the maternal vagina and cervix into the amniotic space during labor. Less commonly, babies develop pneumonia and sepsis some 24 to 48 hours after birth. These infants were well at delivery, but were colonized with a pathogenic organism during the birth process. Following birth, bacteria multiply for a time locally, as in the nasopharynx, and then disseminate to create systemic illness.

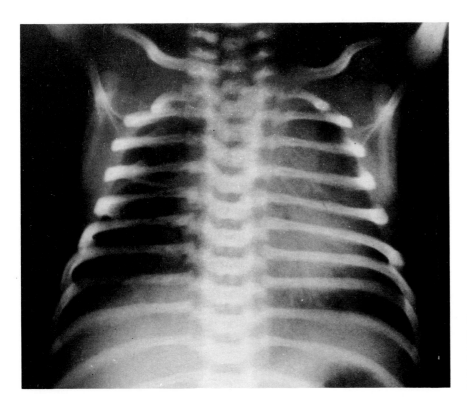

Figure 28—11. Chest radiograph typical of transient tachypnea of the newborn. Note the presence of adequate to increased lung volumes, perihilar congestion, and fluid in the minor fissure of the right lung.

There are many reports that describe various constellations of perinatal events thought to increase the risk of pneumonia. Often these reports are not in agreement with one another. Important risk factors for newborn sepsis or pneumonia include maternal cervical or rectal colonization with group B streptococci; premature labor or a low-birth-weight infant; prolonged rupture of the membranes longer than 18 hours; and evidence of maternal chorioamnionitis during labor, such as fever, high white blood cell count, or abdominal tenderness. Maternal urinary tract infection is also an important risk factor. Premature birth not only is a powerful risk factor for pneumonia but also for a fatal outcome with pneumonia.

The clinical findings in pneumonia are virtually the same as those for SDD or TTNB. When faced with an infant displaying the typical signs of respiratory difficulty, it is not possible to differentiate with certainty among SDD, TTNB, and pneumonia. The chest radiograph in infants with pneumonia may show only a diffuse haze, may resemble SDD in all respects, or may show a typical localized infiltrate. It is not possible to definitively distinguish pneumonia from SDD or TTNB on a single chest radiograph; this is especially true when the study is obtained in the first few hours after birth. As a result of the similarity in clinical and radiographic appearance of pneumonia and SDD, these two entities must always be considered when either of them is being considered. The inability to distinguish between these diseases with confidence is why virtually all children with respiratory symptoms that are not a mere reflection of transition to extrauterine life are appropriately treated with antibiotics.

The treatment of neonatal pneumonia consists of antibiotic therapy as well as support of respiratory function. Treatment decisions are made on the basis of both ABG determinations and serial examinations with assessment of interval improvement or worsening. Among babies with pneumonia who require mechanical ventilation, there are two clues that favor the diagnosis of pneumonia over that of SDD. Infants with pneumonia generally have a higher pulmonary compliance and so require less pressure from the ventilator. Purulent, copious secretions in the endotracheal tube favor the diagno-

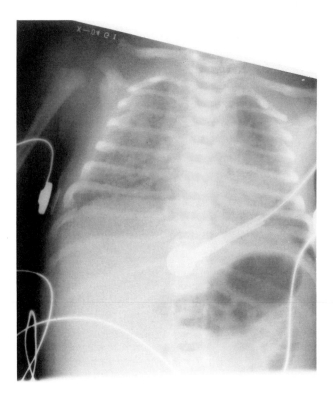

Figure 28—12. Chest radiograph of an infant with meconium aspiration syndrome. Note the diffuse, fluffy densities extending out to the periphery of the lung.

Aspiration may result in obstruction of airways and lead to sections of lung with low ventilation/perfusion ratios, and filling of alveoli with liquid, thereby, creating an intrapulmonary shunt with arterial desaturation. Moreover, there is a later inflammatory reaction to inhalation of any of these substances that results in an additional component of impaired lung function several hours after the initial event.

Risk factors for aspiration include fetal distress, a postdate gestational age, meconium staining of the amniotic fluid, and placental abruption. Initiation of positive-pressure ventilation of a meconium-stained infant before proper tracheal suctioning can cause meconium aspiration syndrome. Infants who aspirate exhibit respiratory difficulty that creates a clinical picture identical with that seen with other neonatal respiratory disorders. The chest radiograph may show just diffuse haziness or, in severe cases, may reveal bilateral "white out." The fluffy, diffuse densities of meconium aspiration syndrome are rather specific for that disorder (Fig. 28—12).

Treatment of these syndromes is supportive. More severely affected children will exhibit respiratory failure and require mechanical ventilation. The prognosis depends on the severity of the aspiration and is generally worse if the inhaled substance was meconium.

sis of pneumonia, as opposed to SDD. This latter condition is generally accompanied by scant, mucoid pulmonary secretions.

The prognosis for pneumonia in full-term infants is good unless the disorder is accompanied by septic shock or is so overwhelming as to make adequate oxygenation impossible. Preterm infants have a higher mortality, which varies with the degree of prematurity.

PERINATAL ASPIRATION SYNDROMES

Before the onset of labor, fetuses intermittently make breathing movements, which are essential for normal lung development. During these movements the net flux of material remains outward from lungs to amniotic fluid. However, certain conditions or events that occur during labor can result in deep gasping movements by the fetus. If at the time of such a gasp the fetal hypopharynx is filled with meconium-stained fluid, blood, infected secretions, or amniotic fluid, aspiration may occur.

PERSISTENT PULMONARY HYPERTENSION OF THE NEWBORN

A high pulmonary vascular resistance caused by constriction of pulmonary arterioles and a consequent high pulmonary artery pressure is characteristic of the fetal circulation. Also characteristic of this circulation is shunting of blood from right to left across the foramen ovale and ductus arteriosus (see Fig. 28—6). Although this circulatory pattern is appropriate for a fetus, it is very detrimental to a newborn because it will result in an intracardiac shunting of unsaturated blood into the systemic arterial circulation. If the shunt is large enough it will preclude adequate tissue oxygenation, and a metabolic acidosis will result from tissue hypoxia. This condition has also been called *persistent fetal circulation*.

Persistent pulmonary hypertension of the newborn (PPHN) can occur alone without any pulmonary disease in its so-called idiopathic form. However, PPHN most often occurs in the setting of, and

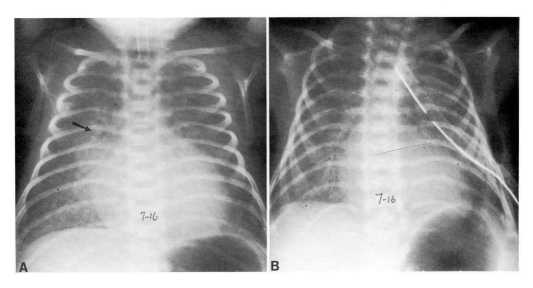

Figure 28–13. (A) Recovering hyaline membrane disease with patent ductus arteriosus. There is evidence of roentgenographic improvement in hyaline membrane disease with less alveolar atelectasis, but there is increased pulmonary vascularity consistent with a left-to-right shunt through the ductus arteriosus. Clinical signs were consistent with a large patent ductus arteriosus (*arrow* points to enlarged pulmonary vessel). (B) This film of the same patient was taken immediately after ligation of a large patent ductus arteriosus. There is decreased pulmonary vascularity and heart size.

complicates the management of, other lung diseases (for example, see Fig. 28–13). Common settings in which PPHN may supervene are SDD in infants of advanced gestational age; pneumonia, especially when the cause is group B streptococci; and meconium aspiration syndrome. Congenital diaphragmatic hernia is also associated with PPHN. Rarely, an infant who initially is thought to have TTNB will have a course complicated by the development of PPHN.

Infants with PPHN in the setting of lung disease initially show the signs of their primary pulmonary illness; PPHN becomes apparent when they fail to respond to the usual therapy or when their course is particularly severe. Babies with the idiopathic form of PPHN have a clear chest radiograph and resemble those with cyanotic congenital heart disease. The diagnosis may be suggested by the history, physical examination, and clinical course. Certain diagnosis requires echocardiographic study, to exclude structural heart disease, and a demonstration of a right-to-left shunt by contrast saline injection, along with other characteristic findings of pulmonary artery hypertension.

Treatment of this disorder virtually always requires mechanical ventilation with an FiO_2 of 1.0.

Support of the systemic circulation with fluid therapy and the use of vasoactive drugs is often required. Administration of sodium bicarbonate to reverse a metabolic acidosis or create a metabolic alkalosis may be required.

The specifics of ventilatory management of these children are controversial. There are some data to suggest that hyperventilation to produce $PaCO_2$ values in the range of 20 to 25 mmHg and arterial pH values greater than 7.55 will reverse pulmonary artery vasoconstriction; this approach to management has been called hyperoxic hyperventilation. Others have pointed out the high mortality that exists with this treatment approach (most reports are approximately 50%) and the lung damage that this type of management engenders. These authors have advised a minimal intervention approach to management that avoids deliberate hyperventilation and advocates managing the mechanical ventilator in a more conventional manner, while using an FiO_2 of 1.0, supporting the systemic circulation, and maintaining a normal arterial pH. No direct comparisons of results with these differing approaches have been made.

In the last few years another approach to treatment of infants with PPHN, that of extracorporeal membrane oxygenation (ECMO), has been available at several medical centers. This approach has been reserved for those infants who, by criteria that vary among institutions, are failing conventional management and are perceived as having fatal disease. The use of ECMO involves the creation of a temporary cardiopulmonary bypass by placing catheters in the right carotid artery and right atrium. Venous blood is removed from the right atrium to a pump and then directed across a membrane oxygenator, where gas exchange occurs. Oxygenated blood is then returned to the aortic arch by way of the right carotid artery catheter (venoarterial bypass). This technique involves permanent ligation of the right carotid artery when the baby is removed from ECMO. With this system, arterial Po_2 can be raised into the physiologic range, and the lungs can be "put to rest" to heal for several days. Reporting institutions generally state that 2 to 5 days of therapy are required before it is possible to return the patients to the mechanical ventilator and more conventional management.

Persistent pulmonary hypertension of the newborn is a very serious condition, with many centers reporting a mortality rate near 50%. Children who recover generally do well in terms of their development but not infrequently have residual chronic lung disease. Treatment with ECMO is currently one of the most controversial areas in newborn medicine. Proponents of ECMO argue that this therapy can save 80% of those babies who would die if managed by conventional means alone. Controversy stems in large part from the lack of uniform criteria by which to judge an individual patient as a failure of conventional management who will ultimately die without ECMO. Institutions that have critically examined criteria to predict mortality with conventional management have found that those criteria that predict mortality with, for example, 80% accuracy vary from one institution to another and change over time within the same institution. Another area in which more data are needed to determine the benefits and risks of ECMO is that of long-term neurodevelopmental outcome. This area is of special concern because of the permanent loss of the right carotid artery, which this therapy involves. Studies of ECMO survivors in relation to long-term neurodevelopmental outcome are ongoing, and it is as yet difficult to draw firm conclusions. A better method of predicting failure of conventional management and more outcome data need to be available to resolve these controversies. The ultimate place of ECMO technology in neonatology has yet to be decided.

PULMONARY AIR LEAK SYNDROMES

The pulmonary air leak syndromes include pneumothorax, pulmonary interstitial emphysema, pneumomediastinum, and pneumopericardium. Pulmonary air leaks begin with the rupture of an overdistended alveolus. This rupture gives rise to air within the pulmonary interstitium, which is able to traverse along the tissue planes that accompany vessels and lymphatics until it reaches the mediastinum. If the air remains within the mediastinum, the result is a *pneumomediastinum*. Rarely, in infants the air will dissect into the pericardial space and create a *pneumopericardium*. Most commonly, the air will break through the mediastinum and a *pneumothorax* will result (Fig. 28–14).

In babies who are free of pulmonary disease, pneumothorax may occur as a consequence of the high airway pressures, often greater than 60 cmH₂O, which accompany the onset of respirations immediately following birth. In fact, an incidence of spontaneous pneumothorax of 1% has been found in this setting. These are most often asymptomatic and of no significance. Treatment is required only rarely, as when there is a mediastinal shift indicating the presence of tension.

The use of positive-pressure ventilation at birth with meconium aspiration syndrome, SDD, and pneumonia, all increase the frequency of pneumothorax. Incidences of pneumothorax as high as 20%

Figure 28–14. Pneumopericardium. Air completely encircles the heart and is causing tamponade. Even though the endotracheal tube is down the right mainstem bronchus, no perforation of the tracheobronchial tree was present at postmortem examination.

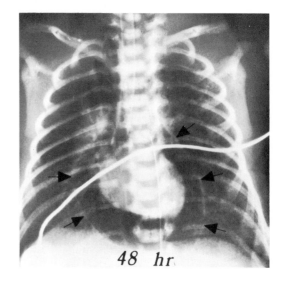

48 hr

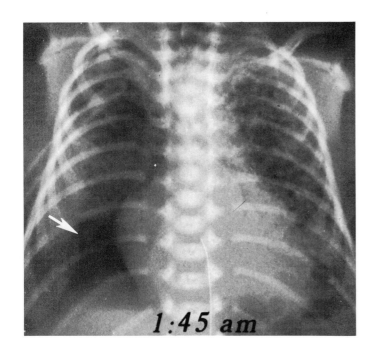

Figure 28—15. Pneumothorax and interstitial emphysema: Pneumothorax is seen on the right, with a chest tube in place. Note the accumulation of air anteriorly and medially (*arrow*) because of noncompliance of the lungs and their inability to collapse concentrically. Interstitial pulmonary emphysema involves the left lung; a left pneumothorax occurred shortly after this film was taken.

to 50% have been found in children with meconium aspiration syndrome. Other aspiration syndromes are also associated with an increased risk of pneumothorax. Transient tachypnea of the newborn also predisposes to pneumothorax and represents one of the major morbidities of this disease.

The underlying pathogenesis in all of these conditions is the presence of abnormal pulmonary mechanics that require the infant to generate high intrathoracic pressures to effect gas exchange. The increased pressures predispose to alveolar rupture. In meconium aspiration syndrome, there is also increased resistance to expiratory (and inspiratory) flow because of the partial obstruction of airways by meconium. The resulting incomplete expiratory flow leads to progressive alveolar distention, which further increases the risk of alveolar rupture. The incidence of pneumothorax is increased whenever mechanical ventilation is used. In preterm infants undergoing mechanical ventilation for SDD, an incidence as high as 40% has been reported.

In contrast with the pneumothoraces that occur spontaneously, those that occur in the setting of lung disease generally do result in compromise of arterial blood gas levels and cardiac output; consequently, drainage with tube thoracotomy is required. This is especially true in patients undergoing mechanical ventilation, in whom pneumothorax will often be a catastrophic event owing to the presence of tension in the thorax, with a conse-

quent mediastinal shift. Arterial blood gas levels deteriorate with pneumothorax because of right-to-left intrapulmonary shunting of blood through the atelectatic lung. Cardiac output is compromised with tension pneumothorax because the high intrathoracic positive pressure and shifting of the mediastinum lead to compression of the great veins. Compression of the great veins diminishes cardiac return and, subsequently, cardiac output falls.

Most often, a *pneumomediastinum* is a silent abnormality and usually is not a cause of respiratory or cardiac dysfunction. Its pathogenesis is analogous to that of a spontaneous pneumothorax. It does have the potential to decompress to form a pneumothorax and, accordingly, deserves careful observation. Generally, it is unwise to attempt to drain a pneumomediastinum. *Pneumopericardium* is rare and is essentially always seen in children who are undergoing mechanical ventilation. It may be asymptomatic, or it may cause the picture of cardiac tamponade. Drainage may be lifesaving in the latter event.

Pulmonary interstitial emphysema (PIE) begins when air dissects out of the alveolar bases or ducts and remains as cysts of air within the perivascular tissues of the lung, rather than following tissue planes to the hilum and leading to pneumothorax. These cysts range in size from 0.1 to 1.0 cm and extend radially from the hilar regions outward (Fig. 28–15). This type of air leak is strongly associated with use of mechanical ventilation. Two types of PIE are recognized: diffuse and localized. Early onset of diffuse and bilateral PIE in infants undergoing mechanical ventilation for SDD is a poor prognostic sign. Localized PIE does not have the same significance for outcome. Beyond reducing the amount of pressure used for ventilation to that which is absolutely essential, no specific management is usually required. On occasion, PIE will be asymmetric, with one side markedly more affected and hyperinflated, whereas the contralateral side is atelectatic. In such cases, positioning the severely affected side down may be of benefit as the weight of the mediastinum and atelectatic lung may prevent progression or lead to reversal of the air leak. Selective intubation of the main stem bronchus leading to the atelectatic side has been reported to be of benefit in specific cases.

A new approach to the management of severe PIE has recently been allowed by the development of mechanical ventilators that operate at very high rates. These ventilators, as a group, are called high-frequency ventilators, and several different types exist. In investigations involving infants with severe progressive PIE and deteriorating ABG levels, both high-frequency oscillatory ventilation and high-frequency jet ventilation have shown promise.

CONGENITAL HEART DISEASE

There are three basic modes of presentation by which newborns with *congenital heart disease* (CHD) can come to attention: (1) cyanosis, (2) congestive heart failure, and (3) low cardiac output states. When cyanosis is the mode of presentation, the infant will be noted to be dusky in room air but generally will not have the grunting, flaring, and retracting characteristic of infants with lung disease. If an ABG is obtained, the PaO_2 will typically be in the 30- to 60-mmHg range. The presence of cyanotic CHD is made more likely by demonstrating that the PaO_2 does not rise significantly in 100% oxygen. A rise in PaO_2 in response to a high FiO_2 would greatly favor the diagnosis of lung disease. Also, lung disease should be accompanied by abnormal lung parenchyma on a chest radiograph, and this is not seen in infants with CHD.

As a second type of presentation, infants may come to attention because of congestive heart failure. Infants presenting with congestive heart failure will exhibit the typical signs of respiratory difficulty in a newborn, but will also have an enlarged liver on examination and cardiomegaly with pulmonary edema seen on a chest x-ray film. Some of

Table 28–12 Presentations of Congenital Heart Disease

CYANOSIS

Pulmonary atresia
Tricuspid atresia
Ebstein's anomaly
Transposition of the great vessels
Total anomalous pulmonary venous return
Pulmonary stenosis
Tetralogy of Fallot
Aortic coarctation

CONGESTIVE HEART FAILURE

Common atrioventricular canal
Truncus arteriosus
Atrial septal defect with patent ductus arteriosus
Ventricular septal defect

LOW CARDIAC OUTPUT STATES

Hypoplastic left heart syndrome
Aortic coarctation
Aortic stenosis
Interrupted aortic arch

these infants may also exhibit cyanosis, and the two presentations of cyanosis and congestive heart failure are not mutually exclusive.

Congenital heart disease may also appear as a low cardiac output state, as when there is obstruction to left ventricular outflow. In its extreme form, this represents cardiogenic shock. Respiratory signs occur late in this type of presentation. Lethargy, poor feeding, poor systemic perfusion, and metabolic acidosis are the early indications of disease.

The immediate newborn history, physical examination, chest radiograph, and a comparison of arterial blood gas levels obtained while the baby is breathing room air or 100% oxygen should differentiate between CHD and lung disease. Table 28–12 lists the specific lesions categorized by their typical mode of presentation. Some diseases may have more than one possible presentation; only the more common diseases are listed. The specific issues of diagnosis and therapy are beyond the scope of this discussion.

APNEA

Apnea is the cessation of effective airflow for longer than 20 seconds or for long enough to produce arterial desaturation, with or without bradycardia. Apneic episodes are very common in preterm infants, occurring in approximately 50% of infants whose birth weights are less than 1500 g. The apneic episodes may be secondary to environmental circumstances or to another disease process, or they may occur as a reflection of an immature respiratory control system. These latter episodes are referred to as idiopathic apnea or prematurity. Table 28–13 lists the specific causes of apnea. Idiopathic apnea of prematurity is the most common cause of apneic events in preterm infants, but it remains a diagnosis of exclusion. Specific causes must be sought in infants who develop new apnea.

The immaturity of respiratory control that gives rise to apnea or prematurity may take several forms. Central apnea results when, because of insensitivity of peripheral chemoreceptors or poor central integration of information from these receptors, there is cessation of central respiratory drive. Obstructive apnea results when immaturity of upper airway reflex events allows collapse of the airway, leading to absence of airflow, despite continued respiratory effort. However, the predominant type of apnea in infants is *mixed apnea*, wherein elements of both impaired central control and obstruction from poor reflex activity are operative.

Table 28–13 Specific Causes of Apnea

Infection
  Sepsis
  Meningtis
  Necrotizing enterocolitis
Decreased oxygen delivery
  Hypoxemia
  Anemia
  Shock
  Left-to-right shunting (as through a PDA)
CNS disease
  Asphyxia and cerebral edema
  Hemorrhage
  Seizures
  Malformations
Drugs
  Maternal narcotics
  Fetal narcotics
Metabolic diseases
  Hypoglycemia
  Hypocalcemia
  Hyponatremia
  Hypernatremia–dehydration
  Hyperammonemia
Thermal instability
Idiopathic apnea of prematurity

Although idiopathic apnea of prematurity is common (present in approximately 50% of babies less than 1500g), it is not necessarily benign. Doppler flow studies of the anterior cerebral artery have demonstrated reverse diastolic flow when apneic episodes have led to heart rates slower than 100 BPM. Some reports have associated recurrent episodes of apnea accompanied by cyanosis with a less favorable developmental outcome.

Several approaches to treatment are available. Removal of any underlying precipitant is the first step. A common example of this would be the finding of a borderline low PaO_2 in a child with apnea. Often, correction of this situation with small amounts of supplemental oxygen will greatly reduce the frequency of apneic episodes. Treatment with nasal CPAP has been advocated. It is possible that this is effective, either because it improves oxygenation or because it "stents" open the soft tissues of the upper airways and improves the course of children with obstructive apnea.

The methylxanthines theophylline and caffeine have both been used to treat apnea in preterm infants. It is widely believed that these agents act to stimulate central respiratory drive, although definitive proof of their mechanism of action is lacking. Methylxanthines increase the mean inspiratory flow rate (a measure of respiratory drive), increase respiratory flow rate output, and also lead to an approximate 20% increase in metabolic rate. This latter finding is a disadvantage of therapy with these agents. Theophylline has variable kinetics in small infants, and it is important to monitor serum levels. Theophylline levels of 5–10 μg/mL and caffeine levels of 8–20 μg/mL are recommended. Generally, apnea of prematurity remits when the children are approximately 34-weeks gestational age, and it is possible to discontinue drug therapy, although continued cardiorespiratory monitoring for a period during and after discontinuance is prudent.

CONGENITAL DIAPHRAGMATIC HERNIA

Congenital diaphragmatic hernia (CDH) is an infrequent but life-threatening neonatal disorder. These newborns come to attention either because of the typical signs of respiratory distress or because of profound cyanosis that does not remit with oxygen therapy. The chest radiograph will usually show loops of bowel in the thorax, although films obtained before significant amounts of air have been swallowed may show a unilateral "white out" with a mediastinal shift. In this latter case, repeat films will show the typical appearance of bowel in the thorax (Fig. 28–16). Approximately 80% of diaphragmatic hernias are left-sided. In several reported series 20% to 25% of children with CDH have associated major congenital abnormalities. These anomalies have included trisomies, several types of congenital heart disease, tracheoesophageal fistula, and genitourinary malformations.

Although definitive repair of this lesion involves surgery, the preoperative management is important. A nasogastric tube attached to suction is used for gastric decompression. In symptomatic infants elective endotracheal intubation is required and should be followed by muscle relaxation and sedation. This approach provides minimal inflation of the gastointestinal tract and aims to minimize lung and heart compression by preventing the gastrointestinal tract from filling with air. These patients should be mechanically ventilated with an FIO_2 of 1.0 and with great care given to minimize inspiratory pressures, as pneumothorax is common in this setting and is associated with a less favorable prognosis.

Surgical repair of this lesion is important, but survival is dictated by the degree of pulmonary hypoplasia that is present. In CDH both lungs are hypoplastic, although the ipsilateral lung is more hypoplastic than the contralateral lung. The earlier in gestation the diaphragmatic hernia appears, the greater the degree of pulmonary hypoplasia, and the less the chances for survival. Arterial blood gas abnormalities in CDH, in part, are due to decreased lung surface area, but a more important determinant is right-to-left shunting of blood across fetal channels. This shunting of blood is a consequence of both the anatomic hypoplasia itself and the pulmonary vasoconstriction that frequently follows surgical repair of these infants.

After surgical repair, infants can be separated into three groups. The first group consists of those children who will do well and have an uncomplicated course. The second group of children have a degree of pulmonary hypoplasia that is fatal, and their arterial blood gas levels are incompatible with life, despite extensive efforts to support them. The third group of infants do well for several hours after surgery (the so-called "honeymoon period") and then experience extensive right-to-left shunting of blood across fetal channels caused by an elevation in pulmonary vascular resistance. The management of this third group of children is similar to that for PPHN.

The overall mortality rate for diaphragmatic hernia has remained unchanged at 50% for the past

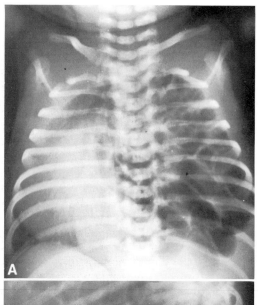
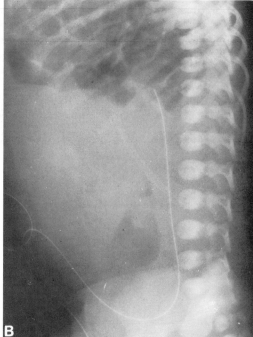

Figure 28–16. (*A*) Anteroposterior view of a diaphragmatic hernia. This full-term newborn had respiratory distress from birth. Hearth tones were heard on the right. Note the multiple loops of bowel in the left pleural space, with herniation of the heart and mediastinum toward the right. (*B*) Lateral view of the same diaphragmatic hernia. Physical examination of the abdomen revealed a scaphoid configuration. The only air below the level of the diaphragm is in the stomach. Note the multiple loops of small bowel in the chest.

5 years. The availability of ECMO technology may alter this in the future, although there are now inadequate data to determine the usefulness of ECMO in these children.

The occurrence of pulmonary hypoplasia is not limited to the setting of CDH. It is also seen in the oligohydramnios malformation sequence, with Potter's syndrome, and with several other chromosomal or malformation syndromes.

ESOPHAGEAL ATRESIA WITH TRACHEOESOPHAGEAL FISTULA

An abnormality of separation between the trachea and esophagus during the fourth to sixth week of intrauterine life leads to this anomaly, the incidence of which is approximately 1:3000 live births. Several anatomic arrangements are possible, as shown in Figure 28–17. Data indicate that 35% of children with tracheoesophageal fistula (TEF) also have a preterm delivery. Approximately 50% of infants with TEF have a recognizable constellation of anomalies that include vertebral abnormalities, imperforate anus, abnormalities of the radius, and congenital heart disease. This constellation of anomalies is refered to as the VATER or VACTERL complex.

Polyhydramnios, caused by the inability of the fetus to swallow amniotic fluid, is a clue to the presence of this defect. The combination of polyhydramnios and prematurity further suggests this condition. Although these infants are generally well at the time of delivery, they rapidly come to attention because of inability to handle oral secretions or as a result of choking and coughing during feedings. Over time, lung damage occurs because of reflux of gastric secretions directly into the lungs. Diagnosis is usually made when a nasogastric tube is seen (on a chest radiograph) to coil in the esophageal pouch rather than enter the stomach.

Immediate management of this condition includes placing the infant in the reverse Trendelenburg position to minimize reflux of gastric contents into the lungs and placing a catheter with constant suction in the proximal esophageal pouch to eliminate upper airway compromise. Adequate temperature control, ventilatory stability, and hydration should be assured. Surgical treatment is definitive and is always required; the procedure of choice depends on the exact characteristics of the defect. The prognosis is generally good except when premature birth or associated congenital anomalies add their own morbidities and morality risk.

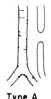

Type A
Esophageal atresia without tracheo-esophageal fistula.
Frequency 8%

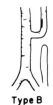

Type B
Esophageal atresia with proximal tracheo-esophageal fistula.
Frequency 1%

Type C
Esophageal atresia with distal tracheo-esophageal fistula.
Frequency 86%

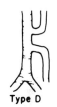

Type D
Esophageal atresia with both proximal and distal tracheo-esophageal fistulae.
Frequency 1%

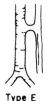

Type E
Tracheo-esophageal fistula without esophageal atresia (H-type).
Frequency 4%

Figure 28–17. Tracheoesophageal anomalies: type and incidence. (Reproduced by permission from Sunshine P et al: Gastrointestinal disorders. In Fanaroff MB, Martin RJ (eds): Berman's Textbook of Neonatal–Perinatal Medicine: Diseases of the Fetus and Infant, 3rd ed. St Louis, The CV Mosby Company, 1983)

BRONCHOPULMONARY DYSPLASIA

Bronchopulmonary dysplasia (BPD), or chronic lung disease of infancy, is a pulmonary disorder that has emerged in parallel with the increasing survival of prematurely born infants with respiratory disease. Its occurrence is closely linked to gestational age at birth, with younger, smaller babies at higher risk. The risk of developing BPD is also strongly associated with the presence of SDD. Although no single "cause" has been agreed on, the need for positive-pressure ventilation, with high

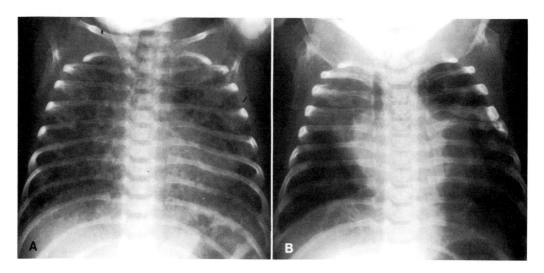

Figure 28—18. (A) Bronchopulmonary dysplasia in a 2-month-old child with severe hyaline membrane disease and prolonged oxygen and ventilatory therapy. Bilateral diffuse interstitial fibrosis and cystic change are present, consistent with stage IV bronchopulmonary dysplasia of Northway (see text). (B) Bronchopulmonary dysplasia in a 2½-month-old patient who had severe hyaline membrane disease, prolonged ventilator and oxygen therapy, and ligation for persistent patent ductus arteriosus. There is now advanced bronchopulmonary dysplasia, with areas of cystic overexpansion of the lower lobes and considerable interstitial fibrosis, not well seen because of the marked cystic changes. The heart is enlarged by cor pulmonale.

concentrations of oxygen seems to be intimately involved in the pathogenesis of this disorder.

Attempts to study BPD have been hampered by the lack of a uniformly accepted definition. Most commonly, the onset of BPD is insidious. Typically, the diagnosis is first considered when a premature baby who is recovering from respiratory disease but continues to require mechanical ventilation and supplemental oxygen ceases to improve or begins to worsen during the second or third week of life. If at an age of 28 days an infant recovering from lung disease continues to require supplemental oxygen, exhibits tachypnea and retractions, with crackles heard by auscultation, and has an abnormal chest radiograph, a diagnosis of BPD may be made (Fig. 28–18). A more recently proposed definition would require these same findings to be present at a corrected gestational age of 36 weeks. There are data to suggest that this latter definition may be the more useful one.

The incidence of BPD varies among reporting authors. This variation in reported occurrence ranges between 6% and 62%, with an average of approximately 30% in infants with birth weights less than 1500g and SDD. Most of the variation in incidence is due not to actual differences in outcome of patients but, rather, to differing popula-

tions reported on and to different definitions of BPD. The frequency of BPD is strongly linked to gestational age, as is shown in Table 28–14.

Although there is no generally agreed upon single cause for BPD, it is generally agreed that the high concentrations of inspired oxygen and positive-pressure ventilation interact with an immature lung such as to lead to the alterations that constitute BPD. Pathologically, BPD is characterized by

Table 28—14 Frequency of Bronchopulmonary Dysplasia as a Function of Birth Weight

BIRTH WEIGHT (g)	INFANTS WITH BPD (%)
701–800	76.1
801–900	68.8
901–1000	46.4
1001–1250	26.0
1251–1500	12.9

(Adapted from Avery ME, Tooley WH, Keller JB et al: Is chronic lung disease in low birth weight infants preventable? Pediatrics 79:26–30, 1987)

several findings. The alveolar structure is abnormal, with fibrosis of alveolar septae and with areas of alveolar overdistention immediately adjacent to areas of atelectasis. Some acini are destroyed. Pulmonary edema is universally present. The small conducting airways exhibit increased thickness of the submucosal muscular layer and abnormal extension of the muscular layer down the bronchial tree. Additionally, there is excessive production of mucus and alteration in function of the mucociliary escalator. A newly emerging feature of this disease is the frequent involvement of the large airways, manifested as tracheomalacia, bronchomalacia, inspissation of secretions, and occlusion of airways by growth of granulation tissue. The microscopic examination of the pulmonary vascular bed shows abnormal muscular thickening and abnormal extension of the muscular layer down through succeeding generations of vessels. Pulmonary artery hypertension is commonly present. Cor pulmonale may occur in children who are severely affected.

These anatomic abnormalities have pathophysiologic consequences. The presence of atelectatic alveoli leads to venous admixture and hypoxemia, whereas the result of emphysematous overdistention in other lung units with high ventilation/perfusion ratios is carbon dioxide retention. Pulmonary fibrosis and pulmonary edema both decrease lung compliance. As a result of the small-airways abnormalities, there is increased resistance to airflow caused by anatomic narrowing of the lumen and the presence of excessive quantities of mucus. Reactive airways disease is a consequence as well. Abnormalities of the large conducting airways may lead to persistent wheezing or stridor. Persistent elevation of pulmonary artery pressures has the potential to lead to cor pulmonale, with heart failure as the ultimate consequence.

As a result of these abnormalities, children with BPD have hypoxemia and hypercarbia, an elevated respiratory rate, retractions, and crackles on examination. They generally have an increased work of breathing. The increased work of breathing often leads to growth failure, despite a caloric intake that would be adequate for normal children. Patients with BPD may have acute worsening of their respiratory condition if their fluid intake leads to a worsening of their pulmonary edema. Another cause of acute deterioration is reactive airways disease.

Treatment of these children is difficult and complicated. Most aspects of therapy have not undergone rigorous trials to establish proof of benefit. Babies with BPD generally require prolonged administration of supplemental oxygen and, often, require prolonged mechanical ventilation. Diuretic agents that ameliorate the abnormalities of pulmonary mechanics related to pulmonary edema are frequently used, but have not been shown to improve the ultimate outcome. Abnormalities in electrolyte balance are common among children treated with diuretics. Fluid restriction may be helpful, but the associated caloric restriction can be a problem because of the frequent requirement for a supranormal caloric intake to achieve growth. Often the feeding of formulas with increased caloric density is helpful in producing weight gain.

Therapy with bronchodilators, such as theophylline or various inhaled β-adrenergic agents, has produced beneficial changes in pulmonary mechanics, but whether this corresponds to improvement in longer-term outcome is not known with certainty. Therapy with corticosteroids recently has been proposed to be of benefit for ventilator-dependent infants with BPD. Currently, data indicate that there *is* a benefit from corticosteroids for the duration of therapy, with improvement in lung compliance and resistance and a need for less support from the mechanical ventilator. However, data also show that these improvements tend to reverse when the corticosteroids are stopped. Also, several series have shown a concerning incidence of sepsis among children given corticosteroids for the amelioration of BPD. At present, the use of these drugs for this purpose cannot be considered routine.

Bronchopulmonary dysplasia has a mortality rate of approximately 30%. Most deaths occur before discharge from the hospital. Children who survive to discharge not infrequently require home oxygen therapy, diuretic therapy, bronchodilator therapy, and special formulas, but have a prognosis for recovery that is good. Hospital readmissions during the first year of life are common and generally occur in association with viral respiratory tract infections. Growth failure is common in babies with BPD and, generally, growth improves simultaneously with improvement in lung function as indicated by clinical assessment.

Pulmonary function testing is able to detect abnormalities for many years in children who have recovered from BPD. The children generally do not have exercise intolerance and are able to keep up with their peers. Respiratory symptom questionnaires have, in some studies, detected a higher incidence of symptoms, such as cough and wheezing, in children who have recovered from BPD. Provocation with methacholine inhalation in the pulmonary function testing laboratory and assessment of response to inhaled bronchodilators has supplied evidence that there is a higher than anticipated incidence of reactive airways in children with BPD. Physician-diagnosed reactive airways disease (asthma) is not uncommon in these children. Despite these findings the great majority of children discharged with BPD will gradually recover, wean from oxygen and medications, and have pulmonary function that permits participation in normal childhood activities.

PRACTICAL ASPECTS OF NEONATAL RESPIRATORY THERAPY

OXYGEN ADMINISTRATION

Oxygen is a drug critical for the survival of newborns with respiratory problems. As with other drugs, it must be administered in the proper dosage to avoid unintended effects. Therapy with oxygen is complicated in that the appropriate "dosage" varies widely from one patient to another and even from one time to another for the same patient. Whatever the mode of delivery, oxygen therapy requires continuous monitoring of the FIO_2, continuous monitoring of the temperature of the delivered gas, and ongoing assessment of the adequacy of therapy.

Two organs seem to be at risk for adverse effects during oxygen therapy—the retina and the lungs. The toxic effects of oxygen on the retina are related to the PaO_2 that is achieved. The effect of oxygen on the retina depends on the stage of development of the retinal vessels and the duration of exposure to excessive levels of oxygen. Preterm infants are most at risk, and the more premature a baby is, the greater the risk. Currently, most infants with significant retinopathy of prematurity were born with birth weight less than 1000 g. To prevent retinal damage the PaO_2 must be kept below the level that stimulates vasoconstriction of retinal vessels. Vasoconstriction for very short periods seems to be reversible, whereas this may no longer be so after prolonged periods. The exact values for PaO_2 that are dangerous are not known with certainty. However, current recommendations are to maintain the PaO_2 below the 80-mmHg level.

The toxic effects of high concentrations of inspired oxygen on the lungs are well described in animals, in which a specific sequence of pathologic changes can be observed. Infants who require therapy with high concentrations of inspired oxygen are at greater risk for the development of BPD.

METHODS OF OXYGEN DELIVERY

Hood Oxygen Therapy

For infants who are breathing without the need for positive airway pressure, hood oxygen delivery systems provide the most precise control of FIO_2, temperature, and humidification of gases delivered. Hood oxygen delivery requires flow rates of fresh gas that are adequate to expel carbon dioxide and maintain the intended FIO_2. The minimum flow rate that will ensure that an infant will not rebreathe expired gases is 8 L/min. The hood chosen should fit comfortably around the infant's neck, but have only a minor leak. The use of a blender system with hood oxygen delivery is preferred because it offers easier control of FIO_2 and reduces the level of noise within the hood. Blender systems also permit quicker and more precise alterations in the delivered FIO_2. The FIO_2 and temperature should be continuously monitored as close to the baby's face as possible. It is important to recognize that radiant warmers and phototherapy lights can alter the temperature within the hood.

Newborns are not able to precisely control their body temperatures, in part because of their large surface area/body mass ratio. As a result they are best cared for in a thermoneutral environment—that is, the environment that allows the lowest possible oxygen consumption. The range of temperatures that leads to a thermoneutral environment for a newborn varies with age after birth and with weight. This means that each newborn has an ideal ambient temperature that will avoid cold stress, the need to burn calories, and the need to increase oxygen consumption to maintain body temperature. Failure to maintain a thermoneutral environment is the most common cause of hypothermia and can substantially worsen an infant's condition. Circulation of cold gas across the face and head of an infant can disrupt a thermoneutral environment and lead to hypothermia.

Nasal Cannula and Face Mask

Oxygen may be delivered by nasal cannula to larger infants who are in the convalescent stage of a respiratory illness or who have BPD. The use of this delivery system during an acute illness is not appropriate. For successful use, the FIO_2 that is required by the infant should be 0.35 or less. Nasal cannula flow rates should be no greater than 1.0 L/min, because excessive drying of the nasal mucosa and gastric distention can result at higher flow rates. The most important use of nasal cannula oxygen therapy is as part of a home oxygen therapy program, allowing early discharge of infants with BPD.

Face masks for oxygen delivery are available in sizes that are appropriate for newborns. These are only occasionally useful, as for short-term administration of oxygen during transport or special procedures. It is important to realize that the flow rate chosen must be sufficient to prevent the rebreathing of exhaled gases. Delivery of oxygen at liter per minute flow rate gives no information on the alveolar Po_2. Therefore, when infants are transferred from one delivery system to another (oxygen hood, mask, or nasal cannula), the adequacy of therapy must be assured by pulse oximetry or blood gas determination.

Continuous Positive Airway Pressure Delivery

Continuous positive airway pressure can be delivered in several ways, no one of which is clearly superior to the others for all circumstances. Most commonly, CPAP is delivered by nasal prongs (Hudson prongs), but is can also be delivered by a single nasopharyngeal tube or by an endotracheal tube. Nasal prongs are subject to displacement but do not become obstructed very frequently and do not increase expiratory resistance. A disadvantage to this delivery system is the loss of CPAP and FIO_2 that may occur during mouth breathing or crying. Nasopharyngeal tubes are more secure in their placement but can become plugged with secretions, resulting in loss of pressure and FIO_2. An endotracheal tube has the advantages of security of placement and very constant pressure and FIO_2 delivery, but it has the disadvantages of requiring endotracheal intubation, creating increased resistance to airflow, with the possibility of inducing respiratory fatigue and the need for repeated tracheal suctioning. The use of face masks, head chambers, and negative-pressure devices is of historical interest only.

The most efficient way to create CPAP is by using a mechanical ventilator in the CPAP mode. This has the additional advantage of in-line monitoring of FIO_2 and alarm systems. It is possible, however, to construct a CPAP system using a gas flow system, water "pop-off," and a screw valve attached to an anesthesia bag, as shown in Figure 28–19. A major disadvantage of such a system is the need for additional equipment to continuously

Figure 28—19.   System for applying CPAP by endotracheal tube: A, gas inflow; B, oxygen monitor; C, Norman elbow; D, endotracheal tube connectors; E, endotracheal tube; F, Sommers T-piece; G, corrugated tubing; H, anesthesia bag; I, screw clamp; J, pressure manometer; K, T-connector; L, pressure exhaust tube; M, underwater seal. (Thibeault DW, Gregory GA (eds): Neonatal Pulmonary Care, 2nd ed. Norwalk, Conn, Appleton & Lange, 1987, with permission)

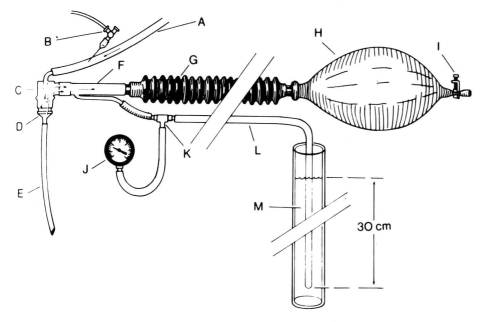

monitor FIO_2 and to alarm for unwanted pressure changes.

Mechanical Ventilators

Reference is made to the previous section concerning mechanical ventilation of the newborn for issues concerning patient management. This section deals with the ventilator itself. Virtually all neonatal ventilators in use today are of the time-cycled, pressure-limited type. A constant gas flow between 5 and 15 L/min is present at the junction between the endotracheal tube and the ventilator. The baby is able to draw on this constant flow during spontaneous breaths, without rebreathing exhaled gases. Inspiration occurs by mechanical obstruction of the expiratory limb of the gas flow circuit and lasts for a period chosen by the operator of the ventilator. This is the *inspiratory time,* the time-cycled component of this type of ventilation. The operator of the ventilator also limits the peak pressure that the ventilator is allowed to generate during inspiration. This is the assigned *peak inspiratory pressure.* Note that the volume of gas that enters the ventilator circuit and the infant is unassigned and unknown. The infant's tidal volume, therefore, is unknown.

Newborns can and do breathe spontaneously both in between and during inspirations given by the mechanical ventilator. It is important to note that some infant ventilators only supply a continual flow of gas in between mechanical inflations. Examples of this type of ventilator include the Bourns BP 200, Bear Cub BP 200, and various Healthdyne models. Attempts by the infant to spontaneously breath during mechanical inspiration, in the absence of gas flow, may result in carbon dioxide retention. Ventilators that supply a true continual flow throughout the respiratory cycle include the BABYbird, BABYbird 2A, Sechrist IV 100B, and the Infant Star.

Several other features are highly desirable for infant ventilators. A digital display of airway pressures, ventilator rate, inspiratory time, and expiratory time makes operation easier. Ventilator pressure alterations are more precise when a digital display exists than when pressures must be read from a cycling manometer. One very useful feature is a digital display of the mean airway pressure. This allows more accurate assessment of changes in an infant's condition and allows better comparison of results of different ventilatory strategies. Independent control of inspiratory time is essential. It is also essential that the ventilator be able to deliver rates as high as 150 BPM.

Certain safety features are an advantage. Not only should the ventilator alarm when a function is violated, such as loss of pressure, but, in some way, it should communicate to the operator which function is involved. Alarms are important for high peak inspiratory pressure, high end-expiratory pressure, and for loss of either of these pressures. An additional important alarm function is that of rate–time incompatibility. This occurs when the combination chosen of rate and inspiratory time is impossible to achieve (e.g., a rate of 100 BPM, with an inspiratory time of 1.0 second). An alarm that notifies the operator of airway obstruction is an advantage.

Infants have small tidal volumes, and their inspiratory time is often short: therefore, the circuit for the infant ventilator should have as low a compliance and as small a dead space as possible. As with other oxygen delivery systems, the delivered gas should be humidified and maintained at a constant temperature. If the temperature is allowed to vary, the compressible volume of the gas will change, and this may affect the volume delivered to the infant. The gas temperature should be measured as close to the infant as possible, because other patient equipment (a radiant warmer, for example) may alter gas temperature.

Aerosol Administration

Administration of β-adrenergic agonists improves pulmonary function in children with BPD, at least as assessed over the course of several hours. Spontaneously breathing infants may receive these drugs through a nebulizer after dilution with normal saline. Racemic epinephrine may also be given in this manner to extubated infants who are having difficulty with upper airway swelling. Intubated infants can be removed from the mechanical ventilator, a nebulizer placed in line between an anesthesia circuit and the baby, and the medication may be administered by manual inflations. When using this technique, care must be taken not to increase the FIO_2 or the inflating pressures beyond those with which the infant is being ventilated.

Ribavirin, an antiviral agent used in the treatment of respiratory syncytial virus (RSV) infections, comes with the manufacturer's warning against its use in children who are receiving mechanical ventilation. Ribavirin is usually administered for 12 to 18 hr/day for 3 to 7 days by a special-

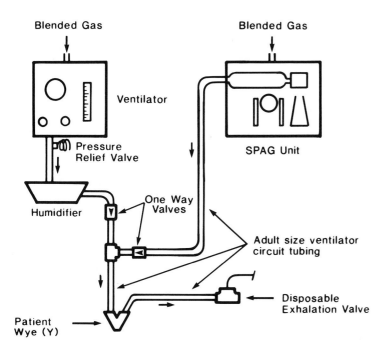

Figure 28–20. Apparatus used at New England Medical Center for administration of ribavirin during mechanical ventilation with a time-cycled, pressure-limited ventilator. The entire circuit is inspected every 2 hours for precipitation, and the exhalation valve is replaced at least every 4 hours.

ized delivery system called a small-particle aerosol generator (SPAG; see Chap. 17). The manufacturer warns against administration during mechanical ventilation because the drug may crystallize in the expiratory limb and the exhalation valve, thereby leading to the delivery of inordinately high airway pressures. However, some authors have reasoned that children ill enough to require mechanical ventilation are the ones who are most in need of treatment with this agent. Several descriptions of results of protocols for treatment during ventilation have been published. Given its potential for teratogenicity ribavirin therapy must still be considered investigational and should be done under the auspices of an institutional review board-approved protocol for human investigation and with informed consent for participation of the child in a research protocol.

The mechanics for administration of ribavirin during mechanical ventilation at our own institution are shown in Figure 28–20. Specific modifications made include use of adult-sized ventilator tubing, humidifier temperature maintained at 35° to 37° C, and use of a double-alarm system. Additionally, the entire circuit is inspected every 2 hours, and the disposable exhalation valve is replaced every 4 hours, or sooner if crystallization is seen. At a minimum, the entire circuit is replaced every 8

hours. Continuous pulse oximetry is used during this therapy.

Chest Physical Therapy

Chest physical therapy (CPT) or bronchopulmonary segmental drainage uses three techniques—percussion, vibration, and postural drainage—to loosen secretions and move then into a larger airway for removal. It is helpful for a prescribing physician to specify the frequency, mode, and area of concentration of this therapy. The duration of therapy is chosen by the amount of secretions and on how well the baby tolerates the procedure. For maximal effectiveness, the lobe or segment of the lung at which therapy is directed should be known to the person performing the CPT. It is also important for the therapist to know the anatomic location of each bronchus and the position that drains each bronchus. Therapy should emphasize the area most involved, and that area should be in the most vertical (superior) position, to facilitate movement of secretions from smaller to larger airways. Drainage from one area usually means drainage into another area and, consequently, the opposite lobe or segment should also be treated if all positions are not being done.

Percussion uses mechanical energy applied to

the chest wall to detach secretions from airway walls and allow drainage. A common way to do this is with an infant resuscitation mask with the 15-mm adapter occluded to make a cushion of air. Speed and force of percussion need not be excessive; a relaxed rhythmic rate will achieve adequate segmental drainage. Each area should be percussed for 3 to 5 minutes.

Chest physical therapy given to adults includes vibration during expiration. The high respiratory rate typical of newborns precludes exclusive expiratory-phase vibration. Commonly, a mechanical vibrator is used; a padded electric toothbrush will function very well for this purpose also. Two minutes of vibration to each area is recommended.

Sometimes CPT constitutes a significant stress for ill infants. This is often manifested as arterial desaturation during therapy, which may continue after therapy is completed. For this reason CPT should not be given within one-half hour of feedings. Percussion is not recommended for infants weighing less than 1500 g because of the possibility of bruising and rib fracture. Most infants will generally do well with vibration only, although a few will tolerate changes in position as the sole form of CPT.

Monitoring

Management of newborns receiving oxygen therapy requires accurate and continuous monitoring to ensure both the adequacy and safety of therapy. Both hyperoxia and hypoxia must be avoided. Arterial blood gas levels are the gold standard for patient management, but even when an indwelling arterial line is present this information will be available only intermittently. It has been demonstrated that the use of transcutaneous Po_2 monitors and pulse oximeters has the potential to reduce the amount of time spent with undesirable oxygenation.

Transcutaneous monitors measure the partial pressure of oxygen and sometimes carbon dioxide that diffuses through the skin. This is accomplished by heating the skin to produce local vasodilatation and to facilitate diffusion. The transcutaneous Po_2 ($tcPo_2$) approximates the PaO_2 closely and, for a given infant, the differences between these two values should be constant over several hours time. For safety considerations, as well as for concerns about accuracy, these devices should be used in strict compliance with the manufacturer's guidelines. This is of particular concern for skin temperature and the interval between changing of sites with recalibration. During the warmup time,

readings are unreliable. It is especially important that the membrane be in good contact with the skin and that bony areas be avoided. Several conditions, including hypothermia, poor peripheral perfusion, hypovolemia, and subcutaneous edema, as well as the drug tolazoline, will make $tcPo_2$ values less reliable.

Pulse oximetry is a recent advance in the monitoring of oxygenation. A color difference between oxygenated and deoxygenated hemoglobin makes this method of monitoring possible. Extinction is a measure of how dark or absorptive a given material, here hemogobin, is at a specified wavelength of light. Oximetry is based on an empirically derived extinction curve for hemoglobin in human subjects. The extinction at 660 nm is compared with the extinction at 940 nm, and this ratio is translated into a percentage saturation of hemoglobin by comparison with an internal calibration curve. The value given on the digital display is oxygen saturation or SaO_2.

The pulse oximeter is extremely accurate. When the ECG-determined heart rate agrees with the pulse oximeter heart rate and the oximeter waveform is regular and of good amplitude, the accuracy of a pulse oximeter is ± 2%. The response time of the oximeter is very short, measured in seconds. This high degree of accuracy and the short response time are advantages of oximetry over $tcPo_2$ monitoring.

Despite the usefulness of this technique, there are several limitations to pulse oximetery. The oximeter will be unable to give accurate data if it cannot detect an adequate waveform. This sometimes represents a problem in location of the oximeter lead. This problem can be minimized by using the oximeter in exact accordance with the manufacturer's recommendations. When an infant has significant compromise of cardiac output, as during cardiogenic or hypovolemic shock, the oximeter may be unable to detect arterial pulsations and, thus, be unable to determine saturation values.

Another limitation of pulse oximetry relates to the shape of the oxyhemoglobin dissociation curve. Adult hemoglobin becomes essentially 100% saturated at a PaO_2 of 75 mmHg and fetal hemoglobin at the significantly lower value of 55 mmHg. Thus, a pulse oximeter will be unable to discriminate between the newborn with a PaO_2 of 60 mmHg and the newborn with a PaO_2 of 250 mmHg. Hyperoxia can be avoided when it is important to do so, as with preterm infants, by administering oxygen to obtain an oxygen saturation of 93% to 95%. This allows the oxygen content of the blood to be nearly maximal while ensuring that the PaO_2 will not be dangerously high.

Capnography or end-tidal carbon dioxide determination is currently undergoing evaluation to determine its role in neonatal respiratory management. End-tidal carbon dioxide is the carbon dioxide in the last portion of an expired breath; these terminal gases have their origins in the alveolar space. When the lung consists of multiple homogeneous units, end-tidal carbon dioxide reflects alveolar PCO_2 accurately. Under most circumstances, alveolar PCO_2 equals arterial PCO_2. Expired gas is analyzed for absorption of infrared light and the carbon dioxide content is read at a specific wavelength. Thus, these devices have the potential to continuously determine and display arterial PCO_2. However, the assumption that the lung is made of homogeneously emptying smaller units is often untrue when lung disease, which tends to be heterogeneous, is present. The relation between end-tidal carbon dioxide and alveolar carbon dioxide concentrations then becomes uncertain. Other assumptions made in the use of end-tidal carbon dioxide monitoring include a constant rate of carbon dioxide production by the baby and constant pulmonary capillary blood flow. In certain disease states, either of these assumptions may be untrue as well. These considerations have limited the use of this type of monitoring to intraoperative monitoring of infants with healthy lungs. Whether further refinements in this technique will lead to greater applicability remains to be seen.

BIBLIOGRAPHY

American Heart Association–American Academy of Pediatrics: Neonatal resuscitation. In Chameides L (ed): Textbook of Pediatric Advanced Life Support, pp 69–76. American Heart Association, 1988

Bartlett RH, Roloff DW, Cornell RG et al: Extracorporeal circulation in neonatal respiratory failure: A prospective randomized study. Pediatrics 76:479–487, 1985

Bland RD: Pathogenesis of pulmonary edema after premature birth. Adv Pediatr 34:175–222, 1987

Bohn D, Tamura M, Perrin D et al: Ventilatory predictors of pulmonary hypoplasia in congenital diaphragmatic hernia, confirmed by morphologic assessment. J Pediatr 111:423–431, 1987

Boyden EA: Growth and development of the airways. In Hodson WA (ed): Development of the Lung, pp 3–35. New York, Marcel Dekker, 1977

Bucciarelli RL, Egan EA, Gessner IH, Eitzman DV: Persistence of fetal cardiopulmonary circulation: One manifestation of transient tachypnea of the newborn. Pediatrics 58:192–197, 1976

Carson BS, Losey BW, Bowes WA, Simmons MA: Combined obstetric and pediatric approach to prevent meconium aspiration syndrome. Am J Obstet Gynecol 126:712–715, 1976

Fiascone JM, Rhodes TT, Grandgeorge SR, Knapp MA: Bronchopulmonary dysplasia: A review for the pediatrician. Curr Probl Pediatr 19:169–227, 1989

Fox WW, Duara S: Persistent pulmonary hypertension in the neonate: Diagnosis and management. J Pediatr 103:505–514, 1983

Fox WW, Gewitz MH, Dinwiddie R et al: Pulmonary hypertension in the perinatal aspiration syndromes. Pediatrics 59:205–211, 1977

Fox WW, Murray JP, Martin RJ: Transient tachypnea. In Fanaroff AA, Martin RJ (eds): Behrman's Neonatal–Perinatal Medicine: Diseases of the Fetus and Infant, pp 447–448. St Louis, CV Mosby, 1983

Givner LB, Baker CJ: The prevention and treatment of neonatal group B streptococcal infections. Adv Pediatr Infect Dis 3:65–90, 1988

Gregory GA: Continuous positive airway pressure. In Thibeault DW, Gregory GA (eds): Neonatal Pulmonary Care, 2nd ed, pp 349–366. Norwalk, Conn, Appleton–Century–Crofts, 1986

Gross I: Regulation of fetal lung maturation. In Ballard P (ed): Respiratory Distress Syndrome, pp 51–64. London, Academic Press, 1984

Halliday HL, McClure G, Reid MAC: Transient tachypnea of the newborn: Two distinct clinical entities? Arch Dis Child 56:322–325, 1981

Hansen J, James S, Burrington J, Whitfield J: The decreasing incidence of pneumothorax and improving survival of infants with congenital diaphragmatic hernia. J Pediatr Surg 19:385–388, 1984

Jobe A: Surfactant and the developing lung. In Thibeault DW, Gregory GA (eds): Neonatal Pulmonary Care, 2nd ed, pp 75–100. Norwalk, Conn, Appleton–Century–Crofts, 1986

Jobe A, Ikegami M: Surfactant for the treatment of respiratory distress syndrome. Am Rev Respir Dis 136:1256–1275, 1987

Madansky DL, Lawson EE, Chernick V, Taeusch HW: Pneumothorax and other forms of pulmonary air leak in newborns. Am Rev Respir Dis 120:729–737, 1979

Mannino FL, Merritt TA: The management of respiratory distress syndrome. In Thibeault DW,

Gregory GA (eds): Neonatal Pulmonary Care, 2nd ed, pp 349–366. Norwalk, Conn, Appleton–Century–Crofts, 1986

Martin MJ, Miller RJ, Carlo WA: Pathogenesis of apnea in preterm infants. J Pediatr 109:733–741, 1986

O'Brodovich HM, Mellins RB: Bronchopulmonary dysplasia: Unresolved neonatal lung injury. Am Rev Respir Dis 132:694–709, 1985

Payne NR, Burke BA, Day DL et al: Correlation of clinical and pathologic findings in early onset neonatal group B streptococcal infection with disease severity and prediction of outcome. Pediatr Infect Dis J 7:836–848, 1988

Peabody JL, Hay WW, Anderson JV: Proceedings of the Broadmoor Symposium: The uses, benefits and limitations of pulse oximetry in neonatal medicine—an education and research oriented program. J Perinatol 7:306–349, 1987

Perlman JM, Volpe JJ: Episodes of apnea and bradycardia in the preterm newborn: Impact on cerebral circulation. Pediatrics 76:333–338, 1985

Reid LM: Structural development of the lung and pulmonary circulation. In Ballard P (ed): Respiratory Distress Syndrome, pp 3–18. London, Academic Press, 1984

Reynolds M, Luck SR, Lappen R: The "critical" neonate with diaphragmatic hernia: A 21 year perspective. J Pediatr Surg 19:385–388, 1984

Spitzer AR, Fox WW: The use and abuse of mechanical ventilation in respiratory distress syndrome. In Stern L (ed): Hyaline Membrane Disease, pp 145–174. Orlando, Fla, Grune & Stratton, 1984

Sullivan JL: Iron, plasma antioxidants, and the 'oxygen radical disease of prematurity.' Am J Dis Child 142:1341–1344, 1988

Sunshine P, Sinatra FR, Mitchell CH, Santulli TV: Esophageal atresia and tracheoesophageal fistula. In Fanaroff AA, Martin RJ (eds): Behrman's Neonatal–Perinatal Medicine: Diseases of the Fetus and Infant, pp 496–498. St Louis, CV Mosby, 1983

Teitel D, Rudolph AM: Perinatal oxygen delivery and cardiac function. Adv Pediatr 32:321–348, 1985

Wung JT, James LS, Kilchevsky E, James E: Management of infants with severe respiratory failure and persistence of the fetal circulation, without hyperventilation. Pediatrics 76:488–494, 1985

TWENTY-NINE

Respiratory Care for the Infant and Child

Robert M. Lewis
Stephen L. Thompson
Allen I. Goldberg

It is quite common for practitioners to feel insecure in caring for infants and children. In part, this stems from lack of knowledge of how the infant and child differ physiologically and anatomically from the adult. The lungs and related structures in children are not only different from adults, but undergo substantial change from birth to adulthood. The study of developmental physiology and anatomy, then, is essential to understanding disease and therapy in pediatrics.

Our objective in this chapter is to summarize differences in respiratory physiology and anatomy, discuss how these differences affect patterns of respiratory illness, and how they suggest differing therapeutic approaches in the child. Next, we will review the application of common respiratory care techniques to the child, and, finally, we will review in detail some of the more important pediatric respiratory diseases. We hope that this information, coupled with carefully guided clinical training, will prepare the respiratory care professional or student for the challenges of pediatric care.

RESPIRATORY ANATOMY AND PHYSIOLOGY IN INFANTS AND CHILDREN

The lungs, chest, and airways of infants and children differ from the adult's in their size, structure, and function. These differences influence the epi-demiology, pathophysiology, therapy, and outcome of respiratory illness. We will explore some of these differences, and their clinical significance.

AIRWAYS

General Considerations

The airways of the infant and small child are smaller and less rigid than the adult's. Both these factors encourage obstruction and collapse. Gas flow through tubes is described by Poiseuille's law, which states:

$$\text{Resistance} = \frac{8LN}{\pi R^4}$$

N refers to the viscosity of the gas and L to the length of the tube, two factors that do not change in response to airway obstruction. Likewise, the constants 8 and π do not vary with disease. Omitting these for simplicity, resistance is inversely proportional to the radius of the tube raised to the fourth power. As Figure 29–1 illustrates, a small amount of edema can greatly increase airway resistance when the lumen of the airway is already small; airway resistance increases little in response to an equal amount of edema when the airway lumen is large. The radii of all airways, from the trachea to the bronchioles, are smaller in the infant and child, ranging from one-third to one-half the adult size, and increasing gradually throughout childhood.[64]

Figure 29—1. Relative effects of airway edema in the infant and adult. The normal infant and adult airways are presented on the *left*, edematous airways (1-mm circumferential) on the *right*. Note that resistance to flow is inversely proportional to the radius of the lumen to the fourth power for laminar flow, and radius of the lumen to the fifth power for turbulent flow. The net result in the infant is a 75% reduction in cross-sectional area, a 16-fold increase in resistance, compared with a 44% reduction in cross-sectional area and a threefold increase in resistance in the adult. (Coté CJ, Todres ID: The pediatric airway. In Ryan JF, Todres ID, Coté CJ, Goudsouzian NH (ed): A Practice of Anesthesia for Infants and Children, p 39. Orlando, Grune & Stratton, 1986)

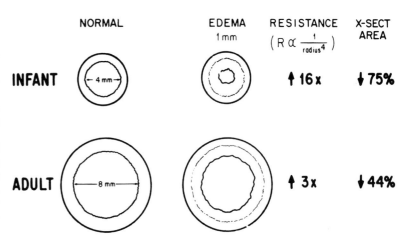

When faced with an airway obstruction, the young child in respiratory distress is likely to require greater airway pressure changes to move air. A laryngeal obstruction, for example, will prompt the patient to generate greater (more negative) inspiratory pressures to move air past the obstruction. This will result in a pressure drop inside the airways. Inside the thorax, the pressures in the airways will be less negative than intrapleural pressure. Hence, the transmural pressure gradient will favor intrathoracic airway dilatation during inspiration.

Those airways outside the thorax will respond differently. Here, the pressure drop inside the airways during inspiration is not balanced by greater negative pressures in the surrounding tissues. Rather, the supporting tissues of the neck are at atmospheric pressure. Therefore, the transmural pressure gradient favors collapse. Paradoxically, the infant's attempt to overcome increased upper airway resistance results only in further collapse of the airway. This process is exacerbated by the fact that the larynx and trachea of the developing child are less cartilaginous and more prone to collapse.[237]

These same concepts apply to intrathoracic airways obstruction. These airways, however, are more likely to collapse during exhalation. The foregoing mechanisms result in dilatation of the intrathoracic airways during inspiration, minimizing the effects of any obstruction. During expiration, when intrapleural pressure becomes positive, pressure surrounding the airways becomes greater than the pressure within. If the airway is critically narrow because of inflammation or bronchospasm, airway collapse can easily occur. Given that infants' and children's airways are already small and lack

adequate supportive structures, peripheral airway obstruction can lead to severe distress in children.

Figure 29–2 illustrates the relationship between changes in intrapleural pressures and airway collapse.

The Upper Airway

The infant is regarded as an "obligate" nose breather until aged 3 to 5 months.[237] This results, in part, from the relatively large tongue in infants, and the lack of teeth, which permits more complete mouth closure. Nasal obstruction, as seen in viral infections, which is not usually a significant cause of respiratory distress in the older child and adult, can be life-threatening in the infant.[237] In addition, the infant's relatively large head and short neck predispose to flexion and airway obstruction. Unlike the older child or adult, the infant may lack the muscle strength and control to change head position to relieve obstruction.

The infant's larynx is structurally different than the adult's, and appears more prone to obstruction. It has the same number of tissue layers with the same cell size as the adult.[237] Hence, the response to trauma will be similar in magnitude to that in the adult. That is, we could expect a similar amount of edema formation, but in a larynx about one-third the diameter of the adult's. The larynx is at its smallest diameter at the level of the cricoid ring.[52] This cartilaginous structure completely surrounds the larynx. An increase in the thickness of the laryngeal wall must take place at the expense of the internal lumen of the airway, rather than expansion of its outer wall.

These factors suggest that upper airway ob-

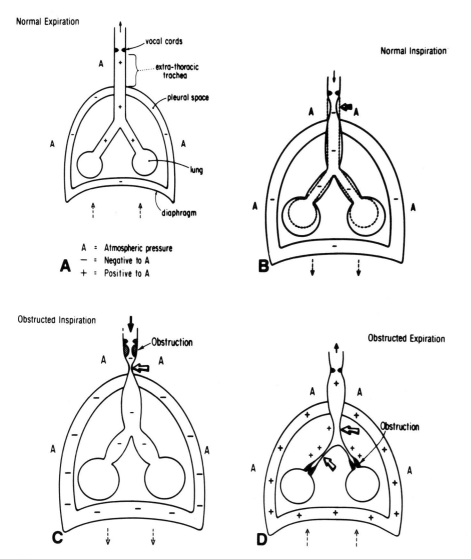

Figure 29—2. (*A*) The normal sequence of events at end-expiration is a slight negative intrapleural pressure stenting the airways open. In infants, the highly compliant chest does not provide the support required; thus, airway closure occurs with each breath. Intraluminal pressures are slightly positive in relation to atmospheric pressure, resulting in air being forced out of the lungs. With descent of the diaphragm and contraction of the intercostal muscles, a greater negative intra-thoracic pressure relative to intraluminal and atmospheric pressure is developed (*B*). The net result is stretching longitudinally of the larynx and trachea, dilatation of the intrathoracic trachea and bronchi, movement of air into the lungs, and some dynamic collapse of the extrathoracic trachea (*arrow*). The dynamic collapse is due to the highly compliant trachea and the negative intraluminal pressure in relation to atmospheric pressure. When airway obstruction is present (*C*), more severe dynamic collapse of the extrathoracic trachea occurs, just below the level of obstruction. This collapse is greatest at the thoracic inlet where the largest pressure gradient exists between negative intratracheal pressure and atmospheric pressure (*arrow*). (*D*) Breathing against an obstructed lower airway (as with bronchiolitis or asthma) results in greater positive intrathoracic pressures, with dynamic collapse of the intrathoracic airways (manifested by prolonged expiration or wheezing [*arrows*]). (Coté CJ, Todres ID: The pediatric airway. In Ryan JF, Todres ID, Coté CJ, Goudsouzian NH (eds): A Practice of Anesthesia for Infants and Children, p 41. Orlando, Fla, Grune & Stratton, 1986)

struction can occur quite readily in the child. Clinical experience demonstrates that acute or chronic upper airway obstruction is a frequent occurrence in children.

The Lower Airways

From birth to adulthood, the bronchioles of the developing lung experience a twofold increase in their diameter, but a threefold increase in bronchiolar wall thickness, and a four- to fivefold increase in the amount of supporting tissues surrounding the airways.[308] The walls of the airways will be thicker (and presumably stronger) in the older child and adult, than in the younger child and infant. In addition, the amount of bronchial smooth muscle (which provides some degree of bronchial wall stability[72]), although present in children, is less in proportion to the size of the airway than in adults.[64]

The relative weakness of the airways allows for greater changes in size in response to pressure changes. During inspiration, for example, airways may widen to a greater extent than occurs in the adult, accounting for the slightly greater dead space/body size ratio observed in younger children.[308] These factors, coupled with the smaller size of the airways, mean that the developing airways are more prone to collapse, not only with pathologic changes secondary to disease, but also during normal events, such as crying.

The lining of the airway walls in the developing lung has a much higher concentration of mucous glands than the mature lung. For example, a 4-year-old has twice the number of mucous glands per square millimeter of bronchial surface area as the adult.[64] Although the amount of mucus produced by the lung of a 4-year-old is generally quite small in comparison with an adult with chronic bronchitis, this smaller quantity of mucus obstructs the lumen of a smaller airway, greatly increasing airway resistance.

In addition to the small size and collapsibility of all the airways, Hogg and coworkers noted that in children under age 5 the small airways (those smaller than 2 mm in diameter) contribute as much as 50% of the total airway resistance. In contrast, small airways contribute between 10% and 20% of the total airways resistance in the adult.[138]

This implies that an obstruction resulting in a 50% increase in small-airway resistance would result in a 25% increase in total airway resistance. In contrast, a similar degree of obstruction in the adult would result in only a 10% increase in total airway resistance. We might then expect small-air-

way disorders to produce a greater symptomatic response in small children than in adults. In fact, respiratory pathogens that affect the bronchioles, such as respiratory syncytial virus, cause significant distress in the infant, but only mild symptoms in the adult.

Other investigators have disputed the claim that the small airways contribute such a large amount to the total airways resistance in the healthy child younger than 5.[302] Nonetheless, the small size of the infant's and child's bronchioles makes even a small amount of obstruction result in a significant increase in resistance, regardless of the contribution of the small airways to total airway resistance in the healthy child.

ALVEOLAR STRUCTURE AND FUNCTION

Alveolar Size and Number

The alveolar portion of the lung increases in size throughout childhood. During the first 2 to 3 years of life, this takes place mainly as a result of the development of new alveoli. Thereafter, the growth of the lungs occurs largely as a result of increased alveolar size.[57,305] Although most alveoli are formed in the first 2 to 3 years of life, it is not known at what age alveolar multiplication ceases. Some investigators believe that some new alveoli appear throughout childhood and adolescence.[237]

Knowledge of the normal growth pattern in the alveolar portion of the lung might assist in decisions for the timing of, for example, surgical interventions to correct space-occupying lesions in the chest. Correction before alveolar multiplication ceases might allow greater regeneration of lung tissue following pneumonectomy. There is evidence that considerable new alveolar growth occurs following pulmonary resections performed in infancy,[324] but not in adulthood.

Lung Volumes

Regardless of the relative contribution of increases in alveolar number or size, lung volumes increase throughout childhood, generally in proportion to height.[237] Furthermore, their relationships to one another is relatively constant throughout life. For example, the functional residual capacity (FRC), after the first few weeks of life, is about 40% of the total lung capacity (as in the adult) and correlates well with height.[308] Likewise, alveolar surface area (in proportion to weight, not height) is generally constant throughout life at 1 m²/kg.[216] Since one of the main functions of the FRC is to serve as a reservoir for oxygen (allowing oxygen uptake during expiration, periods of apnea, and airway obstruction), and alveolar surface area determines, in part, the rate of oxygen transfer from the lung to the blood, we might conclude that the infant or young child is as resistant to hypoxemia during these events as the adult. However, oxygen consumption per unit weight is increased in infants and small children and may be as much as 200% the adult value.[64] This rate of oxygen consumption suggests that the young child would deplete the oxygen reserves much faster than the adult. When viewed from this perspective, then, the FRC and alveolar surface area of the lung may prove inadequate to protect against hypoxemia during brief apneic episodes, as may occur during endotracheal intubation when muscle relaxants are used.

Alveolar Ventilation

Alveolar ventilation parallels oxygen consumption. That is, in the infant, alveolar ventilation is about twice that (based on weight) of the adult and gradually decreases throughout childhood.[237] Furthermore, the infant's and child's resting minute ventilation is closer to the maximum observed in healthy infants. For example, when crying—perhaps the most strenuous activity the infant can perform—ventilation only doubles. In contrast, an adult can increase ventilation 15 times in response to vigorous exercise.[324] These data imply that the infant and child are less well equipped to meet the increased ventilatory demands that accompany respiratory disease and conditions that increase oxygen consumption, such as fever.

Alveolar Structure

Structures that allow collateral ventilation—the pores of Kohn and canals of Lambert—may not be present in substantial quantities in the developing lung and may not contribute significantly to collateral ventilation until the age of 12 or 13.[64] This may facilitate alveolar collapse when airways are completely obstructed or alveolar overdistension when airway resistance is increased.

Elastic fibers are relatively deficient in the developing lung until the age of 12, at which time, elastic fibers are noted to be spread throughout the entire alveoli. Until this time, lung elastic recoil pressure is low in comparison with adults. The appearance of these fibers correlates with the increasing elastic recoil noted at this age.[237]

CHEST WALL AND VENTILATORY MUSCLES

Infants and children have a much higher chest wall compliance than the adult.[216] This means the chest wall will change shape easily in response to intrapleural pressure changes. In part, this lack of rigidity stems from decreased muscle mass and relatively cartilaginous ribs. Increasingly negative intrapleural pressures, as may occur when lung volume is low owing to atelectasis, pulmonary edema, adult respiratory distress syndrome (ARDS), or other cause, or during a maximal inspiratory effort, would be counterbalanced by the relative rigidity of the chest wall in the adult, and further loss of lung volume would be minimized. However, the flexible chest wall of the infant and child cannot offer much resistance to the negative intrapleural pressures seen in these conditions and, hence, loss of lung volume may be greater.

This lack of rigidity is also expressed in the indrawing of the soft tissues between the ribs (retractions) during inspiration in children with respiratory distress. (Increased intrapleural pressures from forced exhalation may cause intercostal bulging.) The use of energy to move the intercostal tissue, rather than air, during breathing increases the work load the young child faces when lung mechanics are altered. This may predispose the infant and young child to fatigue and respiratory failure.

In addition to the greater work load from increased chest wall compliance, there is evidence that the histologic structure of the infant diaphragm may predispose to fatigue. A high proportion of high oxidative diaphragmatic muscle fibers are necessary for the diaphragm to perform an increased work load over a prolonged period. This type of muscle fiber increases with age, until, at 1 year, the infant has the same proportion as the adult.[149]

In addition to increased vulnerability to fatigue, the small infant may have a decreased maximum diaphragmatic strength. Scott et al. found that the amount of pressure the infant diaphragm could generate was less than that of the adult, up until the age of 6 months.[262]

INTERACTIONS BETWEEN CHEST WALL, ALVEOLI, AND AIRWAYS

The chest wall, alveoli, and airways interact to produce the FRC and the closing capacity. The relatively high chest wall compliance of the child should produce a low functional residual capacity, as the chest offers little resistance to collapse. This tendency is opposed by other mechanisms, however. The increased respiratory frequency of children may terminate expiration at a higher lung volume than lung mechanics alone would dictate. Partial closure of the glottis may also be used to maximize end-expiratory volume.[324]

The low elasticity of the developing lung and airways may be responsible for the increased closing capacity noted in children.[213] *Closing capacity* refers to the volume at which airways begin to close during expiration. In the young, healthy adult, closing capacity is less than FRC;[213] that is, airways remain open throughout a normal inspiration and expiration. All lung units are available to participate in ventilation. However, in some disease states and in normal children, closing capacity may be greater than the FRC, especially in the supine position.[213] Consequently, some airway closure occurs during tidal breathing, with incomplete filling and emptying of some alveoli. This results in a ventilation–perfusion mismatch and may account for the slightly lower PaO_2 observed in young children. Low lung elasticity may be responsible for this phenomenon, as elastic fibers in the lung help to hold airways open.

The higher closing capacity noted in children may be of little significance in healthy children, but may have implications for children with small-airway obstructions. When airway lumen is decreased, higher pressures must be generated to maintain gas flow. Higher pressures during expiration promote airway collapse. This phenomenon, coupled with an already high closing capacity, could lead to a closing capacity much greater than tidal volume. Accordingly, many lung units would remain closed throughout the total respiratory cycle, worsening ventilation–perfusion mismatching, and hypoxemia.

PULMONARY VASCULATURE

The pulmonary arteries and arterioles contain a layer of smooth muscle, which constricts or dilates to match perfusion with ventilation. The differences between the adult and newborn in the amount and location of this muscle are well described and form the basis of our understanding of such significant neonatal disorders as persistent pulmonary hypertension of the newborn. Chief among these differences is the increased thickness of the muscular layer of the pulmonary artery and arterioles.[57] After birth, however, the thickness of this layer decreases. Furthermore, as new pulmonary arterioles develop in the first few years of life, they appear with relatively little or no smooth mus-

cle. As a result, pulmonary arterioles closest to the alveoli contain relatively little smooth muscle. This suggests that the vasoconstrictive response to alveolar hypoxia (which would redirect blood flow to better oxygenated alveoli) will be weak in young children. Only when the pulmonary vascular bed is complete does muscularization take the appearance, in amount and distribution, of the adult lung.[57]

MISCELLANEOUS FACTORS

Sleep State

The effects of sleep state on respiratory function have been studied extensively in the newborn and adult, and to a lesser extent, in children with lung diseases. In brief, drops in oxygen saturation, in part owing to chest wall instability and also changes in ventilatory pattern, are noted to occur during sleep, especially rapid eye movement sleep. Infants and children spend a larger amount of time sleeping than adults; therefore, the cumulative affects of sleep-related respiratory function changes may be greater in children than in adults.[237]

Position Change

Conscious adults and older children can voluntarily adjust their position to alleviate respiratory distress. For example, adults and children with chronic lung disease may position themselves in the sitting position to maximize accessory muscle function. Small infants are unable to do so. Likewise, infants are not able to sit up and dangle their legs, which may be beneficial to patients with pulmonary edema, nor can they turn their heads to the side when vomiting, increasing the risk for aspiration.

Response to Pain

Children are more likely to respond to pain by crying than are adults. Crying increases ventilatory work and oxygen consumption, and may lead to hypoxemia in infants with lung disease.[63] In children with near total airway obstruction, such as epiglottitis, painful procedures are avoided whenever possible, since crying may provoke total airway obstruction.

Cognitive Development

Small children lack the capacity to realize that entering a swimming pool or bathtub requires the ability to swim. Consequently, drowning accidents are quite common in the very young. Likewise, young children may not realize the dangers associated with ingestion of toxic or caustic substances, or the dangers associated with placing small objects in the mouth, and lack an appreciation of hygiene. As a result, foreign body aspiration and ingestion of caustic materials accounts for significant respiratory-related mortality and morbidity in children.

REACTION OF THE DEVELOPING LUNG AND AIRWAY TO INJURY

Specific respiratory problems will be dealt with later. However, some of the general patterns of how the developing lung responds to injury are worth considering here.

Insults to the respiratory system from infections, aspiration, congenital defects, and other causes often lead to airway function abnormalities in later life. Premature birth is associated with increased resistance in the small airways in later childhood, and is noted whether or not the infant was treated with oxygen or positive pressure.[47] Infections of the respiratory system, such as bronchiolitis[114] and croup,[113] are also associated with increased airway reactivity in later childhood and

with an increased likelihood of chronic lung disease as adults. Aspiration syndromes, as may occur following repair of tracheoesophageal fistula,[198] likewise are associated with an increased risk of bronchial hyperreactivity in later childhood, as are aspiration of foreign bodies,[104] and near-drowning.[166]

SEX-RELATED DIFFERENCES IN LUNG STRUCTURE AND FUNCTION

Boys have a higher frequency of severe respiratory ailments than girls. Although the reason for this is unclear, it may be related to differences in lung structure and function between boys and girls. Although boys generally have larger lungs than girls,[305] there is evidence to suggest boys' airways may be smaller. Infant girls have expiratory flow rates roughly 25% higher than boys.[302] This difference persists into later childhood. In addition, flow rates improve following maximal inspiration in girls, but not in boys, suggesting boys have altered bronchial muscle tone.[300]

Table 29–1 summarizes some of the differences in pulmonary function between infants and adults. Table 29–2 summarizes factors that predispose the infant and young child to respiratory problems.

Table 29—1   Comparison of Normal Values of Lung Function in Newborns and Adults

	NEWBORN	ADULT	FOLD CHANGE
Tidal volume (mL)	20 (5–7 mL/kg)	450 (6 mL/kg)	22
Alveolar ventilation (ml/min)	400	4200	10
(ml/m²/min)	2.3	2.3	1
Dead space, V_D/V_T ratio	0.3	0.33	1
Anatomical dead space (ml)	7.0	150	20
(ml/kg)	2.5	2	2
Respiratory quotient	0.8	0.8	1
Oxygen consumption (ml/min)	18	250	14
(ml/kg/min)	6.0–6.7	3.5	0.5
CO_2 output (ml/kg/min)	6	3	0.5
Body surface area (m²)	0.21	1.70	8
Body weight (kg)	3	70	23
Lung weight (gm)	50	800	15
FRC (mL)	90	2400	24
(ml/kg)	30	34	1
Lung surface area (m²)	2.8	64–75	30
(m²/kg)	1	1	1
Respiratory rate	34–36	12–14	2–3

(Modified from Doershuk CF, Fisher BJ, Matthews LW: Pulmonary physiology of the young child. In Scarpelli EM, ed: Pulmonary Physiology of the Fetus, Newborn, and Child, p. 174. Philadelphia, Lea & Febiger, 1975)

Table 29—2 Anatomical and Physiological Features of the Developing Respiratory System

PHYSIOLOGICAL/ANATOMICAL FEATURE	CLINICAL IMPLICATIONS
Upper Airway	Prone to obstruction
Nose breather*	
Large tongue	
No teeth*	
Large tonsils/adenoids	
Teeth easily dislodged†	Trauma/aspiration with intubation
Airways	Prone to collapse, obstruction
Small, weak	
Little bronchial smooth muscle*	Poor response to bronchodilators
Alveoli	Increased closing capacity
Less elasticity	
Chest Wall	Prone to collapse, retractions
Less muscle mass	
Soft ribs/sternum	
Ventilatory Muscles	Prone to fatigue
Few high oxidative muscle fibers*	
Pulmonary Vasculature	Insufficient vasoconstriction
Less muscular†	
Increased Oxygen Consumption	Decreased oxygen reserves

* Primarily infants.
† Primarily children beyond infancy.

THE CHILD WITH RESPIRATORY DISTRESS: INITIAL ASSESSMENT AND THERAPY

Any child presenting with respiratory distress must be rapidly evaluated for the necessity of resuscitative measures such as oxygen therapy, endotracheal intubation, ventilatory support, or a combination thereof. For the unconscious patient, standard cardiopulmonary resuscitation protocols should be followed to determine the adequacy of ventilation and circulation and the need for aggressive measures (discussed later).

Those not requiring resuscitation may still require immediate aggressive therapy. The unconscious patient, as well as those presenting with extreme lethargy, irritability, or restlessness, with any signs of respiratory distress such as cyanosis, increased respiratory rate, retractions, nasal flaring, or grunting, should immediately be given oxygen by mask. The adequacy of ventilation should be assessed by visual observation of the chest, as well as by auscultation. If ventilation is present, but appears inadequate, the head should be extended, and an oral airway inserted. If no immediate improvement is noted, bag-and-mask ventilation should be instituted and continued as the diagnostic workup proceeds. Similar measures are needed for the infant or child who appears to have adequate ventilation at times, but exhibits intermittent apnea.

Children who are alert with respiratory distress will require oxygen if cyanotic, and oxygen may be required for those with severe distress, regardless of cyanosis. Most of these children, however, will not require immediate placement of an artificial airway or ventilatory assistance (except as indicated later). Ultimately, oxygen therapy and ventilatory support must be guided by blood gas analysis; however, therapy need not be delayed until these are available.

Following initial therapy for severe distress, a more thorough assessment must be performed and further therapy planned. A variety of conditions can cause respiratory distress in children, some of which are listed in Table 29–3.

Assessment of respiratory status involves the use of one's eyes and ears, hands; occasionally, the nose; and most importantly, the brain. Experienced practitioners can rapidly integrate information from all the senses and quickly distinguish between, for example, a patient with epiglottitis and one with asthma. It is useful, however, to break the assessment process down into its individual components and see how they are applied to each of the elements of the respiratory system in the child with respiratory distress.

Evaluation of the Upper Airway

Upper airway obstructions are more common in infants and children than in adults. An untreated airway obstruction can be rapidly lethal. The respiratory care practitioner should be able to quickly assess the status of the child's upper airway and begin initial therapy.

Elsewhere we have explained that the diseased upper airway tends to narrow or collapse during inspiration. Accordingly, upper airway obstructions tend to produce more noticeable symptoms on inspiration. Inspiratory time may be prolonged, and inspiration is generally noisier than expiration.

Table 29–3 Principal Causes of Respiratory Distress in Children

YOUNG INFANT	OLDER INFANT AND CHILD
Pneumonia	Pneumonia
Bacterial	Bacterial
Viral	Viral
Aspiration	Other
Chlamydial	Asthma
Bronchiolitis	Upper airway obstruction
Sepsis	Croup
Upper airway obstruction	Epiglottitis
(especially congenital anomalies)	Peritonsillar abscess
Congenital heart disease	Foreign body aspiration
Intrathoracic anomalies	Congenital or acquired heart disease
Diaphragmatic lesions	Near-drowning
Vascular rings	Smoke inhalation
Lobar emphysema	Central nervous system dysfunction
Cystic fibrosis	Trauma
Infantile botulism	Infection
Metabolic acidosis	Seizures
Gastroenteritis and dehydration	Thoracic trauma
Salicylism	Sepsis
Miscellaneous causes	Cystic fibrosis
	Neuromuscular diseases
	Guillain–Barré syndrome
	Spinal cord injury
	Metabolic acidosis
	Diabetes mellitus
	Salicylism
	Miscellaneous causes

(Thompson AE: Respiratory distress. In Fleisher GR, Ludwig S (ed): Textbook of Pediatric Emergency Medicine, p 273. © 1988, Williams & Wilkins Co., Baltimore)

Stridor, the high-pitched crowing sound heard on inspiration in children with croup or epiglottitis, for example, is a classic sign of laryngeal obstruction.

An obstruction that is fixed, that is, one that does not allow the normal change in size of the airway lumen with the respiratory cycle, may produce abnormal noises in both inspiration and expiration. For example, foreign bodies in the upper airway may produce an inspiratory wheeze or stridor or, at times, a wheeze or stridor on both inspiration and expiration.

Coarse rhonchi may be heard with nasal congestion, secondary to upper respiratory infections, or after crying. If unaccompanied by other signs of respiratory distress, these noises may be innocuous. Coarse rhonchi may also be produced by soft-tissue obstruction, such as the tongue, which may partially obstruct the airway in the unconscious child or in the child with congenital abnormalities, such as micrognathia (small jaw) or a large tongue (macroglossia). These differing types of obstructions can be distinguished by noting the change in symptoms after position change or suctioning. Noises produced by the tongue often improve or clear with prone positioning (or placement of an oral airway), but not with suctioning. In contrast, rhonchi produced by upper airway secretions improve or clear with suctioning.

Respiratory sounds, such as wheezing or stridor, may be present only during a maximal inspiration, as occurs with coughing or crying, and may be absent during tidal breathing. This suggests a less severe obstruction. At times, however, stridor may appear to be minimal when obstruction is particularly severe, and the patient becomes fatigued, with decreased air exchange.

Children with painful upper airway obstructions, such as epiglottitis, may be unable to swallow and, hence, may drool. Drooling is common in healthy infants, but is suspect in an older child.

The therapist should note the relationship, if any, to posture and signs of upper airway obstruction. Some children will assume a posture that minimizes the obstruction. A child with epiglottitis, for example, will assume the classic "tripod" posture and, perhaps, thrust the jaw forward. Others may extend their heads somewhat, or otherwise alter their head position in an unusual way. Children who assume certain positions or postures should not be forced to lie flat or otherwise change their position, as respiratory distress may worsen.

The child should be inspected for anomalies that may cause obstruction. These include macroglossia, micrognathia, and unusually narrow nostrils.

Finally, the character of the voice, cough, or cry can assist in the evaluation of the upper airway. Since these maneuvers involve movement of the larynx, a weak or hoarse cry suggests laryngeal inflammation. Figure 29–3 illustrates the diagnostic approach to the child with stridor.

General Principles of Management of Upper Airway Obstruction

Management of specific diseases, such as foreign body aspiration or croup, will be discussed in detail later. In general, the choice of treatment will be dictated by the severity of symptoms, the nature and location of the obstruction, and the natural history of the disease.

Oral airways should be used to relieve symptomatic obstruction by the tongue or other soft tissue, as in the unconscious patient, following anesthesia or seizures, as well as in the child with micrognathia. In these latter patients, placement in the prone position may also be useful. When using an oral airway, care should be used to select the proper size. Extremely small oral airways, as would be used for a premature infant, might be contained in a pediatric resuscitation cart. Such an airway placed inappropriately in the mouth of a 3- or 4-year-old child could easily lodge in the trachea or larynx. An oral airway, if used properly for the correct conditions, should immediately provide substantial relief. If symptoms persist, the airway may be improperly placed, or the condition may be misdiagnosed. Finally, the use of an oral airway may produce difficulties in swallowing, increasing the risk for aspiration. Frequent suctioning, or prone positioning, may be necessary. In general, oral airways provide only a temporary solution to soft-tissue upper airway obstruction, and more definitive solutions should be considered for severe or long-lasting conditions. Artificial oral airways are generally poorly tolerated in the alert child.

Supraglottic, laryngeal, or tracheal obstructions will not be relieved by oral airways. Mild cases of croup may be managed conservatively with humidity therapy. Moderate cases may benefit from racepinephrine (racemic epinephrine) therapy, as will obstructions following intubation or bronchoscopy. More severe cases of croup may require intubation.

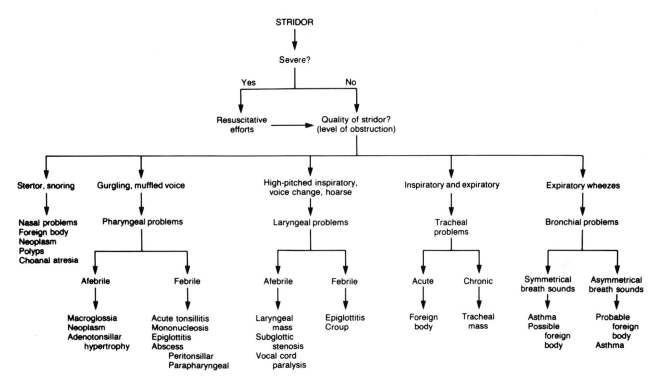

Figure 29—3. The diagnostic approach to stridor. (Handler SD: Stridor. In Fleisher GR, Ludwig S (eds): Textbook of Pediatric Emergency Medicine, p 301. © 1988, Williams & Wilkins Co, Baltimore)

Past experience with epiglottitis dictates that the patient be intubated as soon as the diagnosis is made, or is strongly suspected, even if symptoms do not seem especially severe. Racepinephrine is not useful, and any procedures that are frightening or painful may prompt crying, and complete obstruction.

Laryngotracheal foreign bodies should await experienced endoscopic management, as attempts to remove the object may worsen the obstruction. If complete obstruction occurs, abdominal or chest thrusts, and back blows may be used, as will be described further.

Blood gas values may be useful in evaluating upper airway obstructions such as croup or laryngomalacia, which generally do not lead to sudden, complete obstruction, and which at times are associated with lower airway or alveolar dysfunction. Complete sudden obstruction is possible in such conditions as epiglottitis or foreign body aspirations, and blood gas values are not useful in any sort of prospective or prognostic evaluation of this risk.

EVALUATION OF THE WHEEZY INFANT (LOWER AIRWAY OBSTRUCTION)

For reasons already discussed, the lower (or intrathoracic) airways are prone to obstruction during the expiratory phase. Obstructions requiring urgent therapy are almost always manifested by significant symptoms on expiration, such as wheezing, prolonged expiratory phase, or a forced expiration. Nonspecific signs of respiratory distress, such as retractions, nasal flaring, tachypnea, and cyanosis, may be present. At times, patients with diffuse lower airway obstruction may manifest grunting, usually associated with alveolar diseases. However, the interruption of expiratory airflow associated with grunting may also serve to prevent airway collapse.

Obstruction can be secondary to mucus, edema, inflammation, or bronchospasm. Foreign body aspiration, tumors, and congenital defects may also cause wheezing. The age of the patient and his or her past medical history may help to determine the exact nature and location of the ob-

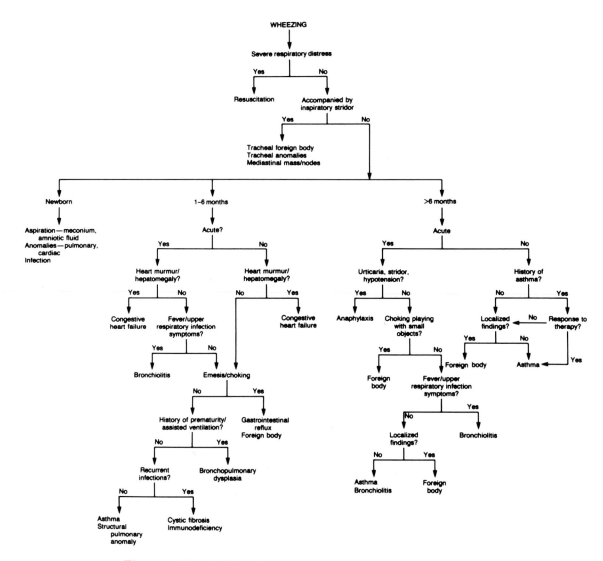

Figure 29—4. The diagnostic approach to the wheezing infant or child. (Thompson AE: Wheezing. In Fleisher GR, Ludwig S (eds): Textbook of Pediatric Emergency Medicine, p 273. © 1988, Williams & Wilkins Co, Baltimore)

struction. Foreign body aspiration would be unusual in an 8-year-old, but the sudden onset of respiratory distress and wheezing in a 2-year-old should bring this possibility to mind. Likewise, a 6-month-old infant with wheezing and symptoms of an upper respiratory infection should be considered for the diagnosis of bronchiolitis. Figure 29–4 illustrates the diagnostic approach to the wheezing child, and Table 29–4 describes some of the many causes of wheezing in children.

In assessing the child with wheezing, it must be determined to what extent the obstruction has af-

fected ventilation and oxygenation, whether the wheezing is responsive to bronchodilators, and to what extent, if any, the lung has been affected by atelectasis or consolidation. The latter two complications are more frequent in younger children and infants.

Therapy is directed first toward correction of hypoxemia, if present. Usually, oxygen by mask is preferred during initial evaluation and treatment. Later, the child can be placed in an oxygen hood or tent, or other oxygen devices, such as cannulae and ventimasks can be used if indicated. Usually, the

Table 29—4   Causes of Wheezing in Childhood: Pathophysiologic Classification

Infection
  Bronchiolitis
  Pneumonia
Bronchospasm
  Asthma
  Anaphylaxis
  Organophosphate poisoning
  Smoke inhalation
Aspiration
  Foreign body aspiration
  Gastroesophageal reflux
  Defective deglutition
  Tracheoesophageal fistula
Mechanical obstruction
  Intrinsic narrowing
    Developmental anomalies: tracheal stenosis tracheomalacia, bronchial stenosis, bronchomalacia
    Endobronchial tumor or granuloma
  Extrinsic compression
    Developmental anomalies: bronchogenic cysts, pulmonary cysts, lobar emphysema, vascular ring
    Mediastinal mass: lymphoma, thyoma, teratoma
    Enlarged lymph nodes
Miscellaneous
  Cystic fibrosis
  Immunodeficiency
  Pulmonary hemosiderosis
  Bronchopulmonary dysplasia
  Pulmonary edema/congenital heart disease
  Immotile cilia syndrome

(Rosenthal BW: Wheezing. In Fleisher GR, Ludwig S (ed): Textbook of Pediatric Emergency Medicine, p 344. © 1988, Williams & Wilkins Co., Baltimore)

child with lower airway obstruction is brought for treatment before severe hypercarbia develops. On occasion, however, the child may need to be intubated and ventilated in the emergency room.

Once hypoxemia and hypercarbia have been treated or ruled out, therapy may be directed at reversing the airway obstruction. Unless foreign body aspiration is suspected, a trial of bronchodilators may be useful. Although the efficacy of bronchodilators has been established, even in some infants less than 1 month of age,[32,33] the most common acute lower respiratory disorders, such as bronchiolitis, are often nonresponsive to these agents. In fact, wheezing unresponsive to bronchodilators in an infant under 6 months strongly suggests the diagnosis of bronchiolitis. In contrast,

most episodes of wheezing in children beyond infancy usually respond to bronchodilators.

Lower airway obstruction, when accompanied by atelectasis or consolidation, may lead to significant hypoxemia and respiratory failure. Infants sick enough to require hospitalization for bronchiolitis are often hypoxemic,[119] and apnea is not uncommon, especially in the "ex-preemie."[5,45] Therefore, apnea monitoring might be needed. Work of breathing has been reported to be up to six times normal in patients with bronchiolitis, and respiratory failure is not uncommon. Therapists should be especially vigilant for signs of respiratory failure in lower airway disease in those whose symptoms are severe; those with a history of prematurity, bronchopulmonary dysplasia, cystic fibrosis, or other chronic lung disease; and in very young infants.

Infants and young children presenting with signs of acute respiratory infection may have a communicable disease. It is common practice, during times of the year when respiratory syncytial virus infections are common, that infants likely to have respiratory syncytial virus infection are isolated until viral studies are completed. Careful handwashing, and when appropriate, use of mask and gown are necessary to control infection.

Where appropriate, definitive pharmacologic therapy should be started. In asthma and other bronchospastic disorders, this includes bronchodilators, and perhaps steroids. In selected cases of bronchiolitis, ribavirin therapy may be helpful. When bacterial infection is suspected, antibiotics will be used. Until such therapy is effective, the patient should be observed for signs of respiratory deterioration and treated accordingly.

Chest physical therapy is usually not effective in acute lower airway obstruction secondary to asthma or bronchiolitis. Some children may have worsening respiratory distress in response to the position changes and percussion. Chest physical therapy may be helpful, however, as the acute process resolves, or when mucus obstruction is the likely cause of distress, as in cystic fibrosis.

Care should also be exercised when applying humidity therapy. Although drying of secretions is part of the pathophysiology of most lower airway diseases, some patients react with further bronchospasm and edema when exposed to aerosols, especially those generated by ultrasonic nebulizers.

Intubation and mechanical ventilation may be necessary for some patients with acute lower airway obstruction. Mechanical ventilation in the patient with lower airway obstruction poses significant risks for pulmonary air leak. Hyperinflation is invariably present in asthma and bronchiolitis, the functional residual capacity at times being 200% of normal.[43] As airway resistance is increased, the time required for adequate exhalation also increases. Failure to allow adequate exhalation may lead to pneumothorax. Judicious use of positive end-expiratory pressure (PEEP) or continuous positive airway pressure (CPAP) may be useful to prevent airway collapse on exhalation, although further overdistension is possible.

Once the acute phase has passed and symptoms have improved, infants may still require oxygen therapy and close observation, as hypoxemia may persist for some time after lower respiratory infections.[119]

ALVEOLAR DISORDERS

In this category, we will discuss atelectasis and pneumonia, the two most common disorders affecting the alveolar portion of the lung in infants and children.

Atelectasis

Atelectasis in children is almost always secondary to some other insult to the lung, be it foreign body aspiration, neuromuscular disease, postoperative respiratory dysfunction, or cystic fibrosis. In early infancy, the right upper lobe is most often affected by atelectasis. Because of the small size of this lobe, it often is not possible to detect atelectasis by auscultation. Although restrictive pulmonary diseases, such as atelectasis, have (in theory) their own specific set of signs and symptoms, these are often masked by coexisting problems in the airways, as in the infant with bronchopulmonary dysplasia or asthma. Generally, a chest x-ray film is necessary to confirm the diagnosis. A patient who has more severe symptoms of a respiratory disease than expected should be assessed for atelectasis.

When atelectasis is associated with diseases that are generally short-term in nature, or respond readily to treatment, such as an acute exacerbation of asthma, if may be prudent to allow the atelectasis to resolve as the primary disease process improves. However, if respiratory function has deteriorated, or atelectasis persists after other symptoms have improved, specific treatment may be warranted. Chest physical therapy is the most widely used therapy specifically for atelectasis, since it can be used even in the uncooperative patient. In older children, incentive spirometry may be helpful. When atelectasis does not resolve, or frequently re-

curs, the existence of an underlying congenital, genetic, or acquired disorder must be suspected. Conditions causing recurrent or chronic atelectasis include foreign body aspiration, congenital heart and vascular defects, and cystic fibrosis.

Consolidation and Pneumonia

Like atelectasis, pneumonia often coexists with lower airway obstruction, such as asthma. Where appropriate, antimicrobial therapy should be instituted. Pending resolution of the disease, respiratory care is primarily supportive. Hypoxemia and respiratory failure should be watched for and treated, along with apnea in the young infant. There is no evidence that chest physiotherapy helps in the clearing of consolidation. However, it may be useful in the clearance of bronchial secretions that sometimes accompany pneumonia. Effectiveness of chest physical therapy should be assessed by improvement of symptoms of bronchial obstruction. When pneumonia coexists with other chronic lung diseases that benefit from chest physical therapy, such as cystic fibrosis, treatment should be continued.

RESPIRATORY CARE PROCEDURES APPLIED TO THE PEDIATRIC PATIENT

CHEST PHYSICAL THERAPY

Chest physical therapy (CPT) is a series of mechanical and physical maneuvers that promote the movement and expectoration of tracheobronchial secretions and improve and maintain the distribution of ventilation in the lungs.[103] Typical pediatric chest physical therapy maneuvers include percussion, vibration, postural drainage, and breathing exercises. Breathing exercises are limited to those children who can understand verbal instructions.

There have been few documented studies performed to gauge the effectiveness of chest physical therapy (see later discussion of cystic fibrosis). As a result, there continues to be much controversy on this subject.[155] One study has shown that infants who receive chest physical therapy after extubation required fewer reintubations as a consequence of right upper lobe atelectasis.[83] In contrast, another study reported an increased risk of postoperative atelectasis in children who received chest physical therapy following correction of congenital heart defects.[251] In the following section we will discuss each CPT modality separately.

Percussion

The mechanism of action in percussion is not known, but it is thought that "clapping" the chest sends a pressure wave through the chest wall to the lung, thereby loosening secretions. This, in conjunction with postural drainage (see postural drainage section), will move secretions to the point in the tracheobronchial tree from which they can be expectorated. In infants and small children, it is very difficult to use an adult-sized hand to perform this maneuver. Therefore, it becomes necessary to utilize an alternative, such as a percussion cup or a resuscitation mask that has the opening taped closed.

Vibration

Vibration applied to the chest wall is thought to promote movement of secretions from small to large airways. Vibrations are performed by placing the hands over the chest wall. With the arms straight, a tremor like movement is created that is coordinated with the patient's exhalation. It may be difficult to coordinate vibrations with exhalations in infants and younger children who have higher respiratory rates. With newborns or infants, it may be helpful to utilize mechanical alternatives, such as an electric toothbrush with the bristles covered, since the size of an adult hand makes it difficult to perform vibrations effectively on a small thorax. Devices designed to administer vibrations during CPT in infants are also available commercially. Vibrations are usually done in conjunction with percussion and postural drainage, but in some cases (e.g., brittle rib cage due to rickets), it can be done in conjunction with postural drainage only.

Postural Drainage

Postural drainage is performed by placing the patient in various positions to utilize gravity in aiding the drainage of pulmonary secretions. These positions relate directly to the direction that the major bronchi radiate off of the trachea and main stem bronchi. Infants and younger children can often be positioned in the practitioner's lap, provided they are not bound to a multitude of life-support equipment. Older children may require help to move into the various positions. Postural drainage may be hazardous in any condition that increases the risk of increased intracranial pressure (e.g., head trauma). Other patients with cardiac or respiratory failure may manifest hypoxemia or respiratory dis-

tress in the head-down position. Therapy may need to be performed with the bed flat in these patients.

Patience and understanding are extremely important when attempting to perform any procedure such as CPT on a child, no matter what age. Children who are old enough to communicate will want to know what is being done to them, if it will hurt, and how long it will take. To gain a child's confidence, it is best not to appear or to be rushed, and to take the time to explain everything that will be done in language that the child can understand. Communication occurs between adults and children of any age (even preverbal) through body language, tone of voice, and style of touch, and caretakers should consider these factors when trying to alleviate patient (and parent) fear and anxiety. In some cases, this can also be accomplished by demonstrating CPT (or any other procedure) on a nearby patient already familiar and comfortable with the procedure. The parents of the child may be present, and may be more apprehensive about the therapy than their child. Careful and thorough explanations of the methods and goals of therapy should be given.

The most difficult CPT maneuvers to perform on children remain those that require understanding of verbal instructions, such as breathing exercises or cough instruction. In those cases for which the child is unable to understand breathing exercises, these obviously become fruitless, and coughing may be accomplished by suctioning the upper airway. This will usually cause the young child to cry, which will cause the child to take deep breaths and cough. The age and maturity of the child should determine the practitioner's approach to the delivery of therapy.

INCENTIVE SPIROMETRY

Successful application of incentive spirometry requires the child be able to follow instructions. There are a variety of incentive spirometers currently on the market for adult use that can be used successfully in children. However, since children have smaller lung volumes than adults, volume goals must be adjusted downward accordingly. Some incentive spirometers come with pediatric adaptations, such as clown's faces that light up when the goal is reached. As with CPT, it is imperative that the patient and his or her parents be given an explanation of the therapy, especially when a therapist will not be present to supervise incentive spirometry. Having the parents supervise this therapy allows them to be active participants in their child's care, as well as help ensure success.

AEROSOL AND HUMIDIFICATION THERAPY

As with adults, it is imperative that pediatric patients receive increased humidity with the administration of dry gases, such as oxygen. Lack of proper humidification can lead to problems, such as atelectasis and bronchial obstruction caused by dried retained secretions, increased insensible water loss from the respiratory tract, and mucociliary dysfunction.[226] Nonheated "bubble" humidifiers, commonly used with low-flow oxygen therapy, provide little humidity (about 14 mgH_2O/L[193]) and, more importantly, frequently leak, reducing delivered FIO_2.[276] Heated humidification devices available vary from the "pass-over" type (which provides the least amount of added humidity of the heated types) to the "wick" type (which can provide, in most situations, 100% relative humidity at 37° C). The major difference between these two types is the degree of interface between the gas and the water surfaces, which is greater in the latter unit and increases the absolute humidity.[266] Heated humidifiers are preferred when artificial airways are in place. In very young children, gases may need to be heated (even though the patient does not have an artificial airway) to maintain a neutral thermal environment. In infants, the temperature of inspired gas can affect body temperature and metabolic rate. For safety, it is essential that a means to measure circuit temperature, preferably with a high-temperature alarm, be incorporated into the patient circuit to protect against thermal injury from the inhalation of hot gases.[157]

Aerosols are liquid particles suspended in air and are used to increase ambient humidity and deliver medications by inhalation.[147] Aerosols can be generated with an ultrasonic nebulizer or a mechanical jet nebulizer. In an infant or young child, fluid overload can result from the overzealous administration of aerosols. Aerosols can also carry microorganisms into the pulmonary tract.[235] Another hazard of aerosols has been seen when delivering aerosolized water to children with reactive airways such as asthma. This can cause a significant decrease in forced vital capacity and other expiratory flow rates.[10]

OXYGEN THERAPY

Delivery of oxygen therapy is one of the major tasks of the pediatric respiratory care practitioner. The indications for use in children are identical with those for adults:

- Reverse hypoxemia
- Decrease the work of breathing
- Decrease myocardial work[266]
- Differentiate cardiac disease from pulmonary disease[112]

Along with the beneficial effects of oxygen, there are serious hazards also. These are:

- Pulmonary oxygen toxicity
- Retinopathy of prematurity (of concern in the premature neonatal population)
- Nitrogen washout absorption atelectasis
- Oxygen-induced hypoventilation

In addition, caretakers, parents, and visitors must be warned against using friction toys (such as toy cars) that may generate sparks. Severe burns or death can result from the use of such toys in an oxygen-enriched atmosphere.

The methods of oxygen administration in children will depend on the age of the child, the desired FIO_2, and the degree of visibility, access, and mobility required. For infants and very young children, the oxygen hood provides a reliable FIO_2 while allowing access to the patient.[193] In addition, hoods are preferable to masks, which are poorly tolerated by infants and younger children. Adequate flow rates and aeration of the area inside and around the head hood are necessary to assure that carbon dioxide does not accumulate.[193] Excessive flows, however, increase the noise level in the head hood.

For infants and children requiring long-term therapy, an oxygen cannula may be used. This device allows greater mobility and visibility, and allows the infant to feed without interrupting oxygen delivery. The infant also is able to see, and hence react to, the environment more readily when not confined to a head hood. These factors may all aid in the child's development.[115,157,174,202] As children age, they become more compliant with the administration of oxygen by face masks and face tents. Estimation of the FIO_2s delivered with low-flow devices is difficult and may be much higher than values expected from adult standards.[103] Transcutaneous or pulse oximetry can be used to guide low-flow oxygen delivery.

ARTIFICIAL AIRWAYS

The indications for, and technique of, placement of an artificial airway depend, in part, on anatomic factors unique to the developing child. In the infant and young child, the larynx is located more anterior and as much as three to six vertebrae higher in the neck in comparison with adults. The cricoid cartilage is the most narrow part of the infant's and young child's airway. By the age of 5 a child's larynx will descend to the adult position, and the vocal cords will become the most narrow portion of the airway.[73]

The sizes and styles of tubes will vary, not only with the size of the patient, but also with the laryngeal anatomy. As previously mentioned, the larynx of a child up to the age of 5 will have a narrow cricoid ring in which the tube "wedges." Endotracheal tubes for the child younger than 5 years of age should not be cuffed. Of special note, the tube should not completely occlude the airway during positive-pressure ventilation, because excessive pressure on the tracheal wall can lead to submucosal ischemia, mucosal breakdown, and eventual subglottic stenosis.[140,175] Older children may require a cuff to seal their airway for positive-pressure mechanical ventilation (see Table 29–5 for correct endotracheal tube size).

Endotracheal Intubation

Endotracheal intubation may be required for the following reasons:[30]

Table 29–5 Endotracheal Tube Sizes for Children

AGE	SIZE (MM ID)
Premature	
1000 g	2.5
1000–2500 g	3.0
Neonate to 6 mo	3.0–3.5
6 mo–1 yr	3.5–4.0
1–2 yr	4.0–5.0
Beyond 2 yr	$\frac{\text{Age (yr)} + 16}{4}$

(Coté CJ, Todres ID: The pediatric airway. In Ryan JF, Todres ID, Coté CJ, Goudsouzian NH (ed): A Practice of Anesthesia for Infants and Children, p 46. Orlando, Fla, Grune & Stratton, 1986)

- To facilitate mechanical ventilation
- To aid in the removal of tracheal secretions by suctioning
- To bypass upper airway obstruction (e.g., epiglottitis)
- To protect against aspiration

Preparation of Equipment. Equipment utilized for pediatric intubation varies little from that utilized in adults. Multiple sizes of endotracheal tubes, suction catheters, anatomic masks, and laryngoscope blades and handles to accommodate different-sized children should be available. These include the following:

- Suction
- Oxygen
- Manual resuscitator and proper-fitting masks
- Laryngoscope with proper handle, blade, bulbs, and batteries
- Appropriate size ET tube (syringe if tube is cuffed)
- McGill forceps if necessary (i.e., for nasal intubation)
- Waterproof tape and tincture of benzoin
- Teflon-coated stylet

Stylets facilitate insertion of the endotracheal tube, but can cause perforation of the larynx if allowed to protrude beyond the end of the tube. In addition, it must be assured that the laryngoscope light bulb is securely connected. A bulb that comes loose during intubation can cause significant airway obstruction.

Preparation and Care of the Patient During Laryngoscopy

Unlike in adults, it is difficult to visualize the vocal cords for endotracheal intubation by hyperextending the child's neck. It is easier to visualize the larynx by placing the child's head in a neutral or "sniffing" position.[108]

Protecting the child from the hazards of intubation is an essential component of successful intubation. Hazards of intubation can include apnea, trauma, hypertension, bradycardia, hypoxemia, coughing, vomiting, aspiration, and pulmonary infection.[1,25,30,106,112,188,222]

Although children under aged 6 months do not have teeth, one must be careful not to injure the gum tissue during laryngoscopy. Children older than this age will have teeth, and careful attention to prevent dental damage must be taken when intubating.[7]

During the intubation procedure, the patient should be protected from hypoxemia by preoxygenation and ventilation. Also useful are laryngoscope blades especially designed to deliver continuous low-flow oxygen into the larynx during laryngoscopy. These are available commercially, or a standard laryngoscope blade can be modified.

Some clinicians advocate gentle pressure on the cricoid ring during intubation and manual ventilation. This prevents gastric inflation.

Pharmacotherapy to Facilitate Intubation

Neuromuscular-blocking agents are frequently used during insertion of endotracheal tubes in children. The two types of neuromuscular-blocking agents are depolarizing (e.g., succinylcholine) and nondepolarizing (e.g., d-tubocurarine or pancuronium). Infants and children may need proportionately larger doses of succinylcholine than adults to achieve paralysis. This is probably due to their proportionately increased blood volume and extracellular fluid volume. As a result, twice as much succinylcholine (per kilogram) is needed to produce half the neuromuscular blockade seen in adults.[50] The duration of action and mechanism of metabolism are similar for children and adults. One noticeable difference in children is that, because of their smaller muscle mass, the fasciculations commonly seen with succinylcholine administration in adults are diminished in young children.[50] Fasciculations are associated with increased intragastric pressure and increased risk of aspiration of gastric contents during intubation. To prevent fasciculations, subparalytic doses of a nondepolarizing agent can be given before administration of a depolarizing agent.[215]

Nondepolarizing agents are also used in infants and young children as a means to control a patient's spontaneous respiratory efforts during mechanical ventilation. Such control may be desirable when treating severe respiratory failure. The use of a neuromuscular-blocking agent results in apnea, which requires the presence of a person skilled in ventilation of the apneic patient by bag and mask. The patient who is pharmacologically paralyzed is at increased risk for hypoxemia and cardiac arrest should accidental extubation occur. The effects of a nondepolarizing-blocking agent are essentially the same as those seen in adults; however, the duration of action may be longer because of a lower glomerular filtration rate and prolonged renal clearance in

children. Pancuronium accumulates with repeated administration; therefore, paralysis can be maintained with smaller doses.[7] Another nondepolarizing-blocking agent, d-tubocurarine, may result in hypotension, perhaps secondary to histamine release; consequently, it is rarely used.[50,215] The potency and duration of action of these drugs can be increased by the presence of hypothermia, antibiotics, or decreased renal function.

Depolarizing agents cannot be reversed. Such drugs will eventually be metabolized by endogenous pseudocholinesterase. The nondepolarizing agents can be reversed by utilizing the anticholinesterase drugs (e.g., neostigmine). To prevent side effects of anticholinesterase drugs (bradycardia, increased gastric motility) atropine should also be given simultaneously.

Sedatives (e.g., thiopental, diazepam) are also utilized during endotracheal intubation in patients who are conscious and alert.

Alternate Techniques

In children with abnormal airways (e.g., micrognathia), special techniques may be required to accomplish intubation. One such technique is the so-called retrograde technique.[22,316] This procedure requires the percutaneous passage of a guide wire upward through the trachea toward the larynx and through the mouth. An endotracheal tube is then passed over the guide wire toward the larynx, and into the trachea.[22,316]

Another technique to secure a different airway is the use of a flexible fiberoptic bronchoscope. This can be used for visualization of the laryngeal area, for suctioning, as well as for checking tube placement and repositioning the tube if necessary.[7] Esophageal obturators are seldom used in pediatrics because children have widely varying lengths of esophagus. Use of an inappropriate size would result in placement of the obturator in the stomach, causing gastric insufflation, or above the level of the carina, thereby compressing and obstructing the trachea.[260]

Care of the Intubated Child

Care of the intubated child centers on preventing accidental extubation, preventing or minimizing the short- and long-term complications of intubation, and assuring continued airway patency. Also, intubation renders the child speechless, and alternative means of communication (as well as feeding and hydration) need to be established.

The first step in preventing unplanned extubation is to properly secure the tube. Light-weight ventilator or CPAP tubing may decrease the risk of unplanned extubation, as will arm restraints and, if necessary, sedation.

Continued airway patency is maintained through adequate humidification and suctioning.

The most common long-term sequela of extended endotracheal intubation is subglottic stenosis.[7,153,159] Repeated or prolonged intubations may increase the risks. Additional hazards include palatial groves and defective dentition.

Another hazard often seen with uncuffed ET tubes is migration of the tube up or down in the trachea in response to head position changes. Turning the child's head to either side will cause the tip of the tube to travel cephalad. Neck and head extension will also cause this to occur. Conversely, neck and head flexion will cause the tube to move toward the carina.[7]

Extubation

A child who has been intubated should be considered for extubation as soon as the indication for intubation has resolved. Feeding should be withheld for several hours before extubation, and gastric tubes aspirated to ensure an empty stomach. After informing the patient (if appropriate), the patient is then preoxygenated, suctioned, and then oxygenated again. The tape securing the tube should be loosened, and, if a cuff is present, it should be deflated. The child should be given a positive-pressure breath with a manual resuscitator. At peak inspiratory pressure, the tube is removed. This sequence will lessen the chance of aspiration and will mimic a cough. It is imperative once a child is extubated that the respiratory care practitioner watch for signs of subglottic stenosis or edema (e.g., stridor) and other signs of respiratory distress (e.g., tachypnea and intercostal retractions).[30] At the authors' institution, we occasionally give extubated patients aerosolized dexamethasone and racepinephrine postextubation and, for some patients, we also perform chest physical therapy to the right upper lobe every 2 hours for 24 hours following extubation. In very young children the right upper lobe frequently becomes atelectatic postextubation.[83]

Tracheostomy

The most common indication for the performance of a tracheostomy in children is a congenital or acquired upper airway obstruction.[81] Other indications include surgical procedures of the neck, pro-

vision of an airway for long-term mechanical ventilation, and long-term upper airway obstruction, such as subglottic stenosis.[7,81]

A tracheostomy is an invasive surgical procedure that carries special risks. Early complications include accidental decannulation, pneumonia, pneumothorax, subcutaneous emphysema, obstructed tube, hemorrhage, stomal infection, tracheitis, and pneumomediastinum.[39,100,218,230,254,319] Late complications include tracheocutaneous fistula, accidental decannulation (a serious life-threatening situation that can be prevented with appropriate monitoring and observation), tracheal granuloma, excessive stomal granulation, obstructed tube, hemorrhage, stomal infection, and tracheomalacia.[319]

In a child with a tracheostomy, great care must be taken to maintain the patency of the airway, especially in the immediate postoperative period. A chest x-ray examination should be performed after insertion to check for free air in the pleural space (pneumothorax) and subcutaneously (subcutaneous emphysema). The tracheostomy tube should be secured properly so that the tube will not move out of the airway, but not so tightly that it will cause pressure necrosis around the skin of the neck. Proper tracheobronchial toilet should be maintained, with heated humidity provided (since the nose and mouth are bypassed), and removal of secretions by suctioning.[7]

Pediatric tracheostomy tubes are made of several different types of material, including metal (silver) and plastic (silastic and polyvinyl chloride).

As with removal of an endotracheal tube, elective decannulation of a tracheostomy tube is performed when the indication is no longer present. It is more difficult to decannulate children than adults because of the small size of the child's airways, coupled with the nonrigid nature of their trachea, which is more prone to collapse. In addition, the smaller airway may be compromised by granuloma tissue or subglottic stenosis. If respiratory distress occurs, the tube should be replaced, and bronchoscopy performed to determine the nature of the distress.[7]

MECHANICAL VENTILATION

Mechanical ventilation in pediatrics is a conglomerate of techniques borrowed from the newborn infant and the adult (see Chap. 21). Mechanical ventilators can be classified into two groups: (1) manually operated (e.g., resuscitation bags) and (2) automatically operated (e.g., all pneumatically or electrically operated ventilators).

Manually Operated Devices

Manual resuscitators are used when changes in ventilatory demands are expected to occur rapidly, as during cardiopulmonary resuscitation. Manually operated ventilators or resuscitation bags are either self-inflating (e.g., the Laerdal or Puritan Manual Resuscitator [PMR]) bags or flow-inflating bags (e.g., rubber anesthesia bags) with nonrebreathing elbows. The major advantage of self-inflating bags is that ventilation can more easily be performed by inexperienced personnel. They are also available in a wide variety of sizes from newborn (0.5 L) to adult (3.0 L). Disadvantages include jamming of the exhalation valve, an inability to produce PEEP without external attachments, and difficulty in control of delivered FIO_2.[30]

Flow-inflating bags need to be operated by experienced personnel familiar with such equipment. There are no valves in most flow inflators, which allows the use of maneuvers such as inspiratory peak pressure plateau and PEEP. The major variable to pressures generated with flow-inflating bags is the gas flow entering the system. The user can estimate lung compliance more readily with flow-inflating bags, since resistance to ventilation is due to the inherent characteristics of the lungs and airways, not the elastic properties of the bag itself (as with many self-inflating devices). The FIO_2 can readily be adjusted by utilizing an appropriate pressurized gas source with a blending system.

A disadvantage with flow-inflating devices is the need for a readily available compressed gas source. Both types of devices carry the risks of barotrauma (e.g., pneumothorax), from overinflation, and acute respiratory acidosis, resulting from underventilation.[30]

Automatic Ventilators

Automatically operated mechanical ventilators can be classified into two groups:

1. Negative-pressure ventilators
2. Positive-pressure ventilators

Negative-pressure ventilators. Negative-pressure ventilators can be used in children with neuromuscular disorders and "normal" lungs who are unable to adequately breathe spontaneously. The iron lung is the most common form of negative-pressure ventilator. Lighter more portable units have been devised, such as the chest cuirass and body jacket. These are also available in pediatric sizes.

The major advantage of negative-pressure ventilation is that it does not require intubation or tracheostomy. Disadvantages of negative-pressure ventilators are that they usually are not capable of ventilating diseased lungs (e.g., decreased compliance, increased airway resistance), they are cumbersome, and they allow very limited access to the patient by caretakers.[194]

Positive-pressure ventilators. Positive-pressure ventilation is currently the preferred method of mechanical ventilation in both pediatrics and adult care. Positive-pressure ventilation is more invasive, as it usually requires an artificial airway. Other side effects include barotrauma, decreased venous return, and decreased cardiac output.

Indications. The indications for positive-pressure mechanical ventilation in pediatrics are the same as for adults and neonates (Table 29–6). They are[266]

- Acute respiratory acidosis
- Impending respiratory failure
- Apnea

Selection and Use of Equipment

Most ventilators utilized in pediatrics are either neonatal ventilators, some of which can be upgraded to meet the increased flow demands of older children, or adult ventilators that are capable of delivering lower tidal volumes and higher rates.[103]

The special problems in ventilation of small children result from

- Low lung compliance
- Small tidal volumes
- High respiratory rates
- Low inspiratory flow requirements secondary to high airway resistance[209]
- Low dead space requirements
- Low compressible volume requirements

The major advantages of pressure preset ventilators are direct control of inspiratory pressures, to decrease the risk of barotrauma, and compensation for tidal volume loss around the uncuffed artificial airway. A major disadvantage of these ventilators is variable volume delivery and the inability to recognize changes in the patient's compliance or resistance.

A major advantage to volume-present ventilators is limitation of volume change with changing

Table 29—6 Guidelines for Initiating Positive Pressure Ventilation

---

PROVISION OF ADEQUATE ALVEOLAR VENTILATION

1. Select rate—physiologic norm for age
2. Select tidal volume—10–15 ml/kg
3. Select inspiratory time (I/E ratio)—age-dependent should result in I/E ratio of 1:2
4. Obstructive diseases—prolong expiratory time, avoid prolonged inspiratory time
5. Immediately assess for signs of adequate ventilation (e.g., chest excursion, breath sounds)
6. Measure $PaCO_2$; adjust IMV rate and/or tidal volume as needed to maintain level between 35 and 45 torr
7. Decrease IMV rate to level tolerated as determined by $PaCO_2$

MAINTENANCE OF ADEQUATE OXYGENATION

1. FIO_2: 1.0 (infants less than 34-wk gestational age must be monitored for PaO_2 closely and FIO_2 adjusted to maintain appropriate PaO_2)
2. PEEP: 3 cmH$_2$O, or higher level if needed, and ability to tolerate hemodynamic effects is anticipated
3. Immediately assess for signs of adequate oxygenation (e.g., color) and circulatory depression (e.g., hypotension, diminished peripheral pulses)
4. Measure PaO_2
  Decrease FIO_2 maintaining $PaO_2 > 70$ torr
  Restrictive disease (low FRC, low compliance)—increase PEEP as needed to achieve $PaO_2 > 70$ torr at $FIO_2 = 0.4$–0.5
  Consider direct monitoring of cardiac output if PEEP > 15 cmH$_2$O; adjust PEEP further to maintain Qs/Qt $< 20\%$
5. Decrease PEEP while maintaining $PaO_2 > 70$ torr

(Modified from Gioia FM, Stephenson RL, Alterwitz SA: Principles of respiratory support and mechanical ventilation. In Rogers MC (ed): Textbook of Pediatric Intensive Care, p 135. © 1987, The Williams & Wilkins Co., Baltimore)

impedance. Since ventilator volume output is constant, inspiratory pressures will reflect increases or decreases in the patient's compliance or resistance, or both. A disadvantage of volume ventilators is that inspiratory pressures can increase sharply in response to changes in lung mechanics, which can increase the risk of barotrauma.[238] This problem highlights the need for pressure alarms and pressure "pop-offs."

Most infant ventilators (i.e., time-cycled, pressure-preset ventilators) currently on the market are capable of ventilating small children. However, volume ventilators are preferred in the larger child.

Selection of Ventilator Settings

Tidal volume, inspiratory and expiratory time, ventilator frequency, and PEEP must be adjusted when volume ventilators are used.

Tidal Volume. Under most circumstances, a volume of 10–15 mL/kg will provide adequate ventilation. The use of adult ventilators to deliver the small tidal volumes that children require poses special problems, many of which relate to the ventilator circuit compliance.

Importance of Ventilator Circuit Compliance. When adult ventilators are adapted for use in children, effort must be made to achieve a low and stable ventilator circuit compliance. When ventilator circuit compliance is high, a large and variable portion of the preset volume remains compressed in the circuit and, therefore, is not delivered to the patient. The preset volume does not predict the tidal volume received by the patient. Likewise, when ventilator circuit compliance changes over time, (secondary to water evaporation from the humidifier) large changes in delivered tidal volume and airway pressure can occur.[116]

A low circuit compliance can be achieved by using small-bore rigid tubing (e.g., ⅜-in. Tygon) in conjunction with humidifiers that have low compressible volume (internal compliance), with a water-feed system that maintains near constant levels of water to avoid major changes in system compressibility.

Ventilator circuit compliance can easily be calculated and used to estimate the actual delivered tidal volume. This can be done by having the ventilator deliver a known volume into the ventilator circuit (with the patient connection occluded) while observing the pressure generated (with no PEEP applied). The volume is divided by the observed pressure, yielding compliance.

Once the compliance of the ventilator circuit is known and a prediction of the expected ventilatory pressures made, the amount of volume that will be compressed in the circuit during inspiration can be calculated. If the circuit compliance is 1.5 mL/cmH$_2$O pressure, for example, then 1.5 mL would be compressed in the ventilator circuit for every centimeter H$_2$O pressure generated by the ventilator. If an inspiratory pressure of 20 cmH$_2$O (without PEEP) is anticipated, then 30 mL [ventilator circuit compliance (1.5) multiplied by expected inspiratory pressure (20)] should be added to the desired delivered tidal volume, and the ventilator's preset tidal volume adjusted accordingly.

Once these determinations have been made, the patient can be connected to the ventilator. Adequacy of ventilation is then assessed by observation of chest excursion, breath sounds, monitoring of exhaled or transcutaneous carbon dioxide, and pulse or transcutaneous oximetry. Inspiratory and expiratory time and respiratory rate are adjusted according to criteria described in the following. Later, the adequacy of ventilation should be confirmed with arterial blood gases.

If, after connecting the patient to the ventilator, the observed inspiratory pressures are substantially different from those expected, then the delivered tidal volume will be different as well. The following formula can be used to determine the actual delivered tidal volume.

Delivered tidal volume = Preset tidal volume − [(Peak-inspiratory pressure − End-expiratory pressure) × Circuit compliance]

The ventilator volume is then adjusted accordingly. When a substantial portion of the inspired volume leaks around the endotracheal or tracheostomy tube, calculated delivered tidal volumes will be greater than actual delivered volumes, and clinical criteria take precedence over calculations in the evaluation of ventilation.

Alternatively, a volume monitor can be used to measure the delivered tidal volume. Measurements must be taken at a point between the ventilator circuit and the endotracheal tube, and the measuring device must not contribute substantially to dead space. A commercially available volume monitor (Bear Neonatal Volume Monitor) meeting these requirements is now available. However, it is accurate only at low-flow rates (20 L/min or less)[240] and may not be useful for children beyond early infancy.

In no case should measurements made distal to the exhalation valve be relied upon to indicate tidal volume delivery. Volumes measured at this point include the volume of gas compressed in the circuit, as well as that exhaled by the patient.

Scott et al. have demonstrated that the compliance of the ventilator tubing also influences the degree of hyperinflation ("auto-PEEP") seen during mechanical ventilation.[263] When tubing compliance is low, inadvertent expiratory hyperinflation is significantly reduced.

Ventilator compliance also determines, in part, the ability of a ventilator to respond to changes in patient lung compliance. Ventilator pressure is determined, not by patient compliance alone, but rather, by the sum of patient and ventilator compliance.[170] When ventilator compliance is low in relation to patient compliance (i.e., low ventilator/patient compliance ratio), the sum of the two compliances is determined largely by the patient's compliance. Changes in patient compliance are then largely reflected in changes in the sum of the ventilator and patient compliance, with a proportional response in ventilator pressure.

Conversely, when ventilator circuit compliance is high in relation to patient compliance, then ventilator compliance is the primary determinate of the sum of the two. A large change in patient compliance will have little impact on the sum of patient and ventilator compliance. The corresponding change in ventilator pressure will be diminished (see display for further explanation of this concept).

Ventilator Frequency, Inspiratory and Expiratory Times. The selection of inspiratory and expiratory times, and respiratory rate, should be guided by an understanding of the interrelationship between airway resistance and lung compliance. This relationship is quantified by the time constant, which is derived by the following equation:

$$TC = R \times C$$

where TC = time constant (sec)
R = resistance (cmH$_2$O/L/sec)
C = compliance (L/cmH$_2$O

In normal healthy infants

C = 0.005 L/cmH$_2$O
R = 30 cmH$_2$O/L/sec
TC = (30 cmH$_2$O/L/sec × (0.005 L/cmH$_2$O)
= 0.15 sec.

The time constant determines the rate of pressure and volume change in the lung. Figure 29–5 shows that approximately 63% of the pressure (and volume) change occurs in one time constant, 95% in three time constants, and 99% in five time constants.

HOW VENTILATOR COMPLIANCE DETERMINES VENTILATOR RESPONSE TO CHANGES IN LUNG COMPLIANCE

Any volume delivered by a ventilator is distributed between the ventilator circuit and the patient in proportion to their respective compliances. Since the ventilator must inflate both the circuit and the patient's lungs, the pressure generated by the ventilator is determined by the sum of ventilator circuit and patient compliance. For example, given

$$Compliance = \frac{Volume}{Pressure,}$$

and assuming

Ventilator tidal volume = 150 mL
Ventilator compliance = 5 mL/cmH$_2$O pressure
Patient compliance = 1 mL/cmH$_2$O pressure

Then the pressure required to deliver the volume is determined by the tidal volume divided by the compliance of the ventilator and patient combination (here, 150 divided by 6, or 25 cmH$_2$O pressure). The volume delivered to the patient is equal to the patient's compliance multiplied by the airway pressure (1 × 25 = 25 mL), and that remaining in the ventilator circuit is 5 × 25 = 125 mL. The sum of the two equals the original ventilator tidal volume. In this illustration, only 16% of the ventilator tidal volume is delivered to the patient.

How does a high ventilator/patient compliance ratio affect the response of the ventilator to changes in patient compliance? Assume that ventilator compliance and preset volume remain unchanged, but the patient's compliance is reduced by 50% (from 1 to 0.5 mL/cmH$_2$O pressure). The sum of both ventilator and patient compliance is decreased by the same amount, from 6 to 5.5 mL/cmH$_2$O pressure. Recalculating the above equations

$$Ventilator\ pressure = \frac{150\ (Tidal\ volume)}{5.5\ (Sum\ of\ compliances)} = 27\ cmH_2O\ pressure$$

Despite the large (50%) drop in patient compliance, pressure increased only 2 cmH$_2$O (8%), because the sum of patient and ventilator compliance changed little [0.5 mL/cmH$_2$O pressure (also 8%)]. With 27 cmH$_2$O pressure, only 13.5 mL can be delivered to the patient [*Volume = Pressure* (27) × *Patient compliance* (0.5)]. Tidal volume has decreased 46% and has produced a negligible increase in pressure.

When ventilator compliance is low relative to patient compliance, as the following equations illustrate, the ventilator is better equipped to respond to patient compliance changes. For example, assume

Ventilator tidal volume = 37.5 mL
Ventilator compliance = 0.5 mL/cmH$_2$O pressure
Patient compliance = 1 mL/cmH$_2$O pressure

Then, ventilator pressure (tidal volume divided by the sum of compliances) equals 25 cmH$_2$O, with 25 delivered to the patient, and 12.5 delivered to the circuit. Should patient compliance decrease by 50%, then

$$Ventilator\ pressure = \frac{37.5\ (Tidal\ volume)}{1.0\ (Sum\ of\ compliances)} = 37.5\ cmH_2O\ pressure$$

At this pressure, 19 mL can be delivered to the lung, representing a loss of only 24%. Considerably less volume is lost, in comparison with the previous example (46%), and pressure increase is much more noticeable.

These concepts also apply when lung mechanics improve. That is, when ventilator compliance is low, an increase in patient compliance will (appropriately) result in decreased airway pressures and less of an (inappropriate) increase in delivered tidal volume.

Airway pressure changes should be interpreted with these concepts in mind. Small changes in pressure may signal large changes in patient compliance, especially when high-compliance ventilator circuits are used in small infants.

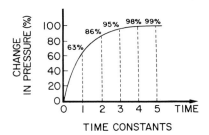

Figure 29—5. Relationship between time constants and change in alveolar pressure: Volume changes parallel pressure changes. Terminating expiration during mechanical ventilation before three time constants have elapsed can result in significant increases in end-expiratory volume and pressure. (Carlo WA, Martin RJ: Principles of neonatal assisted ventilation. Pediatr Clin North Am 33:221, 1986)

From the foregoing data, one time constant equals 0.15 second, and the time needed to deliver 95% of total volume would equal 0.45 seconds. The same rules govern expiration. However, since airway resistance is higher during expiration, expiratory time constants (and expiratory time) will be longer than inspiratory time and time constants.

Time constants increase as compliance or resistance increase. Compliance may increase as a restrictive lung disease resolves. In addition, larger lungs (in older children) are more compliant. Hence, an older child will require longer inspiratory and expiratory times (and a lower respiratory rate) than a younger child. A child with an acute restrictive disease may tolerate higher respiratory rates (with shorter inspiratory times and expiratory times) than one with more compliant lungs.

Increased airway resistance is characteristic of many pediatric pulmonary diseases, such as asthma and bronchiolitis. Time constants are thus elevated in these disorders. An understanding of time constants is essential in understanding ventilatory strategies for pediatric respiratory disorders. Although resistance and compliance data are not always available for individual patients, an understanding of the disease process should adequately predict whether the time constant is increased or decreased from normal.

The consequences of failing to allow adequate inspiratory or expiratory time include hyperinflation and hypoventilation, which have been well documented in the adult and newborn.[41,233,275]

Scott et al. have shown that small endotracheal tubes also contribute to expiratory hyperinflation.[264] Children with upper airway obstruction, such as croup, may require smaller-than-normal endotracheal tubes and, therefore, may be at increased risk for expiratory air-trapping, especially if lung compliance is normal. Use of prolonged expiratory time should be considered if signs of air-trapping are present.

Finally, Greenough[110] and Field,[80] in separate studies, have documented that respiratory rate and inspiratory time can be manipulated to synchronize infant's breathing with the ventilator, thereby avoiding the use of muscle relaxants in some cases. Additionally, Greenough has suggested that shorter inspiratory times (0.5 seconds) are more effective than longer times (1.0 seconds) in weaning infants from mechanical ventilation.[109]

Positive End-Expiratory Pressure. PEEP is utilized to increase the patient's arterial oxygenation. PEEP can improve lung compliance and ventilation–perfusion ($\dot{V}/\dot{Q}$) matching, which in turn improves gas exchange and oxygenation.[103] However, use of PEEP is associated with increased risk of barotrauma and decreased cardiac output.

Various criteria have been proposed by investigators treating respiratory failure in adults to select the optimal level of PEEP. Some advocate that sufficient PEEP should be applied to reduce intrapulmonary shunt to some preselected value (e.g., 15%), in the hope of altering the basic pathophysiologic mechanisms of severe ARDS. This approach usually results in the application of high levels of PEEP, with pharmacologic support of cardiac output often being necessary.[98] Others suggest only that an amount of PEEP necessary to reduce the FIO_2 to nontoxic levels be applied, hoping this approach will minimize cardiovascular consequences of high level PEEP.[53] Only recently have these two approaches been compared. Carroll et al. compared the effects of PEEP that was titrated to reduce shunt to a minimum with PEEP that was titrated to relieve hypoxemia at a nontoxic FIO_2.[38] More aggressive therapy (PEEP adjusted to reduce shunt) produced greater mortality and morbidity than the less aggressive approach. None of the patients in this study, however, had severe hypoxemia.

Yet another approach suggests that PEEP be adjusted to produce the highest systemic oxygen transport.[294] This approach balances the beneficial effects of PEEP (increased PaO_2) against the cardiovascular side effects (decreased cardiac output). This level of PEEP may correlate with highest pulmonary compliance.

Do these studies have any relevance to children? Recently, Witte et al. studied the effects of different levels of PEEP in children with hypoxemic respiratory failure.[322] The amount of PEEP required to produce a significant increase in PaO_2 was higher (9 cmH_2O) than the minimal level (4 cmH_2O) required to relieve hypoxemia in Carroll's study in adults. Witte found that this level of PEEP depressed cardiac output and, hence, systemic oxygen transport. However, she suggests use of volume expansion or ionotropic agents to offset the depressed cardiac output. Interestingly, she was unable to show any relation between the level of PEEP that produced the highest oxygen transport and pulmonary compliance. Likewise, the response to PEEP did not vary with age.

Mode of Ventilation. The same modes of ventilation used for adults have been used in pediatric ventilation: assist–control, intermittent mandatory ventilation (IMV), and pressure support. However, little objective evidence exists to compare their efficacies in children.

Assist–Control. Assist–control ventilation may pose difficulties when applied to the pediatric patient. Slow response times, coupled with high compliance ventilator circuits (which dampen the transmission of airway pressure changes to the ventilator's assist mechanism), may result in assisted breaths being out-of-phase with the child's inspiratory efforts, as well as an increase in the work of breathing. Spontaneous ventilatory efforts in children may be prompted not only by physiologic needs, but also by crying and anxiety, for which a ventilator response would be inappropriate.

Intermittent Mandatory Ventilation. IMV is widely used in pediatrics, in part as a response to the poor performance of the assisted mode of ventilation. IMV allows children to breath spontaneously between the mandatory positive-pressure breaths. This allows the patient to exercise ventilatory muscles preparing them to gradually assume the entire work of breathing.

In recent years, it has become clear that systems used to produce flow for spontaneous breathing during IMV may increase the work of breathing.[44,101,148] However, there is no clear agreement on whether demand valves or continuous flow systems produce the least added work of breathing. No study has yet appeared comparing the advantages and disadvantages of flow and demand IMV or CPAP systems in children. Given their rapid respiratory rates, small endotracheal tube size, and small tidal volumes (which may not be detected by some ventilator's triggering mechanisms), we prefer to use continuous-flow systems, especially with older-model ventilators, and when ventilating small children, regardless of ventilator type.

Newer ventilators, such as the Siemens Servo 900C, are capable of delivering rates of 120/min (with resulting short expiratory times). Since an external continuous-flow IMV circuit could potentially add to expiratory resistance, we delete the external IMV circuit when using high respiratory rates (and short expiratory times).

Pressure Support. Pressure-support ventilation has been advocated as a means to decrease work of breathing and improve patient comfort during mechanical ventilation. With pressure support, airway pressure is maintained constant during a patient's initiated breath, and inspiration is terminated when inspiratory flow reaches 25% of its peak value. As long as the patient continues active inspiration, inspiratory flows should remain high, and the pressure-supported breath continues. When the patient ceases to actively inspire, or actively expires, inspiratory flows are reduced, and inspiration is terminated. Inspiratory time and tidal volume are thus patient controlled. Given the high resistance of pediatric endotracheal tubes, inspiratory flow may drop abruptly, terminating inspiration prematurely. While using a Siemens Servo 900C, Perlman[234] and Czervinski,[54] in separate studies, showed that reduction of ventilator working pressure prevents premature termination of pressure support, presumably by limiting ventilator peak flow. A ventilator working pressure of no more than 20 cmH_2O above the desired level of pressure support is recommended.[54]

Summary. Ventilator settings are selected to provide adequate ventilation and oxygenation and to minimize work of breathing and barotrauma. Table 29–6 provides guidelines for selection of settings.

Weaning

Once the indication for ventilator commitment is no longer present and clinical condition permits, the patient is ready to be weaned from ventilation. Table 29–7 is a set of criteria that can be used to make this decision.

Withdrawing the child from mechanical ventilation can be accomplished by reducing the rate and pressures on time-cycled ventilators until the patient is breathing by CPAP. With volume ventilators, tidal volume is usually not adjusted during the weaning period. While breathing by CPAP, the patient's ability to breath spontaneously is tested without removing the artificial airway.[266] For diffi-

Table 29–7 Criteria to Wean Children from the Ventilator

GAS EXCHANGE

$PaO_2 > 60$ mmHg with $FiO_2 < 0.35$
Alveolar to arterial oxygen gradient < 350 mmHg
$PaO_2/FiO_2 > 200$

VENTILATION

Vital capacity > 10–15 mL/kg body weight
Negative inspiratory force (NIF) < -30 mmHg

(McWilliams BC: Mechanical ventilation in pediatric patients. Clin Chest Med 8:597, 1987)

cult-to-wean patients, who exhibit hypoventilation after more than a brief period when breathing with CPAP, this mode can be used intermittently, for gradually increasing lengths of time, to increase ventilatory muscle strength and endurance. The patient should be returned to IMV before frank respiratory muscle fatigue is evident.

SPECIAL TECHNIQUES

Hyperventilation

Hyperventilation (maintaining by mechanical ventilation a pH > 7.50 and a $Pco_2 < 30$ mmHg) can be used in children to reduce intracranial pressure and pulmonary vascular resistance. The most common indication is to treat persistent pulmonary hypertension of the newborn (PPHN—also known as persistent fetal circulation [PFC]). In addition, hyperventilation is used to reduce pulmonary artery pressures and right ventricular workload following repair of congenital heart defects.[207]

In contrast with the pulmonary circulation, in which alkalosis and hypocarbia secondary to hyperventilation cause vasodilatation, alkalosis and hypocarbia causes *cerebral* vasoconstriction.[79,88] Hyperventilation has thus been used to treat elevated intracranial pressure.[29]

Phrenic Pacing

Phrenic nerve pacing has been utilized for a variety of patients, including those with high cervical (C-1, C-2) spinal cord lesions and central hypoventilation syndrome. To successfully accomplish phrenic pacing, both the diaphragm and phrenic nerve need to be intact and capable of external stimulation.[26] The major benefit of phrenic pacing is that it allows the patient more freedom in their

activities of daily life. It is also a more physiologic form of ventilation, since it uses the patient's diaphragm as the pressure generator for inspiration. This would, in effect, classify phrenic pacers as negative-pressure generators.[144]

Patients breathing with phrenic pacing should be considered "ventilator-dependent" and need appropriate backup emergency equipment should the phrenic pacers fail. In infants and small children, it is necessary to pace both hemidiaphragms simultaneously because of a highly mobile mediastinum.[144] As children grow, it becomes possible to pace each hemidiaphragm unilaterally, thereby resting one side while stimulating the other. Continuous pacing in infants usually must be alternated with time on a positive-pressure ventilator. Children who are being paced also require a tracheostomy because of pacing-related upper airway obstruction. During pacing, the vocal cords fail to actively abduct during inspiration, causing passive vocal cord adduction (secondary to decreased intratracheal pressures during inspiration) and obstruction.[28]

High-Frequency Ventilation

High-frequency ventilation (HFV) has been used in various applications since 1967.[279] It may allow the delivery of "adequate ventilation" at lower mean airway pressures than conventional ventilation. It also provides a way to reduce the cardiac side effects of positive-pressure ventilation (e.g., decreased cardiac output)[279] and improve ventilation–perfusion matching.[194]

High-frequency ventilation in pediatrics has been primarily used in neonates with respiratory distress syndrome,[91,182] pulmonary interstitial emphysema,[91] and meconium aspiration. Other indications for the use of HFV are ventilation during bronchoscopy and laryngoscopy,[278] bronchopulmonary fistulae, and severely compromised right ventricular function.[194]

Hazards of HFV include necrotizing tracheobronchitis.[23,178]

More research is needed to further define the role of HFV in treating pediatric lung disease, as well as to discover ways of decreasing the side effects previously mentioned. As of this writing, this technique is still considered experimental.

Extracorporeal Membrane Oxygenation

With extracorporeal membrane oxygenation (ECMO), a modified heart–lung pump is used to maintain normal gas exchange in severe respiratory failure refractory to conventional ventilator therapy. Currently, it is most widely used in the newborn. The overall survival rate in the neonatal-aged group has been reported at 75%, with the highest rate of survival reported at 91% for the disorder of persistent fetal circulation.[225] Hemorrhage is a major complication of ECMO, owing to the use of systemic heparinization.[127,265] Newborns with significant intraventricular hemorrhage (IVH) are not candidates for ECMO, since heparinization may increase the risk of further hemorrhage.[301]

Extracorporeal membrane oxygenation has been used in older children with limited success. The literature has reported an overall survival rate of 26%; however, it was noted that most of these patients were moribund when first started on ECMO.[12,127,159,283] It has been used in pediatric patients to treat acute respiratory failure (e.g., bronchiolitis) and support cardiac function following cardiac surgery and transplants.[225] Contraindications for use in children would include irreversible lung damage, brain damage, and major multiple congenital anomalies.[301]

Survival may depend on the condition of the patient before commitment to ECMO. The cost of this therapy is high, but may actually reduce the patient's overall length of hospital stay and, therefore, cut the patient's overall hospital costs.[301]

Since the right common carotid artery and jugular vein are used for cannulation, these must be permanently ligated following withdrawal of the catheter. One study did not show any right-sided brain lesions as a result of this ligation.[34] However, another study showed significant problems associated with ligation of the right common carotid artery.[261a] Further study of long-term survivors continues to be warranted,[34,66,307] and its role in children has yet to be defined. It is still experimental and should be confined to centers with specialized ECMO teams.

MONITORING

Most of the major cardiovascular monitoring tools that are available for adults can be utilized in pediatrics if modifications are made for size and age differences. Pediatric intensive care units (PICUs) should have the capability to monitor heart and respiratory rates, systemic central venous and pulmonary artery pressures, and temperature. The placement of these and other monitoring capabilities in the ICU can, however, result in an unjustifiably high number of patients being admitted to the PICU for monitoring only. Pollack et al. showed that 57% of 822 admissions to their PICU required only monitoring and routine care that could have been performed outside of the PICU, thus occupying beds and resources that could have been used more wisely.[239]

Despite advances in noninvasive monitoring of oxygen and carbon dioxide, arterial blood gas analysis remains the respiratory care practitioner's most important diagnostic tool. However, a sole reliance on arterial blood gas values does not permit the caretakers to detect rapid changes in oxygenation or ventilation. In addition, although modern blood gas analyzers require only small quantities of blood, excessive sampling for arterial blood gas analysis can be a significant source of blood loss for small children.

Recent advances in technology have made it possible to continuously monitor patients noninvasively. Transcutaneous P_{O_2} and P_{CO_2}, pulse oximetry (measuring arterial oxygen saturation), and end tidal carbon dioxide monitors have increased the clinician's capabilities to detect sudden changes in a patients condition.

Invasive monitoring through arterial catheters poses substantial risks as well as benefits. For example, radial artery catherization in children carries the following risks:[69,199,202]

- Ischemia of the tissue distal to the puncture site
- Hemorrhage
- Infection
- Embolism

Continuous direct measurement of arterial blood pressure provides more accurate and timely information than noncontinuous indirect measurement by a sphygmomanometer. An arterial line also gives the practitioner access to arterial blood, which can be analyzed for pH and blood gases. Studies have shown that percutaneous arterial cannulation in children can be a safe and appropriate procedure if correct technique and pediatric-sized equipment is used.[185]

Electrocardiographic (ECG) monitoring is routinely used, and monitors used in pediatrics should also incorporate an apnea or respiratory monitor, with display of rate and waveform. Most respiratory monitors actually measure chest wall movement and, therefore, can be influenced by chest wall motion secondary to the cardiac impulse. This may cause the monitor to record an inappropriately high respiratory rate and, perhaps, fail to detect periods of apnea. Likewise, apnea secondary to airway obstruction (when the chest continues to move, but airflow is absent) may not be detected by such monitors.[27] High and low heart rate and respiratory rate alarms can be set to warn of any tachycardic, bradycardic, or apneic event. However, heart rate changes in children are a late sign of cardiovascular problems.[74]

Temperature monitoring is especially important in pediatrics. In infants, it is vital to maintain a neutral thermal environment, since oxygen consumption increases at temperatures outside this range. Older patients can better maintain normal core temperatures because of their larger size, greater insulation (fat), and ability to shiver. Any deviations from normal are usually caused by some physiologic disturbance (e.g., infection). Hyperthermia and hypothermia will both increase a patient's oxygen consumption, further taxing a stressed respiratory system.[74]

Measurement of pulmonary artery systolic, diastolic, and mean pressures, as well as pulmonary capillary wedge pressures (pulmonary artery occluding pressure), and cardiac output can be performed with pediatric pulmonary artery catheters. Measurement and control of pulmonary hypertension that occurs with some congenital cardiac anomalies is one indication for use of pulmonary artery catheters.[18] The persistence of pulmonary hypertension contributes to postoperative mortality in patients following repair of such defects.[40]

The same risks associated with arterial catheters apply to pulmonary artery catheters. In addition, pulmonary artery catheterization can cause pneumothorax, arrhythmias, pulmonary artery rupture, infarction, and embolization.[296]

When monitoring patients with intracardiac right-to-left shunts, (such as a ventricular septal defect) rupture of the inflatable balloon can cause cerebral air embolism. In such patients, inflation of the balloon with carbon dioxide, which is more rapidly absorbed, may be preferable.[296]

Manipulation of the catheter may to be more difficult in children than in adults.[286] Also, the catheter may migrate through intracardiac or other central right-to-left shunts. This can be recognized by inability to wedge the catheter.[296]

Intracranial Pressure Monitoring

Intracranial pressure (ICP) monitoring has become an important tool in the management of children who sustain neurologic insults or impairment. In-creased intracranial pressure, a common consequence of head injury, Reye syndrome, and anoxic events (such as drowning), can cause a decrease in cerebral blood flow, with increased central nervous system damage.

Intracranial pressure monitoring can be performed with either an intraventricular catheter or a subarachnoid bolt.[35] Any child who has suffered a severe head injury, or is a victim of near-drowning, should be monitored early in their clinical course.[35,189,215] Infection is the major hazard of ICP monitoring.[35]

The treatment for increased ICP includes the following:[35]

> Keeping the head in midline and elevated 30° to 45°
> Keeping an endotracheal airway in place with hyperventilation
> Use of muscle paralysis
> Use of osmotic diuretics
> Use of steroids
> Removal of cerebrospinal fluid
> Use of hypothermia
> Use of barbiturate coma

The latter two therapies carry significant risks. Barbiturate use, to the point of coma, generally requires considerable cardiovascular support to overcome depressed cardiac output.[59] Hypothermia can cause arrhythmias, immune suppression, and has increased the risk of pneumonia in some patients.[93]

Respiratory care procedures can pose increased risks to the neurologically injured child. Positive-pressure ventilation can aggravate increased ICP, and attempts should be made to keep airway pressures to a minimum.[59] Suctioning, intubation, and similar procedures may also acutely increase ICP, even when therapy to reduce ICP has already been instituted. Administration of a short-acting barbiturate may be beneficial.[59]

Noninvasive Blood Gas Monitoring

The most common forms of noninvasive monitoring used in the PICU include those devices that continuously assess oxygen and carbon dioxide levels. Transcutaneous monitoring is used to monitor P_{O_2} and P_{CO_2} on the surface of the skin. The transcutaneous P_{O_2} electrode is a heated Clark electrode that can be placed on the surface of the skin. In most patients with adequate cardiac output and tissue perfusion, the transcutaneous P_{O_2} will accurately reflect the PaO_2. In older children, the transcutaneous P_{O_2} is decreased relative to the PaO_2.[309,327]

Transcutaneous P_{CO_2} recording has been used with varying results. The accuracy of the transcutaneous P_{CO_2} electrode depends on the temperature of the electrode and the arterial carbon dioxide tension. Martin et al. found that hypercapnea and normocapnea tended to make the transcutaneous P_{CO_2} read higher than the actual $PaCO_2$.[186]

Most transcutaneous monitors sold today feature a combined sensor that allows the practitioner to monitor the transcutaneous P_{O_2} and P_{CO_2} simultaneously. This entails just one electrode placement and one calibration.

The most serious hazard of using these monitors is burning of the skin, which can occur because heated electrodes are used at 44 to 45° C. The electrode site needs to be changed frequently to prevent skin burns.[255] Another hazard is assuming that measured values are identical with arterial values. Whenever starting a monitor for any patient, corresponding arterial P_{O_2} and P_{CO_2} should be obtained by a blood gas analysis to compare these values with those obtained by the transcutaneous monitor. It is important that these monitors be used by skilled personnel who are aware of all the limitations and hazards of these devices.

Pulse oximetry is a new technique being utilized in pediatric medicine. It has proved itself to be an accurate monitor for assessment of arterial oxygen saturation in children.[197,294,329] Unlike transcutaneous P_{O_2} monitors, pulse oximetry appears to produce reliable measurements of oxygen saturation, regardless of age or skin thickness.[203] It is useful in children who have cyanotic heart disease or who are undergoing cardiac catheterization or cardiac surgery.[24] Pulse oximetry can be used to wean patients from oxygen, without resorting to invasive arterial blood gas monitoring.[154] Pulse oximetry is a more appropriate monitor to measure oxygenation in sick newborn infants than transcutaneous P_{O_2}.[71]

Capnography (End-Tidal Carbon Dioxide Monitoring)

End tidal carbon dioxide monitors use infrared wavelength light to determine carbon dioxide concentrations in exhaled gas.[37] A sampling adaptor is attached to the patient's airway between the endotracheal tube connector and the ventilator circuit. Gas is continuously aspirated from the sampling adaptor at the patient's airway and the concentration of carbon dioxide measured.

Capnography has some limitations that will give rise to erroneous values. These include sudden hypercapnea, large amounts of dead space, and tachypnea (>40 bpm).[126] With this type of monitor, the appropriate-sized adaptor must be used for smaller patients, to obtain accurate values. The use of too large an adaptor can contribute to the patient's dead space. End tidal carbon dioxide monitors have also been used to measure V_D/V_T ratios if the arterial P_{CO_2} level is available.[328] A recording of the end-tidal CO_2 waveform is useful. The presence of an end-tidal plateau in the carbon dioxide value indicates the capnographer has measured "alveolar" carbon dioxide and, hence, a value that more closely reflects arterial $PaCO_2$.[86]

CARDIOPULMONARY RESUSCITATION

Several studies have been performed concerning the etiology of cardiac arrest in children.[75,223] These studies demonstrate the diverse causative factors (e.g., sudden infant death syndrome, near-drowning, airway problems, trauma, and abuse) of cardiac arrest. Also, they indicate that children rarely suffer primary cardiac arrest. Rather, they suffer secondary cardiac arrest caused by the primary insult (hypoxemia) of respiratory arrest.[223] The most common arrythmia was asystole, which presumably led to a higher mortality in pediatric cardiac arrest.[75]

The procedures for the recognition of cardiac arrest and performance of basic life-support measures are essentially the same as those for adults, with modification because of anatomic differences. The sequence of cardiopulmonary resuscitation (CPR) remains the same as that for adults: airway, breathing, and circulation. Some changes made in the 1986 AHA standards[285] include two initial breaths of 1.0 to 1.5 seconds instead of "four quick breaths." This was recommended to eliminate the high peak pressures during the four quick breaths that caused gastric insufflation.[195,196] In addition, during compression, the fingers are now placed one-fingerbreadth below the intermammary line.[285]

To establish a patent airway, perform either a head-tilt, head-tilt with chin-lift, head-tilt with neck-lift, or the jaw thrust.[260] Once the airway is patent, the rescuer should look, listen, and feel for breathing by placing their ear over the child's mouth and nose, and looking for movement of the chest and abdomen. If no respirations are detected, then two breaths are delivered (being careful not to deliver too large a tidal volume). If air does not enter the lungs (i.e., no visible chest expansion) there is either an obstruction or the maneuvers to establish an airway have not been properly performed. The rescuer must then attempt to reestablish the airway, and attempt to ventilate the patient again. If there is still no chest expansion, an obstruction must be present. Procedures for dislodging foreign bodies must be applied, as described later in the discussion of foreign body aspiration.

After the airway has been established and two breaths have been given, the pulse should be assessed. In older children, the carotid artery can be palpated to ascertain pulselessness. In infants, carotid arteries are difficult to palpate, as the infants necks are short and fat. Therefore, to accurately assess pulselessness in infants, the brachial pulse can be palpated.[285]

If no pulse is found, external cardiac compressions are begun. In infants, compress at a rate of 100/min with two fingers on the sternum, one-fingerbreadth below the intermammary line. The depth of compression should be ½ to 1 in. One can also encircle the chest with the hands and compress the sternum with the thumbs.[306] The fingers should support the back of the infant in this technique. The latter method has been recommended as it tends to improve cardiac output during CPR.[56]

For older children, one deepens the compression depth and slows the compression rate. Toddlers should receive a depth of 1 to 1½ in. at a rate of 80/min. Compressions are with the heel of one hand at a two-finger distance above the xiphoid process. Older children should receive compressions the same as an adult. It should be noted that the compression/ventilation ratio in infants and small children is 5:1, regardless of whether it is a one- or two-person rescue.[260]

Advanced life-support requires vascular access for administration of cardiac and vascular support drugs, such as epinephrine, sodium bicarbonate, and atropine. It is also possible to administer drugs by an intraosseous infusion or by the endotracheal tube.[252,282] Table 29–8 lists the drugs used during pediatric CPR, with their appropriate dosages.

Oral endotracheal intubation should be performed, as soon as possible, since it permits more effective ventilation and protection from aspiration.

The results of pediatric CPR have been no better than those of adults.[70] It was suggested that better outcomes might result from early recognition and monitoring of children at risk, earlier intervention with basic and advanced life-support, better education for both medical personnel and the general public, and more research into pediatric cardiopulmonary resuscitation.[70]

Table 29–8 Cardiovascular Resuscitation Drugs for Children

MEDICATION	INITIAL DOSE
Sodium bicarbonate (1 mEq/mL)	1–2 mEq (1–2 mL)/kg
Epinephrine (1:10,000)	10 μg (0.1 mL)/kg*
Atropine (1.0 mg/mL)	0.02 mg (0.2 mL)/kg*
Calcium chloride (10%)	20 mg (0.2 mL)/kg
Lidocaine (2%)	1 mg (0.05 mL)/kg
Dopamine (40 mg/mL)	
60 mg (1.5 mL)/100 mL D5W = 600 μg/mL	1 mL/kg per hr = 10 μg/kg per min†
Epinephrine (1:1000)	
6 mg (6 mL)/100 mL D5W = 60 μg/mL	1 mL/kg per hr = 1 μg/kg per min‡
Isoproterenol (1:5000)	
0.6 mg (3.0 mL)/100 mL D5W = 6 μg/mL	1 mL/kg per hr = 0.1 μg/kg per min§
Lidocaine (4%)	
120 mg (3 mL)/100 mL D5W = 1200 μg/mL	1 mL/kg per hr = 20 μg/kg per min#
Defibrillation	2 watt-sec/kg

* May be given by endotracheal tube.
† Moderate dose: predominantly β-effects.
‡ High dose: α- and β-effects.
§ Low dose
# Moderate dose
(Holbrook PR, Pollack MM, Mickell J, Fields AI: Cardiovascular resuscitation drugs for children. Crit Care Med 8:762, © by Williams & Wilkins 1980)

MAJOR RESPIRATORY DISORDERS IN INFANTS AND CHILDREN

ASTHMA

Asthma is a condition characterized by increased responsiveness of the airways to various stimuli. It is manifested by widespread narrowing of the airways that changes in severity, either spontaneously or as the result of therapy.[273] The increased responsiveness of the airways characteristic of asthma has lead many to use the term "reactive airway disease" or similar nomenclature to describe asthma.

Etiology

A variety of irritants or stimuli can provoke an asthmatic episode. These stimuli include allergens, such as molds and pollens; irritants, such as smoke and air pollution; infections (especially viral); exercise; changes in atmospheric conditions; gastroesophageal reflux; and aspirin and related drugs.[250] Table 29–9 lists some of the common precipitating causes of asthma in children. Often, a specific precipitating factor cannot be identified.

Epidemiology and Natural History

Asthma in childhood is widespread, with as many as 10% of children suffering from asthmalike symptoms at one time or another.[273] Most children with asthma first develop symptoms before the age of 5, with one-third having symptoms before the age of 3.[273] It is the leading cause of chronic illness in children, one of the leading causes of hospital admission, and also one of the leading causes of school absence.[43] Asthma often overlaps or coexists with other conditions, such as cystic fibrosis, bronchopulmonary dysplasia, and congenital abnormalities of the tracheobronchial tree, such as tracheoesophageal fistula.[160]

Pathology and Pathophysiology

Pulmonary function during an acute asthmatic episode is characterized by increased airways resistance, manifested by decreased expiratory flow rates and hyperinflation. Increased airway resistance is caused by diffuse bronchospasm, edema, and mucous plugging of the airways.[137] These changes are thought to be secondary to a diffuse inflammatory response of the airways to irritants.[249] In addition to these functional changes, bronchial smooth-muscle hypertrophy is often noted in the lungs of patients dying of asthma.[137]

Widespread airways obstruction leads to maldistribution of ventilation, with resultant hypoxemia. Generally, minute ventilation is increased and $PaCO_2$ is low.[43] The expiratory phase of respiration is prolonged, and wheezing is usually present, along with other signs of respiratory distress. If the attack is unusually severe, or treatment inadequate, respiratory failure may develop.

Evaluation of the Patient with an Acute Asthmatic Attack

The severity of an asthmatic episode can be gauged by physical examination, measurement of blood gas levels and pulmonary function studies, and by the response to therapy.

Table 29–9 Precipitants of Asthmatic Symptoms in Various Age Groups

PRECIPITANT	INFANCY	EARLY CHILDHOOD	LATER CHILDHOOD	ADULTHOOD
Viral infections	+ + + +*	+ + +	+(+)	+ + +
Exercise	+	+ +	+ + +	+ + +
Irritants	+	+ +	+ + +	+ + +
Foods	+ +	+	(+)	(+)
Indoor inhalants	+(+)	+ + +	+ + +	+ + +
Pollens		+ +	+ + +	+ +(+)
Emotions	(+)	+	+	+

* Relative importance denoted, in order, by + + + +; + + +; + +(+); + +; +(+); +; (+).
(Pearlman DS, Bierman CW: Asthma (bronchial asthma). In Bierman CW, Pearlman DS (ed): Allergic Diseases from Infancy to Adulthood, 2nd ed, p 551. Philadelphia, WB Saunders Co, 1988)

Physical Examination.   The presence and character of wheezing should be assessed. Initially, wheezing may be quite noticeable during the expiratory phase, even without a stethoscope. With more severe obstruction, wheezing may be heard on inspiration. As obstruction becomes critical, wheezing may seem less noticeable, as airflow is minimal. In addition, the depth of ventilation should be noted. The presence of cyanosis and changes in sensorium (secondary to hypoxemia or hypercarbia) should also be assessed. Retractions and use of accessory muscles also reflect the severity of the obstruction.

Scoring systems that are based on the findings of the physical examination have been developed. One of the more popular is the Clinical Asthma Evaluation Score devised by Wood et al.[325] A score of 5 or more signals impending respiratory failure, and a score of 7 or more, existing respiratory failure (Table 29–10).

Another useful tool is the assessment of the pulsus paradoxus. This refers to a difference in systolic blood pressure between inspiration and expiration. As airway obstruction worsens, inspiratory pressures become more negative. This, in turn, temporarily reduces systolic blood pressure. When the pulus paradoxus is 10 to 15 mmHg[43,181] hospitalization should be considered.

Measurement of Pulmonary Function.   Since airflow obstruction is the principle physiologic derangement in asthma, measurement of expiratory flow variables is useful. Depending on equipment available, the peak-expiratory flow rate (PEFR) the forced-expiratory volume in 1 second (FEV1), or other variables, may be monitored and used to follow the response to therapy. A PEFR or an FEV1 value less than 35%[181] of predicted may warrant hospital admission.

Other Laboratory Studies.   For patients who have been receiving theophylline therapy, measurement of serum theophylline levels is necessary. The use of theophylline will be discussed further.

Blood gas analyses are necessary in the evaluation of the moderately or severely symptomatic patient. The $PaCO_2$ is especially important, since it reflects the ability of the patient to adequately compensate for the underlying airway obstruction. Typically, very mild cases of asthma demonstrate normal or only slightly decreased $PaCO_2$. As the obstruction progresses, hyperventilation is evident. With worsening obstruction or fatigue, the $PaCO_2$ may return to normal because the patient is no longer able to maintain increased minute ventilation. Since most patients with asthma are able to maintain a considerable degree of hyperventilation, any patient with a "normal" $PaCO_2$, who also has other signs of respiratory distress, should be considered as having impending respiratory failure.[43] Finally, as respiratory failure becomes overt, the $PaCO_2$ is elevated.

Metabolic acidosis is not uncommon in severe asthma, especially when an associated viral infection that causes dehydration is present.[181] This condition may worsen as work of breathing is increased. Metabolic acidosis may also impair the response to β_2-stimulant agents.[164]

Clinical Response

The response to initial therapy of the acute asthmatic episode must be evaluated to determine the need for hospital admission and further therapy.

Table 29–10   Clinical Asthma Evaluation Score

	0	1	2
PaO_2 (torr)	70–100 in room air	<70 in room air	<70 in 40% O_2
Cyanosis	None	In room air	In 40% O_2
Inspiratory breath sounds	Normal	Unequal	Decreased to absent
Accessory muscles used	None	Moderate	Maximal
Expiratory wheezing	None	Moderate	Marked
Cerebral function	Normal	Depressed or agitated	Coma

A score of 5 or more is thought to indicate impending respiratory failure.
A score of 7 or more with an arterial carbon dioxide tension ($PaCO_2$) of 65 torr indicates existing respiratory failure.
(Wood DW, Downes JJ, Lecks HI: A clinical scoring system for the diagnosis of respiratory failure. Am J Dis Child 123:227, 1972. Copyright 1972 American Medical Association)

When a series of treatments with adrenergic agents, such as epinephrine injections or albuterol aerosols, have failed to provide substantial relief, the diagnosis of status asthmaticus is made. Risk factors for status asthmaticus are outlined in Table 29–11. Generally, these children are admitted to the hospital and should be observed for the development of respiratory failure; 15% to 20% of children seen in the emergency room with asthmatic symptoms may require admission.[97] Mansmann and associates have proposed additional criteria for hospitalization (see Table 29–12).[181]

Treatment

Management of acute asthma has the following goals: correction of hypoxemia, relief of bronchial obstruction, and prevention or treatment of respiratory failure. In addition, the management of the acute episode should end with a program to continue treatment if necessary in the home. This involves patient and family education designed to prevent or minimize further acute attacks.

Hypoxemia. In most cases, treatment of hypoxemia is easily accomplished with low to moderate oxygen concentrations. When hypoxemia is refractory to moderate oxygen therapy, the patient should be assessed for the presence of complications, such as pneumothorax, pneumonia, or atelectasis. Oxygen therapy is also useful in preventing hypoxemia and arrhythmias associated with use of sympathomimetic agents.[164]

Airway Obstruction (β_2-Agents). Administration of β_2-selective sympathomimetic agents, by aerosol or injection, is the mainstay of the treatment of the

Table 29–11 Risk Factors for Status Asthmaticus

Asthma since infancy
Males with severe chronic asthma
Barrel-chest deformity
Short stature
Underweight
Steroid dependency
Poor coping style
Sudden changes in asthma pattern
Previous episodes of status asthmaticus

(Mansmann HC, Bierman CW, Pearlman DS: Treatment of acute asthma in children. In Bierman CW, Pearlman DS (ed): Allergic Diseases from Infancy to Adulthood, 2nd ed, p 573. Philadelphia, WB Saunders Co, 1988)

Table 29–12 Indications for Hospitalization for Treatment of Acute Severe Asthma

---

HISTORICAL REASONS

Recurrent status asthmaticus
Previous respiratory failure
Previous use of intravenous isoproterenol
Previous use of controlled ventilation

CLINICAL FINDINGS

Distrubance of consciousness
Exhaustion
Sternocleidomastoid contraction
Supraclavicular retractions
Pulsus paradoxus > 15 mmHg
PEFR < 35% of predicted
FEV_1 < 35%
$PaCO_2$ > 40 mmHg
PaO_2 > 60 mmHg
Electrocardiographic abnormalities
Diaphoresis
Unresponsiveness to initial therapy in the first hour
Emergency treatment over 2 successive days

(Mansmann HC, Bierman CW, Pearlman DS: Treatment of acute asthma in children. In Bierman CW, Pearlman DS (eds): Allergic Diseases from Infancy to Adulthood, 2nd ed, p 574. Philadelphia, WB Saunders Co, 1988)

bronchospastic component of asthma. These agents are discussed in more detail in Chapter 19.

Considerable debate exists over the age at which bronchodilators are effective. Clinical trials in asthma and other obstructive respiratory disorders in children under 2 years of age have yielded mixed results. Lenny and Milner assessed respiratory resistance in children with wheezing, who received nebulized albuterol, and found no significant fall in airway resistance in those under 18 months of age. However, among those over 20 months of age, 90% had a greater than 20% fall in airway resistance.[168] Prendiville et al.[242] actually found a decrease in expiratory flow rates when albuterol was given to a group of wheezy infants younger than 15 months of age. Stokes et al.[292] showed that albuterol produced a 22% increase in the work of breathing in a group of infants with bronchiolitis. In contrast, Henry et al. found that ipratropium bromide reduced work of breathing per minute by 18%,[131] but, in another study, found that this drug produced no effect on the clinical symptoms and course of infants with bronchiolitis.[132]

In contrast with these studies, Mallol et al. found significant improvements in symptoms and duration of hospitalization in infants under 1 year of age when given nebulized fenoterol, compared with placebo treatment.[176] In another study by the same investigators in infants with a mean age of 10 months, fenoterol was superior to ipratropium bromide, and both were superior to placebo.[177] Both drugs were administered by metered-dose inhaler. Tal et al. showed significant improvement in symptoms when albuterol combined with dexamethasone was administered to infants under 12 months of age. Use of either agent alone failed to show improved results, when compared with placebo.[299] Prendiville et al.[241] demonstrated an improvement in central airway resistance following nebulization of ipratropium bromide in a group of wheezy infants. However, no change occurred in the function of peripheral airways, the site of obstruction in bronchiolitis and asthma. Finally, Cabal et al. demonstrated decreased airway resistance and improved compliance, oxygenation, and ventilation in a group of premature infants with bronchopulmonary dysplasia, some as young as 1-day-old, following administration of isoetharine or metaproterenol.[32,33]

Various reasons have been proposed to explain these discrepancies. Silverman[274] and Tabachnik and Levison[295] have proposed that the relative lack of bronchial smooth muscle in infants may explain, in part, the failure of bronchodilators to show results in some studies. Mucosal edema and mucous plugging, rather than bronchospasm, is proposed as the mechanism of obstruction in very small infants with wheezing. Furthermore, pulmonary function studies are difficult to perform and interpret in small infants, and isolated improvements in single pulmonary function indicators may not correspond with clinical benefit. In addition, it is difficult to give aerosol treatments to young infants, and some centers may be more successful in doing so than others.

In practice, nebulized bronchodilators are widely used in wheezing disorders of infancy. In several recent reviews and texts,[311,274,164] it is recommended that a trial of bronchodilators be employed, based on anecdotal reports of marked improvement in some patients. However, it should be understood that many infants will not respond and may require other forms of therapy, or closer observation.

Dosage and Frequency of Administration. Considerable variability exists in dosage recommendations for use of β_2-agents in children among recent studies, texts, or reviews. Some recommend dosing aerosolized agents by weight, others suggest a standard dose for all patients, and others recommend dosing by weight for some agents and a standard dose for others.[43,97,181,231,241,244,253,274,292] The relative advantages and disadvantages of these approaches toward drug dosages in children have not been directly compared. Recommendations from one recent review are given in Table 29–13.

Several studies suggest that more frequent administration of lower doses of β_2-agents may be more effective than larger, less frequent, doses. Robertson et al. found a greater and more rapid bronchodilator response when, following administration of a 0.15 mg/kg dose of albuterol, subsequent treatments were given every 20 minutes, but with one-third the standard dose.[253] Similar results were achieved by Heimer et al., who used metaproterenol metered-dose inhalers.[128] Both investigators speculate that the initial dose dilated large airways, allowing the subsequent dose to penetrate deeper into the lung. When all of the medication is inhaled at once, only the larger, better-ventilated airways are dilated.

Shapiro et al. found a paradoxic decrease in FEV1 when 0.3 mL of metaproterenol was used, in

Table 29–13 Dosages of Commonly Used β-Adrenergic Agents

AGENT	DURATION (HG)	DOSE (MAX)	SOLUTION (%)
Metaproterenol	3–5	0.01 mL/kg up to 0.3 mL qid	5.0
Isoproterenol	1–2	0.01 mg/kg up to 0.5 mL q 2 hr	0.5
Isoetharine	2–3	0.02 mL/kg up to 0.5 mL q 2–4 hr	1.0
Albuterol	4–6	0.1 mL/kg up to 1 mL qid	0.5
Terbutaline	4–6	0.3 mL/kg up to 1 mL qid	1.0
Fenoterol	4–6+	0.01 mL/kg up to 1 mL qid	0.5

(Rachelefsky GS, Siegel SC: Asthma in infants and children—Treatment of childhood asthma: Part II. J Allergy Clin Immunol 76:409, 1985)

contrast with 0.2 mL, in a group of asthmatic children.[267] These findings suggest that increasing frequency, rather than increasing the dose, may optimize β_2-therapy.

Use of Metered-Dose Inhalers in Children. Several recent reports demonstrate that metered-dose inhalers can be used in infants and young children. Mallol et al.[177] demonstrated improvement in symptoms (compared with placebo) in infants (average age of 10 months) treated with bronchodilators delivered by metered-dose inhalers, using a makeshift expansion chamber. Sly et al.[280] demonstrated improved flow rates in children aged 3 to 6 years following use of an albuterol metered-dose inhaler, with an "Aerochamber" device. No improvement was shown in a similar group of patients with placebo. Since neither of these studies compared meter-dose inhalers directly with conventional nebulizers, it is impossible to determine which form of therapy is superior in these age groups. Further study is needed to define the role of metered-dose inhalers in the management of acute and chronic asthma in infancy and early childhood. The use of metered-dose inhalers by mask and spacing devices would greatly improve the management of infantile asthma outside the hospital setting, allowing rapid relief of symptoms, without the use of nebulizers and air compressors.

Other Methods of Administration. Although aerosolized administration of bronchodilators is preferred because of the lower incidence of side effects and rapid onset of action,[295] at times it may be advisable to administer sympathomimetic agents by injection. Mansmann and coworkers[181] have recommended that subcutaneous injections of terbutaline or epinephrine be used if the FEV1 or PEFR is less than 25% of predicted. In some settings, preparation and administration of bronchodilators by injection may be more convenient than aerosol therapy.

Oral administration of bronchodilators is not recommended for treatment of an acute attack because of the longer onset of action. However before discharge, it may be advisable to begin oral therapy if the child is to receive such therapy at home.

Other Drugs. When a series of treatments with β_2-agents fails to relieve symptoms, the diagnosis of status asthmaticus may be made. In addition to admitting the child to the hospital, other agents may be added to the treatment regimen, such as theophylline and steroids.

Aminophylline (intravenous theophylline) is often used in patients who do not satisfactorily respond to β_2-agents. Serum levels must be carefully monitored, as aminophylline has a narrow therapeutic index; that is, toxic serum levels (above 20 μg/mL) are close to therapeutic levels (10–20 μg/mL).[316] In addition, theophylline can potentiate the side effects of β_2-agents.[316] The respiratory therapist should be alert for the signs of theophylline toxicity (Table 29–14).

Table 29—14 Clinical Symptoms of Theophylline Toxicity

MILD	MODERATE	SEVERE
Tachycardia	Diarrhea	Hematemesis
Nausea or vomiting	Jitteriness	Hypotension
Wakefulness	Agitation	Arrhythmias
Respiratory alkalosis	Headache	Altered consciousness
	Abdominal pain	Abdominal distension
	Hypertension	Hyperthermia
	Hypothermia	Leukocytosis
		Metabolic symptoms
		Hypokalemia
		Hyperglycemia
		Acidosis
		Hyperinsulinemia
		Hypophosphatemia
		Hypcalcemia
		Hypomagnesemia
		Seizures

(Albert M: Aminophylline toxicity. Pediatr Clin North Am 34: 61, 1987)

Ipratropium bromide and atropine, both anticholinergic agents, have been used in the treatment of asthma. Atropine has more systemic side effects than ipratropium bromide[43] and is not widely used. Mallol et al. found that ipratropium bromide produced more improvement in symptoms than a placebo, but less than fenoterol.[177] In another study by the same group, adding ipratropium bromide to feneterol produced no additional benefit, compared with fenoterol alone, in a group of mildly ill infants.[176] Prendiville et al.[241] and Stokes et al.[292] demonstrated improvement in selected pulmonary function indicators, but no clinical benefit could be demonstrated in a large group of infants with bronchiolitis treated with ipratropium bromide. Currently, ipratropium bromide should be considered for those patients who are poorly controlled with conventional therapy.[210]

Steroids are usually recommended for patients who require hospital admision.[43,84,181,244] Studies have shown improvement in flow rates and arterial oxygenation over the course of hours or days in the treatment of severe asthma.[271] Common agents used include hydrocortisone, dexamethasone, and betamethasone,[97] usually intravenously, except in mild cases. When given for short periods, side effects are negligible.[43]

Cromolyn sodium is a widely used agent in the treatment of chronic asthma. However, its use should be suspended during acute exacerbations. Cromolyn sodium lacks immediate effects on pulmonary function and, in at least one form of administration (an inhaled dry powder), it can be irritating.[272]

Prevention and Treatment of Respiratory Failure. Respiratory failure can occur in as many as 5% of patients with status asthmaticus.[277] Various criteria have been proposed to establish the diagnosis of impending or existing respiratory failure in asthma. Clinical criteria include decreased respiratory efforts and air movement because of exhaustion,[43] deterioration in mental status,[43] severe hypoxemia,[43] and hypercarbia ($PaCO_2$ 55 mmHg[181] to 65 mmHg[325]). An asthma score of 7 or greater also indicates respiratory failure.[325] When the $PaCO_2$ is below these levels, but rising by 5 mmHg/hr,[181] or the asthma score is 5 or more, the patient is considered to be in impending respiratory failure.[325] (see Table 29–10)

Pharmacologic Prevention and Treatment. Since mechanical ventilation is associated with significant mortality and complications,[230] treatments have been devised to prevent respiratory failure in

those at risk. Continuous intravenous isoproterenol infusion is the most widely used of these techniques. Use of this technique requires admission to an intensive care unit, because the complications are high, and patients considered as candidates for isoproterenol infusion are a great risk for respiratory failure. Advocates of this therapy report a reduction in the need for mechanical ventilation, one reporting only one treatment failure in 16 years.[180]

Complications of this technique include arrhythmias and myocardial ischemia and necrosis.[180,230] These complications are more common in children past their early teens, and Mansmann has recommended against its use in this aged group.[180]

The isoproterenol infusion is begun at a rate of 0.1 μg/kg per minute, and increased by the same amount every 10 to 15 minutes until the $PaCO_2$ decreases by at least 10% of the preinfusion level[67] or is below 55 mmHg.[164] The infusion rate should be decreased or terminated if tachycardia develops (200/min),[164] or if significant arrhythmias are present.

Some investigators have modified aspects of this protocol. Herman and coauthors suggest aminophylline be continued during isoproterenol infusion, claiming this allows a lower dose of isoproterenol to be used.[135] The original protocols developed by Downes and associates recommended discontinuation of aminophylline, fearing potentiation of side effects.[67] In addition, Mansmann[180] recommends vigorous control of arterial pH, to enhance responsiveness to isoproterenol.

More recently, the use of continuously nebulized terbutaline has been reported. Moler et al. used continuously nebulized terbutaline as an alternative to isoproterenol infusion in a group of 19 patients with impending respiratory failure, and all experienced significant clinical and blood gas improvement, with no side effects.[204] Aggarwal and Portnoy noted similar improvement with continuously nebulized terbutaline, including one patient with a $PaCO_2$ of 85 mmHg, which dropped to below 40 with treatment.[2] No side effects were noted in this study. Figure 29–6 depicts an apparatus designed to administer continuously nebulized medications.

In Canada, Bohn et al. have reported good results with intravenous albuterol (not available in the United States).[21] Their protocol stressed the vigorous correction of respiratory acidosis with sodium bicarbonate.[21,22] Although sodium bicarbonate results in an increase in carbon dioxide production, the enhanced responsiveness to albuterol, associated with normalized pH, results in im-

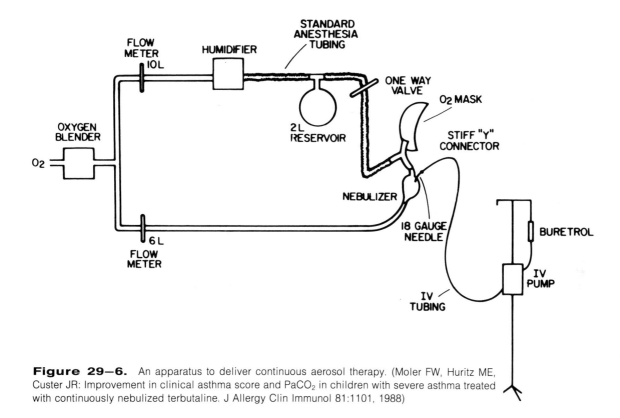

Figure 29—6. An apparatus to deliver continuous aerosol therapy. (Moler FW, Huritz ME, Custer JR: Improvement in clinical asthma score and $PaCO_2$ in children with severe asthma treated with continuously nebulized terbutaline. J Allergy Clin Immunol 81:1101, 1988)

proved $PaCO_2$. The use of halothane has also been reported in an attempt to avoid mechanical ventilation.[224]

Mechanical Ventilation. A few children will require mechanical ventilation, either because measures such as continuous isoproterenol infusion have failed, or if the patient presents with severe respiratory failure, coma, or cardiorespiratory arrest.

Selection of appropriate settings can be difficult, since the ventilator must be adjusted to deliver an adequate tidal volume and minute volume, yet avoid hyperinflation and barotrauma. To allow adequate expiratory time, large tidal volumes (15–20 mL/kg) and a slower rate (50% of normal for age) have been recommended.[164] High tidal volumes may increase peak inspiratory pressure, however.

Stemple and Kurland recommend decreased inspiratory flow rates to reduce peak airway pressures.[289,164] However, experience in neonatal ventilation suggests that the decreased expiratory time associated with this maneuver may increase lung volumes and peak tracheal pressures, even if airway pressures are reduced.[41] Mansmann[180] recom-

mends the use of expiratory retard, to prevent expiratory airways collapse. Others have reported success in preventing airway collapse and improving ventilation when very high levels (25 cmH_2O) or PEEP are used.[243] However, still others recommend against using PEEP, because of the risks of hyperinflation, altered lung mechanics, and barotrauma.[43,164]

Darioli et al. reported successful results in ventilating adult asthmatics utilizing hypoventilation.[55] This approach, which does not require the normalization of $PaCO_2$, may potentially decrease the risk for barotrauma. Bohn[20] has adopted this approach in children, using low tidal volumes and respiratory rates of 8–10/min.

BRONCHIOLITIS

Pathology and Pathophysiology

Bronchiolitis is a diffuse inflammatory condition of the small airways that results in airway obstruction, hyperinflation, respiratory distress, and altered gas exchange. Clinically, bronchiolitis is manifested by signs of upper respiratory infection, such as runny nose, coughing, and sneezing. Signs of lower airway obstruction then become prominent, with respiratory distress, tachypnea and tachycardia, wheezing, and hyperinflation on chest x-ray films. The diagnosis of bronchiolitis is generally reserved for those under 2 years of age, with most clinically significant cases occurring in infants under 6 months of age.[43]

Most cases of bronchiolitis are caused by viruses, with respiratory syncytial virus being most common. Adenoviruses and parainfluenza viruses also cause some cases of bronchiolitis.[228]

Examination of the lungs of infants dying of bronchiolitis show the disease is characterized by diffuse necrosis of the ciliated bronchiolar epithelium and edema of the submucosal membranes. The airways are completely or partially filled with cellular debris.[43]

Pulmonary function studies show a marked increase in lung volumes, inspiratory and (especially) expiratory resistance, and work of breathing.[43] Hypoxemia is almost universal among hospitalized infants and persists several weeks after apparent recovery.[119] Manifestations of apnea are seen in as many 16% to 20% of infants with respiratory syncytial virus infections, the incidence being greatest among those with a history of prematurity, and among the very young.[5,45]

Aside from these immediate complications, there is also evidence that infection with respiratory syncytial virus in infancy is associated with subsequent pulmonary function abnormalities in later life. Persistent lung function abnormalities, such as decreased expiratory flow rates and increased lung volumes, have been found in children 12 months after resolution of the disease[293] and as late as 10 years.[114]

Clinically, it is impossible to distinguish bronchiolitis from an asthmatic infant's first attack. Some investigators suggest that many cases of bronchiolitis are, in effect, asthmatic episodes caused by respiratory syncytial virus infection. It is also not known whether the viral infection itself caused the subsequent pulmonary function abnormalities and increased frequency of asthmalike symptoms, or if a genetic predisposition to reactive airway disease caused both the bronchiolitis and the later abnormalities.[190]

Etiology and Epidemiology

Bronchiolitis is quite common, occurring in 11% of those under 1 year old, and 6% of those aged 1 to 2 years. Like most childhood respiratory illnesses, boys are more frequently and more severely affected than girls.[43]

Most cases, however, are not severe, with only 2% to 5% of cases requiring hospitalization; of these, 80% are less than 6 months old.[43] Those requiring hospitalization, however, are at increased risk for respiratory failure and other significant complications. Recent reports cite an incidence of respiratory failure among hospitalized infants ranging from 17%[192] to 41%.[90] Infants younger than 2 months have a higher rate of respiratory failure (40%) than those over 2 months (14%).[192] Mortality is increased among those with underlying cardiopulmonary or immune system disorders. A death rate of 37% from respiratory syncytial virus bronchiolitis among infants with congenital heart disease has been reported. This figure rises to 73% when pulmonary hypertension is present. In contrast, mortality among hospitalized infants with respiratory syncytial virus, and without underlying disease, is only 1.5%.[175]

Respiratory syncytial virus infections typically occur in the winter (especially December through March), and the incidence varies widely from year to year.[130] Transmission occurs quite readily, even in the hospital setting, where, presumably, isolation and infection control techniques are practiced. Studies have documented an infection rate of up to 45% among previously uninfected hospitalized infants.[43] It is believed that much of this infection is transmitted by infected hospital personnel, who likewise have a high rate of infection during epidemics.[117]

Respiratory syncytial virus is spread through contact with contaminated secretions, either by direct contact with aerosols (after coughing or sneezing), or autoinoculation after touching contaminated surfaces. The virus enters the body through the nose or eyes, rather than the mouth.[117]

The most effective means of control of respiratory syncytial virus infection is the cohorting of patients and staff. That is, infected infants are cared for in a separate room. Where possible, staff caring for infants with respiratory syncytial virus should not also be assigned to care of uninfected infants (especially those with medical conditions known to increase the mortality from respiratory syncytial virus infection).

The routine use of masks and gowns has not been shown to decrease the risk of respiratory syncytial virus infection in patients[118] or staff.[118,208] However, theoretically, they may be of value when staff must care for both infected and noninfected infants. Likewise, gloves are of little value, since the virus lives longer on gloves than on skin.[117]

The routine use of eye–nose goggles may offer the best means of reducing staff and patient infection with respiratory syncytial virus. A recent trial showed that use of such goggles reduced the incidence of infection by two-thirds.[96]

Careful handwashing is key to preventing nosocomial respiratory syncytial virus infection. Respiratory care practitioners and others must be especially careful to do so after contact with infants who have known or suspected respiratory syncytial virus infection and, especially, before caring for children known to be at risk for increased mortality from infections. During the winter months, all infants with acute respiratory symptoms should be considered as having respiratory syncytial virus (for purposes of infection control) until proved otherwise.

Treatment

Most infants with bronchiolitis require supplemental oxygen and respond well to concentrations of 40% to 50%.[226] Mist therapy is often employed, but its efficacy has not been systematically studied. Infants treated with mist should be evaluated closely for worsening of symptoms, as inhalation of aerosols (especially ultrasonically generated aerosols) can provoke bronchospasm in some infants.

The use of bronchodilators in bronchiolitis is controversial (see discussion on the use of bronchodilators in young infants with asthma). Several studies have shown positive results, with improved lung mechanics, blood gas values, and symptoms,[176,177,259] whereas others have not.[132,168,242,292] A trial of bronchodilators may be useful. However, the infant should be closely monitored.

Ribavirin Therapy. The antiviral agent ribavirin is often used in the treatment of bronchiolitis caused by respiratory syncytial virus. Administration of ribavirin by aerosol requires the use of a special nebulizer [small-particle aerosol generator (SPAG), also referred to as a Collison generator] supplied by the drug's manufacturer. Generally, the drug is administered through an oxygen hood or tent for 18–20 hr/day over a period of 3 or more days. (see Chap. 17)

Clinical studies have shown modest improvements in symptoms of respiratory distress and in arterial oxygenation.[11,121,122,297] It has been recom-

mended that patients with underlying cardiopulmonary disease, immunodeficiency, or unusually severe respiratory syncytial virus infection be considered for ribavirin therapy.[49,120]

Usually, laboratory evidence of respiratory syncytial virus infection is obtained before initiation of therapy. This may result in delay of therapy for 24 hours or more, which may influence the efficacy of treatment. Some reports advocate initiating therapy upon admission when the presence of respiratory syncytial virus infection is strongly suspected.[120]

Several recent commentaries on ribavirin have cautioned against widespread use of the drug until further studies are available.[248,288,314] They point to the relatively few patients studied and the lack of substantial clinical benefit in the existing studies. So far, ribavirin has not been shown to decrease the need for mechanical ventilation or other aggressive therapy, decrease mortality, nor decrease the length of hospital stay.

Use of Ribavirin with Mechanical Ventilators. Although widely done, the use of ribavirin with infants undergoing mechanical ventilation is not approved by the US Food and Drug Administration, because of the risk of aerosol precipitation in ventilator circuits and valves, causing ventilator malfunction. However, several reports have described protocols for administration of ribavirin to ventilated infants.

Ribavirin has been administered successfully with both pressure and volume ventilators. With either device, careful monitoring is essential to detect ribavirin precipitation in ventilator tubing and valves.

Because of the small size of many infants with bronchiolitis, many institutions prefer to use pressure ventilators. Outwater et al. described their method of administering ribavirin with a Healthdyne infant pressure ventilator. To prevent drug precipitation, disposable exhalation valves were used and were changed every 4 hours. The remainder of the circuit was changed every 8 hours.[227]

Flow from the SPAG unit may increase inspiratory and expiratory pressures. With pressure ventilators, ventilator flow can be decreased to compensate. However, with volume ventilators, the use of a pressure pop-off is recommended to prevent any flow from the SPAG unit from entering the circuit during inspiration (Fig. 29–7).[90] In either case, a one-way valve is typically inserted between the SPAG unit and the ventilator to prevent loss of ventilator volume to the SPAG unit during inspiration. Outwater et al. also use one-way valves to prevent

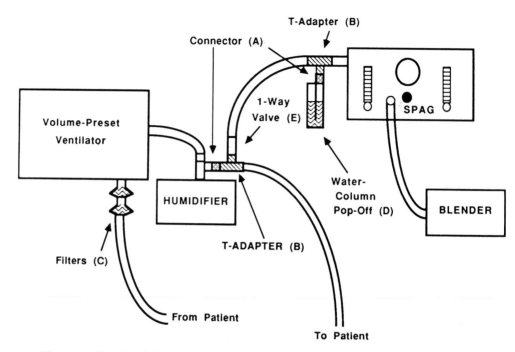

Figure 29—7. Schematic view of circuit employed to deliver ribavirin during volume preset ventilation. (*A*) Silicone rubber coupling (3443, Puritan Bennett Corp., Overland Park, Kan.); (*B*) disposable aerosol T-adapter (1077, Hudson Oxygen, Temecula, Calif.); (*C*) bacteria filter (MG-303-01, Marquest, Englewood, Colo., or BB-50T, Pall, East Hills, N.Y.); (*D*) water-column pressure relief (pop-off) valve (037-00, Aquapak, Arlington Heights, Ill. or CP 0700, Corpak Co., Wheeling, Ill.); (*E*) one-way valve (001671, Inspiron, Cucamonga, Calif.). (Frankel LR, Wilson CW, Demers RR et al: A technique for the administration of ribavirin to mechanically ventilated infants with respiratory syncytial virus infection. Crit Care Med 15:1051, © by Williams & Wilkins Co, 1987)

retrograde flow from the SPAG into the ventilator.[227] These one-way valves must be frequently inspected and changed to prevent obstruction by precipitated ribavirin.

The use of humidifiers that employ heated wires to decrease condensation may help prevent ribavirin precipitation and obstruction of valves and filter.[90] The use of particle filters has been recommended to prevent ribavirin from entering those ventilators (like the Siemens Servo Ventilators) that use internal expiratory valves.[90]

Factors Potentially Affecting Drug Delivery. For sufficient ribavirin to be delivered to the patient, there must be sufficient volume in the portion of the inspiratory tubing between the endotracheal tube and the insertion point of the tubing from the SPAG unit. The introduction of the SPAG flow into the circuit near the humidifier should permit sufficient ribavirin to accumulate in the inspiratory limb before inspiration. High ventilator flow rates also decrease ribavirin delivery, since gas from the ventilator (which does not contain ribavirin) reduces the concentration of ribavirin in the inspired air.[284] Finally, sufficient expiratory time should be allotted to permit an adequate amount of aerosol to enter the ventilator circuit.

Modification of Ventilators to Permit Ribavirin Administration. Ventilators may differ in their response to the added flow from the SPAG unit and to the incorporation of valves and filters. Before patient use, procedures should be developed and tested to ensure that

- Inspiratory and expiratory pressures can be controlled
- Ventilator pressure alarms and pop-offs are not affected
- Sufficient flow is provided for spontaneous breathing
- The ventilator is protected from ribavirin precipitation
- Environmental exposure to ribavirin is prevented or minimized

Finally, policies should be directed toward ensuring that the patient and the ventilator are continuously observed.

Teratogenic and Mutagenic Risks of Ribavirin. The risks to health care personnel exposed to ribavirin aerosols are uncertain. Reviewing the available animal and human data, Demers suggests ribavirin poses little or no risk to health care personnel, and no special precautions are warranted.[60] In contrast, Witek and Schachtner contend that the available data suggest measures should be taken to prevent exposure of health care personnel to ribavirin aerosols, perhaps even prohibiting women of childbearing age from working with this agent.[321] The Centers for Disease Control likewise suggest measures for controlling occupational ribavirin exposure.[42] This may be easily accomplished when ribavirin is administered by mechanical ventilation. However, limitation or prevention of ribavirin exposure when tents are used may prove more difficult.

Treatment of Respiratory Failure in Bronchiolitis. Infants who demonstrate hypercapnia, hypoxemia, severe respiratory distress, or apnea are candidates for intubation and mechanical ventilation. Ventilatory strategy is determined primarily by the increased airway resistance seen in bronchiolitis. Good results have been achieved with prolonged expiratory time to prevent lung overdistension. This may require the use of lower respiratory rates, as well as higher peak inspiratory pressures or tidal volumes.[90,226]

End-expiratory lung volumes are increased in bronchiolitis and, therefore, the use of CPAP or PEEP might be expected to be disadvantageous. Nonetheless, Outwater and Crone have reported favorable results with the use of moderate levels of PEEP in treating severe bronchiolitis.[226] Nasal CPAP has reduced the need for mechanical ventilation in some studies,[14] but not in others.[226]

CYSTIC FIBROSIS

Epidemiology and Etiology

Cystic fibrosis is a genetically inherited disorder that results in widespread dysfunction of the exocrine and mucus-secreting glands. These include the mucous glands of the lung, as well as other organs such as the pancreas. The specific gene locus for cystic fibrosis has recently been identified. Although many body systems and functions are affected in cystic fibrosis, the most clinically impor-

tant effects of the disease are those involving the lung and the gastrointestinal system.

Reports of the prevalence of cystic fibrosis in the population vary widely, but 1 case in 2000 live births is the most commonly cited figure.[125] However, there is considerable variability among ethnic groups, and the prevalence is very low among blacks and Asians.

Pathology and Pathophysiology

The initial cause of pulmonary dysfunction in cystic fibrosis is believed to be secondary to secretion of abnormal mucus in abnormal amounts. This leads to small-airway obstruction, impaired mucociliary clearance, maldistribution of ventilation, and, in many infants with cystic fibrosis, an apparent predisposition to lower respiratory tract infections and atelectasis. Thorough pulmonary function studies cannot be done in early infancy, but a modest decrease in PaO_2[318] and an increase in airway resistance and expiratory lung volumes[236] can be detected in some infants.

Eventually, the lower respiratory tract becomes infected with bacteria, such as *Staphylococcus aureus* and *Haemophilus influenzae*. Later, *Pseudomonas aeruginosa* and, occasionally, *Pseudomonas cepacia* can be found. At first, sputum cultures may be positive only occasionally for these organisms. However, as the disease progresses, infection becomes chronic. Eventually, chronic pulmonary infection leads to diffuse airway disease and obstruction, with bronchiectasis being an almost universal feature of advanced cystic fibrosis. Table 29–15 describes the effects of *P. aeruginosa* and *P. cepacia* on pulmonary function in cystic fibrosis.

Table 29—15 Effect of Colonization with *Pseudomonas* Species on Pulmonary Function in Cystic Fibrosis

COLONIZATION STATUS	% PREDICTED VALUES		
	FVC	FEV$_1$	FEF$_{25\%-75\%}$
Neither	90 ± 2.5	85 ± 2.9	82 ± 4.0
P. aeruginosa	80 ± 1.3	73 ± 1.4	69 ± 2.0
P. cepacia	70 ± 2.8	62 ± 3.2	54 ± 4.5
Both	68 ± 4.5	62 ± 1.4	53 ± 7.1

(Isles A, MacLusky I, Corey M et al: *Pseudomonas cepacia* infection in cystic fibrosis: An emerging problem. J Pediatr 104:206, 1984)

As the obstructive process continues, serial pulmonary function studies will show progressive decreases in expiratory flow rates, increases in residual volume and functional residual capacity, and a decline in vital capacity. As pulmonary function becomes more deranged, hypoxemia is apparent. Carbon dioxide retention is a late feature of the disease and is a poor prognostic sign.[236]

The rate at which the disease progresses varies from child to child. Some have severe disease evident in early infancy and die soon after. Others have stable lung function, with few symptoms throughout most of childhood, and begin to rapidly deteriorate in adolescence. Others do well into early adulthood, and a small group have such minimal symptoms they escape diagnosis until well into adulthood.[318]

Females generally have poorer lung function than males, especially after adolescence. The reasons are not clear, but some have suggested a greater reluctance to cough (especially in public) among girls compared with boys.[171]

Gastrointestinal effects can be seen in the pancreas, intestines, and liver, among other organs. Most patients suffer from a deficiency in pancreatic enzymes. Before effective therapy for this aspect of the disease was developed, many patients with cystic fibrosis would die of malnutrition secondary to malabsorption in early infancy. Pancreatic enzymes may now be taken orally, with significant improvement in nutritional status. Nonetheless, in most patients with cystic fibrosis, some degree of malabsorption persists, and nutritional status is less than optimal. The child will often be significantly smaller than children without cystic fibrosis. Deficiencies in the fat-soluble vitamins are also common.

Another gastrointestinal complication of cystic fibrosis, meconium ileus, is present in some patients (10% to 12%)[236] at birth. This condition is caused by excessively thick meconium, and results in bowel obstruction. These infants may require surgery for correction of the obstruction. Intestinal obstruction occurs occasionally in older patients as well.

Diagnosis

Early diagnosis of cystic fibrosis is important, as early, aggressive treatment may postpone the development of significant pulmonary dysfunction. All newborns with meconium ileus should be tested for cystic fibrosis. In infants, persistent pulmonary symptoms, such as chronic, loose cough, or frequent lower respiratory infections will suggest the diagnosis. In other infants, gastrointestinal symptoms, such as large, foul-smelling stools, or a failure to gain weight at the expected rate, are present. A combination of gastrointestinal and respiratory symptoms are often present.

To definitively diagnose cystic fibrosis, the level of sodium or chloride in the sweat must be measured ("sweat test"). Sweat glands, like all other excreting glands in cystic fibrosis, function abnormally, causing the sweat to have much higher concentrations of sodium and chloride. If concentrations of sodium or chloride are above 60 mEq/L, the diagnosis of cystic fibrosis can be made. Following initial diagnosis, therapy is directed toward correcting malnutrition and respiratory symptoms, and toward preventing the decline in pulmonary function.

Treatment

Bronchial Hygiene. The use of chest physical therapy, even in infants without respiratory symptoms, is almost universal in cystic fibrosis. However, since pulmonary function studies are difficult to perform in this aged group, little is known about the exact effects of chest physical therapy in early cystic fibrosis. In the later stages of the disease, when large quantities of mucopurulent secretions are continuously present, the beneficial effects of chest physical therapy are easier to document.

In attempting to assess the value of daily chest physical therapy, Desmond et al.[61] demonstrated a decline in expiratory flows and vital capacity following a period of 3 weeks without chest physical therapy. At the end of this period, a single treatment reversed much, but not all, of the decline. After resuming daily therapy for 3 weeks, pulmonary function studies returned to their previous level. Although this study emphasizes the importance of daily chest physical therapy, it also suggests that when therapy is not performed regularly, an occasional treatment may be beneficial. This may be important when counseling patients who do not perform therapy on a regular basis.

It is not altogether clear which component of chest physical therapy (percussion, postural drainage, or coughing) is responsible for the benefits seen. Rossman et al.[257] compared the effects of spontaneous coughing; coughing directed by a therapist; postural drainage, with and without percussion (both without directed coughing); and a combination of percussion, postural drainage, and directed coughing. Her study demonstrated that a vigorous cough, with or without percussion and postural drainage, produced significantly greater clearance of mucus from the lung than treatment without vigorous coughing. Surprisingly, she was unable to detect any difference in clearance of mucus or sputum production when percussion was added to simple postural drainage (without coughing).

There are several interesting implications of Rossman's work. First, it suggests vigorous, directed coughing may be as beneficial as the more time-consuming conventional chest physical therapy. This could provide an alternative for those patients who are unable or unwilling to perform chest physical therapy on a regular basis. Second, it suggests that simple postural drainage may be helpful, even if percussion is not performed. This could be helpful in treating those patients who cannot tolerate percussion, or in the home, when no one is available to perform percussion.

It would be unwise, however, to abandon conventional therapy solely on the basis of this study. Rossman evaluated only a limited number of indices (clearance of mucus from the lung and sputum volume) immediately after therapy. Also, all patients were considered clinically stable at the time of treatment, and results may have been different if acutely ill patients had been studied. Nonetheless, the study highlights the value of vigorous coughing as well as postural drainage, and suggests valuable options for those not able to perform standard chest physical therapy.

Another appealing adjunct or alternative to chest physical therapy is vigorous physical exercise. Zach et al.[330] studied pulmonary function changes during a 17-day exercise program in children with cystic fibrosis. Forced vital capacity and expiratory flow rates improved significantly during this period. No chest physical therapy or aerosol inhalation was performed during the study period. This program required full-time attendance in a summer camp-type setting, with several hours of activity each day, and would not be practical for the child attending school, or the young working adult with cystic fibrosis. Another study by Holzer et al.[141] could not demonstrate any benefit when an exercise program was designed for children in their homes. They suggest that constant supervision may be necessary for exercise programs to be successful. In contrast, Blomquist et al.[19] found that, in a group of patients somewhat older than those studied by Holzer, compliance in an unsupervised treatment program was good. Age may have been a factor in influencing compliance, as well as the type of phys-

ical activity used [calisthenics and jogging (Holzer[141]) versus sports activity (Blomquist[19])]. Finally, Andreasson et al.[6] reported improved pulmonary function in a study of vigorous exercise over a 30-month period in children with cystic fibrosis. During the latter part of this period, improvement in pulmonary function was noted, even though chest physical therapy was stopped. The authors of this study attribute the benefits seen, in part, to the deep breathing associated with exercise, which they claim aids in the opening and clearing of peripheral airways.

A subgroup of patients with cystic fibrosis may not be able to tolerate strenuous exercise. Those with a forced vital capacity less than 60% of predicted or an FEV1 of less than 35% of predicted should undergo testing to determine the cardiopulmonary response to exercise before undertaking an exercise program. Also, vigorous exercise could lead to salt depletion in some patients with cystic fibrosis, who cannot control salt loss.[46] Since patients with more severe disease have generally been excluded from these studies, they should not be interpreted as presenting an alternative to chest physical therapy in this group of patients.

Other Therapies

Mist Tent Therapy. Before the mid-1970s, placing the child with cystic fibrosis in a mist tent at night was standard therapy. However, many clinicians abandoned this approach after studies revealed no beneficial effect.[171] Other forms of aerosol therapy have been used, including acetylcysteine, phenylephrine, bronchodilators, and antibiotics.[171]

Bronchodilator Therapy. Previously, it was recognized that bronchodilator therapy could lead to deterioration of expiratory flow rates in some patients with cystic fibrosis.[165] In advanced cystic fibrosis, the bronchial walls are weakened by bronchiectasis, and some degree of bronchial smooth-muscle tone may be necessary to prevent collapse of the airways. Bronchodilator administration may relax smooth muscle to such an extent that airway collapse occurs, especially when coughing.[72]

Other children with cystic fibrosis, however, respond favorably to bronchodilators.[222] A small group of patients also have asthma, and others have intermittent bronchospasm during periods of acute exacerbation of the disease. Children with cystic fibrosis considered candidates for bronchodilator therapy should be evaluated with pulmonary function studies before treatment is initiated.[72,318]

Aerosolized Antibiotics. Administration of aerosolized antibiotics has been used increasingly in the last few years. Usually, antibiotics such as gentamicin, amikacin, or tobramycin are selected for their antipseudomonal activity. Because there are no effective oral antibiotics for this organism, aerosolized antibiotics may permit home treatment of chronic pseudomonal infection. Because these drugs may be irritating to the respiratory tract, a bronchodilator is often given before treatment.

The indications for aerosolized antibiotics have not been clearly defined. Although Schaad et al.[258] found that inhaled amikacin decreased the frequency of pseudomonal colonization of sputum among cystic fibrosis patients, they were unable to demonstrate improvement in pulmonary function or overall clinical status. Likewise, other studies[290] have failed to show significant improvement. Patients in these studies were hospitalized and receiving intravenous antibiotics.

In contrast, Hodson et al.[136] studied the effects of inhaled carbenicillin and gentamicin in a placebo-controlled study, and found significant improvement in pulmonary function and hospitalization rates in the treated group. Her patients were at home and not receiving intravenous therapy during the study. Similarly, others have found clinical benefit from inhaled antibiotics in outpatients.[163] Also, Cooper et al.[51] found aerosolized antibiotics to be as effective as intravenous antibiotics in inpatients being treated for acute pulmonary exacerbations.

Nebulizer brand and flow rate may significantly affect the deposition of antibiotics in the lung. Newman et al.[212] compared various nebulizers and air compressors and found significant variation in particle size and drug deposition. Nebulizers that produce particle sizes smaller than 5 μm can deposit significantly more antibiotics into the lung, with more homogeneous distribution, than those that produce substantially larger particles.[212]

Chest physical therapy should precede aerosolization of antibiotics.[212] This should improve aerosol distribution, which is dependent on the degree of airway obstruction.[4]

Nutritional Therapy. With advancing disease, the interrelationship between nutritional and pulmonary status becomes apparent. The gastrointestinal defects in cystic fibrosis impair absorption of nutrients, and the increased work load imposed by altered lung mechanics increases energy expenditure.[312] In addition, infection may impose additional demands on the short supply of available nutrients. As a result, most children with cystic fibrosis eventually fall far behind their peers in weight and height.[236] The possible interrelationships between advancing pulmonary disease and malnutrition are shown in Figure 29–8.

In an attempt to improve nutritional status and, hopefully, pulmonary function, aggressive approaches to nutritional supplementation have been tried. Approaches range from simple dietary counseling[287] to intravenous alimentation,[268] gastros-

Figure 29—8. Model defining interrelationships between deteriorating lung function and nutritional status in patients with cystic fibrosis (Levy LD, Durie PR, Pencharz PB, Corey ML: Effects of long-term nutritional rehabilitation on body composition and clinical status in malnourished children and adolescents with cystic fibrosis. J Pediatr 107:225, 1985)

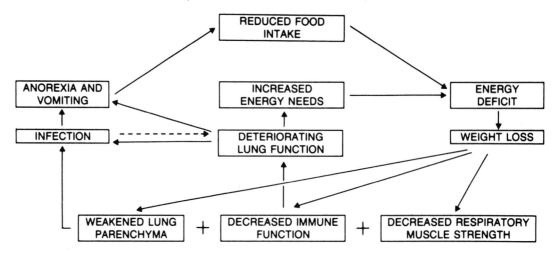

tomy tube,[169] or nasogastric tube feedings.[269] Improved growth and stabilization of pulmonary status have been shown in selected patients with such treatment.[169,268,269]

Treatment of Acute Exacerbations. Regardless of the type of therapy employed to prevent decline in pulmonary function, most patients eventually require hospitalization for acute exacerbations of respiratory symptoms. Signs and symptoms suggesting the need for hospitalization in cystic fibrosis are presented in Table 29–16. Usually, intravenous antibiotics are administered, along with aggressive chest physical therapy and nutritional therapy. It is not clear which of these therapies, or other factors, are responsible for the improvement in pulmonary function usually seen. Some authors have suggested that antibiotic therapy is not warranted in acute exacerbations of cystic fibrosis. Several placebo-controlled studies have failed to demonstrate a beneficial role for antibiotics, in general,[107] or for antipseudomonal drugs in particular.[15] Pointing out that antibiotic therapy rarely eliminates *pseudomonas* from the sputum of cystic fibrosis patients, these investigators suggest that improved performance of chest physical therapy in the hospital setting is responsible for the improvement seen.[107,211] Other studies, however, have shown clinical improvement with antibiotic use in acute exacerbations of cystic fibrosis.[143,320] Regardless,

Table 29–16 Some Indications for Hospitalization of Cystic Fibrosis Patients

Diagnostic and educational (initial admission)
Increasing pulmonary dysfunction
  Fever
  Weight loss
  Increasing coughing or coughing spells
  Increased respiratory rate
  Increased sputum production
  Rales
  Worsening appearance in chest x-ray film
  Elevated white blood cell count
  Deterioration in pulmonary function indicators
  Hemoptysis
  Pneumothorax
  Cor pulmonale
Other system complications
  Gastrointestinal
  Electrolyte imbalance, and such

(Lloyd–Still JD: Textbook of Cystic Fibrosis, p 188. Boston, John Wright, 1983)

many clinicians feel antibiotic therapy is beneficial, and research is currently directed to the type and frequency of antibiotic administration.[211]

Recently, favorable results with home intravenous antibiotic therapy have been reported.[65,102] Less interruption of school, work, or social activities associated with home, rather than hospital, therapy might lead patients and physicians to accept more frequent courses of antibiotic therapy and perhaps improved outcome.

Another approach recently reported in the care of the cystic fibrosis patient is the "prophylactic" hospital admission and treatment of patients at times when symptoms are not particularly severe. One study reported improved survival in patients with chronic pseudomonal infection who were hospitalized for intravenous antibiotic therapy every 3 months, regardless of the severity of symptoms.[232]

Environmental Factors in the Control of Pseudomonal Infections. It appears that pseudomonal infection is inevitable in the cystic fibrosis patient. Nonetheless, it seems reasonable to implement measures to delay this eventuality as long as possible. This is especially true for *P. cepacia*, a newly recognized pathogen seen in some cystic fibrosis centers, which is highly antibiotic-resistant and is associated with a high mortality.[145,298]

Conflicting results have been reported by investigators trying to establish means of controlling these organisms. Some have obtained a decrease in colonization rates by *P. aeruginosa* and *P. cepacia* when colonized patients were segregated from those free of these organisms.[232,303] This segregation was maintained both in inpatient and outpatient facilities, and in cystic fibrosis summer camps. Others have been unable to document an increase in infection rates when these patients are cared for together, and have been unable to find environmental reservoirs for *Pseudomonas* species in their institutions.[124] They have suggested such measures may be unnecessary. It seems reasonable, nonetheless, to remind caretakers of basic infection control procedures when caring for cystic fibrosis patients.

Complications of Cystic Fibrosis

A small subgroup of patients with cystic fibrosis may suffer from pneumothorax or hemoptysis. Both complications occur more often in older patients.[171]

Hemoptysis is associated with severe bronchiectasis, and the bronchial artery hypertension seen in this condition may be a contributing factor in the development of hemoptysis. Small amounts of blood-streaking in the sputum can usually be managed conservatively, with antibiotic therapy, bed rest, and cessation of chest physical therapy. Sometimes, vitamin K may be administered. This vitamin is essential for proper functioning of the blood-clotting mechanisms and, like other fat-soluble vitamins, may be deficient in some cystic fibrosis patients.[172]

More significant hemoptysis may be acutely life-threatening. Bronchial artery embolization may be helpful in some of these patients. Under fluoroscopy, the bleeding vessels are identified. A catheter is advanced to a point upstream of the bleeding, and a foamlike substance released, which occludes the artery, preventing further bleeding. The complication rate is high, and many patients experience recurrence of bleeding.[78,245]

Pneumothorax also is a problem in about 20% of cystic fibrosis patients; frequently it is a recurrent problem. If pneumothoraces persist, surgical procedures designed to produce plural adhesions are performed, and usually result in prevention of recurrent.[245]

Care of End-Stage-Disease

The vast majority of deaths in cystic fibrosis are due to pulmonary disease, with hypoxemia, pulmonary hypertension, cor pulmonale, and hypercarbia being common features. Pulmonary hypertension and cor pulmonale may be related to nocturnal oxygen desaturation and cor pulmonale may be related to nocturnal oxygen desaturation, which occurs commonly in advanced cystic fibrosis.[89,291] Nocturnal oxygen therapy has been recommended for such patients before the development of overt symptoms of right heart failure.[318] However, despite the fact that nocturnal oxygen therapy improves oxygen saturation during sleep,[281] other investigators have been unable to show any affect on morbidity and mortality in end-stage cystic fibrosis.[331]

Mechanical ventilation is usually avoided in end-stage cystic fibrosis. However, some clinicians have reported favorable results with aggressive treatment of severe respiratory failure in young infants with cystic fibrosis and severe bronchiolitis.[236]

GASTROESOPHAGEAL REFLUX

Etiology

Gastroesophageal reflux results from the failure of the normal mechanisms that keep gastric contents in the stomach. Some degree of reflux is normal at all ages, but reflux associated with respiratory or other symptoms is considered pathologic.

Gastroesphageal reflux has been increasingly recognized over the last decade as a common cause of acute and chronic respiratory problems in infants and children.[76,134] In addition, reflux is often present in children with respiratory diseases of other origin, such as asthma[76,133] and bronchopulmonary dysplasia.[142]

For reflux to occur, three factors must be present: First, pressure inside the stomach must be greater than in the esophagus. Second, gastric contents must be able to reach the gastroesophageal junction and be of a consistency enabling them to flow freely. Finally, the lower esophageal sphincter must be sufficiently relaxed.[219] The degree of relaxation or contraction of the lower esophageal sphincter is reflected in the pressure it creates at the gastroesophageal junction, and it is referred to as the *lower esophageal sphincter pressure.*

To effectively treat or prevent reflux, it would be useful to know how changes in intragastric, intraesophageal, or esophageal sphincter pressures occur, and which one(s) of these mechanisms is usually responsible for reflux. Intragastric pressures may increase in response to crying, coughing, or any maneuver that involves contraction of abdominal muscles. Esophageal pressure may drop in response to decreases in intrathoracic pressure, as occurs with deep inspiration. These types of pressure changes occur normally in all infants and children, yet only a few have clinically significant reflux. It seems reasonable, then, to assume that the strength of the lower esophageal sphincter might be involved. This sphincter closes the lower esophagus, to prevent retrograde egress of gastric contents. However, only a small group of patients with gastroesophageal reflux can be shown to have an abnormally weak lower esophageal sphincter. Momentary relaxation of the sphincter can occur, however, and result in reflux,[317] but this also occurs during vomiting, a quite common event in otherwise asymptomatic infants. In practice, it is not always possible to identify specific abnormalities that cause the reflux.

Pathophysiology of Respiratory Complications

Gastroesophageal reflux in infants is usually associated with frequent vomiting.[17] In those patients who are unable to immediately swallow or otherwise expel the vomitus, aspiration may result. Repeated aspiration may result in acute or chronic pulmonary symptoms.[133] In addition, some investigators have linked reflux to apnea and sudden infant death syndrome.[134]

Although direct aspiration of gastric contents into the lungs seems the most logical explanation for pulmonary disease seen with reflux, many of the respiratory symptoms, especially bronchospasm and laryngospasm, may be produced simply by acid irritation of the esophagus. These observations may explain the high incidence of reflux in patients with asthma and apnea or "near-miss sudden infant death syndrome."[219]

In some cases, the treatment of asthma may have caused, or worsened reflux. Theophylline and other bronchodilators may relax the lower esophageal sphincter muscle in much the same way they relax bronchial smooth muscle.[219] Table 29–17 discusses the interactions between reflux and respiratory disease and treatment.

Diagnosis

Several methods are available to diagnose gastroesophageal reflux. One method involves placing a pH probe in the esophagus. A drop in esophageal pH below 4 reflects movement of gastric contents into the esophagus. If the number of episodes or the total amount of time the pH is less than 4 varies significantly from normal, the diagnosis of reflux can be made. Other methods of diagnosis include barium esophagrams and technetium scans.[17]

Treatment

Once the diagnosis of gastroesophageal reflux is made, the infant may be treated with modifications of position and feeding. Frequently, the infant will be placed in an infant seat (i.e., supine, 60° elevation), either continuously or after feedings.[133] This allows gravity to assist in keeping gastric contents out of the esophagus. However, it has also been suggested that this form of therapy may worsen reflux, especially if the infant is allowed to slump forward in the infant seat.[220,246] This could cause an increase in intragastric pressure, which will outweigh any benefits of gravity.

The effects of posture on reflux may be related to the position of the gastroesophageal junction relative to gastric contents. As Figure 29–9 illustrates, in the supine position, flat or seated, the gastric contents remain in contact with the gastroesopha-

Figure 29–9. Representation of the position of the gastreosophageal junction with a patient in various positions. (Ramenofsky ML, Leape LL: Continuous upper esophageal pH monitoring in infants and children with gastroesophageal reflux, pneumonia, and apneic spells. J Pediatr Surg 16:374, 1981)

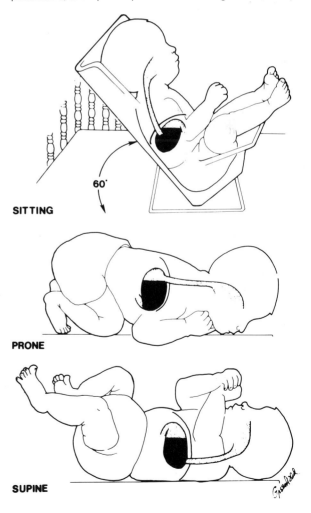

SITTING

PRONE

SUPINE

Table 29–17 Reflux and Respiratory Disease Interactions

RESPIRATORY DISORDERS THAT MAY BE CAUSED BY GASTROESOPHAGEAL REFLUX

- Aspiration
- Bronchospasm
- Laryngospasm and apnea

RESPIRATORY DISORDERS, ACTIVITIES, OR THERAPIES THAT MAY CAUSE GASTROESOPHAGEAL REFLUX

- Forced expiration (crying, coughing, wheezing)
- Forced inspiration (hiccups, upper airway obstructions)
- Bronchodilators
- Supine positioning (during chest physical therapy)

(Modified from Orenstein SR, Orenstein DM: Gastroesophageal reflux and respiratory disease in children. J Pediatr 112:847, 1988)

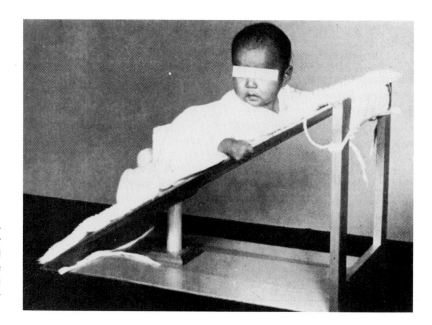

Figure 29—10. An apparatus that facilitates positional therapy. The padded peg or saddle maintains the child on the inclined plane. Usually a sheet is wrapped around the infant and board to keep the child from falling off. (Herbst JJ, Minton SD, Book LS: Gastroesophageal reflux. J Pediatr 98:859, 1981)

geal junction, thus facilitating reflux. Head-up, prone positioning in a specially designed infant seat is now recommended by some experts[133,219] (Fig. 29—10).

The consistency of feedings may also be altered in an attempt to prevent reflux. Usually cereal is added to formula to thicken the feedings.[219] Like positioning therapy, this aspect of treatment is controversial, with some investigators claiming thickened feedings are of no value in treating reflux,[9] whereas others claim it has a positive role.[218]

In some infants, drugs that increase the strength of the lower esophageal sphincter (such as metoclopramide) may be used. Antacids, and drugs that decrease acid formation such as cimetidine, are sometimes used if esophagitis is present secondary to acid reflux.[219]

When conservative therapy fails, surgery may be needed. The most commonly used procedure is the Nissen fundoplication (Fig. 29—11). In this procedure, the upper portion of the stomach is wrapped around the intra-abdominal esophagus. This tightens the lower esophageal opening and allows intragastric pressures to be readily transmitted to the esophageal wall. The esophagus will then close in response to increased intragastric pressures, rather than open. A gastrostomy tube is usually inserted to facilitate feeding.

Relief of respiratory symptoms usually occurs, except when preexisting central nervous system damage is present. In these children, chronic respi-

Figure 29—11. A completed Nissen fundoplication. The upper part of the stomach (the fundus) is wrapped around the lower (intra-abdominal) esophagus, to prevent reflux. (Randolph J: Experience with the Nissen fundoplication for correction of gastroesophageal reflux in infants. Ann Surg 198:579, 1983)

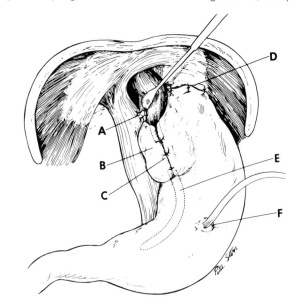

ratory problems secondary to aspiration of secretions often persists.[146]

Common respiratory care procedures may worsen gastroesophageal reflux. Chest physical therapy, when head-down and supine positioning are used, can increase reflux. Crying or coughing, which may follow suctioning or painful procedures, will increase intra-abdominal pressures, with a similar effect. The supine position often used in ventilated patients may also promote reflux.[219]

Complications can be minimized by performing therapy as long after feedings as possible. However, since many infants with reflux are treated with frequent, or continuous, feedings, it may be necessary to withhold feedings for a period before therapy. While performing chest physical therapy, any head-down or supine, flat positioning should be avoided. Prone and side positioning can generally be performed safely, but care should be taken to avoid compression of the abdomen while doing so. Since treatments often require interruption of feeding (in children who are likely to be malnourished) and may worsen reflux, attempts should be made to limit the frequency and duration of therapy.

Also, gatrostomy or nasogastric feeding tubes may aggravate reflux.[219] Because these devices are often used to treat children with reflux, caretakers must be aware of the potential for increased reflux.

FOREIGN BODY ASPIRATION

Etiology and Epidemiology

Airway or esophageal foreign body aspiration is one of the leading causes of death in young children. Recent figures show that foreign body aspiration is the leading cause of accidental death in children under 1 year of age, and is the fourth leading cause of accidental death in those under 4.[151]

Advances have been made through education and consumer legislation in recent years. Legislation such as the Consumer Products Safety Act of 1979, which regulates the manufacture of toys designed for children under 3, as well as extensive education, may have contributed to the decline in mortality from foreign body aspiration from 1012 in 1969 to 341 in 1982.[151]

Food is the item most often aspirated into the tracheobronchial tree, with peanuts frequently being the item most often cited in series reported from the United States. Carrots and popcorn are also fre-

quently cited. In contrast, coins are the objects most frequently impacted in the esophagus.[179]

Numerous studies have demonstrated that most cases of serious foreign body aspiration occur in children between the ages of 1 and 3.[151,179,191] This, in part, may be due to the lack of molar teeth, which results in incomplete chewing of solid food. Additionally, some infants this age may have poor coordination of breathing and swallowing and often may eat while talking or running.[191] Also, boys aspirate more often than girls.[191]

Recognition and Management

Complete obstruction of the trachea or larynx can cause sudden death, and is recognized by the complete absence of vocalization and air movement, despite respiratory efforts. Emergency treatment, as advocated by the American Heart Association, consists of back blows and chest thrusts in infants. In the child over 1 year of age, only the "Heimlich" maneuver (abdominal thrust) should be performed. Back blows and chest thrusts are omitted. Blind finger sweeps are avoided in all children, as this maneuver may inadvertently push the object deeper into the airway. These maneuvers can also be performed when airway obstruction is not complete, but the obstruction appears life-threatening.[285]

In the hospital setting, laryngoscopy can relieve complete laryngeal or tracheal obstruction by foreign bodies. If removal is difficult, an endotracheal tube may be used to push the object into one of the main stem bronchi, allowing ventilation of the other lung.[68]

Less severe obstruction can be evaluated by the degree of air entry, stridor, and cyanosis. If the obstruction is near complete, stridor may be diminished or absent.

If the obstruction does not appear life-threatening, only supportive care (e.g., oxygen, positioning to relieve symptoms) should be given until endoscopy can be performed. Employment of other techniques to dislodge the object can cause the obstruction to worsen. This is especially true of so-called hygroscopic foreign bodies, which may increase in size from water absorption while in the airway. These objects were small enough to enter the airway, but may, after the passage of time, be too large to pass through the glottis.

Laryngeal foreign bodies may interfere with phonation and swallowing, and, hence, hoarseness, aphonia, and drooling may be symptoms. These reactions may serve to differentiate laryngeal foreign body from tracheal foreign body. Although laryngeal obstructions, such as croup or epiglottitis, are often associated with stridor, Gay et al. noted stridor in only three of six patients with subglottic foreign bodies, whereas wheezing was present in five. Other signs and symptoms of laryngeal, tracheal, and bronchial foreign bodies are listed in Table 29–18.[151]

Foreign bodies that lodge in the bronchi may also be life-threatening, but usually the object lodges in one or the other of the main stem bronchi, allowing adequate ventilation of the unaffected side. Because symptoms are less severe, diagnosis may be more difficult and delayed.

The signs and symptoms of foreign body aspiration may mimic more common conditions, such as asthma, croup, and pneumonia. This often results in a considerable delay between the aspiration event and definitive diagnosis and management. McGuirt et al. reported an average delay of 12 days between aspiration and definitive treatment, with one delay of 10 months. The possibility of a foreign body should be considered in any child who fails to respond to standard therapy for croup, asthma, pneumonia, or other persistent respiratory problem.

A careful history is important in establishing the diagnosis. Often, when questioned, the parents will report a sudden coughing episode that developed while the child was eating, playing with small toys, and such, and that subsided spontaneously. Frequently, the child is brought in for evaluation of the complications of foreign body aspiration, such as recurrent cough and wheezing (suggestive of asthma). Pneumonia or atelectasis which often accompany foreign body aspiration, usually have other etiologies. Because these symptoms of foreign body aspiration are also characteristics of other, more common disorders, the diagnosis of foreign body aspirations will be missed or delayed if a careful history is not taken.

The physical examination may reveal signs of complete or partial bronchial obstruction. Complete bronchial obstruction leads to atelectasis or pneumonia, or both, with resulting unilateral decrease in breath sounds. When partial obstruction is present, unilateral wheezing and hyperinflation may be present. Unilateral wheezing may be difficult to appreciate in some small children, as breath sounds are easily transmitted to the unaffected side. Although most children will have some signs and symptoms that help establish the diagnosis, a significant few will have no clear-cut evidence of foreign body aspiration on physical examination.[179,191]

On occasion, a foreign body can be directly demonstrated with a standard chest radiograph. This is especially true of objects containing metal. However, most aspirated objects are vegetable matter, and are not radiopaque.

Chest radiographs can be used to indirectly point to the presence of a foreign body. However, since intrathoracic obstructions produce greater increases in airway resistance on expiration, expiratory lung volumes will be increased. An expiratory chest film that shows unilateral hyperinflation strongly suggests unilateral bronchial obstruction, such as a foreign body. Congenital defects, and occasionally, tumors, can also produce unilateral expiratory hyperinflation.

Since it may be difficult to obtain an adequate expiratory film in a tachypneic infant or child, bilateral decubitus films may be needed. Placing the child on their side causes the heart and other mediastinal structures to compress the dependent lung. If airway resistance is normal, a considerable loss of lung volume should be evident. However, the presence of a foreign body limits loss of lung volume (Fig. 29–12 and 12–7 illustrate typical lateral decubitus films in foreign body aspiration). A fluoroscopic examination may also be used to observe unilateral expiratory hyperinflation.

Table 29—18 Signs and Symptoms of Foreign Bodies in the Airway

| SIGNS/SYMPTOMS | LOCATION OF FOREIGN BODY | | |
	Larynx	Trachea	Bronchi
Hoarseness	X		
Aphonia	X		
Odynophagia	X		
Drooling	X		
Audible slap		X	
Cough	X	X	X
Hemoptysis	X	X	X
Stridor	X	X	X
Wheeze	X	X	X
Dyspnea	X	X	X
Airway obstruction	X	X	X
Sudden death	X	X	X

X indicates presence of sign or symptom.
(Kenna MA, Bluestone CD: Foreign bodies in the air and food passages. Pediatri Rev 10:25, 1988. Reproduced by permission of Pediatrics in Review)

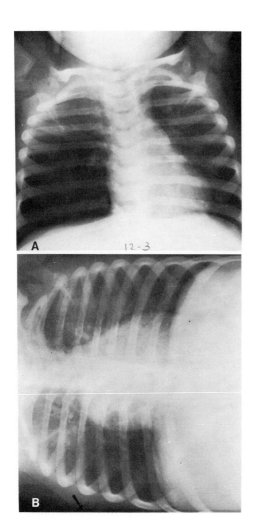

Figure 29—12. (*A*) Foreign body aspiration in an 18-month-old child who aspirated a piece of crayon. Air is trapped in the middle and lower lobes on the right, as compared with the left and right upper lobes. There is mild cardiac and mediastinal shift toward the left because of air-trapping on the right. (*B*) Right lateral decubitus view. In the dependent position, the right middle and lower lobes do not empty the air as does the right upper lobe. The *arrow* indicates a board on which the child is resting.

X-ray films may fail to confirm the diagnosis in a limited number of cases. If symptoms of foreign body aspiration persist, the child may require a bronchoscopic examination to confirm or rule out foreign body aspiration.

Treatment

Removal of the foreign body with a rigid broncho-scope is the preferred treatment of tracheobron-chial foreign bodies. This instrument is preferred because it allows ventilation as well as visualiza-tion of the airway. Other methods, such as chest physical therapy, should be avoided. Dislodged bronchial foreign bodies may obstruct the trachea and larynx, causing complete airway obstruc-tion.[161]

Following endoscopy, treatment is directed to-ward any residual abnormality, such as atelectasis or pneumonia, that may have developed. A few children may require racepinephrine to treat sub-glottic edema associated with endoscopy. Persis-tence of symptoms following bronchoscopy sug-gests the presence of an additional foreign body.

Prevention

Education, in addition to appropriate legislation concerning the manufacture of children's toys, pac-ifiers, and similar objects, is the key to reducing death from foreign body aspiration. Infants and children in the hospital should be protected from unnecessary risk. Millunchick and McArtor re-cently reported fatal aspiration of a makeshift paci-fier, similar to those used in many nurseries and pediatric wards. These are usually made from the nipple and plastic collar used for infant formulas (Fig. 29—13).[200]

Although most pacifiers manufactured in the United States are safe, hospitalized infants may be seen using unsafe pacifiers brought from home that have been manufactured outside the United States. Of particular concern are those with detachable nipples, which can be aspirated.[162] Caretakers should take advantage of opportunities to educate parents in the prevention of aspiration.

EPIGLOTTITIS

Etiology and Pathophysiology

Epiglottitis is an acute infection of the epiglottitis and surrounding structures, which results in severe airway obstruction. The epiglottis is grossly en-larged, interfering with airflow and swallowing. Most often, infection with *Haemophilus influenzae* (type B) can be demonstrated as the cause. If not properly treated, epiglottitis can cause sudden le-thal airway obstruction. Therefore, prompt recogni-tion and appropriate management are essential.

Clinical Presentation

The child with epiglottitis typically presents with severe respiratory distress, fever, stridor, and gen-

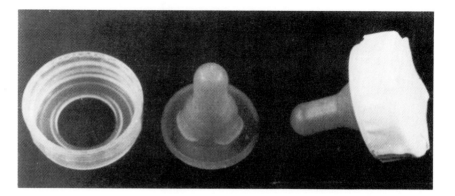

Figure 29—13. Example of a makeshift pacifier. Nipple can become detached and aspirated. (Millunchick EW, McArtor RD: Fatal aspiration of a makeshift pacifier. Pediatrics, 77:369, 1986, reproduced with permission of Pediatrics)

erally appears "toxic." Often, but not always, the child assumes an upright posture, with the jaw thrust forward and mouth open, and is drooling (Fig. 29–14). These latter signs may be secondary to the inability to swallow oral secretions. In addition, some investigators have noticed an absence of

Figure 29—14. Typical appearance of a child with epiglottitis. (Davis HW et al: Acute upper airway obstruction: Croup and epiglottitis. Pediatr Clin North Am 28:859, 1981)

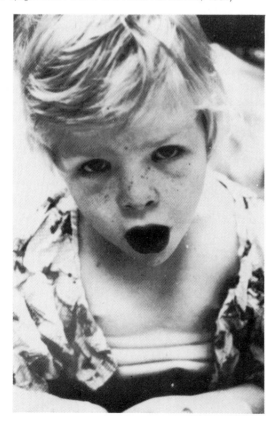

spontaneous cough in patients with epiglottitis, in contrast with other causes of upper airway obstruction and respiratory distress.[188]

Since this presentation has some characteristics of severe viral laryngotracheobronchitis (LTB), it is important to be able to differentiate between the two on clinical, historical, and epidemiologic bases. Distinguishing features of the two conditions are presented in Table 29–19.[8]

The diagnosis of epiglottitis often can be made on clinical and historical grounds and confirmed by direct visualization at intubation. Lateral neck x-ray films may also help establish the diagnosis. The grossly enlarged epiglottis is easily recognized (Fig. 29–15). Endoscopy and intubation of any patient with severe airway obstruction, however, should not be delayed for diagnostic procedures. If symptoms are severe and obstruction is thought to be imminent, the child should be brought to the operating room or the intensive care unit and intubated, even if the diagnosis is not firmly established.

Although some have advocated the use of pharyngoscopy or other procedures to visualize the epiglottis in the emergency room,[188] other experts recommend against this practice, because manipulation of glottic structures and depression of the tongue in this condition can provoke laryngospasm and obstruction.[62,95] In any case, procedures such as this should be performed only by those experienced in difficult intubations, with necessary equipment for intubation or tracheostomy at hand.

Management

Adherence to carefully thought-out protocols is essential in the successful management of epiglottitis. Most important is the designation of a team of pediatric airway experts, consisting of pediatric anesthesiologists, laryngologists, surgeons, and inten-

Table 29—19 Clinical Characteristics Differentiating Laryngotracheobronchitis LTB from Epiglottitis

CHARACTERISTIC	LTB	EPIGLOTTITIS
Age	6 mo–3 yr	2–6 yr
Onset	Gradual	Rapid
Etiology	Viral	Bacterial
Swelling site	Subglottic	Supraglottic
Symptoms		
Cough–voice	Hoarse cough	No cough
		Muffled voice
Posture	Any position	Sitting
Mouth	Closed, nasal flaring	Open, chin forward drooling
Fever	Absent to high	High
Appearance	Often not acutely ill	Anxious, acutely ill
X-ray film	Narrow subglottic area	Swollen epiglottic and supraglottic structures
Palpation of larynx	Nontender	Tender
Recurrence	May recur	Rarely recurs
Seasonal incidence	Winter	None

(Backofen JE, Rogers MC: Upper airway disease. In Rogers MC (ed): Textbook of Pediatric Intensive Care, p 190. © 1987, Williams & Wilkins Co, Baltimore)

sivists. This team should be immediately notified as soon as the diagnosis of epiglottitis is suspected. Additionally, the methods of airway management, anesthetic techniques, and other details of management should be determined in advance.

Definitive management of epiglottitis consists of establishment of an artificial airway, most commonly a nasotracheal tube. Before placing the airway, the child should be considered at risk for sudden airway obstruction. A person experienced in difficult airway management should continually be in attendance, and appropriate equipment should accompany the child on the trip to the intensive care unit, operating room, or x-ray department. Routine procedures, such as blood drawing or intravenous line insertion, should be deferred. It is also advisable to allow the parents to stay with the child to reduce unnecessary anxiety and crying. Oxygen is essential to prevent asphyxia, should complete obstruction occur.

Intubation usually takes place in the operating room or the intensive care unit and is performed under general anesthesia. Tracheostomy is rarely necessary; however, personnel and equipment required to do so should be available. Usually, a cuffless tube 0.5 to 1.0 mm smaller than normal for the child's age is used. Initially, the child may be orally intubated, and after stabilization, a nasotracheal tube is inserted.

Postintubation Care. After intubation, blood drawing, intravenous line insertion, and other procedures can be performed safely. Since epiglottitis is a result of a bacterial infection, antibiotics should be administered. *Haemaphilus influenzae* almost invariably can be detected in the bloodstream in a patient with epiglottitis: therefore, blood cultures are used to determine the appropriate antibiotic.

Afterward, care is directed toward maintaining airway patency, and most importantly, preventing accidental extubation. The risk of extubation can be minimized by the use of arm splints and restraints.[31]. Some clinicians also recommend the use of sedatives[8,62,111,167] in some or all patients, although others fear this may increase the duration of intubation.[31] A more radical approach is advocated by Kimmons and Peterson, who routinely paralyze, sedate, and ventilate all children with epiglottitis.[153]

There appears to be an inverse relationship between the risk of spontaneous extubation and duration of intubation. Kimmon's accidental extubation rate for children managed by his protocol was zero, with an average duration of intubation of 51 hours.[153] Vernon et al., who do not use ventilation and paralysis routinely, and rely on restraints to prevent extubation, reported an extubation rate of only 2%, with a mean duration of intubation of 41 hours.[313] Butt et al., who do not use sedatives, re-

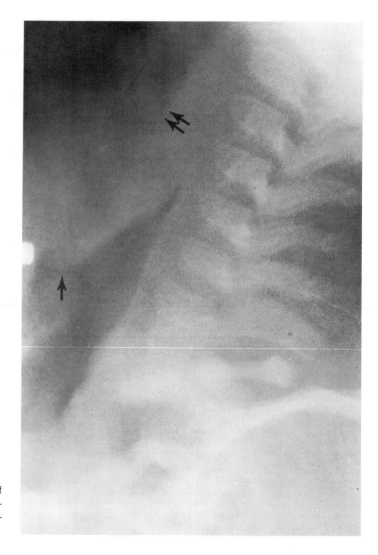

Figure 29—15. Epiglottitis seen in a lateral view of the airway. The *single arrow* indicates the markedly swollen epiglottis. The *double arrow* indicates a normal subglottic airway.

ported an extubation rate of 10%, with a mean duration of intubation of 18 hours.

Because endotracheal intubation can reduce the functional residual capacity and PaO$_2$, the routine use of low-level CPAP is advocated by some.[62] Furthermore, pulmonary edema and pneumonia may coexist with epiglottitis, necessitating mechanical ventilation or positive airway pressure in some patients.[8]

Others, however, fear unnecessary attachments to the endotracheal tube may increase the risk of extubation, and have achieved good results using heat and moisture exchangers ("artificial noses")[31] or mist tents and hoods.[111,313] The latter devices may impair visualization of the child, however.

Management of Accidental Extubation. Although the child with epiglottitis who has not had an endotracheal tube inserted is considered at grave risk for obstruction, many children who self-extubate after even a few hours do surprisingly well. The presence of an endotracheal tube in the swollen supraglottic area compresses these structures, creating a groove, through which the child can breathe, at least temporarily. Reintubation can proceed under relatively controlled circumstances, and may be accomplished more easily than originally.[111] Of those who spontaneously extubate, many will not require reintubation, especially if antibiotics were started promptly, and the patient has been intubated for more than 8 hours.[31] Nonetheless, children who self-extubate need close observation and rapid evaluation of the need for reintubation, especially those who have been intubated for fewer than 24 hours.

Criteria for Extubation. A variety of criteria have been proposed to determine when extubation can be safely performed. Some institutions rely on direct visualization of the epiglottis,[8,153] whereas others rely on clinical criteria, such as resolution of fever and general improvement in appearance.[31] Additionally, because endotracheal tubes 0.5 to 1.0-mm smaller than usual are used, resolution of epiglottic swelling should produce a noticeable leak around the tube at low airway pressures. This is considered by some to be a reliable indicator of the feasibility of extubation.[8,62]

Complications. Although it is abundantly clear that epiglottitis can be managed successfully by nasotracheal intubation, nonetheless some reports on the management of epiglottitis at major pediatric centers cite instances of death or severe neurologic sequelae from cardiorespiratory arrest. Most of these involve patients who experienced obstruction before or immediately upon arrival at a medical facility (2/60 in Vernon,[313] 6/349 in Butt,[31] 2/48 in Faden[77]). Some, however developed cardiorespiratory arrest after admission to local hospitals and were managed without intubation (3/7 in Vernon).[313]

Laryngeal trauma,[31] and some cases of aspiration pneumonia[31,153] from difficult intubation have been reported, as well as pneumothoraces.[153,313]

Management Without Intubation. Although the routine use of intubation or tracheostomy appears well established, some reports have appeared describing successful management of large series of patients without intubation. Glicklich et al. reported a management protocol in which most patients treated for epiglottitis at their institution were successfully managed without intubation.[105] Steroids and intermittent bag–mask ventilation were used instead, and no deaths were reported. Butt reported that 13% (45/349) of their patients with less severe obstruction were successfully managed with antibiotics and observation in the intensive care unit without intubation,[31] and Kimmons and Peterson reported 17% (7/41) of their patients were similarly managed successfully.[153]

It is not clear what is gained by this approach, since all patients so managed require admission to the intensive care unit. Furthermore, the complication rate of conventional management of endotracheal intubation is low, it immediately relieves respiratory distress, and it permits the use of sedation, if warranted.

Although nonintubation has apparently been successful in some hands, it has not been so in others. Rapkin reported no mortality in a small group of patients managed with an artificial airway (tracheostomy) as soon as the diagnosis was established, in contrast with a 20% mortality in a group closely observed, but not routinely tracheostomized.[247] Likewise, Margolis et al. experienced 13% mortality or severe neurologic impairment with observation and elective tracheostomy, but no mortality or serious complications when all patients were tracheostomized at diagnosis.[183] More current series (see foregoing) also report a high mortality in a small group of patients managed without intubation.[313]

CROUP (LARYNGOTRACHEOBRONCHITIS)

Etiology, Pathology, and Clinical Presentation

Laryngotracheobronchitis is an acute, infectious disorder of the subglottic airway, and is the most common cause of stridor in the pediatric patient. Most commonly, children between the ages of 6 months and 3 years are affected, and, like most respiratory problems, boys are more often affected than girls. Parainfluenza viruses are responsible for most cases of laryngotracheobronchitis, and the disorder is most common in late fall and late spring.[129]

Airway obstruction is caused by inflammation and occasionally spasm of the subglottic larynx and trachea, with the bronchi also being affected at times. Frank respiratory distress is usually preceded by symptoms of acute upper respiratory infections, such as runny nose and perhaps fever. As the larynx, trachea, and bronchi become affected, the classic signs of "croup" (barking cough, stridor, and respiratory distress) become evident.

Usually the diagnosis can be established on clinical and historical ground. However, lateral neck x-ray films are used at times to distinguish between laryngotracheobronchitis and other conditions, such as epiglottitis. A subglottic narrowing, variably referred to as a "steeple" or "pencil" sign is often seen.

The symptoms of laryngotracheobronchitis often overlap with those of epiglottitis. Distinguishing features of the two disorders are listed in Table 29–19.

Although most children with croup are successfully managed without hospitalization, a small group require more intensive therapy, including, on occasion, intubation (or tracheostomy) and mechanical ventilation. The need for therapy is generally guided by the severity of symptoms. Inhalation of cold mist is the mainstay of inpatient management, although its efficacy has not been documented. Often, use of oxygen tents or "croupettes" interfere with observation of the child, and increase patient anxiety. In addition, most mist units require the use of oxygen, which may mask signs of hypoxemia when the patient is breathing room air.

Corticosteroids are often used, but their role in the treatment of laryngotracheobronchitis is controversial.[94,310] Racepinephrine is also widely used to provide temporary relief of the symptoms of upper airway obstruction. Its use should be restricted to inpatients, however, since severe symptoms often return 1 to 2 hours after treatment ("rebound" effect). In addition, racepinephrine can cause tachycardia. The usual dose is 0.25 mL for infants under 1 year of age, and 0.5 mL for those older than 1 year. The volume of diluent should be at least 2.0 mL.[62] Therapy is usually given every 2 to 4 hours, but can be repeated as often as every 30 minutes.[8]

Increasing restlessness, cyanosis, stridor, and retractions as well as increasing need for racepinephrine treatments, suggest the need for intubation. Unlike other upper airway obstructions, arterial blood gas determinations are useful in assessing the need for an artificial airway, since obstruction is gradual. A $PaCO_2$ of 45 mmHg or more, or a PaO_2 of 70 mmHg or less when breathing room air, signifies severe disease,[87] and a $PaCO_2$ of 55 mmHg or more indicates the need for an artificial airway.

A tube 0.5- to 1-mm (internal diameter) smaller than normal for size or age should be used to prevent damage to inflamed laryngeal tissues. Most infants can be extubated after several days. Those with persistent obstruction should be evaluated for the presence of underlying airway abnormalities, such as subglottic stenosis.

REFERENCES

1. Aberdeen E, Downes JJ: Artificial airways in children. Surg Clin North Am 54:1155, 1974
2. Aggarwal J, Portnoy J: Continuous terbutaline inhalation for treatment of severe asthma [Abstract]. J Allergy Clin Immunol 77:185, 1986
3. Albert S: Aminophylline toxicity. Pediatr Clin North Am 34:61, 1987
4. Alderson PO, Secker–Walker RH, Strominger DB et al: Pulmonary deposition of aerosols in children with cystic fibrosis. J Pediatr 84:479, 1974
5. Anas N, Boettrich C, Hall CB, Brooks JG: The association of apnea and respiratory synchytial virus infection in infants. J Pediatr 101:65, 1982
6. Andréasson B, Jonson B, Kornfält R et al: Long-term effects of physical exercise on working capacity and pulmonary function in cystic fibrosis. Acta Paediatr Scand 76:70, 1987
7. Backofen JE, Rogers MC: Emergency management of the airway. In Rogers MC (ed): Textbook of Pediatric Intensive Care, pp 57–82. Baltimore, Williams & Wilkins, 1987
8. Backofen JE, Rogers MC: Upper airway disease. In Rogers MC (ed): Textbook of Pediatric Intensive Care, pp 171–198. Baltimore, Williams & Wilkins 1987
9. Bailey DJ, Andres JM, Danek GD, Pineiro–Carrero VM: Lack of efficacy of thickened feeding as treatment for gastroesophageal reflux. J Pediatr 110:187, 1987
10. Barker R, Levison H: Effects of ultrasonically nebulized distilled water on airway dynamics in children with cystic fibrosis and asthma. J Pediatr 80:396, 1972
11. Barry W, Cockburn F, Cornall R et al: Ribavirin aerosol for acute bronchiolitis. Arch Dis Child 61:593, 1986
12. Bartlett RH, Gazzaniga AB, Wetmore NE et al: Extracorporeal membrane oxygenation (ECMO) in the treatment of cardiac and respiratory failure in children. Trans Am Soc Artif Intern Organs 26:578, 1980
13. Battersby EF, Hatch DJ, Towey RM: The effects of prolonged naso-endotracheal intubation in children. Anaesthesia 32:154, 1977
14. Beasley JM, Jones SEF: Continuous positive airway pressure in bronchiolitis. Br Med J 283:1506, 1981
15. Beaudry PH, Marks MI, McDougall D et al: Is antipseudomonas therapy warranted in acute respiratory exacerbations in children with cystic fibrosis? J Pediatr 97:144, 1980
16. Berquist WE: Gastroesophageal reflux in children: A clinical review. Pediatri Ann 11:135, 1982
17. Berquist WE, Fonkalsrud EW, Ament ME: Effectiveness of Nissen fundoplication for gastroesophageal reflux in children as measured by 24-hour intraesophageal pH monitoring. J Pediatr Surg 16:872, 1981
18. Blackstone EH, Kirklin JW, Bradley EL et al: Optimal age and results in repair of large ventricular septal defects. J Thorac Cardiovasc Surg 72:661, 1976
19. Blomquist M, Freyschuss U, Wiman L-G, Strandvik B: Physical activity and self treatment in cystic fibrosis. Arch Dis Child 61:362, 1986
20. Bohn D: Personal communication.
21. Bohn D, Kalloghlian A, Jenkins J et al: Intravenous salbutamol in the treatment of status asthmaticus in children. Crit Care Med 12:892, 1984
22. Borland LM, Swan DM, Leff S: Difficult pediatric endotracheal intubation: A new approach to the retrograde technique. Anesthesiology 55:577, 1981

23. Boros SJ, Mammel MC, Lewallen PK et al: Necrotizing tracheobronchitis: A complication of high frequency ventilation. J Pediatr 109:95, 1986

24. Boxer RA, Gottesfeld I, Singh S et al: Non-invasive pulse oximeter in children with cyanotic congenital heart disease. Crit Care Med 15:1062, 1987

25. Brook I: Bacterial colonization, tracheobronchitis and pneumonia following tracheostomy and long-term intubation in pediatric patients. Chest 76:420, 1979

26. Brouillette RT, Ilbawi MN, Hunt CE: Phrenic nerve pacing in infants and children: A review of experience and report on the usefulness of phrenic nerve stimulation studies. J Pediatr 102:32, 1983

27. Brouillette RT, Morrow AS, Weese–Mayer DE, Hunt CE: Comparison of respiratory inductive plethysmography and thoracic impedance for apnea monitoring. J Pediatr 111:377, 1987

28. Brouillette RT, Thach BT: A neuromuscular mechanism maintaining extrathoracic airway patency. J Appl Physiol 46:772, 1979

29. Bruce DA, Berman WA, Schut L: Cerebrospinal fluid pressure monitoring in children: Physiology, pathology and clinical usefulness. Adv Pediatr 24:233, 1977

30. Burgess WR, Chernick V: Respiratory Therapy in Newborn Infants and Children, 2nd ed. New York, Thieme Inc, 1986

31. Butt W, Shann F, Walker C et al: Acute epiglottitis: A different approach to management. Crit Care Med 16:43, 1988

32. Cabal L, Larrazabal C, Ananda K et al: Bronchial reactivity in preterm infants with RDS. Pediatr Res 20:424A, 1986

33. Cabal LA, Larrazabal C, Ramanathan R et al: Effects of metaproterenol on pulmonary mechanics, oxygenation, and ventilation in infants with chronic lung disease. J Pediatr 110:116, 1987

34. Campbell LR, Bunyapen C, Holmes GL et al: Right common carotid artery ligation in extracorporeal membrane oxygenation. J Pediatr 113:110, 1988

35. Caniano DA, Nugent SK, Rogers MC, Haller JA: Intracranial pressure monitoring in the management of the pediatric trauma patient. J Pediatr Surg 15:537, 1980

36. Carlo WA, Martin RJ: Principles of neonatal assisted ventilation. Pediatr Clin North Am 33:221, 1986

37. Carlon GC, Ray C, Miodownik S et al: Capnography in mechanically ventilated patients. Crit Care Med 16:550, 1988

38. Carroll GC, Tuman KJ, Braverman B: Minimal positive end-expiratory pressure (PEEP) may be "Best PEEP." Chest 93:1020, 1988

39. Carter P, Benjamin B: Ten year review of pediatric tracheotomy. Ann Otol Rhinol Laryngol 92:398, 1983

40. Cartmill TB, DuShane JW, McGoon DC, Kirklin JW: Results of repair of ventricular septal defect. J Thorac Cardiovasc Surg 52:486, 1966

41. Cartwright DW, Willis MM, Gregory GA: Functional residual capacity and lung mechanics at different levels of mechanical ventilation. Crit Care Med 12:422, 1984

42. Centers for Disease Control: Assessing exposures of health care personnel to aerosols of ribavirin. MMWR 37:560, 1988

43. Chantarojanasiri T, Nichols DG, Rogers MC: Lower airway disease: Bronchiolitis and asthma. In Rogers MC (ed): Textbook of Pediatric Intensive Care, pp 199–236. Baltimore, Williams & Wilkins, 1987

44. Christopher KL, Neff TA, Bowman JL et al: Demand and continuous flow intermittent mandatory ventilation systems. Chest 87:625, 1985

45. Church NR, Anas NG, Hall CB, Brooks JG: Respiratory syncytial virus related apnea in infants. Am J Dis Child 138:247, 1984

46. Coates AL: Exercise in CF: Does it help? Does it tell us anything? Pediatr Pulmonol Suppl 1:71, 1987

47. Coates AL, Bergsteinsson H, Desmond K et al: Long-term pulmonary sequelae of premature birth with and without idiopathic respiratory distress syndrome. J Pediatr 90:611, 1977

48. Colgan FJ, Stewart S: An assessment of cardiac output by thermodilution in infants and children following cardiac surgery. Crit Care Med 5:220, 1977

49. Committee on Infectious Diseases: Ribavirin therapy of respiratory syncytial virus. Pediatrics 79:475, 1987

50. Cook DR: Muscle relaxants in infants and children. Anesth Analg 60:335, 1981

51. Cooper DM, Harris M, Mitchell I: Comparison of intravenous and inhalation antibiotic therapy in acute pulmonary deterioration in cystic fibrosis. Am Rev Respir Dis 131:A242, 1985

52. Coté CJ, Todres DI: The pediatric airway. In Ryan JF, Todres ID, Coté CJ, Goudsouzian NH (eds): A Practice of Anesthesia for Infants and Children, pp 35–58. Orlando, Grune & Stratton, 1986

53. Craig KC, Pierson DJ, Carrico CJ: The clinical application of positive end-expiratory pressure in the adult respiratory distress syndrome (ARDS). Respir Care 30:184, 1985

54. Czervinski MP, Shreve J, Lester KB, Teague WG: Effects of working pressure on respiratory pattern and airway pressure during pressure support ventilation in infants with chronic lung disease. Respir Care 33:930, 1988

55. Darioli R, Perret C: Mechanical controlled hypoventilation in status asthmaticus. Am Rev Respir Dis 129:385, 1984

56. David R: Closed chest cardiac massage in the newborn infant. Pediatrics 81:552, 1988

57. Davies G, Reid L: Growth of the alveoli and pulmonary arteries in childhood. Thorax 25:669, 1970

58. Davis HW, Gartner JC, Galvis AG et al: Acute upper airway obstruction: Croup and epiglottitis. Pediatr Clin North Am 28:859, 1981

59. Dean JM, Rogers MC, Traystman RJ: Pathophysiology and management of the intracranial vault. In Rogers MC (ed): Textbook of Pediatric Intensive Care, pp 527–556. Baltimore, Williams & Wilkins, 1987

60. Demers B: Ribavirin—No evidence of teratogenic or mutagenic properties [Letter]. Respir Care 33:212, 1988

61. Desmond KJ, Schwenk WF, Thomas E et al: Immediate and long-term effects of chest physiotherapy in patients with cystic fibrosis. J Pediatr 103:538, 1983

62. Dickison AE: The normal and abnormal pediatric airway: Recognition and management of obstruction. Clin Chest Med 8:583, 1987

63. Dinwiddie R, Patel BP, Kumar SP, Fox WW: The effects of crying on arterial oxygen tension in infants

recovering from respiratory distress. Crit Care Med 7:50, 1979

64. Doershuk CF, Fisher BJ, Mattews LW: Pulmonary physiology of the young child. In Scarpelli EM (ed): Pulmonary Physiology of the Fetus, Newborn and Child, pp 166–182. Philadelphia, Lea & Febiger, 1975

65. Donati MA, Guenette G, Auerbach H: Prospective controlled study of home and hospital therapy of cystic fibrosis pulmonary disease. J Pediatr 111:28, 1987

66. Donn SM: Neonatal extracorporeal membrane oxygenation. Pediatrics 82:276, 1988

67. Downes JJ, Wood DW, Harwood I et al: Intravenous isoproterenol infusion in children with severe hypercapnia due to status asthmaticus: Effects on ventilation, circulation, and clinical score. Crit Care Med 2:63, 1973

68. Downes JJ, Goldberg AI: Airway management, mechanical ventilation and cardiopulmonary resuscitation. In Scarpelli EM, Auld PAM, Goldman HS (eds): Pulmonary Disease of the Fetus, Newborn and Child, pp 99–131. Philadelphia, Lea & Febiger, 1978

69. Ducharme FM, Gauthier M, Lacroix J, LaFleur L: Incidence of infection related to arterial catheterization in children: A prospective study. Crit Care Med 16:272, 1988

70. Duncan PG, Friesen R: Appraisal of pediatric cardiopulmonary resuscitation. Anesthesiology 53:S152, 1980

71. Durand M, Ramanathan R: Pulse oximetry for continuous oxygen monitoring in sick newborn infants. J Pediatr 109:1052, 1986

72. Eber E, Oberwaldner B, Zach MS: Airway obstruction and airway wall instability in cystic fibrosis: The isolated and combined effects of theophylline and sympathomimetics. Pediatr Pulmonol 4:205, 1988

73. Eckenhoff JE: Some anatomic considerations of the infant layrnx influencing endotracheal anesthesia. Anesthesiology 12:401, 1951

74. Edmonds JF, Barker GA, Conn AW: Current concepts in cardiovascular monitoring in children. Crit Care Med 8:548, 1980

75. Eisenberg M, Bergner L, Hallstrom A: Epidemiology of cardiac arrest and resuscitation in children. Ann Emerg Med 12:672, 1983

76. Euler AR, Byrne WJ, Ament ME et al: Recurrent pulmonary disease in children: A complication of gastroesophageal reflux. Pediatrics 63:47, 1979

77. Faden HS: Treatment of *Haemophilus influenzae* type B epiglottitis. Pediatrics 63:402, 1979

78. Fellows KE, Khaw KT, Schuster S, Shwachman H: Bronchial artery embolization in cystic fibrosis; technique and long-term results. J Pediatr 95:959, 1979

79. Ferrara B, Johnson DE, Chang PN, Thompson TR: Efficacy and neurologic outcome of profound hypocapneic alkalosis for the treatment of persistent pulmonary hypertension in infancy. J Pediatr 105:457, 1984

80. Field D, Milner AD, Hopkin IE: High and conventional rates of positive pressure ventilation. Arch Dis Child 59:1151, 1984

81. Filston HC, Johnson DG, Crumrine RS: Infant tracheostomy. Am J Dis Child 132:1172, 1978

82. Finer NN, Boyd J: Chest physiotherapy in the neonate. A controlled study. Pediatrics 61:282, 1978

83. Finer NN, Moriartey RR, Boyd J et al: Post extubation atelectasis: A retrospective review and a prospective controlled study. J Pediatr 94:110, 1979

84. Fireman P: Status asthmaticus in children. In Middleton E Jr, Reed CE, Ellis EF (eds): Allergy Principles and Practice, 2nd ed, pp 997–1002. St Louis, CV Mosby, 1983

85. First aid for the choking child, 1988. Pediatrics 81:740, 1988

86. Fisher DM, Swedlow DB: Estimating $PaCO_2$ by end tidal gas sampling in children. Crit Care Med 9:287, 1981

87. Fleisher GR: Infectious disease emergencies. In Fleisher GR, Ludwig S (eds): Textbook of Pediatric Emergency Medicine, pp 415–470. Baltimore, Williams & Wilkins, 1988

88. Fox WW, Duara S: Persistent pulmonary hypertension in the neonate—diagnosis and management. J Pediatr 103:505, 1983

89. Francis PWJ, Muller NL, Gurwitz D et al: Hemoglobin desaturation: Its occurrence during sleep in patients with cystic fibrosis. Am J Dis Child 134:734, 1980

90. Frankel LR, Wilson CW, Demers RR et al: A technique for the administration of ribavirin to mechanically ventilated infants with severe respiratory syncytial virus infection. Crit Care Med 15:1051, 1987

91. Frantz ID, Werthammer J, Stark AR: High frequency ventilation in premature infants with lung disease: Adequate gas exchange at low tracheal pressure. Pediatrics 71:483, 1983

92. Freed MD, Keane JF: Cardiac output measured by thermodilution in infants and children. J Pediatr 92:39, 1978

93. Frewen TC, Swedlow DB, Watcha M et al: Outcome in severe Reye syndrome with early pentobarbital coma and hypothermia. J Pediatr 100:663, 1982

94. Fried MP: Controversies in the management of supraglottitis and croup. Pediatr Clin North Am 26:931, 1979

95. Fulginiti VA: Acute supraglottitis (epiglottitis): To look or not [Editorial]? Am J Dis Child 142:597, 1988

96. Gala CL, Hall CB, Schnabel KC et al: The use of eye–nose goggles to control nosocomial respiratory syncytial virus infection. JAMA 256:2706, 1986

97. Galant SP: Therapeutic approaches to acute asthma in children. In Tinkelman DG, Falliers CJ, Naspitz CK (eds): Childhood Asthma, pp 231–248. New York, Marcel Dekker, 1987

98. Gallagher TJ, Civetta JM, Kirby RR: Terminology update: Optimal PEEP. Crit Care Med 6:323, 1978

99. Gay BB Jr, Atkinson GO, Vanderzalm T et al: Subglottic foreign bodies in pediatric patients. Am J Dis Child 140:165, 1986

100. Gerson CR, Tucker GF: Infant tracheotomy. Ann Otol Rhinol Laryngol 91:413, 1982

101. Gibney RTN, Wilson RS, Pontoppidan H: Comparison of work of breathing on high gas flow and demand valve continuous positive airway pressure systems. Chest 82:692, 1982

102. Gilbert J, Robinson T, Littlewood JM: Home intravenous antibiotic therapy in cystic fibrosis. Arch Dis Child 63:512, 1988

103. Gioia FR, Stephenson RL, Alterwitz SA: Principles of respiratory support and mechanical ventilation. In Rogers MC (ed): Textbook of Pediatric Intensive Care, pp 113–170. Baltimore, Williams & Wilkins, 1987

104. Givan D, Scott P, Jeglum E et al: Lung function and airway reactivity of children 3–10 years after foreign body aspiration. Am Rev Respir Dis 123(suppl):158, 1981

105. Glicklich M, Cohen RD, Jona JZ: Steroids and bag and mask ventilation in the treatment of acute epiglottitis. J Pediatr Surg 14:247, 1979

106. Goitein KJ, Rein AJJT, Gornstein A: Incidence of aspiration in endotracheally intubated infants and children. Crit Care Med 12:19, 1984

107. Gold R: Mild to moderate chest exacerbations: Do antibiotics help? Pediatr Pulmonol Suppl 1:38, 1987

108. Gregory GA: Respiratory care of the child. Crit Care Med 8:582, 1980

109. Greenough G, Grenall F, Gamsu HR: Inspiratory times when weaning from mechanical ventilation. Arch Dis Child 62:1269, 1987

110. Greenough G, Grenall F, Gamsu HR: Synchronous respiration: Which ventilator rate is best? Acta Paediatr Scand 76:713, 1987

111. Griffith JA, Perkin RM: Management of acute epiglottitis in pediatric patients [Letter]. Crit Care Med 15:283, 1987

112. Gurthie RD, Hodson WA: Clinical diagnosis of pulmonary insufficiency: History and physical. In Thiebealt DW, Gregory GA (eds): Neonatal Pulmonary Care, 2nd ed, pp 175–194. Norwalk, Conn, Appleton–Century–Crofts, 1986

113. Gurwitz D, Corey M, Levison H: Pulmonary function and bronchial reactivity in children after croup. Am Rev Respir Dis 122:95, 1980

114. Gurwitz D, Mindorff C, Levison H: Increased incidence of bronchial reactivity in children with a history of bronchiolitis. J Pediatr 98:551, 1981

115. Hack M, Mostow A, Miranda SB: Development of attention in pre-term infants. Pediatrics 58:669, 1976

116. Haddad C, Richards CC: Mechanical ventilation of infants: Significance and elimination of ventilator compressure volume. Anesthesiology 29:365, 1988

117. Hall CB, Douglas RG Jr: Modes of transmission of respiratory syncytial virus. J Pediatr 99:100, 1981

118. Hall CB, Douglas RG Jr: Nosocomial respiratory syncytial viral infections: Should gowns and masks be used? Am J Dis Child 135:512, 1981

119. Hall CB, Hall WJ, Speers DM: Clinical and physiological manifestations of bronchiolitis and pneumonia: Outcome of respiratory syncytial virus. Am J Dis Child 133:798, 1979

120. Hall CD, McBride JT: Vapors, viruses, and views: Ribavirin and respiratory syncytial virus. Am J Dis Child 140:331, 1986

121. Hall CB, McBride JT, Gala CL et al: Ribavirin treatment of respiratory syncytial viral infection in infants with underlying cardiopulmonary disease. JAMA 254:3047, 1985

122. Hall CB, McBride JT, Walsh EE et al: Aerosolized ribavirin treatment of infections with respiratory syncytial viral infection: A randomized double-blind study. N Engl J Med 308:1443, 1983

123. Handler SD: Stridor. In Fleisher GR, Ludwig S (eds): Textbook of Pediatric Emergency Medicine, pp 300–305. Baltimore, Williams & Wilkins, 1988

124. Hardy KA, McGowan KL, Fisher MC, Schidlow DV: *Pseudomonas cepacia* in the hospital setting: Lack of transmission between cystic fibrosis patients. J Pediatr 109:51, 1986

125. Harris CJ, Nadler HL: Incidence, genetics, heterozygote, and antenatal detection of cystic fibrosis. In Lloyd–Still JD (ed): Textbook of Cystic Fibrosis, pp 1–8. Boston, John Wright, 1983

126. Healey CJ, Fedullo AJ, Swinburne AJ, Wahl GW: Comparison of non-invasive measurements of carbon dioxide tension during withdrawal from mechanical ventilation. Crit Care Med 15:764, 1987

127. Heiden D, Meikle CH, Rodvien R, Hill JD: Platelets, hemostasis and thromboembolism during treatment of acute respiratory insufficiency with extracorporeal membrane oxygenation: Experience with 28 clinical perfusions. J Thorac Cardiovasc Surg 70:664, 1975

128. Heimer D, Shim C, Williams MH: The effects of sequential inhalations of metaproterenol aerosol in asthma. J Allergy Clin Immunol 66:75, 1980

129. Hen J Jr: Current management of upper airway obstruction. Pediatr Ann 15:274, 1986

130. Henderson FW, Clyde WA Jr, Collier AM et al: The etiologic and epidemiologic spectrum of bronchiolitis in pediatric practice. J Pediatr 95:183, 1979

131. Henry RL, Hiller EJ, Milner AD et al: Nebulised ipratropium bromide and sodium cromoglycate in the first two years of life. Arch Dis Child 59:54, 1984

132. Henry RL, Milner AD, Stokes GM: Ineffectiveness of ipratropium bromide in acute bronchiolitis. Arch Dis Child 58:925, 1983

133. Herbst JJ: Gastroesophageal reflux. J Pediatr 98:859, 1981

134. Herbst JJ, Minton SD, Book LS: Gastroesophageal reflux causing respiratory distress and apnea in newborn infants. J Pediatr 95:763, 1979

135. Herman JJ, Noah ZL, Moody RR: Use of intravenous isoproterenol for status asthmaticus in children. Crit Care Med 11:716, 1983

136. Hodson ME, Penketh ARL, Batten JC: Aerosol carbenicillin and gentamicin treatment of *Pseudomonas aeruginosa* infections in patients with cystic fibrosis. Lancet 2:1137, 1981

137. Hogg JC: Pathology of asthma. In Middleton E Jr, Reed CE, Ellis EF (eds): Allergy Principles and Practice, 2nd ed, pp 833–842. St Louis, CV Mosby, 1983

138. Hogg JC, Williams J, Richardson JB et al: Age as a factor in the distribution of lower airway conductance and in the pathologic anatomy of obstructive lung disease. N Engl J Med 282:1283, 1970

139. Holbrook PR, Mickell J, Pollack MM, Fields AI: Cardiovascular resuscitation drugs for children. Crit Care Med 8:588, 1980

140. Holinger PH, Kutnick SL, Schild JA, Holinger LD: Subglottic stenosis in infants and children. Ann Otol 85:591, 1976

141. Holzer FJ, Schnall R, Landau LI: The effect of a home exercise programme in children with cystic fibrosis and asthma. Aust Paediatr J 20:297, 1984

142. Hrabovsky EE, Mullett MD: Gastroesophageal reflux and the premature infant. J Pediatr Surg 21:583, 1986

143. Hyatt AC, Chipps BE, Kumor KM et al: A double-

blind controlled trial of anti-pseudomonas chemotherapy of acute respiratory exacerbations in patients with cystic fibrosis. J Pediatr 99:307, 1981

144. Ilbawi MN, Idriss FS, Hunt CE et al: Diaphragmatic pacing in infants: Techniques and results. Ann Thorac Surg 40:323, 1985

145. Isles A, Maclusky I, Corey M et al: *Pseudomonas cepacia* infection in cystic fibrosis: An emerging problem. J Pediatr 104:206, 1984

146. Jolley SG, Herbst JJ, Johnson DG et al: Surgery in children with gastroesophageal reflux and respiratory symptoms. J Pediatr 96:194, 1980

147. Kacmerak RM, Mack CW, Dimas S: Essentials of Respiratory Therapy, 2nd ed, p 391. Chicago, Year Book Medical, 1985

148. Katz JA, Kraemer RW, Gjerde GE: Inspiratory work and airway pressure with continuous positive airway pressure delivery systems. Chest 88:519, 1985

149. Keens TG, Bryan AC, Levison H et al: Developmental pattern of muscle fiber types in human ventilatory muscles. J Appl Physiol 44:909, 1978

150. Keep PJ, Manford MLM: Endotracheal tube sizes for children. Anaesthesia 29:181, 1974

151. Kenna MA, Bluestone CD: Foreign bodies in the air and food passages. Pediatr Rev 10:25, 1988

152. Kilham H, Gillis J, Benjamin B: Severe upper airway obstruction. Pediatr Clin North Am 34:1, 1987

153. Kimmons HC Jr, Peterson BM: Management of acute epiglottitis in pediatric patients. Crit Care Med 14:278, 1986

154. King T, Simon RH: Pulse oximetry for tapering supplemental in hospitalized patients. Chest 92:713, 1987

155. Kiriloff LH, Owens GR, Rogers RM, Mazzocco MC: Does chest physical therapy work? Chest 88:436, 1985

156. Klaus MH, Kennell JH: Parent–infant Bonding, 2nd ed, p 74. St Louis, CV Mosby, 1982

157. Klein EF Jr, Graves SA: "Hot pot" tracheitis. Chest 65:225, 1974

158. Koka BV, Jeon IS, Andre JM et al: Postintubation croup in children. Anesth Analg 56:501, 1977

159. Kolobow T, Stool EW, Sacks KL, Vurek GG: Acute respiratory failure: Survival following ten days support with a membrane lung. J Thorac Cardiovasc Surg 69:947, 1975

160. König P: Asthma: A pediatric pulmonary disease and a changing concept. Pediatr Pulmonol 3:264, 1987

161. Kosloske AM: Tracheobronchial foreign bodies in children: Back to the bronchoscope and a balloon. Pediatrics 66:321, 1980

162. Kravath RE: A lethal pacifier. Pediatrics 58:853, 1976

163. Kun P, Landau LI, Phelan PD: Nebulized gentamicin in children and adolescents with cystic fibrosis. Aust Paediatr J 20:43, 1984

164. Kurland G, Leong AB: The management of status asthmaticus in infants and children. Clin Rev Allergy 3:37, 1985

165. Landau LI, Phelan PD: The variable effect of a bronchodilating agent in cystic fibrosis. J Pediatr 82:863, 1983

166. Laughlin JJ, Eigen H: Pulmonary function abnormalities in survivors of near drowning. J Pediatr 100:26, 1982

167. Lazoritz S, Saunders BS, Bason WM: Management of acute epiglottitis. Crit Care Med 7:285, 1979

168. Lenny W, Milner AD: At what age do bronchodilator drugs work? Arch Dis Child 53:532, 1978

169. Levy LD, Durie PR, Pencharz PB, Corey ML: Effects of long-term nutritional rehabilitation on body composition and clinical status in malnourished children and adolescents with cystic fibrosis. J Pediatr 107:225, 1985

170. Lewis RM: Automatic increases in mean airway pressure during mechanical ventilation. Respir Care 27:675, 1982

171. Lloyd–Still JD: Pulmonary manifestations. In Lloyd–Still JD (ed): Textbook of Cystic Fibrosis, pp 165–198. Boston, John Wright, 1983

172. Lloyd–Still JD: Growth, nutrition and gastrointestinal problems. In Lloyd–Still JD (ed): Textbook of Cystic Fibrosis, pp 227–262. Boston, John Wright, 1983

173. Lough MD, Williams TJ, Rawson JE: Newborn Respiratory Care, pp 174–175. Chicago, Year Book Medical, 1979

174. Louhimo I, Grahne B, Pasila M, Suutarinen T: Acquired laryngotracheal stenosis in children. J Pediatr Surg 6:730, 1971

175. MacDonald NE, Hall CB, Suffin SC et al: Respiratory syncytial viral infection in infants with congenital heart disease. N Engl J Med 307, 1982

176. Mallol J, Barrueto L, Girardi G et al: Use of nebulized bronchodilators in infants under 1 year of age: Analysis of four forms of therapy. Pediatr Pulmonol 3:298, 1987

177. Mallol J, Barrueto L, Girardi G, Toro O: Bronchodilator effects of fenoterol and ipratropium bromide in infants with acute wheezing: Use of an MDI with a spacer device. Pediatr Pulmonol 3:352, 1987

178. Mammel MC, Ophoven JP, Lewallen PK et al: High frequency ventilation and tracheal injuries. Pediatrics 77:608, 1986

179. Manning PB, Wesley JR, Polley JRTZ, Coran AG: Esophageal and tracheobronchial foreign bodies in infants and children. Pediatr Surg Int 2:346, 1987

180. Mansmann HC: A 25-year perspective of status asthmaticus. Clin Rev Allergy 1:147, 1983

181. Mansmann HC, Biermann CW, Pearlman DS: Treatment of acute asthma in children. In Bierman CW, Pearlman DS (eds): Allergic Diseases from Infancy to Adulthood, 2nd ed, pp 571–586. Philadelphia, WB Saunders, 1988

182. Marchak BE, Thompson WK, Duffty P et al: Treatment of RDS of high frequency oscillatory ventilation: A preliminary report. J Pediatr 99:287, 1981

183. Margolis CL, Ingram DL, Meyer JH: Routine tracheostomy in *Hemophilus influenzae* type b epiglottitis. J Pediatr 81:1150, 1972

184. Marquez JM, Douglas ME, Downs JB et al: Renal function and cardiovascular responses during positive airway pressure. Anesthesiology 50:393, 1979

185. Marshall AG, Erwin DC, Wyse RKH, Hatch DJ: Percutaneous arterial cannulation in children. Anaesthesia 39:27, 1984

186. Martin RJ, Beoglos A, Miller MJ et al: Increasing arterial carbon dioxide tension: Influence on transcutaneous carbon dioxide tension measurements. Pediatrics 81:684, 1988

187. Mattila MAK, Suutarinen T, Sulamaa M: Prolonged endotracheal intubation or tracheostomy in infants and children. J Pediatr Surg 4:674, 1969

188. Mauro RD, Poole SR, Lockhart CH: Differentiation of epiglottitis from laryngotracheitis in the child with stridor. Am J Dis Child 142:679, 1988

189. Mayer T, Walker ML: Emergency intracranial pressure monitoring in pediatrics. Clin Pediatr 21:391, 1982

190. McConnochie KM: Bronchiolitis: What's in the name? Am J Dis Child 137:11, 1983

191. McGuirt WF, Holmes KD, Feehs R, Browne JD: Tracheobronchial foreign bodies. Laryngoscope 98:615, 1988

192. McMillan JA, Tristman DA, Weiner LB et al: Prediction of hospitalization in patients with respiratory syncytial virus infection: Use of clinical parameters. Pediatrics 81:22, 1988

193. McPherson SP: Respiratory Therapy Equipment, 3rd ed. St Louis, CV Mosby, 1985

194. McWilliams BC: Mechanical ventilation in pediatric patients. Clin Chest Med 8:597, 1987

195. Melker RJ: Asynchronous and other alternative methods of ventilation during CPR. Ann Emerg Med 13:758, 1984

196. Melker RJ, Banner MJ: Ventilation during CPR: Two rescuer standards reappraised. Ann Emerg Med 14:397, 1985

197. Mihm FG, Halperin BD: Non-invasive detection of profound arterial desaturation using a pulse oximetry device. Anesthesiology 62:85, 1985

198. Milligan DWA, Levison H: Lung function in children following repair of tracheoesophageal fistula. J Pediatr 95:24, 1979

199. Milliken J, Tait GA, Ford–Jones EL et al: Nosocomial infections in a pediatric intensive care unit. Crit Care Med 16:233, 1988

200. Millunchick EW, McArtor RD: Fatal aspiration of a makeshift pacifier. Pediatrics 77:369, 1986

201. Miranda SB: Visual abilities and pattern preferences of premature infants and full term neonates. J Exp Child Psychol 10:189, 1970

202. Miyasaka K, Edmonds JF, Conn AW: Complications of radial artery lines in the paediatric patient. Can Anaesth Soc J 23:9, 1976

203. Mok J, Pintar M, Benson L et al: Evaluation of non-invasive measurements of oxygenation in stable infants. Crit Care Med 14:960, 1986

204. Moler FW, Hurwitz ME, Custer JR: Improvement in clinical asthma score and PaCO₂ in children with severe asthma treated with continuously nebulized terbutaline. J Allergy Clin Immunol 81:1101, 1988

205. Moodie DS: Measurement of cardiac output by thermodilution in pediatric patients. Pediatr Clin North Am 27:513, 1980

206. Moore RA, McNicholas K, Gallagher JD, Niguidula F: Migration of pediatric pulmonary artery catheters. Anesthesiology 58:102, 1983

207. Morray JP, Lynn AM, Mansfield PB: Effect of pH and Pco₂ on pulmonary and systemic hemodynamics after surgery in children with congenital heart disease and pulmonary hypertension. J Pediatr 113:474, 1988

208. Murphy D, Todd JK, Chao RK et al: The use of gowns and masks to control respiratory illness in pediatric hospital personnel. J Pediatr 99:746, 1981

209. Mushin WW, Rendall–Baker L, Thompson PW, Mapleson WW: Automatic Ventilation of the Lung, 2nd ed, p 167. Oxford, Blackwell Scientific, 1980

210. Naspitz CK, Tinkelman DG: Therapeutic approaches to acute asthma in children. In Tinkelman DG, Falliers CJ, Naspitz CK (eds): Childhood Asthma, pp 249–280. New York, Marcel Dekker, 1987

211. Nelson JD: Management of acute pulmonary exacerbations in cystic fibrosis: A critical appraisal. J Pediatr 106:1030, 1985

212. Newman SP, Woodman G, Clarke SW: Deposition of carbenicillin aerosols in cystic fibrosis: Effects of nebuliser system and breathing pattern. Thorax 43:318, 1988

213. Nichols DG, Rogers MC: Developmental physiology of the respiratory system. In Rogers MC (ed): Textbook of Pediatric Intensive Care, pp 83–112. Baltimore, Williams & Wilkins, 1987

214. Nugent SK, Laravuso R, Rogers MC: Pharmacology and use of muscle relaxants in infants and children. J Pediatr 94:481, 1979

215. Nussbaum E, Galant SP: Intracranial pressure monitoring as a guide to prognosis in the nearly drowned, severely comatose child. J Pediatr 102:215, 1983

216, O'Brodovich HM, Chernick V: The functional basis of respiratory pathology. In Kendig EL, Chernick V (eds): Disorders of the Respiratory Tract in Children, 4th ed, pp 3–45. Philadelphia, WB Saunders, 1983

217. Okafor BC: Tracheostomy in the management of pediatric airway problems. Ear Nose Throat J 62:50, 1983

218. Orenstein SR, Magill HL, Brooks P: Thickening of infant feedings for therapy of gastroesophageal reflux. J Pediatr 110:181, 1987

219. Orenstein SR, Orenstein DM: Gastroesophageal reflux and respiratory disease in children. J Pediatr 112:847, 1988

220. Orenstein SR, Whitington PF, Orenstein DM: The infant seat as treatment for gastroesophageal reflux. N Engl J Med 309:760, 1983

221. Orlowski JP, Ellis NG, Amin NP, Crumrine RS: Complications of airway intrusion in 100 consecutive cases in a pediatric ICU. Crit Care Med 8:324, 1980

222. Ormerod LP, Thomson RA, Anderson CM, Stableforth DE: Reversible airway obstruction in cystic fibrosis. Thorax 35:768, 1980

223. O'Rourke PP: Out of hospital cardiac arrest in pediatric patients: Outcome. Crit Care Med 12:283, 1984

224. O'Rourke PP, Crone RK: Halothane in status asthmaticus. Crit Care Med 10:341, 1982

225. Ortiz RM, Cilley RE, Bartlett RH: Extracorporeal membrane oxygenation in pediatric respiratory failure. Pediatr Clin North Am 34:39, 1987

226. Outwater KM, Crone RK: Management of respiratory failure in infants with acute viral bronchiolitis. Am J Dis Child 138:1071, 1984

227. Outwater KM, Meissner C, Peterson MB: Ribavirin administration to infants receiving mechanical ventilation. Am J Dis Child 142:512, 1988

228. Pagtakhan RD, Wohl MEB, Chernick V: Bronchiolitis. Semin Resp Med 2:123, 1979

229. Palva A, Jokinen K, Niemela T: Tracheostomy in children. Arch Otolaryngol 101:536, 1975

230. Parry WH, Martorano F, Cotton EK: Management of life-threatening asthma with intravenous isoproterenol infusions. Am J Dis Child 130:39, 1976

231. Pearlman DS, Bierman CW: Asthma (bronchial asthma). In Bierman CW, Pearlman DS (eds): Allergic

Diseases from Infancy to Adulthood, 2nd ed, pp 546–570. Philadelphia, WB Saunders, 1988

232. Pedersen SS, Jensen T, Høiby N et al: Management of *Pseudomonas aeruginosa* lung infection in Danish cystic fibrosis patients. Acta Paediatr Scand 76:955, 1987

233. Pepe PE, Marini JJ: Occult positive end-expiratory pressure in mechanically ventilated patients with airflow obstruction: The auto-PEEP effect. Am Rev Respir Dis 126:166, 1982

234. Perlman ND, Schena J, Thompson J, Crone RK: Effects of ETT size, working pressure and compliance on pressure support ventilation. Respir Care 33:926, 1988

235. Pierce AK, Sanford JP: Bacterial contamination of aerosols. Arch Intern Med 131:156, 1973

236. Phelan PD, Landau LI, Olinsky A: Cystic fibrosis. In Phelan PD, Landau LI, Olinsky A (eds): Respiratory Illness in Children, 2nd ed, pp 239–294. Oxford, Blackwell Scientific, 1982

237. Polgar G, Weng TR: The functional development of the respiratory system. Am Rev Respir Dis 120:625, 1979

238. Pollack MM, Fields AI, Holbrook PR: Pneumothorax and pneumomediastinum during pediatric mechanical ventilation. Crit Care Med 7:536, 1979

239. Pollack MM, Ruttimann UE, Glass NL, Yeh TS: Monitoring patients in pediatric intensive care. Pediatrics 76:719, 1985

240. Post DJ, Kita R, Myers TF, Paveza G: Neonatal volume monitoring: A new device. Respir Care 33:890, 1988

241. Prendiville A, Green S, Silverman M: Ipratropium bromide and airways function in wheezy infants. Arch Dis Child 62:397, 1987

242. Prendiville A, Green S, Silverman M: Paradoxical response to nebulised salbutamol in wheezy infants, assessed by partial expiratory flow-volume curves. Thorax 42:86, 1987

243. Qvist J, Anderson JB, Pemberton M, Bennike KA: High level PEEP in severe asthma. N Engl J Med 307:1347, 1982

244. Rachelefsky GS, Siegel SC: Asthma in infants and children—treatment of childhood asthma: Part II. J Allergy Clin Immunol 76:409, 1985

245. Raffensperger JG: Surgical problems in cystic fibrosis. In Lloyd–Still JD (ed): Textbook in Cystic Fibrosis. pp 371–382. Boston, John Wright, 1983

246. Ramenofsky ML, Leape LL: Continuous upper esophageal pH monitoring in infants and children with gastroesophageal reflux, pneumonia and apneic spells. J Pediatr Surg 16:374, 1981

247. Rapkin RH: Tracheostomy in epiglottitis. Pediatrics 52:426, 1974

248. Ray CG: Ribavirin: Ambivalence about an antiviral agent. Am J Dis Child 142:488, 1988

249. Reed CE: Basic mechanisms of asthma: Role of inflammation. Chest 94:175, 1988

250. Reed CE, Townley RG: Asthma: Classification and pathogenesis. In Middleton E Jr, Reed CE, Ellis EF (ed): Allergy Principles and Practice 2nd ed, pp 811–832. St Louis, CV Mosby, 1983

251. Reines HD, Sade RM, Bradford BF, Marshall J: Chest physiotherapy fails to prevent post operative atelectasis in children after cardiac surgery. Ann Surg 195:451, 1982

252. Roberts JR, Greenberg MI, Knaub MA et al: Blood levels following intravenous and endotracheal epinephrine administration. JACEP 8:53, 1979

253. Robertson CF, Smith F, Beck R, Levison H: Response to frequent low doses of nebulized salbutamol in acute asthma. J Pediatr 106:672, 1985

254. Rodgers BM, Rooks JJ, Talbert JL: Pediatric tracheostomy: Long term evaluation. J Pediatr Surg 14:258, 1979

255. Rooth G, Huch A, Huch R: Transcutaneous oxygen monitors are reliable indicators of arterial oxygen tension (if used correctly). Pediatrics 79:283, 1987

256. Rosenthal BW: Wheezing. In Fleisher GR, Ludwig S (eds): Textbook of Pediatric Emergency Medicine, pp 344–350. Baltimore, Williams & Wilkins, 1988

257. Rossman CM, Waldes R, Sampson D, Newhouse MT: Effect of chest physiotherapy on the removal of mucus in patients with cystic fibrosis. Am Rev Respir Dis 126:131, 1982

258. Schaad UB, Wedgewood-Krucko J, Suter S, Kraemer R: Efficacy of inhaled amikacin as adjunct to intravenous combination therapy (ceftazidime and amikacin) in cystic fibrosis. J Pediatr 111:599, 1987

259. Schena J, Crone RK, Thompson JE: The use of aminophylline in severe bronchiolitis [Abstract]. Crit Care Med 12:225, 1984

260. Schleien CL, Rogers MC: Cardiopulmonary resuscitation in infants and children. In Rogers MC (ed): Textbook of Pediatric Intensive Care, pp 57–82. Baltimore, Williams & Wilkins, 1987

261. Schumacher RE, Barks JDE, Johnston MV et al: Right-sided brain lesions in infants following extracorporeal membrane oxygenation. Pediatrics 82:155, 1988

262. Scott CB, Nickerson BG, Sargent CW et al: Developmental pattern of maximal transdiaphragmatic pressure in infants during crying. Pediatr Res 17:707, 1983

263. Scott LR, Benson MS, Pierson DJ: Effect of inspiratory flowrate and circuit compressible volume on auto-PEEP during mechanical ventilation. Respir Care 31:1075, 1986

264. Scott LR, Benson MS, Bishop MJ: Relationship of endotracheal tube size to auto-PEEP at high minute ventilation. Respir Care 31:1080, 1986

265. Sell LL, Cullen ML, Whittlesey GC et al: Hemorrhagic complications during extracorporeal membrane oxygenation: Prevention and treatment. J Pediatr Surg 21:1087, 1986

266. Shapiro BA, Harrison RA, Kacmerak RM, Cane RD: Clinical Application of Respiratory Care, 3rd ed, p 92. Chicago. Year Book Medical, 1985

267. Shapiro GC, Furukawa CT, Pierson WE et al: Double-blind, dose response study of metaproterenol inhalant solution in children with acute asthma. J Allergy Clin Immunol 79:378, 1987

268. Shepherd R, Cooksley WGE, Cooke WDD: Improved growth and clinical, nutritional, and respiratory changes in response to nutritional therapy in cystic fibrosis. J Pediatr 97:351, 1980

269. Shepherd RW, Holt TL, Thomas BJ et al: Nutritional rehabilitation in cystic fibrosis: Controlled studies of effects on nutritional growth retardation, body protein turnover and course of pulmonary disease. J Pediatr 109:788, 1986

270. Shiley Incorporated Product Literature, 17600 Gillette Avenue, Irvine, CA 92714–5751.

271. Siegel SC: Overview of corticosteroid therapy. J Allergy Clin Immunol 76:312, 1985

272. Siegel SC, Katz RM, Rachelefsky GS: Asthma in infancy and childhood. In Middleton E Jr, Reed CE, Ellis EF (eds): Allergy Principles and Practice, 2nd ed, pp 863–900. St Louis, CV Mosby, 1983

273. Siegel SC, Rachelefsky GS: Asthma in infants and children: Part I. J Allergy Clin Immunol 76:1, 1985

274. Silverman M: Bronchodilators for wheezy infants? Arch Dis Child 59:84, 1984

275. Simbruner G: Inadvertent positive end-expiratory pressure in mechanically ventilated newborn infants: Detection and effect on lung mechanics and gas exchange. J Pediatr 108:589, 1986

276. Simmons D, Elliot CG, Greenway L, Turner K: Results of change to dry low flow oxygen delivery. Respir Care 33:921, 1988

277. Simmons FER, Pierson WE, Bierman CW: Respiratory failure in childhood status asthmaticus. Am J Dis Child 131:1097, 1977

278. Sjostrand U: High frequency positive pressure ventilation (HFPPV): A review. Crit Care Med 8:345, 1980

279. Sjostrand UH, Eriksson IA: High rates and low volumes in mechanical ventilation—not just a matter of ventilatory frequency. Anesth Analg 59:567, 1980

280. Sly RM, Barbera JM, Middleton HB, Eby DM: Delivery of albuterol aerosol by aerochamber to young children. Ann Allergy 60:403, 1988

281. Spier S, Rivlin J, Hughes D, Levison H: The effect of oxygen on sleep, blood gases, and ventilation in cystic fibrosis. Am Rev Respir Dis 129:712, 1984

282. Spivey WH: Intraosseous infusions. J Pediatr 111:639, 1987

283. Splaingard ML, Frazier OH, Jefferson LS et al: Extracorporeal membrane oxygenation: Its role in the survival of a child with adenoviral pneumonia and myocarditis. South Med J 76:1171, 1983

284. Staib SG, Friel D: Evaluation of the delivery system of ribavirin via a SPAG-2 generator and a pressure ventilator. Respir Care 32:944, 1987

285. Standards and guidelines for cardiopulmonary resuscitation (CPR) and emergency cardiac care (ECC). JAMA 255:2905, 1986

286. Stanger P, Heymann MA, Hoffman JIE, Rudolph AM: Use of Swan-Ganz catheter in cardiac catheterization of infants and children. Am Heart J 83:749, 1972

287. Stark LJ: The behavioral approach to nutrition support. Pediatr Pulmonol Suppl 1:61, 1987

288. Steele RW: Antiviral agents for respiratory infections. Pediatr Infect Dis J 7:456, 1988

289. Stempel D, McCarthy M, Morray JP: Status asthmaticus. In Morray JP (ed): Pediatric Intensive Care. pp 191–200. Norwalk, Appleton & Lange, 1987

290. Stephens D, Garey N, Isles A et al: Efficacy of inhaled tobramycin in the treatment of pulmonary exacerbations in children with cystic fibrosis. Pediatr Infect Dis J 2:209, 1983

291. Stokes DC, McBride JT, Wall MA et al: Sleep hypoxemia in young adults with cystic fibrosis. Am J Dis Child 134:741, 1980

292. Stokes GM, Milner AD, Hodges IGC et al: Nebulised therapy in acute severe bronchiolitis in infancy. Arch Dis Child 58:279, 1983

293. Stokes GM, Milner AD, Hodges IGC, Groggins RC: Lung function abnormalities after acute bronchiolitis. J Pediatr 98:871, 1981

294. Suter PM, Fairley HB, Isenberg MD: Optimum end-expiratory airway pressure in patients with acute pulmonary failure. N Engl J Med 292:284, 1975

295. Swedlow DB, Stern S: Continuous non-invasive oxygen saturation monitoring in children with a new pulse oximeter [Abstract]. Crit Care Med 11:228, 1983

296. Tabachnick E, Levison H: Infantile bronchial asthma. J Allergy Clin Immunol 67:339, 1981

297. Tabata BK, Kirsch JR, Rogers MC: Diagnostic tests and technology for pediatric intensive care. In Rogers MC (ed): Textbook of Pediatric Intensive Care, pp 1401–1432. Baltimore, Williams & Wilkins, 1987

298. Taber LH, Knight V, Gilbert BE et al: Ribavirin aerosol treatment of bronchiolitis associated with respiratory syncytial virus infection in infants. Pediatrics 72:613, 1983

299. Tablan OC, Chorba TL, Schidlow DV et al: *Pseudomonas cepacia* colonization in patients with cystic fibrosis: Risk factors and clinical outcome. J Pediatr 107–382, 1985

300. Tal A, Bavilski C, Yohai D et al: Dexamethasone and salbutamol in the treatment of acute wheezing in infants. Pediatrics 71:13, 1983

301. Taussig LM, Cota K, Kaltenborn W: Different mechanical properties of the lung in boys and girls. Am Rev Respir Dis 123:640, 1981

302. Technology for Respiratory Therapy, Vol 7, #7, Jan 1987

303. Tepper RS, Morgan WJ, Cota K et al: Physiological growth and development of the lung during the first year of life. Am Rev Respir Dis 134:513, 1986

304. Thomassen MJ, Demko CA, Doershuk CF et al: *Pseudomonas cepacia:* Decrease in colonization in cystic fibrosis patients. Am Rev Respir Dis 134:669, 1986

305. Thompson AE: Respiratory distress. In Fleisher GR, Ludwig S (eds): Textbook of Pediatric Emergency Medicine, pp 272–278. Baltimore, Williams & Wilkins, 1988

306. Thurlbeck WM: Postnatal human lung growth. Thorax 37:564, 1982

307. Todres ID, Rogers MC: Methods of external cardiac massage in the newborn infant. J Pediatr 86:781, 1975

308. Towne BH, Lott IT, Hick DA, Healy T: Long term follow-up of infants and children treated with extracorporeal membrane oxygenation (ECMO): A preliminary report. J Pediatr Surg 20:410, 1985

309. Tooley WH: The respiratory system. In Rudolph AM (ed): Pediatrics, pp 1359–1444. Norwalk, Appleton & Lange, 1987

310. Tremper KK: Transcutaneous PO_2 measurement. Can Anaesth Soc J 31:664, 1984

311. Tunnesson WW, Feinstein AR: The steroid–croup controversy: An analytic review of methodologic problems. J Pediatr 96:751, 1980

312. Twarog FJ: Treatment of the wheezing infant. In Tinkelman DG, Falliers CJ, Naspitz CK (eds): Childhood Asthma, pp 183–202. New York, Marcel Dekker, 1987

313. Vaisman N, Pencharz PB, Corey M et al: Energy expenditure of patients with cystic fibrosis. J Pediatr 111:496, 1987

314. Vernon DD, Sarnaik AP: Acute epiglottitis in chil-

dren: A conservative approach to diagnosis and management. Crit Care Med 14:23, 1986

315. Wald ER, Dashefsky B, Green M: In re ribavirin: A case of premature adjudication? J Pediatr 112:154, 1988

316. Waters DJ: Guided blind endotracheal intubation for patients with deformities of the upper airway. Anaesthesia 18:158, 1963

317. Weinberger M, Hendeles L: Theophylline use: An overview. J Allergy Clin Immunol 76:277, 1985

318. Werlin SL, Dodds WJ, Hogan WJ, Arndorfer RC: Mechanisms of gastroesophageal reflux in children. J Pediatr 97:244, 1980

319. Wessel HU: Lung function in cystic fibrosis. In Lloyd–Still JD (ed): Textbook of Cystic Fibrosis, pp 199–216. Boston, John Wright, 1983

320. Wetmore RF, Handler SD, Potsic WP: Pediatric tracheostomy experience during the past decade. Ann Otol Rhinol Laryngol 91:628, 1982

321. Wientzen R, Prestidge CB, Kramer RI et al: Acute pulmonary exacerbations in cystic fibrosis: A double-blind trial of tobramycin and placebo therapy. Am J Dis Child 134:1134, 1980

322. Witek TJ, Schachter EN: Concern about ribavirin [Letter]. Respir Care 33:506, 1988

323. Witte MK, Galli SA, Chatburn RL, Blumer JL: Optimal positive end expiratory pressure therapy in infants and children with acute respiratory failure. Pediatr Res 24:217, 1988

324. Wohl MEB, Chernick V: Bronchiolitis. Am Rev Respir Dis 118:759, 1978

325. Wohl MEB, Mead J: Age as a factor in respiratory disease. In Kendig EL, Chernick V (eds): Disorders of the Respiratory Tract in Children, 4th ed, pp 135–145. Philadelphia, WB Saunders, 1983

326. Wood DW, Downes JJ, Lecks HI: A clinical scoring system for the diagnosis of respiratory failure. Am J Dis Child 123:227, 1972

327. Wyse SD, Pfitzner J, Rees A et al: Measurement of cardiac output by thermal dilution in infants and children. Thorax 30:262, 1975

328. Yahav J, Mindorff C, Levison H: The validity of the transcutaneous oxygen tension method in children with cardiorespiratory problems. Am Rev Respir Dis 124:586, 1981

329. Yamanaka MK, Sue DY: Comparison of arterial-end-tidal P_{CO_2} difference and dead space/tidal volume ratio in respiratory failure. Chest 92:832, 1987

330. Yelderman M, New W: Evaluation of pulse oximetry. Anesthesiology 59:349, 1983

331. Zach MS, Oberwaldner B, Häusler F: Cystic fibrosis: Physical exercise versus chest physiotherapy. Arch Dis Child 57:587, 1982

332. Zinman R, Corey M, Coates AL et al: Nocturnal oxygen therapy in the treatment of cystic fibrosis patients. Pediatr Pulmonol Suppl 1:73, 1987

THIRTY

Respiratory Care of the Surgical Patient

Harry L. Anderson III
Robert H. Bartlett

Respiratory complications are the single largest cause of morbidity and mortality in surgical patients. Much of the surgeon's time is spent preventing or treating such conditions. Respiratory complications may occur in any patient subjected to anesthesia and surgery, but the patient who needs an operation on the chest or the lung itself is at particularly high risk. In this chapter we shall review the definitions of postoperative pulmonary complications, the pathophysiology of pulmonary insufficiency as seen in surgical patients, and the current guidelines for prevention and treatment.

As a corollary, a segment of this chapter is entitled "Surgical Care of the Respiratory Patient." This serves to introduce common surgical procedures such as thoracostomy, bronchoscopy, and tracheostomy. Conditions of the chest wall, pleural space, lung parenchyma, and airways that commonly require operative management are also discussed. More detailed information on any of these topics can be found in a relatively recent monograph.[3]

Major changes in pulmonary function occur after anesthesia and major surgical procedures. These changes occur in all patients and progress to clinically obvious pulmonary insufficiency in a small percentage. If patients with preexisting chronic or acute lung disease must undergo surgery, the effects of the operation must be appreciated earlier and more readily, because the patient has less pulmonary reserve.

Abnormal lung function owing to the basic disease (e.g., pancreatitis, massive transfusion, fat embolism from fracture) or postoperatively owing to the normal response to surgery may be present in varying degrees and goes under many names. The clinical picture may range from minor atelectasis, hypoventilation, or positional ventilation–perfusion abnormalities, to the syndromes of adult respiratory distress (ARDS), or so-called wet lung.

The terms atelectasis and ARDS are merely part of a continuum of physiologic change. It is not helpful to isolate segments of this continuum with specific names. In the following discussion, we shall focus on the alterations in pulmonary structure and function that accompany anesthesia and major operations and then discuss how these changes might add to, or be affected by, other factors that affect lung function.

POSTOPERATIVE CHANGES IN LUNG FUNCTION

USUAL AND CUSTOMARY POSTOPERATIVE CHANGES

After any major operation, changes occur in function as a result of alveolar atelectasis. These changes occur in all patients, but are generally not routinely detected.[23] Aside from shallow tidal ventilation and some decreased breath sounds at the lung bases, the patient shows no signs of respiratory abnormality. On direct measurement lung volumes are decreased [particularly residual volume, expiratory reserve volume, functional residual capacity (FRC), and vital capacity]. Compliance is decreased because of the decrease in FRC. The work of breathing is increased for the same reason (i.e., more pressure is required to inhale a given volume into the decreased lung air space). Further evidence that alveoli are not being ventilated is absolute or relative arterial hypoxemia, which occurs with the patient breathing room air or 100% oxygen, indicating that nonventilated alveoli are being perfused (transpulmonary shunting).

These changes in lung function are present immediately after an operation, slowly worsen over the next 1 to 2 days, and then return to normal in most patients. The extent and duration of abnormality are related to the site of operation and anesthesia, quality of postoperative care, and preexisting pulmonary status. These changes in pulmonary function for a typical laparotomy patient are shown in Figure 30–1.

The extent and the duration of these abnormalities are greatest for operations on the thorax and upper abdomen and progressively decrease as the site of operation moves more distally and more superficially on the body structures. These changes may occur after only 1 to 2 hours of general anesthesia if careful attention is not paid to maximal lung inflation during anesthesia.[11] They are superimposed on the patient's preexisting lung status. If, for example, the patient requires an operation for pancreatitis 2 weeks after the onset of disease, he may already have pleural effusions, increased pulmonary capillary permeability, and existing transpulmonary shunting and will not tolerate any further deterioration of lung function. Likewise, the patient with preexisting chronic obstructive lung disease with high airway resistance, maximal work of breathing, and minimal functional lung tissue preoperatively may proceed to carbon dioxide retention if the work of breathing is only slightly increased after an operation.

Several factors contribute to these changes in pulmonary function, but shallow breathing with in-

Figure 30–1. Usual and expected changes in pulmonary function after an abdominal operation. Note the transient nature of the abnormalities, all of which have returned to normal by the fifth postoperative day (see text). (Bartlett RH: Post-traumatic pulmonary insufficiency. In Cooper P, Nyhus L (eds): Surgery Annual. New York, Appleton–Century–Crofts, 1971)

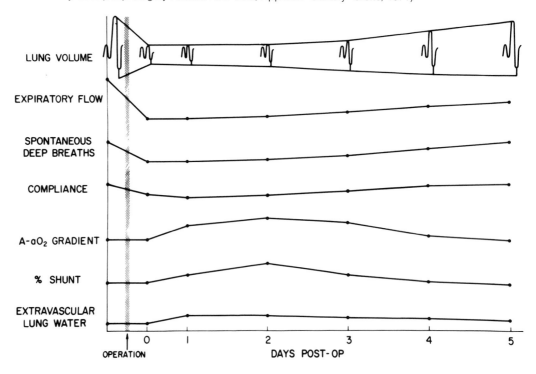

complete alveolar inflation is the common denominator. If spontaneous deep breaths to maximal lung inflation are eliminated from the pattern of breathing, alveolar collapse begins within 1 hour and progresses rather rapidly to produce significant transpulmonary shunting. Several studies have shown that patients postoperatively lack the normal pattern of spontaneous deep breaths[25,42] because of severe pain, anesthetics, or narcotic drugs. Further evidence supporting this observation is that the postoperative changes in lung function can be returned toward normal by instituting maximal inflation, deep-breathing exercises at regular intervals.[6] In part, these alterations may result from reduced diaphragmatic activity after surgery, which returns to normal after 24 hours.[17] Finally, excessive tracheobronchial secretions, aspiration of oral or gastric contents, and intraoperative fluid overload or blood transfusion may be additional contributing factors to the foregoing postoperative changes.

POSTOPERATIVE PULMONARY COMPLICATIONS

If the pattern of decreased lung volume and shunting progresses rather than returns to normal, it becomes clinically evident within 2 to 4 days after an operation. Decreased lung volume is detectable as decreased breath sounds on physical examination, and atelectatic areas may be visible on chest x-ray film. Shunt-produced hypoxemia leads to an increased ventilatory rate and the sensation of dyspnea.

Severe hypoxemia may cause cyanosis. Atelectasis causes fever and pooling of mucous secretions in nonventilated areas, leading to an apparent increase in sputum production. This sequence of events is diagrammed in Figure 30–2, in which physiologic changes that become clinically obvious as pulmonary "complications" are compared with the normal pattern of lung changes and recovery after surgery. Against this background of changes

Figure 30–2. Progression from the normal response (see Figure 30–1) to pulmonary failure after an abdominal operation. The *shaded* areas outline the expected *normal* postoperative course. (Bartlett RH: Post-traumatic pulmonary insufficiency. In Cooper P, Nyhus L (eds): Surgery Annual. New York, Appleton–Century–Crofts, 1971)

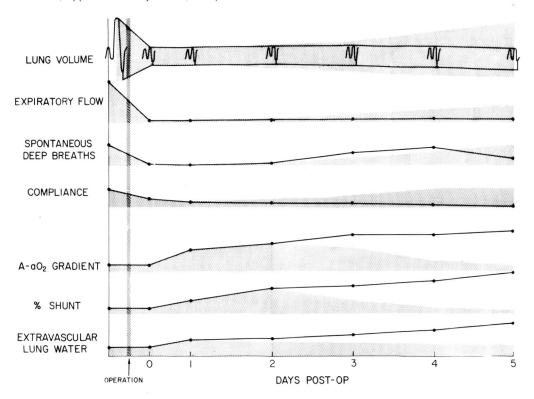

that normally accompany major operations, a more complete picture of pulmonary pathophysiology in the surgical patient can be drawn.

PATHOGENESIS AND PATHOPHYSIOLOGY

Abnormal patterns of breathing postoperatively are a major factor in the development of postoperative respiratory complications. In any specific patient, however, other factors that actually cause lung damage may be more important causes of pulmonary insufficiency (Fig. 30–3). These factors can be divided into (1) ventilatory or airway mechanisms; (2) humoral or hydrostatic mechanisms acting at the *capillary* level; and (3) direct lung trauma. Bacterial infection or progressive fibrosis are the final common pathways of severe pulmonary insufficiency resulting from any of these mechanisms.

VENTILATORY FACTORS

Abnormal ventilation (Table 30–1) will cause altered pulmonary function as outlined in the foregoing. The abnormal pattern of tidal breathing without spontaneous deep breaths after an operation is a good example of this phenomenon. A patient lying on his back in bed will preferentially ventilate the superior lobes, whereas the blood flow will preferentially go to dependent lobes. This ventilation–perfusion imbalance itself will result in hypoxemia. If it progresses over time, dependent alveoli begin to collapse in the pathogenetic pathway, as outlined earlier. Alveolar collapse will occur in any patient who remains in one position for a prolonged period and in whom the pattern of breathing is that of shallow tidal ventilation. It should be emphasized that 600-mL breaths delivered with a mechanical ventilator will lead to alveolar collapse, in the same fashion as shallow spontaneous breathing, if regular maximal inflations are not carried out.

Figure 30–3. Interaction of factors involved in the development of posttraumatic pulmonary insufficiency (Bartlett RH: Post-traumatic pulmonary insufficiency. In Cooper P, Nyhus L (eds): Surgery Annual. New York, Appleton–Century–Crofts, 1971)

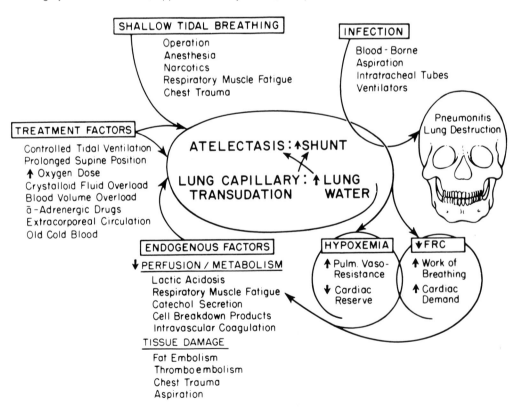

Table 30—1   Ventilatory Factors Resulting in Pulmonary Insufficiency

CAUSES

Shallow incomplete inflation
  Spontaneous breathing
  Mechanical ventilation
  Obstructed airways
  Diaphragm dysfunction
Absorptive atelectasis
  ↑ FiO_2
Alveolar damage (↓ surfactant)
  Infection
  Aspiration
↑ Lung water

EFFECTS

Transpulmonary shunting
Hypoxemia
Hyperventilation
↓ Compliance
↑ Work of breathing
↑ Risk of infection
↑ Lung water (?)

Foreign materials inhaled by means of the airway may contribute to pulmonary insufficiency in surgical patients. Aspiration of blood, gastric juice, or other gastric contents damages the respiratory mucosa and may reach the alveolar level, causing direct damage to alveoli and capillaries. Vomiting with aspiration is a constant concern in patients who have suffered acute trauma, head injury patients, patients requiring gastric feedings, and patients undergoing general anesthesia.

When vomiting occurs and aspiration is even suspected, vigorous treatment measures should be undertaken immediately. (This will be discussed in a later section.) Tissue may also be damaged by inhalation of toxic vapors; in surgical patients this is most commonly smoke inhalation, often associated with surface burn injury. The pathogenesis of pulmonary lesions from smoke inhalation, with or without burn, is also discussed later.

CAPILLARY FACTORS

The second category of conditions that may lead to lung damage is that which occurs at the capillary level (Table 30–2). Increased pulmonary hydrostatic pressure, decreased plasma oncotic pressure, or increased capillary permeability may all occur in the surgical patient. All will cause increased pulmonary extravascular water and deterioration of lung function.

Hydrostatic and Humoral Factors

In Figure 30–4, the factors regulating fluid flux in the lung are shown, although the actual mechanisms are not as simple as illustrated.[35] For example, interstitial pressure itself, the oncotic effects of interstitial protein, and the effects of lymph flow are not illustrated. However, fluid flux is a net function of the hydrostatic pressure that tends to force fluid out of the vascular space, on the one hand, and the oncotic pressure that tends to pull fluid in, on the other hand.

High hydrostatic pressure or low oncotic pressure will result in accumulation of fluid in the extravascular space. If the pulmonary endothelium is damaged, fluid may leak into the extracellular space at normal hydrostatic or oncotic pressures. The mechanisms and the effects of increased extravascular water are shown in Table 30–2. Pulmonary vascular resistance increases owing to periarteriolar cuffing. Ventilation–perfusion imbalance is created by peribronchiolar and alveolar compression. Shunting occurs if the alveoli become com-

Table 30—2   Capillary Factors Resulting in Increased Lung Water and Pulmonary Insufficiency

CAUSES

↑ Capillary filtration pressure
  ↑ Hydrostatic pressure
    LV failure
    ↑ Pulmonary vascular resistance
    ↑ Pulmonary artery pressure (?)
  ↓ Oncotic pressure
    Hypoproteinemia
    Crystalloid overload
Pulmonary capillary damage
  Airway
  Blood borne
  Direct trauma
  Atelectasis (?)

EFFECTS

↑ Pulmonary vascular resistance
↑ Small airway resistance
↓ FRC, compliance
↑ Risk of infection
V̇/Q̇ imbalance, hypoxemia

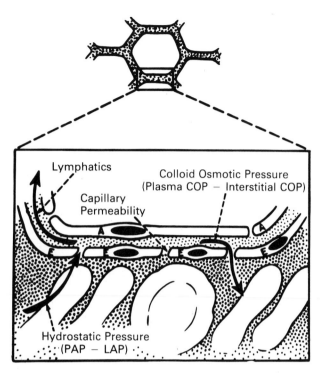

Figure 30—4. Forces that control fluid flux at the alveolar-capillary membrane. COP, colloid osmotic pressure; LAP, left atrial pressure; PAP, pulmonary artery pressure; A, alveolar epithelium; E, capillary endothelium.

pletely collapsed or filled with fluid. Finally, boggy atelectatic areas of the lungs are ideal breeding grounds for bacterial pulmonary infection.

Well-intentioned therapy done in the normal course of treatment or resuscitation may cause increased lung water. Examples are replacement of blood or plasma loss with *crystalloid solution* that must equilibrate into the entire extracellular space, including the lung. Inappropriate exogenous fluid replacement or overload of this type, along with endogenous production of the water of metabolism during hypermetabolic states, combine to make increased total body extracellualar fluid the major cause of pulmonary extravascular water collection. This fact is compounded by the decreased oncotic pressure that results when protein is lost or replaced with noncolloid-containing fluids. When plasma proteins are diluted in this way, lung interstitial proteins are diluted also; thus, the oncotic gradients stay unchanged, whereas the entire extracellular space expands.[15]

The pulmonary capillary endothelium is the first major vascular bed to "see" any toxic substance arising from peripheral organ metabolism or perfusion of ischemic or infected tissue. The venous effluent from an underperfused tissue (whether localized to a single organ, as in arterial embolism, or the entire body, as in any type of shock) arrives directly at the lung where pulmonary capillary damage occurs. *Humoral substances,* such as lysosomal enzymes and bacterial endotoxin, or particulate materials, such as microemboli, major thromboemboli, platelet aggregates, and fat particles, may lodge in the pulmonary capillary bed.

As these materials are cleared, leaky pulmonary capillaries are left behind, resulting in the accumulation of extravascular water. If the material trapped in pulmonary capillaries includes large amounts of platelets, secondary effects caused by platelet breakdown products, notably serotonin, are also seen. In major thromboembolism, for example, hypoxemia occurs because of ventilation–perfusion imbalance owing to bronchial spasm, presumably secondary to serotonin released from platelets.

The pulmonary effects of materials released into the venous blood in shock and sepsis entrain a particularly vicious circle. Increased pulmonary vascular resistance and hypoxia resulting from the capillary damage lead to decreased cardiac output and peripheral oxygen delivery, adding to the shock state, and perpetuating the pulmonary lesion. Shock and sepsis similarly produce a generalized, systemic capillary leak. It is the capillary leak in the lungs, however, that appears earliest as respiratory dysfunction.

Left ventricular failure with increased left atrial pressure will result in pulmonary transcapillary transudation, which may be subtle or grossly obvious, as in conventional heart failure with overt pulmonary edema. Left ventricular pressures may waver at the point of high left atrial pressures for short periods, even minutes, resulting in a transient increase in lung water, and then return to a balanced state. This situation may not lead to severe pulmonary edema, in itself, but probably places the lung in a more vulnerable position in the presence of coexisting minor capillary damage.

PREVENTION OF PULMONARY COMPLICATIONS

PREOPERATIVE MEASURES

With an understanding of the pathogenesis and mechanisms of potential lung damage in surgical patients, as outlined in the foregoing, one can draw up guidelines to prevent pulmonary complications (Tables 30–3 and 30–4).

If a patient is scheduled for an elective operative procedure, as much time as is necessary should be spent measuring lung function, correcting abnormalities when present, and changing conditions that may predispose to pulmonary complications. This is particularly true in patients with preexisting cardiopulmonary disease. Preoperative patients are advised to train for a major operation as one would train for an athletic event. The respiratory muscles should be exercised and specific breathing maneuvers learned.

Factors that may decrease the efficiency of ventilation should be corrected, including cessation of smoking, elective weight loss in grossly obese patients, and treatment of existing bacterial infection (chronic bronchitis) with culture-specific antibiotics, where indicated. Patients with a known tendency to bronchospasm should become accustomed to bronchodilator treatment preoperatively, and the effect of bronchodilators on pulmonary mechanics should be directly measured, particularly in patients with known bronchospastic disorders, such as asthma.

An excellent test of preoperative lung function is to measure arterial blood gas levels while the patient breathes room air. These are useful as a measure of overall lung function and as a baseline for postoperative comparisons.

If the patient is hypoxemic breathing room air; if he has a history of asthma, intermittent bronchospasm, wheezing, or any other significant lung disorder; or if the proposed operation is to be on the lung itself, pulmonary mechanics should be measured (lung volumes and flows). These measure-

Table 30–3 Treatment Modalities Used to Prevent Alveolar Collapse

Maximum inflation
  Yawn maneuver
  Continuous positive-pressure breathing (CPPB)
  Intermittent positive-pressure breathing (IPPB)
  Incentive spirometry
  Mechanical ventilation (IPPV) and intubation
    Large tidal volume
    "Sighs" and IMV
    Positive end-expiratory pressure (PEEP)
Airway cleaning
  Chest physiotherapy
↓ FIO_2
↓ Lung water

Table 30–4 Treatment Modalities Used to Prevent Accumulation of Lung Water

Capillary filtration pressure
  Avoid left ventricular failure
  Maintain oncotic pressure
Pulmonary capillary damage
  Prevent
    Endotoxemia
    Shock
    Ischemia
    Disseminated intravascular coagulation
  Avoid
    ↑ Airway pressure (?)
    ↑ FIO_2
Maintain alveolar inflation

ments should be made with and without bronchodilators, if indicated. If the values are abnormally low (less than 80% of predicted), training and exercise in specific breathing maneuvers should be carried out and function testing repeated until the ventilation is normal or has reached a stable plateau. Conversely, if the patient has no history of respiratory problems and has a normal examination of the chest (including x-ray), no further pulmonary function testing is indicated.

Although much has been written about specific flow or volume tests or their correlation with postoperative pulmonary complications, abnormal pulmonary function is rarely a contraindication to surgery, except when the operation involves resection of lung tissue itself.

The flow and volume tests that correlate best with postoperative lung function are vital capacity, timed vital capacity, and maximal breathing capacity.[20] These tests are completely effort-dependent, so that the surgical patient with abdominal or chest pain, poor abdominal muscle function from disease, or general debility from cancer or infection may perform poorly on these tests, for reasons completely unrelated to lung function. Routine preoperative flow and volume testing of all patients is costly and unnecessary.

Included in preoperative preparation should be efforts to minimize pulmonary extravascular water leakage intraoperatively and postoperatively. This includes adequate nutrition (and parenteral supplementation, if necessary) to assure a normal total serum protein concentration and, therefore, a normal plasma oncotic pressure. Left ventricular function should be assisted pharmacologically if signs of left ventricular failure exist. Prophylactic digitalis should be used in elderly patients, primarily to avoid rapid atrial fibrillation postoperatively, rather than for general toning of the left ventricle.

The patient with preexisting lung disease requires special consideration. Preparation related to bronchospasm or chronic bronchitis has been discussed. The patient with acute pulmonary insufficiency, increased lung water, and atelectasis secondary to an acute disorder, such as pancreatitis or systemic sepsis, will often improve during the operation and during the postoperative mechanical ventilation.

The patient with severe, chronic obstructive lung disease should be improved as much as possible with bronchodilators, treatment of bronchitis, if present, nutrition, and breathing and coughing training. If the pulmonary disorder is very severe [PaO_2 (air) < 50 torr, or carbon dioxide retention], prolonged postoperative intubation and mechanical ventilation should be anticipated and the patient advised accordingly.

INTRAOPERATIVE MEASURES

Intraoperatively, several procedures may minimize the risk of postoperative pulmonary complications. The operation may directly *improve* pulmonary function (e.g., by repairing a mitral valve or a large abdominal wall hernia) or may improve factors that, of themselves, are causing pulmonary insufficiency (such as draining of an empyema, removing a foreign body, or resecting dead tissue).

The surgeon plans his operative procedure to simultaneously treat the patient and to avoid factors that may cause postoperative complications of any sort. For the pulmonary system, this includes the following: Abdominal incisions should be planned to minimize postoperative pain and to maintain the strength of the abdominal wall for forced inspiration; and transverse incisions should be used whenever possible, particularly in patients with chronic heavy sputum production who will have to cough excessively after operation.

Gastrostomy should be considered to avoid prolonged nasogastric intubation. Bone fragments should be manipulated as gently as possible to avoid possible marrow embolism. Veins under negative pressure (e.g., in the brain) must be managed carefully to avoid air embolism. Prolonged periods of vascular stasis should be avoided as much as possible and systemic heparinization used whenever vascular occlusion is unavoidable.

When gastrointestinal function is impaired by surgery, a few minutes spent in assuring good postoperative nutrition (hence, good postoperative oncotic pressure and muscular function) will always be well spent, such as inserting a centrally placed venous catheter for hypertonic glucose administration. If the patient has a history of pulmonary embolism or existing deep venous thrombosis in the legs, prophylactic inferior vena cava plication should be considered when abdominal procedures are done.[8]

A large portion of the intraoperative prevention of pulmonary complications is carried out by the anesthesiologist. Maintaining large tidal volume ventilation (10–15 mL/kg) during surgery has been emphasized repeatedly. Particularly during long procedures, alveoli will begin to collapse unless regularly hyperinflated, at least every hour. The anesthesiologist contributes greatly toward preventing pulmonary complications by avoiding crystalloid fluid overload during the operation. Minimal blood and protein losses can be replaced with crystalloid during surgery. More significant amounts of blood or protein loss should be replaced with like components. All replacement therapy should closely match real or anticipated deficits, thereby avoiding pulmonary insufficiency from fluid overload.

Mechanical ventilation should be continued postoperatively until the adequacy of spontaneous ventilation has been clearly established. The action of paralytic drugs should be reversed completely and a vital capacity at least twice the tidal volume documented before extubation.

ROUTINE POSTOPERATIVE MEASURES

Postoperatively, both the surgeon and the patient must participate in preventing pulmonary complications. In the recovery room, the endotracheal tube should be maintained in place as long as necessary, as noted in the foregoing. Patients with preexisting pulmonary dysfunction or those at high risk of pulmonary complications may need to be left intubated and maintained by mechanical ventilation for hours or days after surgery.

Abundant evidence suggests that the well-ventilated alveolus is less susceptible to humoral damage at the capillary level than is the atelectatic alveolus.[2] In our institution, elderly, debilitated patients, patients with major cardiac procedures, and patients with extensive trauma, multiple fractures, pancreatitis, dead tissue, or severe peritonitis are commonly left intubated and maintained by mechanical ventilation 12 hours or more postoperatively. When the patient is fully alert and awake, when his perfusion and cardiac status are stable, and when the blood and extracellular fluid volumes are demonstrated to be normal, *then* the patient is ready for spontaneous ventilation and extubation.

Deep-breathing exercises, clearing of sputum and mucus, and avoidance of prolonged periods in the supine position must begin in the recovery room. Profound hypoventilation, ventilation–perfusion imbalance, and resultant hypoxemia are the rule in the patient awakening from anesthesia. For this reason, it is common practice to administer moderate amounts (5–10 L/min) of supplemental oxygen to all patients in the recovery room. This is a wise precaution for the first 1 or 2 hours after anesthesia, but this practice is really prophylactic only against hypoxic arrhythmias and may actually be slightly detrimental to lung function by suppressing whatever deep breathing may result from moderate degrees of hypoxemia. Consequently, supplemental oxygen should not be administered for more than a few hours, unless serial blood gas analyses so dictate.

Airway cleaning, suctioning, expectorant drugs, mist inhalation, and mucolytic agents are all useful in patients with preexisting chronic bronchitis or thick, tenacious tracheobronchial secretions. However, these maneuvers and agents may not be necessary in patients who maintain the lung adequately inflated by *emphasis on inspiratory maneuvers*. A compulsion to force patients to cough dominates much of the thinking on postoperative pulmonary care. Coughing maneuvers are painful in thoracotomy or laparotomy patients and should not be necessary if the lung remains well ventilated.

Breathing maneuvers, and devices designed to encourage those maneuvers, are important adjuncts to postoperative care. Because shallow breathing, the lack of spontaneous deep breaths, and alveolar collapse are the steps that lead to postoperative pulmonary complications, respiratory maneuvers must be those that emphasize maximal lug inflation.[7,38] Emphasis on breathing out (coughing, tracheal stimulation, "blow bottles") will do nothing to accomplish alveolar inflation, save the preparatory inspiration the patient may take before the maneuver. The more emphasis that is placed on the inhaled volume and inspiratory pressure, the more effective the maneuver will be.

Postoperative breathing maneuvers are compared in Figure 30–5. As can be seen, spontaneous deep-breathing exercise fulfills these criteria best. Inflation with a mechanical ventilator (intermittent positive-pressure breathing; IPPB) is useful theoretically, but in controlled studies, it has not been shown to decrease the incidence of pulmonary complications.[7] The reasons for the failure of IPPB lie not in the theory, but in the usual method of practice. Regular alveolar inflation must be carried out at frequent intervals, preferably every hour, to be effective. The IPPB treatment is usually done for periods of minutes with long hours between "treatments."

Maximal inhaled volumes must be assured; however, the volumes delivered by IPPB are regulated by pressure. The more the atelectasis, the lower the compliance, and the less volume is delivered by the ventilator to reach the cycling pressure of the IPPB device. Hence, the desired inhaled volume is not assured. Finally, many patients involuntarily swallow with each blast of the ventilator in the mouth, resulting in gastric distention, compression of the diaphragm, and further compromise of pulmonary function.

Several authors have emphasized the ineffectiveness of routine IPPB in preventing pulmonary complications.[9,10] This does not mean that IPPB is not a useful method of treatment. On the contrary, in patients who are too obtunded, in those too weak to carry out spontaneous breathing maneuvers, or in those with already established atelectasis, IPPB is very useful. In those circumstances, however, the device should be used frequently, preferably each hour, and monitored by direct measurement of exhaled volumes, with maximum volume inflation attempted with each breath. "Pressure support" on the ventilator is, in essence, IPPB for intubated patients.

Deep inspiratory maneuvers can be done spontaneously, but are better done with the use of a device that will record the volume inhaled and "reward" the patient for his efforts. Such a device is the *incentive spirometer*. When using this device, the patient can see his inspired volume with each breath, and the total breathing excursions in a period of time are recorded on a counter. Consequently, the physician, respiratory therapist, and patient can all be assured that the proper maneuver is being done, and frequently enough to maintain alveolar inflation. The regular use of deep-breathing exercises using an incentive spirometer has decreased the incidence of pulmonary complications

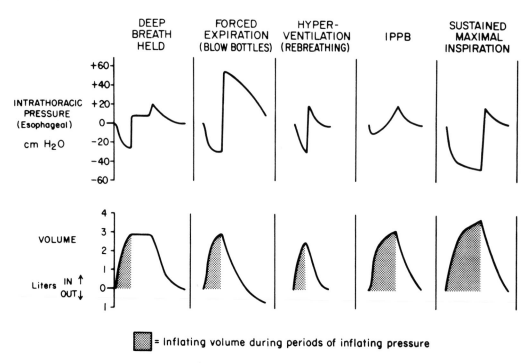

= Inflating volume during periods of inflating pressure

Figure 30—5. A comparison of respiratory maneuvers used to inflate the lung. The best maneuver has the largest volume inhaled during periods of inflating (negative) pressure (shown as *shaded area*). (Bartlett RH, Brennan MD, Gazzaniga AB et al: Studies on the pathogenesis and prevention of postoperative-pulmonary complications. Surg Gynecol Obstet 137:925, 1973)

from about 30% to about 10%.[6] Incentive spirometry may not, however, be of value in the patient at low risk for the development of pulmonary complications.[32]

Another method of preventing postoperative atelectasis is the application of continuous positive airway pressure (CPAP) with a tight-fitting mask. Initial reports of this technique show improved alveolar inflation.[19] The potential complications of mask CPAP (gastric distention, vomiting and aspiration, patient discomfort) did not occur in the initial series, but remain a cause for concern. This technique, perhaps combined with "mask" IPPB, may prove useful in patients who are extubated but who cannot, or will not, breathe deeply.

Whatever method is used to accomplish maximal inflation must be carefully taught to the patient *preoperatively*. Most patients cannot learn breathing exercises in a painful, narcotized, postoperative state. Reviews and discussion of postoperative pulmonary prophylaxis are available.[5,27,33]

Frequent change of position and early ambulation will minimize fluid collection in the dependent portions of the lung. Postoperative nutrition

should be maintained. If the patient must go without oral intake for more than 4 or 5 days, total parenteral nutrition is advisable for several reasons, not the least of which is to maintain the strength of the respiratory effort. Fluids must be managed carefully to avoid overloading the extracellular space and diluting the serum proteins.

Pulmonary thromboembolism from deep veins of the leg or pelvis is a constant threat in the postoperative patient. Patients older than 40 years of age and patients with cancer constitute a particularly high-risk group. Several methods have been proposed to prevent deep venous thrombosis, including anticoagulation, drugs that inhibit platelet function, applying pressure to the legs with plastic wraps or stockings, and frequent active or passive lower leg exercises.

Regularly exercising the muscles is the easiest of these maneuvers, has the fewest complications, and is advised for all postoperative patients. Again, early ambulation will also promote venous flow in the deep veins of the leg.

Even if all the foregoing steps are followed, postoperative pulmonary complications will still occur in about 15% of thoracotomy patients, less than 10% of laparotomy patients, and in progressively smaller numbers of patients with extremity, head and neck, or pelvic surgery. Pulmonary complications usually occur because the patient cannot pursue maximum inflation exercises or because some combination of fluid infusion and pulmonary capillary damage has led to interstitial pulmonary edema. Early vigorous treatment of such complications will almost always reverse the situation. Rarely, a postoperative patient progresses to severe pulmonary insufficiency, requiring further intensive care.

TREATMENT OF POSTOPERATIVE PULMONARY INSUFFICIENCY

Treatment of pulmonary insufficiency in the surgical patient, as in any patient, has two primary goals: to expand collapsed alveoli and maintain or return lung volumes to normal, and to decrease extravascular water in the lung and return pulmonary capillary permeability to normal, the end result being adequate delivery of oxygen to tissues to satisfy metabolic needs. Systemic oxygen delivery (based on the cardiac output multiplied by oxygen content of blood) is approximately five times the oxygen consumption in the normal human. This relationship of oxygen delivery to oxygen consumption is normally maintained at 5:1, even at higher metabolic rates. This is usually accomplished by increasing cardiac output (and thereby increasing oxygen delivery), since the hemoglobin content of blood and, thus, oxygen content of blood, is not subject to homeostatic control in the short-term.

When oxygen delivery falls (e.g., decreased cardiac output, anemia, or inadequate saturation of hemoglobin with oxygen) or oxygen consumption increases (e.g., sepsis or increased muscle activity), or both, the ratio of delivery to consumption falls. As the ratio drops below 2:1, oxygen consumption becomes dependent on delivery: anaerobic metabolism and hemodynamic instability ensues—the threshold of shock.

In treating postoperative pulmonary insufficiency, the aim is to maintain oxygen delivery in excess of oxygen consumption by a ratio greater than 2:1, while returning lung function to normal. Respiratory care should be directed at optimizing oxygen delivery while minimizing iatrogenic damage by the ventilator to the lungs as healing occurs.

TREATMENT AIMED AT ALVEOLAR INFLATION

Treatment aimed at alveolar inflation is outlined in Table 30–5. The cornerstone is to establish large-volume inflation by merely instituting breathing exercises, perhaps with the assistance of an incentive spirometer. In most patients, atelectasis can be treated successfully by merely intensifying breathing exercise efforts. If adequate volumes cannot be generated by the patient in this manner, then mechanical assistance is necessary, initially with IPPB with a mechanical ventilator, without intubation. As mentioned earlier, this must be done with direct volume measurements and often requires high pressures with the IPPB device (40 cmH$_2$O). Efforts at alveolar inflation must be combined with cleaning and dilating the airway, where necessary.

When an area of lung is not ventilated, mucus secreted in the bronchi draining from that lung segment becomes thickened and impacted, which hinders efforts at reexpansion. This mucus should be cleared by chest physical therapy (percussion) and postural drainage.

Hydration and nebulized bronchodilator and mucolytic drugs through the airway may be used. Coughing will help to expel mucus from airways that have been inflated distally. Coughing will not dislodge mucus from airways, leading to nonventilated areas of lung. In this situation mucus must be removed directly with tracheal suction or bronchoscopy. We prefer bronchoscopy as the initial step in managing any postoperative patient with major atelectasis.

Table 30–5   Treatment Modalities Used to Reverse Alveolar Collapse

Maximum inflation
Yawn
CPPB
IPPB
Mechanical ventilator
Volume-limited
Pressure-limited
Airway cleaning
Suctioning
Chest physical therapy
Use least possible FiO$_2$
Decrease lung water
Treat lung infection
Optimize nutrition

Tracheal suctioning will exacerbate hypoxia if not done properly. The catheter is passed through the nose, verified as passing through the larynx by a change in voice, and connected to oxygen at 5 L/min. Then, 5 mL of saline is injected and the oxygen reconnected for several coughing breaths. Suction is applied for no longer than 15 seconds, and oxygen is resumed. This process is continued until the suction return is clear (1–5 minutes). Electrocardiographic monitoring should be done during and after suctioning. Atropine is given for bradycardia.

Routine endotracheal suctioning is practiced on many surgical services. In adults, the value of this technique lies primarily in stimulation of deep breathing associated with the vigorous coughing that it produces. If that is the intent, then deep breathing can be easily accomplished by other means without the potential vagal complications associated with tracheal suctioning. In other words, *routine* tracheal suctioning has no rational place in the care of postoperative adult patients.

In infants, the size of the airway is such that a very small amount of mucus (which would be insignificant in a larger patient) may cause major tracheal or bronchial occlusion. Infants breathe rapidly with a large ventilation of dead space, leading to drying of the tracheal secretions, and may have difficulty coughing material from the lower trachea or from the bronchi. Consequently, routine endotracheal suctioning can be valuable in the postoperative management of infants, following operations on the thorax or upper abdomen.

In both infants and adults, if adequate ventilation cannot be established with the aforementioned methods, endotracheal intubation and continuous mechanical ventilation are instituted. As with bronchoscopy, we favor this type of management. We consider mechanical ventilation to be indicated when the inspiratory force during a Müller maneuver is less than 20 cmH$_2$O, when the vital capacity is less than twice the tidal volume, or if the patient is severely hypoxemic (PaO$_2$ less than 50 mmHg breathing room air). If any one of these indications exist and cannot be reversed by the aforementioned measures, intubation and mechanical ventilation are carried out. The same criteria apply for extubating the patient. Intubation with spontaneous breathing and CPAP (5 to 10 cmH$_2$O) without mechanical ventilation are standard therapy in the respiratory distress syndrome of the newborn and are commonly used when that condition is complicated by a surgical procedure. Continuous positive airway pressure is reportedly useful in some adults with respiratory insufficiency associated with absence of surfactant. Generally, if the patient requires intubation, the use of the mechanical ventilator is also indicated.

The principles just outlined for spontaneous respiration apply equally well to mechanical ventilation. Emphasis is placed on maximum alveolar inflation with every breath. The goal is to return the FRC to normal and to maintain it there. The use of large tidal volumes will assure that alveoli distal to narrowed airways are well inflated with each breath. The use of positive end-expiratory pressure (PEEP) will offset the effects of decreased surfactant and minimize absorption atelectasis when high concentrations of oxygen are needed. Mechanical ventilation must be regulated by volume, either by using a volume ventilator or by continuously measuring exhaled volume when using a pressure-cycled ventilator. Inspiratory pressure is determined by the inspired volume and the FRC. With a severely decreased FRC, inspiratory pressures of 60 to 80 cmH$_2$O may be necessary to deliver ventilatory volumes of 10 mL/kg. As alveoli become reinflated (FRC increases), the peak pressure needed to deliver this volume decreases.

Mechanical ventilation must be maximized to provide adequate oxygen delivery while, at the same time, minimizing barotrauma to the lungs. Relying on arterial PO$_2$ as the sole indicator of adequacy of oxygen delivery may be misleading in patients with low cardiac output, anemia, or high metabolic rates, or in patients with an abnormal hemoglobin with a high affinity for oxygen.[16] A more reliable indicator of the adequacy of oxygen delivery to tissues is the (mixed) venous oxyhemoglobin saturation (S$\bar{\text{v}}$O$_2$). When measured at the pulmonary artery by Swan–Ganz catheter, the S$\bar{\text{v}}$O$_2$ gives a measure of that portion of delivered oxygen that is not utilized by tissues and, thus, it is a unique indicator of changes in oxygen delivery (increased cardiac output, increased hematocrit) versus consumption. *An S$\bar{\text{v}}$O$_2$ between 65% and 75% results from oxygen delivery/consumption ratios of about 3 : 1 or 4 : 1, and thus denotes adequate delivery of oxygen to tissues.*

With the S$\bar{\text{v}}$O$_2$ as additional information to the PaO$_2$, inspired oxygen concentration may be regulated to the lowest level necessary to provide adequate oxygen delivery. Increased peak inspiratory pressures may, on one hand, increase alveolar recruitment and, hence, oxygenation and ventilation (increasing both PaO$_2$ and S$\bar{\text{v}}$O$_2$), but may also decrease venous return, cardiac output and, hence, systemic oxygen delivery, thereby decreasing S$\bar{\text{v}}$O$_2$

(at constant metabolic rate). Sustained peak airway pressures at or exceeding 50 cmH$_2$O (at least in sheep) lead to progressive pulmonary dysfunction and, therefore, are probably best avoided.[22]

Positive end-expiratory pressure helps to maintain alveolar inflation and should be used whenever FRC is decreased. When PEEP is used, tidal volume is decreased to avoid high peak inspiratory pressure. The increase in mean intrathoracic pressure, as with increased peak inspiratory pressure, impedes venous return and decreases cardiac output. Therefore, a level of PEEP, and a tidal volume and rate are selected to give optimal alveolar inflation and oxygen delivery, while minimizing peak inspiratory pressure. Continuous S$\bar{v}$O$_2$ monitoring simplifies the assessment of alterations in PEEP in maximizing oxygen delivery, developing the so-called best-PEEP curve. Selectively increasing PEEP increases arterial oxygenation, while at the same time decreasing cardiac output (by impediment to venous return) at higher levels. The *best-PEEP* is, therefore, the best compromise (highest S$\bar{v}$O$_2$ or oxygen delivery/consumption ratio) between these opposing variables. Usually this is also the PEEP level associated with the best pulmonary compliance.[36]

The respiratory rate should be regulated by the patient's respiratory center, if possible. The ventilator is set at a very low rate (5–8 breaths/min) and the patient allowed to breathe at a more rapid rate, triggering the ventilator to regulate the PaCO$_2$ at 40 mmHg (assist–control mode). In a comatose patient or a patient in whom the assist mode cannot be used, the rate should be set to maintain the PaCO$_2$ at 40 mmHg. With large tidal volumes and minimal lung dysfunction, this may require the addition of a rebreathing volume (dead space) between the ventilator and the patient to avoid hypocapnea. Direct access to the airway allows adequate humidification, delivery of nebulized drugs, and easy access for tracheal cleaning and suctioning when appropriate.

Airway access is gained by direct endotracheal intubation in all patients except those with laryngeal trauma or possible cervical spine injury. With the exception of these latter conditions, emergency tracheostomy for airway access is never indicated. Tracheostomy is always safer when done over an endotracheal tube in a previously intubated patient. Tracheal intubation should always be carried out before tracheostomy. The endotracheal tube is uncomfortable and precludes the patient from moving about easily and from eating. Tracheostomy provides easier access to the airway and allows the patient to move about and eat and drink without difficulty; it may, however, have a higher incidence of direct tracheal complications. These various factors balance out after 48 to 72 hours of ventilator management by endotracheal tube, and tracheostomy is usually advised if mechanical ventilation is needed beyond that time. Further support for early tracheostomy arises from data showing increased incidence of pulmonary infection in trauma patients with prolonged endotracheal intubation, with a much lower incidence of pulmonary infection after early tracheostomy. Prophylaxis of pulmonary infection might best be afforded by placement of tracheostomy early in the course of expected prolonged mechanical ventilation.[39]

Whether airway access is maintained by means of direct endotracheal intubation or tracheostomy, several principles are important in avoiding tracheal damage, including avoiding high-pressure, low-volume occlusive cuffs that may damage the tracheal mucosa; inserting a shock-absorbing piece of tubing between the ventilator and the patient; and putting a swivel connector in the circuitry to avoid torsion of the tube when the patient moves.

Monitoring of the patient receiving mechanical ventilation requires frequent blood gas analysis. If the patient requires ventilator support for longer than 24 hours, the best practice is to place an indwelling arterial cannula, preferably in a radial or ulnar artery, to avoid repeated arterial punctures.

Swan–Ganz pulmonary artery catheterization allows central fluid status monitoring, cardiac output measurement, and sampling of mixed venous oxygen saturation (*continuous* S$\bar{v}$O$_2$, if the catheter is of the fiber-optic variety). Pulmonary artery catheterization should be performed whenever an inspired oxygen concentration of 100%, high peak airway pressures or PEEP levels greater than 5 cmH$_2$O are necessary to achieve adequate oxygenation.

TREATMENT OF INCREASED LUNG WATER

Lung water can be decreased by decreasing the entire extracellular fluid space, decreasing the hydrostatic pressure in the pulmonary capillary bed, and increasing the plasma oncotic pressure, without increasing the oncotic pressure in the interstitial fluid of the lung (Table 30–6). Evidence exists for improved survival in patients with ARDS when a negative fluid balance is maintained.[31] Mechanical positive-pressure ventilation is *not* listed as a means to decrease lung water. In fact, positive-pressure ventilation with PEEP actually increases lung

Table 30—6 Treatment Modalities Used to Reverse Established Increases in Lung Water

---

↓ Capillary filtration pressure
  Inotropic drugs
    ↓ Pulmonary artery pressure
  Diuresis, dialysis, hemofiltration
↑ Oncotic pressure
  Concentrated albumin
  Packed red blood cells
  Dehydration
Treat pulmonary capillaries
  ↓ F_IO_2
  ↓ Airway pressure
  Steroids (?)
  Platelets (?)
  Lung inflation

---

water slightly, probably by stretching the pulmonary tissue. Mechanical ventilation will improve gas exchange in patients with pulmonary edema by overcoming $\dot{V}/\dot{Q}$ imbalance associated with bronchiolar or alveolar thickening, but will not decrease lung water itself.

Patients with simple atelectasis do not need treatment for increased lung water, except by avoiding fluid overload and cardiac failure. Increased lung water requires treatment when diffuse interstial fluid collection is evident by x-ray film and by the hospital course. For example, the patient who has had an episode of septicemia, one who has had an episode of disseminated intravascular coagulation or fat embolism, one with peritonitis or reperfusion of ischemic tissue, or one who received 4 L of Ringer's lactate solution during a 3-hour operation would be likely to have increased lung water in association with other pulmonary problems.

Decreasing pulmonary hydrostatic pressure by improving left ventricular function is done pharmacologically and can, and should, be done in all patients with major pulmonary insufficiency. If the patient has received large infusions of citrate in the form of banked blood or plasma substitutes, a transient myocardial depression may occur, which can be reversed with calcium infusion. A long-acting inotropic drug, such as digoxin, should be instituted and may be supplemented with a short-acting inotrope, such as dopamine.

The effectiveness of this treatment can be determined only by measuring cardiac output and left atrial (or pulmonary capillary wedge) pressure directly. This requires insertion of a pulmonary artery catheter. Pulmonary artery and wedge pressure monitoring and mixed venous blood sampling are nearly as important as direct arterial blood gas sampling in managing the patient with pulmonary insufficiency who has a major increase in lung water. The exact position of the pulmonary artery catheter must be carefully determined and the pressure tracing properly interpreted, which requires continuous display on a monitor and careful selection of the end-expiratory point for pressure readings.

Total extracellular fluid volume is reduced by forced diuresis or dialysis if the patient is in renal failure. Diuresis is induced with a potent diuretic, such as furosemide or mannitol. The course of diuresis is followed with careful measurement of body weight daily and measurement of fluid intake and output hourly. Usually, the postoperative patient with pulmonary insufficiency will be found to be 4- to 5-kg overloaded, primarily with extracellular fluid. Positive fluid balance and weight gain in respiratory failure may correlate with poor outcome.

Adequate treatment of increased lung water must include removing the excess extravascular fluid (returning the patient to his baseline, or "dry" weight) and possibly establishing continued diuresis until the patient is in 1 to 3 L of negative water balance and is maintained in this condition.[28,34] Net weight loss and lower cumulative fluid intake and output differences correlate with survival in ARDS.[31] This major decrease in total extracellular fluid volume will be accompanied by a minor decrease in pulmonary extracellular fluid volume, but this change may be enough to improve pulmonary function greatly. Use of diuretic drugs will remove water, sodium, and potassium at different rates; consequently, all must be monitored carefully and frequently. Usually water is removed in excess of electrolyte so that with extreme forced diuresis a hypernatremic, hyperosmotic state will result. Serum sodium concentrations should be monitored closely. Diuresis has reached its limit when the serum sodium is between 140 and 150 mEq/L and the patient has reached dry weight.

Diuresis is combined with colloid loading to increase plasma oncotic pressure transiently, which forces the movement of fluid from the extravascular to the intravascular space. This should be done concomitantly with diuresis because most agents used for colloid loading, such as albumin, have a molecular weight between 50,000 and 100,000 and will gradually find their way into the extracellular space within 4 to 12 hours after infusion. The advantages of colloid loading come during the first 1 or 2 hours after infusion and before the colloid joins the lymphatic system and is subsequently metabolized.

Although some animal studies suggest a deleterious effect of albumin loading in pulmonary insufficiency,[21] treatment of human subjects with colloid loading (and diuresis), particularly with packed red blood cells, is usually highly successful. Transfusion of packed red blood cells also is a means of increasing oxygen-carrying capacity by raising hemoglobin content. These techniques should be used when capillary integrity has been restored, as determined by response to small initial doses of colloid.[4,29]

SPECIFIC CONSIDERATIONS

GASTRIC ASPIRATION

Vomiting with subsequent aspiration is a dreaded complication for the surgeon and the anesthesiologist. Elective operations are always done after 12 hours of fasting so that the stomach will be empty. However, emergency procedures or elective procedures in patients with intestinal obstruction may be associated with vomiting at any time during the procedure. The patient is most likely to vomit during the induction of anesthesia. Whenever an emergent procedure is planned, a nasogastric tube should be placed first and the stomach emptied as much as possible. Anesthesia should be induced abruptly and followed immediately by endotracheal intubation, or intubation should be achieved before induction of anesthesia. Even with these precautions, aspiration of gastric contents will occur occasionally. If aspiration is suspected before or during the operation, an endotracheal tube should be passed, the balloon inflated, and the trachea irrigated and aspirated vigorously. If aspiration is documented by return of gastric contents from the trachea, a short course of steroids and large-volume ventilation may avoid subsequent aspiration pneumonitis.[13]

Postoperatively, the patient who has aspirated should always be suctioned vigorously, with saline lavage until clear. Any patient who may have aspirated food particles (some would say any patient who aspirates) should undergo bronchoscopy with a conventional rigid bronchoscope, careful examination of all bronchi, vigorous lavage, and suctioning. Most patients who have aspirated should be maintained with large-volume mechanical ventila-

tion until physiologic and x-ray film studies indicate that any lung damage is resolving.

FAT EMBOLISM

A small percentage of patients with extensive fractures develop the clinical syndrome of fat embolism, which is due to pulmonary embolization of neutral fat globules from the marrow cavity and is often associated with embolization of megakaryocytes and other marrow cells. Hypoxemia and bilateral patchy pulmonary infiltrates, beginning 12 to 36 hours after trauma, are typical of this lesion. Associated findings include a falling hematocrit, hemolysis, high fever, cerebral symptoms, petechiae (particularly in the anterior axillary folds, sclerae, and eyelids), and possibly fat globules in the urine, blood, or sputum. Pulmonary capillary damage occurs in this condition, apparently caused by sterile inflammation from fatty acids released as the triglyceride particles break down in the lung parenchyma.

Steroids have been shown to decrease the inflammation and, thereby, mortality from this lesion, although they must be given early and in large doses. Intubation and mechanical ventilation are indicated as soon as the syndrome has been diagnosed. Care must be taken to maintain the patient's fluid balance as "dry" as possible, since the pulmonary capillaries leak, even at normal hydrostatic pressures. This is often difficult to achieve in patients who have multiple-system trauma and may have active bleeding or oliguria at the same time that the pulmonary lesion develops. Intravenous heparin and alcohol, suggested by some, have not proved to be useful drugs in the clinical treatment of this disorder.

SMOKE INHALATION

Several investigators have demonstrated a generalized increase in capillary permeability (including that of the pulmonary capillaries) after a small body surface burn. The more extensive the burn, the greater the capillary leakage. For reasons outlined earlier in this chapter, the pulmonary capillary bed shows signs of increased capillary permeability first, in the form of increased lung water. This phenomenon has confused clinicians caring for patients with smoke inhalation syndrome for many years. The problem was recently clarified by Zawacki,[41] who found smoke inhalation injury to be a relatively mild pulmonary insult, but a major insult when combined with body surface burn, as is often the case in humans.

The toxic materials in smoke are carbon monoxide, heat, various aldehydes and other organic materials, and other organic compounds in the vapor state. Materials that are totally combustible (such as natural gas or gasoline) burn to carbon dioxide and water, producing certain toxic organic compounds and causing minimal lung damage when inhaled in smoke.[1] On the other hand, wood, paint, upholstery, and the like, burn incompletely, yielding various toxic vapors in addition to the usual products of combustion. These vapors are damaging to the respiratory epithelium and alveoli. Heat in smoke is a minimal factor that causes lung damage because air is such a poor heat conductor. Deep lung damage from heat is unusual unless the thermal injury is conveyed by hot steam.

Carbon monoxide is the major toxic material in smoke. It does not damage the lungs, but renders the brain hypoxic by association with hemoglobin, creating potentially lethal brain damage. Patients with smoke inhalation injury without a surface burn usually pass through a period of mild pulmonary insufficiency and recover completely, unless irreversible brain damage or metabolic acidosis has occurred because of carboxyhemoglobinemia. Patients with the same degree of smoke insufficiency, with combined atelectasis and decreased lung water, usually requiring intubation, mechanical ventilation, and efforts to reduce lung water as outlined earlier.

BACTERIAL PNEUMONITIS AND PULMONARY THROMBOEMBOLISM

Because these problems so often complicate otherwise uneventful surgery, the reader is urged to review the topics of bacterial pneumonitis (see Chap. 18) and pulmonary thromboembolism (see Chap. 36).

CHEST TRAUMA

Direct injury to the chest may cause damage to the chest wall, lung parenchyma, diaphragm, airway, and other intrathoracic structures, such as the heart and great vessels. These injuries are usually associated with hemothorax or pneumothorax. Life-threatening hypoventilation may result from injuries to the chest wall or from alveolar collapse caused by fluid or blood in the pleural space. Emergency treatment includes placement of a large chest tube to empty the pleural space and to reexpand the lung and mechanical ventilation if spontaneous breathing is inadequate.

Blunt trauma to the chest may be caused by any direct blow, but it is most commonly associated with motor vehicle accidents. Most rib fractures do not require specific treatment, other than intercostal nerve block to relieve pain. Fractured ribs should, however, always suggest more serious injuries to internal organs. Fracture of the ribs or sternum may create a segment of the chest wall that moves inward in response to the negative pressure created during spontaneous inspiration. This is referred to as paradoxic motion, and the floating segment of the chest wall is referred to as a *flail segment* or *flail chest*. A small amount of paradoxic motion with no physiologic side effects does not require specific treatment. Hypoxemia or carbon dioxide retention associated with the flail chest injury indicates lung contusion and requires intubation and ventilation.

If air or fluid is detected in the pleural space, a large chest tube should be placed (Fig. 30–6). If a patient with minor chest injuries requires immediate surgery for other problems (such as a ruptured spleen or head injury), prophylactic chest tubes should be placed on both sides to eliminate the possibility of a tension pneumothorax or hemothorax developing during anesthesia. Mechanical ventilation is required for patients with major flail segments and with lung contusion or chest injury complicating other serious multiple-system injuries. The use of corticosteroids for 1 or 2 days in severe lung contusion decreases mortality and morbidity in both experimental animals and patients.[37] The risk of infection should be balanced against possible benefits of this treatment in patients with multiple injuries. Operation is rarely necessary for blunt injury to the chest, but may be needed for injury to the heart, aorta, bronchus, esophagus, or diaphragm. An operation to stabilize rib and sternal fractures should be considered in any patient with multiple fractures or a large flail segment.

Penetrating trauma occurs from gunshot wounds, stab wounds, and some crushing injuries. Any hole between the pleural space and skin will result in a "sucking chest injury." In this circumstance air is inhaled into the pleural space during inspiration, filling the pleural space and eliminating the pressure gradient that would normally cause the lung to inflate, resulting in atelectasis of that lung. If the chest wall injury prevents the egress of air (a "flap valve" effect), a tension pneumothorax results, with hypoventilation and

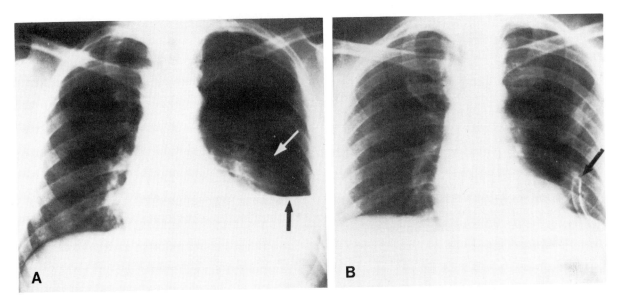

Figure 30—6. Chest x-rays showing (*A*) hemopneumothorax with collapse of the lung and (*B*) same patient after treatment with chest tube.

blockage of venous return. Bleeding into the pleural space from the chest wall or lung complicates this problem.

Penetrating chest injury is treated by placing a chest tube to drain accumulated air and blood. This maneuver, along with appropriate replacement of blood lost, will usually quite promptly return cardiac output and respiration to normal. Bleeding from the lung itself will usually subside because the pulmonary circulation is a low-pressure system. Air leaks from the lung usually seal within 1 or 2 days. Prolonged major leaks should suggest injury to a large bronchus, trachea, or esophagus that requires surgical repair. Massive bleeding (more than half the blood volume in 12 hours or less) suggests injury to the heart, a major vessel, or an intercostal artery and should be treated by thoracotomy and direct repair. The possibility of penetrating injury through the diaphragm involving abdominal viscera should always be considered.

RESPIRATORY CARE AFTER THORACOTOMY AND PULMONARY RESECTION

The principles of pathogenesis, prevention, and management of pulmonary problems after thoracic operations are those described in the early part of this chapter. Some patients require resection of part or all of the lung for infection, cancer, congenital abnormalities, or (rarely) trauma. If the remaining lung is normal, removal of lung tissue does not cause a major physiologic deficit. However, pulmonary resection creates unique problems because the "empty" space that was formerly occupied by the lung tissue must be managed very carefully or poor healing and infection may result. If pleural space infection, leak from a supposedly closed bronchus, or pulmonary failure occur after pulmonary resection, challenging ventilatory problems result.

SURGICAL CARE OF THE RESPIRATORY PATIENT

The *pleural space* is the space between the parietal and visceral pleural surfaces. Normally, it is filled with a few cubic centimeters of clear fluid that serves to lubricate the surfaces as they slide past each other during normal breathing. In abnormal conditions, the pleural space can fill with air (pneumothorax), blood (hemothorax), plasma, serum or lymph (hydrothorax, chylothorax, or pleural effusion), or pus (pyothorax or empyema). Anything in the pleural space compresses the underlying lung and causes atelectasis. Any fluid (with or without air) in the pleural space is subject to infection by direct contamination or blood-borne bacteria. Fluid detected by examination and x-ray film should be removed to establish a diagnosis and to prevent subsequent infection.

Aspiration of fluid or air from the chest is called *thoracentesis* and usually is done to remove fluid. Placement of a tube to establish more permanent drainage of the pleural space is called *thoracostomy, closed thoracostomy* or *tube thoracostomy.*

Pleural effusion may be associated with systemic edema or with pulmonary edema caused by congestive heart failure or lung capillary leakage. In addition, infection, infarction, or cancer in the lung itself may result in accumulation of fluid in the pleural space. If a pleural effusion becomes infected with bacteria, an inflammatory reaction results that creates an abscess in the pleural space (an empyema). An empyema will usually form in the most dependent area of the pleural space and will become walled off from the remaining space by acute inflammation at the walls of the abscess, which seals the visceral and parietal pleura together around the abscess (pleural symphysis). An empyema, like any other abscess, is treated by establishing external drainage, usually with a chest tube or (if the empyema is chronic and walled off) by removing segments of ribs overlying the empyema to allow free external drainage.

Pneumothorax may occur from trauma or operation on the lung or after rupture of lung tissue (spontaneous pneumothorax). Pneumothorax is treated by placement of a chest tube to remove the air from the pleural space. When air is removed, the leaking area of lung is brought into apposition with the parietal pleura, which usually results in spontaneous healing or sealing of the air leak. If the air leak from the lung is major (more than half the tidal volume with each breath) or prolonged (more than 5 days), the condition is referred to as a bronchopleural fistula and requires operation for repair.

SPECIFIC PROCEDURES

Thoracentesis for removal of fluid is done with the patient in a sitting position, inserting the needle where fluid has been detected, usually in the posterior axillary line. The skin, rib periosteum, and pleura are the only pain-sensitive structures in the chest wall. These areas are liberally anesthetized with local anesthetic, and a needle (mounted on a syringe with a stopcock) is advanced into the pleural space and fluid removed. Thoracentesis should be a painless procedure. Meticulous sterile conditions must be maintained (Fig. 30–7).

Tube thoracostomy is also done under local anesthesia (Fig. 30–8). A tube is placed in the third or fourth interspace in the midaxillary line and directed to the apex of the pleural space. A tube placed to remove blood, with or without air, is

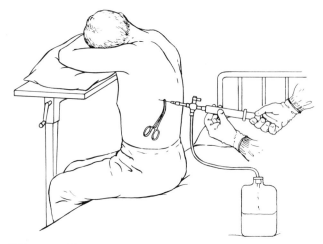

Figure 30–7. Technique for thoracentesis.

placed in the sixth or seventh interspace in the midaxillary or posterior axillary line and then directed posteriorly. Local anesthesia is used for chest tube placement. Regional anesthesia by intercostal block should be done for placement of large chest tubes. In adults, an incision large enough to insert one finger is made two interspaces below the point at which the chest tube will enter the pleural space. Subcutaneous tissue and muscle are bluntly dissected with a large clamp and with the finger. The clamp is forced into the pleural space, followed by an exploring finger to be sure that the lung is not adherent. The tube is advanced to the desired position, the clamp on the tube removed, and the air or fluid in the pleural space drained into a valved system. In small children a finger-sized hole is too large, and a smaller dissection should be done. *Trocars* are large pointed rods or tubes that have been used for introducing chest tubes. These instruments commonly result in injury to the lung and should never be used for tube thoracostomy.

Once the chest tube has been properly positioned, it should be attached to a system that allows free egress of fluid or air, but prevents aspiration of external air into the chest. This is commonly accomplished with a water-seal valve. In addition, suction may be applied to the chest tube to facilitate air or fluid removal.

An alternative to large-bore tube thoracostomy for simple traumatic pneumothorax is catheter aspiration (CASP). A 16-gauge catheter is placed in the affected hemithorax and attached to a stopcock and syringe, to allow aspiration of the pneumothorax. In one series, 16 of 17 patients with simple traumatic pneumothorax showed resolution of the

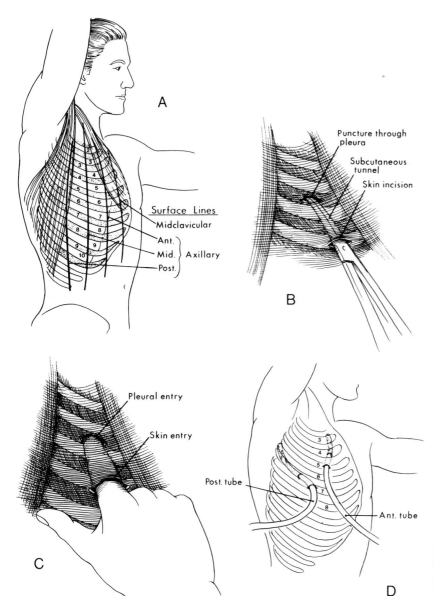

A

Surface Lines
Midclavicular
Ant.
Mid. } Axillary
Post.

B

Puncture through
pleura
Subcutaneous
tunnel
Skin incision

C

Pleural entry

Skin entry

D

Post. tube

Ant. tube

Figure 30—8. Technique of chest tube placement. (*A*) Landmarks; (*B*) dissecting with hemostat; (*C*) exploring with finger; (*D*) proper tube placement.

pneumothorax, after which the catheter was removed, and the patient was sent home. This method of outpatient treatment of simple pneumothorax is significantly less expensive than conventional tube thoracostomy treatment in hospital.[24]

Bronchoscopy is a procedure that involves placement of a viewing instrument into the trachea and bronchi to diagnose or treat lung and airway problems. The respiratory therapist may be called on to assist with bronchoscopy and, therefore, should be familiar with this technique.[30] The *flexi-*

ble bronchoscope (see Chap. 26) is made up primarily of fiberoptic bundles that carry illuminating light into the bronchus and reflected light back to the lens, which enables direct visualization of the airways. The tip of the bronchoscope can be manipulated with a series of levers. Parallel channels of the bronchoscope can carry irrigating fluid and flexible biopsy forceps and can be used for suctioning at the end of the instrument. The flexible bronchoscope is small and maneuverable and can be used through an endotracheal tube in ventilated patients; it can reach far into the segmental and subsegmental bronchi. The *rigid bronchoscope* is a long, straight metal tube with a light at the tip. The rigid bronchoscope can be used to manipulate the wall of the trachea and bronchi; the large lumen allows aspiration of large particles, but vision is limited to the lobar and some segmental bronchi. Hence, the rigid bronchoscope is used if large particles must be cleared from the airways or if fixation or mobility of the tracheal wall is in question.

During bronchoscopy the mouth, pharynx, larynx, and airways are anesthetized with topical anesthetic. The bronchscope is passed into the lower airways, and appropriate studies and lavage are carried out. The assistant to the bronchoscopist must be sure that all equipment is in proper working order, adjust the light or power source, and supply local anesthesia, irrigating solution, and suction, as needed.

Tracheostomy is an operation in which a tube is placed through the skin of the neck into the trachea.[26] This is needed if the upper airway is occluded or if the patient requires prolonged ventilatory support. Although endotracheal intubation can be maintained for weeks at a time, there are many advantages to direct tracheostomy for pro-

longed ventilator support (less resistance, easier tracheal suctioning, less damage to the larynx, and the ability of the patient to eat by mouth). The major advantage of tracheostomy over endotracheal intubation is that it is much more comfortable for the patient and, consequently, does not require prolonged sedation. If the operation is properly done, the advantages of tracheostomy far outweigh any advantages of prolonged intubation. We now favor tracheostomy for airway access in any patient who needs mechanical ventilation for more than a few days (Fig. 30–9).

With the rare exceptions of cervical spine injury and laryngeal occlusion, tracheostomy is always an elective operation done with an endotracheal tube in place. Tracheostomies are conventionally done through the second tracheal cartilage. This operation can be easily done in a well-equipped intensive care unit under local anesthesia and requires excellent lighting, suction, exposure, and hemostasis. Tracheostomy done through the cricothyroid membrane was formerly an emergency procedure only. This operation is quicker and easier to do, but it may damage the cricoid cartilage or vocal cords. It has recently been shown that this

Figure 30—9. Potential complications of endotracheal intubation and tracheostomy. Balloon cuff complications are common to both.

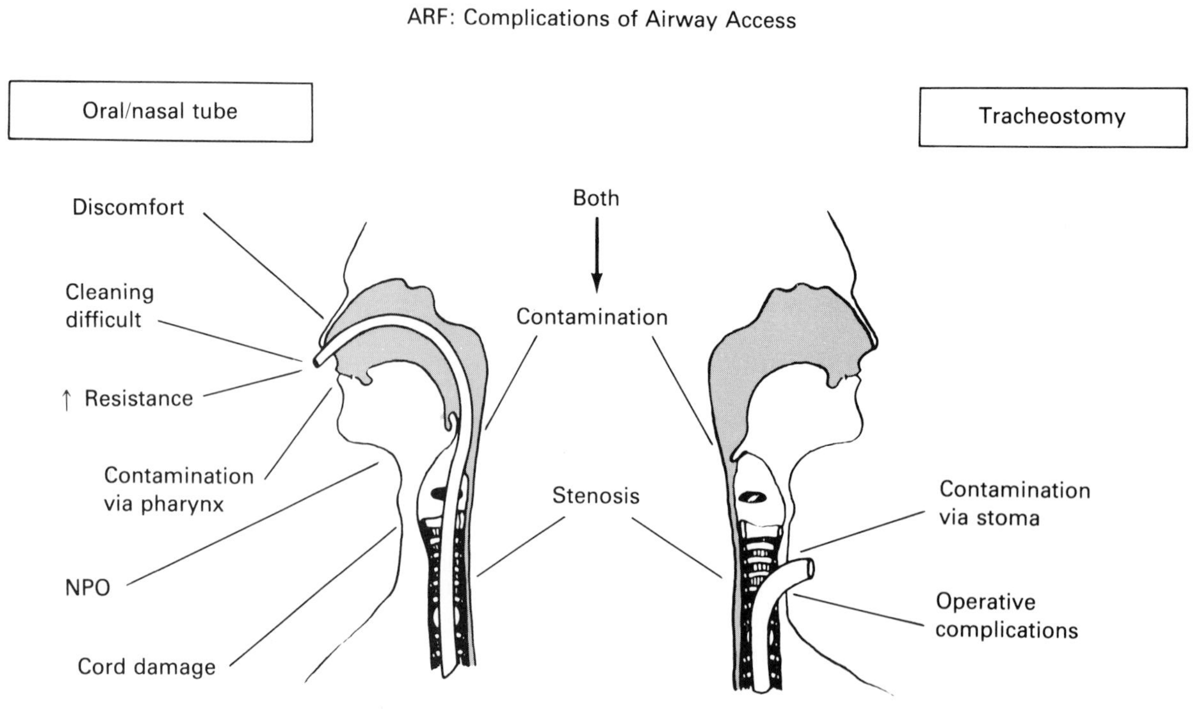

ARF: Complications of Airway Access

type of tracheostomy is acceptable for chronic and elective airway access, as long as damage to the cricoid cartilage is avoided.[12] Currently available is a percutaneous device for subcricoid placement of a tracheostomy at the bedside, eliminating the need for costly operating room time, equipment, and personnel.[14] Usually, tracheostomy is done because the patient has pulmonary failure and needs ventilator support. This requires coordination between the surgeon and the nurse or respiratory therapist. Often, the endotracheal tube balloon is punctured as the trachea is entered, so that the tracheostomy tube must be prepared and available as soon as the trachea has been opened. Under direct vision and with the patient breathing by ventilator, the endotracheal tube is pulled back until the tracheal lumen has been exposed. The tracheostomy tube is placed, the endotracheal tube completely removed, and the ventilator attached to the tracheostomy tube. When the ventilator is attached to the tracheostomy tube, the operative field is contaminated. It is not necessary to use separate sterile ventilator tubing for this transition.

EXTRACORPOREAL MEMBRANE OXYGENATION

When acute pulmonary insufficiency becomes severe and prolonged enough to carry a high mortality risk with continued therapy, extracorporeal membrane oxygenation (ECMO) may provide total life-support for all organs while new and innovative treatment is pursued. This technique is an extension of cardiopulmonary bypass, in which an artificial lung and pumping system are substituted for the lungs and heart during cardiac surgery. ECMO may more appropriately be designated ECLS, for extracorporeal life-support because, with current technology respiratory, cardiac, nutritional, and renal function can all be sustained artificially while on bypass.

During cannulation for ECMO, large catheters are placed into the heart or great vessels under local anesthesia. A diagram of a typical ECLS system is shown in Figure 30–10. The patient is anticoagulated with heparin, and venous blood is drained from the patient, oxygen is added, and carbon diox-

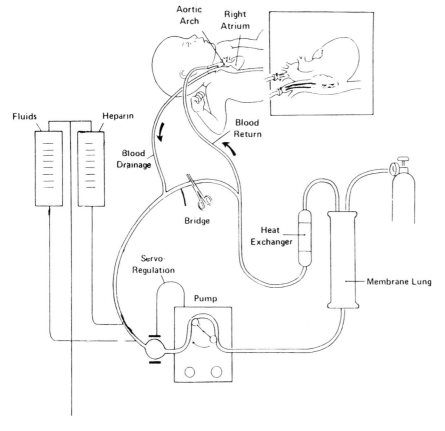

Figure 30–10. Extracorporeal life-support system for respiratory failure.

ide removed; the arterialized blood is then pumped back into the patient. In this way the artificial lung takes over the function of the normal lung, essentially allowing removal of the patient from the ventilator, even though severe lung disease exists. Ventilator settings may thus be decreased to noninjurious levels, allowing pulmonary healing to occur and allowing eventual decannulation from the bypass circuit.

Extracorporeal life-support had been evaluated extensively in adults with severe acute respiratory failure during the 1976–1978 National Institutes of Health (NIH) sponsored multicenter trial. The results of this comparative study between ECLS and conventional ventilator treatment showed 90% mortality in both groups,[40] owing to fibrosis or infection in the lung. Because of these initial results, ECLS research in the United States had stopped. A resurgence of ECLS for adult respiratory failure has occurred following success with adult ECLS, primarily by Gattinoni in Milan, Italy. Although concentrating on bypass for carbon dioxide removal (ECOR, or extracorporeal CO_2 removal) and CPAP for oxygenation, survival in this group of patients was approximately 50%.[18] Several centers are again reinvestigating ECLS as a modality in the treatment of adult respiratory failure.

Extracorporeal life-support has become the standard treatment for respiratory failure for near-term and term neonates who fail to respond to optimal therapy. Currently, over 50 centers in the United States and abroad conduct ECLS, with 2500 neonates treated thus far. Survival now nears 95% in patients who would otherwise experience a 90% mortality with conventional ventilatory management. ECLS for neonates involves right common carotid artery and right internal jugular vein ligation for cannulation. Techniques using venovenous (i.e., no arterial cannulation) access for oxygenation of blood may soon replace more conventional venoarterial bypass.

SUMMARY

Respiratory care in the surgical patient includes prevention and treatment of the single largest cause of complication and death—respiratory insufficiency and failure. Ventilation–perfusion imbalance leading to total alveolar collapse is found, to some extent, in almost every surgical patient. An increase in pulmonary extravascular water volume frequently complicates this situation. Prevention

and treatment of pulmonary insufficiency, therefore, are aimed at achieving and maintaining normal FRC, normal hemodynamics, and normal pulmonary capillary permeability.

REFERENCES

1. Achauer BM, Allyn PA, Furnas DW et al: Pulmonary complications of burns: The major threat to the burned patient. Ann Surg 177:311, 1974
2. Bartlett RH: Post-traumatic pulmonary insufficiency. In Cooper P, Nyhus L (eds): Surgery Annual. New York, Appleton–Century–Crofts, 1971
3. Bartlett RH: Respiratory care in surgery. Surg Clin North Am 16(6), Philadelphia, WB Saunders, 1980
4. Bartlett RH: Cardiopulmonary complications of pancreatitis. In Dent TL (ed): Pancreatic Disease. New York, Grune & Stratton, 1981
5. Bartlett RH: Postoperative pulmonary prophylaxis: Breathe deeply and read carefully [Editorial]. Chest 81:1, 1982
6. Bartlett RH, Brennan MD, Gazzaniga AB et al: Studies on the pathogenesis and prevention of postoperative pulmonary complications. Surg Gynecol Obstet 137:925, 1973
7. Bartlett RH, Gazzaniga AB, Geraghty TR: Respiratory maneuvers to prevent postoperative pulmonary complications. A critical review. JAMA 224:1017, 1973
8. Bartlett RH, Yahia C: Management of septic chemical abortion with acute renal failure. N Engl J Med 281:747, 1969
9. Baxter WD, Levine RS: An evaluation of intermittent positive pressure breathing in the prevention of postoperative pulmonary complications. Arch Surg 98:795, 1969
10. Becker A et al: The treatment of postoperative pulmonary atelectasis with intermittent positive pressure breathing. Surg Gynecol Obstet 111:517, 1960
11. Bendixen HH, Hedley–Whyte J, Laver MR: Oxygenation in surgical patients during general anesthesia with controlled ventilation. N Engl J Med 269:991, 1963
12. Brantigan CO, Growe B: Cricothyroidotomy: Elective use in respiratory problems requiring tracheostomy. J Thorac Cardiovasc Surg 71:72, 1976
13. Broe PJ, Toung TJK, Cameron JL: Aspiration pneumonia. Surg Clin North Am 60:1551, 1980
14. Ciaglia P, Firsching R, Syniec C: Elective percutaneous dilational tracheostomy: A new simple bedside procedure; Preliminary report. Chest 87:715, 1985
15. Demling RH, Manohar M, Will JA et al: The effect of plasma oncotic pressure on the pulmonary micro-circulation after hemorrhagic shock. Surgery 86:323, 1979
16. Dudell G, Cornish JD, Bartlett RH: What constitutes adequate oxygenation? Pediatrics 85:39, 1990
17. Ford GT, Whitelaw WA, Rosenal TW et al: Diaphragm function after upper abdominal surgery in humans. Am Rev Respir Dis 127:431, 1983
18. Gattinoni L, Presenti A, Mascheroni D et al: Low-fre-

quency positive pressure ventilation with extracorporeal CO_2 removal in severe acute respiratory failure. JAMA 256:881, 1986

19. Greenbaum DM, Millen JE, Eross B et al: Continuous positive pressure without tracheal intubation in spontaneously breathing patients. Chest 69:615, 1976

20. Hodgkin JE, Dines DE, Didier EP: Preoperative evaluation of the patient with pulmonary disease. Mayo Clin Proc 48:114, 1973

21. Holcroft JW, Trunkey DD, Lim RC: Further analysis of lung water in baboons resuscitated from hemorrhage shock. J Surg Res 20:291, 1976

22. Kolobow T, Moretti MP, Fumagalli R et al: Severe impairment in lung function induced by high peak airway pressure during mechanical ventilation: An experimental study. Am Rev Respir Dis 135:312, 1987

23. Lee AB, Kinney JM, Turino G et al: Effects of abdominal operations on ventilation and gas exchange. J Natl Med Assoc 61:164, 1969

24. Obeid FN, Shapiro MJ, Richardson HH et al: Catheter aspiration for simple pneumothorax (CASP) in the outpatient management of simple traumatic pneumothorax. J Trauma 25:882, 1985

25. Okinaka AJ: The pattern of breathing after operation. Surg Gynecol Obstet 125:785, 1967

26. Orringer M: Endotracheal intubation and tracheostomy. Surg Clin North Am 60:1447, 1980

27. Pontoppidan H: Mechanical aids to lung expansion in non-intubated surgical patients. Am Rev Respir Dis 122:109, 1981

28. Powers SR, Shah D, Ryon D et al: Hypertonic mannitol in the therapy of acute respiratory distress syndrome. Ann Surg 185:619, 1977

29. Puri V, Weil MH, Michaels S et al: Pulmonary edema associated with reduction in plasma oncotic pressure. Surg Gynecol Obstet 151:344, 1980

30. Ratliff JL: Bronchoscopy in respiratory care. Surg Clin North Am 60:1497, 1980

31. Sammons RS, Berdine GG, Seidenfeld JJ et al: Fluid balance and the adult respiratory distress syndrome. Am Rev Respir Dis 135:924, 1987

32. Schwieger I, Gamulin Z, Forster A et al: Absence of benefit of incentive spirometry in low-risk patients undergoing elective cholecystectomy: A controlled randomized study. Chest 89:655, 1986

33. Shapiro BA: IPPB therapy is indicated preoperatively and postoperatively in some patients with pulmonary disease. In Eckenhoff JG (ed): Controversy in Anesthesiology. Philadelphia, WB Saunders, 1979

34. Skillman JJ, Parikh BM, Tanenbaum BJ: Pulmonary arteriovenous admixture: Improvement with albumin and diuresis. Am J Surg 119:440, 1970

35. Staub NC: State of the art review: Pathogenesis of pulmonary edema. Am Rev Respir Dis 109:358, 1974

36. Suter PM, Fairley HB, Isenberg MD: Optimum end-expiratory pressure in patients with acute pulmonary failure. N Engl J Med 292:284, 1975

37. Trinkle JK, Richardson JD, Franz FL et al: Management of flail chest without mechanical ventilation. Ann Thorac Surg 19:355, 1975

38. Vandewater JM: Preoperative and postoperative techniques in the prevention of pulmonary complications. Surg Clin North Am 60:1339, 1980

39. Walker WE, Kapelanski DP, Weiland AP et al: Patterns of infection and mortality in thoracic trauma. Ann Surg 210:752, 1985

40. Zapol WM, Snider MT, Hill SD et al: Extracorporeal membrane oxygenation in severe acute respiratory failure: A randomized prospective study. JAMA 242:2193, 1979

41. Zawacki BE, Jung RC, Joyce J et al: Smoke, burns, and the natural history of inhalation injury in fire victims. Ann Surg 185:100, 1977

42. Zikria BA, Spencer JL, Kinney JM et al: Alterations in ventilatory function in breathing patterns following surgical trauma. Ann Surg 179:1, 1974

THIRTY-ONE

Acute Respiratory Failure

Roger C. Bone

Acute respiratory failure (ARF) persists as one of the most life-threatening processes affecting acutely ill patients in the critical care setting today.[1–3]

All age groups are susceptible to this disease process. Therefore, knowledge of the potential multiple-organ complications, and expertise in the disease process itself, are essential for possible prevention and treatment of acute respiratory failure.

The purpose of this chapter is to outline a systemized approach defining the etiology as well as the laboratory patterns with which acute respiratory failure develops.

HISTORY

Acute respiratory failure was not easily discernible preceding the 1950s because of the difficult task of controlling oxygen therapy and measuring arterial blood oxygen and carbon dioxide partial pressures.[4–6] Barbiturate overdose and bulbar and anterior horn cell poliomyelitis were the principal causes of acute respiratory failure.[4,7]

The Salk vaccine obliterated poliomyelitis. The utilization of effective airway management and advances in continuous mechanical ventilation quickly improved the treatment of barbiturate overdose, which was initially managed with central nervous system (CNS) stimulants and gastric lavage.

The advent of the 1960s brought improvements in the analysis of arterial blood gases and the use of controlled oxygen therapy in the treatment of acute respiratory failure. Only then, did the genuine incidence of this condition become evident.

The contemporary period of treatment commenced as physicians became cognizant that acute respiratory failure and significant hypoxemia could result from a myriad of causes, including shock, sepsis, burns, trauma, and acute pulmonary complications.[8,9]

It was apparent by the late 1960s that a coordinated approach to treatment was needed and that the critical care units had become intrinsic components of most large hospitals. By 1970, these advances augmented the number of patients treated for acute respiratory failure. One-third to one-half of all patients in the intensive care setting received artificial ventilation at some point during their hospital course.[7] It was during this time that clinicians had a greater understanding of this disease process. Survival was prolonged with improved supportive care, and it became increasingly apparent that multiorgan failure caused more deaths than progressive hypoxemia. It was during this time that acute left ventricular failure and complications of acute respiratory failure, including disseminated intravascular coagulation, sepsis, hypotension, stress ulceration, opportunistic infections, acute renal failure, and cardiac arrhythmias, were identified by numerous authors.[10,11] These critically ill patients required total life-support and were vulnerable to a high incidence of iatrogenic complications.[12,13]

The extremely high cost of caring for critically ill patients became a nucleus for debate. In today's atmosphere of frugal financial spending for health care, this debate will undoubtedly continue.[14,15]

DEFINITION OF ACUTE RESPIRATORY FAILURE

Acute respiratory failure is present when gas exchange by the pulmonary system is unable to keep pace with the metabolic demands of the body.[16] Unfortunately, there is no comprehensive definition that encompasses all the causes of ARF. Some authors distinguish ARF from acute ventilatory failure, which is a mechanical limitation to the movement of air in and out of the alveoli. For the purpose of this chapter, I will not make this distinction, since acute ventilatory failure is often a secondary component of ARF. The hallmark of both processes involves a maldistribution of ventilation and perfusion.[17] Disruption in the *function* of the respiratory system is often used by other authors to describe ARF. In this definition, the respiratory system is considered to consist of the CNS control center, with efferent and afferent nervous pathways, as well as the nerves, muscles, pleura, and lungs themselves.[4,7,8,18] The term ARF is used in the latter context in this discussion.

Although no uniform definition of *acute respiratory failure* exists that includes all causative factors, it is best described as a condition resulting in an abnormally low arterial oxygen tension, with or without an abnormally high carbon dioxide tension.[4,7,14,19,20] A useful definition that applies to most causes of ARF is when at least two of the four following criteria are present:

1. The patient is acutely dyspneic
2. The PaO_2 is less than 50 mmHg when breathing room air
3. The $PaCO_2$ is greater than 50 mmHg
4. The arterial pH shows significant respiratory acidemia

Although these figures are somewhat arbitrary, what is really being defined are values for PaO_2 and $PaCO_2$ that are lower or higher than those expected in the conditions under which the arterial blood gases are measured. There are two types of ARF: Type 1 is manifested by an abnormally low PaO_2 with a $PaCO_2$ that is either low or normal. Type 2 is represented by hypoxemia as well as hypercapnia.

Type 1 patients usually present with acute lung injury, such as the adult respiratory distress syndrome (ARDS).[9,21] Type 2 includes respiratory failure predominately in patients with chronic obstructive pulmonary disease (COPD), central causes of alveolar hypoventilation, or chest bellows dysfunction.

Limited clinical information is gained by classifying a process as either type 1 or type 2 respiratory failure. Nothing is revealed about the specific disease entity involved, the severity of that disease, or its prognosis. These represent clinical evaluations that are based on history, physical examination, and chest x-ray films, as well as arterial blood gas analysis. Therefore, it should be considered that type 1 and type 2 respiratory failure represents two manifestations of ARF, and these are not specific disease entities.

ETIOLOGIES

Acute respiratory failure results from a defect in the functioning of some portion of the respiratory system. The causes of ARF can be considered as one of the seven weak links in the interconnecting chain (Fig. 31–1). It is imperative to be aware of the diverse nature of the major causes that constitute each of the links in the chain (Table 31–1). As indicated in this table, certain etiologies will result in only type 2 failure. Diseases involving the brain, spinal cord, neuromuscular system, or thorax, and pleura result pathophysiologically in alveolar hypoventilation and, therefore, produce only type 2 failure. Conversely, the recognition of type 1 failure suggests a disease involving a component of the lungs themselves.

DIAGNOSIS AND TREATMENT

Acute respiratory failure may occur as a result of malfunction in one or more of the seven systems shown in Figure 31–1. Table 31–1 outlines an abbreviated approach to diagnosis (by blood gas abnormalities only) and treatment.

Respiratory failure from alveolar and airway disease in adults can be subdivided into that characterized by hypoxemia and hypercapnia (predominantly patients with COPD) and that characterized by hypoxemia alone (predominantly patients with acute lung injury, ARDS).

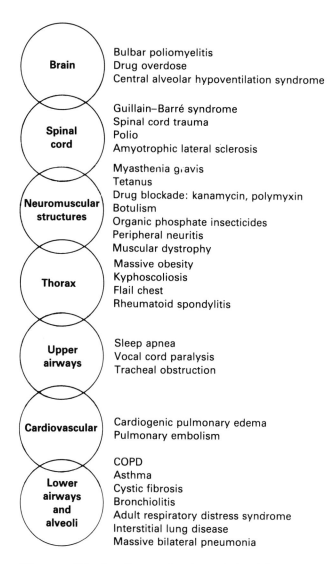

Brain	Bulbar poliomyelitis Drug overdose Central alveolar hypoventilation syndrome
Spinal cord	Guillain–Barré syndrome Spinal cord trauma Polio Amyotrophic lateral sclerosis
Neuromuscular structures	Myasthenia gravis Tetanus Drug blockade: kanamycin, polymyxin Botulism Organic phosphate insecticides Peripheral neuritis Muscular dystrophy
Thorax	Massive obesity Kyphoscoliosis Flail chest Rheumatoid spondylitis
Upper airways	Sleep apnea Vocal cord paralysis Tracheal obstruction
Cardiovascular	Cardiogenic pulmonary edema Pulmonary embolism
Lower airways and alveoli	COPD Asthma Cystic fibrosis Bronchiolitis Adult respiratory distress syndrome Interstitial lung disease Massive bilateral pneumonia

Figure 31–1. Causes of acute respiratory failure.

TREATMENT OF HYPOXEMIC, HYPERCAPNIC RESPIRATORY FAILURE

The major risk of the use of high concentrations of oxygen in the patient with hypercapnic respiratory failure is the iatrogenic precipitation of progressive hypercapnia from relief of the hypoxic drive to breathing.[22] The correct dose of oxygen to use in respiratory failure is that which satisfies tissue needs for oxygen, but does not produce carbon dioxide narcosis or oxygen toxicity. Thus, the proper concentration of oxygen is that which produces an adequate, but not excessive, arterial oxygen tension (generally thought to be between 50 and 60 mmHg).

Since the introduction of the concept of controlled oxygen therapy by Barach[23] and its practical implementation by Campbell,[24,25] the administration of progressive increments of inspired oxygen has become the usual therapy for patients with ARF secondary to chronic obstructive lung disease and its exacerbations. Most such patients respond to an increased fraction of inspired oxygen (FIO_2) by an improvement in arterial hypoxemia and, in conjunction with other therapy, an improvement in clinical status. However, some patients experience progressive hypercapnia and acidosis, with resultant confusion, stupor, or coma, even when the FIO_2 is only moderately increased. These latter patients may require an artificial airway and mechanical ventilation.

The rationale for controlled oxygen therapy is that most patients with chronic obstructive lung disease who develop ARF have reversible problems, such as airways infection, bronchospasm, retained secretions, congestive heart failure, or other conditions that have resulted in decreased alveolar ventilation. Low concentrations of oxygen are used to produce an acceptable PaO_2, whereas other therapy is directed toward reversing the factors that precipitated the respiratory failure. The goal is to maintain adequate oxygenation, without significantly worsening respiratory acidosis. Thus, adequate oxygenation may result from improvement of the PaO_2 from 40 to 60 mmHg, rather than to absolute "normal" PaO_2 values. This leads to a substantial increase in oxygen delivery to the tissue, since such PaO_2 values are on the steep portion of the oxyhemoglobin dissociation curve.

Air-entrainment oxygen masks, such as venturi masks, can deliver a precise dose of oxygen. These devices use the Bernoulli principle, by passing oxygen through a restriction, and entraining room air, to provide precise concentrations of oxygen ranging from 24% to 50%, depending on the mask. If the original PaO_2 when breathing room air is known, a reasonable estimate of the PaO_2 that will be achieved in patients with hypercapnic respiratory failure resulting from a specific venturi mask is shown in Figure 31–2.[26,27] If use of the venturi mask is not available or feasible, then a nasal cannula at flow rates of 0.25–2 L/min can be used to treat hypoxemia (low-flow oxygen therapy). Arterial blood gases should be measured at frequent intervals, usually every 30 minutes for the first 1 to 2 hours, or until it is certain that an acceptable PaO_2 has been achieved, without the precipitation of hypercapnia and respiratory acidosis. Simultaneously, bronchodilators, antibiotics, and other

Table 31—1 Acute Respiratory Failure

CAUSES	DIAGNOSIS AND TREATMENT

BRAIN

Clinical examples
  Bulbar poliomyelitis
  Drug overdose
  Central alveolar hypoventilation
    syndrome

A. Arterial blood gases show a decreased PaO_2 and increased $PaCO_2$.
B. Adequate oxygenation is no problem if patient is given assisted ventilation.
C. Special situations
  1. For bulbar poliomyelitis, assisted ventilation is usually necessary.
  2. For narcotics, propoxyphene (Darvon), and pentazocine (Talwin), naloxone HCl (Narcan) in a dose of 0.4 mg (1 mL) may be given to reverse respiratory depression. This dose can be repeated in 2 to 3 minutes.
  3. For central alveolar ventilation, phrenic nerve pacing has been used, but upper airway obstruction has been noted after phrenic pacing.

SPINAL CORD

Clinical examples
  Guillain–Barré
  Spinal cord trauma
  Poliomyelitis

A. Arterial blood gases show a decreased PaO_2 and increased $PaCO_2$.
B. Adequate oxygenation is no problem if patient is given assisted ventilation.
C. Special situations
  1. For spinal cord disease, intubation and mechanical ventilation should be instituted when patient's vital capacity <1000 mL or < 10 mL/kg body weight, or both.
  2. Rocking beds, pneumatic belts, cuirass ventilation, and "iron lung" may be attractive alternatives to long-term, if not permanent, intubation and mechanical ventilation.

NEUROMUSCULAR STRUCTURES

Clinical examples
  Myasthenia gravis
  Tetanus
  Drug-induced neuromuscular
    blockage (e.g., curare,
    neomycin, kanamycin, strep-
    tomycin, polymyxin)
  Botulism
  Organic phosphate insecticide
    poisoning

A. Arterial blood gases show a decreased PaO_2 and increased $PaCO_2$.
B. Adequate oxygenation is no problem if patient is given assisted ventilation.
C. Special situations
  1. Intubation and mechanical ventilation should be instituted when patient's vital capacity <1000 mL or <10 mL/kg body weight.
  2. In myasthenia gravis, intubation and assisted ventilation should also be instituted when patient is unable to clear secretions from airway and saliva from mouth.
  3. In tetanus, good debridement of wound, penicillin, and human tetanus antitoxin are used. Diazepam (Valium) is often used for sedation and pancuronium bromide (Pavulon) for paralysis.
  4. Neomycin, kanamycin, and steptomycin produce a competitive blockage at the myoneural end plate, which may be reversed by neostigmine. Polymyxin B, colistin, and possibly kanamycin produce a noncompetitive blockage, which may be helped by intravenous calcium gluconate.
  5. In botulism, treatment includes antitoxin.
  6. In organic phosphate insecticide poisoning, atropine, 1 to 2 mg IM and 2-PAM (pyridine aldoxime methiodide) may combat the cholinesterase inhibition.

THE THORAX AND ABDOMEN

Clinical examples
  Kyphoscoliosis
  Massive obesity
  Muscular dystrophy
  Flail chest
  Rheumatoid spondylitis

A. Arterial blood gases show decreased PaO_2 and increased $PaCO_2$.
B. Adequate oxygenation is no problem if patient is given assisted ventilation.
C. Special situations
  1. Patients with kyphoscoliosis usually have severe spinal deformity before hypoventilation occurs.
  2. Massive obesity is a major risk factor for accentuating other causes of respiratory failure.
  3. In flail chest associated with chest contusion or ARDS, intubation with mechanical ventilation and PEEP are often indicated.

(continued)

Table 31—1 (continued)

CAUSES	DIAGNOSIS AND TREATMENT

UPPER AIRWAYS

Clinical examples
  Obstructive sleep apnea
  Vocal cord paralysis
  Tracheal obstruction
  Epiglottitis/laryngotracheitis
  Large tonsils and adenoids
  Postextubation laryngeal
    edema

A. Arterial blood gases show decreased PaO_2 and increased $PaCO_2$.

B. Adequate oxygenation is no problem if patient is given assisted ventilation.

C. Special situations
  1. Obstructive sleep apnea is usually improved by tracheostomy.
  2. Epiglottitis/laryngotracheitis and postextubation laryngeal edema may be helped by antibiotics (e.g., ampicillin) for infection. Corticosteroids are used for laryngeal edema and aerosolized racemic epinephrine as a decongestant to reduce edema.
  3. Tracheal obstruction by tumor or stricture may be corrected surgically.

CARDIOVASCULAR AND THROMBOEMBOLIC

Clinical examples
  Cardiogenic pulmonary edema
  Pulmonary embolism

A. Arterial blood gases show a decreased PaO_2 and a decreased $PaCO_2$ (respiratory alkalosis).

B. Oxygen mask or high-flow oxygen by nasal cannula often needed to treat hypoxemia.

C. Intubation and mechanical ventilation usually not needed unless acidotic or impending cardiovascular collapse.

D. Special situations
  1. Pulmonary edema secondary to left ventricular failure is treated with diuretics, digoxin, unloading agents, and fluid and salt restriction.
  2. Pulmonary embolism is treated with heparin or fibrinolytic agents, or both.

ALVEOLI AND LOWER AIRWAYS

Clinical examples
  Chronic obstructive pulmonary
    disease
  Asthma
  Cystic fibrosis
  Bronchiolitis
  Adult respiratory distress
    syndrome
  Interstitial lung disease

A. Arterial blood gases in chronic obstructive lung disease usually show a decreased PaO_2 and increased $PaCO_2$. In asthma, usually a decreased PaO_2 and $PaCO_2$ are seen except in late stages, when a a decreased PaO_2 and increased $PaCO_2$ are seen. In ARDS, a decreased PaO_2 and $PaCO_2$ are seen except in late stages, when an elevated $PaCO_2$ can be seen.

B. Special situations.
  1. For COPD and ARDS, see text and Chap. 32.
  2. For asthma, cystic fibrosis, bronchiolitis, and interstitial lung disease, see text and chapters on these topics.

---

measures are used as indicated to treat the primary cause of ARF.

The patient should be managed in an intensive care unit, since life-threatening changes in oxygenation and acid–base balance may occur on a minute-to-minute basis. Most patients with COPD respond favorably to this regimen, and adequate oxygenation is usually achieved without the precipitation of severe hypercapnia. Despite these precautions, if the patient does hypoventilate and significant hypercapnia does occur, care should be taken to avoid complete removal of oxygen. At this time, mechanical ventilation should probably be considered.

The likelihood of carbon dioxide narcosis developing despite controlled oxygen therapy can be predicted with some certainty (Fig. 31–3) and is a function of admission PaO_2 and pH. Experience has shown that not all patients need to be intubated simply because they have a slightly increased $PaCO_2$ after being given oxygen. Slight carbon dioxide retention should be considered a tolerable, adaptive response to oxygen administration (Fig. 31–4).[28] At least initially, a major therapeutic goal in hypoxemia, hypercapnic respiratory failure is to avoid endotracheal intubation and mechanical ventilation, if possible. The reasons for this are (1) the complications of intubation are more frequent with

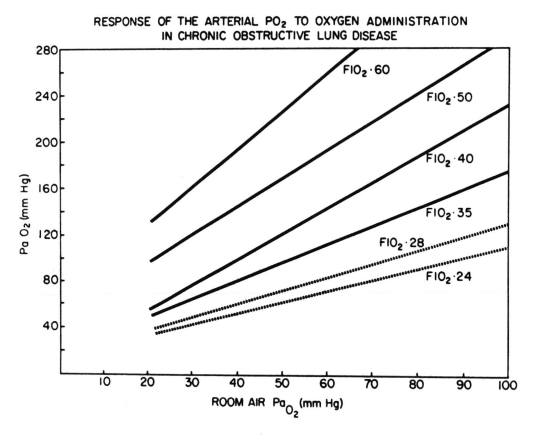

Figure 31—2. Regression lines for different inspired percentages of oxygen (FiO$_2$). Each line gives the expected arterial oxygen tension (PaO$_2$) for oxygen therapy based on the patient's room air PaO$_2$ and applied FiO$_2$. The relationships were determined with patients in acute respiratory failure (*dashed lines*) and stable patients (*solid lines*).

Figure 31—3. Arterial oxygen tension (PaO$_2$) and pH at admission. Patients developing somnolence on controlled oxygen therapy were generally severely hypoxemic or had a combination of moderate hypoxemia and acidemia. This figure demonstrates the importance of hypoxemia and acidemia as risk factors for the development of carbon dioxide narcosis with controlled oxygen therapy. The line separating high- from low-risk patients was found by discriminant analysis (pH = 7.66 − 0.00919 PO$_2$). Δ = intubated patients; ● = nonintubated patients. (Bone RC, Pierce AK, Johnson RL Jr: Controlled oxygen administration in acute respiratory failure in chronic obstructive pulmonary disease: A reappraisal. Am J Med 65:896, 1978, with permission)

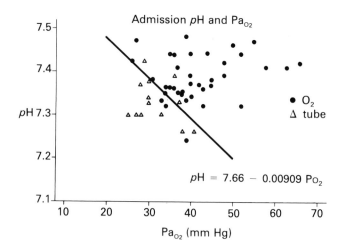

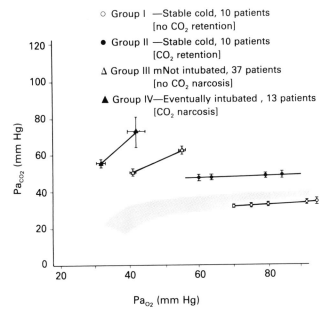

○ Group I —Stable cold, 10 patients
[no CO_2 retention]

● Group II —Stable cold, 10 patients
[CO_2 retention]

△ Group III mNot intubated, 37 patients
[no CO_2 narcosis]

▲ Group IV—Eventually intubated , 13 patients
[CO_2 narcosis]

Figure 31–4. Mean values for admission PaO_2–$PaCO_2$ plotted with PaO_2 and $PaCO_2$ at point of greatest hypercapnia after oxygen administration in four separate groups of patients with chronic obstructive pulmonary disease. The hatched area represents a normal human response to various inspired oxygen tensions during (*lower portion*) and after (*upper portion*) acclimatization to high altitudes. Horizontal and vertical bars indicate standard error of the mean for the PaO_2 and $PaCO_2$, respectively. (Bone RC, Pierce AK, Johnson RL Jr: Controlled oxygen administration in acute respiratory failure in chronic obstructive pulmonary disease: A reappraisal. Am J Med 65:896, 1978, with permission)

hypoxemic, hypercapnic respiratory failure; (2) the need for ventilatory support, once applied, is usually more prolonged, and weaning is difficult; and (3) the physiologic profile of these patients make it more likely that they can be managed without artificial support.

If intubation is performed, however, it should be done with a high-compliance, low-pressure cuffed endotracheal tube. Usually, ventilator tidal volumes of 8–12 mL/kg are sufficient. The inspiratory flow rate should be regulated carefully to allow adequate time for full expiration to avoid air-trapping. In most cases, an inspiratory/expiratory (I/E) ratio of 1:3 is satisfactory. The respiratory rate may have to be decreased to achieve this. Again, the goal of ventilator therapy is not normalization of blood gases. If chronic carbon dioxide retention has been present before illness, decreasing the arterial $PaCO_2$ to levels that result in a normal pH is acceptable for

initial treatment. However, when weaning the patient from ventilator support, it may be best to allow the $PaCO_2$ to increase back up to its stable level. All changes from admission baseline in arterial $PaCO_2$ and pH should be made gradually, since rapid changes may cause significant alkalosis, with resultant cardiac arrhythmias, convulsions, or both.

The monitoring of vital signs, tidal volume, respiratory rate, compliance, arterial blood gases, electrocardiogram, and fluid and electrolyte balance is routine for all patients. Careful monitoring of such patients is particularly important during sleep because there is often greater bronchosecretion, poorer secretion clearance, worse oxygen desaturation, worse pulmonary hypertension, and cardiac arrhythmias. In selected patients, particularly those in whom left ventricular failure is suspected, a flow-directed pulmonary artery catheter may be used, but the data must be interpreted with caution, particularly in patients with COPD who are breathing by ventilator. Rapid swings in the intrapleural pressure in such patients will cause reliance on the mean pulmonary artery pressure to be in error. The pulmonary wedge pressure should be read at end-expiration, and, even then, its values should be compared closely with the patient's clinical condition before alterations are made.

TREATMENT OF HYPOXEMIC, NORMOCAPNIC RESPIRATORY FAILURE

The prototype of hypoxemic, normocapnic respiratory failure is the adult respiratory distress syndrome (ARDS),[9,29] discussed in detail in Chapter 32. The reader is referred to this chapter for pertinent details of the pathophysiology and treatment of this condition, in which mortality may be greater than 75% in patients needing long-term oxygen therapy with an FIO_2 of 0.50 or greater.

The ARDS may be largely preventable if it is anticipated and appropriate measures are instituted in the immediate postinjury period. Respiratory failure in ARDS is self-perpetuating, since hypoventilation and alveolar closure, as may occur postinjury, lead to further atelectasis and hypoxemia. Simple measures in the postoperative or postinjury period that may abort respiratory failure at an early phase are listed in Table 31–2.

The treatment of all causes of ARDS includes providing adequate tissue oxygenation by respiratory and circulatory support.[30] Regardless of the inciting agent in ARDS, once the alveolocapillary membrane has been damaged, the clinical prob-

Table 31—2 Prophylactic Measures to Prevent ARDS

1. Restore circulatory blood volume promptly after shock.
2. Leave endotracheal tube in place until postoperative patient is fully awake and ventilation adequate.
3. Encourage sighing (deep breathing) in postinjury period.
4. Change patient position frequently.
5. Use blood filters for blood transfusion exceeding 4 units.
6. Use enteral alimentation or hyperalimentation early for major injury with adequate nutrition.

lems are similar. The therapeutic goal in all causes of ARDS is to support the patient until the integrity of the alveolocapillary membrane had been reestablished. The critical factors in treatment of ARDS are (1) optimal distention of alveoli to increase functional residual capacity, (2) maintenance of tissue perfusion, and (3) control of the primary problem. Because the basic physiologic event in this syndrome is alveolar collapse, major efforts are made to obtain optimal distention of alveoli.

A major problem in ARDS is the potential development of oxygen toxicity. The toxic effects of increased oxygen concentrations were described by Smith in 1899.[31] Continuous exposure of animals to 100% oxygen leads to death within a few days. Pulmonary oxygen toxicity in humans was demonstrated by Barber and colleagues in a prospective study of ten patients with irreversible brain damage.[32] One group of patients received air and the other, 100% oxygen. Greater impairment of pulmonary physiology was detected in the oxygen-treated patients. The pathologic changes of oxygen toxicity include endothelial proliferation and perivascular edema. Later, pulmonary fibrosis occurs.

Because of the danger of oxygen toxicity, patients with ARDS should be treated with the lowest concentration of oxygen that provides adequate oxygenation. Clinical manifestations of oxygen toxicity have not been shown to develop if the inspired oxygen concentration is less than 50%.

DIAGNOSIS OF DETERIORATION OF RESPIRATORY STATUS IN VENTILATOR PATIENTS

In patients who develop worsening respiratory failure while on ventilator support, the cause for such deterioration may not always be apparent. The use of static and dynamic pressure–volume curves has

Figure 31—5. Causes of acute respiratory distress in patients receiving assisted ventilation. After acute respiratory distress in patients treated with mechanical ventilation, static compliance curves and curves for dynamic characteristics compared with the same curves plotted before respiratory distress will assist in differential diagnosis of causes for acute respiratory distress. Idealized curves obtained before and after respiratory distress categorized by their pattern of abnormality are shown. *Solid curves* represent static compliance curves, and *dashed curves* represent curves for dynamic characteristics. *Asterisk* indicates cardiogenic and noncardiogenic pulmonary edema (adult respiratory distress syndrome). (Bone RC: Diagnosis of causes for acute respiratory distress by pressure-volume curves. Chest 70:740, 1976, with permission)

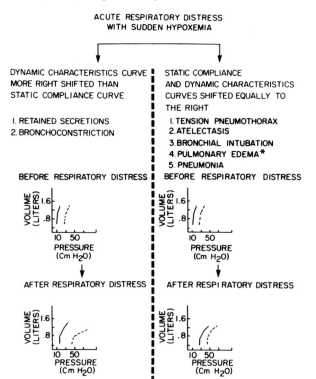

been advocated to separate airways obstructive problems, such as retained secretions and broncho-constriction, from parenchymal disorders, such as atelectasis, pulmonary edema and other causes of increased lung water, and pneumonia (Fig. 31–5).[33] The technology involved is simple and noninvasive and will identify the presence of complicating factors in the already ill patients.

TERMINOLOGY OF MECHANICAL VENTILATION

In this chapter, only three terms will be used from the multiple eponyms available. *Intermittent positive-pressure ventilation* (IPPV) usually implies that a mechanical respirator forces a ventilating gas mixture into the lungs. Exhalation is passive and results from the recoil of the lung and chest wall. Flow ceases at end-expiration when alveolar pressure equals atmospheric pressure.

Positive end-expiratory pressure (PEEP) refers to positive pressure of selected magnitude at end-expiration, that is maintained throughout expiration (Figs. 31–6 and 31–7). With *continuous positive airway pressure* (CPAP), above-ambient pressure is maintained throughout the respiratory cycle in the spontaneously breathing patient.

A PEEP of significant magnitude used in a normal lung will markedly decrease cardiac output because of a decrease in preload to the heart. When alveolar pressure exceeds pulmonary arterial pressure, no blood flow occurs, as shown in Figure 31–8, and a zone 1 alveolus is produced. As long as ARDS results in uniform disease, less alveolar pressure is transmitted to the blood vessels. However, if the disease is patchy or excessive levels of PEEP are

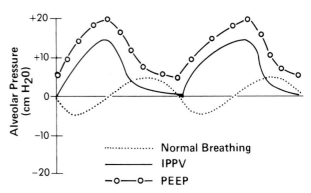

Figure 31—7. With spontaneous breathing, alveolar pressure is negative in inhalation and positive in exhalation. With IPPV, when alveolar pressure returns to atmospheric and a slight negative alveolar pressure is generated by the patient (not shown in figure), the ventilator forces a certain predetermined volume into the lung. With PEEP, if the patient is controlled, inspiration begins when the alveolar pressure reaches a preset level of PEEP (5 cmH$_2$O in this example). (Bone RC: Treatment of severe hypoxemia due to the adult respiratory distress syndrome. Arch Intern Med 140:85, 1980. Copyright 1980, American Medical Association, with permission)

used, either maldistribution of pressure or excessive alveolar pressure can decrease cardiac output or cause regional lung damage, such as alveolar rupture and pneumothorax.

Recruitment of collapsed alveoli by PEEP may take 30 minutes or longer. Discontinuance of PEEP prematurely results in rapid alveolar collapse. Thus, PEEP should be maintained until alveoli are sufficiently stable to remain open without it. General principles for the use of ventilator therapy in ARDS are outlined later. The future of improve-

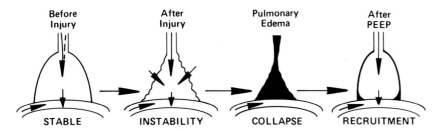

Figure 31—6. The ARDS is characterized by an unstable alveolus, resulting in alveolar collapse and perfusion of unventilated alveoli (intrapulmonary shunt). With PEEP, the increase in alveolar pressure at end-expiration prevents partial or complete collapse of unstable alveoli. PEEP may also recruit unstable alveoli. The net beneficial result is a reduction in intrapulmonary shunt owing to an improvement in ventilation—perfusion relationship in diseased lung units. (Bone RC: Treatment of severe hypoxemia due to the adult respiratory distress syndrome. Arch Intern Med 140:85, 1980. Copyright 1980, American Medical Association, with permission)

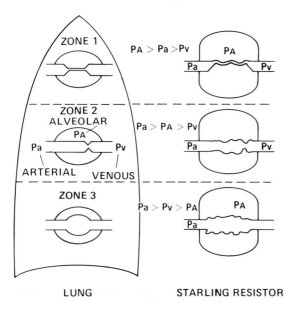

Figure 31—8. The pulmonary capillary bed has flow characteristics of a Starling resistor. In the Starling resistor, when chamber pressure exceeds downstream pressure, flow is independent of downstream pressure. However, when downstream pressure exceeds chamber pressure, flow is determined by the upstream—downstream difference. Alveolar pressure is the same throughout the lung. Pulmonary arterial pressure increases down the lung. There may be a region at the top of the lung (*zone 1*) where pulmonary arterial pressure falls below alveolar pressure. Thus, zone 1 will occur whenever alveolar pressure exceeds pulmonary arterial pressure. This may occur when the pulmonary arterial pressure is decreased, as in hypovolemia, or when alveolar pressure is increased, as with the application of PEEP. Zone 1 produces an alveolar dead space. In *zone 2*, pulmonary arterial pressure increases and exceeds alveolar pressure. In zone 2, blood flow is determined by the difference between arterial and alveolar pressure. In *zone 3*, blood flow is determined by the arteriovenous pressure difference. (Bone RC: Treatment of severe hypoxemia due to the adult respiratory distress syndrome. Arch Intern Med 140:85, 1980. Copyright 1980, American Medical Association, with permission)

ment in survival depends probably on a pharmacologic decrease in inflammation.

OPTIMAL COMPLIANCE AND MONITORING

Frequent determination of static compliance of the lungs and chest wall may allow one to pick tidal volumes and PEEP that put the lung in the range of optimal compliance (Fig. 31–9). In this range, the incidence of pulmonary barotrauma (pneumothorax, pneumomediastinum, and subcutaneous emphysema) is least, and tissue oxygen delivery may be maximal.

Several studies have shown that despite an increased PaO_2, significant reduction in cardiac output and mixed venous oxygen retention may occur from PEEP (Fig. 31–10). In the patent with severe ARDS, improvement in tissue oxygenation is the goal. Since oxygen delivery is the product of cardiac output and arterial oxygen content, cardiac output or some index of change in cardiac output should be made as PEEP is altered. If cardiac output or mixed venous oxygen tension ($P\bar{v}O_2$) decreases as PEEP is increased, a reduction in oxygen delivery to the tissue may have occurred. If PEEP results in decreased cardiac output, the patient may be hypovolemic and cardiac filling pressure too low to be maintained in the presence of PEEP; hence, fluid loading is indicated. Alternatively, the patient may have primary cardiac dysfunction and require inotropic agents. A properly positioned pulmonary artery catheter allows measurement of the pulmonary capillary wedge pressure (PCWP), which reflects the filling pressure of the left ventricle. When PEEP is used, the positive alveolar pressure can influence the reliability of the PCWP. This results from transmission of PEEP to the microvasculature. If the transmitted alveolar pressure exceeds left atrial pressure, the vessels may be collapsed, as demon-

Figure 31—9. Static pressure–volume relationship of the lungs and thorax in ARDS. Each observation represents the inflation hold manometer pressure on the ventilator (*horizontal axis*) obtained for the tidal volume indicated on the *vertical axis*. Static compliance = tidal volume/inflation hold pressure − PEEP pressure. In this example, PEEP pressure is 10 cmH2O. Compliance for tidal volumes is indicated by ● = 25 mL/cmH2O; ○ = 30 mL/cmH2O; ▲ = 25 and 20 mL/cmH2O. (Bone RC: Treatment of severe hypoxemia due to the adult respiratory distress syndrome. Arch Intern Med 140:85, 1980. Copyright 1980, American Medical Association, with permission)

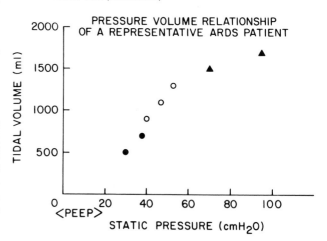

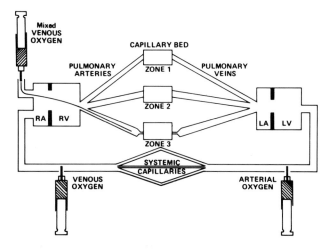

Figure 31—10. Oxygen can be obtained from the arterial, peripheral venous, or mixed venous blood. Arterial blood provides essential information about lung function. In certain circumstances, the PaO_2 may increase, despite a deterioration in oxygen delivery to tissue. For example, the application of PEEP in a relatively hypovolemic patient with ARDS might increase PaO_2, but depress cardiac output. In this situation, the arterial–mixed venous oxygen content difference may increase, reflecting the decreased cardiac output. A decreased $P\bar{v}O_2$ (taken from a pulmonary artery catheter) gives important information about decreased tissue oxygenation, despite improvement of arterial oxygenation. (Bone RC: Treatment of severe hypoxemia due to the adult respiratory distress syndrome. Arch Intern Med 140:85, 1980. Copyright 1980, American Medical Association, with permission)

strated in zone 1 of the Starling resistor model (see Fig. 31–8). In this case, the PCWP may be artificially high because it reflects alveolar pressure.

INDICATIONS FOR EXTUBATION

The numerous criteria underscore the fact that none are foolproof. Each roughly assesses baseline ventilation and oxygen transfer capability and reserve. Regardless of the criteria for extubation, maintenance of satisfactory arterial blood gas concentrations during a trial of spontaneous ventilation must be achieved by means of a T-tube attached to the airway or from the reservoir of an intermittent mandatory ventilation (IMV) apparatus. With IMV weaning, the patient breathes spontaneously while still being administered a preset diminishing number of assisted breaths per minute. Although use of IMV is popular, whether or not it is a superior method of weaning awaits

controlled trials of weaning methods. By decreasing mean intrathoracic pressure, IMV might decrease the incidence of pneumothorax or the depression of cardiac output that results from a high ventilating pressure or high levels of PEEP. Because cessation of mechanical ventilation may result in increased airway closure, CPAP of 2 to 10 cmH_2O may be used to decrease microatelectasis on transition from mechanical to spontaneous ventilation.

REFERENCES

1. Ashbaugh DG, Petty TL: Sepsis complicating the acute respiratory distress syndrome. Surg Gynecol Obstet 135:865, 1972
2. Harris (Pingleton) SK, Bone RC, Ruth WE: Gastrointestinal hemorrhage in a respiratory intensive care unit. Chest 72:301, 1977
3. Kramar S, Kham F, Patel S et al: Renal failure in the respiratory intensive care unit. Crit Care Med 7:263, 1979
4. Balk R, Bone RC: Classification of acute respiratory failure. Med Clin North Am 67:551, 1983
5. Campbell EJ: Respiratory failure thirty years ago. Br Med J 2:657, 1979
6. Hectman HB: Historical background. In Hectman HB (ed): Acute Respiratory Failure. Etiology and Treatment, pp 1–18. Boca Raton, Fla, CRC Press, 1979
7. Bone RC: Acute respiratory failure: Classification, differential diagnosis, and introduction to management of respiratory failure. In Burton GG, Hodgkin JE (eds): Respiratory Care: A Guide to Clinical Practice, 2nd ed. Philadelphia, JB Lippincott, 1984
8. Sheriff NS, Khan F, Logo BJ: Acute respiratory failure. Current concepts of pathophysiology and management. Med Clin North Am 57:1539, 1973
9. Ashbaugh DG, Bigelow DB, Petty TL: Acute respiratory distress in adults. Lancet 2:319, 1967
10. Ammundsson T, Kilburn K: Complications of acute respiratory failure. Ann Intern Med 70:487, 1969
11. Pingleton SG: Complications associated with the adult respiratory distress syndrome. Clin Chest Med 3:143, 1982
12. Boysen PG, Broome JA: Noninvasive monitoring of lung function during mechanical ventilation. Crit Care Clin 3:527, 1988
13. Zwillich CW, Pierson DJ, Creagh CE et al: Complications of assisted ventilation. Am J Med 57:161, 1974
14. Pontoppidan H, Griffin B, Lowenstein E: Acute respiratory failure in the adult. N Engl J Med 287:690, 1972
15. Butler PW, Bone RC, Field TF: Technology under Medicare diagnosis related groups prospective payments. Implications for medical intensive care. Chest 87:229, 1985
16. Neuth CJL: Recognition and management of respiratory failure. Pediatr Clin North Am 26:617, 1979
17. Bone RC, Fisher, CJ, Clenner TP et al: A controlled clinical trial of high-dose methylprednisone in the treatment of severe sepsis and septic shock. N Engl J Med 317:653, 1987
18. Martin L: Respiratory failure. Med Clin North Am 61:1369, 1977

19. Bone RC: Acute respiratory failure and chronic lung disease: Recent advances. Med Clin North Am 65:563, 1981

20. Garrard CS: Guidelines for treating respiratory failure. Drug Ther 71:91, 1980

21. Esbenshade AM, Newman JH, Landis PM et al: Respiratory failure after endotoxin implication in sheep: Lung mechanics and lung fluid balance. J Appl Physiol Biol 53:976, 1982

22. Bone RC: Treatment of respiratory failure due to advanced chronic obstructive lung disease. Arch Intern Med 140:1018, 1980

23. Barach AL: Physiological methods in diagnosis and treatment of asthma and emphysema. Ann Intern Med 12:454, 1938

24. Campbell EJM: Management of respiratory failure. Br Med J 2:1328, 1964

25. Campbell EJM, Gabbis T: Mask and tent for providing controlled oxygen concentration. Lancet 1:468, 1966

26. Bone RC, Pierce AK, Johnson RL: Controlled oxygen administration in acute respiratory failure in chronic obstructive pulmonary disease: A reappraisal. Am J Med 65:869, 1978

27. Mithoefer JC, Keighley MB, Karetzky M: Response of the arterial Po_2 to oxygen administration in chronic pulmonary disease. Ann Intern Med 74:328, 1971

28. Rahn HJ, Otis AB: Man's response during and after acclimatization to high altitude. Am J Physiol 157:445, 1949

29. Murray JF: Mechanism of acute respiratory failure. Am Rev Respir Dis 115:1071, 1977

30. Bone RC: Treatment of severe hypoxemia due to the adult respiratory distress syndrome. Arch Intern Med 140:85, 1980

31. Smith JL: Pathological effects due to increased oxygen in air breathed. J Physiol 24:19, 1899

32. Barber RE, Lee J, Hamilton WK: Oxygen toxicity in man—a prospective study in patients with irreversible brain damage. N Engl J Med 283:1478, 1970

33. Bone RC: Diagnosis of causes for acute respiratory distress by pressure–volume curves. Chest 70:740, 1976

THIRTY-TWO

Adult Respiratory Distress Syndrome

Leonard D. Hudson

The adult respiratory distress syndrome (ARDS) has emerged as an important clinical syndrome in the last two decades. This syndrome represents a complication that occurs in a variety of critically ill and injured patients. It may represent a single organ injury (e.g., as occurs with aspiration of gastric contents) or one of several injured organs (i.e., part of a systemic process). This is often the case when it complicates clinical sepsis or septic shock. Even when multiple-organ system failure is present, the lung injury of ARDS often is the most clinically prominent of the several failing organ systems. This may relate both to the pathogenesis and the clinical presentation of organ failure. If the multiple-organ injury is due to blood-borne mediators, the lung may be one of the most severely injured organs, since all of the blood is filtered through the pulmonary circulation. Also, often lung injury is more clinically apparent than injury to other organs because of the accompanying dyspnea, respiratory distress, and severe hypoxemia, with its attendant clinical manifestations.

DEFINITION

Adult respiratory distress syndrome is difficult to define succinctly because it is a clinical syndrome with several components. More importantly, it also represents a pathophysiologic concept in which the lung abnormalities are due to diffuse acute lung injury. It was first described as a clinical syndrome, with the term ARDS, in 1967 by Ashbaugh and coworkers at the University of Colorado.[1] Similar syndromes had been described previously, but were always related to specific clinical settings. The Denver group described a clinical syndrome occurring in a variety of surgical and medical patient settings involving critically ill or injured patients. Their clinical definition of the syndrome included obvious respiratory distress with tachypnea, severe hypoxemia (with intrapulmonary shunting as the major pathophysiologic mechanism), and diffuse infiltrates on chest roentgenogram. From their early description, they hypothesized that the pathophysiology involved acute diffuse lung injury with (1) increased permeability pulmonary edema, and (2) surfactant depletion or inactivation, leading to diffuse microatelectasis.[1] Subsequent investigations have supported this hypothesis.[2–6]

Several other terms have been applied to the same syndrome. These include descriptive pathologic terms, such as congestive atelectasis or diffuse alveolar damage; terms implying pathogenesis, such as alveolar capillary leak syndrome; or a combination of the two (increased permeability edema). Several others name the syndrome for the specific clinical situation in which it occurs such as shock lung, pump lung, posttraumatic pulmonary insufficiency, and DaNang lung—used during the Vietnam war for posttraumatic ARDS.

Adult respiratory distress syndrome is best thought of as representing a spectrum of acute diffuse lung injury.[7–10] However, a certain minimum physiologic or clinical effect should be present before the term ARDS is used. Several workers have attempted to define this syndrome by specific arterial blood gas and chest roentgenographic criteria.[11–13] Common blood gas criteria have included a PaO_2/FiO_2 ratio less than 150,[11] a PaO_2/FiO_2 ratio less than 200,[12] or a PaO_2/PaO_2 ratio less than 0.20.[13] Most definitions have required bilateral alveolar-filling infiltrates, and some have required infiltrates involving all four quadrants of the lung fields.[11–13] Some definitions have required a normal pulmonary artery wedge pressure or, at least, one that was not increased sufficiently to explain the abnormalities solely on the basis of left-sided congestive heart failure.[11,12] Since the placement of a pulmonary artery balloon flotation catheter may not be justified in many patients, the definition should be modified to require either a normal pulmonary artery wedge pressure or no clinical evidence or setting that would suggest left heart failure.[8,10]

Several clinical settings are associated with pulmonary abnormalities that might qualify for the foregoing definition of ARDS, but controversy existing over the designation of ARDS is warranted. High-altitude pulmonary edema (HAPE) is one such example. This condition fits all of the foregoing criteria; however, the course of the illness differs markedly from ARDS associated with most other clinical situations, with rapid improvement on either breathing a supplemental oxygen mixture or taking the victim to low altitude.[14] Because of this difference in clinical course, it does not seem to be clinically useful to include HAPE as a classic form of ARDS. Whether or not to include diffuse infections, such as *Pneumocystis carinii* pneumonia, as a form of ARDS is also controversial. Certainly, the clinical presentation may meet all of the defined criteria, and the hypoxemia may respond to the application of positive end-expiratory pressure (PEEP).

The term ARDS should probably be further modified by the suspected cause or associated condition for any given clinical situation. Thus, it should be stated that the patient has ARDS secondary to aspiration of gastric contents, ARDS associated with septic shock, or ARDS associated with severe blunt trauma to the lower extremities and the abdomen. This allows each clinical practitioner to make a decision on whether or not the use of the term ARDS is consistent with their own understanding and usage.

EPIDEMIOLOGY

A variety of clinical settings have been associated with ARDS. Until recently, these associations have been made from retrospective reviews of patients with ARDS.[15] Recently, studies have attempted to define clinical risk factors for ARDS and prospectively follow patients with these risks for the development of ARDS to determine the incidence of this syndrome (Table 32–1).[13,16,17] The two most important risk factors are septic shock and severe multiple trauma. Septic shock is synonymous with sepsis syndrome or clinical sepsis.[18] *Sepsis syndrome* is defined by (1) several clinical findings indicating infection or inflammation such as abnormal white blood count, fever, or known infection (but not necessarily requiring positive blood cultures), plus (2) evidence of associated hemodynamic abnormalities manifest either by hypotension, otherwise unexplained metabolic acidosis, or a measured low systemic vascular resistance.[11,16] Sepsis syndrome defined in this way is associated with the highest incidence of ARDS for any single risk factor—approximately 40%.[17] On the other hand, bacteremia itself (but not necessarily associated with any particular clinical syndrome) is associated with a relatively low incidence of ARDS, approximately 4%.[13] Trauma, using the findings of (1) multiple long-bone or unstable pelvic fractures in an intensive care unit (ICU) patient, (2) localized lung contusion, or (3) the requirement of greater than 15 units of blood for emergency resuscitation as markers of severe trauma, is associated with a 15% to 25% incidence of ARDS.[17] However, if these markers are found in combination, the incidence increases to 40% to 50%. Other commonly occurring clinical situations associated with approximately a 10% risk of ARDS include aspiration of gastric contents and drug overdose requiring mechanical ventilation. Less common clinical risks include severe pancreatitis, inhalation injuries, and near-drowning.[15] Severe head trauma, without other associated trauma, was not found to be a particularly significant risk factor.[17] Many other clinical situations have been associated with ARDS in either single-case reports or small series.[15] Obviously, the frequency of the clinical risk factors and, to some extent, the incidence of ARDS development will depend on the population of patients seen at any given medical center.

The clinical risk factors that have been studied to date appear to be synergistic in their effect on the frequency of ARDS development.[13,17] When any of the clinical risks are added together, the likelihood of ARDS more than doubles (see Table 32–1). An

Table 32—1 Incidence of ARDS Following Single or Multiple Risks in Study at Harborview Medical Center, Seattle, Washington

CLINICAL CONDITION	INCIDENCE OF ARDS				
	As Single Risk (No.)	(%)	As Multiple Risk (No.)	(%)	Total (%)
Sepsis syndrome	39/94	41	15/31	48	43
Aspiration	6/62	10	15/45	33	20
Drug overdose	8/76	11	7/18	39	16
Near-drowning	3/6	50	4/6	67	58
Multiple transfusions	18/53	34	18/36	50	40
Pulmonary contusion	13/72	18	23/65	35	26
Multiple fractures	5/52	10	18/48	38	23
Head injury	6/100	6	8/28	29	11
Total	98/520	19	58/138	42	156/658 24

(Maunder RJ, Hudson LD: The adult respiratory distress syndrome. In Simmons DH (ed): Current Pulmonology, Vol 7, pp 97–116. Chicago, Year Book Medical Publishers, 1986)

exception to this is sepsis syndrome. Other risks added to sepsis syndrome are associated with a smaller increase in the ARDS risk, presumably because sepsis syndrome itself already is associated with such a high likelihood of the development of ARDS.

The time from recognition of the clinical risk to the onset of ARDS varies from occurring simultaneously to up to 72 hours.[13,17] About half the cases of ARDS develop within 24 hours of recognition of the clinical risk; the development of ARDS is rare once 72 hours have elapsed, unless a second clinical risk, such as sepsis syndrome, has developed in the meantime. Often the recognition of clinical sepsis or sepsis syndrome is accompanied with some degree of acute lung injury (manifest by hypoxemia) and often full blown ARDS.[19] Lesser degrees of lung injury may progress over the next several hours to full-blown ARDS.[19] This relatively short interval between recognition of sepsis syndrome and development of ARDS may be because once all the criteria for sepsis syndrome are met, the process has been ongoing for some time. Risks that involve direct lung injury by aspiration, such as near-drowning or aspiration of gastric contents, also are usually associated with a short interval to development of ARDS. Recognition of the clinical risks are useful to enable monitoring of the patient for development of progressive lung injury, with early intervention. It is hoped that once the mechanisms leading to lung injury are better understood, recognition of clinical risks that have a high likelihood of ARDS development will permit early intervention

that might prevent or modify the development of lung injury.

The breathing of high oxygen tensions has been associated with ARDS-like lung injury in several animal species.[20–23] However, considerable interspecies variation in susceptibility to oxygen toxicity exists, and these data are difficult to extrapolate to humans. Determination of the human susceptibility to oxygen toxicity is further complicated because fractions of inspired oxygen (FiO_2) of the magnitude probably required for injury—greater than 0.7—are used only in patients who already have relatively diffuse lung abnormalities. In addition, some animal model studies have reported that prior lung injury both protects against (the majority) and increases susceptibility to lung injury, perhaps depending, in part, on the type, mechanism, or timing of the prior injury.

PATHOPHYSIOLOGY

MORPHOLOGIC CHANGES

The lungs of patients with ARDS are heavy and congested owing to the presence of protein-rich edema fluid.[24,25] The early description by the Denver group described the lungs at autopsy as having the appearance of liver.[1] Hyaline membranes are apparent on microscopic examination, caused by the aggregation of fibrin and other proteins in the alveolar space. Hyaline membrane formation is a nonspecific finding and is identical with that seen in premature infants with infant respiratory distress syndrome (RDS). In fact, this similar morphologic appearance, in part, was responsible for the choice of the term ARDS. Alveolar flooding is present as well as microatelectasis. Inflammatory cells, particularly neutrophils, are present within the alveolar space. This accumulation of neutrophils may reflect the possible role of malignant intravascular inflammation in the pathogenesis of the diffuse alveolar injury or may simply be a response to that injury.

Ultrastructural abnormalities, demonstrated by electron microscopy, include early cytopathic changes of type I pneumocytes.[24,25] Pulmonary vascular endothelial cells are also affected, but these changes are less striking. As the course of the syndrome progresses, proliferation of type II pneumocytes is seen.[24,25] Deposition of collagen can be demonstrated within several days following injury.[26] The collagen accumulation is nonspecific, being similar in appearance to other more chronic scarring processes of the lung.[26]

PHYSIOLOGIC CHANGES

The primary physiologic abnormalities associated with ARDS involve impaired gas exchange and altered lung mechanics. The severe hypoxemia is due to pulmonary venoarterial shunting owing to the alveolar flooding and collapse. In addition, increased dead space occurs; although the arterial $PaCO_2$ may remain normal, this is at the expense of increased minute ventilation requirements.

Low lung volumes, measured experimentally as low functional residual capacity, are uniformly present and correlate with the oxygenation abnormality. Lung compliance usually is significantly reduced, again presumably caused by alveolar flooding and microatelectasis. Pulmonary hypertension has been reported as a common finding in some series in the later stages of ARDS.[27,28] An abnormality in the relationship between tissue oxygen utilization and oxygen availability has also been described in patients with ARDS.[29,30] Usually, tissue oxygen utilization is independent of oxygen supply, but oxygen consumption has been shown to be dependent upon supply in ARDS subjects as well as in other experimental situations.

PRESUMED PATHOPHYSIOLOGY

The foregoing described morphologic and physiologic abnormalities are due to two consequences of acute diffuse lung injury: (1) capillary endothelial and alveolar epithelial injury, with increased permeability;[12,31–35] and (2) abnormal surfactant.[2–6] The first stage of the increased permeability pulmonary edema is leakage of protein-rich fluid into the interstitial space. The interstitial edema is associated with only mild gas exchange abnormalities. In response to the interstitial edema, the lung lymphatic drainage increases severalfold in an attempt to keep the lung "dry."[36] When the protective lymphatic drainage mechanism is overwhelmed and if alveolar epithelial injury has also occurred, then fluid leaks into the alveolar space with subsequent intrapulmonary shunting of blood and profound hypoxemia.

The exact pathophysiology of the surfactant abnormality is less well known. The reduced surfactant could be due to inactivation by the presence of increased protein in the alveolar space. Also, surfactant secretion by the alveolar type II pneumocytes might be diminished. Whatever the etiology, the abnormality in surfactant is associated with the development of a diffuse microatelectasis. Although the surfactant abnormality is a secondary phenomenon in ARDS, as opposed to a more primary role in infant respiratory distress syndrome, its effect on the course of the syndrome is quite likely to be extremely significant. The relatively prolonged clinical course, with slow therapeutic response compared with that seen with cardiogenic pulmonary edema, could be due either to persistence of the microatelectasis or to continuing injury or failure of the permeability defect to heal.

MECHANISMS AND MEDIATORS OF INJURY

The source of injury in ARDS can either be direct (alveolar) or indirect (blood borne). Direct injury is due to aspiration or inhalation of toxic substances, such as acid gastric contents, irritating gases, or high fraction of inspired oxygen with production of toxic oxygen radicals. Most ARDS cases occur with an indirect or blood-borne injury such as occurs with sepsis syndrome or trauma. Over the last decade, considerable research attention has been focused on elucidation of the mechanisms of this injury and the mediators involved. Although considerable progress has been made, the exact mechanisms responsible for lung injury have not yet been determined. The most prevalent theory is that the injury is due to uncontrolled or malignant intravascular inflammation. Inflammation usually is a beneficial process and is a necessary part of the healing response of the body to any type of insult. In ARDS

Table 32—2 Proposed Mediators of Acute Lung Injury

Formed blood elements
  Neutrophils
  Platelets
Chemoattractants
  Complement fragments
  Leukotriene-B$_4$
  Platelet-activating factor
  Bacterial peptides
  Macrophage-derived chemotactic factor
Neutrophil-related mediators of cell damage
  Oxygen radicals (H$_2$O$_2$, O$_2^-$, ·OH)
  Proteolytic enzymes including neutrophil elastase
  Phospholipase products
Miscellaneous (including cytokines)
  Tumor necrosis factor (TNF)
  Interleukin-1
  Endotoxin
  Kallikrein
  Coagulation factors

it is hypothesized that the inflammatory process itself is injurious.

Many possible mediators of injury have been proposed.[31,37–53] Some of these are shown in Table 32–2. It is likely that no single mediator is responsible for the injury and that either a cascade of mediators or parallel but interactive pathways are involved.

Many investigators believe that neutrophils play a central role in the pathogenesis of ARDS.[40,53–63] Evidence for this hypothesis comes from studies of patients with ARDS,[62,63] as well as from investigations in animal models. It has been demonstrated that neutrophils accumulate in the lungs of patients with ARDS as well as in the lungs of animals with sepsis or endotoxemia.[58] Neutrophils can synthesize and release products that are capable of tissue injury, including proteolytic enzymes, toxic oxygen species, and phospholipid products. These factors are involved in bacterial killing, but they can also cause tissue injury. In addition, many of the other mediators that have been found in animal models or in patients with ARDS have neutrophil chemotactic properties. Finally, a variety of studies have found that depletion of circulating neutrophils in experimental animals can prevent or markedly reduce the lung injury.[64–69] However, other studies have shown that the depletion of neutrophils was *not* protective.[70–75] These studies, coupled with the description of

ARDS developing in patients with marked neutropenia,[76–79] have challenged the concept that neutrophils are always involved in the injury process.[80] I sense that a probable consensus of current workers in the field favors the view that neutrophils play a central role in many, but not all, cases of ARDS.

Several of the potential mediators shown in Table 32–2 have been studied to determine whether their presence in patients at risk predicts the development of ARDS. Measurements of these substances have been made in the sera of patients with clinical conditions indicating a high risk for development of ARDS. The factors studied include activated complement, decreased fibronectin, and arachidonic acid metabolites.[17,81] Abnormal levels were present in patients who subsequently went on to develop ARDS, but abnormalities of similar magnitude were also present in patients, with the same clinical risk factors, who did not go on to develop full-blown lung injury. Therefore, none of these implicated mediators have yet been found to be helpful in predicting the development of ARDS. These studies also indicate that the mediators studied are, by themselves, not sufficient to cause ARDS. However, an important pathogenetic role for these mediators is still possible.

MANAGEMENT OF THE PATIENT WITH ADULT RESPIRATORY DISTRESS SYNDROME

All of the respiratory care treatment modalities discussed in this chapter are covered in detail in other chapters of this text. Discussion in this chapter will be limited to their application to patients with ARDS, including indications and goals of therapy. The reader should look to the other relevant chapters for information on all the technical aspects of their application and a more complete discussion of potential complications.

OXYGENATION AND MECHANICAL VENTILATION

Intrapulmonary shunting of blood is the primary physiologic abnormality in ARDS, and much of the respiratory therapeutic efforts are primarily aimed at correcting the hypoxemia. The goals of therapy are (1) to provide adequate tissue delivery of oxygen (the product of arterial oxygen content and cardiac output), while (2) avoiding potentially toxic levels of F$_I$O$_2$. The first of these goals requires achieving nearly complete oxygen saturation of the hemoglobin (>90%), since oxygen content is primarily dependent upon oxyhemoglobin saturation. This usually can be achieved by a PaO_2 above 60 mmHg. Whether or not a further margin of safety is prudent depends on the patient's clinical status, including the degree of hemodynamic stability. Avoiding or minimizing the risk of oxygen toxicity raises the question: What FIO_2 level is toxic to the lung? Although an FIO_2 of 0.8 or higher has been demonstrated to cause direct injury to lung tissue, there is no clear agreement on what level of FIO_2 is not toxic to lung parenchyma. Smaller concentrations of oxygen have been shown to have other toxic pulmonary effects in animal models, including a decrease in mucociliary function and impaired bacterial clearance. The clinical importance of these effects in patients with ARDS remains unclear.

Administration of Supplemental Oxygen

Parenchymal oxygen toxicity is related to both dose and length of exposure. Although human oxygen toxicity data are sparse, high levels of oxygen administered for relatively short periods (hours to 1 or 2 days) are considered relatively safe. Therefore, initially, a high FIO_2 should be administered to achieve adequate arterial oxygenation. Then, the level of FIO_2 should be decreased to the lowest level that still provides adequate arterial oxygen saturation. If this level is still in a potentially toxic range, other methods to improve oxygenation, primarily application of PEEP, should be attempted. Some clinicians feel this potentially toxic level is any $FIO_2 > 0.4$, whereas others accept a level of 0.7 as relatively safe. Currently, I like to see the FIO_2 at or below 0.6 in patients with ARDS. However, firm oxygen toxicity data in humans indicating the superiority of any given FIO_2 level over another are lacking.

Role of Mechanical Ventilation

There are three potential roles for using mechanical ventilation in patients with ARDS: (1) improvement in oxygenation, (2) decrease in work of breathing and improved patient comfort and, infrequently, (3) treatment of respiratory acidosis.

Improvement of oxygenation with mechanical ventilation has not been studied in a consistent way in patients with ARDS. However, clinicians have commented on the observation that oxygenation can improve with mechanical ventilation alone before the application of PEEP. We noticed this in a study of early application of PEEP in patients at high risk for developing ARDS.[11] We required treatment of both the control group and the experimental group with mechanical ventilation (a minimum of 4 breaths per minute); mechanical ventilation was started in the experimental group before applying PEEP. One of the entry criteria was that the patient be above a certain level of oxygenation to be certain that the patient had not already developed full-blown ARDS. We frequently found that patients at risk did not meet this criterion (i.e., had more severe hypoxemia) while breathing spontaneously. Once mechanical ventilation was started, the next blood gas analysis often showed improvement in oxygenation. Presumably, this improvement in oxygenation was due to a correction of atelectasis that may not be apparent on the chest x-ray film. Investigators from the University of Florida have shown, in animal models of near-drowning, that the combination of both mechanical ventilation and PEEP was necessary to improve oxygenation in animals with freshwater,[82] but not saltwater, drowning.[83] They hypothesized that freshwater resulted in a more severe abnormality of surfactant and more severe atelectasis than aspiration of saltwater.

Carbon dioxide removal is commonly considered to be normal in patients with ARDS, but, in fact, it is not. Dead space measurements are elevated[84–86] and, although arterial PCO_2 usually is normal or low, the minute ventilation required to achieve this usually is markedly increased. The subjective discomfort associated with maintaining a high minute ventilation (e.g., > 20 L/min) often is reduced with mechanical ventilation.

The modes of ventilation most commonly employed in patients with ARDS are intermittent mandatory ventilation (IMV) or assist–control (A/C), each mode having its strong advocates. The proponents of IMV point to the physiologic advantages associated with the spontaneous portion of the breathing. The major physiologic advantage in this situation is enhanced venous return, as opposed to the tendency for decreased venous return and, thus, decreased cardiac output with both mechanical ventilation breaths and PEEP. Assist–control proponents argue that, in patients with severe ARDS, a high mandatory rate of IMV is necessary to adequately reduce the work of breathing and, consequently, the beneficial physiologic effects of IMV are not achieved. If metabolic demands and, therefore, minute ventilation demands, increase in a patient with already very high minute ventilation requirements, a patient breathing by IMV may not be able to adequately respond to these changes. This is more easily achieved in the patient breathing with the A/C mode, who simply needs to trigger the ventilator breaths at a more rapid rate. It should be noted that some patients who are using A/C continue to actively inhale, using their muscles of respiration throughout inhalation, despite the fact that a ventilator breath has been triggered.[87] This effect can often be countered by appropriate manipulation of the ventilator settings, particularly increasing the inspiratory flow rate. Many, if not most, patients with ARDS can be safely and effectively managed with either IMV or A/C. In patients with extremely high minute ventilation, I prefer A/C for the arguments given in the foregoing.

Inverse ratio ventilation (IRV) is a form of mechanical ventilation in which the inflation is held for a longer proportion of the respiratory cycle (see Chaps. 21 and 22). Inverse ratio ventilation has been effective in some patients with very severe ARDS whose oxygenation is inadequate, despite conventional mechanical ventilation and PEEP.[88,89] However, one group demonstrated that improved oxygenation was associated with an increase in mean airway pressure.[89] Because of this, the disadvantages of IRV are similar to those of PEEP, especially a potential reduction in cardiac output. When IRV is employed, the patient must be carefully monitored, and the application of IRV should be considered as an individual therapeutic trial. Thus, application of IRV requires experience and constant attention, with very careful monitoring. Currently, we limit a trial of IRV to the situation in which other more conventional (or familiar) forms of ventilation, such as IMV with PEEP or A/C with PEEP, are failing.

Use of high-frequency ventilation in animal models of acute lung injury was associated with improved oxygenation and decreased pathologic changes.[90,91] However, a multicenter controlled trial of high-frequency jet ventilation (HFJV) in patients with ARDS found no advantage over conventional ventilation with PEEP.[92] Another crossover trial of HFJV in a variety of patients being successfully ventilated with conventional ventilation also found no significant clinical advantage to HFJV.[93] These authors found that HFJV was not able to provide adequate alveolar ventilation in 7 of the 65 patients studied. All 7 of their ventilatory failures with jet ventilation occurred in the 22 patients with ARDS in their study population.

Extracorporeal Membrane Oxygenation and Carbon Dioxide Removal

Oxygen can be added and carbon dioxide removed from the blood by diverting some of the body's blood to a circuit outside of the body that contains a membrane providing a diffusion gradient across the membrane for oxygen and carbon dioxide. A multicenter National Institutes of Health (NIH)-sponsored study of extracorporeal membrane oxygenation (ECMO) in patients with severe ARDS found no difference in survival rates between patients randomized to treatment with ECMO versus treatment with conventional mechanical ventilation and PEEP, despite that ECMO was technically successful in improving arterial oxygenation.[94] More recently, Gattinoni and colleagues from Italy reported improved survival in a group of patients treated with extracorporeal carbon dioxide removal, compared with a historical control group treated with conventional methods.[95] Their method differed from that used in the ECMO trial in that mechanical ventilation was minimal. The lungs were kept inflated by four mechanical breaths per minute at a low tidal volume and a low level of PEEP; oxygenation was achieved primarily by passive diffusion or convection, using an elevated FIO_2. Carbon dioxide was removed through an extracorporeal membrane. These investigators hypothesize that conventional mechanical ventilation actually causes further injury to the already injured lungs of the ARDS patient. They believe that survival was enhanced in their patients by placing the lungs "at rest" and preventing or minimizing this additional injury. Currently, this method is being studied in a randomized controlled fashion in an NIH-sponsored study.[96] The number of patients studied, to date, is too small to allow conclusions. However, interestingly, both the extracorporeal carbon dioxide removal group and the conventional ventilation group (following a strict protocol for management) show improved survival, compared with the historical control group from the original ECMO trial, the same historical control group used by the Italian investigators.

Positive End-Expiratory Pressure

A positive pressure applied throughout exhalation, termed PEEP when applied with mechanical ventilation, and continuous positive airway pressure (CPAP), when applied during spontaneous ventilation, is a mainstay in the management of the patient with ARDS. Its successful use in these patients and in a relevant animal model was first described in reports from the Denver group who named this syndrome.[1,97,98] PEEP clearly increases lung volume, restoring the decreased functional residual capacity (FRC) toward normal, with an accompanying improvement in arterial oxygenation.[99–101] A major controversy exists whether PEEP is "therapeutic" to the lung injury process in the ARDS patient or simply supportive. By supportive, I mean that PEEP helps to achieve the oxygenation goals reviewed in the foregoing, but has no significant effect on the underlying disease process—that is, PEEP supports improved gas exchange, while the body's defense processes repair the lung injury. If PEEP were therapeutic, in addition to its effect on improved oxygenation, one would expect its application to result in (1) improved survival, (2) shortened duration of illness, or (3) some other manifestation of lessened severity of illness. To date, no experimental evidence has indicated that PEEP is therapeutic (i.e., it favorably alters the basic lung injury process). Although this possibility remains, the consensus of clinical investigators in this field (although with some articulate exceptions) consider PEEP and mechanical ventilation to be supportive. The answer to this controversy is extremely important in that it dictates the logical approach to PEEP application. If PEEP is simply supportive, then the lowest level of PEEP should be employed that provides adequate arterial oxygenation and allows a reduction in the FIO_2 to a nontoxic range. However, if PEEP is therapeutic, then higher levels of PEEP would be indicated, levels that, in themselves, carry a somewhat higher risk of adverse effects and that may require other potentially adverse countertherapies, such as a greater intravenous volume administration.

The available evidence favoring the supportive nature of PEEP includes three controlled trials, one in patients at high risk for developing ARDS,[11] one in patients with an early mild form of acute lung injury and moderate hypoxemia,[102] and another trial in patients with postoperative respiratory failure.[103] A ramdomized controlled trial of the early application of PEEP in patients known to be at high risk for ARDS failed to affect the incidence of ARDS development.[11] However, this study is controversial because previous studies of early PEEP application concluded that some protective effect was present.[104,105] Another study in patients with a mild degree of lung injury (i.e., with an oxygenation abnormality that did not meet the criteria for ARDS) found no difference in outcome from application of

PEEP to simply provide adequate oxygenation, compared with application of high levels of PEEP to reduce the shunt to 15% or less.[102] A controlled trial in postoperative patients in a surgical intensive care unit randomized those patients developing a $PaO_2/FIO_2 < 200$ to receive either "recruitive PEEP" [titrated to a goal of halving the baseline venous admixture ($\dot{Q}va/\dot{Q}T$)] or "supportive PEEP" (to maintain $PaO_2 > 60$ mmHg, while lowering FIO_2 to 0.5).[103] Although these patients did not necessarily meet diagnostic criteria of ARDS, other than abnormal oxygenation, the two groups of patients were similar by comparison of demographic and physiologic features. Patients receiving recruitive PEEP, when compared with patients receiving supportive PEEP, had a significantly increased incidence of hypotension (55% versus 0%), pneumothorax (20% versus 0%), and death during PEEP treatment (27% versus 4%). After PEEP treatment, deaths in each group were similar (19% and 15%). These authors concluded that the use of PEEP to achieve their "recruitive" goals in this group of patients (postoperative respiratory failure, but not necessarily ARDS) may be harmful. In addition, application of PEEP in animal models of acute lung injury have failed to affect the lung lesions or resolution of injury.[106,107]

The major adverse effects of PEEP in patients with ARDS are a fall in cardiac output[101,108,109] and the potential risk of barotrauma, particularly pneumothorax, resulting from alveolar rupture.[103,110] The decrease in cardiac output can be due to either a decrease in venous return[101,109,111,113] or an increase in pulmonary vascular resistance.[109,112,114,115] The decrease in venous return is related to an increase in intrathoracic pressure. This pressure is transmitted, in part, from the alveolar space to the pleural space and affects the potentially collapsible great veins returning through the thorax to the right atrium. The degree of transmission of the alveolar pressure to the pleural space is in part related to the lung compliance. The stiffer the lung, the less pressure is transmitted. However, even in patients with ARDS with very stiff lungs, some degree of the increased alveolar pressure with PEEP is transmitted to the pleural space and can affect venous return.

Another variable in the effect on venous return is the volume status of the patient. Patients who are hypovolemic have an increased propensity to develop a decrease in venous return and, thereby, a reduction in cardiac output at lower levels of PEEP application than in patients who are euvolemic.[109,112] Accordingly, the philosophy of PEEP application must be reconciled with the fluid management philosophy in the ARDS patient.

The increased lung volume resulting from PEEP results in stretching of alveolar capillaries and a reduction in their lumen, and, thereby, a potential increase in pulmonary vascular resistance. This increase in pulmonary vascular resistance can also reduce cardiac output. Although there is some evidence that this phenomenon does occur in ARDS patients with PEEP application, the predominant effect has been primarily with high levels of PEEP (20 cmH$_2$O or greater).[115] At the lower levels of PEEP that are more commonly employed, the reduction in venous return appears to be the predominant mechanism in the reduced cardiac output.[113]

The potential reduction in cardiac output is extremely important in considering the goals of PEEP therapy because of its effect on tissue oxygen delivery. One of the overall goals in the ARDS patient is to maintain or increase the tissue oxygen delivery. Tissue oxygen delivery is a function of the product of arterial oxygen content (primarily dependent upon arterial oxygen saturation) and cardiac output. If arterial oxygenation improves with PEEP, but there is a greater reduction in cardiac output, then oxygen delivery to the tissues will be impaired, and the patient will be potentially harmed. Some investigators have defined the goal of PEEP therapy—so-called optimal-PEEP or best-PEEP—as the PEEP level at which tissue oxygen delivery is maximal.[116] Although there is some validity to the rationale behind this concept, use of the absolute peak value for arterial oxygen content multiplied by cardiac output as a marker of the optimal PEEP level oversimplifies the clinical situation. First, the arterial oxygen content is very dependent upon the FiO$_2$ that is administered. If arterial oxygen desaturation is present on the baseline or control arterial blood gas value, then PEEP is likely to significantly improve arterial oxygen content by increasing arterial oxygen saturation. In this situation, the value for tissue oxygen delivery might increase, even if there is a subsequent reduction in cardiac output, as long as the relative percentage increase in arterial oxygen content is greater than the percentage decrease in cardiac output. However, if the FiO$_2$ is increased before PEEP application—for example, to 1.0—raising the arterial Po$_2$ above 60 and, therefore, raising the arterial oxygen saturation to greater than 90%, PEEP is unlikely to cause a major change in the arterial oxygen content, since the oxygen saturation of the hemoglobin is already nearly complete.

In this situation, PEEP application could result in a marked improvement in PaO$_2$, allowing reduction of the FiO$_2$ to a nontoxic level, but would have relatively little effect on oxygen saturation and arterial oxygen content. If a small, and possibly clinically unimportant, fall in cardiac output also occurred, the value for tissue oxygen transport might decrease. However, the PEEP level at which this occurred might be judged to be more beneficial than the previous level for which the calculated tissue oxygen delivery was slightly higher. This also raises the question of what magnitude of change in any of these values is clinically important. This is a judgment that must be made by the clinician understanding the underlying physiologic principles.

Another consideration is whether tissue oxygenation is already adequate. If arterial oxygen saturation is well above 90% at an FiO$_2$ of, say 0.5, and there is no evidence of extrapulmonary organ dysfunction, then further increases in PEEP to increase the arterial oxygen content by the relatively minor effect of increasing dissolved oxygen in the serum (associated with a substantial increase in arterial PaO$_2$) seems to be an artificial goal of therapy, unless clinical improvement could be demonstrated. No convincing evidence of clinical improvement in this situation has yet been demonstrated. Thus, the most rational goal for PEEP therapy seems to be an arbitrary level of adequate arterial oxygenation, chosen by the clinician, and an arbitrary value of FiO$_2$ that is likely to be nontoxic, also chosen by the knowledgeable clinician. A reasonable goal is an arterial oxygen saturation of 90% or greater at an FiO$_2$ of 0.5 or 0.6.[117,118] At the same time, it is extremely important that PEEP not result in a clinically important decrease in tissue oxygen delivery, and, therefore, the possibility of a reduction in cardiac output must be constantly kept in mind during PEEP application.

Measurement of mixed venous oxygen saturation (S$\bar{v}$O$_2$) has been advocated as a means of assessing tissue oxygen delivery. This can be done either by drawing blood from the pulmonary artery through a pulmonary artery catheter or by using special pulmonary artery catheters that include an oximeter in the tip and continuously monitor mixed venous oxygen saturation. Monitoring S$\bar{v}$O$_2$ to follow tissue oxygen delivery assumes that the tissues will increase their extraction of oxygen in response to a reduction in tissue oxygen delivery and, thus, the mixed venous oxygen saturation will fall. There are two problems with using this method to monitor optimal PEEP application. The first has already been discussed in principle—that is, that systemic oxygen delivery may not be changed much with a PEEP application that is successful in allowing reduction in the FIO_2. Thus, $S\bar{v}O_2$ would not be expected to change in this circumstance. The second deals with the use of monitoring $S\bar{v}O_2$ to detect a reduction in tissue oxygenation associated with PEEP application. Although a reduction in mixed venous oxygenation almost certainly means a decrease in tissue oxygenation, as discussed in the foregoing assumption, it has now been well described that tissue oxygen delivery may be reduced in a variety of clinical circumstances and by several different mechanisms, without a concomitant change in $S\bar{v}O_2$. Usually, oxygen consumption is independent of oxygen delivery. In ARDS and sepsis, as well as other clinical situations, oxygen consumption may become dependent on oxygen delivery.[29,30] Therefore, when tissue oxygen delivery is reduced, tissue oxygen consumption or extraction may also decrease, resulting in no change in $S\bar{v}O_2$. Therefore, one cannot rely on monitoring of $S\bar{v}O_2$ to detect a reduction in oxygen delivery. In fact, maintenance of a constant value may provide a false sense of security. Because of

this, we have elected not to routinely monitor $S\bar{v}O_2$ in patients with ARDS in our unit.

The other potential adverse effect of PEEP is barotrauma.[103,108,110,119,120] Although there is little actual evidence demonstrating that barotrauma is directly related to PEEP application, most clinicians still feel that this is a potential adverse effect. It seems reasonable that total static compliance might be associated with risk for alveolar rupture,[108,110,120] although there are no prospective studies to show this and, because of the dangers involved, there are likely to be none. The rationale for this relationship is based on the reasonable assumption that a persistent and progressive fall in total static compliance with PEEP therapy is associated with major regions of the lung being near their maximal distention. When this occurs, further increases in pressure result in relatively minor increases in volume; hence, compliance (change in volume per change in pressure) decreases.

Suter and associates suggested another use for measuring compliance, suggesting that maximal oxygen delivery occurs at the point of maximal pulmonary compliance.[116] However, it is not intuitively apparent why cardiac output and compli-

Table 32–3 Elements of a PEEP Trial

A. Set the goals of PEEP therapy
  1. Adequate arterial oxygenation (e.g., $PaO_2 \geq 60$ mmHg and O_2 saturation $\geq 90\%$)
  2. Level of FIO_2 that is probably nontoxic (e.g., $FIO_2 < 0.5$; desired value may vary with the degree of initial shunt—i.e., the level of FIO_2 required initially)
B. Determine means of monitoring
  1. Beneficial effects
    a. Increase in PaO_2
    b. Adequate O_2 saturation
  2. Toxic effects
    a. Decrease in cardiac output
      1) Systemic blood pressure, mentation, urine output—versus
      2) Cardiac output measurement (requires pulmonary artery catheter—see Table 32–4)
    b. Risk of alveolar rupture
      1) Total static compliance
C. Increase PEEP by increments of 5 cmH$_2$O (in rare instances 2.5 cmH$_2$O)
  1. 15 to 30 minutes duration at each new increment
  2. Repeat monitoring measurements after each incremental change
D. Stop PEEP trial when:
  1. Selected goals are achieved (the goal for a reduction in FIO_2 requires a clinical judgment—has the PaO_2 increased adequately to permit the FIO_2 to be decreased to the selected goal? Then reduce FIO_2 to test this judgment), or
  2. Evidence of possible toxicity occurs
    a. Significant reduction in indicators reflecting cardiac output or in the thermodilution cardiac output measurement
    b. Significant decrease in compliance
E. If toxicity occurs before desired goal is achieved, reassess the clinical situation and determine need for other therapy, for example, intravenous volume administration if cardiac output has fallen
F. After the PEEP level has been selected, consider adjustment of the other ventilator settings, especially tidal volume (V$_T$/compliance curve, see text)

---

ance should both fall at the same PEEP level, and other investigators have been unable to confirm Suter's findings.[121]

How then should PEEP be applied in a practical fashion to patients with ARDS? I still encourage the use of a PEEP trial that should include several elements.[122] These elements are shown in Table 32–3. The two major clinical decisions to be made before starting the PEEP trial are first, selecting the goals of therapy as already discussed, and, second, selecting the appropriate means of monitoring for both determining when these goals have been achieved and avoiding the potentially adverse effects. Arterial blood gas levels should be measured in all patients during PEEP application and total static compliance should be measured in all patients receiving mechanical ventilation and PEEP application. Therefore, the major decision is whether to follow clinical findings that reflect cardiac output, including systemic blood pressure, mental status changes, and change in urine output, or whether to place a pulmonary artery balloon flotation catheter and measure cardiac output by the thermodilution technique. Guidelines to be considered in the decision to place a pulmonary artery catheter are listed in Table 32–4.

Once the level of PEEP to be maintained has been selected by a systematic PEEP trial, the other ventilator settings should be reviewed and adjusted, if necessary. This particularly includes changing the FIO_2 and tidal volume (V_T). The FIO_2 should be reduced to the lowest level that still achieves adequate arterial saturation. This can often be done using a pulse oximeter, without need for further blood gas measurements until the FIO_2 is selected that is likely to be maintained. Consideration should be given to a reduction in V_T at this point. The PEEP trial can be performed with a V_T of approximately 10 mL/kg or one chosen by plotting V_T against compliance and choosing the V_T with the highest compliance. Some indirect evidence supports a relationship between high tidal volumes and the risk of barotrauma.[110] Since the application of PEEP increases resting lung volumes (functional residual capacity), possibly, in part, by reversal of microatelectasis, it might be possible to use a lower V_T than that required before PEEP administration, to reduce the risk of barotrauma. On the other hand, changing V_T might result in a change in oxygenation (i.e., change the optimal PEEP level). Therefore, if V_T is lowered, arterial blood gas levels should be checked before and after the change. Again, it seems reasonable to use the total static compliance measured with inflation hold at vary-

Table 32–4 Guidelines Favoring Pulmonary Artery Balloon Flotation Catheter Placement Before (or During) PEEP Trial in ARDS Patients

1. Clinical evidence of shock or possible hypovolemia (e.g., hypotension, mental status change without other explanation, oliguria)
2. Unknown vascular volume status in patient at risk for hypovolemia (e.g., trauma victim with significant blood loss)
3. Known cardiac disease (possible need for higher cardiac filling volumes and pressures to achieve optimal cardiac output)
4. PEEP level > 15 cmH$_2$O in euvolemic patients

ing V_Ts to make this adjustment. The V_T associated with the highest total static compliance can be used as a determinant of the final V_T.

FLUID MANAGEMENT

Intravascular fluid management must be carefully approached in ARDS patients. Excessive fluid will easily leak into the injured lungs with their increased permeability, worsening pulmonary edema and further impairing gas exchange. This can occur at only mild to moderate elevations in intravascular pressure or even at normal pulmonary vascular pressures. On the other hand, hypovolemia may result in a decrease in cardiac output and impairment of tissue oxygen delivery and may increase the risk of developing renal injury and acute renal failure. Simmons and coworkers from San Antonio, in a retrospective review of prospectively collected data, showed a correlation of progressive weight gain in patients who ultimately die of ARDS, as opposed to progressive weight loss in those who ultimately survive.[123] This correlation must be interpreted with some caution, as it may be a reflection of the patient's underlying physiologic state, rather than a result of inappropriate fluid therapy. For example, patients who ultimately die of ARDS often have continuing sepsis, with diffuse intravascular leak and widespread third-spacing of fluid. These patients may require greater amounts of intravascular volume administration simply to maintain adequate systemic blood pressure. We have recently confirmed the San Antonio group's finding of an association between positive fluid balance and increasing mortality in patients with ARDS. However, when analyzed by multiple logistic regression, this factor was negligible when considered along with other variables.[124]

A controversy over whether to administer colloid or crystalloid intravenous solutions to patients with ARDS has continued for nearly two decades. Proponents of both sides can quote literature to support their views. It is our practice to primarily administer crystalloid solutions or, when volume is needed and the hematocrit is below normal, to administer blood. This is based on the evidence that, at least early in ARDS, large-molecular-weight substances, including albumin, can leak from the vascular space through the injured vascular and epithelial barriers and can be recovered from the alveolar space. The rationale behind administration of colloids is that they should stay in the intravascular space and draw fluid from the edematous lungs back into the intravascular space where it can be removed through the kidneys. However, if the colloids that are administered leak into the lungs, not only will there be no beneficial effect, but, in fact, the colloids may tend to hold additional fluid in the interstitium and alveolar space of the lung. If a clinically practical marker of repair of the lung permeability defect were available, then it would make sense to administer colloid solution once the permeability defect was repaired, or at least when particularly large-molecular-weight substances might remain in the vascular space. However, such a practical clinical tool is currently unavailable. Thus, we continue to rely primarily on crystalloid solution and blood administration.

Some workers measure serum colloid osmotic pressure and recommend administration of albumin or colloid when this measurement is low and thereby could be contributing to the development of alveolar edema. We have not followed this practice in patients with ARDS, based on the same reasoning as above, that is, even in the face of low serum colloid osmotic pressure, the administered colloid presumably would not stay intravascularly, but would leak into the alveolar space of the lung. Also, in patients with full-blown ARDS, the effect of serum colloid osmotic pressure is probably relatively small compared with the permeability defect from the acute lung injury.

Currently, we attempt to maintain a euvolemic state in ARDS patients. Our desired goal is to use the least amount of fluid administration that will maintain an adequate cardiac output. Guidelines for determining which patients might benefit from the placement of a pulmonary artery balloon flotation catheter are similar to those given in Table 32–4.

TREATMENT OF THE UNDERLYING DISEASE PROCESS

All of the therapy that has been described in the foregoing is supportive. The illness or injury that precipitated the acute respiratory failure must be controlled to limit the lung injury and allow healing to occur. Many of the illnesses or injuries that precipitate ARDS are self-limited and, in themselves, require only supportive therapy. A notable exception is that of infection, with associated sepsis syndrome. Since infection is a potentially treatable process, it should be carefully considered in the differential diagnosis of any patient with ARDS. This includes patients who have some other apparent reason for ARDS, since infection can coexist with other clinical risk factors and, in fact, is often a complication of some of those disease processes. It is particularly important to consider the possibility of an intra-abdominal source of sepsis, since surgical intervention may be required for adequate drainage, in addition to appropriate antibiotic therapy.

CORTICOSTEROID THERAPY

Several controlled trials have recently defined the role of corticosteroid therapy in the prevention and early treatment of ARDS. None of these studies have shown a beneficial effect of corticosteroids. Two studies have evaluated corticosteroid therapy in patients at risk for ARDS. Weigelt and coworkers studied surgical patients at significant risk for developing ARDS as well as already having mild oxygenation abnormalities.[125] Corticosteroids used for 2 days not only failed to prevent the development of ARDS, but were associated with a trend for more severe gas exchange abnormalities than in the control group and also a significantly higher incidence of complicating infections during the first week of therapy. Luce and coworkers studied patients with sepsis syndrome as a risk for ARDS and again failed to affect the development of this syndrome.[19] A multicenter trial of corticosteroid administration following onset of ARDS showed no change in any outcome variable.[126] In addition, two large multicenter controlled trials found that corticosteroid therapy does not improve survival in sepsis syndrome.[127,128] One of the multicenter groups also evaluated the development and course of ARDS in patients with sepsis syndrome and found no benefit associated with corticosteroid use.[129] Thus, corticosteroids are not warranted as routine therapy in patients with ARDS or at risk for ARDS.

Ashbaugh and Maier have anecdotally reported significant improvement following corticosteroid therapy in patients with late or "chronic" ARDS.[130] This group of patients had ARDS for at least a week, and often longer, and showed evidence of progressive pulmonary fibrosis, with gradually deteriorating gas exchange. In their series of ten patients, an open-lung biopsy reasonably ruled out pulmonary infection as a cause for this clinical course and demonstrated significant pulmonary fibrosis and active inflammation. Corticosteroids in this clinical situation have not been studied in a controlled prospective trial, and their role remains to be determined.

Some investigators have had the clinical impression that corticosteroids were particularly helpful when administered for fat embolism syndrome.[131,132] A controlled trial of prophylactic corticosteroids in patients with multiple fractures suggested that fat embolism syndrome might be prevented by corticosteroids, although the number of patients with "fulminant" fat embolism syndrome was small.[133] Subsequently, a randomized controlled trial of corticosteroids administered to patients with fractures showed prevention of a clinical fat embolism syndrome in the treatment group, compared with the control group.[134] However, this study described a very mild clinical syndrome that was of little clinical consequence; no deaths occurred, even in the control group patients who developed their definition of fat embolism syndrome. None of the patients developed what I would consider a full-blown ARDS picture. Therefore, I cannot recommend corticosteroids for prevention of fat embolism with ARDS, and we do not follow this practice in our trauma unit. Whether corticosteroids would be helpful in treatment of ARDS caused by isolated fat embolism has not been tested.

PROPOSED SPECIFIC THERAPY IN PATIENTS WITH ADULT RESPIRATORY DISTRESS SYNDROME

One of the exciting aspects resulting from both recent investigative interest in the mechanisms of injury in ARDS and advances in basic science investigations unrelated to ARDS, is the wide array of potential therapeutic agents that might be available for clinical trials in ARDS patients in the near future. Proposed new therapies include nonsteroidal anti-inflammatory agents, anti-endotoxin agents, surfactant replacement, antioxidant agents, and other blockers of specific potential mediators of injury.

Ibuprofen has been studied in animal models, with encouraging results.[135,136] Preliminary safety studies have been performed in humans, and preparations are being made for a controlled trial of this agent.

Surfactant replacement administered intratracheally by aerosolization has been successful in reversing physiologic abnormalities in premature infants with infant respiratory distress syndrome (RDS)[137,138] and in prevention of infant RDS.[139] However, surfactant depletion is a likely primary abnormality in infant RDS as opposed to a secondary effect in adult patients with ARDS. Nonetheless, surfactant might be expected to result in physiologic improvement in ARDS patients as well.[6] Several different surfactant replacement agents are either available or on the horizon. These include agents both with and without the protein moiety associated with surfactant; whether this is needed for maximal therapeutic effect remains controversial. In addition, there are practical problems in delivery of surfactant in adults. Relatively large volumes are required to achieve diffuse distribution at a level that is likely to be effective. Any further concentration of the currently available agents render them too viscous to be adequately delivered by aerosolization. Despite these questions, plans are currently underway for clinical studies of artificial surfactant agents, and this is one of the most promising of the potential therapies.

Antibodies directed against endotoxin are currently being studied in patients with septic shock, with prevention of ARDS being one of the end points under evaluation. Previous studies of a polyclonal antibody against endotoxin, by Zeigler and coworkers, resulted in statistically significant improvements in survival of patients with septic shock[140] and also prevented the development of septic shock in surgical patients at high risk.[141] Whether ARDS was prevented was not studied. However, the antibody used in those studies was not commercially available. The studies that currently are underway are using antibodies that can be prepared commercially in sufficient quantities to be used clinically if they are found to be effective. Preliminary results suggest benefit from treatment with a monoclonal antibody against endotoxin in patients with septic shock.[142]

Toxic oxygen radicals and proteases are among the agents thought to produce the injury in ARDS.[38,42,44,45] α_1-Protease inhibitor is currently available and preliminary studies of its safety in humans are being carried out in preparation for a clinical trial of its therapeutic effectiveness. Antioxidant agents are also currently available, although whether they can be delivered in sufficient levels to intracellular sites at which the oxygen radicals presumably act is a major question that may limit their usefulness.

REFERENCES

1. Ashbaugh DG, Bigelow DB, Petty TL, Levine BE: Acute respiratory distress in adults. Lancet 2:319–323, 1967
2. Petty TL, Reiss OK, Paul GW et al: Characteristics of pulmonary surfactant in adult respiratory distress syndrome associated with trauma shock. Am Rev Respir Dis 115:531–536, 1977
3. Petty TL, Silvers GW, Paul GW et al: Abnormalities in lung elastic properties and surfactant function in adult respiratory distress syndrome. Chest 75:571–574, 1979
4. Hallman M, Spragg R, Harrell JH et al: Evidence of lung surfactant abnormality in respiratory failure: Study of bronchoalveolar lavage phospholipids, surface activity, phospholipase activity and plasma myoinositol. J Clin Invest 70:673–683, 1982
5. von Wichert P, Kohl FV: Decreased dipalmitoyllecithin content found in lung specimens from patients with so-called shock lung. Intensive Care Med 3:27–30, 1977
6. Mason RJ: Surfactant in adult respiratory distress syndrome. Eur J Respir Dis 71(suppl 153):229–236, 1987
7. Rinaldo JE: The prognosis of the adult respiratory distress syndrome: Inappropriate pessimism? Chest 96:470–471, 1986
8. Murray JF, Matthay MA, Luce JM, Flick MR: An expanded definition of the adult respiratory distress syndrome. Am Rev Respir Dis 138:720–723, 1988
9. Rocker DM, Pearson D, Wiseman MS, Shale DJ: Diagnostic criteria for adult respiratory distress syndrome: Time for reappraisal. Lancet 1:120–123, 1989
10. Petty TL: ARDS: Refinement of concept and redefinition. Am Rev Respir Dis 138:724, 1988
11. Pepe PE, Hudson LD, Carrico CJ: Early application of positive end-expiratory pressure in patients at risk for the adult respiratory distress syndrome. N Engl J Med 311:281–286, 1984
12. Calindrino FS Jr, Anderson DJ, Mintun MA, Schuster DP: Pulmonary vascular permeability during the adult respiratory distress syndrome: A positron emission tomographic study. Am Rev Respir Dis 138:421–428, 1988
13. Fowler AA, Hamman RF, Good JT et al: Adult respiratory distress syndrome: Risk with common predispositions. Ann Intern Med 98:593–597, 1983
14. Schoene RB: Pulmonary edema at high altitude: Review, pathophysiology, and update. Clin Chest Med 6:256–263, 1985
15. Hudson LD: Causes of the adult respiratory distress syndrome: Clinical recognition. Clin Chest Med 3:195–212, 1982
16. Pepe PE, Potkin RT, Holtman-Reus D, Hudson LD, Carrico CJ: Clinical predictors of the adult respiratory distress syndrome. Am J Surg 144:124–130, 1982
17. Maunder RJ: Clinical prediction of the adult respiratory distress syndrome. Clin Chest Med 6:413–426, 1985
18. Hudson LD: Multiple systems organ failure: Lessons learned from the adult respiratory distress syndrome (ARDS). Crit Care Clin 5:697–705, 1989
19. Luce JM, Montgomery AB, Marks JD et al: Ineffectiveness of high-dose methylprednisolone in preventing parenchymal lung injury and improving mortality in patients with septic shock. Am Rev Respir Dis 138:62–68, 1988
20. de los Santos R, Seidenfeld JJ, Anzueto A et al: One hundred percent oxygen lung injury in adult baboons. Am Rev Respir Dis 136:657–661, 1987
21. Crapo JD, Barry BE, Foscue HA, Shelburne J: Structural and biochemical changes in rat lungs occurring during exposure to lethal and adaptive doses of oxygen. Am Rev Respir Dis 122:123–143, 1980
22. Barber RE, Lee J, Hamilton WK: Oxygen toxicity in man: A prospective study in patients with irreversible brain damage. N Engl J Med 283:1478–1484, 1970
23. de Lemos R, Wolfsdorf J, Nachman R et al: Lung injury from oxygen in lambs. Anesthesiology 30:609–618, 1969
24. Meyrick B: Pathology of the adult respiratory distress syndrome. Crit Care Clin 2:405–428, 1986
25. Bachofen M, Weibel ER: Structural alterations of lung parenchyma in the adult respiratory distress syndrome. Clin Chest Med 3:35–56, 1982
26. Raghu G, Striker LJ, Hudson LD, Striker GE: Extracellular matrix in normal and fibrotic human lungs. Am Rev Respir Dis 131:281–289, 1985
27. Zapol WM, Snider WT: Pulmonary hypertension in severe acute respiratory failure. N Engl J Med 296:476–480, 1977
28. Zapol WM, Jones R: Vascular components of ARDS: Clinical pulmonary hemodynamics and morphology. Am Rev Respir Dis 136:471–474, 1987
29. Danek SJ, Lynch JP, Weg JG, Dantzker DR: The dependence of oxygen uptake on oxygen delivery in the adult respiratory distress syndrome. Am Rev Respir Dis 122:387–395, 1980
30. Mohsenifar Z, Goldbach P, Tashkin DP, Campisi DJ: Relationship between O_2 delivery and O_2 consumption in the adult respiratory distress syndrome. Chest 84:267–271, 1983
31. Fein A, Weiner-Kronish JP, Niederman M, Matthay MA: Pathophysiology of the adult respiratory distress syndrome: What have we learned from human studies? Crit Care Clin 2:429–453, 1986
32. Anderson RR, Holliday RL, Driedger AA et al: Documentation of pulmonary capillary permeability in the adult respiratory distress syndrome accompanying human sepsis. Am Rev Respir Dis 119:869–877, 1979
33. Holter JF, Weiland JE, Pacht ER et al: Protein permeability in the adult respiratory distress syndrome: Loss of size selectivity of the alveolar epithelium. J Clin Invest 78:1513–1522, 1986
34. Sibbald WJ, Driedger AA, Hoffat JD et al: Pulmonary microvascular clearance of radiotracers in human

cardiac and noncardiac pulmonary edema. J Appl Physiol 50:1337–1347, 1981

35. Rinaldo JE, Borovetz HS, Mancini MC et al: Assessment of lung injury in the adult respiratory distress syndrome using multiple indicator dilution curves. Am Rev Respir Dis 13:1006–1010, 1986

36. Vreim CF, Staub NC: Protein composition of lung fluids in acute alloxan edema in dogs. Am J Physiol 230:376–379, 1976

37. Niedermeyer ME, Sheller JR, Brigham KL: Pathogenesis of the adult respiratory distress syndrome. Curr Pulmonol 5:229–254, 1984

38. Cochrane CG, Spragg R, Revak S: Pathogenesis of the adult respiratory distress syndrome: Evidence of oxidant activity in bronchoalveolar lavage fluid. J Clin Invest 71:754–761, 1983

39. Hechtman H, Valeri R, Shepro D: Role of humoral mediators in the adult respiratory distress syndrome. Chest 86:623–627, 1984

40. Henson P, Larson G, Webster R et al: Pulmonary microvascular alterations and injury induced by complement fragments, synergistic effect of complement activation, neutrophil sequestration, and prostaglandins. Ann NY Acad Sci 384:287–300, 1982

41. Idell S, Cohen A: Bronchoalveolar lavage in patients with the adult respiratory distress syndrome. Clin Chest Med 6:459–472, 1985

42. Idell S, Kucich U, Fein A et al: Neutrophil elastase-releasing factors in bronchoalveolar lavage from patients with adult respiratory distress syndrome. Am Rev Respir Dis 132:1098–1105, 1985

43. Matthay MA: Pathophysiology of pulmonary edema. Clin Chest Med 6:301–314, 1985

44. Lee CT, Fein AM, Lippman M et al: Elastolytic activity in pulmonary lavage fluid from patients with the adult respiratory distress syndrome. N Engl J Med 304:192–196, 1981

45. McCord J: Oxygen radicals and lung injury: The state of the art. Chest 83 (suppl):355, 1983

46. McGuire W, Spragg R, Cohen A et al: Studies on the pathogenesis of adult respiratory distress syndrome. J Clin Invest 69:543–553, 1982

47. Worthen S, Henson P: Mechanisms of acute lung injury. Clin Lab Med 3:601–617, 1983

48. Jacobs ER, Bone RC: Mediators of septic lung injury. Med Clin North Am 67:701–715, 1983

49. Brigham KL: Mechanisms of lung injury. Clin Chest Med 3:9–24, 1982

50. Rinaldo JE, Rogers RM: Adult respiratory-distress syndrome: Changing concepts of lung injury and repair. N Engl J Med 306:900–908, 1982

51. Rinaldo JE, Gadek JE, Repine J et al: Adult respiratory distress syndrome: Mechanisms of injury and new approaches to therapy. Am Rev Respir Dis 134:825–826, 1986

52. Brigham KL, Duke SS: Prostaglandins in lung disease: Adult respiratory distress syndrome. Semin Respir Med 7:11–16, 1985

53. Reynolds HY: Lung inflammation: Normal host defense or a complication of some diseases? Annu Rev Med 38:295–323, 1987

54. Tate R, Repine J: Neutrophils and the adult respiratory distress syndrome. Am Rev Respir Dis 128:552–557, 1983

55. Weiland J, Davis W, Holter J et al: Lung neutrophils in the adult respiratory distress syndrome: Clinical and pathophysiologic significance. Am Rev Respir Dis 133:218–225, 1986

56. Zimmerman G, Renzetti A, Hill R: Functional and metabolic activity of granulocytes from patients with adult respiratory distress syndrome. Am Rev Respir Dis 127:290–300, 1983

57. Zimmerman GA, Renzetti AD, Hill HR: Granulocyte adherence in pulmonary and systemic arterial blood samples from patients with adult respiratory distress syndrome. Am Rev Respir Dis 129:798–804, 1984

58. Brigham KL, Meyrick B: Interactions of granulocytes with the lungs. Circ Res 54:623–635, 1984

59. Harlan JM: Leukocyte–endothelial interactions. Blood 65:513–524, 1985

60. Hogg JC: Neutrophil kinetics and lung injury. Physiol Rev 67:1249–1295, 1987

61. Holman RG, Maier RV: Superoxide production by neutrophils in a model of adult respiratory distress syndrome. Arch Surg 123:1491–1495, 1988

62. Powe JE, Short A, Sibbald WJ et al: Pulmonary accumulation of polymorphonuclear leukocytes in the adult respiratory distress syndrome. Crit Care Med 10:712–718, 1982

63. Warshawski FJ, Sibbald WJ, Driedger AA, Cheung H: Abnormal neutrophil–pulmonary interaction in the adult respiratory distress syndrome: Qualitative and quantitative assessment of pulmonary neutrophil kinetics in humans with in vivo [111]Indium neutrophil scintigraphy. Am Rev Respir Dis 133:797–804, 1986

64. Heflin AC, Brigham KL: Prevention by granulocyte depletion of increased vascular permeability of sheep lung following endotoxemia. J Clin Invest 68:1253–1260, 1981

65. Flick MR, Perel A, Staub NC: Leukocytes are required for increased lung microvascular permeability after microembolization in sheep. Circ Res 48:344–351, 1981

66. Tahamont MV, Malik AB: Granulocytes mediate the increase in lung microvascular permeability after thrombin embolism. J Appl Physiol 54:1489–1495, 1983

67. Shasby DM, Fox RB, Harada RN et al: Reduction of the edema of acute hyperoxic lung injury by granulocyte depletion. J Appl Physiol 52:1237–1244, 1983

68. Shasby DM, Vanbenthysen KM, Tate RM et al: Granulocyte mediate acute edematous lung injury in rabbits and in isolated rabbit lungs perfused from phorbol myristate acetate: Role of oxygen radicals. Am Rev Respir Dis 125:443–447, 1982

69. Eiermann GJ, Dickey BF, Thrall RS: Polymorphonuclear leukocyte participation in acute oleic acid-induced lung injury. Am Rev Respir Dis 128:845–850, 1983

70. Winn R, Maunder R, Chi E, Harlan J: Neutrophil depletion does not prevent lung edema endotoxin infusion in goats. J Appl Physiol 62:116–121, 1987

71. Busch C, Llindquist D, Saldeen T: Respiratory insufficiency in the dog induced by pulmonary microembolism and inhibition of fibronolysis: Effect of defibrinogenation, leucopenia, and thrombocytopenia. Acta Clin Scand 140:255–266, 1974

72. Pingleton WW, Coalson JJ, Guenter CA: Significance of leukocytes in endotoxic shock. Exp Mol Pathol 22:183–194, 1975

73. Schwartz BA, Niewohner DE, Hoidal JR: Neutrophil

depletion does not protect rats from hyperoxic lung injury [Abstract]. Clin Res 31:746A, 1983

74. Millen JE, Glauser FL, Smeltzer D et al: The role of leukocytes in ethchlorvynol-induced pulmonary edema. Chest 73:75–78, 1978

75. Julien M, Heuffel JM, Flick MR: Oleic acid lung injury in sheep. J Am Physiol 60:433–440, 1986

76. Maunder RJ, Hackman R, Riff E et al: Occurrence of the adult respiratory distress syndrome in neutropenic patients. Am Rev Respir Dis 133:313–316, 1986

77. Laufe MD, Simon RH, Flint A, Keller JB: Adult respiratory distress syndrome in neutropenic patients. Am J Med 80:1022–1026, 1986

78. Ognibene FP, Martin SE, Parker MM et al: ARDS in patients with severe neutropenia. N Engl J Med 315:547–551, 1986

79. Braude S, Apperley J, Kraus T et al: Adult respiratory distress syndrome after bone marrow transplantation: Evidence for a neutrophil-independent mechanism. Lancet 2:1239–1242, 1985

80. Glauser FL, Fairman RP: The uncertain role of the neutrophil in increased permeability pulmonary edema. Chest 88:601–607, 1985

81. Jacobs ER, Bone RC: Clinical indicators in sepsis and septic adult respiratory distress syndrome. Med Clin North Am 70:921–932, 1986

82. Ruiz BC, Calderwood HW, Modell JH, Brogdon JE: Effect of ventilatory patterns on arterial oxygenation after near-drowning with fresh water: A comparative study in dogs. Anesth Analg 52:570–576, 1973

83. Modell JH, Calderwood HW, Ruiz BC et al: Effects of ventilatory patterns on arterial oxygenation after near-drowning in sea water. Anesthesiology 40:376–383, 1974

84. Lamy M, Fallat RJ, Koeniger E et al: Pathologic features and mechanisms of hypoxemia in adult respiratory distress syndrome. Am Rev Respir Dis 114:267–284, 1976

85. Dantzker DR, Brook CJ, DeHart P et al: Ventilation–perfusion distributions in the adult respiratory distress syndrome. Am Rev Respir Dis 120:1039–1052, 1979

86. Ralph DD, Robertson HT, Weaver MP et al: Distribution of ventilation and perfusion during positive end-expiratory pressure in the adult respiratory distress syndrome. Am Rev Respir Dis 131:54–60, 1985

87. Marini JJ, Rodriquez RM, Lamb V: The inspiratory workload of patient-initiated mechanical ventilation. Am Rev Respir Dis 134:902–909, 1986

88. Gurevitch MJ, VanDyke J, Young ES et al: Improved oxygenation and lower peak airway pressure in severe adult respiratory distress syndrome: Treatment with inverse ratio ventilation. Chest 89:211, 1986

89. Gattinoni L, Marcolin R, Caspani ML et al: Constant mean airway pressure with different patterns of positive pressure breathing during the adult respiratory distress syndrome. Bull Eur Physiopathol Respir 21:275–279, 1985

90. Kolton M, Cattran EB, Kent G et al: Oxygenation during high-frequency ventilation compared with conventional mechanical ventilation in two models of lung injury. Anesth Analg 61:323–332, 1982

91. Hamilton PP, Onayemi A, Smyth JA et al: Comparison of conventional and high-frequency ventilation, oxygenation, and lung pathology. J Appl Physiol 55:131–138, 1983

92. Carlon GC, Howland WS, Ray C et al: High frequency jet ventilation: A prospective randomized evaluation. Chest 84:551–559, 1983

93. MacIntyre NR, Follett JV, Deitz JL et al: Jet ventilation at 100 BPM in adult respiratory failure. Am Rev Respir Dis 134:897–901, 1986

94. Zapol WM, Snider MT, Dill JD et al: Extracorporeal membrane oxygenation in severe acute respiratory failure. JAMA 242:2193–2196, 1979

95. Gattinoni L, Pesenti A, Mascheroni D et al: Low-frequency positive-pressure ventilation with extracorporeal CO_2 removal in severe acute respiratory failure. JAMA 256:881–886, 1986

96. Morris AH, Menlove RL, Rollins RJ et al: A controlled clinical trial of a new 3-step therapy that includes extracorporeal CO_2 removal for ARDS. Trans Am Soc Artif Organs 34:48–53, 1988

97. Ashbaugh DG, Petty TL, Bigelow DB et al: Continuous positive pressure breathing (CPPB) in adult respiratory distress syndrome. J Thorac Cardiovasc Surg 57:31–41, 1969

98. Uzawa T, Ashbaugh DG: Continuous positive-pressure breathing in acute hemorrhagic pulmonary edema. J Appl Physiol 26:427–432, 1969

99. McIntyre BW, Laws AK, Ramachandran PR: Positive expiratory pressure plateau: Improved gas exchange during mechanical ventilation. Can Anaesth Soc J 16:477–486, 1969

100. Kumar A, Falke KJ, Geffin B et al: Continuous positive-pressure ventilation in acute respiratory failure. N Engl J Med 283:1430–1436, 1970

101. Powers S, Mannal R, Neclerio M et al: Physiologic consequences of positive end-expiratory pressure (PEEP) ventilation. Ann Surg 173:265–272, 1973

102. Nelson LD, Civetta JM, Hudson-Civetta J: Titrating positive end-expiratory pressure therapy in patients with early, moderate arterial hypoxemia. Crit Care Med 15:14–19, 1987

103. Carroll GC, Tuman KJ, Braverman B et al: Minimal positive end-expiratory pressure (PEEP) may be "best PEEP." Chest 93:1020–1025, 1988

104. Schmidt GB, O'Neil WW, Kotb K et al: Continuous positive airway pressure in the prophylaxis of the adult respiratory distress syndrome. Surg Gynecol Obstet 143:613–618, 1976

105. Weigelt JA, Mitchell RA, Snyder WH: Early positive end-expiratory pressure in the adult respiratory distress syndrome. Arch Surg 114:497–501, 1979

106. Luce JM, Robertson HT, Huang TW et al: The effects of expiratory positive airway pressure on the resolution of oleic acid-induced lung injury in dogs. Am Rev Respir Dis 125:716–722, 1982

107. Luce JM, Huang TW, Robertson HT et al: The effects of prophylactic expiratory positive airway pressure on the resolution of oleic acid-induced injury in dogs. Ann Surg 197:327–336, 1983

108. Craig KC, Pierson DJ, Carrico CJ: The clinical application of positive end-expiratory pressure (PEEP) in the adult respiratory distress syndrome (ARDS). Respir Care 30:184–201, 1985

109. Luce JM: The cardiovascular effects of mechanical ventilation and positive and expiratory pressure. JAMA 252:807–811, 1986

110. Pierson DJ: Alveolar rupture during mechanical ventilation: Role of PEEP, peak airway pressure and distending volume. Respir Care 33:472–486, 1988

111. Cournand A, Motley HL, Werko L: Physiological studies of the effects of intermittent positive pressure breathing on cardiac output in man. Am J Physiol 152:162–174, 1948

112. Harken AH, Brennan MF, Smith B, Barsamian EH: The hemodynamic response to positive end-expiratory ventilation in hypovolemic patients. Surgery 76:786–793, 1974

113. Potkin RT, Hudson LD, Weaver LJ, Trobaugh G: Effect of positive end-expiratory pressure on right and left ventricular function in patients with the adult respiratory distress syndrome. Am Rev Respir Dis 135:307–311, 1987

114. Kirby RR, Perry JC, Calderwood HW, Ruiz BC, Lederman DS: Cardiorespiratory effects of high positive end-expiratory pressure. Anesthesiology 43:533–539, 1975

115. Jardin F, Farcot J, Boisante L et al: Influence of positive end-expiratory pressure on ventricular performance. N Engl J Med 304:387–392, 1981

116. Suter PM, Fairley HB, Isenberg MD: Optimum end-expiratory airway pressure in patients with acute pulmonary failure. N Engl J Med 292:284–289, 1975

117. Putterman C: Adult respiratory distress syndrome: Current concepts. Resuscitation 16:91–105, 1988

118. McDonnell TJ, Voelkel NF, Petty TL: Adult respiratory distress syndrome and its management. Compr Ther 13:33–40, 1987

119. Pierson DJ, Horton CA, Bates PW: Persistent bronchopleural air leak during mechanical ventilation: A review of 39 cases. Chest 90:321–323, 1986

120. Bone RC: Complications of mechanical ventilation and positive end-expiratory pressure. Respir Care 27:402–407, 1982

121. Hudson LD, Tooker J, Haisch CE, Carrico CJ: Does compliance reflect optimal oxygen transport with positive end-expiratory pressure [Abstract]? Chest 67:156, 1977

122. Maunder RJ, Rice CL, Benson MS, Hudson LD: Managing positive end-expiratory pressure: The Harborview approach. Respir Care 31:1059–1065, 1986

123. Simmons RS, Berdine GG, Seidenfeld JJ et al: Fluid balance and the adult respiratory distress syndrome. Am Rev Respir Dis 135:924–929, 1987

124. Maunder RJ, Kubilis PS, Anardi DM, Hudson LD: Determinants of survival in the adult respiratory distress syndrome [Abstract]. Am Rev Respir Dis 139(4, pt 2):A220, 1989

125. Weigelt JA, Norcross JF, Borman KR, Snyder WH III: Early steroid therapy for respiratory failure. Arch Surg 120:536–540, 1985

126. Bernard GR, Luce JM, Sprung CL et al: High-dose corticosteroids in patients with the adult respiratory distress syndrome. N Engl J Med 317:1565–1570, 1987

127. Bone RC, Fisher CJ Jr, Clemmer TP et al: A controlled clinical trial of high dose methylprednisolone in the treatment of severe sepsis and septic shock. N Engl J Med 317:653–658, 1987

128. Veterans Administration Systemic Sepsis Cooperative Study Group: Effect of high-dose glucocorticoid therapy on mortality in patients with clinical signs of systemic sepsis. N Engl J Med 317:659–665, 1987

129. Bone RC, Fisher CJ Jr, Clemmer TP et al: Early methylprednisolone treatment for septic syndrome and the adult respiratory distress syndrome. Chest 92:1032–1036, 1987

130. Ashbaugh DG, Maier RV: Idiopathic pulmonary fibrosis in adult respiratory distress syndrome. Arch Surg 120:530–535, 1985

131. Ashbaugh DG, Petty TL: The use of corticosteroids in the treatment of respiratory failure associated with massive fat embolism. Surg Gynecol Obstet 123:493–500, 1966

132. Fischer JE, Turner RH, Herndon JH, Riseborough EJ: Massive steroid therapy in severe fat embolism. Surg Gynecol Obstet 132:667–672, 1971

133. Alho A, Saikku K, Eerola P et al: Corticosteroids in patients with a high risk of fat embolism syndrome. Surg Gynecol Obstet 147:358–362, 1978

134. Schonfeld SA, Ploysongsang Y, DiLisio R et al: Fat embolism prophylaxis with corticosteroids: A prospective study in high-risk patients. Ann Intern Med 99:438–443, 1983

135. Rinaldo JE, Pennock B: Effects of ibuprofen on endotoxin-induced alveolitis. Am J Med Sci 291:29–38, 1986

136. Sprague RS, Stephenson AH, Dahus TE et al: Effects of ibuprofen on the hypoxemia of established ethchlorvynol-induced unilateral acute lung injury in anesthetized dogs. Chest 92:1088–1093, 1987

137. Collaborative European Multicenter Study Group: Surfactant replacement therapy for severe neonatal respiratory distress syndrome: An international randomized clinical trial. Pediatrics 82:683–691, 1988

138. Horbar JD, Soll RF, Sutherland JM et al: A multicenter randomized placebo-controlled trial of surfactant therapy for respiratory distress syndrome. N Engl J Med 320:959–965, 1989

139. Merritt TA, Hallman M, Bloom BT et al: Prophylactic treatment of very premature infants with human surfactant. N Engl J Med 315:785–790, 1986

140. Zeigler EJ, McCutchan JA, Fierer J et al: Treatment of gram-negative bacteremia and shock with human antiserum to a mutant *Escherichia coli*. N Engl J Med 307:1225–1230, 1982

141. Baumgartner JD, McCutchan JA, Ziegler EJ, Glausner MP. Prevention of gram-negative shock and death in surgical patients by antibody to endotoxin core glycolipid. Lancet 2:59–63, 1985

142. Ziegler E, Fisher C, Sprung C et al: Prevention of death from Gram-negative bacteremia and sepsis by HA-1A, a human monoclonal antibody specific for lipid A of endotoxin: Results of phase III trial. Clin Res 38:304A, 1990

THIRTY-THREE

Respiratory Care in the Coronary Care Unit

Steve G. Peters
John T. Wheeler
Douglas R. Gracey

Recent advances have changed the approach to the patient with acute myocardial ischemia. Accordingly, the present-day respiratory care practitioner must not only be aware of the physiologic relationship between the heart and the lungs, but also appreciate how respiratory care might appropriately be tailored to the patient in the coronary care unit. This chapter will review aspects of medical management in coronary intensive care, relationships between cardiac and pulmonary disease, and aspects of respiratory care specifically applied to the patient with heart disease.

CLINICAL ASPECTS OF CORONARY DISEASE

In recent years, cardiovascular diseases have accounted for approximately 1 million deaths annually in the United States, roughly half of which are due to coronary disease.[1] Of sudden deaths because of coronary heart disease, 60% to 70% occur outside a hospital, which has been the major impetus for widespread training in cardiopulmonary resuscitation (CPR) and basic life support techniques. Cardiac arrest in this setting is most often due to ventricular fibrillation, with or without evidence of acute myocardial infarction.

Approximately one-half of the patients with symptomatic or clinically apparent myocardial infarction survive to be admitted to the hospital. The coronary unit typically serves as the site for acute management of cardiac ischemia, including myocardial infarction, and new or unstable angina. The coronary unit may also be used for monitoring and management of unstable or life-threatening cardiac dysrhythmias and for patients with heart failure related to ischemia, cardiomyopathy, severe hypertension, or valvular disease.

Risk factors for the development of coronary disease include age, male sex, hypertension, hypercholesterolemia, diabetes mellitus, cigarette smoking, and family history.[1] Recent psychological stress and lower socioeconomic status are implicated as risk factors for coronary disease and sudden death. Each of these factors is assessed in the history, physical examination, and laboratory testing of the patient.

The classic symptom of myocardial ischemia is *angina pectoris*; that is, chest discomfort, which may be sensed as pain, pressure, or tightness across the central area of the chest or the epigastrium. There may be a similar sensation or radiation of discomfort to the neck, jaw, shoulders, arms, or back. Typical symptoms may occur with exertion and improve within minutes after resting or using nitroglycerin.

The symptoms of *myocardial infarction* include a new or unstable pattern of chest pain, pain occurring with minimal activity or at rest, or prolonged pain not relieved by rest or nitroglycerin. Dyspnea is frequently noted. Nausea may also be present and may mimic a gastrointestinal disorder. Light-headedness or palpitations may indicate a dysrhythmia or decreased cardiac output or both conditions. A recent history of orthopnea or peripheral edema may suggest the presence of left or right ventricular failure, respectively. The pattern of the chest pain, including quality of the discomfort, duration, location, radiation, and aggravating and alleviating factors, may be useful in differentiating cardiac ischemia from such disorders as aortic dissection, pericarditis, pulmonary embolism, pneumonitis, pleuritis, or chest wall pain. Gastrointestinal discomfort caused by esophageal spasm, ulcer disease, pancreatitis, or gallbladder disease may also be confused with pain from myocardial ischemia.

Physical examination of the patient with uncomplicated myocardial infarction may be nonspecific. Tachynpnea, tachycardia, diaphoresis, and hypertension or hypotension may be present. The cardiac examination may be normal. A fourth heart sound may indicate filling of a noncompliant left ventricle during atrial contraction. A systolic murmur of mitral regurgitation may indicate papillary muscle dysfunction or rupture of chorda tendineae.

When acute cardiac ischemia or infarction is suspected, a prompt electrocardiogram (ECG) is typically the initial diagnostic study. ST-segment depression and T-wave flattening or inversion are changes associated with ischemia, although these findings may be chronic or nonspecific. New ST-segment elevation or Q waves are associated with infarction. It is important to recognize that the electrocardiogram may also appear normal during an acute ischemic event. Serial electrocardiograms improve the accuracy for a diagnosis of myocardial infarction.

Laboratory testing typically centers upon assessment of serum levels of cardiac enzymes. Acutely, the myocardial or MB fraction of creatine kinase (CKMB) is most useful. The CKMB rises 4 to 6 hours after myocardial infarction, peaks at approximately 24 hours, and remains elevated for 48 to 72 hours. An MB fraction of less than 5% of the total CK may not be significant, and this distinction is especially helpful in postoperative patients who may have elevated CK levels and experience acute symptoms of myocardial infarction.

Recent advances have provided a variety of diagnostic imaging tools for assessing cardiac function. Two-dimensional echocardiography provides important information on ventricular size and function, regional wall motion abnormalities, mural thrombus formation, valvular function, and abnormalities of the pericardium. Doppler studies have recently been developed to estimate intracardiac pressure gradients, pulmonary artery pressure, and cardiac output.[2]

Radionuclide-scanning studies have also gained an increasing role in assessing areas of infarction, myocardial perfusion, and ventricular function. Technetium Tc99m pyrophosphate, injected within several days of acute infarction, is incorporated into areas of myocardial cellular damage. Technetium Tc99m scanning may be used to establish whether an infarct has occurred, to localize the area, and to estimate size.[3] Myocardial perfusion may be assessed by thallium 201 scintigraphy. This isotope accumulates in proportion to blood flow, so that defects may identify areas of ischemia or infarction. Thallium 201 scanning is most often combined with exercise testing to provide additional diagnostic and prognostic information. An increased uptake of thallium by the lungs during exercise is a sign of left ventricular dysfunction and is associated with a higher risk of subsequent cardiac complications.[4] A radionuclide ventriculogram with multiple-gated acquisition (MUGA scan) provides an assessment of ventricular function and ejection fraction. Such scanning is also frequently coupled with exercise; a decreased ejection fraction with exercise following myocardial infarction carries an adverse prognosis.[3]

Coronary angiography remains the standard for defining coronary anatomy, and the site and degree of obstructing lesions. Angiography has recently been combined with techniques of thrombolytic therapy and coronary angioplasty. These therapeutic maneuvers will be discussed in the following sections.

MANAGEMENT OF ACUTE MYOCARDIAL ISCHEMIA

The respiratory care practitioner should be aware of the drugs and other interventions commonly used in the coronary care setting and of the cardiovascular and respiratory physiologic effects. Table 33–1 summarizes several drugs that are most commonly employed in the acute medical management of the patient with myocardial infarction.

Oxygen is usually administered at low-flow rates (e.g., 2–4 L/min) by nasal cannulae. There is evidence that supplemental oxygen may reduce myocardial ischemia and improve arrhythmias and ventricular function if hypoxemia is present.[5–8] Although a similar benefit has not been proved for

Table 33—1 Medical Management of Acute Myocardial Infarction

DRUGS	ACTION, RATIONALE	COMMENTS, SIDE EFFECTS
Oxygen	Improve hypoxemia; reduce ischemic injury	May require ABG monitoring, especially in COPD patient with hypoxic respiratory drive
Morphine	Pain relief, sedation; reduced preload	Observe for hypotension, respiratory depression (especially in COPD). Vagotonic; bradycardia may require atropine
Nitroglycerin	Coronary vasodilation ↓ Left ventricular volume ↓ Myocardial ischemia ↓ Peripheral resistance	Hypotension; tachycardia
Lidocaine	Prevention of ventricular dysrhythmias	Altered mental status, seizures, nausea; decrease dose with CHF, hepatic failure
Inotropic agents	Treat hypotension; increase contractility, cardiac output ± vasodilation (decrease afterload) *Examples*: dopamine ± nitroprusside, dobutamine	May increase O_2 consumption; monitor BP closely
β-Adrenergic blockers	Decrease heart rate, contractility, O_2 consumption; decrease overall mortality, reinfarction rate *Examples*: propranolol, metroprolol, timolol, atenolol	May induce hypotension, bradycardia, CHF, bronchospasm

patients with normal arterial oxygenation, low-flow oxygen is initially used for most patients. Arterial blood gas values might be reasonably obtained from all patients with acute myocardial infarction. In particular, patients with chronic obstructive pulmonary disease (COPD) should be monitored to document improvement in hypoxemia without significant carbon dioxide retention.

Relief of pain and anxiety is an important early goal. Morphine is most frequently used, typically titrated in increments of 2–8 mg to achieve pain relief and sedation. Morphine may also increase venous capacitance and decrease pulmonary artery pressures.[9] Hypotension, respiratory depression, bradycardia, and nausea are potential side effects.

Nitrates, by the sublingual or oral route and, more recently, by continuous intravenous infusion, have the potentially beneficial effects of increasing coronary blood flow and reducing preload and afterload by venous and arterial dilatation, thereby decreasing left ventricular work and oxygen demand. However, hypotension and reflex tachycardia may also occur, so that nitroglycerin must be used with caution, and the patient must be monitored closely. Furthermore, hypoxemia has been observed following intravenous nitroglycerin, the presumed mechanism being loss of regional hypoxic vasoconstriction and worsening of ventilation–perfusion mismatch.[11]

Lidocaine has been effective in the prevention of primary ventricular fibrillation following myocardial infarction.[12] Side effects may occur in a significant number of patients receiving recommended doses, in the range of 2–4 mg/min following a bolus of approximately 1 mg/kg body weight, especially if left ventricular failure or hepatic congestion is present. These adverse effects may include nausea, mental status changes, speech disturbances, dizziness, or seizures. The routine use of lidocaine is therefore debated, but prophylactic treatment is commonly given, with observation for side effects and dose adjustment if necessary.

Hypotension or ventricular failure following myocardial infarction may require treatment with inotropic agents. These agents generally increase myocardial contractility and cardiac output, but may have varying effects on systemic vascular resistance. Dopamine is a β-agonist with α-adrenergic effects at doses above approximately 10 μg/kg per minute, with resultant increase in vascular resistance at these higher dose levels. Nitroprusside is often added for its effects in reducing arterial resistance and venous return. Durrer et al. observed a decreased incidence of left heart failure and decreased mortality in patients given nitroprusside during the first 24 hours after hospitalization for acute myocardial infarction.[13] Cohn et al. found a benefit in mortality only for patients with persistent ventricular failure.[14] Dobutamine increases cardiac output, but also decreases systemic and pulmonary arterial pressures, so this agent is often used alone when ventricular failure occurs in the presence of elevated vascular resistance.[15] Amrinone is a newer agent, with positive inotropic and peripheral vasodilator properties, that also may be useful in the treatment of left ventricular failure.[16]

A variety of β-blocking agents may be used in the acute management of the patient with myocardial ischemia and in long-term management following myocardial infarction. In large trials, timolol, atenolol, propranolol, and metoprolol have decreased overall mortality, reinfarction rates, and sudden death rates.[17,18] Side effects may include hypotension, bradycardia, and congestive failure. Significant bronchospasm may also occur, despite the relative β_1-selectivity of the newer agents. Therefore, these drugs must be used cautiously in patients with chronic obstructive lung disease or reactive airways. Concomitant treatment with β-adrenergic inhalers may be tried, but the relative risks and benefits must be weighed for the individual patient.

Calcium channel blocking agents, such as nifedipine, verapamil, and diltiazem may be useful in the long-term management of the patient with coronary disease, particularly with coexisting hypertension. Nifedipine is an effective systemic and coronary vasodilator, but reflex tachycardia commonly occurs. Verapamil is also a potent vasodilator and, in addition, it slows atrioventricular conduction and heart rate and may depress myocardial contractility. Diltiazem is a coronary vasodilator with weaker effects on the systemic arterial bed. Heart rate is usually slowed slightly. In a multicenter trial of diltiazem following nontransmural myocardial infarction, the rate of reinfarction was reduced by approximately 50% compared with placebo.[19] Overall mortality was unchanged. Studies of the varying physiologic effects of these drugs and their role in the acute management of myocardial ischemia are ongoing.

HEMODYNAMIC MONITORING

Important information may be gained by the use of a balloon flotation pulmonary artery catheter for the management of hemodynamically unstable patients with acute myocardial infarction. The respiratory care practitioner should have knowledge not only of the technical aspects of hemodynamic mon-

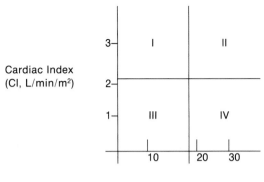

Figure 33—1. Hemodynamic subsets: Classes I–IV are divided according to CI greater or less than 2.2 L/min/m², and PCWP greater or less than 18 mmHg. Clinical correlations and potential treatment include the following: *I*, no pulmonary congestion or hypoperfusion: treatment supportive (see text); *II*, congestion without hypoperfusion: diuretics, peripheral vasodilators; *III*, hypoperfusion, normal to decreased PCWP: volume expansion; *IV*, hypoperfusion and congestion: diuretics, vasodilators, inotropes. (Adapted from Forrester JS et al: Medical therapy of acute myocardial infarction by application of hemodynamic subsets. N Engl J Med 295:1404–1413, 1976)

itoring, but also of the clinical applications (see Chap. 27). Recent controversy has surfaced over the potential overuse of the pulmonary artery catheter in critically ill patients; however, in selected situations the data may directly affect therapy.

Forrester et al. have categorized subsets of hemodynamic data useful for the medical management of patients following acute myocardial infarction.[20,21] These are shown in Figure 33–1, plotting cardiac index (CI) against pulmonary capillary wedge pressure (PCWP). The hemodynamic and clinical subclasses are separated by a CI greater or less than approximately 2.2 L/min/m², and PCWP greater or less than approximately 18 mmHg. In class I (CI $\geq$ 2.2 L/min/m², PCWP $\leq$ 18 mmHg) there is generally no evidence of tissue hypoperfusion or pulmonary congestion. Treatment may include oxygen, morphine, nitrates, and β-blockers as discussed previously, but no other specific intervention may be required. In Class II (CI $\geq$ 2.2 L/min/m², PCWP greater than 18 mmHg) perfusion may be adequate, but signs of pulmonary edema or congestion may develop. Treatment might include diuretics and peripheral vasodilators. Class III patients (decreased cardiac output with PCWP $\leq$ 18 mmHg) may benefit from expansion of intravascular fluid volume and, possibly, from inotropic agents. The goal of therapy is to increase cardiac output, without overstimulation of the heart and an adverse increase in myocardial oxygen demand. Class IV patients (low cardiac output and pulmonary edema) may require a combination of diuretics, vasodilators (afterload reduction), and inotropic agents. A significantly higher mortality is associated with clinical evidence of hypoperfusion or a measured decrease in cardiac output as observed in groups III and IV patients.

THROMBOLYTIC THERAPY AND CORONARY ANGIOPLASTY

Major recent developments in acute coronary care include the use of thrombolytic agents and *percutaneous transluminal coronary angioplasty* (PTCA). The goals of these techniques are early reperfusion following coronary occlusion, limitation of infarct size, preservation of ventricular function, and decreased mortality. Coronary thrombosis has been observed in approximately 87% of patients with acute transmural infarction.[22] Thrombus (clot) formation occurs through the coagulation cascade, whereas thrombolysis is mediated by the fibrinolytic system. Fibrinolysis depends upon the conversion of plasminogen to plasmin, an enzyme with proteolytic activity against fibrin thrombi, as well as fibrinogen and other clotting factors. The thrombolytic agents streptokinase (SK), urokinase, and

tissue plasminogen activator (t-PA) have different modes of action, but all induce the formation of plasmin from plasminogen. The t-PA produces relatively more plasmin from plasminogen bound to fibrin, rather than from circulating plasminogen. Therefore, this agent is felt to be more clot-specific in its action.[23]

Many clinical trials have attempted to analyze the efficacy of thrombolytic therapy in acute coronary thrombosis. Table 33–2 summarizes several large studies of thrombolytic therapy and recent studies examining the role of PTCA. Trials of intravenous SK compared with placebo have shown reduction in mortality and improvement in ventricular function if thrombolytic therapy is given within several hours of the onset of symptomatic infarction.[24–27] Subsequent studies have shown greater reperfusion rates for t-PA than for SK.[28,29] Furthermore, t-PA induced less systemic fibrinolysis than SK.

The major risk of thrombolytic therapy is bleeding. It is important to realize that these agents may lyse any recently formed clot. Significant hemorrhage may occur from previous arterial or venous puncture sites. Surgery within the previous 3 weeks, recent trauma, lesions of the central nervous system, poorly controlled hypertension, and gastrointestinal bleeding are contraindications to thrombolytic therapy.

Coronary angioplasty has been introduced as a technique to dilate residual stenotic areas following thrombolytic therapy. In this procedure, a bal-

Table 33—2   Thrombolytic Therapy Trials

STUDY (REF)	TREATMENT	NO. PTS	RESULTS	COMMENTS
GISSI[24]	IV SK vs placebo	11,806	18% reduction in mortality at 21 days	Rx within 12 hr of symptoms; 47% decrease mortality if Rx within 1 hr
ISAM[25]	IV SK vs placebo	1741	20% reduced mortality (not significant)	SK group showed higher ejection fraction, smaller CK rise
ISIS-2[26]	IV SK vs placebo	4000	33% reduced mortality	Rx within 4 hr of symptoms
White et al[27]	IV SK vs placebo	219	81% reduced mortality	Ejection fractions higher in SK group
TIMI[28]	IV SK vs t-PA	214	Reperfusion 60% t-PA 35% SK	Mortality 5% t-PA 8% SK
European[29] Cooperative	IV SK vs t-PA	129	Reperfusion 70% t-PA 55% SK	Less systemic fibrinolysis with t-PA than SK
O'Neill et al[30]	Intracoronary SK vs PTCA	56	Recanalization 83% t-PA 85% SK	Less residual stenosis after PTCA; PTCA associated with better ejection fraction and wall motion
Guerci et al[31]	IV t-PA vs placebo, then PTCA vs none after arteriogram day 3	138	Patency 66% t-PA 24% placebo PTCA improved ejection fraction with exercise, decreased post-infarction angina	t-PA improved ejection fraction, decreased prevalence of congestive failure

loon catheter is passed through an area of focal coronary artery stenosis identified by angiography. The balloon is then inflated to dilate the narrowed region. The role of this procedure is currently under investigation. Practical treatment protocols must take into account the limited availability of PTCA on an emergency basis. O'Neil et al. compared intracoronary SK to PTCA in 56 patients treated within 12 hours of symptoms of myocardial infarction.[30] Similar recanalization rates were observed, but PTCA produced less residual stenosis, better ejection fractions, and improved ventricular wall motion. Guerci et al. studied patients given intraveous t-PA or placebo, who were randomized after 3 days to receive PTCA or no further therapy.[31] Compared with placebo, t-PA produced greater coronary patency, greater mean ejection fraction, and a reduction in episodes of congestive heart failure. PTCA improved ejection fraction with exercise, and decreased postinfarction angina. A current multicenter thrombolysis and angioplasty in myocardial infarction (TAMI) study includes treatment with intravenous t-PA, followed by PTCA either on an emergency basis or after several days. Preliminary results show reperfusion in 72% of patients treated with t-PA, and in 94% with the addition of PTCA have been reported.[32] Further data are expected on the importance of the timing of PTCA relative to the acute infarct and thrombolytic therapy.

With the emergence of thrombolytic therapy and PTCA in the management of acute myocardial infarction, the role of emergency *coronary artery bypass grafting* (CABG) has become more limited. Current indications for early CABG include left main coronary artery disease, extensive three-vessel disease, and multiple lesions not suitable for PTCA. Also, emergency CABG may be necessary if attempted PTCA is unsuccessful, or if it results in sudden worsening of coronary obstruction.[33] The role of CABG versus medical management in the long-term care of the patient with ischemic heart disease remains controversial and will not be reviewed in detail here. In young patients with severe heart disease, cardiac transplantation is also emerging as a potential therapy.

INTERACTIONS OF THE HEART AND LUNGS

Changes in cardiac function may affect pulmonary function and alter gas exchange. With left ventricular dysfunction, an increase in pulmonary venous pressure may lead to interstitial edema and increased small-airway resistance. Alveolar filling by fluid ensues in more severe pulmonary edema. Lung volumes and lung compliance decrease. Bronchospasm may also occur, so that a mixed restrictive and obstructive pattern may be found by pulmonary function tests.[34] Small-airway closure at higher-than-normal lung volumes has been reported, even in uncomplicated cases in the first 2 weeks following myocardial infarction.[35] Arterial hypoxemia is frequently observed, although severe desaturation is typically found only in the presence of pulmonary edema or other respiratory complication, such as atelectasis or pnumonitis. With biventricular cardiac failure, pleural effusions are also a common cause for altered lung mechanics and gas exchange.

Lung disease may also have profound effects on cardiac function. Diffuse parenchymal or vascular disease, or any cause of chronic hypoxemia, may lead to increased pulmonary vascular resistance, pulmonary hypertension, and eventual right heart failure or cor pulmonale. This is commonly observed in patients with severe COPD. Cardiac arrhythmias, particularly atrial premature contractions, atrial tachycardias, and ventricular premature contractions, are frequently observed in monitored COPD patients.[36] Patients with COPD are also frequently at risk for coronary artery disease because of the common etiologic factor of tobacco use. Left ventricular function may be normal in patients with severe COPD, but concurrent left ventricular dysfunction has been attributed to coexisting coronary disease and ischemia.[37]

Acute alterations in lung mechanics also affect cardiac function. Hemodynamic changes associated with negative- and positive-pressure breathing are discussed elsewhere in this text. Briefly, increases in intrathoracic pressure, which may occur with positive-pressure breathing, or with applied positive end-expiratory pressure (PEEP), may decrease venous return to the right heart and, thereby, decrease right ventricular filling and cardiac output.[38] Pulmonary vascular resistance and right ventricular afterload are also increased in this setting, further limiting right ventricular output. These physiologic changes are also found in cases of airway obstruction with hyperinflation, increased intrathoracic pressure, and intrinsic PEEP (PEEP$_i$); i.e., alveolar pressure greater than atmospheric at end-expiration owing to high resistance and incomplete lung emptying. These changes may be overcome, to some extent, by increasing intravascular volume, but at the risk of subsequent fluid overload and worsening congestive failure. At high lung volumes, there may also be an increase in juxtacardiac pressure, such that left ventricular end-diastolic volume is reduced, leading to a further fall in cardiac output.

Mechanical ventilation may become necessary in patients with acute myocardial ischemia or infarction complicated by congestive failure or coexisting pulmonary disease. In the absence of ventilatory failure, spontaneous breathing may allow greater cardiac output as outlined in the foregoing. Chin et al. observed a higher cardiac index in patients supported with continuous positive airway pressure and spontaneous breathing, compared with continuous positive-pressure mechanical ventilation or intermittent mandatory ventilation with PEEP.[39] However, assisted ventilation can decrease the work and oxygen cost of breathing and permit greater sedation and rest for the patient. Improved ventilation, inflation of unstable alveoli, and increased functional residual capacity may also improve oxygenation. Räsänen et al. noted symptomatic and electrocardiographic evidence of ischemia as mechanical ventilation was withdrawn in patients with acute myocardial infarction.[40] Patients requiring mechanical ventilation should be monitored carefully as weaning is carried out. Gradual weaning techniques, such as intermittent mandatory ventilation or pressure support, or a combination thereof, have the potential advantage of allowing a transition to spontaneous ventilation without abrupt stress or patient discomfort.

High-frequency ventilation (HFV) has been employed in patients with left ventricular dysfunction and following cardiac surgery and may provide adequate ventilation and oxygenation at lower airway pressures than conventional mechanical ventilation.[41–43] However, the outcome of HFV versus conventional support has not been studied in a controlled fashion.

RESPIRATORY THERAPY MANEUVERS AND ACUTE MYOCARDIAL ISCHEMIA

In the patient with acute myocardial ischemia or infarction, the potential benefits of any intervention aimed at preventing or treating respiratory complications must be weighed against the possible immediate harm to the patient. Chest physical therapy (CPT) may induce increases in heart rate, blood pressure, oxygen consumption, and carbon dioxide production. Klein et al. have recently reported that in mechanically ventilated patients,

short-acting narcotics attenuated the hemodynamic responses to CPT, but not the effects on oxygen consumption and carbon dioxide production.[44] Additional maneuvers, such as endotracheal suctioning, even for brief periods may cause significant desaturation and adverse hemodynamic effects, particularly if mechanical ventilation or PEEP must be interrupted. Nasotracheal suctioning of the spontaneously breathing patient is a particularly noxious procedure that should be avoided.

Treatment with sympathomimetic bronchodilators, systemically or by aerosol, must also be carefully evaluated for potential risks and benefits. Adverse effects on cardiac rhythm or myocardial oxygen consumption might occur. However, in the patient with significant and reversible bronchospasm, the improvements in ventilation–perfusion relationships, oxygenation, and work of breathing, typically outweigh any effects of cardiac stimulation, and these medications should not be withheld.

CARDIOPULMONARY RESUSCITATION

Algorithms for the management of sudden cardiorespiratory arrest are outlined in Chapter 34. Cardiac arrest related to myocardial infarction most often occurs within the first 24 to 48 hours of hospitalization. In-hospital mortality of approximately 80% has been observed, although long-term survival rates may be similar for patients discharged following acute myocardial infarction, with or without a history of resuscitation from cardiac arrest.[45]

The basic components of cardiopulmonary resuscitation are external chest compression and artificial ventilation. The respiratory care practitioner is frequently a part of the CPR provider team, and may also face complications of CPR in the patient who survives resuscitation. The most commonly observed complication of CPR has been injury to the sternum and ribs from chest compressions.[46,47] A flail chest is less common, but may require temporary support with positive-pressure ventilation.[48] Mediastinal hemorrhage, pneumothorax, or hemothorax may occur. Traumatic injury to abdominal viscera may also occur during CPR, with significant hemorrhage or rupture of the stomach, liver, or spleen. Burn injuries of the chest wall may complicate attempts at defibrillation.

Complications of airway management are frequent and include regurgitation and aspiration, injuries to the mouth and pharynx, laryngeal trauma, endotracheal tube misplacement, and esophageal injury.[46] In an attempt to avoid gaseous distention of the stomach during bag–mask or mouth-to-mouth ventilation, it has been suggested that a longer inspiratory time (therefore slower flow rate and lower peak pressure) be used, and that cricoid pressure be applied during ventilation.[49]

SUMMARY

New developments and technology are changing the initial evaluation and treatment of the patient with acute myocardial ischemia. Coexisting cardiac and respiratory diseases are common, and management requires an understanding of cardiopulmonary interactions. Thoughtful respiratory care is an integral part of the successful management of the patient admitted to the coronary care unit.

REFERENCES

1. Standards and guidelines for cardiopulmonary resuscitation (CPR) and emergency cardiac care (ECC). JAMA 255:21:2905–2914, 1986
2. Nishimura RA, Miller FA, Callahan MJ et al: Doppler echocardiography: Theory, instrumentation, technique and application. Mayo Clin Proc 60:321–343, 1985
3. Willerson JT: Radionuclide assessment and diagnosis of acute myocardial infarction. Chest 93:(suppl 1):7S–9S, 1988
4. Gill JB, Ruddy TD, Newell JB et al: Prognostic importance of thallium uptake by the lungs during exercise in coronary artery disease. N Engl J Med 317:1485–1489, 1987
5. Valentine PA, Fluck DC, Mounsey JPD et al: Blood-gas changes after acute myocardial infarction. Lancet 2:837–841, 1966
6. Al Bazzaz FJ, Kazemi H: Arterial hypoxemia and distribution of pulmonary perfusion after uncomplicated myocardial infarction. Am Rev Respir Dis 106:721–728, 1972
7. Ayres SM, Grace WJ: Inappropriate ventilation and hypoxemia as causes of cardiac arrhythmias. Am J Med 46:495–505, 1969
8. Ishikawa K, Hayashi T, Kohashi Y et al: Reduction of left ventricular size following oxygen inhalation in patients with coronary artery disease as measured by biplane coronary cineangiograms. Jpn Circ J 48:225–232, 1984
9. Hoel BL, Bay G, Refsum HE: The effects of morphine on the arterial and mixed venous blood gas state and on the hemodynamics in patients with clinical pulmonary congestion. Acta Med Scand 190:549–554, 1971
10. Zelis R, Mansour EJ, Capone RJ, Mason DT: The cardiovascular effects of morphine: The peripheral capacitance and resistance vessels in human subjects. J Clin Invest 54:1247–1258, 1974
11. Berthelsen P, St Haxholdt O, Husum B, Rasmussen JP: PEEP reverses nitroglycerin-induced hypoxemia following coronary artery bypass surgery. Acta Anaesth Scand 30:243–246, 1986
12. Lie KI, Wellens HJ, van Capelle FJ, Durrer D: Lidocaine in the prevention of primary ventricular fibrillation. A double blind randomized study of 212 consecutive patients. N Engl J Med 291:1324–1326, 1974
13. Durrer JD, Lie KI, van Capelle FJL, Durrer D: Effect of sodium nitroprusside on mortality in acute myocardial infarction. N Engl J Med 306:1121–1128, 1982
14. Cohn JN, Franciosa JA, Francis GS et al: Effect of short-term infusion of sodium nitroprusside on mortality rate in acute myocardial infarction complicated by left ventricular failure. N Engl J Med 306:1129–1135, 1982
15. Gillespie TA, Ambos HD, Sobel BE, Roberts R: Effects of dobutamine in patients with acute myocardial infarction. Am J Cardiol 39:588–594, 1977
16. Taylor SH, Verma SP, Hussian M et al: Intravenous amrinone in left ventricular failure complicated by acute myocardial infarction. Am J Cardiol 56:29B–32B, 1985
17. Yusuf S: The use of beta-adrenergic blocking agents, IV nitrates and calcium channel blocking agents following acute myocardial infarction. Chest 93(suppl):25S–28S, 1988
18. Yusuf S, Peto R, Lewis J et al: beta Blockade during and after myocardial infarction: An overview of the randomized trials. Prog Cardiovasc Dis 27:335–371, 1985
19. Gibson RS, Boden WE, Theroux P et al and the Diltiazem Reinfarction Study Group: Diltiazem and reinfarction in patients with non-Q-wave myocardial infarction. Results of a double-blind, randomized, multicenter trial. N Engl J Med 315:423–429, 1986
20. Forrester JS, Diamond G, Chatterjee K, Swan HJC: Medical therapy of acute myocardial infarction by application of hemodynamic subsets (pt 1 of 2). N Engl J Med 295:1356–1362, 1976
21. Forrester JS, Diamond G, Chatterjee K, Swan HJC: Medical therapy of acute myocardial infarction by application of hemodynamic subsets (pt 2 of 2). N Engl J Med 295:1404–1413, 1976
22. DeWood MA, Spores J, Notske R et al: Prevalence of total coronary occlusion during the early hours of transmural myocardial infarction. N Engl J Med 303:897–902, 1980
23. Marder VJ, Sherry S: Thrombolytic therapy: Current status (pt 1 of 2). N Engl J Med 318:1512–1520, 1988
24. Gruppo Italiano Per Lo Studio Della Streptochinasi Nell'Infarcto Miocardio (GISSI): Effectiveness of intravenous thrombolytic treatment in acute myocardial infarction. Lancet 1:397–401, 1986
25. The ISAM Study Group: A prospective trial of intravenous streptokinase in acute myocardial infarction (ISAM). N Engl J Med 314:1465–1471, 1986
26. International Study of Infarct Survival (ISIS) Steering Committee: Intravenous streptokinase given within 0–4 hours of onset of myocardial infarction reduced mortality in ISIS-2. Lancet 1:502, 1987
27. White HD, Norris RM, Brown MA et al: Effect of intravenous streptokinase on left ventricular function and early survival after myocardial infarction. N Engl J Med 317:850–855, 1987
28. The TIMI Study Group: The thrombolysis in myocar-

dial infarction (TIMI) trial. N Engl J Med 312:932–936, 1985

29. Verstraete M, Bory M, Collen D et al: Randomized trial of intravenous recombinant tissue-type plasminogen activator versus intravenous streptokinase in acute myocardial infarction. Lancet 1:842–847, 1985

30. O'Neill W, Timmis G, Bourdillon P et al: A prospective randomized clinical trial of intracoronary streptokinase versus coronary angioplasty therapy of acute myocardial infarction. N Engl J Med 314:812–828, 1986

31. Guerci AD, Gerstenblith G, Brinker JA et al: A randomized trial of intravenous tissue plasminogen activator for acute myocardial infarction with subsequent randomization to elective coronary angioplasty. N Engl J Med 317:1613–1618, 1987

32. Topol EJ et al, TAMI Study Group: A multicenter randomized trial of intravenous recombinant tissue plasminogen activator and emergency coronary angioplasty for acute myocardial infarction: Preliminary report from the TAMI study. Circulation 74:11–23, 1986

33. Cohn LH: Surgical treatment of acute myocardial infarction. Chest 93(suppl):13S–16S, 1988

34. Light RW, George RB: Serial pulmonary function in patients with acute heart failure. Arch Intern Med 143:429–433, 1983

35. Hales CA, Kazemi H: Small-airways function in myocardial infarction. N Engl J Med 290:761–765, 1974

36. Holford FD, Mithoefer JC: Cardiac arrhythmias in hospitalized patients with chronic obstructive pulmonary disease. Am Rev Respir Dis 108:879–885, 1973

37. Steele P, Ellis JH, Van Dyke D et al: Left ventricular ejection fraction in severe chronic obstructive airways disease. Am J Med 59:21–28, 1975

38. Robotham JL: Cardiovascular disturbances in chronic respiratory insufficiency. Am J Cardiol 47:941–949, 1981

39. Chin WDN, Cheung HW, Driedger AA et al: Assisted ventilation in patients with pre-existing cardiopulmonary disease. The effect on systemic oxygen consumption, oxygen transport, and tissue perfusion variables. Chest 88:503–511, 1985

40. Räsänen J, Nikki P, Heikkilä: Acute myocardial infarction complicated by respiratory failure. The effects of mechanical ventilation. Chest 85:21–28, 1984

41. Yeston NS, Grasberger RC, McCormick JR: Severe combined respiratory and myocardial failure treated with high frequency ventilation. Crit Care Med 13:208–209, 1985

42. Räsänen J: Conventional and high frequency controlled mechanical ventilation in patients with left ventricular dysfunction and pulmonary edema. Chest 91:225–229, 1987

43. Shinozaki T, Deane RS, Perkins FM et al: Comparison of high-frequency lung ventilation with conventional mechanical lung ventilation. Prospective trial in patients who have undergone cardiac operations. J Thorac Cardiovasc Surg 89:269–274, 1985

44. Klein P, Kemper M, Weissman C et al: Attenuation of the hemodynamic responses to chest physical therapy. Chest 93:38–42, 1988

45. Goldberg RJ, Gore JM, Haffajee CI et al: Outcome after cardiac arrest during acute myocardial infarction. Am J Cardiol 59:251–255, 1987

46. Krischer JP, Fine EG, Davis JH, Nagel EL: Complications of cardiac resuscitation. Chest 92:287–291, 1987

47. Enarson DA, Gracey DR: Complications of cardiopulmonary resuscitation. Heart Lung 5:805–807, 1976

48. Enarson DA, Didier EP, Gracey DR: Flail chest as a complication of cardiopulmonary resuscitation. Heart Lung 6:1020–1022, 1977

49. Melker RJ: Recommendations for ventilation during cardiopulmonary resuscitation: Time for a change? Crit Care Med 13:882–883, 1985

THIRTY-FOUR

Cardiopulmonary Resuscitation

James M. Hurst
Richard D. Branson
Kenneth Davis, Jr.
Jay A. Johannigman

Cardiac arrest is a generic term used to describe the sudden loss of vital signs. Most arrests are either cardiac or pulmonary in origin. Primary cardiac arrest is often the result of lethal arrhythmias, such as ventricular fibrillation or tachycardia, occurring in individuals with ischemic heart disease. Cardiac arrest occurring secondary to respiratory arrest may be the result of a drug overdose, aspiration, drowning, or hypoventilation. Metabolic disorders, such as hyperkalemia or hypocalcemia, are a third, and less frequent, cause of cardiac arrest.

Although the evolution of cardiopulmonary resuscitation (CPR) can be traced back as far as the 16th century and Vesalius' description of resuscitation of animals,[1] the current method of CPR is attributed to the work of Kouvenhoven and associates of Johns Hopkins.[2] *Basic life-support* (BLS) is the term used by the American Red Cross in place of CPR. Basic life-support consists of the initiation of emergency ventilation–oxygenation and circulatory support. *Advanced cardiac life-support* (ACLS) is the attempt to restore, maintain, and stabilize cardiopulmonary function by means of pharmacotherapy or electrical defibrillation after the initiation of BLS.

Recently, the silver anniversary of contemporary CPR was celebrated. A national conference was convened to review and revise the standards and guidelines for cardiopulmonary resuscitation and emergency cardiac care. This chapter is designed to be in compliance with the American Heart Association (AHA) guidelines. As such, the most current algorithms for the management of various cardiac dysrhythmias are reproduced near the end of this chapter (see Figs. 34–9 through 34–15). The remainder of the chapter will be dedicated to providing the reader with a basic understanding of when to initiate emergency cardiac care (ECC) and cardiopulmonary resuscitation (CPR) and a basic understanding of the physiologic principles involved.

SCOPE OF THE PROBLEM

In 1984, cardiovascular disease accounted for nearly 1 million deaths, representing 50% of deaths from all causes. Of these cardiovascular deaths, approximately one-half were due to coronary heart disease, most of which were sudden deaths.[3] It is estimated that two-thirds of sudden deaths of coronary heart disease occur outside of the hospital. Therefore, emphasis has been placed on early (field) intervention. Education of the lay community provides the potential for the ultimate coronary care unit capable of acting on the sudden arrest victim. With increasing education and earlier intervention, resuscitation has been successful in up to 40% of cases. This suggests that with an effective education program, as many as 150,000 sudden coronary deaths per year may be prevented. Based on these statistics, the American Heart Association has continued to support an aggressive campaign to educate and train the lay public. The goals of education are twofold: (1) to educate the public to recognize risk factors associated with heart disease and (2) to provide training in the techniques of CPR (BLS).

TRAINING AND EVALUATION OF RESCUERS

In 1977, surveys indicated that approximately 12 million adults had been trained in CPR. Estimates anticipated that an additional 60 to 80 million would be trained in the ensuing years. Some areas of the country have been highly motivated and dedicated to training the lay public in CPR. For example, it is estimated that more than one-third of the adult nonmedical population of Seattle had been trained in CPR by 1983.

It is of paramount importance that appropriate methodology that provides simplistic, yet accurate, widespread training for CPR be sought. When considering lay rescuer CPR, it is important that emphasis be placed on the training of families, neighbors, and office workers of individuals who are at high risk for developing cardiac events. Appropriate educational methods are necessary to obviate the many reasons why potential rescuers fail to get involved during emergency situations. Reasons why potential rescuers fail to get involved include (1) lack of motivation, (2) fear of doing harm, (3) inability to remember exact sequences, (4) poor skill retention, and more recently, (5) the fear of acquiring disease.

It is clear that emphasis should be placed on one-rescuer CPR when dealing with the lay public. The two-rescuer method of CPR adds to the complexity of the repetitive sequences and, therefore, decreases retention. Likewise, obstructed airway maneuvers and infant resuscitations should be targeted to individuals who are in high-risk environments (day care centers, restaurants, and such).

All health care professionals, regardless of their setting, be it hospital, private offices, home health care, or special care units, should be taught all skills of CPR, including single-rescuer, two-rescuer, infant resuscitation, obstructed airway management, and basic cardiovascular pharmacology, so that the optimum return of vital organ function may be provided in the shortest period.

Since repetition of learned acts is a vital part of the learning process, the in-hospital code team or cardiac arrest teams should provide simulations in both patient care and nonpatient care areas so that these skills will be maintained.

CARDIOPULMONARY RESUSCITATION (CODE) TEAMS IN THE INSTITUTIONAL SETTING

Depending on the institution, the composition of the code team will vary. In teaching institutions, a medical resident, cardiology fellow, surgical resident, respiratory therapist, and anesthesiologist are traditionally involved. In nonteaching institutions, immediate response generally rests with the emergency medicine physicians, who, in most institutions, are present in-house 24 hours a day. In addition to the foregoing members, our own institution has adopted the practice of providing a pharmacist who responds with the code team. This enables the appropriate administration of drugs and, generally, the immediate recognition of adverse drug reactions and combinations before they occur.

A modern, well-equipped cardiac arrest cart is essential for proper function of the CPR team. Several such carts should be kept in strategic patient care areas throughout the hospital. In remote locations a "roving" crash cart should be available. At our institution the "roving crash cart" is located in the central pharmacy. During activation of the code team, when the pharmacist responds to nonpatient care areas, the roving crash cart accompanies him. We have found this to be a successful addition to the CPR team. Accurate record keeping, a constant review of the sequence of events during the emergency response, and review of the written records are mandatory.

Activation of the CPR team should be kept as simple as possible. Depending on the institution, the use of an overhead paging system or group of pagers with a common frequency should be employed. When a cardiac arrest occurs, a single call will activate the members of the CPR team simultaneously. Notification of a security officer will enable a designated elevator to be secured from general use so that the CPR team may be transported without delay.

BASIC LIFE-SUPPORT

ESTABLISHING THE NEED FOR RESUSCITATION

The first step in the resuscitation of a victim is establishing need; is the patient unresponsive? Simple maneuvers, such as shaking the patient and asking "Are you OK?" are the first steps in the resuscitation procedure. Observation for the presence of respiratory effort as well as listening and feeling for the movement of air at the nose and mouth establishes the need for intervention. If there is no evidence of conscious respiratory effort, the rescuer must activate the emergency medical service (EMS) or hospital code team and initate CPR (BLS).

AIRWAY CONTROL

Once the need for BLS is determined, establishment of adequate airway control is the immediate concern. In the unconscious victim, absence of sufficient muscle control will allow the tongue to fall posteriorly, obstructing the hypopharynx. Initial attempts to maintain a patient airway include the head-tilt neck-lift, head-tilt chin-lift, and jaw-thrust maneuvers.

In nontraumatic cardiac arrest, in which there is no question of the integrity of the cervical spine, the first attempt at opening the airway should consist of the head-tilt chin-lift maneuver (see Figs. 20–7A and 34–1). The preferred method of airway control, it is easily learned and simple to perform. One hand is placed on the forehead to provide backward displacement and extend the neck. The opposite hand grasps the chin and lifts directly upward, keeping the mouth slightly open. This maneuver aligns the airway structures in such a way as to assure patency.

An alternative method is the head-tilt neck-lift (Fig. 34–2). With this maneuver the rescuer should place one hand beneath the patient's neck and lift while tilting the patient's head backward with the other hand. This maneuver stretches the anterior neck structures, displacing the tongue from the posterior pharyngeal wall. It is estimated that the hypopharynx may be successfully opened in 70% to 80% of unconscious patients by these methods.

In patients with suspected neck injury, the jaw-thrust technique provides an alternative means of establishing an airway. With this technique the victim's lower jaw is grasped and lifted with both hands, displacing the mandible forward while tilting the head slightly backward. The mouth should be held partially open (Fig. 34–3). It should be emphasized that airway control takes precedence over potential cervical injury.

If airway patency cannot be achieved with these maneuvers, a high index of suspicion should exist for partial or complete airway obstruction. Severe or even complete airway obstruction is indicated by hyperactivity of the accessory respiratory

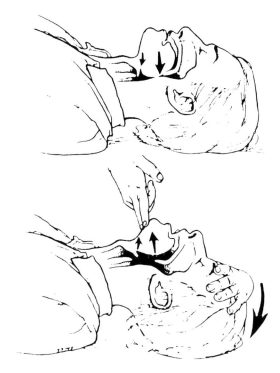

Figure 34–1. Head-tilt chin-lift maneuver for opening the airway. *Top:* Airway is obstructed by posterior movement of the tongue. *Bottom:* Relief of obstruction with the head-tilt chin-lift maneuver. (Reproduced with permission. © Textbook of Advanced Cardiac Life Support, p 27. Dallas, TX, American Heart Association, 1987)

muscles of the neck, supraclavicular, and intercostal areas. If airway obstruction is complete, airflow sounds will be absent. If incomplete, various degrees of noise intensity may be produced, depending on the severity of obstruction. Crowing, gurgling, wheezing, or snoring may be indications of partial airway obstruction. The experienced respiratory therapist can frequently suspect an obstruction at either the bronchial, laryngeal, or hypopharyngeal level depending on the character of the noise.

In cases of partial obstruction, if the victim is conscious, he or she should be encouraged to breathe deeply and attempt to cough or spit out the obstruction. When a conscious patient exhibits complete airway obstruction (cyanosis, inability to cough or talk), or uses the international distress signal for choking (clutching both hands at the neck), several techniques may be attempted. These techniques include back blows, chest thrusts, abdominal thrusts, and subdiaphragmatic abdominal thrusts (Heimlich maneuver) (see Fig. 20–8).[4] All of these techniques are controversial, although the

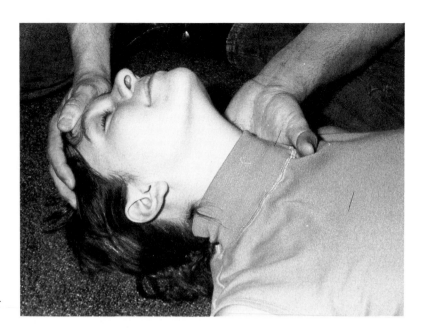

Figure 34—2. Head-tilt neck-lift maneuver for opening the airway.

Figure 34—3. Jaw-thrust maneuver for use in cases of suspected cervical spine injury.

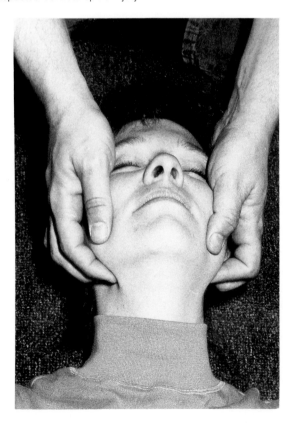

AHA and American Red Cross have recently recommended the Heimlich maneuver in place of back blows. Theoretically, all these techniques increase intrathoracic pressure, simulating a normal cough, expelling the obstruction. Success of these techniques have been described anecdotally, but scientific evidence is lacking. With these maneuvers, the increases in intrathoracic pressure (with a closed airway) and airflow through the trachea (with an open airway) are significantly less than with normal coughing. Effectiveness may also be reduced after a coughing spell, since this results in a low lung volume.

Complications of the Heimlich maneuver have been reported. These include gastric rupture, pneumomediastinum, aortic injury, liver rupture, and regurgitation. Despite the relative paucity of evidence supporting these techniques, in a deteriorating situation of complete obstruction, any organized attempt at expelling the foreign body is warranted.[5–9]

The previously described methods of airway control are always available, very effective, and should not be overlooked during the initial phases of CPR–BLS. In addition, there are a wide variety of airway adjuncts for maintaining and for securing an adequate airway.

Pharyngeal Intubation

Oropharyngeal and nasopharyngeal tubes, often referred to as oral and nasal airways, are used to hold the tongue forward and provide an open passageway past the lips and teeth (see Figs. 20–15, 20–17, and 34–4). When properly placed, "airways" relieve the rescuer of the necessity for providing continuous chin-lift or jaw-thrust maneuvers. However, even with the airway in place, the head should remain tilted slightly backward.

Oral airways should be used only in unconscious victims, as they may provoke gagging and regurgitation in the victim with intact airway reflexes. Nasal airways are more readily tolerated by the semiconscious or stuporous victim and are easier to place. Oral airways, however, provide a larger air passage.

Esophageal Obturator Airway

The esophageal obturator airway (EOA) (see Fig. 20–19) consists of a large-bore tube with a blind-end tip, a cuff that inflates in the esophagus, and a series of ventilation holes (located approximately one-third the way down the tube at the hypopharyngeal level) that allow positive-pressure ventilation to inflate the lungs, while a face mask seals the mouth and nose. The EOA is intended for emergency field use in comatose, apneic patients in whom endotracheal intubation cannot be performed. The EOA is placed blindly into the esophagus and the cuff inflated to prevent gastric insufflation and regurgitation. The mask is sealed tightly around the nose and mouth while ventilation is provided through the side holes (Fig. 34–5).

Initially, the EOA was felt to be a replacement for endotracheal (ET) intubation.[10,11] However, the EOA does not allow true control of the airway, and clinical studies have shown it to be inferior to ET

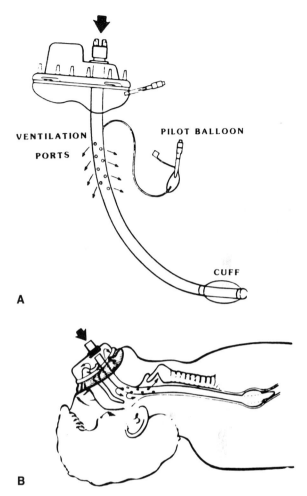

Figure 34–5. (*A*) Esophageal obturator airway. (*B*) Correct placement of the esophageal obturator airway. *Arrows* depict the movement of inspired and expired gas.

Figure 34–4. A nasal airway (*top*) and oral airway (*bottom*).

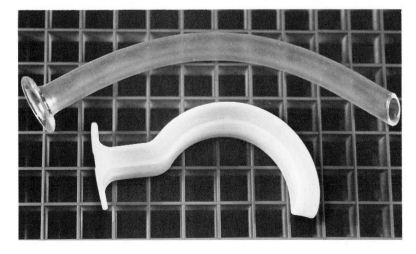

intubation.[12,13] Problems with the EOA include difficulty in maintaining a tight seal at the mask, inability to control laryngospasm, and inability to suction the tracheobronchial tree. Complications of EOA use have been reported frequently. In 10% of cases, inadvertent tracheal intubation may occur, which, if unrecognized will result in death. Other complications include esophageal and gastric laceration or perforation, vomiting with subsequent gastric aspiration, and precipitation of laryngospasm.[14,15]

If a patient arrives in the emergency department with an EOA, the staff should be familiar with its structure and operation. The EOA should never be removed or the cuff deflated until endotracheal intubation has been accomplished and control of the airway assured. Removal of the EOA is usually followed by regurgitation; therefore, adequate suction should be available.

The EOA should be used only by trained emergency personnel in the rare event that ET intubation cannot be accomplished. As such, it is preferable to teach ET intubation, rather than the use of the EOA.

The esophageal gastric tube airway (EGTA) is a modification of the EOA that has an open-end tube for continuous removal of gastric contents. Consequently, ventilation is delivered to the mask and travels through the natural airway to the lungs. If the airway is obstructed, use of the EGTA is contraindicated.

Tracheal Intubation

Endotracheal intubation remains the preferred method of airway control. It permits complete isolation of the airway and facilitates oxygenation, ventilation, and suctioning.

Responsibility for endotracheal intubation should lie with the most experienced member of the resuscitation team. Most often, this is either an anesthesiologist, anesthetist, or respiratory therapist. Regardless of who is responsible, a regular training schedule, including both mannequin and operating room practice should be in place to assure continued proficiency.

Equipment for Endotracheal Intubation

The equipment necessary to perform endotracheal intubation should be located within every crash cart and checked daily to assure its presence and proper function. This should include a laryngoscope handle, a variety of laryngoscope blades (various sizes), endotracheal tubes, Magill forceps, syringes (to inflate the cuff), water-soluble lubricant, and suction catheters.

Laryngoscope and Laryngoscope Blades. The laryngoscope and attached blade is used to directly expose the glottis. The handle contains batteries that provide the electrical source for the light bulb located at the distal portion of the blade. When the handle and blade are snapped together, the bulb should illuminate. If it does not, the batteries, connection, and light bulb should all be checked. Often the bulb may need to be tightened into its receptacle to make contact. It is good practice to check that the bulb is secure beforehand, rather than encountering darkness or losing the bulb into the tracheobronchial tree. There are a variety of blades, the two major groups being curved (MacIntosh) and straight (Miller). The curved blade is inserted above the epiglottis into the vallecula to expose the vocal cords, whereas the straight blade is placed more distally and lifts the epiglottis directly (Fig. 34–6). Technically speaking, neither is superior, and blade choice should be made according to clinician preference.

Endotracheal Tube. The endotracheal tube is an open-ended, thermoliable, polyvinyl chloride tube, with a standard 15-mm connector at the proximal end, an inflatable cuff at the distal end, an inflating tube, and a pilot balloon. After placement, a syringe is connected to the pilot balloon and the cuff is inflated until an adequate seal is obtained. Endotracheal tubes from 6.0 to 9.5 mm, in 0.5-mm increments, should be stocked in the crash cart at all times. Choosing the appropriate ET tube size is guided by clinical experience. In adults, sizes 8.0 to 8.5 mm (for men) and 7.0 to 7.5 mm (for women)

Figure 34–6. Proper laryngoscope placement for straight (*left*) and curved blades (*right*).

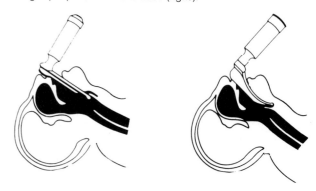

are commonly used. Of course, in certain instances (airway edema, malformation, and such) appropriate tube size will vary. The malleable stylette can be placed inside the ET tube and pre-formed to assist entry into the larynx. The tip of the stylette should always be recessed one-half inch from the distal opening of the tube to prevent trauma or puncture of the airway. Magill forceps may be used to remove foreign bodies from the airway as well as to assist in directing the ET tube towards the larynx.

Procedure. Before beginning the intubation attempt, the patient should be oxygenated and adequately ventilated to assure tolerance of the procedure. The patient should be placed in the "sniffing" position and, when possible, maintained in this manner by an assistant. The laryngoscope blade is inserted into the right side of the mouth, sweeping the tongue to the left, and advanced midline, while simultaneously lifting the mandible at a 45 ° angle toward the ceiling. Once the vocal cords are visualized the tube should be inserted, maintaining sight of the cords at all times. After placement, auscultation of breath sounds and visual inspection of chest movement should be accomplished to assure correct positioning of the tube. If available, a chest radiograph is the definitive method for checking placement.

During the emergency situation, orotracheal intubation is preferred to nasotracheal because it is more simple and easy, it allows use of a larger tube, and it is generally less traumatic.

Percutaneous Transtracheal Ventilation. PTV is a temporary airway and ventilatory support technique that is used when ET intubation is impossible and the necessary equipment for cricothyroidotomy or tracheostomy is unavailable. PTV is accomplished by inserting a large-bore cannula through the cricothyroid membrane. The cannula should be connected to a syringe and during insertion aspirated slightly. When the syringe fills with air (which will be humid and should fog the sides of the syringe) entrance into the trachea is confirmed. Intermittent insufflation of oxygen through the cannula provides adequate oxygenation and ventilation in most cases. With this system, expiration occurs passively through the natural airway. If complete upper airway obstruction is present, lung volume will gradually increase (unless the obstruction is dislodged) until only slight chest excursions are seen during insufflation. This may result in extensive barotrauma and signals the need for cricothyroidotomy or tracheostomy.

Cricothyroidotomy and Tracheostomy. In the face of the inability to provide an adequate airway or in the face of significant maxillofacial trauma in which orotracheal or nasotracheal intubation may be contraindicated, cricothyroidotomy remains the procedure of choice if surgical access to the airway is deemed necessary. An incision is made at the location level of the cricoid cartilage. In the absence of significant anterior cervical trauma, the cricoid cartilage and cricothyroid membrane are readily identifiable landmarks. A transverse incision is made and a puncture is made through the cricothyroid membrane. The knife handle is then turned and inserted into the incision and rotated 90°. The airway can thus be opened and a small tracheostomy tube placed.

Tracheostomy has been advocated as a procedure to be undertaken when other methods fail to achieve an adequate airway. This procedure is not to be undertaken lightly, since its complications far exceed those of a cricothyroidotomy.

BREATHING SUPPORT

Once a patient airway has been established, ventilation of the lungs should be attempted. The simplest, most readily available method of ventilation is the mouth-to-mouth technique. The rescuer should pinch the patient's nose, take a large breath, cover the victim's mouth with his or her own, and expire a volume of approximately 800 mL over a 1.5-second period. The amount of volume delivered should be gauged by observing adequate chest excursion. In the adult, breathing should continue every 5 seconds.

Expired gas resuscitation in infants is provided every 3 seconds (20 BPM) and volume should be limited to that which causes the chest to rise. Depending on size, ventilation may be provided through the nose or mouth, or both simultaneously. This technique reduces resistance to inflation and provides a tighter seal. The expired gas of the rescuer contains between 16% to 18% oxygen and 2% to 4% carbon dioxide. This will normally provide an alveolar oxygen tension of 80 torr. The actual PaO_2 will depend upon ventilation–perfusion matching and cardiac output.[17]

A recent change in the methods for providing ventilatory assistance during respiratory and cardiac arrest has occurred. In conscious individuals, the lower esophageal sphincter functions as a pressure-sensitive valve that prevents gastric insufflation, regurgitation, and aspiration. In the anesthetized patient, when static airway pressure is less than 19 cmH₂O, the likelihood of gastric insufflation and regurgitation is low.[18] A recent study has demonstrated a 30% decrease in total lung compliance and a fall in lower esophageal sphincter pressure from 28 cmH₂O to 4 cmH₂O during 15 minutes of electrically induced cardiac arrest without CPR. The previous recommendations of four "ventilator breaths" after airway opening have been felt to increase the incidence of gastric insufflation and the likelihood of regurgitation aspiration. The major strategy during CPR is to prolong inflation and decrease the risk of gastric insufflation. Studies have indicated that the use of a longer inspiratory time, which produces a lower flow rate and a lower peak inspiratory pressure, may achieve these goals. Therefore, the current recommendations of a 1.5-second inspiratory time (I/E = 1:3), which should average 12 breaths/min, should be the goal of respiratory assistance.[19,20]

Mouth-to-Adjunct Ventilation

The decade of the 1980s has resulted in relative paranoia over the possibility of contracting disease. As such, potential rescuers and health care professionals may be reluctant to perform mouth-to-mouth breathing. Industry has capitalized on these events and provided a wide variety of devices to assist in expired gas resuscitation. These are generically put into two groups: (1) mouth-to-airway and (2) mouth-to-mask devices.

Mouth-to-airway devices include (1) the S-tube, (2) double Guedel airways, and (3) the Brooke airway. Each acts as an oral airway for the patient, but allows ventilation without mouth-to-mouth contact. Mouth-to-mask devices are more popular and have found their way to the bedside of virtually every hospitalized patient (see Figs. 20–13 and 34–7). The initial mouth-to-mask device was the Laerdal pocket-mask described by Safar.[21] This was a simple mask that contained a nipple for supplemental delivery of oxygen. The newest generation of mouth-to-mask devices includes a filter (which protects both rescuer and victim), an oxygen inlet, an exhalation valve (which directs the victims expired gases away from the rescuer), and a lightweight, transparent face mask. These devices have recently been reviewed by Hess et al.[22] In general, if a tight seal is able to be maintained, mouth-to-mask ventilation may be easier to learn and perform than mouth-to-mouth resuscitation.

Figure 34—7. Mouth-to-mask device.

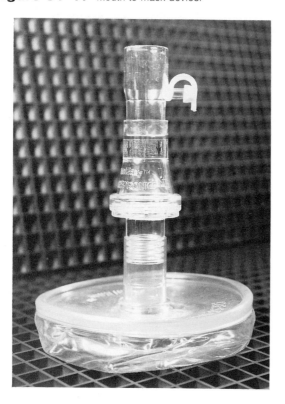

Bag–Valve–Mask Ventilation

Bag–valve devices, more commonly known as manual resuscitators or AMBU bags, consist of a self-inflating bag (SIB), a nonrebreathing valve (NRV), air-inlet valve, oxygen inlet, and oxygen reservoir. On the tail of the SIB is an air inlet (where ambient air fills the bag during refill) and, when available, an oxygen inlet and reservoir. At the top end is an NRV, which directs gas from the bag to the patient and expired gas from the patient to the atmosphere. Whenever possible oxygen should be supplied to the resuscitator to provide the highest FiO₂ to the patient.

An adequate bag–valve–mask unit should satisfy the following criteria: (1) self-refilling capability, (2) a valve system that will not permit rebreathing and will not jam at a high oxygen flow (15 L/min), (3) capabilities to perform satisfactorily at extremes of temperature and uncommon environmental conditions, (4) the availability of both adult and pediatric sizes, (5) no pressure pop-off valve except in pediatric sizes, (6) adequate oxygen to ensure the delivery of an FiO₂ of 0.95 with the standard 15/22-mm connecting fittings, (7) the face mask should be made of transparent material viable enough to ensure a tight facial seal, (8) performance characteristics that make is suitable for mannequin practice, (9) capability of delivering positive end-expiratory pressure from 0 to 12 cmH₂O and (10) the ability to monitor airway pressure. Manual resuscitators may be used with a mask, ET tube, or EOA. When used with an ET, tube operation is easily learned and accomplished. Adequate ventilation with bag–valve–masks (BVM), however, is very difficult for one rescuer. Several studies have demonstrated the inability of physicians, respiratory therapists, nurses, and emergency medical personnel to perform adequate BVM ventilation. As such, when ET intubation is not available, mouth-to-mask is preferred to BVM.

Ventilators and Cardiopulmonary Resuscitation

In general terms, use of an automatic ventilator during CPR is to be discouraged. Because most units may be pressure-limited or pressure-cycled, high airway pressures associated with cardiac compressions may cause premature termination of the breath. The result is hypoventilation with resultant hypercarbia, acidosis, and hypoxemia. When used, portable ventilators should be volume- or time-cycled. These ventilators should also be rugged, durable, and simple to use. We have previously described the successful use of automatic ventilators in paramedic ambulances.[23] However, in our series, only intubated patients were ventilated. The use of ventilators with a mask is more difficult and is not now recommended. When a mechanical ventilator is used with a mask, it should be capable of providing independent adjustment of rate and tidal volume.

Oxygen-Powered Breathing Devices. Oxygen-powered breathing devices are mentioned here only to be condemned. These devices operate from a 50 psi source and are capable of delivering large tidal volumes and extremely high flow rates, with very little operator control or effort. They are associated with barotrauma and, when used with a mask, may produce massive gastric distension.

CLOSED CHEST COMPRESSIONS

Regardless of whether the resuscitation attempt is being run by a one-rescuer or two-rescuer effort, the patient should be placed in the supine position on a flat, nonyielding surface for initiating closed chest compressions. Intermittent pressure should be applied to the lower third of the sternum with

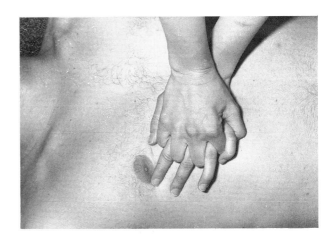

Figure 34–8. Correct hand position for closed-chest compressions.

the base of the palm of the hand (Fig. 34–8). When this maneuver is properly executed, studies have estimated that approximately 20% to 35% of normal cardiac output can be maintained. In 1960, it was generally accepted that blood flow during closed compressions was generated by actual cardiac compression.[2] In 1976, it was demonstrated that the heart merely serves as a conduit.[24] Flow is generated by pressure gradients created between intrathoracic and extrathoracic vascular structures. Forward flow to the arterial side is favored by functional venous valves, one of the more significant being contraction of the diaphragm against the inferior vena cava during chest compressions. Although the predominant mechanism of flow during cardiac compression remains the thoracic pump theory, 25% to 35% of patients may derive some benefit from direct cardiac compressions.

The initial American Heart Association guidelines recommended 60 compressions per minute, with a 50% chest compression/relaxation ratio for the most favorable blood flow during CPR. Recent studies have indicated that a more rapid rate, one approaching 90/min, may be more appropriate than the presently recommended 60/min. Additional studies have indicated that high impulse cardiopulmonary resuscitation with rates of 120–150/min may actually improve coronary blood flow. Although improvement in coronary and cerebral blood flow have been shown to occur, there is inconclusive evidence that the more rapid rates will facilitate cardiopulmonary resuscitation. This fact, coupled with the increase in adverse side effects, such as rib fractures, pneumothoraces, and injury to intra-abdominal structures, have failed to lead to the adoption of the 120 to 150 compressions per minute strategies.

Mechanical Cardiopulmonary Resuscitation Devices. Piston devices or "thumpers" used to provide automatic chest compressions have been used for some time.[25] When operated competently and positioned properly, they are as effective as manual compressions. Their use, however, is limited to unique situations, and routine application is to be discouraged.

Specialized Cardiopulmonary Resuscitation. Several techniques have been advocated that may increase the efficacy of closed-chest compressions. The most popular are simultaneous ventilation–compression (SVC–CPR) and interposed abdominal binding–chest compressions (IAC–CPR). In animal studies, each has been shown to enhance cardiac output and cerebral perfusion pressure. Clinical evidence supporting these techniques, however, is currently lacking.

Precordial Thump. The precordial thump is accomplished by delivering a quick, sharp, single blow to the midportion of the sternum, using the fleshly portion of the fist. Initially, this was recommended in all cases of cardiac arrest as an attempt to "restart" the heart. Current use should be limited to the ICU, where the ECG can be monitored. In this setting, restoration of normal sinus rhythm has been achieved when delivered shortly after the onset of ventricular fibrillation or ventricular tachycardia.

ONE-RESCUER CARDIOPULMONARY RESUSCITATION

Application of the techniques described in the foregoing in proper sequence is what constitutes BLS–CPR. When only one rescuer is present, the recommended sequence is as follows:

1. Establish the need for intervention.
2. Perform the head-tilt chin-lift maneuver (see Fig. 34–1) and check for breathing.
3. If respirations are absent, give two deep lung inflations. Allow 1 to 2 seconds for each inspiration and make sure complete passive expiration occurs.
4. Feel the carotid pulse, if it is present continue inflations every 5 seconds in adults (12 BPM), every 4 seconds in children (15

BPM) and every 3 seconds in infants (20 BPM).
5. If the pulse is absent, begin chest compressions at a rate of 80–100/min.
6. After 15 compressions, stop and provide two more lung inflations. Continue this sequence until the patient recovers, help arrives, or exhaustion prevents further efforts.

TWO-RESCUER CARDIOPULMONARY RESUSCITATION

When two rescuers are present, steps 1 through 3 (foregoing) are repeated and followed by:

4. Begin compressions at 80–100/min, giving a single inflation every fifth breath. If inflations are difficult, the rescuer performing compression may allow a slight pause after every fifth compression to assist in lung inflation.

ELECTRICAL THERAPY

Defibrillation should be applied as soon as possible when the heart is known to be in ventricular fibrillation. Almost all patients can be successfully converted from this rhythm if defibrillation shocks are applied immediately upon recognition. Studies have proved the value of out-of-hospital immediate defibrillation. Therefore, early application of direct current (DC) defibrillation should be taught to all prehospital personnel. The previously advocated practice of "blind" defibrillation, although it remains a standard recommendation, is usually not necessary in the modern environment because of the availability of the so-called quick look paddles common on most defibrillators. Determination of the appropriate current dose (joules) for initial fibrillation is based on the major factors determining thoracic impedence. These include (1) energy level, (2) electrode size, (3) interface between the skin and electrode, (4) number and interval of previous shocks, (5) phase of ventilation, (6) the distance between electrodes, and (7) paddle electrode pressure. Studies have indicated that the initial energy level should be 200 joules. If high thoracic impedence is encountered or suspected, higher energy levels will be needed. Failure to convert the rhythm after two applications of 200 joules should be followed by higher energy levels (360 joules).

Patients who are known to have pacemaker generators should have the defibrillation electrodes placed at least 12 cm from the pacemaker generator. While defibrillation is not generally recommended for the treatment of asystole, fine ventricular fibrillation may masquerade as cardiac standstill. Therefore, failure of appropriate response suggest the possibility that it may be due to fine ventricular fibrillation and a trial of defibrillation should be attempted.

Temporary electrical pacing may be extremely helpful in some clinical situations. The patient whose primary problem is that of impulse formation or conduction, may respond to electrical stimuli. Patients who have profound bradydysrhythmias are also good candidates for temporary electropacing. When cardiac arrest is associated with asystole or electrical mechanical disassociation, pacing is usually ineffective. Since placement of a transvenous or transthoracic pacing wire is an invasive procedure, it is generally relegated to trained medical professionals. With the advent of transcutaneous pacing, pacemakers are now available to a wide variety of personnel, from the prehospital care arena to nonphysician members of the hospital staff. Studies have shown that adequate pacing may be obtained with this modality.

RESUSCITATION PHARMACOLOGY

Drugs are a useful and often necessary adjunct during cardiovascular resuscitation. The term *adjunct* must be stressed because initiation of successful base life-support with adequate ventilation and effective cardiac compression is of primary importance. Utilization of drugs during resuscitation should be considered after sound, effective CPR has been established. The agents used during CPR may be divided into the following categories:

1. Drugs used to restore spontaneous circulation or support circulation following the restoration of spontaneous circulation (epinephrine, norepinephrine, dopamine, dobutamine)
2. Drugs used for control of rhythm and heart rate (lidocaine, bretylium, procainamide, atropine, verapamil)
3. Drugs used to control or correct acid–base imbalance (sodium bicarbonate)
4. Miscellaneous agents (calcium, digitalis, nitroglycerin, nipride)

Catecholamines are a class of agents, with potent cardiovascular effects, that may be conveniently divided into two major classes, α and β, based upon their receptor stimulation. The α-adrenergic properties, which may be of benefit during CPR, include peripheral vasoconstriction. They elevate aortic diastolic pressure, favorably improving coronary perfusion and coronary blood flow. The β-adrenergic effects that may be useful during CPR include increased chronotropy (cardiac rate) and inotropy (cardiac contractility). Adrenergic drugs are categorized according to their relative agonism for α- or β-receptors: pure α-agonists (methoxamine, phenylephrine), pure β-agonists (isoproterenol, dobutamine), or mixed agonists (epinephrine, norepinephrine, dopamine).

By selectively combining the use of one group of agonists with blocking agents, it is possible to selectively study the effects that α- and β-agonists have on successful resuscitation. Results of these studies demonstrate that the agonist properties of adrenergic drugs result in successful resuscitation.

There appears to be little or no added benefit from β-agonist properties. To date, data comparing mixed agonists, such as epinephrine, with selective α-agonists, such as phenylephrine, do not conclusively demonstrate any advantage of one type of catecholamine in terms of vital organ blood flow, long-term survival, or neurologic outcome. Therefore, **epinephrine** should continue to be used at the currently suggested dose and intervals (Table 34–1) as the primary catecholamine during resuscitation. Use of epinephrine promotes successful conversion of ventricular fibrillation and may be of value in resuscitation during cardiac arrest from asystole and electromechanical dissociation.

DRUGS USED FOR CONTROL OF HEART RHYTHM AND RATE

Lidocaine remains the drug of choice for management of ventricular ectopy as well as ventricular tachycardia and ventricular fibrillation. Lidocaine acts predominantly by reducing the variability of ventricular refractoriness and by reducing ventricular automaticity. In animal models, lidocaine also elevates the threshold for ventricular fibrillation. There are several ways to administer lidocaine. It is reliably and predictably absorbed when administered by either the IV or endotracheal route. After an initial 1 mg/kg bolus, additional 0.5 mg/kg boluses can be given every 8 to 10 minutes as necessary to a total dose of 3 mg/kg. After successful resuscitation, a continuous infusion should be begun at 2–4 mg/min.

Table 34—1 Commonly Used Pharmacologic Agents

DRUG AND DOSAGE	MECHANISM	INDICATION
Epinephrine 0.5–1.0 mg IV or ETT q5min	α- and β-agonist	All forms of cardiac arrest
Atropine 0.5 mg IV	Vagolytic	Symptomatic bradycardia
Lidocaine Bolus of 1.5 mg/kg	Decreases automaticity, elevates fibrillation threshold	Ventricular fibrillation, ventricular tachycardia, PVCs
Procainamide 100 mg q5min	Decreases automaticity	PVCs and ventricular tachycardia when lidocaine is not successful
Bretylium 5 mg/kg bolus (may repeat)	Similar to lidocaine	Ventricular fibrillation and ventricular tachycardia not responsive to other Rx
Verapamil 5 mg slow IVP	Calcium channel blocker	Paroxysmal SVT
Sodium bicarbonate 1 mEq/kg	Buffer	When indicated by ABG.
Calcium chloride 2–4 mg/kg of 10% solution	Increases myocardial contractile function	Acute hyperkalemia, acute hypocalcemia
Norepinephrine 2 μg/min	α- and β₁-agonist	Significant hypotension
Dopamine 2–5 μg/kg/min	Dopaminergic agonist	Significant hypotension
Dobutamine 2.5–10 μg/kg/min	α- and β₁-agonist	Low cardiac output
Isoporoterenol 2 μg/min	Pure β-agonist	Atropine-resistant bradycardia
Amrinone load: 0.75 mg/kg 2–20 μg/kg/min	Phosphodiesterase inhibitor	Low cardiac output
Digitalis 10–15 μg/kg	ATPase inhibitor	Rapid response atrial fibrillation or atrial flutter
Sodium nitroprusside 0.5 μg/kg/min	Peripheral vasodilator	Hypertensive emergency
Nitroglycerin 0.3 mg SL q 5	Smooth-muscle dilator	Angina

In recent years, there has been increasing emphasis on the use of **bretylium** in the treatment of resistant ventricular tachycardia and ventricular fibrillation. Bretylium results in the rapid release of catecholamines and effects a brief period of hypertension, tachycardia, and increased contractility. Subsequently, bretylium's blockade of α-adrenergic receptors reduces blood pressure and results in hypotension (a major side effect). Bretylium elevates the ventricular fibrillation threshold and, in some studies, has been shown to have more potent antifibrillatory effects than other agents. The efficacy of bretylium has been demonstrated in several studies, but it has not been demonstrated to be more effective than lidocaine. For this reason, and because of the hypotension associated with the use of bretylium, it should not be used as a first-line agent. The use of bretylium is reserved for situations for which (1) lidocaine and defibrillation have failed to convert ventricular fibrillation, (2) ventricular fibrillation has recurred during lidocaine administration, or (3) lidocaine and procainamide have failed to control ventricular tachycardia. In these settings, 5 mg/kg of bretylium is given IV as a bolus followed by electrical defibrillation. if ventricular fibrillation persists, the dose may be increased to 10 mg/kg and repeated at 15- to 30-minute intervals, up to a maximum dose of 30 mg.

Procainamide, like lidocaine, is effective in suppressing ventricular ectopy. It is recommended when lidocaine has failed to suppress ventricular ectopy or recurrent ventricular tachycardia. Procainamide may be given in a dose of 50 mg IV every 5 minutes until either the arrhythmia is suppressed, hypotension occurs, or the QRS complex is widened by 50% of its original width. The maintenance infusion rate is 1–4 mg/min.

Atropine sulfate is a parasympatholytic drug that reduces cardiac vagal tone. Atropine is useful in treating sinus bradycardia that results in hypotension, hypoperfusion, or frequent ventricular ectopic beats. There is also some data to suggest that atropine may be effective in the therapy of ventricular asystole. The recommended dose of atropine for asystole is 1.0 mg IV. This dose may be repeated every 5 minutes that asystole persists. For bradycardia, the dose is 0.5 mg IV every 5 minutes to a total dose of 2.0 mg.

Verapamil is a calcium channel blocking agent the action of which on the AV node makes it particularly effective in treating supraventricular tachycardia. It may reduce blood pressure and left ventricular function. Therefore, it must be used with caution in patients with congestive heart failure. Verapamil is the agent of choice for the conversion of paroxysmal supraventricular tachycardia in stable patients if maneuvers that increase vagal tone (e.g., carotid massage) are unsuccessful. An initial dose of 5 mg is given. This may be increased to 10 mg if conversion has not occurred within 15 to 30 minutes. Severe bradycardia, hypotension, and congestive heart failure can occur after administration. The hypotension associated with the use of verapamil can often be reversed by the administration of 0.5 to 1.0 g of IV calcium chloride.

SODIUM BICARBONATE

The use of **sodium bicarbonate** to manage the acidosis that may accompany cardiac arrest has, until recently, been an accepted component of the therapeutic armamentarium. The critical role of acidosis in aggravating electrolyte disturbances, antagonizing the effects of catecholamines, and lowering the ventricular fibrillation threshold served as the rationale for aggressive therapy with sodium bicarbonate. In the late 1970s, an increasing body of evidence emphasized the potentially deleterious effects of the use of sodium bicarbonate during resuscitation. The adverse effects potentially attributable to the use of bicarbonate became more apparent and include (1) a pH induced shift in the oxyhemoglobin saturation curve, inhibiting the release of oxygen at the tissue level; (2) a paradoxic central nervous system acidosis, resulting from the inability of bicarbonate to cross the blood–brain barrier; (3) the generation of malignant arrhythmias induced by alkalosis; (4) a marked increase in serum sodium and serum osmolarity; and (5) a direct myocardial depressant effect, produced by bicarbonate itself.

It has also been demonstrated in clinical studies that sound basic life-support measures are capable of preventing acidosis for a prolonged period. It was established that an adequate arterial pH could be maintained by hyperventilation alone, obviating the need for large amounts of buffer. On the basis of this data, the most recent standards have been revised to emphasize the critical role of adequate alveolar ventilation and to restrict the use of bicarbonate. It has been estimated that instituting these effective interventions would require at least 10 minutes; therefore, it is suggested that bicarbonate not be administered during the initial 10 minutes of a resuscitation sequence. Because of the lack of totally definitive data in this area, it is acknowledged that some individuals might wish to use bicarbonate thereafter.

CALCIUM CHLORIDE

Because recent evidence suggests that, during cardiopulmonary arrest, high intramitochondrial calcium levels may result in "mitochondrial poisoning," the general use of calcium during resuscitation is not now recommended. It has also been suggested that the "no-reflow phenomena" may be due to the influx of calcium into anoxic smooth-muscle cells, both in the heart as well as in the arteriolar smooth muscle. This reduces arteriolar diameter and may increase resistance to blood flow, further inhibiting postanoxic neurologic recovery. There remain, however, specific indications for the use of calcium. These include cardiac arrest secondary to the use of calcium channel blockers, hypocalcemia, and possibly cardiac arrest secondary to massive transfusion of blood bank products.

TREATMENT OF COMMON CARDIAC ARRHYTHMIAS

A detailed discussion of arrhythmias and their recognition is beyond the scope of this chapter. In lieu of this, the *treatment* of the seven most common arrhythmias, according to The American Heart Association, are found in Figures 34–9 to 34–15.

(text continues on p 901)

Bradycardia

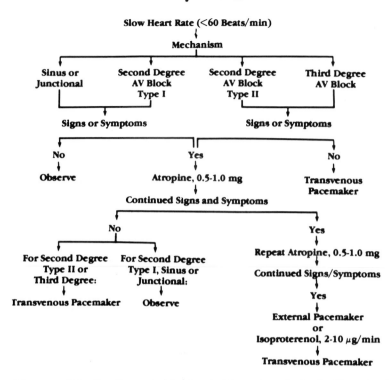

Figure 34—9. Suggested treatment of hemodynamically significant bradycardia is demonstrated: Significant signs and symptoms include hypotension (systolic blood pressure < 90 mmHg), premature ventricular contractions, altered mental status, chest pain, dyspnea, ischemia, or myocardial infarction. The use of isoproterenol should be considered as temporizing therapy only. The algorithm represents suggested management only. Some patients may require care not specified in the figure. (Reproduced with permission. Standards and Guidelines for Cardiopulmonary Resuscitation and Emergency Cardiac Care. Copyright American Heart Association, 1986)

Figure 34—10. Suggested treatment of paroxysmal supraventricular tachycardia (PSVT) is demonstrated: The flow of the algorithm presumes that PSVT is continuing. The algorithm represents suggested management only. Some patients may require care not specified in the figure. (Reproduced with permission. Standards and Guidelines for Cardiopulmonary Resuscitation and Emergency Cardiac Care. Copyright American Heart Association, 1986)

Paroxysmal Supraventricular Tachycardia

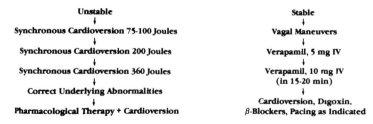

Ventricular Ectopy

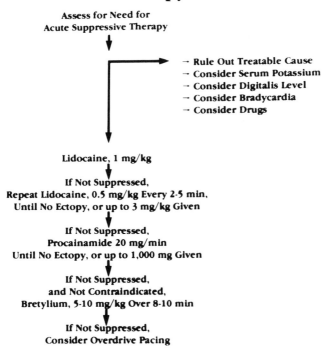

**Assess for Need for
Acute Suppressive Therapy**

→ **Rule Out Treatable Cause**
→ **Consider Serum Potassium**
→ **Consider Digitalis Level**
→ **Consider Bradycardia**
→ **Consider Drugs**

Lidocaine, 1 mg/kg

**If Not Suppressed,
Repeat Lidocaine, 0.5 mg/kg Every 2-5 min,
Until No Ectopy, or up to 3 mg/kg Given**

**If Not Suppressed,
Procainamide 20 mg/min
Until No Ectopy, or up to 1,000 mg Given**

**If Not Suppressed,
and Not Contraindicated,
Bretylium, 5-10 mg/kg Over 8-10 min**

**If Not Suppressed,
Consider Overdrive Pacing**

**Once Ectopy Resolved, Maintain as Follows:
After Lidocaine, 1 mg/kg...Lidocaine Drip, 2 mg/min
After Lidocaine, 1-2 mg/kg...Lidocaine Drip, 3 mg/min
After Lidocaine, 2-3 mg/kg...Lidocaine Drip, 4 mg/min
After Procainamide...Procainamide Drip, 1-4 mg/min (Check Blood Level)
After Bretylium...Bretylium Drip, 2 mg/min**

Figure 34—11. Suggested treatment of ventricular ectopy is demonstrated: The flow of the algorithm presumes that ventricular ectopy is continuing. The algorithm represents suggested management only. Some patients may require care not specified in the figure. (Reproduced with permission. Standards and Guidelines for Cardiopulmonary Resuscitation and Emergency Cardiac Care. Copyright American Heart Association, 1986)

Sustained Ventricular Tachycardia

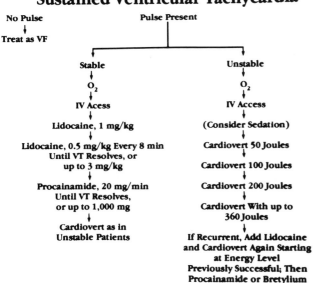

No Pulse
↓
Treat as VF

Pulse Present

Stable
↓
O₂
↓
IV Access
↓
Lidocaine, 1 mg/kg
↓
**Lidocaine, 0.5 mg/kg Every 8 min
Until VT Resolves, or
up to 3 mg/kg**
↓
**Procainamide, 20 mg/min
Until VT Resolves,
or up to 1,000 mg**
↓
**Cardiovert as in
Unstable Patients**

Unstable
↓
O₂
↓
IV Access
↓
(Consider Sedation)
↓
Cardiovert 50 Joules
↓
Cardiovert 100 Joules
↓
Cardiovert 200 Joules
↓
**Cardiovert With up to
360 Joules**
↓
**If Recurrent, Add Lidocaine
and Cardiovert Again Starting
at Energy Level
Previously Successful; Then
Procainamide or Bretylium**

Figure 34—12. Suggested treatment of sustained ventricular tachycardia (VT) is demonstrated: The flow of the algorithm presumes that VT is continuing. Unstable patients include those with chest pain, dyspnea, hypotension (systolic BP < 90 mmHg), congestive heart failure, ischemia, or myocardial infarction. The algorithm represents management only. Some patients may require care not specified in the figure. (Reproduced with permission. Standards and Guidelines for Cardiopulmonary Resuscitation and Emergency Cardiac Care. Copyright American Heart Association, 1986)

Electromechanical Dissociation

Continued CPR
↓
Establish IV Acess
↓
Epinephrine, 1:10,000, 0.5-1.0 mg IV Push
↓
Intubate When Possible
↓
(Consider Bicarbonate)
↓
Consider Hypovolemia,
Cardiac Tamponade,
Tension Pneumothorax,
Hypoxemia,
Acidosis,
Pulmonary Embolism

Figure 34—13. Suggested treatment of electromechanical dissociation (EMD) is demonstrated: The flow of the algorithm presumes that EMD is continuing. The algorithm represents suggested management only. Some patients may require care not specified in the figure. (Reproduced with permission. Standards and Guidelines for Cardiopulmonary Resuscitation and Emergency Cardiac Care, Copyright American Heart Association, 1986)

Figure 34—14. Suggested treatment of ventricular fibrillation (VF) and pulseless ventricular tachycardia (VT) is demonstrated: The flow of the algorithm presumes that VF or pulseless VT is continuing. The algorithm represents suggested management only. Some patients may require care not specified in the figure. (Reproduced with permission. Standards and Guidelines for Cardiopulmonary Resuscitation and Emergency Cardiac Care. Copyright American Heart Association, 1986)

Ventricular Fibrillation
and
Pulseless Ventricular Tachycardia

Witnessed Arrest   Unwitnessed Arrest
↓   ↓
Check Pulse—If No Pulse   Check Pulse—If No Pulse
↓
Precordial Thump
↓
Check Pulse—If No Pulse

CPR Until a Defibrillator Is Available
Check Monitor for Rhythm—if VF or VT
Defibrillate 200 Joules
↓
Defibrillate 200-300 Joules
Defibrillate With up to 360 Joules
CPR If No Pulse
Establish IV Access
↓
Epinephrine, 1:10,000, 0.5-1.0 mg IV Push
↓
Intubate If Possible
Defibrillate With up to 360 Joules
Lidocaine, 1 mg/kg IV Push
↓
Defibrillate With up to 360 Joules
Bretylium, 5 mg/kg IV Push
↓
(Consider Bicarbonate)
Defibrillate With up to 360 Joules
↓
Bretylium, 10 mg/kg IV Push
Defibrillate With up to 360 Joules
↓
Repeat Lidocaine or Bretylium
↓
Defibrillate With up to 360 Joules

Asystole

**If Rhythm Is Unclear and Possibly Ventricular
Fibrillation, Defibrillate as for VF. If Asystole is Present**

↓

Continue CPR

↓

Establish IV Access

↓

Epinephrine, 1:10,000, 0.5-1.0 mg IV Push

↓

Intubate When Possible

↓

Atropine, 1.0 mg IV Push (Repeated in 5 min)

↓

(Consider Bicarbonate)

↓

Consider Pacing

Figure 34—15. Suggested treatment of asystole is demonstrated: The flow of the algorithm presumes that asystole is continuing. The algorithm represents suggested management only. Some patients may require care not specified in the figure. (Reproduced with permission. Standards and Guidelines for Cardiopulmonary Resuscitation and Emergency Cardiac Care. Copyright American Heart Association, 1986)

CEREBRAL RESUSCITATION AFTER CARDIAC ARREST

Safar recently reviewed cerebral resuscitation after cardiac arrest. In this review, he states that cerebral neurons are capable of tolerating a 20-minute period of normothermic ischemic anoxia. Cerebral recovery after a period of 5 minutes of cardiac arrest is hampered by a complex set of secondary derangements, associated with multiple-organ system reperfusion. He has characterized the postresuscitation syndrome as including the following events: (1) secondary cerebral perfusion failure, (2) cerebral reoxygenation injury, and (3) cerebral intoxication from toxic metabolic products from extracerebral organs.

Several complex postcerebral resuscitation protocols have been studied extensively by Safar. These include (1) a brain-oriented extracerebral life-support protocol; (2) intra-arterial hemodilution, hypertension, and artificial circulation; (3) use of barbiturates; (4) use of calcium channel blockers; (5) the use of free radical scavengers; and (6) a multifaceted treatment protocol. Less-than-successful cerebral protection has been shown on experimental animals. Many of the protocols are far too complex and may be clinically impractical in some settings. Therefore, widespread use of these modalities is currently relegated to the laboratory and tightly controlled clinical protocols. The current mainstay of cerebral resuscitation during cardiac arrest is to maintain adequate cerebral blood flow with presently accepted techniques.[26]

OPEN-CHEST CARDIAC MASSAGE

Closed-chest cardiopulmonary resuscitation has been advocated since the 1950s because of the philosophy that it may be applied "to anyone, anytime." Historical data suggests that open-chest cardiac massage may result in a higher mean arterial pressure and greater cerebral blood flow. Some studies have demonstrated that after cardiac arrest of fewer than 4 minutes, internal cardiac massage could maintain normal electroencephalographic activity for periods of up to 1 hour. Likewise, cerebral blood flow was maintained at approximately 50% (as opposed to 25% to 30%) of control values for periods up to 1 hour. Although systolic arterial pressure was not substantially different between open- and closed-chest groups—as in one study—diastolic pressure was three times greater during open cardiac massage. The greater diastolic blood flow, therefore, favors improved coronary blood flow.

Closed-chest CPR results in high intrathoracic venous and intracranial pressure peaks, which may result in low cerebral perfusion pressure and decreased common carotid blood flow. Open-chest CPR results in lower venous and intracranial pressures and higher cerebral perfusion pressures and coronary blood flow. There is ample evidence to support the open-chest CPR is hemodynamically superior to closed-chest CPR.

However, standard CPR remains an effective means of cardiopulmonary resuscitation that may be employed by lay persons as well as trained medical personnel. Although there may be a reasonably well-defined role for open-chest CPR in the patient with traumatic arrest, the precise role of open-chest CPR in nontraumatic cardiac arrest remains to be defined. An important unanswered question is: How long should standard CPR be performed before resorting to open-chest CPR? This is a complex issue and, even given that the complication of open-chest CPR remain very low, it is unlikely that controlled trials comparing open-chest versus closed-chest CPR will be undertaken in the near future.

SURVIVAL FOLLOWING CARDIOPULMONARY RESUSCITATION

The survival following out-of-hospital cardiac arrest is reported to be from 2% to 80% in certain populations. The major determinants of improved survival are witnessed versus unwitnessed arrest, proximity to BLS–ACLS support (EMS system), initial cardiac rhythm, time to reach definitive care, and total resuscitation time. Improvements in these areas will improve out-of-hospital mortality.

In-hospital mortality is effected by underlying disease process, presence of sepsis, prearrest level of consciousness, length of resuscitation, and hemodynamic stability. Those patients who respond to resuscitation in fewer than 15 minutes have a mortality of 40%, whereas those requiring longer than 15 minutes have a mortality of 95%. In all, however, the major determinant appears to be underlying abnormality.

REFERENCES

1. Vesalius A: De Lumani corporis fabrica libri septem. Basel, 1555.
2. Kouwenhoven WB, Jude JR, Knickerbocker GG: Closed chest cardiac massage. JAMA 173:1064, 1960
3. National Center for Health Statistics: Births, marriages, divorces and deaths for January. 34:1, 1985
4. Heimlich HJ: A life-saving maneuver to prevent food choking. JAMA 234:398, 1975
5. Croom EW: Rupture of stomach after attempted Heimlich maneuver. JAMA 250:2602, 1983
6. Chapman JH, Menapace FJ, Howell, RR: Ruptured aortic valve cusp: A complication of the Heimlich maneuver. Ann Emerg Med 12:446, 1983
7. Redding JS: The choking controversy: Critique of evidence on the Heimlich maneuver. Crit Care Med 77:45, 1979
8. Vistine RG, Baick CH: Ruptured stomach after Heimlich maneuver. JAMA 234:415, 1975
9. Palmer E: The Heimlich maneuver misused. Curr Prescrib 5:45, 1979
10. Carlson WJ, Hunter SW, Bonnabeau RC Jr: Esophageal perforation with obturator airway. JAMA 241:1154, 1979
11. Smith JP, Bodai BI, Seifkin A et al: The esophageal obturator airway. JAMA 250:1081, 1983
12. Goldenberg IF, Campion BC, Siebold CM et al: Esophageal gastric tube airway vs endotracheal tube in prehospital cardiopulmonary arrest. Chest 90:90, 1986
13. Smith JP, Bodai BI, Auborg R et al: A field evaluation of the esophageal obturator airway. J Trauma 23:317, 1983
14. Michael TAD: The esophageal obturator airway—a critique. JAMA 246:1098, 1981
15. Johnson KR Jr, Genovesi MG, Lassar KH: Esophageal obturator airway: Use and complications. JACEP 5:36, 1976
16. Jacobs HB: Emergency percutaneous transtracheal catheter and ventilator. J Trauma 12:50, 1972
17. Elam JO, Greene DG, Brown ES: Oxygen and carbon dioxide exchange and energy cost of expired air resuscitation. JAMA 167:328, 1958
18. Ruben HM, Elam JO, Ruben AM: Investigation of upper airway problems in resuscitation. Anesthesiology 22:271, 1961
19. Melker RJ: Asynchronous and other alternative methods of ventilation during CPR. Ann Emerg Med 13:758–761, 1984
20. Melker RH, Banner MJ: Ventilation during CPR. Two-rescuer standards reappraised. Ann Emerg Med 141:197, 1985
21. Safar P: Pocket mask for emergency artificial ventilation and oxygen inhalation. Crit Care Med 2:273, 1974
22. Hess D, Hess C, Oppel A, Rhoads K: Evaluation of mouth to mask ventilation devices. Respir Care 34:191, 1989
23. Hurst JM, Davis K, Branson RD et al: Ventilatory support in the field: A prospective study. Crit Care Med 34:17, 1989
24. Westerfeldt ML, Chandra N, Fisher J: Mechanisms of perfusion in cardiopulmonary resuscitation. In Shoemaker WC, Thompson WL, Holbrook PR (eds): Textbook of Critical Care Medicine, p 31. Philadelphia, WB Saunders, 1984
25. Taylor GI, Resin R, Tucker M: External cardiac compressions: A randomized comparison of mechanical and manual techniques. JAMA 240:644, 1978
26. Safar P: Cerebral resuscitation after cardiac arrest. A review. Circulation 74:138, 1986

THIRTY-FIVE

Respiratory Care of the Patient with Neuromuscular Disease

Douglas R. Gracey

THE NEUROMUSCULAR COMPONENT OF THE RESPIRATORY SYSTEM

The signal that drives the periodic activation of the muscles that control ventilation of the lung originates mainly in the pons and medulla. Rhythmic contraction and relaxation of the muscles of respiration is produced from signals generated in the medullary respiratory center, the apneustic center of the lower pons and the pneumotaxic center of the upper pons. The medullary respiratory center is the primary source of the inspiratory signal to the respiratory muscles. However, only the cortex of the brain can voluntarily control respiration.

The control of ventilation relies on a complex system, with the output of the respiratory center being modified by several sensors that supply input signals. The sensors, which provide feedback to the respiratory center, include the central chemoreceptors, the peripheral chemoreceptors, pulmonary stretch receptors, stretch (J) receptors, irritant receptors, upper airway receptors, joint and muscle receptors, and arterial baroreceptors.

The *central chemoreceptors* are located near the surface of the medulla where the hydrogen ion concentration of the extracellular fluid is monitored. Increases in hydrogen ion concentration stimulate ventilation, and decreases have the opposite effect. The hydrogen ion concentration of the extracellular fluid of the medulla is related to that of the cerebrospinal fluid and local blood flow. The metabolic activity of the brain and brain stem is also important in determining hydrogen ion concentration.

The *peripheral chemoreceptors* are located in the carotid and aortic bodies. The peripheral chemoreceptors respond to a fall in arterial pH and oxygen tension and an increase in arterial carbon dioxide tension by increasing input to the respiratory center and increasing ventilatory drive.

Other receptors are important for airway protective mechanisms, cough, stimulation of respiration with exercise and in other situations that require increased ventilation, production of the sensation of dyspnea, and such.

The efferent or output signal from the respiratory center passes to the anterior horn cells of the spinal cord through three groups of neurons. One group carries the signals for involuntary rhythmic breathing. A second group is responsible for the voluntary control of breathing, such as is necessary for speech. A third group controls nonrhythmic functions, such as cough.

Two types of efferent motor neurons pass from the anterior horn cells to the muscles of respiration. Thick (alpha) efferent neurons go to the neuromuscular junction of the main skeletal muscle fiber, whereas thin (gamma) efferent neurons supply the intrafusal muscle spindle fibers. The muscles of respiration innervated by the thick and thin efferent neurons include the diaphragm, intercostal muscles, abdominal muscles, and the accessory muscles of respiration.

Clinical respiratory compromise can occur with disease at any level of the central or peripheral nervous system, the neuromuscular junction, or with primary muscle disease.

DISEASES OF THE BRAIN

Disease of the brain, and especially the brain stem, can affect the respiratory system. Alterations within the brain itself may produce abnormal respiratory patterns, respiratory failure, inability to protect the airway, inability to clear the airway by coughing, and other respiratory complications.

CEREBRAL BLOOD FLOW-INTRACEREBRAL PRESSURE

Cerebral blood flow is autoregulated by the arterial carbon dioxide tension. Rising arterial carbon dioxide tensions increase cerebral blood flow, whereas lowering the $PaCO_2$ has the opposite effect. This is why patients with *acute cerebral trauma* are frequently hyperventilated with mechanical ventilation immediately after the traumatic event. Hyperventilating the patient to a $PaCO_2$ of about 20 torr significantly reduces cerebral blood flow. Theoretically, it reduces the degree of cerebral edema produced by the trauma and also helps to decrease intracranial pressure. A substantial rise in intracranial pressure can reduce cerebral perfusion pressure to critically low levels and, frequently, patients with head injuries are monitored by continuously measuring intracranial pressure.

In patients with very high intracranial pressures, the brain is forced inferiorly with compression of the brain stem (especially the medulla) into the foramen magnum. This herniation can compromise the blood supply to the brain stem and cause acute inactivation of the respiratory center and death. As noted previously, attempts may be made to reduce cerebral blood flow, and thereby intracranial pressure, by hyperventilating the patient with a mechanical ventilator to reduce the arterial carbon dioxide tension.[1,2] In addition, corticosteroids and certain hypertonic solutions, such as mannitol, may be given intravenously to reduce cerebral edema and intracranial pressure. Significant elevation of intracranial pressure is a contraindication to lumbar puncture because the rapid decompression of cerebral spinal fluid pressure may precipitate herniation of the brain stem into the foramen magnum.

NEUROGENIC PULMONARY EDEMA

Another complication of acute brain injury is *neurogenic pulmonary edema*, secondary to elevated intracranial pressure. The exact mechanisms causing neurogenic pulmonary edema have been debated for some time.[3] One theory is that massive sympathetic neuronal discharge produces transient systemic vasoconstriction, and that a shift of blood volume to the pulmonary vascular bed occurs, with resulting high pulmonary vascular pressures and secondary pulmonary edema. Some authors have implicated sudden pulmonary venous constriction, with transient high pulmonary vascular pressures and secondary pulmonary edema as the cause. Elevation of both systemic and pulmonary arterial pressures occurs within seconds of the injury to the central nervous system. It probably results from massive α-adrenergic sympathetic discharge, caused by stimulation of the hypothalamic centers, and this has also been suggested as the cause of neurogenic pulmonary edema. Whatever the mechanisms, acute noncardiogenic pulmonary edema can result from acute brain injury and may require mechanical ventilation with positive end-expiratory pressure (PEEP) and high inspiratory FIO_2 requirements.

CENTRAL NEUROGENIC BREATHING DISORDERS

Abnormal patterns of breathing commonly result from intracranial disorders and indicate bilateral hemispheric or brain stem injury. Head trauma, intracranial tumors, and vascular events, all can lead to neurogenic breathing disorders. The abnormal breathing patterns associated with damage at different levels of the brain and brain stem include the following (Fig. 35–1):

Cheyne–Stokes Breathing. This disordered-breathing pattern is characterized by alternating patterns of hyperventilation followed by either apnea or marked hypoventilation. Some authors state that the variation is in tidal volume alone, and that true apnea is not part of the periodic-breathing pattern. The cause of Cheyne–Stokes breathing is not well understood, although a number of factors, including enhanced ventilatory response to carbon

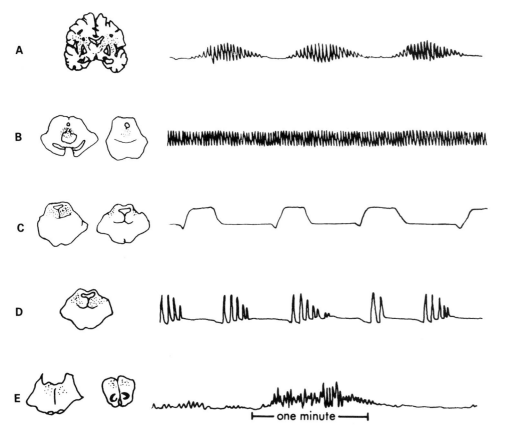

Figure 35—1. Abnormal respiratory patterns associated with pathologic lesions (*shaded areas*) at various levels of the brain. The dotted areas in the brain and brain stem represent the postulated sites of lesions producing the various rhythm abnormalities. Tracings are by chest—abdomen pneumograph: inspiration reads up: (*A*) Cheyne—Stokes respiration; (*B*) central neurogenic hyperventilation; (*C*) apneusis; (*D*) cluster breathing; (*E*) ataxic breathing (see text). (Plum F, Posner JB: The Diagnosis of Stupor and Coma, 2nd ed. Philadelphia, FA Davis, 1972)

dioxide and disordered cerebral blood flow, have been suggested. Severe heart failure is probably the major cause of Cheyne—Stokes respiration. Although the pattern of breathing in Cheyne—Stokes respiration is striking, arterial blood gas abnormalities are not necessarily present. Respiratory alkalosis in this condition is, however, a poor prognostic sign.

Apneustic Breathing. This pattern of breathing is characterized by a prolonged cessation of breathing in an inspiratory position. This disorder indicates damage to the pons.

Central Neurogenic Hyperventilation. This marked hyperventilation persists despite arterial oxygen tensions well in excess of 75 mmHg. Per-

sistent hyperventilation produces minute ventilations in excess of four times normal and is related to damage to the midbrain and upper pontine tegmentum from infarction, trauma, or severe anoxia. As with Cheyne—Stokes breathing, central neurogenic hyperventilation has a high mortality if accompanied by respiratory alkalosis. Central neurogenic hyperventilation is very rare, and stimulatory drugs, such as acetylsalicylic acid, must be excluded as the cause.

Central Neurogenic Hypoventilation. This breathing disorder, which is associated with narcotic suppression of the respiratory center, head trauma, vascular accidents, and central nervous system infections, is characterized by carbon dioxide retention. Chronic obstructive lung disease must be ruled out as the cause of alveolar hypoventilation in these patients.

Central Sleep Apnea. This condition has also been called Ondine's curse. When these patients sleep, they have apneic spells with secondary hypoxemia and respiratory acidosis. Obstructive sleep apnea may accompany central sleep apnea. Whether this condition is congenital or is due to prior infection of the central nervous system, such as encephalitis, is not clear. Central sleep apnea and idiopathic central neurogenic hypoventilation can be treated with the implantation of phrenic nerve pacemakers.[4] Progesterone administration may produce an improvement in idiopathic central neurogenic hypoventilation.

Cluster Breathing. Damage to the low pons or high medulla can produce an abnormal pattern of breathing, characterized by normal breaths separated by irregular pauses.

Ataxic Breathing. This pattern of breathing is seen in narcotic poisoning, hypercarbic stupor, brain stem infarcts, meningitis, and with brain tumors. It is characterized by a totally chaotic pattern of breathing with periodic hyperventilation, inspiratory gasps, and apneusticlike inspiratory pauses. This pattern of breathing indicates low pontine and medullary damage.

MOVEMENT DISORDERS

There are a number of diseases of the extrapyramidal system that can cause respiratory complications. *Parkinson disease* can cause respiratory muscle rigidity just as it does with other muscle groups, and this can compromise respiration. Irregular-breathing patterns and incoordination of swallowing make patients with severe Parkinson disease prone to aspiration, with resulting respiratory embarrassment. *Tardive dyskinesia* is another movement disorder associated with respiratory difficulties.

It is clear from this discussion that numerous conditions can cause malfunction of the signal from the respiratory center to the neuromuscular respiratory apparatus below the brain stem. This category includes: vascular events, such as thrombosis and embolism; suppression by drugs, such as narcotics and anesthetics; trauma; tumors; metabolic abnormalities, such as alkalosis and myxedema; movement disorders; and idiopathic

disorders, such as sleep apnea and central hypoventilation.

DISEASES OF THE SPINAL CORD, ANTERIOR HORN CELLS, AND PERIPHERAL NERVES

TRANSECTION OF THE SPINAL CORD

Trauma is the most common cause of death in young people in their teens and early 20s. Motor vehicle and sports accidents are the most frequent causes of trauma. One of the most devastating sequelae of trauma is spinal cord injury.

The extent of paralysis following spinal cord trauma is related to the degree of injury and the location of the injury. Traumatic transection of the cord above the level of the third cervical segment leads to complete respiratory muscle paralysis and death unless mechanical ventilation is instituted. If the lesion of the cord is below the level of the third cervical segment, diaphragmatic function is spared. However, in quadraplegia with spared diaphragm function, the work of breathing is totally maintained by the diaphragm, which must greatly increase its level of work. In addition, respiratory function is not normal, and the potential for respiratory complications is great. These patients, even with intact diaphragm function, have a compromised ability to cough. Paralysis of the abdominal muscles is one reason for this ineffective cough because, to be effective, part of the cough mechanism requires tensing the abdominal muscles. Although the inspiratory capacity of these quadriplegic patients may be quite good, the actual act of coughing causes paradoxic motion of the abdominal wall, and effective cough pressures are difficult to generate unless the abdomen is supported or assisted with inward pressure by the hands of an attendant. Such patients need to be treated with a respiratory therapy protocol that includes frequent turning and assistance in maintaining adequate clearance of airway secretions.[5] With time, spasticity of the intercostal and abdominal muscles helps to improve the patient's spontaneous cough.

DIAPHRAGM PARALYSIS

Unilateral diaphragm paralysis is not uncommon following cardiovascular surgery, owing to trauma to the phrenic nerve. This paralysis may be temporary or permanent, depending on the cause. In patients with normal pulmonary function, unilateral diaphragm paralysis is usually asymptomatic. However, patients with significant obstructive lung disease or restrictive disease may be extremely symptomatic if they sustain unilateral diaphragm paralysis, and this is one of the causes of inability to wean patients from mechanical ventilation postoperatively. In addition to trauma, there are a number of other causes of diaphragm paralysis, including progressive motor neuron disease (amyotrophic lateral sclerosis), poliomyelitis, tetanus, diphtheria, acute porphyria, Guillain–Barré syndrome, malignancy, and cervical cord trauma. The diaphragmatic paralysis can be unilateral or bilateral, depending on the cause. In many patients, the cause of unilateral paralysis of the diaphragm is never found and is termed idiopathic.[6]

MULTIPLE SCLEROSIS

Although respiratory complications occur with multiple sclerosis, they are rare. This demyelinating disease can affect the cervical spinal cord pyramidal tracts and possibly anterior horn cells. Bulbar involvement with multiple sclerosis can affect the respiratory center and airway protective reflex mechanisms and can produce respiratory failure.[7]

POLIOMYELITIS

Poliomyelitis was the disease that literally launched the field of respiratory care (see Preface). Although polio is uncommon in the developed world today, it is still a problem in developing countries. Mechanical ventilation of large numbers of these patients in the polio epidemics of the 1950s provided a great deal of experience in the acute (short-term) and chronic (long-term) mechanical ventilation of patients. Negative-pressure tank ventilators, "iron lung," cuirass ventilators, and positive-pressure ventilators, all were developed in response to the needs of polio patients.

The poliomyelitis virus attacks the anterior horn cells and may lead to paralysis of the limbs and trunk. If the high cervical cord segments supplying the respiratory muscles are involved, varying degrees of respiratory compromise result. If the brain stem is involved (bulbar poliomyelitis), hypoventilation or apnea may result. Today it is apparent that some patients who had poliomyelitis in the 1950s (and survived with minimal and at times inapparent respiratory muscle and bulbar compromise) are being seen with clinical compromise of their respiratory system function as they grow older.[8] Frequently, these patients required respira-

tory support with negative- and positive-pressure mechanical ventilators, years after their acute poliomyelitis infection.

PROGRESSIVE MOTOR NEURON DISEASE

Also known as *amyotrophic lateral sclerosis* (Lou Gehrig disease), progressive motor neuron disease is a progressive disease of the anterior horn cells of unknown cause. It is the most common motor neuron disease. These patients can develop involvement of the respiratory muscles, especially the diaphragm, early or late in their course and develop progressive respiratory failure. Involvement of the brain stem by this disease produces bulbar dysfunction with difficulty speaking and swallowing. Aspiration is common. Some of these patients elect to undergo tracheostomy for airway care and prolonged mechanical ventilation to prolong their lives.[9] Some neurologists use the term amyotrophic lateral sclerosis to describe patients with upper and lower motor involvement and use progressive motor neuron disease to describe those with mainly lower motor neuron involvement. Some of the patients with predominantly lower motor involvement may have a prolonged course, with late onset of respiratory muscle or bulbar involvement.

GUILLAIN–BARRÉ SYNDROME

Guillain–Barré syndrome, also called Landry–Guillain–Barré syndrome and "French polio," is an acute inflammatory polyneuropathy of unknown cause. Frequently, there has been an antecedent viral illness days or weeks before the onset of this illness. This disease affects all ages, but tends to cluster in incidence in the late teenaged, early 20s, and midlife aged groups.

Typically, these patients first note paresthesias in the distal lower extremities, followed by ascending paralysis. The degree of muscle paralysis may be mild, or there may just be paresis. However, in severe cases, complete paralysis of the voluntary muscles may occur, and severe respiratory muscle involvement results in death, unless support with mechanical ventilation is undertaken. Examination of the spinal fluid reveals increased levels of protein, without an increased number of leukocytes. This finding is classic for Guillain–Barré syndrome. Experience at the Mayo Clinic with 79 acute Guillain–Barré patients showed that one-fourth were admitted to a respiratory intensive care unit, and 17% of the patients required mechanical ventilation.[10] Three of the 79 patients died of complications of the disease or its treatment. The usual complications include aspiration, nosocomial infections, pulmonary embolism, and labile autonomic function. Careful attention to nutritional support, prevention of venous thrombosis and pulmonary embolism, and a physical medicine program are the key to the successful treatment of these patients. On the whole, if the Guillain–Barré patient requires mechanical ventilation, tracheostomy should be performed early, as the mean number of days on the ventilator in the Mayo Clinic study was 37 ± 29 days.

Currently, it is not clear if plasma exchange (plasmaphoresis) is beneficial in treating Guillain–Barré patients. It appears that plasma exchange may speed recovery in acute-onset, rapidly progressive disease, but the studies are not conclusive. Corticosteroids do not appear to be of clear-cut benefit in this disease. From 90% to 95% of these patients recover fully. The remainder are left with residual paresis, which is of variable severity.

ACUTE INTERMITTENT PORPHYRIA

Porphyrins are side products of the synthesis of heme. Acute intermittent porphyria is always listed as a cause of respiratory failure, but it is an exceedingly rare cause. Acute intermittent porphyria is the most important of the group of porphyria cutanea tarda, congenital porphyria, and acute intermittent porphyria. Patients with acute intermittent phorphyria have a hereditary partial deficiency of porphobilinogen deaminase and excrete excessive amounts of δ-aminolevulinic acid and porphobilinogen in the urine.

Attacks of acute intermittent porphyria occur in susceptible individuals when precipitated by the administration of certain drugs (e.g., barbiturates), menstruation and pregnancy, infection, and excessive alcohol use. Neurologic features of acute intermittent porphyria can include motor paralysis or paresis varying from mild limb weakness to quadriplegia. Upper and lower motor neuron lesions have been described. The respiratory muscles can be involved, and acute respiratory failure can occur.[11]

DISORDERS OF NEUROMUSCULAR TRANSMISSION

MYASTHENIA GRAVIS

Myasthenia gravis is due to a defect in neuromuscular transmission and is characterized by muscle weakness that worsens with repetitive effort. The defect is confirmed by electromyography. Repeat compound nerve stimulation causes a decremental response in the amplitude of the evoked muscle action potential. In addition, most patients with myasthenia gravis exhibit acetylcholine receptor antibodies in their serum. There is a significant association between the thymus gland and myasthenia gravis. Regardless of the underlying abnormality, thymectomy can produce substantial improvement of myasthenic weakness in some patients. About 5% of patients with myasthenia gravis have thymomas, 75% show thymic hyperplasia, and 10% have a normal gland. The pharmacologic treatment of myasthenia gravis consists of the administration of anticholinesterase drugs such as pyridostigmine. One test for myasthenia gravis, the Tensilon test, consists of giving edrophonium chloride, a very short-acting anticholinesterase drug, and noting its effects on muscle strength. If the patient exhibits respiratory muscle weakness, the vital capacity and maximum inspiratory and expiratory airway pressures can be measured before and after Tensilon administration. In addition to anticholinesterase drugs, patients with myasthenia gravis are frequently treated with long-term, alternate-day corticosteroids and with a short course of plasma exchange to reduce the level of antibody to the acetylcholine receptor sites.

Myasthenia gravis produces compromise of the respiratory system in a number of ways. First there frequently is weakness of the respiratory muscles, with impairment of cough and vital capacity. Bulbar weakness may be significant and lead to aspiration and pneumonia. Anticholinesterase drugs increase airway secretions, and this may be a problem in patients with impaired ability to cough. Too much anticholinesterase medication produces cholinergic crisis and aggravates muscle weakness. These patients can be exceedingly difficult to manage, and respiratory failure can be precipitated by any number of events.[12] Meticulous respiratory care, including chest physical therapy and monitoring of respiratory muscle strength, are keys to the treatment of these patients.

Patients with myasthenia gravis are extremely sensitive to nondepolarizing myoneural blocking drugs and certain other drugs, such as aminoglycosides. At times, unsuspected cases of myasthenia gravis are precipitated into acute respiratory failure by these medications when in the hospital for treatment of other medical problems.

Some patients who are in prolonged respiratory failure and ventilator-dependent with myasthenia gravis may be weaned from ventilator support after multiple plasma exchanges.[13] Subsequent control of acetylcholine receptor antibody production frequently requires high-dose alternate-day corticosteroids, and even immunosuppression with drugs, such as azathioprine.

LAMBERT–EATON MYASTHENIC SYNDROME

The Lambert–Eaton myasthenic syndrome (LEMS) is a disease of the myoneural junction, usually associated with bronchogenic small-cell carcinoma. It is associated with proximal muscle weakness, easy fatigability, dry mouth, and impotence in men. The electromyogram in LEMS characteristically shows a progressive increase in amplitude of compound muscle action potentials, with rates of nerve stimulation above 10/sec. On clinical examination, these patients may exhibit progressive increase in muscle strength with repeated stimulation of a deep tendon reflex or repeated testing of a weak muscle group. Clinical and electromyographic evidence of LEMS can be transferred by serum from human to laboratory animal, but the specific antibody has not been isolated, and plasma exchange has little affect on the syndrome. Respiratory failure may occur in LEMS.[14]

TETANUS

Clostridium tetani is a gram-positive bacillus that has a spore form. The spores, when introduced into a wound, can germinate, and the bacteria will multiply in anaerobic conditions and produce a toxin. Penicillin kills the organism, and persons who have received a previous series of tetanus toxoid injections with periodic booster shots are not susceptible to tetanus. However, nonimmunized individuals who become infected with *C. tetani* can develop tetanus. The organisms liberate a toxin that eventually fixes to the presynaptic terminals of spinal inhibitory interneurons and interferes with the release of inhibitory transmitter substance. This produces the classic picture of tetanic muscle spasm and rigidity. Trismus may occur, with inability to open the mouth, and rigidity of the facial muscles produces an expression called "risus sardonicus." Opisthotonus, dysphagia, aspiration, and respiratory muscle spasm occur in severe cases, and respiratory failure may ensue.

Treatment consists of antibiotics, usually penicillin, surgical debridement of the infected wound, intravenous human tetanus immune globulin, active immunization with tetanus toxoid, and fluid and nutritional support. In severe tetanus, control of the airway and muscle spasms requires that the patient be paralyzed with pancuronium, sedated with diazepam or narcotics, and mechanically ventilated. Usually, after treatment as outlined, a trial of weaning the patient from pancuronium can be attempted after 1 to several weeks.

BOTULISM

Botulism is a severe paralytic disease caused by toxin produced by *Clostridium botulinum*. The most common source of botulism is from food poisoning, but it can occur from wound infection with the organism. Botulism from food poisoning involves the ingestion of pre-formed toxin in infected food. The toxin binds to the presynaptic neuromuscular junction and prevents acetylcholine release. This results in hypotonia and symmetric paralysis. Ingestion of the toxin first produces gastrointestinal symptoms, followed by symptoms of dry mouth, diplopia, and then descending motor paralysis, including the muscles of respiration.

Treatment consists of ventilatory support, elimination of residual toxin in the gastrointestinal tract, and antitoxin. If the toxin type, designated A through G, has been determined from examination of the patient's serum or stool, specific antitoxin is given.

PHARMACOLOGIC NEUROMUSCULAR TRANSMISSION DEFECT

Depolarizing and nondepolarizing muscle relaxant drugs are frequently used in surgery and the respiratory care unit. Meticulous attention to detail and ventilatory support are required if problems are to be avoided. In addition, a large number of substances such as antibiotics (e.g., aminoglycosides), anticholinesterases (e.g., parathione), phenothiazine intoxication, methyl alcohol, magnesium, and clinical hypokalemia can produce neuromuscular transmission defects and respiratory failure.

ORGANOPHOSPHATE POISONING

Organophosphate insecticide poisoning can occur by ingestion, inhalation, or absorption through mucous membranes. Two forms of organophosphate poisoning affect the respiratory system: acute organophosphate toxicity and an intermediate toxicity syndrome that occurs 1 to 4 days after exposure.

Organophosphate insecticides are potent lipid-soluble anticholinesterases. The anticholinesterase binds to acetylcholinesterase and inhibits hydrolysis of acetylcholine. This leads to decreased respiratory muscle strength and may lead to cholinergic crisis, with respiratory failure requiring mechanical ventilation.

Treatment consists of atropine and the cholinesterase reactivator pralidoxime. The atropine is effective against the central respiratory effects of organophosphate, but has little effect on the neuromuscular junction blockade. Mechanical ventilation may be required for up to 2 weeks, depending on the severity of the poisoning.

DISEASES OF THE MUSCLES

MUSCULAR DYSTROPHIES

There are several types of muscular dystrophy, and respiratory complications are common in most of them. Aspiration pneumonia, ineffective cough, and progressive alveolar hypoventilation occurs as these diseases progress. Myotonic dystrophy and progressive muscular dystrophy can lead to progressive respiratory failure.[15] Patients with Duchenne-type muscular dystrophy usually maintain adequate diaphragm function until late in the course of their disease, but frequently die of respiratory infections or respiratory failure.[16] Limb–girdle type of muscular dystrophy patients appear to have early involvement of the diaphragm, associated with respiratory insufficiency.[17] Fascioscapulohumeral dystrophy does not appear to be associated with serious respiratory dysfunction.

MYOPATHIES

There are several myopathies that may lead to respiratory failure. These are rather rare diseases, but include centronuclear myopathy, progressive congenital myopathy, Issac's syndrome, and acid maltase deficiency. Acid maltase deficiency is a metabolic myopathy in which glycogen accumulates in cells because of an inherited enzyme deficiency. These patients develop a proximal myopathy that includes diaphragmatic dysfunction and hypoventilation. This disease usually appears in childhood, but it can also first appear in adults.[18]

POLYMYOSITIS AND DERMATOMYOSITIS

Polymyositis is an inflammatory disease of the skeletal muscle. Characteristically in polymyositis the muscles of the neck, pharynx, and limb girdle are involved. Weakness is the primary complaint. Dysphagia caused by weakness of the posterior pharyngeal muscles can lead to aspiration pneumonia and also respiratory failure.[19] Similar problems occur in dermatomyositis in which inflammation of both skin and muscle occurs. In both diseases, associated malignancy must be ruled out as the cause of the disease, especially in adults. The incidence of associated malignancy is rare, but rises with aging.

RESPIRATORY CARE IN NEUROMUSCULAR DISEASE

ASSESSMENT OF THE PATIENT

The status of the respiratory muscles can be assessed in several ways. Since the most important respiratory muscle is the diaphragm, assessment of this muscle is of most interest.

The physical examination of the patient may suggest that the patient has a paralyzed diaphragm in that *paradoxic (inward) movement of the abdomen* may be observed during inspiration. This paradox of the abdomen may be subtle or absent in unilateral diaphragm paralysis. Normally the abdomen moves out on inspiration as the descending diaphragm pushes down on the abdominal contents. In addition, the patient with diaphragm paralysis may be observed to have dyspnea when supine or may complain of being unable to lie supine.

The function of the diaphragm may be checked with fluoroscopy. Since unilateral diaphragm paralysis may be missed on fluoroscopy with quiet breathing, it is common practice to ask the patient to sniff while being fluoroscoped. The "sniff test" causes sudden contraction of the diaphragm; if one side is paralyzed, it will be observed to move paradoxically. In addition, each side of the diaphragm can be paced transcutaneously in the neck while observing it fluoroscopically and recording its action potential with esophageal or surface electrodes.

The transdiaphragmatic pressure (P_{di}) can be measured by using pressure transducers to measure intrathoracic and intra-abdominal pressures during a maximum inspiration. The P_{di} in normal individuals is greater than 80 cmH$_2$O. Patients with weak or paralyzed diaphragms will exhibit gradations of pressure less than 80 cmH$_2$O.

The most simple means of measuring diaphragmatic function is to measure the vital capacity (VC) and maximum static inspiratory pressure ($P_{I_{max}}$). Both of these measurements are greatly dependent on diaphragm function and strength.[20] The maximum static expiratory pressure ($P_{E_{max}}$) is less useful in measuring diaphragm function, but is helpful for evaluating the ability to produce adequate cough pressures. In Guillain–Barré syndrome, with ascending paralysis, patients may have an excellent VC and $P_{I_{max}}$, but exhibit a drop in $P_{E_{max}}$. This is usually a sign that the abdominal muscles have become paralyzed. Since the ability to hold the abdominal muscles rigid is key to producing an adequate $P_{E_{max}}$ and also cough, this measurement is of great value in patients with neuromuscular disease.

Arterial blood gas assessments are essential to the evaluation of patients with neuromuscular disease. Abnormalities of the arterial blood gas values will vary from hypoxemia, perhaps only when supine with diaphragm paralysis, to varying degrees of carbon dioxide retention caused by alveolar hypoventilation. As a general rule, the progression of hypoxemia and carbon dioxide retention in neuromuscular disease is gradual, and the carbon dioxide retention is metabolically compensated. Because of this, many chronic neuromuscular disease patients may develop serious pulmonary artery hypertension and cor pulmonale before their hypoxemia and carbon dioxide retention are discovered.

HEAD TRAUMA

Patients with trauma to the skull are frequently unconscious or severely obtunded. Therefore, as a rule, they require endotracheal intubation for protection of the airway and secretion management. If respiratory function is compromised, assisted or controlled mechanical ventilation is required. Since significant hypoxemia or hypercapnia causes an increase in cerebral blood flow and, therefore, increased intracranial pressure (ICP), avoidance of both of these situations is desirable. As noted earlier, the production of hypocapnia with controlled mechanical ventilation may be desirable in some head trauma patients to reduce cerebral blood flow, ICP, and cerebral edema.[1] It is also desirable to avoid high intrathoracic pressures because the resulting compromise of venous return elevates systemic venous pressure, which is transmitted to the CNS and has an adverse effect on cerebral spinal fluid drainage. If PEEP must be used in these patients, it should be used carefully. Monitoring of ICP is very helpful in the management of these patients.

SPINAL CORD TRAUMA

As stated earlier, the degree of respiratory compromise with spinal cord trauma depends upon the level of the trauma. Cord lesions above the level of C-3 cause the loss of diaphragm function, and to maintain life, long-term mechanical ventilation is required. Although lesions below C-3 will leave the patient with diaphragm function, special attention will usually be required to maintain adequate tracheobronchial toilet. The management of the patient with a high spinal cord injury is best done with a protocol; the one used in one neurosurgical intensive care unit is shown in Table 35–1.

Table 35–1 Pulmonary Management After Spinal Cord Injury

IN THE EMERGENCY ROOM

1. Assess respiratory function
   Vital capacity, $P_{I_{max}}$, $P_{E_{max}}$
   Arterial blood gases
   Chest x-ray film
2. Supply oxygen, humidification, mechanical ventilatory support as necessary to maintain PaO_2 above 70 mmHg.
3. Pass a nasogastric tube for gastric decompression and prevention of aspiration.
4. Be aware of the possibility of pulmonary edema following overtransfusion. (In the absence of other injuries, a systolic blood pressure of 90 mmHg may provide adequate perfusion as monitored by a urine output greater than 30 mL/hr. When other injuries have resulted in hypovolemia, a central venous cannula may be inserted.)

IN THE INTENSIVE CARE UNIT

1. Once the cervical spine is stabilized with Crutchfield tongs or other device and on a turning frame, turn the patient prone for 2 hr at 4-hr intervals (e.g., 1, 5, 9 AM; 1, 5, 9 PM) with approval of neurosurgeon.
2. Order chest physical therapy to be done immediately before and after pronation.
   Breathing exercises
   Assisted coughing
   Incentive spirometry
3. In the presence of secretion retention
   Order IPPB with a nebulized bronchodilator to be given before pronation.
   Consider bronchoscopy if lobar collapse is present on chest x-ray film.
   Sputum for Gram stain, culture, and sensitivities.
4. Obtain chest x-ray examination and arterial blood gas assessment the day after admission.
5. Obtain vital capacity, $P_{I_{max}}$, and $P_{E_{max}}$ the day after admission and then twice weekly while in intensive care.

AFTER LEAVING THE INTENSIVE CARE UNIT

1. Order side-to-side turning every 2 hr.
2. Order chest physical therapy (breathing exercises and assisted coughing) and incentive spirometry every 2 hr, except between 10 PM and 6 AM.
3. Obtain vital capacity, $P_{I_{max}}$, and $P_{E_{max}}$ once a week.

LONG-TERM MECHANICAL VENTILATION

The most common reason for long-term mechanical ventilation is neuromuscular disease. In addition, appreciation of the fact that respiratory muscles fatigue when overworked, and function much more efficiently when rested, has led to the use of nocturnal intermittent positive- and negative-pressure-assisted mechanical ventilation in patients such as those with chronic obstructive lung disease.[21-23]

Extensive experience with home negative-pressure ventilation has shown this mode of therapy to be useful in a number of neuromuscular diseases.[24,25] Home positive-pressure-assisted ventilation is now commonly used for patients with amyotrophic lateral sclerosis[9] and muscular dystrophy.[26] Both negative- and positive-pressure home mechanical ventilators have been modernized and made more convenient to use. Recent reports of the ability to maintain patients with neuromuscular disease by nocturnal positive-pressure ventilation, using a nasal mask, are very exciting.[27] This method of nasal positive-pressure ventilation avoids the need for tracheostomy in patients whose only problem is alveolar hypoventilation. Further experience with this method in more centers is needed to fully assess its value and potential.

REFERENCES

1. Bozza Marrubini ML, Rossanda M, Tretola L: The role of artificial hyperventilation in the control of brain tension during neurosurgical operations. Br J Anaesth 36:415–431, 1964
2. James HE, Langfitt TW, Kumar VS, Ghostine SY: Treatment of intracranial hypertension: Analysis of 105 consecutive recordings of intracranial pressure. Acta Neurochir 36:189–200, 1977
3. Theodore J, Robin ED: Speculations on neurogenic pulmonary edema (NPE). Am Rev Respir Dis 113:405–411, 1976
4. McMichan JC, Piepgras DG, Gracey DR et al: Electrophrenic respiration. Report of six cases. Mayo Clin Proc 54:662–668, 1979
5. McMichan JC, Michel L, Westbrook PR: Pulmonary dysfunction following traumatic quadraplegia. JAMA 243:528–531, 1980
6. Piehler JM, Pairolero PC, Gracey DR, Bernatz PE: Unexplained diaphragmatic paralysis: A harbinger of malignant disease? J Thorac Cardiovasc Surg 84:861–864, 1982
7. Boor JW, Johnson RJ, Carnales L, Dunn DP: Reversible paralysis of automatic respiration in multiple sclerosis. Arch Neurol 34:686–689, 1977
8. Lane DJ, Hazleman B, Nichols PVR: Late onset respiratory failure in patients with previous poliomyelitis. Q J Med New Ser 43:551–568, 1974
9. Sivak ED, Gipson WT, Hanson MR: Long-term management of respiratory failure in amyotrophic lateral sclerosis. Ann Neurol 12:18–23, 1981
10. Gracey DR, McMichan JC, Divertie MB, Howard FM Jr: Respiratory failure in Guillain–Barré syndrome: A 6-year experience. Mayo Clin Proc 57:742–746, 1982
11. Goldberg A: Acute intermittent porphyria: A study of 50 cases. Q J Med New Ser 28:183–209, 1959
12. Gracey DR, Divertie MB, Howard FM Jr: Mechanical ventilation for respiratory failure in myasthenia gravis. Two-year experience with 22 patients. Mayo Clin Proc 58:597–602, 1983
13. Gracey DR, Howard FM Jr, Divertie MB: Plasmapheresis in the treatment of ventilator-dependent myasthenia gravis patients: Report of four cases. Chest 85:739–743, 1984
14. Gracey DR, Southorn PA: Respiratory failure in Lambert–Eaton myasthenic syndrome. Chest 91:716–718, 1987
15. McCormack WM, Spalter HF: Muscular dystrophy, alveolar hypoventilation and papilledema. JAMA 197:957–960, 1966
16. Inkley SR, Oldenburg FC, Vigno PJ Jr: Pulmonary function in Duchenne muscular dystrophy related to stage of disease. Am J Med 56:297–306, 1974
17. Newsom–David J: The respiratory system in muscular dystrophy. Br Med Bull 36:135–138, 1980
18. Rosenow EC III, Engel AG: Acid maltase deficiency in adults presenting as respiratory failure. Am J Med 64:485–491, 1978
19. James JL, Park HWJ: Respiratory failure due to polyomyositis treated by intermittent positive-pressure respiration. Lancet 2:1281–1282, 1961
20. Black LF, Hyatt RE: Maximal static respiratory pressures in generalized neuromuscular disease. Am Rev Respir Dis 103:641–650, 1971
21. Sharp JT: Respiratory muscles: A review of old and newer concepts. Lung 157:185–199, 1980
22. Cohen CA, Zagelbaum G, Gross D et al: Clinical manifestations of inspiratory muscle fatigue. Am J Med 73:308–316, 1982
23. Rochester DF, Braun NMT: The respiratory muscles. Basics RD vol 6, no 4, March 1978. American Thoracic Society
24. Splaingard ML, Frates RC, Jefferson LS et al: Home negative pressure ventilation: Report of twenty years experience in patients with neuromuscular disease. Arch Phys Med Rehabil 66:239–242, 1985
25. Holtackers TR, Loosbrock LM, Gracey DR: The use of the chest cuirass in respiratory failure of neurologic origin. Respir Care 27:271–275, 1982
26. Alexander MA, Johnson EW, Petty J, Stauch D: Mechanical ventilation of patients with late stage Duchenne muscular dystrophy: Management in the home. Arch Phys Med Rehabil 60:289–292, 1979
27. Carrey Z, Gottfried SB, Levy RD: Ventilatory muscle support in respiratory failure with nasal positive pressure ventilation. Chest 97:150–158, 1990
28. Leger P, Jennequin J, Gerard M, Robert D: Home positive pressure ventilation via nasal mask for patients with neuromuscular weakness or restrictive lung or chest wall disease. Respir Care 34:73–78, 1989

THIRTY-SIX

Pulmonary Thromboembolic Disease

Myron Stein
Steven E. Levy

Venous thrombosis with subsequent embolization of the lungs (venous thromboembolism) is probably the most common pulmonary disease encountered in the hospitalized patient. The importance of this disease is emphasized by recent estimates that there are approximately 200,000 deaths each year in the United States caused by pulmonary embolism. In 100,000, it is the sole cause of death; in the remaining 100,000, it is the major contributing cause of death. The incidence of symptomatic episodes of pulmonary embolism is estimated to be 630,000 per year, which would make this disease half as common as acute myocardial infarction.

The diagnosis is not established in approximately two-thirds of the patients suffering an embolic episode, and it is in this group of 400,000 patients that most fatalities occur (approximately 120,000). With appropriate therapy, fewer than 10% of patients suffering from pulmonary embolism will die if they survive the initial hour after the embolic event. Thus, the major problem in the management of this disease is recognition and accurate diagnosis. This becomes a particularly difficult problem in the patient with underlying nonembolic pulmonary disease in whom respiratory therapy may be indicated (e.g., the patient with chronic obstructive airway disease, the postoperative patient with atelectasis, or the patient who has aspirated for any of several reasons).

For therapy, the primary goal of thromboembolism treatment is the prevention of further venous thrombosis with anticoagulation, allowing natural thrombolytic mechanisms to lyse the thromboemboli in the pulmonary arteries. The primary role for respiratory therapy in the treatment of the patient with pulmonary thromboembolism is supportive, utilizing the administration of oxygen to correct the arterial hypoxemia that may be typically a consequence of acute pulmonary embolism. Other respiratory therapy modalities, including periodic hyperinflation of the lungs, administration of aerosols, and chest physiotherapy have no proved benefit in pulmonary embolism.

ETIOLOGY AND PATHOLOGY

Pulmonary thromboembolism denotes the passage of a thrombus into a pulmonary artery, with subsequent obstruction of blood supply to lung tissue. In most patients who suffer a symptomatic embolic event, the thrombi initially form in the deep veins of the calves and then propagate proximally into the deep veins of the thighs and pelvis. From these sites the thrombi break off and travel through the venous circulation through the right heart into the lungs. Symptomatic embolic events from thrombi forming in the upper extremities or the right cardiac chambers do occur, but are uncommon.

Pulmonary infarction is an infrequent consequence of thromboembolic obstruction of the pulmonary arteries, occurring in no more than 10% of embolic events. Infarction is characterized by hemorrhagic consolidation of the lung and is often associated with pleuritis and a pleural effusion, which frequently is hemorrhagic. When actual necrosis of lung tissue occurs, the infarction is said to be "complete" and will heal by organization and fibrosis over a period of several weeks. If necrosis does not occur, the infarction is said to be "incomplete" and may resolve in a few days, with restoration of normal lung architecture. The thromboemboli themselves typically are lysed over a period of weeks to months, with restoration of normal pulmonary arterial perfusion to the lung parenchyma. Rarely, the thromboemboli organize, resulting in permanent obstruction of the pulmonary arteries, with serious clinical and hemodynamic consequences (pulmonary hypertension).

The mechanisms of thrombus formation in the venous system involve stasis, alterations in the coagulability of the blood, and damage to the veins. Clinical evidence of venous damage manifested by the signs of thrombophlebitis is not detected in most patients with pulmonary embolism and, even when present, does not usually manifest itself until after the embolic event. Venous stasis is very likely to be important in the genesis of venous thrombosis in the setting of bed rest, prolonged immobility, cardiac failure, pregnancy, obesity, chronic obstructive airway disease, and the postoperative state. Hypercoagulability, although difficult to measure by coagulation studies, is probably important in the setting of hip fracture, the administration of oral contraceptives, hematologic disorders, pregnancy, malignancy, the postoperative state, antithrombin III deficiency, and other rare abnormalities in the coagulation scheme. Patients in respiratory failure may be particularly likely to develop venous thrombosis and pulmonary embolism.

PATHOPHYSIOLOGY

The diagnosis and subsequent treatment of pulmonary thromboembolism must be based upon a firm understanding of the pathophysiologic changes that occur as a consequence of thromboembolic obstruction of the pulmonary arteries. These changes are complex, involving alterations in pulmonary and cardiac hemodynamics, pulmonary gas exchange, pulmonary mechanics, and ventilatory control.

The magnitude of disordered cardiopulmonary function following an embolic event is a function of two factors: (1) the extent of pulmonary arterial obstruction, which will vary depending upon the size and number of the thrombi that impact into the pulmonary arteries; and (2) the functional state of the lungs and the heart before the embolic event. Thus, the patient with preexisting obstructive lung disease or cardiac failure is more likely to manifest serious symptoms and signs following embolization. Moreover, it is the patient with preexisting cardiac or pulmonary disease who is more likely to succumb as a consequence of the embolic event. Individuals with normal heart and lung function can tolerate massive embolization and still survive with appropriate specific and supporting therapy.

A great deal of the current knowledge on the pathophysiology of this disease has been obtained from studies performed on experimental animals subjected to pulmonary embolism. This has been necessary because of the difficulty and risk of performing extensive physiologic studies in acutely ill patients. However, if an appropriate model is used (e.g., embolization of the lungs by venous thrombi formed in vivo), the changes that occur are comparable with those seen in humans. In the following discussion, the extrapolation of these experimental observations will be so noted. A presentation of the pathophysiology of pulmonary thromboembolism must provide a mechanism (or mechanisms) to explain (1) the development of breathlessness with rapid, shallow respirations (tachypnea) and hyperventilation (low arterial $PaCO_2$ with an elevated arterial pH); (2) the development of arterial hypoxemia; (3) the development of pulmonary infarction; and (4) the development of pulmonary hypertension, with right ventricular failure and shock.

Pulmonary hypertension is the most important and dangerous physiologic alteration following pulmonary embolization. It occurs primarily as a consequence of the decrease in the functional cross-sectional area of the pulmonary arterial tree, with an increase in pulmonary vascular resistance. To maintain cardiac output, the right ventricle must generate higher pressures (i.e., pulmonary hypertension). The normal pulmonary artery pressure is 25/10 mmHg, with a mean pulmonary artery pressure no greater than 15 mmHg. Thus, *pulmonary hypertension* can be defined as an increase in mean pulmonary artery pressure above 15 mmHg.

Most patients with symptomatic acute pulmonary embolism manifested by breathlessness are found to have an elevated mean pulmonary artery pressure, usually in excess of 20 mmHg. With increasing pulmonary arterial occlusion, the severity of pulmonary hypertension increases, but is ultimately limited by the maximal function of the right ventricle. The normal, nonhypertrophied right ventricle can generate a mean pulmonary arterial pressure of approximately 35 to 40 mmHg, or systolic pressure of 50 to 55 mmHg. When pulmonary vascular obstruction increases beyond the limits of right ventricular function, the right ventricle fails, with a fall in forward cardiac output and the development of shock (i.e., syncope, peripheral vasoconstriction; diaphoresis; a weak, thready pulse; decreased urine output or oliguria; and changes in sensorium). An important characteristic of this form of shock is the association with an increased central venous or right atrial pressure, in contrast with a variety of other shock states in which the cardiac filling pressures tend to be low (e.g., septic shock and shock caused by blood loss).

Clinical observations demonstrate a rough correlation between the extent of pulmonary arterial obstruction, as determined by pulmonary angiography, and the degree of pulmonary hypertension. Evidence exists suggesting the role of active pulmonary vasoconstriction as a contributing factor in the development of pulmonary hypertension, both in experimental animals and humans. A dog subjected to pulmonary embolization with autologous in vivo thrombi develops active constriction of the pulmonary arteries. The vasoconstriction in the dog is mediated, in part, by the release of serotonin from platelets that have aggregated on the thromboembolus as it passes through the venous circulation into the pulmonary arteries. Additional humoral substances many be involved in humans, including other vasoactive amines and various prostaglandins, leukotrienes, and others. There is no convincing evidence to suggest that reflex pulmonary vasoconstriction occurs. The development of arterial hypoxemia may be of great importance in producing additional pulmonary arterial constriction. Current evidence suggests that, in patients, active pulmonary vasoconstriction plays a less important role in the development of pulmonary hypertension than mechanical obstruction of the pulmonary arteries. The development of right ventricular failure with shock is usually seen only in the event of massive embolization of pulmonary arteries wherein 60% to 70% of the pulmonary arterial bed has been occluded.

Breathlessness (dyspnea), with rapid, shallow respirations (tachypnea), occurs in almost all patients following a symptomatic episode of pulmonary thromboembolism. This symptom is difficult to explain on the basis of the mechanisms that are thought to be operative in other patients with breathlessness and airway or parenchymal lung disease. In the presence of airway or parenchymal lung disease, there are usually significant alterations in lung mechanics, either increased airway resistance or decreased lung compliance. To maintain a normal volume of ventilation, it is necessary to increase the work of breathing to overcome the mechanical alterations, and the increased work load of breathing is in some manner sensed as breathlessness, possibly by receptors in the muscles of the chest wall that can relate the movement of the respiratory system to the excess effort expended.

Although there are changes in lung mechanics following pulmonary embolism, they are usually mild and probably not sufficient, of themselves, to cause breathlessness. Recent experimental studies in animals of the humoral and reflex events that occur immediately after an embolic event may provide an explanation. Located in the alveolar wall are receptors known as juxtapulmonary capillary receptors, or J receptors, that are stimulated by increased interstitial fluid pressure, humoral agents (e.g., serotonin), and microemboli. When these receptors are stimulated, the response is rapid and shallow breathing, which is the typical pattern seen following pulmonary embolism in humans. This pattern of breathing is usually associated with alveolar hyperventilation and a respiratory alkalemia.

Another type of receptor, the irritant receptor, may also be involved. This receptor is located in the airway epithelium and can be stimulated by humoral substances, changes in lung compliance, bronchoconstriction, and irritants such as cigarette smoke. Stimulation of these receptors may cause tachypnea and cough. When these intrapulmonary receptors are stimulated in the experimental animal, there is an increase in afferent nerve impulse activity in the vagus nerve supplying the lung, with subsequent stimulation of respiratory neurons in the medulla of the brain. It is this afferent input to the respiratory center that presumably mediates the development of the rapid, shallow-breathing pattern. It has been suggested, but not proved, that this increased level of vagal discharge to the respiratory center may be sensed as breathlessness. Currently, it is not known how or where the dyspneic sensation develops in the cerebrum. Most patients with pulmonary embolism and sustained breathlessness are found to have pulmonary hypertension when subjected to right heart catherization and pulmonary angiography. This increase in pressure may effect an increase in interstitial fluid pressure in the lung, stimulating the J receptors, with additional stimulation by the humoral substances that are thought to be released. However, these reflex changes are not likely to be the only mechanism in the causation of breathlessness and the abnormal-breathing pattern following pulmonary embolism (to be discussed later).

The physiologic hallmark of pulmonary vascular occlusion is the development of an increase in dead space or "wasted" ventilation. Following occlusion of the pulmonary arteries, the nonperfused lung units cease to accomplish gas exchange, but in the absence of infarction, ventilation continues. Ventilation to these units is "wasted" in a functional sense, because there is little or no carbon dioxide or oxygen exchange. The ventilation/perfusion ratio ($\dot{V}/\dot{Q}$) in these units is near infinity and, as will be described, this alteration in lung function can sometimes be detected by radioisotope lung scanning. A more direct approach is to measure the physiologic dead space/tidal volume ratio (V_D/V_T). With the increase in dead space ventilation, total ventilation of the lungs must increase to maintain normal carbon dioxide and oxygen exchange. The increase in total ventilation may be an additional factor in the development of breathlessness. If ventilation does not increase (e.g., in the patient on a ventilator with a fixed rate and tidal volume), hypercapnia will ensue with hypoxemia.

Although the nonspecific development of high $\dot{V}/\dot{Q}$ lung units is characteristic of acute pulmonary embolism, there are changes that occur that serve to decrease ventilation to the embolized lung units, including bronchoconstriction and pneumoconstriction in these units, possible changes in pulmonary surfactant in these units, and infarction. With cessation of perfusion the carbon dioxide tension in the embolized lung units falls to low levels, resulting in smooth-muscle constriction in the terminal lung units, which causes a shrinkage and stiffening of the embolized lung unit (pneumoconstriction), and smooth-muscle constriction in the bronchi (bronchoconstriction). These alterations in alveolar and airway mechanics effect a shift in ventilation away from the embolized lung units, but never to the extent that the $\dot{V}/\dot{Q}$ ratio is restored to normal.

Within a period of 12 to 24 hours the embolized, nonperfused lung units may become deficient in the production of surfactant—the lipoprotein secretion that serves to maintain the stability of the peripheral lung units. In the absence of adequate amounts of surfactant, the embolized lung units may become stiff and collapse, thereby shifting ventilation away from them. If infarction of the embolized lung units occurs, this will also serve to shift the ventilation to more normally perfused lung units.

These changes in lung mechanics and structure are the result of pulmonary ischemia. In addition, there are humorally mediated changes that are a consequence of changes involving the thromboembolus. In experimental thromboembolism in the canine, pulmonary resistance increases (bronchoconstriction), and pulmonary compliance falls (pneumoconstriction) immediately after embolization, and similar changes probably occur in humans. The observed acute decrease in maximal expiratory flow rate in humans who have angiographically documented pulmonary thromboembolism is probably a consequence of bronchoconstriction, and the decrease in lung volume seen radiographically after an acute pulmonary embolism, manifested by elevation of the diaphragms, may well be the result of the pneumoconstriction. In an experimental animal these changes are due to the release of serotonin from platelets that have aggregated on the thromboembolus as it traverses the venous circulation. The transient nature of the radiographic changes that occur in humans, as well as the changes in animal expiratory flow rates, are consistent with the possibility that they are humorally mediated. The changes can be prevented in the animal by administration of heparin before embolization. In humans, heparin appears to lessen the degree of bronchoconstriction. Even if these changes in lung mechanics occur in humans, it is unlikely that they are the major factor in the development of persistent dyspnea, for they are transient and of mild severity.

These mechanical changes are of more importance in the development of arterial hypoxemia, which is a common occurrence following pulmonary thromboembolism. However, the presence of a normal PaO_2 does not exclude the diagnosis. A variety of mechanisms have been proposed as the cause of arterial hypoxemia, including a decrease in diffusing capacity owing to a reduction in the surface area of the alveolocapillary membrane, abnormally rapid passage of blood through a pulmonary capillary bed decreased in volume, ventilation–perfusion abnormalities, atelectasis, and right-to-left shunting. Alveolar hypoventilation cannot be invoked, since these patients usually hyperventilate.

Obstruction of the pulmonary vascular bed may result in a decrease in the diffusing capacity of the lung, but it is variable in degree and not usually of sufficient magnitude to account for arterial hypoxemia at rest. A shortened transit time may be an important factor in hypoxemia during exercise, but not at rest. Although there is evidence in humans that arterial hypoxemia following embolism can be in part due to right-to-left shunting secondary to atelectasis (which can be partially reversed by deep breathing), most of the evidence favors ventilation–perfusion imbalance as the primary cause of arterial hypoxemia at rest.

Following thromboembolism in a dog, a $\dot{V}/\dot{Q}$ imbalance does develop. The following explanation has been proposed to explain the $\dot{V}/\dot{Q}$ imbalance, and it can also account for the development of atelectasis with right-to-left shunting: After embolism, release of serotonin or of other humoral agents into the pulmonary circulation induces nonuniform constriction of distal airways and terminal lung units, with a decrease in ventilation of these units relative to their perfusion (i.e., low $\dot{V}/\dot{Q}$ ratio and a fall in PaO_2). When these changes are severe, atelectasis can occur with right-to-left shunting. This explanation is supported by the observation that heparin, when given *prior* to the release of thromboemboli in a dog, prevents, to a substantial degree, the changes in lung mechanics and the fall in PaO_2. Therefore, the disturbance in ventilation–perfusion relationships following embolization is characterized by the development of high $\dot{V}/\dot{Q}$ lung units, as manifested by an increase in VD/VT and by development of low $\dot{V}/\dot{Q}$ lung units as manifested by a decrease in arterial PaO_2 and a widened A–a PaO_2 difference (Fig. 36–1).

In a recent interesting series of experiments on dogs, some workers have postulated that postembolic decreases in PaO_2 are due to shifting of perfusion to poorly ventilated areas of lung (low $\dot{V}/\dot{Q}$). However, the experimental models included complex perturbations and, therefore, may not resemble clinical pulmonary embolism in humans. Recent observations by Yann et al. tended to confirm these observations in a few patients with severe acute pulmonary thromboemboli.

There is, as yet, insufficient understanding of the metabolic effects of pulmonary arterial obstruction to explain the development of pulmonary infarction. The lung parenchyma is protected by three sources of oxygen supply: the bronchial arteries, the pulmonary arteries, and the airways. In most clinical situations wherein infarction develops, there is either impairment of the bronchial circulation, as a consequence of previous lung disease, or pulmonary vascular congestion, secondary to cardiac failure, or a combination thereof.

Thromboembolism of a large pulmonary artery alone is not associated with pulmonary infarction.

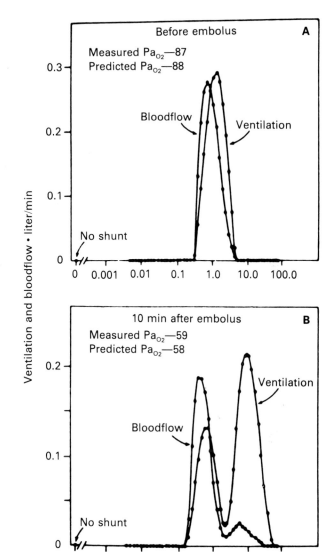

Figure 36–1. Distributions of ventilation/perfusion ratios (*A*) before and (*B*) after experimental pulmonary thromboembolism in a dog. Note that embolization caused a region of high ventilation/perfusion ratios and that the main body of the distribution had its ventilation/perfusion ratio somewhat increased. These changes were sufficient to account for the fall in arterial PaO_2 to 59 mmHg. (Reprinted with permission from West JB: Pulmonary Pathophysiology—The Essentials, p 129. Baltimore, Williams & Wilkins, 1977).

When a peripheral pulmonary artery suffers vascular occlusion, influx of bronchial blood may produce alveolar hemorrhage. In the presence of congestive heart failure and pulmonary hypertension, the hemorrhage does not resolve and tissue necrosis (infarction) results. Pulmonary hemorrhage can resemble infarction on the chest radiograph, but may be transient, lasting 4 to 5 days. Pulmonary infarction is persistent and leaves a scar. Pulmonary hemorrhage or infarction may contribute to dyspnea and tachypnea by incurring painful, shallow respirations owing to pleuritis. The role of endorphins, if any, in mitigating the effects of painful respirations or dyspnea is not known.

The natural history of these pathophysiologic changes is determined primarily by the rapidity with which the thromboemboli lyse. In patients, this is a dynamic process. The thrombi begin to lyse immediately after the embolic event and, within a matter of hours to days, sufficient lysis will occur to allow reperfusion of embolized lung units, with a lessening of the physiologic alterations and, thereby, the symptoms and signs of the embolic event. The rare emboli that fail to lyse result in permanent obstruction of the pulmonary vascular bed. If the residual obstruction is massive, chronic pulmonary hypertension will occur (discussed later).

CLINICAL MANIFESTATIONS

The symptoms and signs of pulmonary thromboembolism are nonspecific, and for this reason the diagnosis is often difficult to establish without resorting to more precise and definitive diagnostic procedures. Those clinical findings that do occur are variable, both in frequency and intensity. They depend upon the extent of pulmonary vascular occlusion, the functional state of the heart and the lungs before embolization, and the development of pulmonary infarction. It is particularly important to distinguish between the clinical findings in the patient with embolization alone and those in the patient having embolization with infarction. Because most embolic events do not result in infarction, the classic clinical picture occurs infrequently and is one of the major reasons that the diagnosis is not made in many patients.

In the absence of infarction, embolization is almost invariably manifested by the abrupt onset of breathlessness. Unless the extent of embolic obstruction is severe, this may be the only subjective manifestation of the embolic event. When massive pulmonary embolization occurs with obstruction of more than 50% to 60% of the pulmonary vascular bed, severe pulmonary hypertension results, and may be manifested by the development of substernal chest pain similar in character to the sensation experienced by patients with myocardial ischemia. The mechanism of the pain is unclear, but may be secondary to subendocardial ischemia.

When as a consequence of severe pulmonary outflow obstruction, the right ventricle fails with a decrease in cardiac output and perfusion to vital organs such as the brain, light-headedness or syncope may occur. It should be emphasized, however, that these latter symptoms are infrequent because massive embolization is uncommon. In most patients breathlessness will be the only symptom of the embolic event. It may be fleeting or persistent, and is usually exacerbated by physical exertion. The embolic event will usually occur in a patient with one or more of the previously described predisposing conditions.

On physical examination, the patient with acute pulmonary embolism will usually manifest an increase in respiratory rate (tachypnea) faster than 20/min, and an increase in heart rate (tachycardia) faster than 90/min. Evidence of pulmonary hypertension as manifested by an increase in the intensity of the pulmonary second sound, or an abnormal splitting of the second sound, with a widened and fixed split, occurs less frequently, and is usually clearly manifested only when the mean pulmonary artery pressure is greater than 25 to 30 mmHg. With massive embolism and a marked increase in pulmonary vascular resistance, there will be evidence of right ventricular overwork and failure, as manifested by a right ventricular gallop and distension of the jugular veins with an elevation of jugular venous pressure. Systemic arterial hypotension, with evidence of peripheral vasoconstriction, may be seen, as well as central cyanosis.

One of the most striking findings in the patient with acute pulmonary embolism without infarction is the absence of any abnormal physical findings on examination of the lungs. It is this combination of acute breathlessness with no apparent pulmonary abnormality that should strongly suggest the diagnosis. Although wheezing has been described in some patients with acute pulmonary embolism, it occurs infrequently and is more likely to be seen in patients who have underlying bronchial disease such as asthma. Evidence of peripheral venous thrombosis on physical examination is seen in less than 50% of patients.

When embolic obstruction of the pulmonary arteries results in the development of *pulmonary infarction*, the clinical picture will be more typical. Cough, hemoptysis, pleuritic pain, and physical findings consisting of signs of pulmonary consolidation with dullness and bronchial breathing, signs of pleuritis, with a friction rub, or signs of pleural fluid will be present. Fever is also a common finding. Most patients who sustain a pulmonary infarct will usually manifest the symptoms and signs of embolization in addition to those of infarction. It is possible, but difficult to prove, that some patients may develop infarction as a consequence of a small peripheral embolus, but it does not obstruct enough of the pulmonary vascular bed to cause pulmonary hypertension with breathlessness.

Leukocytosis, with an increase in sedimentation rate, occurs frequently in the patient with pulmonary infarction, as do elevated lactate dehydrogenase, normal aspartate transaminase, and elevated bilirubin levels, the so-called diagnostic triad. Unfortunately, these findings are nonspecific and of minimal diagnostic value. Arterial hypoxemia occurs frequently in association with alveolar hyperventilation. This again is a nonspecific finding, since most of the diseases with which pulmonary embolism is confused are usually associated with arterial hypoxemia. The measurement of wasted ventilation by determination of the physiologic dead space/tidal volume ratio (V_D/V_T) has been advocated as a useful diagnostic procedure, but again is limited in applicability to those patients who have no other underlying cardiac or pulmonary disease. As is true of many pulmonary function tests, an abnormality may not be specific for a disease, but is a consequence of many conditions that alter lung structure.

In the absence of massive embolism, the electrocardiogram is not particularly helpful, aside from showing tachycardia or nonspecific ST changes. The development of a rightward shift in axis, right ventricular strain, the classic S1-Q3-T3 pattern, or P pulmonale is seen only with massive pulmonary embolism, and then not consistently.

Before the development of lung scanning and pulmonary angiography, the chest roentgenogram was the most useful laboratory diagnostic aid (see Chap. 12). In many patients with embolization without infarction, the chest roentgengram is completely normal. When there are abnormalities, they include diaphragmatic elevation (a manifestation of pneumonconstriction) and avascular lung zones (Westermark's sign). With the development of infarction, pulmonary infiltrates are seen. They are not invariably the typically described triangular-shaped densities abutting on the pleural surface, but may appear as consolidated or atelectatic densities, often with pleural effusions. In contrast to most pneumonias, the radiographic lesions are usually bilateral.

DIAGNOSIS AND DIFFERENTIAL DIAGNOSIS

The diagnosis of pulmonary thromboembolism, with or without infarction, necessitates differentiating this disease from other diseases that can cause similar clinical and laboratory findings. Ultimately, this requires the performance of lung scanning and, in many patients, pulmonary angiography, to be specific or definitive. These techniques, which can visualize the pattern of distribution of pulmonary blood flow (radioisotopic lung scans) and the anatomy of the pulmonary arteries (pulmonary angiography), have made it possible to approach the diagnosis of suspect embolism in a systematic manner.

The first step in the diagnosis of pulmonary embolism and infarction is a high degree of suspicion on the basis of suggestive clinical symptoms and signs. The second step includes the rapid performance of routine laboratory tests, including chest roentgenogram, electrocardiogram, complete blood count, and arterial blood gas analyses with the measurement of pH, $PaCO_2$, and PaO_2. If all of these tests are consistent with the diagnosis, and the clinical picture is very typical, it may not be necessary to proceed with further studies before instituting anticoagulant therapy. This is an infrequent occurrence and the diagnosis should be confirmed by definitive studies.

Most patients who present with breathlessness and nonembolic cardiac or pulmonary disease will have abnormal test results. The differential diagnosis of pulmonary embolism without infarction includes acute myocardial infarction, dissecting aneurysm, bacteremic shock, and anxiety states. In the differential diagnosis of pulmonary infarction, pneumonia, atelectasis, heart failure, and neoplasm also must be considered. Unless contraindicated, it is necessary to perform additional studies to establish the diagnosis.

The third step in evaluating a patient with suspected pulmonary embolism is the performance of a perfusion lung scan. This test is performed by the intravenous infusion of technetium-labeled macroaggregates of human serum albumin, which are of sufficient size that they do not pass through the pulmonary capillaries, but lodge there. As the macroaggregates pass through the right heart, they are mixed uniformly with the blood in the right ventricle, and then distributed throughout the lungs in a pattern that corresponds to regional pulmonary blood flow. When the lungs are scanned with an appropriate imaging device (scintillation camera), the distribution of pulmonary blood flow can be assessed. In contrast with the chest roentgenogram, for which only one or two views of the lungs are required, perfusion lung scanning requires viewing the lungs in the anterior, posterior, oblique, and lateral projections, to evaluate overall perfusion of lungs. *It cannot be emphasized too strongly that an abnormality in the distribution of pulmonary blood flow that may be detected by perfusion lung scanning is a nonspecific finding.* Abnormalities in the distribution of pulmonary blood flow are the usual consequence of any pulmonary or cardiac disease that affects lung structure or function. Thus, perfusion lung scan abnormalities, being nonspecific, never establish a causal diagnosis. This has led to many errors in diagnosis (Fig. 36–2).

The typical defect that is seen on the perfusion lung scan is an area of absent to markedly reduced radioactivity that conforms to a lung segment, lobe, or entire lung. Nonsegmental defects, which cross the boundary between adjacent lung segments, are more typical of nonembolic pulmonary diseases. One of the *most important* considerations in the interpretation of the perfusion lung scan is to correlate radiographic abnormalities, if present, with perfusion lung scan abnormalities. If the perfusion lung scan demonstrates abnormalities that correspond with radiographic abnormalities the scan is considered to be "intermediate" (Fig. 36–3), with the likelihood of pulmonary embolism ranging from 25% to 50%. Thus, the intermediate perfusion lung scan is of limited diagnostic value. Moreover, this is the most frequent scan pattern found in patients with suspect pulmonary embolism who

undergo lung scanning. The demonstration of a perfusion defect is more helpful when the chest roentgenogram is normal. However, even when a typical perfusion defect with a normal chest roentgenogram is observed, the probability of pulmonary embolism may be as low as 50%.

The specificity of perfusion lung scanning can be increased when combined with ventilation lung scanning. The distribution of ventilation can be evaluated by the inhalation of xenon-133, with a subsequent imaging of the lungs with a scintillation camera to determine the distribution of ventilation. If an abnormality in the distribution of perfusion is a consequence of parenchymal lung disease involving airways or alveoli, a defect in ventilation comparable with the perfusion defect will be found. Such a defect, in the presence of a normal chest roentgenogram, is said to be a "matched ventilation–perfusion defect." A matched defect does not usually occur following pulmonary embolization, but does not conclusively rule out pulmonary embolism.

Emboli in the absence of infarction do not usually cause a persistent decrease in ventilation of the embolized lung unit, and the ventilation scan will typically show normal ventilation in the area of diminished perfusion (Fig. 36–4). This type of defect (i.e., areas of diminished perfusion with normal chest roentgenogram) is called a *mismatch*. The specificity of this combined defect is much greater than that of a perfusion defect alone, and it has been shown to be a manifestation of angiographically proven emboli in 80% to 100% of instances when the perfusion defects are of moderate

Figure 36–2. Pulmonary perfusion scintiscans (posterior view). (*A*) Normal perfusion scan; (*B*) perfusion scan showing a lobar defect involving the right upper lobe, consistent with pulmonary embolism, but caused by a bronchogenic carcinoma.

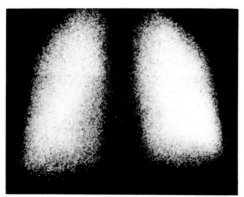

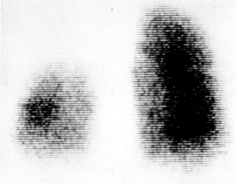

A   B

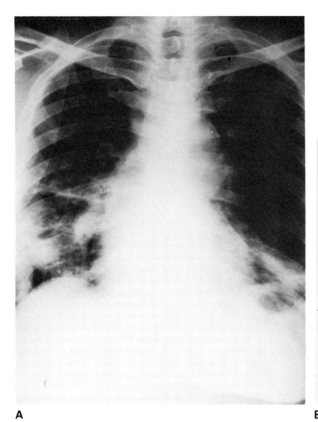

A

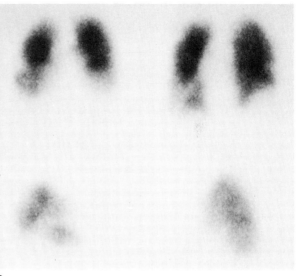

B

Figure 36—3. Findings in a patient with dyspnea, pleurisy, and hemoptysis. (*A*) Chest roentgenogram demonstrating bibasilar atelectatic and infiltrative changes consistent with pulmonary embolism and infarction or pneumonitis; (*B*) pulmonary perfusion scintiscans: *upper left*, anterior view; *upper right*, posterior view; *lower left*, right lateral view; *lower right*, left lateral view. Perfusion defects correspond to the roentgenographic defects. This scan is "intermediate." Pulmonary angiogram (not shown) demonstrated thromboemboli.

size or greater (more than 25% of segmental volume) and multiple. However, it must be emphasized that the scans never provide entirely specific anatomic information. If the diagnosis of pulmonary embolism is still in doubt after ventilation–perfusion scanning, and it is necessary to establish a definitive diagnosis, pulmonary angiography is indicated. It is the only test that can provide specific and definitive evidence for the presence of pulmonary emboli. Scan interpretation criteria that are used in many nuclear medicine facilities are described in Table 36–1.

Pulmonary angiography is a procedure that has minimal risks to the patient unless severe pulmonary hypertension (mean pulmonary artery pressure greater than 45 mmHg), shock, or renal failure are present.

Pulmonary angiography requires the positioning of a suitable catheter in the pulmonary artery (i.e., right heart catheterization). A radiopaque dye is rapidly injected into the pulmonary artery and rapid serial roentgenograms are taken. Findings that are diagnostic of embolism are the presence of a filling defect within the artery and obstruction of the artery (Fig. 36–5). The filling defect results from incomplete filling of the lumen of the thrombus-occluded artery with contrast material. (The obstruction is seen as an abrupt termination of the contrast material within the artery as a consequence of total occlusion by an embolus.) Another advantage of performing pulmonary angiography is that the pulmonary artery pressure can be measured to assess the functional severity of the embolic event. It is also possible at this time to mea-

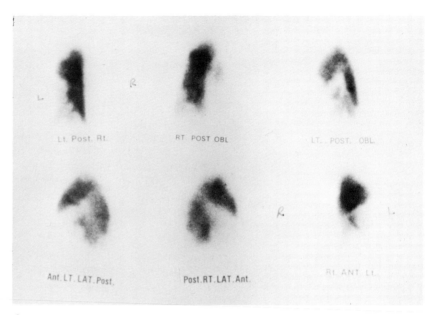

A

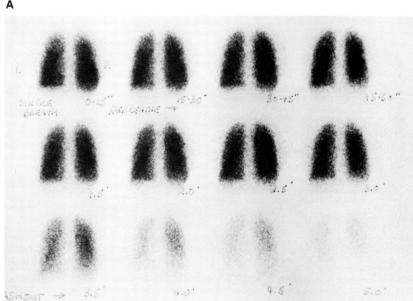

B

Figure 36—4. Pulmonary scintiscans in a patient with chronic dyspnea and recurrent pleurisy with hemoptysis. Chest roentgenogram was normal. (*A*) Perfusion scan: There is absent perfusion to the entire right lung. (*B*) Ventilation scan. Ventilation to both lungs is normal. This V̇/Q̇ scan is a "mismatch" because of pulmonary thromboembolism (see Fig. 36–5).

sure cardiac output and quantitate the pulmonary vascular resistance.

When the lung scan is completely normal in a patient with suspect pulmonary embolism, and has been performed within 48 to 72 hours of the acute episode, the likelihood of pulmonary embolism as a cause of symptoms suggesting embolization (e.g., breathlessness) is very remote. A normal perfusion scan, however, does not exclude the possibility of a small peripheral pulmonary embolus, which might cause infarction with pleurisy, but not breathlessness. This type of embolic event cannot be diagnosed by conventional angiography either, and there is no reliable method of making a definitive diagnosis of this type of pulmonary embolism. Fortunately, life-threatening embolic disease is rarely, if ever, a consequence of small, peripheral emboli. In the Urokinase Pulmonary Embolism Trial, 150

Table 36—1 Interpretation of Ventilation—Perfusion (V—P) Scintigrams

CATEGORY	PATTERN*
Normal	No perfusion defects
Low-probability	Small V—P mismatches
	V—P matches without corresponding roentgenographic changes
	Perfusion defect substantially smaller than roentgenographic density
Intermediate-probability	Severe, diffuse obstructive pulmonary disease with perfusion defects
	Perfusion defect of same size as roentgenographic change
	Single medium or large† V—P mismatches
High-probability	Two or more medium or large V—P mismatches
	Perfusion defect substantially larger than roentgenographic density

* A small perfusion defect involves less than 25% of the expected volume of a pulmonary segment; medium, 25% to 90%; and large, 90% or more.
† Controversy currently exists over the important categorization of single large V—P mismatches. These have been considered either of high or intermediate probability. The more conservative interpretation has been used in this table.
(Biello DR: Radiological (scintigraphic) evaluation of patients with suspected pulmonary thromboembolism. JAMA 257:3257—3259, Copyright 1987, American Medical Association)

patients with angiographically proven emboli had lung scans, and in none was the scan completely normal. Currently, it is felt that a completely normal, well-performed perfusion lung scan rules out the possibility of arteriographically detectable emboli.

In a recent study sponsored by the National Institutes of Health, the ventilation—perfusion scan was evaluated in the diagnosis of pulmonary embolism. This randomized study was performed prospectively in six clinical centers selected competi-

tively. Seven hundred fifty-five patients underwent ventilation—perfusion imaging followed by pulmonary angiography within 12 to 24 hours in the Prospective Investigation of Pulmonary Embolism Diagnosis (PIOPED Investigation). The objective of this study was to determine the sensitivity (true positive ratio) and specificity (true negative ratio) of the ventilation—perfusion filling image. Among 116 patients with high-probability lung scans, pulmonary emboli were present in 102 (88%). However, 105 of 322 (33%) patients with intermediate

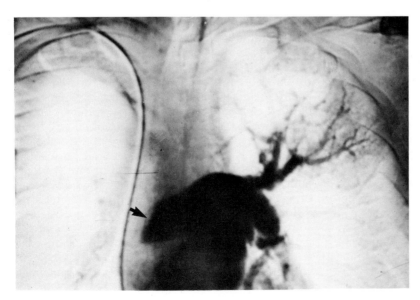

Figure 36—5. Pulmonary angiogram in a patient with V̇/Q̇ mismatch (see Fig. 36—4). Posteroanterior chest film shows the catheter that has been passed through the superior vena cava, through the right atrium and ventricle, and into the pulmonary trunk. The pulmonary trunk, both main pulmonary arteries, and several lobar and segmental arteries in the left lung are opacified by the injected contrast. A large filling defect ("cutoff") in the right main pulmonary artery diagnostic of embolism is seen (*arrow*). Additional filling defects can be seen in the left lower lobe arteries.

scans had pulmonary emboli; 29 of 238 (16%) with low-probability scans; and 5 of 55 (9%) with near-normal/normal scans had pulmonary embolism. The investigators of this inpatient study felt that their observations settled many controversial aspects concerning the role of the lung scan in the diagnosis of pulmonary embolism. Thus, a high-probability lung scan is indicative of pulmonary embolism, but is present in only a few patients with pulmonary embolism. A low-probability lung scan combined with careful clinical evaluations indicated a small likelihood of the diagnosis. A near-normal or normal scan is infrequently associated with pulmonary embolism. An intermediate lung scan is of no aid in making the diagnosis of pulmonary embolism. In brief, this study suggests that it will be necessary to perform more pulmonary angiograms to make conclusive decisions about the diagnosis of pulmonary embolism. The study also concluded that pulmonary angiography, although invasive, was an accurate and safe technique with a mortality of 0.3%.

Other procedures that may be helpful in evaluating the patient with suspected pulmonary embolism are those tests designed to detect deep venous thrombosis. The tests include venography—the "gold standard"—real-time ultrasonography with and without Doppler flow studies, impedance phlebography, and ^{125}I-labeled fibrinogen scanning. The demonstration of deep vein thrombi would not confirm a diagnosis of pulmonary embolism but would provide the justification for anticoagulation therapy.

The most promising noninvasive test is real-time ultrasonography. The demonstration of non-compressible common femoral veins or popliteal veins is a specific finding indicative of venous thrombosis. The absence of this finding effectively rules out venous thrombosis in these veins. Numerous studies have demonstrated that this method is accurate, with a sensitivity for thigh and popliteal deep vein thromboses of 96% and a specificity (i.e., no thrombi when the test is normal) of 99%. However, cautionary notes need to be sounded. First, the studies that have been done were on patients with the clinical suspicion of deep vein thromboses, not pulmonary embolism. Second, the test is highly operator-dependent, and it remains to be determined if the high sensitivity and specificity can be achieved in a community hospital setting. At present, the failure to demonstrate deep vein thrombosis does not exclude the diagnosis of pulmonary embolism.

Alternatively, objective testing for venous thrombosis in patients with clinically suspected pulmonary embolism and abnormal perfusion lung scans may be positive in up to 20% to 30% of patients, obviating the need for additional testing and providing justification for the institution of anticoagulant therapy.

The diagnosis of pulmonary thromboembolism is particularly difficult to establish in the patient with underlying, previously diagnosed pulmonary disease, whether obstructive or restrictive in nature. In such patients, both a ventilation and perfusion scan must be done. In the patient with a normal chest roentgenogram, a matched defect suggests (low-probability) that the symptoms and signs are not a consequence of pulmonary embolism. However, in the presence of pulmonary infiltrates (e.g., the patient with pneumonia, atelectasis, or heart failure), a matched (low-probability) defect might well be due to an embolic event with infarction. If the diagnosis is to be established or excluded with certainty, pulmonary angiography is mandatory.

In summary, the diagnosis of pulmonary embolism (in 10% to 15% of patients) can be established with reasonable certainty on the basis of the clinical evaluation, chest roentgenogram, electrocardiogram, and perfusion lung scan. In some patients, a ventilation scan may add useful information. In many patients pulmonary angiography will be necessary to ensure diagnostic accuracy.

PROGNOSIS AND NATURAL HISTORY

To appreciate the impact and effect of anticoagulant therapy of pulmonary thromboembolism, it is helpful to review the natural history of untreated embolic disease. The mortality following the initial thromboembolic event has been estimated to be about 25%. This figure may be misleading, being both an overestimate and an underestimate. In the patient with compromised cardiopulmonary function, who is at greater risk to develop thromboemboli, there is a greater likelihood that the patient will succumb to the initial embolic event. Those patients who have normal cardiopulmonary function most likely have a lower incidence of mortality following the initial embolic event.

Once the embolic event has occurred and the patient has survived, the chances of recurrence without therapy and subsequent fatality are great, with approximately 50% of patients experiencing a recurrent episode. In approximately half of these embolic episodes a fatality occurs. With anticoagulant therapy the recurrence rate is reduced to approximately 5%, and fewer of the recurrences will be fatal. Thus, the initial outcome of a thromboembolic episode is, in large part, predetermined by the patient's cardiopulmonary status and the extent of embolization. The subsequent response will depend primarily upon the adequacy of anticoagulant therapy. With adequate therapy, resolution by lysis of the thrombi begins immediately and may be reasonably complete within 14 days following the embolic event, with comparable resolution of the cardiopulmonary functional alterations, symptoms, and signs. Recurrent embolism is unlikely unless a predisposing factor persists (e.g., persistent cardiac failure or long-term immobility).

THERAPY

Any discussion of the treatment of pulmonary thromboembolism must include consideration of (1) prophylactic therapy in the patient who is predisposed to venous thrombosis and embolism, (2) therapy of the acute embolic event, and (3) the prevention of further embolism in the patient who has experienced an acute embolic event.

PROPHYLACTIC THERAPY

The optimal therapy of pulmonary thromboembolism would be a reliable and consistent method to prevent venous thrombosis. Toward this end, it is apparent that the correction of any predisposing factor is of great importance (e.g., early ambulation after surgery). However, in many patients this is not easily accomplished (e.g., following a myocardial infarction or hip fracture). Recently, there has been great interest in the development of therapeutic modalities that will prevent venous thrombosis and, thereby, prevent thomboembolism.

The most promising approaches have been directed at the prevention of coagulation with drugs that either prevent the generation of thrombin or inhibit platelet aggregation. In the latter instance, acetylsalicyclic acid (aspirin) and dipyridamole, drugs that can inhibit platelet aggregation, have been used, among others. Controlled studies of each drug used independently have not demonstrated any convincing decrease in the incidence of ^{125}I-labeled fibrinogen-detectable venous thrombi in the legs in the postoperative state.

The most promising results to date have been achieved with the use of heparin in low doses, which prevents the generation of thrombin. When given before and following surgery in a dosage of 5000 units subcutaneously every 12 hours, there was a significant decrease in the incidence of ^{125}I-labeled fibrinogen-detectable calf vein thrombosis in treated patients. When given in this manner, there was little or no effect on coagulation, specifically on the thrombin clotting time. Similar results have been obtained in postmyocardial infarction patients when the heparin was given every 8 hours, although there was a slight prolongation of the activated partial thromboplastin time (APTT). Low-dose heparin, however, has not been effective in the prophylaxis of deep vein thrombosis and pulmonary embolism in patients with hip fractures or following hip surgery. Clinically significant bleeding has not been a problem with the use of low-dose heparin.

Although low-dose heparin appears to be effective in certain situations in preventing venous thrombosis, it is of no value in the treatment of established acute thromboembolic disease. One might anticipate that this type of prophylactic therapy in the patient with chronic obstructive pulmonary disease, particularly when in respiratory failure, might be beneficial in decreasing the incidence of venous thrombosis and pulmonary embolism. In a single reported study, low-dose heparin, 5000 units subcutaneously every 8 hours, produced a significant decrease of pulmonary emboli in respiratory intensive care unit patients. Although the increased incidence of gastrointestinal bleeding encountered in patients in respiratory failure may argue against the routine use of low-dose heparin in such patients, the reported study failed to demonstrate a significant increase in frequency or severity of gastrointestinal hemorrhage. However, low-dose heparin was believed to be contraindicated in a large number of intensive care patients. Also, the duration of therapy and the effectiveness of prophylactic heparin to prevent deaths caused by pulmonary embolism in such patients has not been established.

TREATMENT OF THE EMBOLIC EVENT AND PREVENTION OF FURTHER EMBOLISM

Following an embolic episode, therapy is directed at two goals. First, supportive therapy is used to maintain cadiopulmonary function and relieve breathlessness, pain, and hypoxemia until the thrombi begin to lyse. Second, and most importantly, is the prevention by anticoagulation of further venous thrombosis with embolization. It is in those infrequent instances for which these goals cannot be achieved that surgical therapy may be indicated.

Supportive therapy includes the administration of oxygen in concentrations sufficient to raise the PaO$_2$ to greater than 60 to 70 mmHg, analgesics for relief of severe pleuritic pain if present, and vasoactive drugs if cardiac failure with a depression of cardiac output occurs. Isoproterenol given by intravenous drip (2–4 mg/500 mL of 5% dextrose in water) may be effective in this event because of its pulmonary vasodilator effect and its inotropic effect on the heart. Dopamine may also be effective.

Although digitalization may not be particularly effective therapy, it may be used if there is cardiac failure. There probably is no contraindication to its use as long as the patient is adequately oxygenated.

Three points should be made in regard to oxygen therapy: (1) the arterial hypoxemia responds well to modest increases in inspired oxygen concentrations (e.g., 6–8 L/min by a nasal cannula) because the mechanism of hypoxemia is primarily a $\dot{V}/\dot{Q}$ abnormality; (2) these patients rarely hypoventilate and there is no need to fear respiratory depression as a consequence of raising the arterial oxygen tension; and (3) one should not expect significant relief of breathlessness with oxygen therapy, since the cause of the breathlessness presumably has other origins.

The mainstay of therapy for pulmonary thromboembolism is directed at the prevention of further venous thrombosis. Most patients, if they survive the immediate hemodynamic effects of the embolic event, will recover as the thrombi spontaneously lyse. The prevention of further venous thrombosis is accomplished by anticoagulation. This is initiated with heparin, rather than an oral anticoagulant, because of the rapid action of the former. The oral anticoagulants do not become antithrombotic for at least 4 to 6 days, and it is during this period that the patient is most likely to suffer recurring embolic episodes as a consequence of continuing venous thrombosis. Heparin can be administered by either of two intravenous methods: as a bolus of 5000 to 7500 units every 4 to 6 hours, or by continuous pump infusion with the goal of prolonging the clotting time to 2 to 2.5 times normal. The precise methods of heparin administration, dose, monitoring, and duration of therapy have not been established. When given by continuous pump infusion,

a loading dose of 4000 to 5000 units is given, followed by 1000 units/hr. Regardless of the method, the adequacy of anticoagulation should be assessed by periodic determination of activated partial thromboplastin time (APTT). When given by the bolus method, the APTT should be determined one-half to 1 hour before the next dose of heparin.

With adequate anticoagulation, the likelihood that the patient will experience further venous thrombosis with recurrent embolization is low (i.e., less than 5% to 10%), unless there is a significant predisposing factor, such as intractable cardiac failure or a defect in antithrombin III. Once supportive therapy and anticoagulant therapy have been instituted and the patient is improving, the major decision that remains is the question of how long to continue the anticoagulant therapy. In the patient who can be identified as having definable causes of venous thrombosis that can be reversed (e.g., the postoperative state in an otherwise healthy individual), anticoagulation needs be continued only until the patient is *fully* ambulatory, although many physicians may prefer to continue with an oral anticoagulant for 3 to 4 months. Heparin will usually be administered a minimum of 8 to 10 days. As soon as the patient's hemodynamic and respiratory status has stabilized and has begun to return to normal, ambulation is very important in the prevention of further venous thrombosis and embolization. In the patient with no definable cause for thromboembolism, anticoagulation should be continued empirically for a period of 6 months, changing from heparin to an oral anticoagulant during the first week of therapy. In the patient in whom an irreversible predisposing factor persists (e.g., chronic congestive heart failure, pulmonary hypertension caused by pulmonary embolism, recurrent episodes of pulmonary embolism on cessation of therapy, or an underlying malignancy) anticoagulant therapy probably should be continued indefinitely.

The only absolute contraindication to the use of heparin is a hemorrhagic disorder or active bleeding. The incidence of morbidity and mortality related to hemorrhagic complications associated with heparin therapy must be considered in the treatment of the patient with presumed pulmonary thromboembolism. In the patient in whom the diagnosis is not in question, the risk of not treating is far greater than the risk of treating. However, the complications of heparin therapy are significant, with bleeding occurring in 10% to 20% of patients treated by the bolus method. However, this increased incidence of bleeding may be related to the administration of larger doses of heparin when given by the intermittent bolus method. Women over 65 are even more likely to experience hemorrhagic complications, for reasons that are not clear. Other patients may also have an increased risk of complicating hemorrhage: elderly males, recent gastrointestinal bleeding, liver disease, and abnormal coagulation. For this reason, if there is any question about the diagnosis, pulmonary angiography should be seriously considered before instituting or continuing anticoagulant therapy.

Currently, newer anticoagulant agents including low-molecular-weight heparin (LMWH), are under investigation in the search for safer agents.

Therapy directed at lysis of the thromboemboli (thrombolytic therapy) has been the subject of a number of recent studies. The drugs that have been evaluated are urokinase and streptokinase, both of which activate and accelerate the rate of clot lysis during the first 24 to 48 hours following the initial thromboembolic event. More recently, therapeutic trials with tissue plasminogen activator (t-PA) have been described. During the period of perfusion with the thrombolytic agent, patients receiving thrombolytic therapy may have greater resolution of hemodynamic abnormalities and more rapid restoration of perfusion. However, a comparison of patients treated with anticoagulation only versus anticoagulation plus thrombolytic therapy did not demonstrate any significant difference in the resolution of symptoms, mortality, or cardiopulmonary abnormalities 2 weeks after the embolic event. Moreover, there was a significantly greater incidence of bleeding in the patients treated with thrombolytic drugs. The situation wherein thrombolytic therapy may possibly prove most useful is in the patient with massive pulmonary embolism and shock, thus effecting a "medical pulmonary embolectomy." Recombinant human tissue-type plasminogen activator (rt-PA) and other second-generation thrombolytic agents have been used to lyse thrombi and thromboemboli in humans. Whereas, rt-PA appears more potent experimentally than urokinase and steptokinase in clot lysis, the precise therapeutic role of this newer agent has not been determined. Thrombolytic therapy is also recommended for the patient with onset of deep venous thrombosis of recent origin. Recently, a National Institutes of Health Consensus Conference recommended increasing use of the thrombolytic drugs. The reader is referred to recent reviews for indications, contraindications, monitoring, and continuing controversies regarding these agents.

SURGICAL THERAPY

A surgical approach to the treatment of acute pulmonary thromboembolism is indicated only when anticoagulation fails to prevent current thromboembolism, or in the patient in whom anticoagulation is contraindicated. In these instances vena caval interruption or embolectomy or both, may be employed. Several methods have been developed to interrupt the passage of the venous thrombi through the inferior vena cava, including ligation of the inferior vena cava, plication of the vena cava with sutures or a clip, the placement of a "harp-string grid" of sutures across the vena cava, and the placement of a (Greenfield) filter in the vena cava.

In most instances, regardless of the method used to interrupt the vena cava, subsequent thrombosis at the site of interruption occurs, thereby converting the nonocclusive modalities into a total occlusion. Inasmuch as the patient who fails to respond to anticoagulation therapy usually has underlying cardiac, pulmonary, or other predisposing disease, it is not surprising that when vena caval interruption is indicated, there is significant morbidity and mortality related to the procedure itself. Although recurrent embolization is unlikely to occur during the immediate period following the ligation, recurrent embolization does occur in a significant percentage of patients (i.e., 10% to 20%). This suggests that when medical therapy fails, the ultimate prognosis is poor, with the likelihood of further embolization and mortality being great. Whenever the vena cava is interrupted, continued anticoagulation should be considered, unless contraindicated, to minimize the chances of complications related to venous disease developing in the lower extremities.

Rarely, patients with massive embolism will not succumb immediately, but will survive for a time ranging from several hours to several days, experiencing progressive deterioration of cardiac and pulmonary function. In such patients, if thrombolytic therapy and anticoagulation have failed, *pulmonary embolectomy* may be indicated. Few patients will fall into this category, inasmuch as the natural history of the disease is spontaneous lysis of the thrombi, with improvement in cardiac and pulmonary function with the institution of appropriate therapy. Thus, if the patient can be kept alive for a period of 24 hours, he or she usually will recover. In the event that pulmonary embolectomy is necessary, it should be undertaken only if adequate facilities for open-heart surgery with cardiopulmonary bypass are available. Pulmonary angi-

Table 36—2 Observations in a Patient Before and After Pulmonary Thromboendarterectomy (PTE)

	BEFORE PTE	AFTER PTE
Dyspnea	Present with mild exertion	None with moderate exertion
Vital capacity (L)	5.2	4.1
Total lung capacity (L)	6.9	5.2
Airway mechanics	Normal	Normal
Diffusing capacity (single breath) (mL · min^{-1} · mmHg^{-1})	31	36
PaO$_2$ (mmHg)		
Rest	59	104
Exercise	40	88
Minute volume (L/min)		
Rest	20.0	5.1
Exercise*	117.0	42.5
Physiologic dead space/tidal volume %		
Rest	51	32
Exercise*	61	28

* At similar power output before and after PTE.

ography should always be performed to verify the diagnosis before surgical therapy.

A few patients have been reported in whom there is failure of resolution of the pulmonary emboli. These patients have chronic pulmonary thromboembolism and, if the pulmonary vascular obstruction is great, they may have disabling, chronic pulmonary hypertension. They may experience progressive dyspnea on exercise, hypoxemia increased by exercise, large dead space ventilation, and increases in pulmonary artery pressure (Table 36–2). The normal diffusing capacity observed in the patient described in Table 36–2 may be due to filling of the pulmonary capillary bed by bronchial arteries or retrograde filling from pulmonary veins. Perfusion lung scans and pulmonary arteriograms in this subject demonstrated complete absence of perfusion of the right lung and partial vascular obstruction of the left—findings that did not change over an 8-month period, despite a course of adequate anticoagulation (see Fig. 36–4). Following pulmonary thromboendarterectomy, perfusion lung scans (Fig. 36–6) and exercise tolerance (see Table 36–2) improved dramatically. Four months after the surgical procedure, the patient was jogging 4 miles daily. Although chronic pulmonary embolism is a rare complication, increasing follow-up of pulmonary embolism has lead to discovery of increasing numbers of such patients. It is hoped that the mechanisms involved in failure of thrombus lysis will be uncovered in the near future.

SPECIAL CONSIDERATIONS IN THE PATIENT RECEIVING MECHANICAL VENTILATION WHO HAS SUFFERED A PULMONARY EMBOLUS

Patients with chronic obstructive airway disease are likely to develop pulmonary thromboembolism

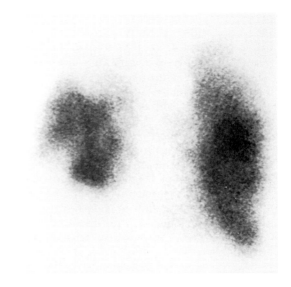

Figure 36—6. Pulmonary perfusion scintiscan in a patient with V̇/Q̇ mismatch (see Figs. 36–4, 36–5) following pulmonary thromboendarterectomy. There has been significant reperfusion of the right lung and improved perfusion to the left lower lobe.

and the diagnosis can be exceedingly difficult. This is particularly true in the patient who is already in respiratory failure and dependent on a ventilator. The clinical findings that should suggest pulmonary embolism would include the abrupt worsening of breathlessness, for which no apparent explanation can be found (i.e., secretions, bronchospasm, pneumothorax, or acute cardiac failure). There usually will be no specific clinical findings that will enable one to make the diagnosis, and reliance must be placed on physiologic studies, lung scanning, and pulmonary angiography. Although not specific, the measurement of wasted ventilation may be very useful in this situation, particularly if previous baseline measurements have been done.

With embolization there will be an abrupt increase in the physiologic dead space/tidal volume ratio. In the patient who has limited ventilatory capacity, or in the patient who is breathing by ventilator and unable to increase minute ventilation, the consequence of the increase in wasted ventilation will be a decrease in "effective" alveolar ventilation with a sudden rise in arterial carbon dioxide tension. The PaO_2 will also fall abruptly and the fall will be out of proportion to the rise in $PaCO_2$.

Thus, the abrupt development of increased breathlessness with tachycardia and tachypnea in a patient breathing on a respirator, with an abrupt increase in $PaCO_2$ in the absence of any change in total minute ventilation, strongly suggests the development of pulmonary embolization. Recognizing the limitations of lung scanning in such a patient, pulmonary angiography is probably the diagnostic procedure of choice. The use of low-dose heparin prophylactically in such patients may prevent this unwanted complication.

BIBLIOGRAPHY

Incidence and Importance

Dalen JE, Alpert JS: Natural history of pulmonary embolism. Prog Cardiovasc Dis 27:259, 1975

Etiology and Pathology

Castleman B: Pathologic observations on pulmonary infarction in man. In Sasahara AA, Stein M (eds): Pulmonary Embolic Disease. New York, Grune & Stratton, 1965

Freiman DG: Pathologic observations on experimental and human pulmonary thromboembolism. In Sasahara AA, Stein M (eds): Pulmonary Embolic Disease, New York, Grune & Stratton, 1965

Kakkar VV, Flanc C, Howe CT, Clarke MD: Natural history of postoperative deep vein thrombosis. Lancet 2:230, 1969

Shackford SR, Moser KM: Deep venous thrombosis and pulmonary embolism in trauma patients. J Intensive Care Med 3:87, 1988

Pathophysiology

McIntyre KM, Sasahara AA: Hemodynamic and ventricular responses to pulmonary embolism. Prog Cardiovasc Dis 27:175, 1974

Moser KM: Venous thromboembolism. Am Rev Respir Dis 141:235, 1990

Stein M, Levy SE: Reflex and humoral responses to pulmonary embolism. Prog Cardiovasc Dis 27:164, 1974

Thomas DP, Gurewich V, Ashford TP: Platelet adherence to thromboemboli in relation to pathogenesis and treatment of pulmonary embolism. N Engl J Med 274:953, 1966

Thomas DP et al: Mechanism of bronchoconstriction produced by thromboemboli in dogs. Am J Physiol 206:1207, 1964

Yann H, Lemaire F, Brun-Buisson J et al: Hypoxemia in pulmonary embolism. Chest 88:829, 1985

Clinical Manifestations

Goodwin JF: Clinical diagnosis of pulmonary thromboembolism. In Sasahara AA, Stein M (eds): Pulmonary Embolic Disease. New York, Grune & Stratton, 1965

Sasahara AA: Clinical studies in pulmonary thromboembolism. In Sasahara AA, Stein M (eds): Pulmonary Embolic Disease. New York, Grune & Stratton, 1965

Simon M: Plain film and angiographic aspects of pulmonary embolism. In Moser KM, Stein M (eds): Pulmonary Thromboembolism. Chicago, Year Book Medical Publishers, 1973

Diagnosis and Differential Diagnosis

Ashburn WL, Moser KM: Pulmonary ventilation and perfusion scanning in pulmonary thromboembolism. In Moser KM, Stein M (eds): Pulmonary Thromboembolism. Chicago, Year Book Medical Publishers, 1973

Becker DM et al: Real-time ultrasonography for the diagnosis of lower extremity deep venous thrombosis. Arch Intern Med 149:1731–1734, 1989

Biello DR: Radiological (scintigraphic) evaluation of patients with suspected pulmonary thromboembolism. JAMA 253:3257, 1987

Hull RP, Hirsh J, Carter CT et al: Diagnostic value of ventilation–perfusion lung scanning in patients with suspected pulmonary embolism. Chest 88:19–28, 1985

Moser KM: Diagnostic measures in pulmonary embolism. Basics RD 3(5), 1975

The PIOPED Investigators: Value of the ventilation–perfusion scan in acute pulmonary embolism. Results of the prospective investigation of pulmonary embolism diagnosis (PIOPED). JAMA 263:2753, 1990

Tow DE, Simon AL: Comparison of lung scanning and pulmonary arteriography in the detection and follow-up of pulmonary embolism. The urokinase pulmonary embolism trial experience. Prog Cardiovasc Dis 27:239, 1975

Tow DE et al: Validity of measuring regional pulmonary blood flow with macroaggregates of human serum albumin. Am J Roentgenol Radium Ther Nucl Med 96:664, 1966

Wagner HN, Strauss HW: Radioactive tracers in the differential diagnosis of pulmonary embolism. Prog Cardiovasc Dis 27:271, 1975

Therapy

Goldhaber SZ, Markis JE, Kessler CM et al: Perspectives in treatment of acute pulmonary embolism with tissue plasminogen activator. Semin Thromb Hemost 13:171, 1987

Moser KM, Daily PO, Peterson K et al: Thromboendarterectomy for chronic major vessel thromboembolic pulmonary hypertension. Ann Intern Med 107:560, 1987

NIH Consensus Conference: Prevention of venous thrombois and pulmonary embolism. JAMA 256:744, 1986

Sasahara AA: Therapy for pulmonary embolism. JAMA 229:1795, 1974

Silverglade AJ: Thromboembolism: Diagnosis and treatment. West J Med 120:219, 1974

Thrombolytic Therapy in Thrombosis: A National Institutes of Health Consensus Development Conference. Ann Intern Med 93:141–144, 1980

Urokinase Pulmonary Embolism Trial Study Group: Phase 1 results. JAMA 214:2163, 1970

Urokinase–Streptokinase Embolism Trial: Phase 2 results. JAMA 229:1606, 1974

THIRTY-SEVEN

Definitions of Airflow Disorders and Implications for Therapy

Thomas L. Petty

Clinical conditions characterized by acute or chronic airflow obstruction are common in all age groups and in both genders. Cardinal symptoms of both acute and chronic airflow obstruction are cough, wheeze, and dyspnea. These are nonspecific symptoms and allow a diagnosis to be made only in the context of other clinical and laboratory information.

Airflow obstruction can be identified by experienced clinicians on the basis of the intensity and quality of breath sounds as assessed by auscultation. Marked prolongation of the expiratory time well beyond the normal 4 to 6 seconds also helps to indicate the degree of advanced states of airflow obstruction. However, objective measurements are by far superior, and critical to the evaluation of patients when one is in pursuit of a diagnosis and to monitor responses to therapy. Simple measurements by spirometry or even disposable devices (e.g., peak flow meters and a vital capacity meter) can be useful in measuring airflow and volume to be able to diagnose the disease states that are defined in the following. For the purposes of this chapter airflow is judged by the simple forced expiratory volume in 1 second (FEV_1), which is obtained by spirometry, and total exhaled volume by the forced vital capacity (FVC).

ASTHMA

Asthma is a heterogeneous disorder characterized by cough, wheeze, dyspnea, and variable degrees of reversible airflow obstruction. Acute intermittent asthma is easy to define and diagnose. Attacks are characterized by the sudden onset of dyspnea, cough, and wheeze, followed by complete or nearly complete cessation of symptoms and a return to normal airflow. Reversible airflow obstruction, which usually follows the use of bronchodilators, may sometimes subside spontaneously, as in exercise-induced asthma. Acute, intermittent, and completely reversible asthma should not be included in the chronic obstructive pulmonary disease (COPD) designation.

ASTHMATIC BRONCHITIS

Asthmatic bronchitis, a term that is reappearing, refers to a different clinical state.[1] The asthmatic symptoms of cough, dyspnea, and wheeze may occur throughout the year, and varying degrees of airflow obstruction are present. Asthmatic bronchitis refers to chronic, persistent asthma, but the designation "bronchitis" is also appropriate because of significant airways inflammation. If major reversibility cannot be achieved by bronchoactive drugs in conjunction with preventive therapy (e.g., avoidance of precipitating attacks) or mediator blockers (i.e., cromolyn), asthmatic bronchitis *should* be included in the COPD spectrum (see later discussion). However, completely reversible chronic asthma should not be "lumped" in the COPD designation, particularly if there is a symptom-free interval. Indeed a degree of fixed airflow obstruction, often with progressive features commonly occurs in asthmatic bronchitis. It should be emphasized that asthmatic bronchitis is actually a form of chronic bronchitis. Asthmatic bronchitis could be described histologically as hypertrophic and desquamative eosinophilic chronic bronchitis,[2] to refer to the eosinophilic inflammatory infiltrates of the conducting airways in protracted and chronic states of bronchial asthma. A polymorphonuclear cell infiltrate may also be present. In addition to chronic and variable airflow obstruction, hyperinflation may be present in asthmatic bronchitis, but not of the degree that occurs in advanced emphysema. Residual volume elevation is common, indicating expiratory air-trapping owing to small airways obstruction. The carbon monoxide diffusion test, which is a useful indicator of the integrity of the air–blood interface (alveolocapillary membrane), is well preserved in asthmatic bronchitis. This test of carbon monoxide transfer is often normal or near normal even in states of severe protracted airflow obstruction from chronic asthmatic bronchitis.

CHRONIC BRONCHITIS

So-called chronic bronchitis is very similar to asthmatic bronchitis. Cough and sputum production for many months over several years are the hallmarks of chronic bronchitis. Historically, *chronic bronchitis* has been defined as a chronic cough with expectoration for at least 3 months and lasting at least 2 years;[3] but only a few patients with chronic cough and expectoration have associated airflow obstruction.[4] Patients with chronic bronchitis, but without airflow obstruction, have been termed *simple bronchitis*. Patients with this symptom complex have a good prognosis, as contrasted with the premature morbidity and mortality that characterize chronic bronchitis with chronic airflow obstruction.[4] Patients with chronic cough and airflow obstruction have been designated as having "chronic obstructive bronchitis," but the less specific term, chronic bronchitis, is commonly used. The pathophysiology of chronic bronchitis is identical to asthmatic bronchitis and is characterized by varying degrees of airflow obstruction caused by a combination of inflammation and increased bronchomotor tone because of so-called nonspecific bronchial hyperreactivity. Thus, neither measurement of airflow obstruction nor of lung compartments can be used to distinguish asthmatic bronchitis from chronic bronchitis. Some authors question if this distinction is important at all.[1,5] Air-trapping (increased residual volume), without

hyperinflation, and a normal or near-normal diffusion test is commonly present in both asthmatic bronchitis and chronic bronchitis. Consequently, it is easy to understand how asthmatic bronchitis and chronic bronchitis are often indistinguishable or mistaken for each other.

EMPHYSEMA

Emphysema is characterized clinically by progressive dyspnea and variable cough. Physiologically, emphysema is characterized by hyperinflation followed by chronic progressive airflow obstruction. The degree of hyperinflation exceeds other states of chronic airflow obstruction. In fact, an increased total lung capacity, associated with reduced elastic recoil is found in the earliest stages of emphysema in studies of excised human lungs.[6] The official diagnosis of emphysema relies on loss of alveolar walls, a designation founded on anatomic studies. More recently, a consensus conference has rede-

Figure 37—1. PA chest x-ray film of patient with advanced emphysema. Aged 61, FEV₁ 0.6, L; postbronchodilator 0.7; total lung capacity, 10.04 L. Notice paucity of lung markings in the outer half of the lung field.

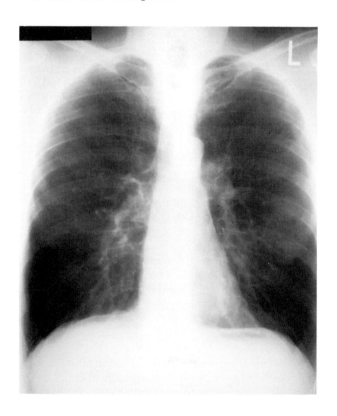

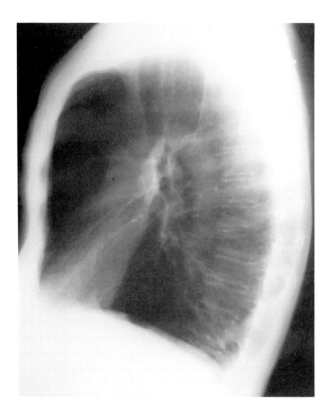

Figure 37—2. Lateral chest x-ray film to accompany Fig. 37–1. Notice the marked enlargement of the retrosternal space and flattened diaphragms.

fined emphysema in more practical and clinical terms.[7] Loss of alveolar surface finally results in a reduction of carbon monoxide uptake, the basis of the single-breath diffusion test. Hence, in advanced states of emphysema, severe degrees of airflow obstruction, air-trapping, marked hyperinflation, and a reduced diffusion test are all present. By this stage of disease, the chest x-ray film shows this degree of hyperinflation, reduced pulmonary markings, signifying loss of lung parenchyma, and flattened diaphragm (Figs. 37–1 and 37–2). Chest roentgenographic criteria for suggesting the diagnosis of emphysema have been offered.[8] It must be emphasized that the chest x-ray examination is most accurate in indicating *advanced* states of emphysema. Airflow obstruction (or limitation) is the key to the diagnosis of emphysema. Therefore, some degrees of reversibility may be expected in response to vigorous treatment, even in advanced emphysema. A small to moderate degree of airflow improvement may be present in emphysema in response to bronchodilating drugs.[9]

Inflammation of both small airways and surrounding alveoli is due to the release of polymorphonuclear elastases.[10] These processes are augmented by cigarette smoke, which can also inactivate the normal antielastase protective material at the air–blood interface.[11] Some of the same airway inflammatory mediators that are included in asthmatic and chronic bronchitis may occur in the pathogenesis of emphysema.

THE CONCEPT OF CHRONIC OBSTRUCTIVE PULMONARY DISEASE

It should be apparent from the foregoing that there are multiple pathways into the final state of COPD, including untreated or unrelenting asthmatic bronchitis, chronic (obstructive) bronchitis, and emphysema. By the time the patient has advanced to irreversible airflow obstruction, particularly at an older age, there is little point in seeking a more specific diagnosis than COPD, if airflow obstruction cannot be substantially reversed by bronchodilators or corticosteroids. By contrast, there is great importance in identifying those patients with major reversibility in response to therapy (the so-called hidden asthmatics), since they have a much better prognosis with systemic therapy than those with fixed and progressive airflow obstruction.

Table 37–1 lists the clinical pulmonary function measurements that help to classify the various disease states that, together, constitute the spectrum of COPD. Patients with other disease states also characterized by chronic airflow obstruction (e.g., cystic fibrosis, bronchiectasis, and bronchiolitis obliterans) and interstitial states with airflow obstruction, such as eosinophilic granuloma and lymphangiomyomatosis (all rare) should not be designated by the label COPD. These other states either have a different prognosis or, sometimes, other forms of therapy that are not appropriate for COPD (e.g., lymphangiomyomatosis).

RESPONSES TO SYSTEMATIC MANAGEMENT

These designations (asthmatic bronchitis, chronic bronchitis, emphysema, and, indeed, COPD) are often used as labels that, at first, may be relatively meaningless. It has already been pointed out that it is nearly impossible to distinguish asthmatic bronchitis from chronic bronchitis. The only feature that sets emphysema apart from these disorders,

Table 37—1 Physiologic Determinants of Diseases Characterized by Acute and Chronic Airflow Obstruction

	MAJOR SYMPTOMS COMPLEX	PATTERN OF AIRFLOW OBSTRUCTION (FEV_1)	TRAPPING RESIDUAL VOLUME	HYPERINFLATION	DIFFUSION
Intermittent asthma	Acute wheezing, dyspnea, with variable cough	Reversible airflow obstruction	Mild, intermittent	Transient	Normal
Asthmatic and chronic bronchitis	Chronic cough, wheeze, with variable degrees of dyspnea	Partly reversible or irreversible airflow obstruction	Moderate, partly reversible	Mild to moderate	Normal and slightly reduced
Emphysema	Dyspnea, variable cough and wheeze	Irreversible airflow obstruction, progressive impairment	Moderate to marked, progressive	Moderate to marked	Reduced
COPD, advanced	Elements of 2 and 3—mostly owing to emphysema and irreversible changes in the conducting airways				

which are characterized by airways inflammation and bronchial hyperreactivity, is hyperinflation and evidence of a functional or anatomic loss of a substantial portion of the air–blood interface, as identified by the reduced transfer of carbon monoxide in the single-breath diffusion test. In fact, all of the pathogenetic processes that result in airways inflammation, bronchial hyperreactivity, small-airways changes, and dissolution of alveolar walls may be related. All are certainly aggravated by the irritant and oxidant effects of inhaled tobacco smoke. Accordingly, stopping all smoking is key to therapy in all of these disease states. However, some patients with asthmatic bronchitis and chronic bronchitis have never smoked.

Consequently, we are likely to label patients with cough, wheeze, and dyspnea "asthmatic" if they are nonsmokers, and we will almost certainly call the same patients "chronic bronchitic" if they smoke. In the past, it was more common to call nonsmoking women asthmatic and smoking men bronchitic, but today the prevalence of smoking in both sexes is becoming more equal. Of course, many people smoke and even cough without airflow obstructive disorders. So we cannot use smoking as a distinguishing feature, although it must be stressed that nearly all patients with emphysema are smokers. Exceptions are patients with hereditary forms of α_1-antiprotease deficiency.[11] Even in this condition, the primacy of protease excess versus antiprotease protection has been questioned recently.[11] Certainly, the protease–antiprotease theory of disease is important, but it probably does not explain all of the pathogenetic mechanisms that result in emphysema.

Today, there is desirable lumping of nearly all chronic, nonspecific, and progressive disease states of airflow obstruction under the designation chronic obstructive pulmonary disease (COPD). This recognizes two important principles. First, it is very difficult to be accurate in the use of more specific terms, at least until systematic, pharmacologically oriented therapy is applied (see following discussion). Secondly, both airway and alveolar components are present in end stages of disease. The COPD designation, though purposely nonspecific, is therefore an appropriate designation for most disease states with chronic irreversible states of airflow obstruction (limitation).

The systematic use of bronchoactive drugs can be helpful in better-defining the disease states described in this chapter. The details of how β-agonists, methylxanthines, anticholinergics, corticosteroids, and a variety of other drugs are used is beyond the scope of this chapter (see Chap. 19). A stepwise approach generally is employed. Therapy for all patients with airflow obstruction disorders should be begun with inhaled β-agonist drugs used regularly around-the-clock. Even patients who do not have demonstrable responsiveness in the laboratory, as judged by simple spirometric tests, should be given at least a 1-month trial of inhaled β-agonists. If patients will not or cannot use inhaled β-agonists, oral β-agonists are a reasonable alternative. However, the oral dose required to achieve equal bronchodilating responses of the conducting air passages may be 20 to 100 times that which provides maximum dilatation by the inhaled route. There are no known advantages of using inhaled and oral β-agonists together.

Methylxanthines also improve airflow, but their mechanism of action is not well understood. Methylxanthines also improve the patients' global functioning state by improving respiratory muscle strength and through a small, but sometimes significant, improvement in cardiac output if associated heart failure is present. A mild respiratory center-stimulating effect of methylxanthines may also be an advantage. Both β-agonists and methylxanthines help improve mucociliary clearance.

The inflammatory nature of both airways and alveolar damage resulting in all states of COPD has been mentioned briefly. Thus, anti-inflammatory agents are used as key pharmacologic strategies, necessary in the control of airways and probably alveolar inflammation. Both inhaled and oral corticosteroid drugs are useful. Oral corticosteroids are generally employed for major exacerbations of disease and in chronic irreversible states of airflow obstruction in patients who are steroid-responsive. Inhaled corticosteroids are useful in maintenance management, but not in acute exacerbations. Cromolyn sodium should be considered a first-line drug in asthmatic states, including chronic asthmatic bronchitis. Cromolyn was extremely effective in adult asthmatics who had various degrees of chronic airflow obstruction, in a recent controlled clinical trial.[12] Cromolyn sodium probably works by preventing the release of pre-formed inflammatory mediators that can damage any portion of the conducting air passages and possibly even alveoli.[13] However, cromolyn has not been useful in patients with more-advanced forms of COPD, including emphysema.

Anticholinergics are returning to the scene as important bronchodilators. Anticholinergic bronchodilators are particularly useful in patients with emphysema.[14] Apparently, the cholinergic autonomic nervous system is more active in states of COPD including emphysema. Perhaps the β-adrenergic nervous system is less responsive because of disease or because of the longstanding use of β-agonistic drugs. If this theory is correct, the cholinergic nervous system would be unopposed in its effect on increased bronchomotor tone. The anticholinergic ipratropium bromide appears to be more effective than the β-agonist agents in patients with advanced COPD.[15] Atropine methylnitrate may be equally effective.[15]

The physician and respiratory care workers should focus upon the patient's symptoms and the fact of airflow obstruction as therapeutic strategies are designed and evaluated. If patients have marked improvement in airflow, the designation "asthmatic" or "chronic bronchitic" seems most appropriate. In states of irreversible airflow obstruction, the nonspecific designation COPD or emphysema is probably best used. But the point of therapy is to attempt to gain reversibility using potent bronchoactive drugs along with minimal, or at least acceptable, side effects. These goals can be achieved in almost all patients with diseases characterized by chronic airflow obstruction.

In summary, states of airflow obstruction are common disorders that compose the spectrum from asthma–chronic bronchitis to emphysema. Asthmatic and chronic bronchitic states are at least potentially reversible by systematic, pharmacologically oriented therapy, focusing on bronchodilators and corticosteroids. Emphysema and the final common pathway COPD are progressive states, unless cessation of smoking can be achieved in early or mild stages of the disease. The future focuses on the great challenge of early identification, classification, and intervention. Thus, all patients with cough, dyspnea, and wheeze should be carefully evaluated by health workers who understand the history, physical examination, and simple pulmonary function hallmarks, which together can help define the disease states characterized by airflow obstruction. Often, a final definition of disease cannot be made until aggressive attempts at the treatment of the airflow obstruction and its attendant symptoms complex have been vigorously pursued by experienced workers.

REFERENCES

1. Burrows B: An overview of obstructive lung diseases. Med Clin North Am 65:455–471, 1981
2. Hogg JC: The pathology of asthma. Chest 87:1525–1535, 1985
3. Ciba Foundation Guest Symposium: Terminology, definitions and classifications of chronic pulmonary emphysema and related conditions. Thorax 14:286–299, 1959
4. Bates DV: The fate of the chronic bronchitic. A report of the ten-year follow-up in the Canadian Department of Veterans Affairs Coordinated Study of Chronic Bronchitis. Am Rev Respir Dis 108:1043–1065, 1973
5. Petty TL: Chronic bronchitis versus asthma—or what's in a name? J Allergy Clin Immunol 62:323–324, 1978
6. Petty TL, Silvers GW, Stanford RE: Mild emphysema is associated with reduced elastic recoil and increased lung size but not with airflow limitation. Am Rev Respir Dis 136:867–871, 1987
7. Snider GL, Kleinerman J, Thurlbeck WM et al: The definition of emphysema (Report of National Heart, Lung and Blood Institute, Division of Lung Diseases Workshop). Am Rev Respir Dis 132:182–185, 1985

APPENDIX **A**

Methodology of Arterial Blood Gas Analysis

Lia Bickford
Cliff Bickford
John E. Hodgkin

The scope and the application of arterial blood gas analysis have taken giant steps forward during the last few years. With the advent of automated equipment, fast, accurate data analysis, with a minimum of human interaction, has become available. The complexity of the newer automated systems has not added to the accuracy of the sensors, but has been applied to such things as autocalibration, membrane integrity checks, drift and stability checks, and calculation of secondary results. The P_{O_2}, pH, and P_{CO_2} electrodes remain relatively unchanged. Thus, push-button simplicity in blood gas analysis does not yet exist, and the present level of sophistication in equipment should never be expected to compensate for unqualified or inexperienced personnel. The demands of the laboratory should determine whether a manual or automated system is most appropriate (Fig. A–1). In the following sections, we shall discuss the types of systems available and their respective applications.

Many factors affect the performance of the three electrodes involved in blood gas analysis. If calibration gases are introduced too rapidly or under too much pressure, the semipermeable membranes could be stretched, which would affect the electrodes' response time. After sampling, incomplete flushing of the cuvettes can cause contamination of the electrode membranes, which will also affect their response. Other factors, such as adjustment time, contamination of buffers, temperature, and electrode maintenance, will affect performance. These factors demonstrate the importance of consistency in calibration techniques and equipment maintenance. Automated equipment was developed to decrease the variability in calibration technique and equipment maintenance that occurs when humans perform these tasks.

OXYGEN ELECTRODE (CLARK ELECTRODE)

The first polarographic electrodes for the measurement of oxygen were developed in the late 1930s. However, the development in the 1950s of an electrode for measuring oxygen in blood and other solutions is attributed to Clark. Thus the P_{O_2} electrode is commonly referred to as a Clark electrode.

Both automated and manual systems use a Clark-type electrode for measuring P_{O_2} (Fig. A–2). The design is slightly different, but the principle for both systems is the same.

Measurements are made on whole blood that has been drawn or injected into a small chamber known as a cuvette. Blood is thereby brought into contact with a thin plastic membrane (usually polypropylene), about 1 mm thick, which covers the tip of the electrode. This membrane has two functions: It serves as a barrier between the blood and the electrode, keeping the electrode and its electrolyte free of contamination: and it is a semipermeable barrier that permits diffusion of oxygen molecules.

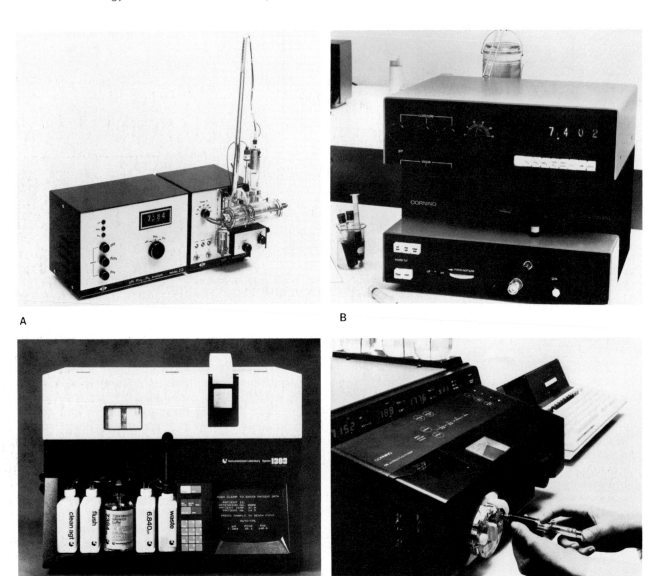

Figure A–1. (*A, B*) Two examples of manual systems. Calibration and service procedures, such as maintenance of liquid levels and flush procedures, must be performed by the operator. (*C, D*). Two examples of automated systems: Calibration and flush procedures are performed automatically at preset intervals. These procedures can be initiated by the operator, but are still controlled by the instrument. Alarms warn the operator of service needs, electrode drift, and other mechanical or electronic malfunctions. (Courtesy of Corning and Instrumentation Laboratory, Inc)

Accordingly, equilibration between blood and electrolyte occurs while variables such as temperature, contamination, and calibration can be closely controlled.

The cuvette is maintained at a thermostatically controlled temperature (usually 37° C), and the sample reaches this temperature within seconds of entry. Oxygen molecules present in the plasma diffuse through the semipermeable membrane until equilibrium between the plasma and the electrode solution occurs. A platinum cathode in contact with the electrolyte solution is supplied with a

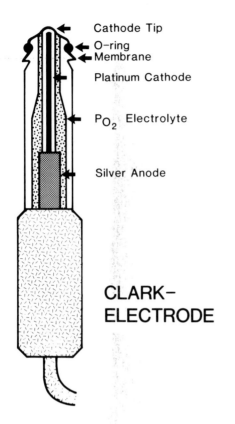

Cathode Tip
O-ring
Membrane
Platinum Cathode

P_{O_2} Electrolyte

Silver Anode

CLARK-ELECTRODE

Figure A—2. Schematic representation of the PO₂ (Clark) electrode.

small voltage (about 700 mV), and oxygen molecules in contact with it undergo hydrolysis. The number of oxygen molecules present in the electrolyte determines the intensity of this reaction, which then determines the number of electrons (voltage) produced. Therefore, the reaction that takes place at the cathode produces a voltage proportional to the concentration of oxygen molecules present in the electrolyte solution (Fig. A–3). The more oxygen molecules present to take on electrons, the greater the electron flow or electrical current produced and the higher the PO₂ reading.

Most glass pH electrodes are of similar design. On one side of a pH-sensitive glass is a solution with a known pH (usually pH 6.840) and, on the other side a solution of unknown pH (blood). The difference in H⁺ concentration between the two solutions produces a potential difference (voltage) that is proportional to the difference in pH between the two solutions (Fig. A–4).

The electrode is similar to two half cells with a liquid junction (saturated potassium chloride). One

half cell is a silver–silver chloride-measuring electrode in contact with a liquid of known pH (usually 6.840). Its function is to convey the potential difference across the pH-sensitive glass to the electronic circuitry. The other half cell is a mercury–mercurous chloride (calomel) reference electrode (anode) that supplies a constant reference voltage. The reference half cell is connected to the measuring half cell by the liquid junction or potassium chloride salt bridge that completes the circuit (Fig. A–5).

PCO₂ ELECTRODE (SEVERINGHAUS ELECTRODE)

The modern-type PCO₂ electrode was first developed by Stowe in the mid-1950s. It was further modified by Severinghaus in 1958; therefore, the PCO₂ electrode is commonly referred to as the Severinghause electrode.

Although physically resembling a PO₂ electrode, the PCO₂ electrode is, in principle, a pH electrode. The tip is covered by a membrane that acts as a diffusion barrier between the blood and the electrolyte. Blood is brought into contact with the membrane by means of a sampling cuvette similar to the PO₂ electrode. Carbon dioxide molecules diffuse across the membrane into the electrolyte solution and react with the buffer (Fig. A–6).

Diffusion proceeds until equilibrium has been reached. The resultant change in H⁺ concentration in the buffer solution is measured by the pH-type electrode and is proportional to the amount of carbon dioxide that has diffused into the buffer (Fig. A–7).

ASTRUP EQUILIBRATION METHOD FOR DETERMINING PCO₂

The Astrup method can be readily applied as a system of quality control on manual equipment. It incorporates the relationship between pH and PCO₂, as depicted in the derivation of the Henderson–Hasselbalch equation and is expressed in the Astrup nomogram as a graphic demonstration of the linear relation between pH and log PCO₂ (Fig. A–8). The procedure consists of placing two small samples of well-mixed whole blood into two separate equilibration chambers known as tonometers. The tonometer is equipped with a motorized shaker so that the blood can be shaken and swirled completely. The blood in the tonometers is equilibrated with gases that contain two known concentrations

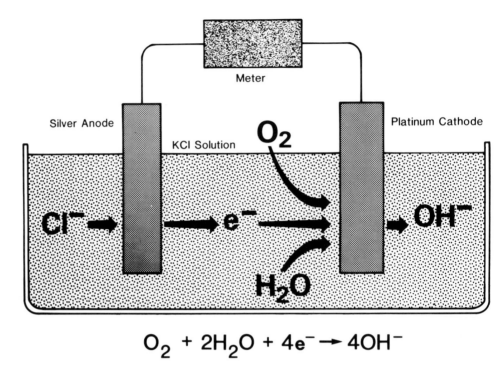

$$O_2 + 2H_2O + 4e^- \longrightarrow 4OH^-$$

Figure A–3. Chloride ion (Cl$^-$) reacts with silver anode to form silver chloride. This is an oxidation reaction that produces electrons (e$^-$). At the cathode, oxygen will react with platinum and water in a reduction reaction, thus using electrons generated at the anode. The resultant flow of electrons can be measured as a current. The more oxygen molecules present in the solution, the greater the flow of electrons (current).

of carbon dioxide (about 4% and 8%), with the balance being oxygen, so that at the end of a 3-minute equilibration period, the blood in the tonometers will have taken on the partial pressure of the equilibrating gas. By measuring the resulting pH of each tonometered sample, one is essentially observing the buffering capacity of the blood. Since the PCO$_2$s of the equilibrated samples are known and the pHs measured, two x–y coordinates are available to be plotted on the nomogram. The two points plotted on the nomogram establish a buffer line that states the relationship for any PCO$_2$ and pH as determined by that particular blood sample. Hence, the actual pH of the patient's whole blood, anaerobically maintained, can be located along this buffer line and the PCO$_2$ subsequently can be read off the vertical axis.

CALCULATION OF ADDITIONAL ACID–BASE PARAMETERS

Calculation of additional acid–base parameters based on pH and PCO$_2$ can be handled manually through the use of nomograms. These nomograms require simple plotting of data points, constructing a line between these points, and reading off the desired values at the appropriate intercepts, thus eliminating the need for mathematical computation.

The Siggaard–Anderson nomogram was originally devised empirically, and it graphically expresses relationships among pH, PCO$_2$, buffer base, base excess, standard bicarbonate, and plasma bicarbonate. To use this nomogram, the Astrup equilibration technique is carried out, and the two sets

I

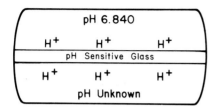

II

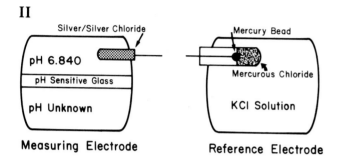

III

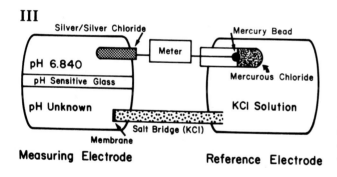

Figure A—4. Principle of pH electrode. (*I*) Voltage develops across pH-sensitive glass when H+ concentrations of the two solutions are unequal; (*II*) two half cells, a measuring electrode, and a reference electrode; (*III*) Diagrammatic representation of a modern pH electrode.

of pH–PCO$_2$ coordinates are plotted on a graph (see Fig. A–8).

Another Siggaard–Andersen nomogram, the alignment nomogram, requires only pH and PCO$_2$ measurements to determine base excess, total carbon dioxide, actual plasma bicarbonate, standard bicarbonate, base excess of the extracellular fluid (BE$_{ECF}$), and T$_{40}$ bicarbonate (Fig. A–9). These and other similar nomograms have been adapted to slide-rule form, which provides quick and easy calculation of data. Use of a computer, of course, simplifies calculation of these additional values.

CO-OXIMETER FOR MEASURING OXYGEN SATURATION

Both Lavoisier and Priestley (in 1774) recognized that the color of blood and atmospheric oxygen were related. Hoppe-Seyler (in 1859) studied the spectra of blood and gave the colored pigment the name hemoglobin. Angström had described the absorbance spectrum of blood 2 years earlier. Vierodt (in 1873) was apparently the first to use the differences in the absorbance spectra of the species of hemoglobin to measure their concentration. Hufner

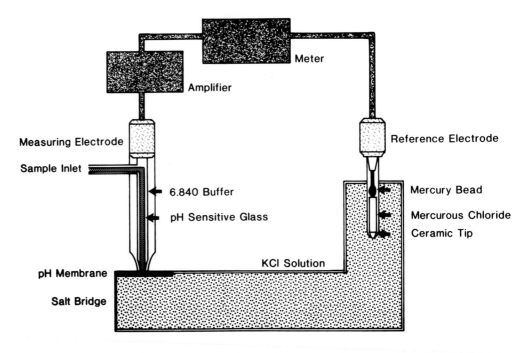

Figure A—5. Schematic representation of a modern micro-pH electrode.

Figure A—6. Diagrammatic representation of the reaction occurring within the PCO_2 electrode.

Unknown CO_2 ⟶ $CO_2 + H_2O \rightleftharpoons H_2CO_3 \rightleftharpoons H^+ + HCO_3^-$

Figure A—7. Schematic diagram of PCO_2 electrode.

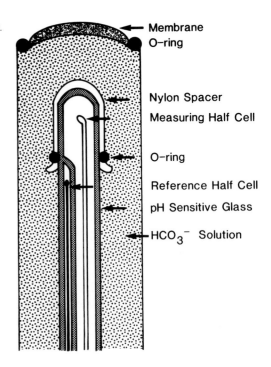

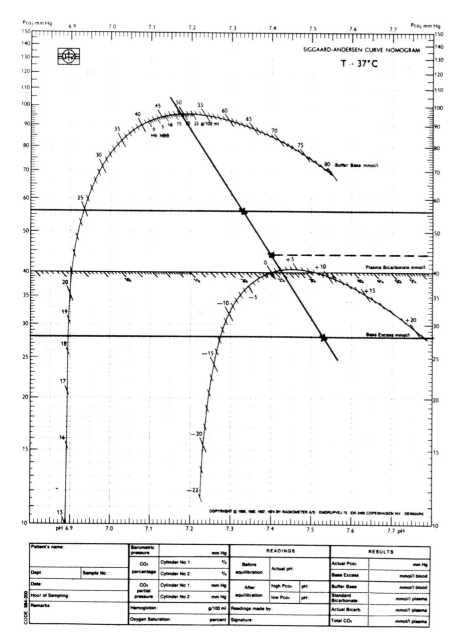

Figure A—8. Siggaard—Andersen curve nomogram: (1) pH values are measured after equilibration, and the two points are plotted versus known PCO_2; (2) a line is drawn between the two points and extended to intersect the buffer base and base excess curves (these values are read directly); (3) an approximate hemoglobin for purposes of quality control can be interpolated by subtracting the value of the BE curve from the BB curve reading directly below BB on the hemoglobin scale; (4) actual pH is plotted along this line, and the PCO_2 is read off the vertical axis; (5) the line itself intersects HCO_3^- at a PCO_2 of 40 mmHg, thus indicating the standard HCO_3^-; (6) to determine actual plasma HCO_3^-, a 45° angle must be constructed through the actual pH until it intersects the HCO_3^- scale. Calculation of buffer base, base excess, and standard bicarbonate uses another modification of the Siggaard—Andersen nomogram. (Reproduced, with modifications, by permission of Siggaard—Andersen O and Radiometer A/S, Copenhagen, 1962)

(in 1900) extensively described a two-wavelength photometric method to determine the percentages of oxyhemoglobin and carboxyhemoglobin.

Haldane (in 1900) developed the concept of oxygen saturation and oxygen capacity and devised a manometric instrument for their measurement. The standard gasometric method, still in use as a reference procedure, was described by Van Slyke and Neill in 1924.[4]

The normal oxyhemoglobin dissociation curve relating PO_2 and oxygen saturation is well documented for normal pH (7.4) and temperature (37° C). By use of proper correction factors, the oxygen saturation measurement can be corrected for curves shifted by varying pH or temperatures. Nomograms exist that allow these corrections to be determined quickly. However, these corrections do not permit any change in the shape of the actual curve. Many

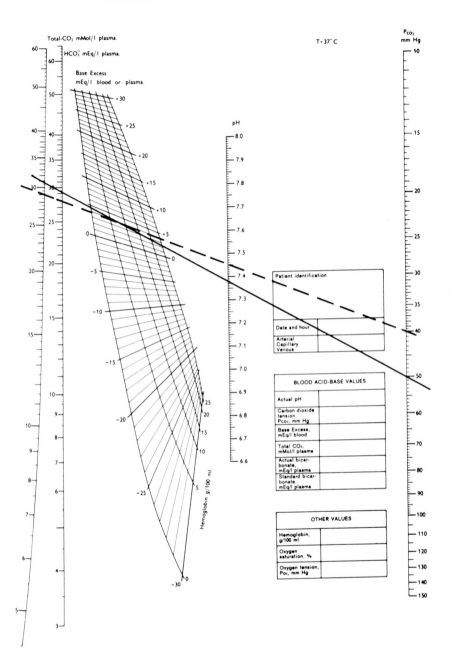

Figure A—9. Siggaard–Andersen alignment nomogram: (1) a line is constructed between pH and PCO₂; (2) actual plasma HCO₃⁻ is read directly at the intersection of the line; (3) BE_b is hemoglobin-dependent and can be read at the intersection of the constructed line and the patient's Hb value; (4) standard HCO₃⁻ can be determined by constructing another line through the BE_b–Hb point, and a PCO₂ of 40 mmHg, and by reading the HCO₃⁻ scale; (5) buffer base can be computed from the equation $BB = 41.7 + (0.42 × Hb) + BE$; (6) BE_ECF is calculated similarly to the BE_b, but the BE_ECF is read off at the intersection of the constructed line and one-third of the patient's Hb value; (7) T₄₀ HCO₃⁻ can be determined by constructing another line through the BE_ECF, Hb/3 point, and a PCO₂ of 40 mmHg, and by reading the HCO₃⁻ scale. (Reproduced, with modifications, by permission of Siggaard–Andersen O and Radiometer A/S, Copenhagen, 1963)

factors can affect the relationship of hemoglobin to oxygen and alter the shape of the PO₂–oxygen saturation curve. For example, a sample with an elevated carboxyhemoglobin level may have an actual oxygen saturation much lower than that predicted from the measured PO₂. The curve may also be affected by factor such as 2,3-DPG, methemoglobin, and various congenital hemoglobins. Therefore, the ability to measure oxygen saturation accurately is preferable to reporting a calculated value.

Oxygen saturation measurements can be made by using a spectrophotometric device such as the IL

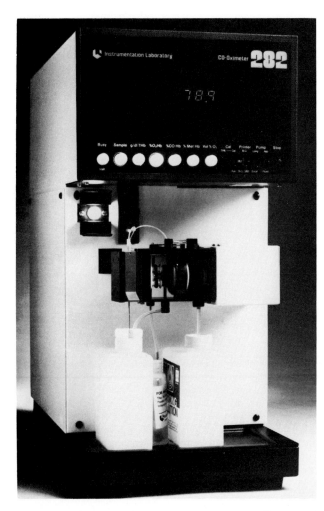

Figure A—10. IL 282 CO-Oximeter Analyzer. (Courtesy of Instrumentation Laboratory, Inc)

282 Co-Oximeter analyzer (Fig. A—10). With this instrument, whole blood is aspirated, mixed with diluent, and hemolyzed. It is then drawn into a cuvette where it is brought to a constant temperature. Monochromatic light at four specific wavelengths passes through the cuvette to a photodetector whose output is used to determine the absorbance pattern of the hemoglobin at these specific wavelengths (Fig. A—11). The instrument electronically computes total hemoglobin, percentage of oxyhemoglobin (O_2Hb), percentage of carboxyhemoglobin (COHb), percentage of methemoglobin (MetHb), oxygen content, and percentage of reduced hemoglobin (RHb). This assumes that RHb, O_2Hb, COHb, and MetHb are the only forms of hemoglobin present. Another form of hemoglobin that absorbs significantly at any of the specific wavelengths can introduce spectral interference—that is, sulfhemoglobin has an absorbance level similar to that of methemoglobin, and thus interference with absorbance at that specific wavelength would affect the measurement of methemoglobin. Other measurements might be affected, but the interference would probably be less because the absorption patterns are not as close as those for sulfhemoglobin and methemoglobin. Methemoglobin is the only measured form that exhibits significant pH sensitivity. For MetHb levels greater than 10%, this sensitivity can cause absorbance variations at the four wavelengths used, which can generate errors in all displayed values. For MetHb levels below 10%, a high degree of accuracy can be achieved for all parameters.

PULSE OXIMETRY

Pulse oximetry is a noninvasive method of measuring arterial oxyhemoglobin saturation in pulsating blood vessels. Pulse oximeters utilize a probe or sensor that is applied to a single site on the body to measure absorption of selected wavelengths of light. Oxygenated and deoxygenated blood can be distinghished through the use of red and infrared light waves. That is, light absorption characteristics of deoxyhemoglobin (Hb), and oxyhemoglobin (O_2Hb) are markedly different in the red and infrared spectra.

Pulse oximeters transmit infrared and red light supplied by light-emitting diodes (LEDs), located in an arm of the probe or sensor, through the ear, finger, or nose. As the light is shined through the pulsating vascular bed of the site, it is partially absorbed. Some of the light is absorbed by the tissues (skin, muscle, adipose), which are constant, and some of the light is absorbed by the blood that flows through the arterioles in a pulsatile fashion characteristic of arterial blood flow. As a result, there is a variable source of absorption. Constant absorption of lightwaves is ignored, and focus is placed on the pulsatile absorption.

Calculation of oxygen saturation can be made at any point(s) in the pulsatile absorption cycle by taking the ratio of the infrared light absorbed to the red light absorbed. It should be noted that if large quantities of either methomoglobin (MetHb) or carboxyhemoglobin (COHb) are present, there will be an error in the computation of oxygen saturation by the pulse oximeter (i.e., the true oxygen saturation will be lower than is being reported).

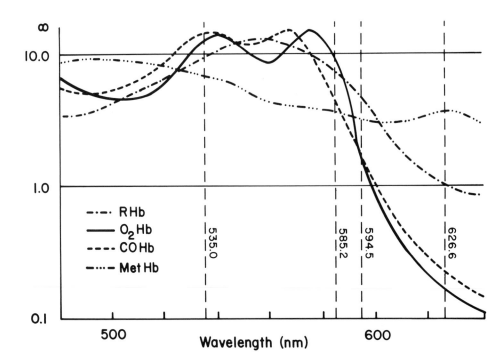

Figure A—11. Many two-wavelength methods have been published for determining either carbon monoxide- or oxygen-bound hemoglobin. The wavelengths that are used vary. Typically, the wavelengths are either at an inflection or at an isosbestic point of two or more of the species. It is common to select one wavelength at which the absorbance difference between species is at a maximum and the other at which this difference approaches zero. Since the absorbance of these species generally changes differently and abruptly as a function of wavelength, the spectrophotometer must have the smallest possible bandwidth, and the center wavelength must be positioned accurately and reproducibly. This figure shows hemoglobin spectra for four species of hemoglobin. Furthermore, in two-wavelength methods, unmeasured species must be absent, or the wavelengths must be chosen to minimize spectral interference from unmeasured species. This has frequently been overlooked in determining oxyhemoglobin in the presence of small but varying levels of endogenous and environmentally generated carbon monoxide. (Courtesy of Instrumentation Laboratory, Inc. from the IL-282 Operators Manual)

Pulse oximetry has become an important adjunct in the care of the critically ill patient receiving oxygen therapy or mechanical ventilation, reducing the number of arterial blood analyses required. It can be an invaluable tool in continuous monitoring of those patients who are at risk of low oxygen transport.

Pulse oximetry has gained widespread application in other settings over the last few years. Applications include use of oximetry to document nocturnal hypoxemia during sleep; during maximal exercise testing to document exercise-induced hypoxemia; to reinforce the benefits of pursed-lip breathing, paced exercise, and relaxation techniques in patients with COPD; and during procedures such as bronchoscopy.

Pulse oximetry has advantages and disadvantages. Advantages include noninvasive monitoring and data that can be obtained quickly and updated continuously. It is a simple technique requiring a minimum of training. The major disadvantage is that it does not detect changes in alveolar ventilation or acid–base status, as does arterial blood gas analysis.

QUALITY CONTROL

As blood gas analysis continues to gain importance in the management of critically ill patients, the need for comprehensive quality control procedures becomes more crucial. Erroneous data are worse than no data. A quality control program encompasses (1) equipment maintenance, (2) calibration techniques, (3) standards and controls, and (4) sampling and analysis protocols. These procedures are all interdependent, and, if any are neglected, the accuracy of data analysis is affected.

EQUIPMENT MAINTENANCE

To help assure optimum performance, one should routinely maintain all instruments (manual or automated). This routine schedule should include all of the operator maintenance recommended for the specific instrument, plus tubing change, membrane change, and electrode cleaning and rotating. The frequency with which the procedures should be performed is largely a function of the age of the instrument, its electrodes, and the work load of the laboratory. Poor electrode performance is often correctable by more frequent membrane changes or cleaning. Electrode banks are useful in extending the life of the electrodes and minimizing the "down time" of the instrument. The electrodes are stored "wet"—that is, with a membrane and electrolyte—and are rotated through the instrument routinely (monthly or biweekly). However, a new membrane and electrolyte should be applied when the electrode is put into service. This system keeps the operator aware of the condition of backup as well as working electrodes. Log books are invaluable in evaluating instrument performance. For example, a sudden increase in membrane changes may indicate that an electrode needs cleaning or replacing, and this can be attended to before the situation becomes critical.

CALIBRATION TECHNIQUES FOR THE PO_2, pH, AND PCO_2 ELECTRODES

An electrode's accuracy and performance are directly related to its calibration. Therefore, the accuracy of data analysis depends directly on exacting attention to detail in the calibration procedure. Each electrode should be calculated by using two different known values: one above and one below the usual range of values measured. The selection of these points will determine the range and relative accuracy of the electrode. Traditionally, 4% to 5% carbon dioxide and 8% to 10% carbon dioxide are the gases used for calibrating the PCO_2 electrode. This provides a low calibration point of about 25 to 35 mmHg and a high calibration point of about 55 to 69 mmHg. These values are derived using the following formula and reflect the expected physiologic ranges of carbon dioxide most frequently measured.

$$(P_B - 47) \times (\% \text{ gas}) = \text{partial pressure in mmHg (or torr)}$$

P_B: barometric pressure in mmHg
47: standard correction factor for water vapor pressure
% gas: The specific calibration gas used—that is, 4% $CO_2 = 0.04$

Once the electrode has been calibrated using these two points, accuracy of measurement between those two points is assumed. Unfortunately, the linearity of the electrode will begin to decrease if measured values exceed the calibration points (Fig. A–12). The degree of nonlinearity depends on the age and maintenance history of the electrode. If blood samples that exceed the standard calibration points are to be analyzed, alternate gases should be used that allow recalibration above and below the expected unknowns. These same principles for calibration apply to the PO_2 electrode. These principles are diagrammatically represented in Figure A–12.

Calibration of the pH electrode involves the use of liquid buffers, as opposed to the gases used for the PCO_2 and PO_2 electrodes. These must be certified buffers accurate to 0.005 pH units. Typically, the buffers used are 6.840 and 7.384. The pH electrode is stable enough and the physiologic range small enough to guarantee linearity above and below these calibration points. However, if samples (e.g., spinal fluid) with anticipated pHs of greater than 7.6 or less than 6.0 are to be measured, the pH electrode should be checked for its expected value. These instruments are designed to measure blood, and to attempt to use them for other purposes could adversely affect their performance by damaging pH-sensitive glass, dissolving membranes, and damaging hydrolics.

Automated machines calibrate themselves automatically at preset time intervals. In most machines this function can be overridden, if desired. Consistency is maintained by introducing the gases and buffer solutions at controlled rates and pressures and by maintaining a constant equilibrium time. If electrode response is not within acceptable limits, the performance is flagged as unacceptable and an alarm is activated on the instrument. The technician must then correct the situation before the machine will perform analysis with that electrode. Other functions, such as buffer levels, are also monitored and any service requirements indicated. Most automated instruments apply correc-

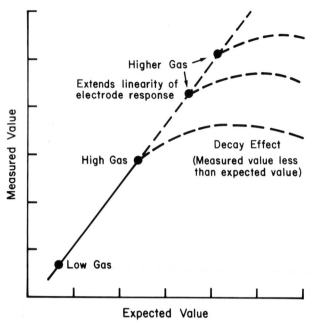

Figure A—12. Diagrammatic representation of the nonlinearity of electrode behavior. If the value to be measured exceeds the high calibration point, the accuracy of that measurement cannot be guaranteed. Some electrodes will maintain their linearity past the high calibration point, whereas others will drop off dramatically. This is a function of the electrodes' age and maintenance and cannot be predicted. If the unknown to be measured is expected to exceed the high calibration point, the instrument should be recalibrated. This recalibration should be performed using a new slope gas that will provide a new high calibration point slightly exceeding the expected unknown. On some automated machines, resetting of the calibration points is not possible or the range is very limited. In these instances, accuracy past the high calibration point can be checked with tonometry. For example, if a shunt study is to be performed on a patient breathing 100% O_2 and the analyzer to be used cannot be recalibrated, blood tonometered with 100% O_2 can be used to check performance. The use of two samples, one at 50% O_2 and one at 100% O_2, would provide further assurance of analyzer performance. In instances such as shunt studies, for which the unknowns to be analyzed could range from below 100 to above 500, a check of more than one point on the calibration curve is advisable to guarantee accuracy of results.

tion factors to the performance of their electrodes. These factors are derived statistically to compensate for the fact that the electrodes are calibrated with a gas, but measure a liquid; however, the best indicator of precision and accuracy in any instrument is its performance on tonometry (to be discussed later).

Calibration of manual equipment requires that the technician introduce the calibration gases into the PO_2 and PCO_2 cuvettes. Buffers must be intro-

duced into the pH cuvette. To control drift of the electrodes, one should perform a complete two-point calibration every 8 hours and a single-point calibration before each sample is analyzed. If the single-point calibration indicates excessive drift between samples, complete recalibration or electrode maintenance is indicated. Strict attention to a standard calibration technique is critical for non-automated equipment because it determines the accuracy and response time of the electrodes.

Typically, drift of all three electrodes is most marked just after the electrode membrane has been changed or a new electrode has been put into service. This problem lessens as the electrode is used. Maximum drift in a stabilized electrode should not exceed 1% to 2% of the reading in 5 minutes.

STANDARDS AND CONTROLS

The term *standards* refers to the gases or buffers with which the electronics of the instrument are set to read in a linear manner and over a reasonable physiologic range. The gases that are used must be certified (guaranteed to be accurate), usually to within ±0.5%. The buffers must be calibration buffers meeting the specifications of the specific instrument. Once the instrument has been properly calibrated with these standards, controls are used to verify the quality of performance. Many problems can go undetected unless the instrument's performance is verified with controls. For example, if the instrument or a portion of it were to become improperly thermostated and calibration were carried out, the electrodes would appear to calibrate properly, but would be set inaccurately for the true concentration present in the standard. The pH buffers themselves are relatively insensitive to temperatures ranging from room temperature to body temperature, and in the event of heat loss from the analyzer the pH buffer may continue to produce the expected value. However, in an actual blood sample the pH is affected by the temperature of the analyzer; that is, if the analyzer is too cold or too hot, this will cause the carbon dioxide measurement to change, and the change in carbon dioxide will affect a change in pH. Thus, even though the buffer was measured correctly, the blood pH measurement could be incorrect if the temperature of the analyzer is incorrect. Similarly, faulty or contaminated standards or misuse of the standards (i.e., poor technique in calibration) can lead to erroneous calibration of the electrodes, which will produce inaccurate blood gas values. Properly used, controls will detect such problems.

Commercially prepared controls are currently available. These controls provide a range of known values typical of those encountered in the clinical setting; pH values range from extreme acidosis to extreme alkalosis. The PO_2 and PCO_2 readings are represented in low, medium, and high ranges. Failure of the instrument to report the appropriate values will alert the user that a problem exists.

Tonometry is a method of equilibrating a gas of known concentration with a liquid. Tonometry for quality control can use either a buffer or whole blood. The choice of buffer or blood should be made after considering the advantages and disadvantages of each. Blood has the same viscosity and gas exchange properties as patient samples; however, because the buffering capacity (principally bicarbonate) of whole blood is unknown, it is impossible to predict how the change in PCO_2 and PO_2 will affect the pH of that same sample. Therefore, whole blood does not permit control of pH. Buffers do provide a control for pH; because the bicarbonate is constant, the pH can be calculated. However, the viscosity and gas exchange properties of buffer solutions are different from those of whole blood. The gas used for tonometry must be checked for accuracy in the same manner as calibration gases. The chief disadvantage of tonometry is that it is technique-dependent and can vary from technician to technician. Small variations in such things as temperature, gas flow rate, sample size, and equilibration time will affect the results. Exacting attention to detail is needed to ensure that the procedure is done *exactly* the same way each time. To obtain reliable results with tonometry, the tonometer must be maintained at 37° C, the gas must be humidified, and the gas flow rate, the sample size, and equilibration time must be in accordance with the manufacturer's instructions. Before the sample is transferred from the tonometer to the blood gas analyzer, the sampling syringe must be purged with the tonometry gas to expel any room air from the syringe. Tonometry is performed at 37° C, which makes the tonometer and the solution in it an excellent culture medium. All equipment used for tonometry should be sterilized or disinfected to prevent bacterial growth. If previously analyzed patient samples are to be the source of blood for tonometry, it may be advisable to add antibiotics to the tonometry system to prevent bacterial growth and its associated oxygen consumption before analysis. Some manufacturers use replacement cups to be disposed of with each sample to ensure cleanliness. Bacitracin and neomycin have been found effective in concentrations of 0.5 μg and 0.01 μg/mL blood, respec-

tively. The expected tonometry value must be calculated daily using the daily barometer reading according to the following formula.

Sample value = (barometric pressure − 47)
  × % gas

47 = standard correction factor for water vapor

% gas = % CO_2 or % O_2 in the tonometry gas—that is, 8% CO_2 = 0.08

The results of all quality control analyses must be documented. This should include the values obtained, control limits, and any corrective action taken if the results were out-of-control limits. A specific log book should be used to record quality control records.

The control limits for a quality control sample are the range within which the control value is expected to fall. Typically, the accepted limit of tolerance is ±2 standard deviations of an established mean, since, in a normal gaussian distribution, 95% of all observations will fall within this range. Each laboratory should establish its own statistics on its instrumentation for all levels of each new lot of material before it is put into routine use. This is necessary whether assayed commercial material, tonometry, or gas buffers are used. The mean and standard deviation should be established by using a minimum of ten determinations.

A written protocol for the staff to follow should a quality control sample be out of range is invaluable. This helps to maintain consistency in equipment maintenance and troubleshooting.

Proficiency testing involves analyzing unknown samples provided by a vendor or professional organization. The analysis results are returned to the testing agency that provides statistical information on the laboratory's performance. The testing agency must provide the state's Laboratory Licensing Board with the results in states where proficiency testing is required for laboratory licensure.

SAMPLING AND ANALYSIS PROTOCOLS

A standardized technique for obtaining and handling blood samples is essential for a good quality control program. Variables such as time between sampling and analysis, metabolism in vitro, air bubbles, and sample size can affect the sample before and during the analysis procedure. Any one or a combination of these factors can lead to results that do not reflect accurately the patient's true physiologic state.

Samples should be analyzed as quickly as possible after sampling to expedite patient care and to reduce the risk of effects on the sample from air bubbles or metabolism. In blood samples iced immediately after sampling, there is no significant change in pH, PCO_2, or PO_2 for up to 2 hours. The most dramatic change in noniced samples occurs during the first 15 minutes after the sample has been taken, and the value most dramatically affected is the PO_2. The magnitude of change is impossible to predict because it depends on the initial level of PO_2 (values over 100 demonstrate the biggest change), white cell metabolism, and the diffusion properties of the sampling syringe.

An air bubble equivalent to 10% of the sample size has been demonstrated to induce a marked change in PO_2.[3] Thus immediate removal of any air bubbles obtained during sample or analysis is important, that is, if verification of results were required owing to equipment failure and an air bubble had been left in the sample after the first analysis, the second analysis could be inaccurate.

Heparin dilution can affect all three measured blood gas values,[1,2] although its effect on PCO_2 is usually greater than on pH or PO_2. Preventing adverse effects from heparin dilution is dealt with most effectively by controlling closely the amount of heparin used and the sample size. When using liquid heparin, one should evacuate the heparin from the sample syringe just before sample analysis. This will leave only the very tip of the syringe and the needle filled with heparin. The blood sample taken should fill at least one half of the volume of the sampling syringe—that is, 2.5- to 3-mL sample in a 5-mL syringe. The larger the sample, the less the dilutional affect of heparin. Very small samples are at higher risk for heparin dilution. In patient populations for whom small sample sizes are important (children and neonates), capillary tubes of 1-mL syringes that use crystalline heparin are advisable. This will keep the sample from clotting without the dilutional effects that could be expected with liquid heparin in such a small sampling device.

QUALITY CONTROL OF THE PATIENT SAMPLE

Even on a properly maintained, calibrated, and controlled blood gas analyzer, an incorrect measurement on any given sample is always possible. To eliminate any possibility of an erroneous reading owing to a temporary technical flaw (e.g., an undetected air bubble in the cuvette), a further measure of quality control is needed to confirm blood gas accuracy. One approach is to analyze the sample simultaneously on two separate analyzers. The likelihood that the same error will occur on two instruments simultaneously is remote.

Another approach for pH and PCO_2 control is to compare the Astrup PCO_2 (see the section on the Astrup Equilibration Method) with the measured PCO_2. Arrived at by two independent methods, this verifies the accuracy of both pH and PCO_2. Another ingredient of quality control inherent in the Astrup method is verification of quality of slope of the buffer line on which all other calculations are based. Since hemoglobin is one of the principal blood buffers participating in establishing this buffer line, incorporated into the Siggaard–Anderson nomogram is a means of calculating the hemoglobin using the data obtained by the buffer line. This calculated hemoglobin can then be compared with the patient's observed hemoglobin, and the values should agree within 2–3 g/dL.

Another estimate of reliability can be obtained on routine PO_2 measurements when used in conjunction with an observed oxygen saturation value, such as that determined by the IL CO-Oximeter. The oxygen saturation, calculated from the patient's observed temperature, pH, and PO_2, can be compared with the measured oxygen saturation. Appreciable discrepancy may suggest an error. If inspection and repetition verify the original measurement, this indicates that the patient either has a shifted oxyhemoglobin disassociation curve or the presence of carboxyhemoglobin, methemoglobin, or sulfhemoglobin. In the hands of experienced technicians, using nomograms or blood gas slide rules, these comparisons can be made very quickly and, in terms of quality control, are well worth the time. For large numbers of procedures, even more desirable is the use of a computer program that can perform the calculations and corrections and present the data to the technician in seconds.

REFERENCES

1. Bageant RA: Variations in arterial blood gas measurements due to sampling techniques. Resp Care 20:565, 1974
2. Hansen JE, Simmons DH: Systematic error in the determination of blood PCO_2. Am Rev Respir Dis 115:1061, 1977
3. Ishikawa S et al: The effects of air bubbles and time delay on blood gas analysis. Ann Allergy 33:72, 1974
4. Manual of Operations, IL 282, p 12. Instrumentation Laboratory, Lexington, Massachusetts, 1980

APPENDIX B

Equations and "Rules of Thumb" for Management of Patients

John E. Hodgkin

OXYGENATION

CALCULATION OF PaO_2 BREATHING ROOM AIR BASED ON AGE

- Predicted normal PaO_2, ages 14 to 84 years, supine[25]

$$PaO_2 = 103.5 - (0.42 \times age) \pm 4$$

This was the formula from Sorbini's data, at 500-m elevation. When the data are corrected for a barometric pressure of 760 mmHg, the formula for predicting the normal PaO_2 at sea level becomes

$$PaO_2 = 109 - (0.43 \times age) \pm 4.$$

- Predicted normal PaO_2, ages 15 to 75 years, seated[20]

$$PaO_2 = 104.2 - (0.27 \times age) \pm 6$$

CALCULATION OF PIO_2

- PIO_2 (dry gas) = barometric pressure (PB) $\times$ FIO_2

- PIO_2 (humidified gas)
1. PIO_2 = (barometric pressure $-$ PH_2O) $\times$ FIO_2

  PH_2O = 47 mmHg (normal water vapor pressure for humidified gas)

2. A rough guide to calculating PIO_2 of humidified gas at or near sea level is as follows.

$$PIO_2 = (PB - PH_2O) \times FIO_2$$

Since PB is 760 mmHg at sea level and normal PH_2O is 47 mmHg, then $PB - PH_2O =$ approximately 700. Thus,

$$PIO_2 = 700 \times FIO_2,$$

or $PIO_2 = 7 \times \% O_2$ in inspired gas.

Example: PIO_2 for an FIO_2 of 0.40 (40% O_2) is

$$PIO_2 = 7 \times 40 = 280$$

CALCULATION OF PAO_2

1. $PAO_2 = PIO_2 - (PaCO_2 \times 1.25)$
   1.25 is a factor for respiratory quotient, assuming a respiratory quotient of 0.8 where oxygen uptake equals 250 mL/min and CO_2 production equals 200 mL/min.
2. Simplified alveolar air equation at sea level, on room air

$$PAO_2 = 150 - PaCO_2$$

CALCULATION OF ALVEOLAR–ARTERIAL OXYGEN TENSION DIFFERENCE

1. $P(A-a)O_2 = PAO_2$ (calculated) $- PaO_2$ (measured)

2. Calculation of approximate normal $P(A-a)O_2$, breathing room air, according to patient's age: The $P(A-a)O_2$ increases approximately 4 mmHg for every increase of 10 years in age.

Example: For an 80-year-old man, the $P(A-a)O_2$ should normally be ≤ 32 mmHg.

DETERMINATION OF THE CAUSE OF HYPOXEMIA

- If $P(A-a)O_2$ is normal, in the presence of hypoxemia, the cause is overall hypoventilation. A reduction in PIO_2 from high altitude will also reduce the PaO_2, with a normal $P(A-a)O_2$. The $P(A-a)O_2$ is increased when hypoxemia is due to $\dot{V}/\dot{Q}$ mismatch, diffusion defect, or shunt. The average $P(A-a)O_2$ in normal adults is 10 to 15 mmHg; however, it widens normally with aging.
- If the sum of the PaO_2 and $PaCO_2$ is between 110 and 130 mmHg, breathing room air, hypoxemia is due to overall hypoventilation. If the sum of the PaO_2 and $PaCO_2$ is <110, breathing room air or supplemental O_2, the cause is $\dot{V}/\dot{Q}$ mismatch, diffusion defect, or shunt. The sum would also be <110 when a reduction in PaO_2 occurs from the decreased PIO_2 of high altitude.

DETERMINATION IF A PATIENT IS BREATHING SUPPLEMENTAL OXYGEN

If the sum of the PaO_2 and $PaCO_2$ is >130 mmHg, the patient is most likely breathing supplemental O_2. In young people (e.g., <16 years of age) the sum may approach 140 mmHg, even though the subject is breathing only room air.

DETERMINATION OF PREDICTED NORMAL PaO_2 AT ALTITUDES ABOVE SEA LEVEL[12,13,18]

$$a/A \; O_2 \; ratio = \frac{\text{Predicted room air } PaO_2 \text{ at sea level}}{PAO_2 \text{ at sea level}}$$

Example: If a patient had a predicted normal PaO_2 of 87 mmHg at sea level, with a PAO_2 of 100 mmHg, the a/A O_2 ratio would be

$$a/A \; O_2 = 87/100$$
$$= 0.87.$$

At 5000 feet elevation, assuming a PB of 632 mmHg, the normal PAO_2 would be approximately 73 mmHg. The predicted normal PaO_2 for this patient,

at 5000 feet elevation, would then be

$$PaO_2 \text{ (normal at 5000 feet)} = PAO_2 \text{ (at 5000 feet)} \\ \times a/A \text{ (at sea level)} \\ = 73 \times 0.87 \\ = 63.5 \text{ mmHg.}$$

CALCULATION OF FIO_2 NEEDED TO ACHIEVE A DESIRED PaO_2, HAVING DETERMINED AN INITIAL PaO_2[12,13,18]

This assumes that such factors as cardiac output, $\dot{V}/\dot{Q}$ matchup, shunt, $PaCO_2$, and O_2 uptake remain constant.

Example: Knowing the patient's FIO_2, $PaCO_2$, and PaO_2, one can calculate the PAO_2 and a/A O_2 ratio.

If a patient has a PaO_2 of 50 mmHg on an FIO_2 of 0.4, and a $PaCO_2$ of 40 mmHg at sea level, the PAO_2 = 235 mmHg and the a/A O_2 ratio is 0.2127. If a PaO_2 of 70 mmHg is desired in this patient, the a/A O_2 ratio can be used to determine the PAO_2 and FIO_2 required to achieve this PaO_2 for this patient.

$$PAO_2 \text{ (required)} = \frac{PaO_2 \text{ (desired)}}{a/A \; O_2 \text{ (calculated)}}$$
$$= \frac{70}{0.2127}$$
$$= 329 \text{ mmHg}$$

Assuming a respiratory quotient of 0.8, this can then be fitted into the alveolar air equation to solve for the FIO_2 needed to produce this PAO_2.

$$PAO_2 = PIO_2 - (PaCO_2 \times 1.25)$$
$$PAO_2 = (PB - PH_2O) \; FIO_2 - (PaCO_2 \times 1.25)$$
$$329 = (760 - 47) \; FIO_2 - (40 \times 1.25)$$
$$329 = (713) \; FIO_2 - 50$$
$$FIO_2 \; (713) = 379$$
$$FIO_2 = \frac{379}{713}$$
$$= 0.53$$

If the FIO_2 is raised from 0.4 to 0.53, assuming things remain stable, the PaO_2 should increase from 50 mmHg to 70 mmHg. Of course, the PaO_2 must always be measured to determine the true PaO_2 on the new FIO_2.

CALCULATION OF OXYGEN UPTAKE ($\dot{V}O_2$) OR CARDIAC OUTPUT ($\dot{Q}$) WITH THE FICK EQUATION

$$\dot{Q} = \frac{\dot{V}O_2}{(CaO_2 - C\bar{v}O_2) \; 10}$$

$\dot{V}O_2$ is in mL/min, CaO_2 and $C\bar{v}O_2$ are in mL O_2/100 mL blood. The factor 10 is necessary to express $\dot{Q}$ in L/min.

CALCULATION OF PHYSIOLOGIC SHUNT

$$\frac{\dot{Q}s}{\dot{Q}T} = \frac{(CcO_2 - CaO_2)}{(CcO_2 - C\bar{v}O_2)}$$

$\dot{Q}s/\dot{Q}T$ = ratio of shunt to cardiac output. CcO_2 represents the end-pulmonary capillary O_2 content in mL O_2/100 mL blood.

For calculation of O_2 content in arterial (CaO_2) and mixed venous ($C\bar{v}O_2$) blood, use the following equations.[24]

$$\begin{aligned}
O_2 \text{ content} &= \text{mL } O_2 \text{ bound to Hb/100 mL blood} \\
&\quad + \text{mL } O_2 \text{ dissolved/100 mL blood} \\
&= [\text{Hb (g/100 mL)} \times O_2 \text{ saturation} \\
&\quad \times 1.39^*] + (PaO_2 \times 0.003)
\end{aligned}$$

For determination of CcO_2, it is best to take carboxyhemoglobin (HbCO) into account.[7] The PaO_2 should first be calculated. If the PaO_2 is greater than 150 mmHg, the PcO_2 is assumed to equal the PaO_2, and the formula is

$$CcO_2 = \text{Hb} [(1.0 - \text{HbCO})(1.39)] + (0.003 \times PaO_2).$$

The following correction factors are recommended for a $PaO_2 \le 150$ mmHg.[7,24]

If $PaO_2 > 125$ and ≤ 150 mmHg,
then $CcO_2 = \text{Hb} [(1.0 - \text{HbCO}) - 0.01] (1.39) + (0.003 \times PaO_2)$

If $PA > 100$ and ≤ 125 mmHg,
then $CcO_2 = \text{Hb} [(1.0 - \text{HbCO}) - 0.02] (1.39) + (0.003 \times PaO_2)$

If HbCO (carboxyhemoglobin) is not measured directly, one could assume that the HbCO is approximately 1.5%.

ESTIMATION OF SHUNT

If a patient is breathing 100% O_2, there is a 5% shunt for every 100 mmHg the PaO_2 is below that expected.

> *Example:* For a patient at sea level, the PaO_2 breathing 100% O_2 should be 550 to 600 mmHg normally. If the PaO_2 is 300 mmHg, one has a 15% shunt, *plus* the normal 3% to 4% shunt everyone has.

---

* Some use the factor 1.34 here; however, there is evidence that 1.39 is more accurate.

This rule of thumb works well down to a PaO_2 of 100 mmHg. Below this level, it is no longer accurate.

ACID–BASE

CALCULATION OF EXTRACELLULAR FLUID BASE EXCESS (BE_{ECF})[9]

$$BE_{ECF} = \Delta HCO_3^- + 10\Delta pH$$

Where $\Delta HCO_3^- $ = actual $HCO_3^- - 24$ and $\Delta pH = $ actual pH $- 7.4$

> *Example:* if the pH = 7.14 and plasma HCO_3^- = 28 mEq/L, then
>
> $$\begin{aligned}
BE_{ECF} &= (28 - 24) + 10(7.14 - 7.40) \\
&= 4 + 10(-0.26) \\
&= 4 - 2.6 \\
&= 1.4 \text{ mEq/L}
\end{aligned}$$

See Chapter 10, Blood Gas Analysis and Acid–Base Physiology, for a detailed explanation of extracellular fluid base excess.

IN ACUTE RESPIRATORY ACIDOSIS

The plasma bicarbonate will increase, rapidly, approximately 1 mEq/L for every 15 mmHg increase in the $PaCO_2$ above 40 mmHg as a result of the bicarbonate–carbonic acid buffer reaction.[2] This small increase in bicarbonate does not represent renal compensation for the CO_2 retention.

IN CHRONIC RESPIRATORY ACIDOSIS

For each mmHg increase in $PaCO_2$, the HCO_3^- increases 0.4 mEq/L.[4,10,16,21]

IN ACUTE RESPIRATORY ALKALOSIS

The plasma bicarbonate will decrease, rapidly, approximately 1 mEq/L for every 5 mmHg decrease in the $PaCO_2$ below 40 mmHg as a result of the bicarbonate–carbonic acid buffer reaction.[2] This decrease in plasma bicarbonate does not represent renal compensation for the acute hypocapnia.

IN CHRONIC RESPIRATORY ALKALOSIS

For each mmHg decrease in $PaCO_2$, the HCO_3^- decreases 0.5 mEq/L.[4,11,1]

IN MAXIMALLY COMPENSATED METABOLIC ACIDOSIS

The $PaCO_2$ will decrease by about 1 mmHg for every 1 mEq/L decrease in plasma bicarbonate.[19]

The level of compensatory hypocapnia expected in metabolic acidosis can be calculated by the following formula.[1]

$$PaCO_2 = 1.54 \times plasma\ HCO_3^- + 8.36 \pm 1.1$$

IN METABOLIC ALKALOSIS

For each mEq/L increase in HCO_3^-, the $PaCO_2$ increases 0.5 to 1.0 mmHg.[5,8,21] The ventilatory response to metabolic alkalosis is less predictable than that seen with metabolic acidosis, and compensatory hypercapnia above 55 to 60 mmHg is unusual.[5,14]

FOR REASONABLY ACCURATE CONVERSION OF pH TO [H⁺][15]

pH	[H⁺] (nM/L)
7.0	100
7.05	90
7.1	80
7.15	70
7.2	60
7.3	50
7.4	40
7.5	30
7.6	25
7.7	20
7.8	15
7.9	12.5
8.0	10

One might note that within the range of 7.2 to 7.5 there is a decrease of 0.01 in pH for every increase of 1 nM/L in the [H⁺].

FOR CALCULATING [H⁺], PCO₂, OR PLASMA BICARBONATE FROM THE OTHER TWO VALUES[17]

$$[H^+] = 24 \times \frac{PaCO_2}{Plasma\ HCO_3^-}$$

TO DETERMINE WHETHER THE CHANGE IN [H⁺] or pH IS APPROPRIATE FOR ACUTE RESPIRATORY ACIDOSIS OR CHRONIC RESPIRATORY ACIDOSIS

- In *acute* retention
  One would expect an increase in [H⁺] of 0.8 nM/L for every increase of 1 mmHg in PCO_2.

  The increase in $PCO_2 \times 0.008$ = the decrease in pH.[3]
- In *chronic* CO_2 retention
  One would expect an increase in [H⁺] of 0.3 nM/L for every increase of 1 mmHg in PCO_2.
  The increase in $PCO_2 \times 0.003$ = the decrease in pH.[3]

ROUGH GUIDELINES FOR PaCO₂–pH RELATIONSHIP IN ACUTE VENTILATORY CHANGES

For every 20 mmHg increase in $PaCO_2$ above 40 mmHg, the pH decreases approximately 0.10 unit.

For every 10 mmHg decrease in $PaCO_2$ below 40 mmHg, the pH increases approximately 0.10 unit.

PaCO₂	pH
80	7.20
60	7.30
40	7.40
30	7.50
20	7.60

DETERMINATION OF PLASMA BICARBONATE FROM pH AND PaCO₂ (ASSUMING AN UNCOMPENSATED ACID–BASE STATUS)

$$Plasma\ bicarbonate = \frac{PaCO_2 \times 24}{difference\ of\ last\ two\ digits\ of\ pH\ and\ 80}$$

Example:
pH = 7.30
$PaCO_2$ = 50

$$Plasma\ bicarbonate = \frac{40 \times 24}{80 - 30}$$
$$= \frac{950}{50}$$
$$= 19\ mEq/L$$

ESTIMATION OF BASE EXCESS FROM pH AND PaCO₂[24]

1. Determine the difference between the measured $PaCO_2$ and 40 mmHg, then move the decimal point two places to the left.
2. If the $PaCO_2$ is above 40 mmHg, subtract one-half of the number calculated in step 1 from 7.40. If the $PaCO_2$ is below 40 mmHg, add the difference to 7.40.

3. Determine the difference between the measured pH and the pH calculated in step 2. Move the decimal point two places to the right and multiply by ⅔.

Example: Patient with $PaCO_2$ of 75 mmHg and pH of 7.30.

1. $75 - 40 = 35$; moving the decimal two places to the left results in 0.35.
2. Since the $PaCO_2$ is > 40 mmHg, $7.40 - (\frac{1}{2}$ of 0.35 $) = 7.22$.
3. $7.30 - 7.22 = 0.08$; moving the decimal point two places to the right and multiplying by ⅔, (i.e., $8 \times \frac{2}{3} = 5$ mEq/L base excess).

DETERMINATION OF BICARBONATE NEEDED IN PATIENTS WITH METABOLIC ACIDOSIS

The HCO_3^- needed* = body wt (kg) × BE × 0.3. BE represents the deficit in buffer base. Three-tenths (0.3) is the factor that represents the extracellular space bicarbonate distribution.

MECHANICAL VENTILATION

CALCULATION OF RESPIRATORY SYSTEM COMPLIANCE IN PATIENTS BREATHING BY VENTILATOR

- Dynamic effective compliance

$$C_{RS} \text{ (dyn)} = \frac{V_T}{\text{peak pressure}}$$

If PEEP being used

$$C_{RS} \text{ (dyn)} = \frac{V_T}{\text{peak pressure} - \text{PEEP}}$$

- Static effective compliance (eliminates airway resistance as a factor).

$$C_{RS} \text{ (st)} = \frac{V_T}{\text{inflation hold pressure}}$$

If PEEP being used

$$C_{RS} \text{ (st)} = \frac{V_T}{\substack{\text{inflation hold} \\ \text{pressure} - \text{PEEP}}}$$

---

* Infuse one-half of this amount IV, recheck an ABG in 15 to 20 minutes, and repeat the calculation.

DETERMINATION OF NEW MINUTE VENTILATION ($\dot{V}E$) REQUIRED TO ACHIEVE A DESIRED $PaCO_2$

- New $\dot{V}E = \dfrac{\text{present } \dot{V}E \times \text{present } PaCO_2}{\text{desired } PaCO_2}$

Example: Present $\dot{V}E = 8$ L/min and $PaCO_2 = 50$ mmHg and a $PaCO_2$ of 40 mmHg is desired

$$\text{New } \dot{V}E = \frac{8 \times 50}{40}$$
$$= 10 \text{ L/min}$$

The new $\dot{V}E$ can be achieved by either increasing the V_T or the respirator rate. Of course, the V_D/V_T ratio is a factor. If the V_T is kept constant, and the ventilator rate is altered to achieve the new $\dot{V}E$, the foregoing equation should be quite precise. If the V_T is increased, the V_D/V_T obviously changes, and the equation will not be quite as accurate.

- Another method for estimating the change in ventilator rate needed to achieve a desired $PaCO_2$ is as follows:[6]

$$\text{New ventilator rate} = \frac{\substack{\text{present ventilator rate} \\ \times \text{ present } PaCO_2}}{\text{desired } PaCO_2}$$

Example: If the $PaCO_2$ is 80 mmHg on a ventilator rate of 12 breaths/min, and one desires a $PaCO_2$ of 60 mmHg, then the

$$\text{new ventilator rate} = \frac{12 \times 80}{60}$$
$$= 16 \text{ breaths/min.}$$

This method assumes, of course, that the tidal volume remains constant.

- Determination of new $\dot{V}E$ required to achieve a desired $PaCO_2$, using alveolar ventilation $(\dot{V}A)$[22]

$$\text{New } \dot{V}A = \frac{\text{present } \dot{V}A \times \text{present } PaCO_2}{\text{desired } PaCO_2}$$

Example: In a 200-lb (lean body weight) patient with a measured tidal volume of 600 mL and a ventilator rate of 10, the $\dot{V}E$ is 600 mL. The anatomic dead space in this patient would be assumed to be 200 mL (1 mL/lb lean body weight). 200 mL × 10 equals 2000 mL of anatomic dead space ventilation per minute. 6000 mL − 2000 mL represents 4000 mL alveolar ventilation per minute. If the measured $PaCO_2$ in this patient is 60 mmHg and a $PaCO_2$ of 40 mmHg is desired, then the

$$\text{new } \dot{V}A = \frac{4000 \times 60}{40}$$
$$= 6000 \text{ ml.}$$

If the new $\dot{V}A$ is to be achieved by increasing the V_T, the V_T would have to be increased from 600 to 800 mL, if the ventilator rate remains at 10/min, to achieve the new $\dot{V}A$ required to alter the $PaCO_2$ from 60 to 40 mmHg. An extra 200 mL of alveolar volume/breath × 10 = an increase in $\dot{V}A$ of 2000 mL/min. In this example, the new $\dot{V}E$ is 8000 mL.

If the new $\dot{V}A$ is to be achieved by increasing the ventilator rate, the rate would have to be increased from 10/min to 15/min, if the V_T remains at 600 mL, to achieve the new $\dot{V}A$ required to alter the $PaCO_2$ from 60 to 40 mmHg. Since in this patient 400 mL of the 600 mL V_T is alveolar volume, then an extra 5 breaths/min will increase the $\dot{V}A$ by 2000 mL/min. In this example, the new $\dot{V}E$ is 9000 mL.

- Determination of new $\dot{V}E$ required to achieve a desired $PaCO_2$, using the V_D/V_T[23]

The minute ventilation–$PaCO_2$–V_D/V_T graph depicted in Figure B–1 is used as follows.

1. Place patient on respirator breathing at a minute ventilation ($\dot{V}E$) of 6 to 8 L/min.
2. After 30 minutes of equilibration, measure the minute ventilation and obtain a simultaneous arterial CO_2 tension ($PaCO_2$).
3. The $\dot{V}E$ and corresponding $PaCO_2$ are plotted on the graph. The dead space/tidal volume ratio (V_D/V_T) is obtained by noting the isopleth that coincides with this point.
4. To obtain the $\dot{V}E$ required to achieve a desired $PaCO_2$, draw a vertical line from the desired $PaCO_2$ on the abscissa to the V_D/V_T isopleth obtained in step 3. From this point, a horizontal line is drawn to the ordinate to obtain the required $\dot{V}E$.
5. The respirator is then adjusted by changing the tidal volume (V_T) or frequency (f) to

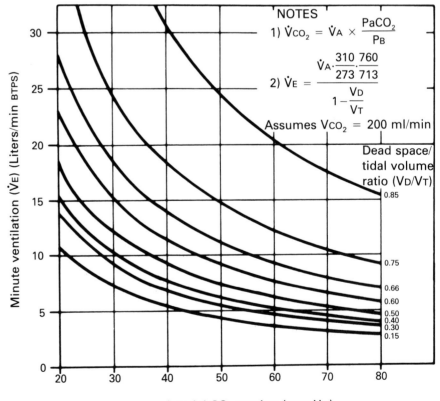

Figure B–1. The relation between minute ventilation ($\dot{V}E$) and arterial PCO_2 ($PaCO_2$) for various isopleths of the ratio of physiological dead space to tidal volume (V_D/V_T). The basic assumptions are noted in the upper right corner. $\dot{V}CO_2$, CO_2 output; $\dot{V}A$, alveolar ventilation; P_B, atmospheric pressure. (Selecky PA et al: A graphic approach to assessing interrelationships among minute ventilation, arterial carbon dioxide tension, and ratio of physiologic dead space to tidal volume in patients on respirators. Am Rev Respir Dis 117:181, 1978)

NOTES

1) $\dot{V}CO_2 = \dot{V}A \times \dfrac{PaCO_2}{P_B}$

2) $\dot{V}E = \dfrac{\dot{V}A \cdot \dfrac{310}{273} \cdot \dfrac{760}{713}}{1 - \dfrac{V_D}{V_T}}$

Assumes $\dot{V}CO_2 = 200$ ml/min

Dead space/tidal volume ratio (V_D/V_T)

0.85
0.75
0.66
0.60
0.50
0.40
0.30
0.15

Minute ventilation ($\dot{V}E$) (Liters/min BTPS)

Arterial CO_2 tension (mm Hg)

achieve the newly determined $\dot{V}_E$ ($\dot{V}_E = V_T \times f$). (After 30 minutes at this new $\dot{V}_E$ the $PaCO_2$ should be remeasured).

6. As the patient's respiratory problem improves, the V_D/V_T will often decrease, indicating a need for a lower $\dot{V}_E$. This new V_D/V_T can be calculated as in step 3 and an appropriate $\dot{V}_E$ determined.

REFERENCES

1. Albert MD, Dell RB, Winters RW: Quantitative displacement of acid base equilibrium in metabolic acidosis. Ann Intern Med 66:312, 1964

2. Armstrong BW, Mohler JG, Jung RC, Remmers J: The in-vivo carbon dioxide titration curve. Lancet 1:759, 1966

3. Avery AG, Nicotra MB, Deaton WJ: Respiratory acid–base balance. Respir Ther p 59, May/June 1977

4. Bia M, Thier SO: Mixed acid base disturbances: A clinical approach. Med Clin North Am 65:347, 1981

5. Bone JM, Cowie J, Lambie A, Robson JS: The relationship between arterial PCO_2 and hydrogen ion concentration in chronic metabolic acidosis and alkalosis. Clin Sci Mol Med 46:113, 1974

6. Bone RC: Mechanical ventilation: Understanding the basics. J Respir Dis, p 57, Jan 1982

7. Cane RD et al: Minimizing errors in intrapulmonary shunt calculations. Crit Care Med 8:294, 1980

8. Cohen JJ, Kassirer JP: Acid base metabolism. In Maxwell MH, Kleeman CR (eds): Clinical Disorders of Fluid and Electrolyte Metabolism, pp 181–232. New York, McGraw–Hill, 1980

9. Collier CR, Hackney JD, Mohler JG: Use of extracellular base excess in diagnosis of acid–base disorders: A conceptual approach. Chest 61:6S, 1972

10. Engel K et al: Quantitative displacement of acid–base equilibrium in chronic respiratory acidosis. J Appl Physiol 24:288, 1968

11. Gennari FJ, Goldstein MB, Schwartz WB: The nature of the renal adaption to chronic hypocapnia. J Clin Invest 51:1722, 1972

12. Gilbert F, Keighly JF: The arterial/alveolar oxygen tension ratio: An index of gas exchange applicable to varying inspired oxygen concentrations. Am Rev Respir Dis 109:142, 1974

13. Gilbert R, Auchincloss J, Kuppinger M, Thomas MV: Stability of the arterial/alveolar oxygen partial pressure ratio. Crit Care Med 7:267, 1979

14. Goldring RM, Cannon PJ, Heinemann HO, Fishman AP: Respiratory adjustment to chronic metabolic alkalosis in man. J Clin Invest 47:188, 1968

15. Jones NL: Blood Gases and Acid–Base Physiology, p 87. New York, Brian C Decker, 1980

16. Kaehny WD: Pathogenesis and management of respiratory and mixed acid–base disorders. In Schrier RW (ed): Renal and Electrolyte Disorders, pp 121–142. Boston, Little, Brown & Co, 1976

17. Kassirer JP, Bleich HL: Rapid estimation of plasma carbon dioxide tension from pH and total carbon dioxide content. N Engl J Med 272:1067, 1965

18. Krider T: Clinical equations for oxygen therapy. In Eubanks DH (ed): AART 1981 Convention Lecture Series: Catch a Star. Dallas, American Association for Respiratory Therapy, 1982

19. Lennon EJ, Lemann J Jr: Defense of hydrogen ion concentration in chronic metabolis acidosis. Ann Intern Med 65:265, 1966

20. Mellemgaard K: The alveolar–arterial oxygen difference: Its size and components in normal man. Acta Physiol Scand 67:10, 1966

21. Narins RG, Emmett M: Simple and mixed acid–base disorders: A practical approach. Medicine 59:161, 1980

22. Rogers RM, Jeurs JA: Physiologic considerations in the treatment of acute respiratory failure. Basics RD, Vol 3, (No 4). New York, American Thoracic Society, 1975

23. Selecky PA, Wasserman K, Klein M, Ziment I: A graphic approach to assessing interrelationships among minute ventilation, arterial carbon dioxide tension, and ratio of physiologic dead space to tidal volume in patients on respirators. Am Rev Respir Dis 117:185, 1978

24. Shapiro BA, Harrison RA, Walton JR: Clinical Application of Blood Gases, 3rd ed, pp 129, 222, 223. Chicago, Year Book Medical Publishers, 1982

25. Sorbini CA, Grassi V, Solinas E: Arterial oxygen tension in relation to age in healthy subjects. Respiration 25:3, 1968

Examples of Pulmonary Function Data

John E. Hodgkin

Patient 1. A 58-Year-Old White Woman with Dyspnea

	PREDICTED	PREBRONCHODILATOR		POSTBRONCHODILATOR	
		Observed	% Predicted	Observed	% Predicted
FVC (L)	2.63	1.81	69	1.57	60
FEV$_1$ (L)	1.95	1.46	75	1.50	77
FEV$_1$/FVC (%)	≥74	81		95	
MVV (L/min)	79	34	43	34	43
FEF$_{25-75\%}$ (L/sec)	2.4	1.5	62	2.0	66
FRC (L)	2.29	1.72	75		
RV (L)	1.42	1.06	75		
TLC (L)	4.05	3.04	75		
RV/TLC (%)	35	35			
D$_L$CO (mL/min/mmHg CO)	18.4	9.3	51		

Interpretation and Discussion

The classic pattern for restrictive disease is present. The FVC and FEV$_1$ are reduced; however, the FEV$_1$/FVC% is normal. The reduction in FEF$_{25-75\%}$ is proportional to the reduction in VC. There is no improvement in spirometric data after inhalation of bronchodilator. All lung volumes are reduced; however, the RV/TLC is normal. The diffusing capacity (D$_L$CO) is reduced, suggesting the presence of interstitial lung disease in light of the restrictive pattern. This group of findings is suggestive of many types of interstitial lung disease. The mediastinoscopy on this patient yielded lymph nodes that revealed noncaseating granulomas on the sections, examined histopathologically, consistent with sarcoidosis.

Patient 2.   A 73-Year-Old White Male Smoker with Shortness of Breath

	PREDICTED	PREBRONCHODILATOR		POSTBRONCHODILATOR	
		Observed	% Predicted	Observed	% Predicted
FVC (L)	2.95	2.08	70	2.02	68
FEV$_1$ (L)	2.01	0.70	35	0.64	32
FEV$_1$/FVC (%)	≥68	34		32	
MVV (L/min)	76	29	38	31	42
FEF$_{25-75\%}$ (L/sec)	2.3	0.2	9	0.2	9
FRC (L)	2.81	5.50	196		
RV (L)	1.83	5.09	278		
TLC (L)	4.78	7.17	150		
RV/TLC (%)	38	71			
DLCO (mL/min/mmHg CO)	23	8	35		

Interpretation and Discussion

This pattern demonstrates obstructive airway disease. The reduction in VC suggests the possible presence of concomitant restrictive disease; however, the increased TLC indicates that the reduced VC is secondary to air-trapping and that there is no evidence for restrictive disease. No improvement occurs after bronchodilator inhalation. The marked reduction in diffusing capacity is compatible with loss of alveolocapillary membrane owing to the patient's severe pulmonary emphysema.

Patient 3.   A 37-Year-Old White Woman with a History of Rheumatic Heart Disease Who Now Complains of Dyspnea

	PREDICTED	PREBRONCHODILATOR		POSTBRONCHODILATOR	
		Observed	% Predicted	Observed	% Predicted
FVC (L)	3.10	1.45	47	1.54	50
FEV$_1$ (L)	2.42	1.30	54	1.37	57
FEV$_1$/FVC (%)	≥78	90		89	
MVV (L/min)	84	59	70	63	75
FEF$_{25-75\%}$ (L/sec)	2.7	2.0	75	2.1	79
FRC (L)	2.62	1.34	51		
RV (L)	1.58	0.76	48		
TLC (L)	4.68	2.43	52		
RV/TLC (%)	34	31			
DLCO (mL/min/mmHg CO)	20.6	14.4	70		

Interpretation and Discussion

These studies show a restrictive pattern. The FEV$_1$ and FVC are reduced; however, the FEV$_1$/FVC% is normal. The lung volumes are reduced, and the RV/TLC is normal. The diffusing capacity is slightly reduced. There is no significant improvement after inhalation of bronchodilator. This patient has mitral stenosis, resulting from rheumatic fever. Pulmonary interstitial edema is manifested by the reduction in TLC and diffusing capacity.

Patient 4. A 62-Year-Old White Woman with Cough and Shortness of Breath

	PREDICTED	PREBRONCHODILATOR		POSTBRONCHODILATOR	
		Observed	% Predicted	Observed	% Predicted
FVC (L)	2.35	2.05	87	2.24	95
FEV$_1$ (L)	1.74	0.73	42	0.84	48
FEV$_1$/FVC (%)	≥74	36		38	
MVV (L/min)	58	28	48	32	55
FEF$_{25-75\%}$ (L/sec)	2.2	0.3	15	0.3	18
FRC (L)	1.98	2.77	140		
RV (L)	1.20	1.72	143		
TLC (L)	3.55	4.22	119		
RV/TLC (%)	34	48			
D$_L$CO (mL/min/mmHg CO)	17.8	16.0	90		

Interpretation and Discussion

This patient's spirogram shows marked obstruction to airflow. There is no improvement after inhalation of bronchodilator. Although the RV and FRC are increased, the TLC is only at the upper limits of normal. The diffusing capacity is normal, suggesting that the patient has predominantly chronic bronchitis, rather than anatomic emphysema. This patient does indeed have severe chronic obstructive pulmonary disease, with chronic bronchitis as the predominant problem.

Patient 5. A 47-Year-Old-White Woman Who Complained of Lethargy. She Was 63 Inches Tall and Weighed 247 Pounds

	PREDICTED	PREBRONCHODILATOR	
		Observed	% Predicted
FVC (L)	2.77	3.15	114
FEV$_1$ (L)	2.11	2.67	127
FEV$_1$/FVC (%)	≥76	85	
MVV (L/min)	101	68	67
FEF$_{25-75\%}$ (L/sec)	2.8	3.1	111

Interpretation and Discussion

The spirographic data are normal, except for the reduction in MVV. This pattern is suggestive of variable effort.

Patient 6. A 52-Year-Old White Man with a 2-Month History of Chronic Nonproductive Cough After a Severe Viral Pneumonia. His Cough Has Been Getting Progressively Better; He is a Nonsmoker

	PREDICTED	PREBRONCHODILATOR		POSTBRONCHODILATOR	
		Observed	% Predicted	Observed	% Predicted
FVC (L)	4.45	3.86	87	4.39	99
FEV_1 (L)	3.29	2.95	90	3.38	101
FEV_1/FVC (%)	≥74	77		77	
MVV (L/min)	126	107	85	144	114
$FEF_{25-75\%}$ (L/sec)	3.6	2.4	67	3.5	98

Interpretation and Discussion

The spirogram is normal, except for the reduced $FEF_{25-75\%}$ on the prebronchodilator study. The postbronchodilator spirometric data are normal. This patient had viral pneumonia and has a slowly resolving bronchiolitis secondary to that infection.

Patient 7. A 26-Year-Old White Man with Persistent "Wheezing" for 4 Months

	PREDICTED	PREBRONCHODILATOR	
		Observed	% Predicted
FVC (L)	4.89	5.33	109
FEV_1 (L)	4.01	1.54	38
FEV_1/FVC (%)	≥82	35	
$FEF_{25-75\%}$ (L/sec)	4.50	1.03	23

Interpretation and Discussion

The pattern suggests obstructive airway disease. Flow–volume curves demonstrated a plateau on both the forced inspiratory and expiratory loops, indicative of a fixed large airway obstruction. A bronchoscopy was performed that demonstrated a mass partially obstructing the trachea. Biopsy of the lesion showed a bronchial adenoma of the cylindroma type. Usual spirographic data do not differentiate between large-airway and small-airway obstruction. In this instance, the lesion was suggested by the characteristic shape of the flow-volume loop.

Patient 8. A 38-Year-Old White Man with a History of Intermittent Attacks of Shortness of Breath Associated with Wheezing

	PREDICTED	PREBRONCHODILATOR		POSTBRONCHODILATOR	
		Observed	% Predicted	Observed	% Predicted
FVC (L)	4.14	5.92	143	6.11	148
FEV$_1$ (L)	3.23	3.77	116	4.26	132
FEV$_1$/FVC (%)	≥78	64		70	
MVV (L/min)	122	140	115	169	138
FEF$_{25-75\%}$ (L/sec)	3.9	2.4	61	3.2	81

Interpretation and Discussion

The mechanics of ventilation are abnormal, demonstrating a reduction in the FEV$_1$/FVC% and the FEF$_{25-75\%}$ in the prebronchodilator study. After inhalation of bronchodilator, the FEF$_{25-75\%}$ is normal. The finding of obstructive airway disease responsive to bronchodilator, in association with a history of intermittent attacks of wheezing along with symptom-free intervals, would be compatible with the diagnosis of bronchial asthma.

Patient 9. A 66-Year-Old White Man with a 15-Year History of Chronic Cough and Sputum Production. On Physical Examination He Had Severe Kyphoscoliosis.

	PREDICTED	PREBRONCHODILATOR		POSTBRONCHODILATOR	
		Observed	% Predicted	Observed	% Predicted
FVC (L)	3.69	2.11	57	2.12	57
FEV$_1$ (L)	2.62	1.05	40	1.09	42
FEV$_1$/FVC (%)	≥71	50		51	
MVV (L/min)	87	31	36	40	46
FEF$_{25-75\%}$ (L/sec)	2.9	0.5	17	0.5	17
FRC (L)	3.04	2.58	85		
RV (L)	1.81	1.56	86		
TLC (L)	5.02	3.56	71		
RV/TLC (%)	36	44			

Interpretation and Discussion

The mechanics of ventilation are abnormal on the spirogram, suggesting possible combined obstructive and restrictive pulmonary disease. A TLC measurement is helpful to determine whether the reduction in vital capacity is due to air-trapping from severe obstructive airway disease or whether it does indeed represent the presence of concomitant restrictive disease. In this case, the TLC is reduced, suggesting that the patient does indeed have restrictive pulmonary disease. The reduction in FEV$_1$/FVC%, along with the fact that the FEF$_{25-75\%}$ is reduced considerably more than the reduction in FVC, confirms that the patient has obstructive airway disease. There is no significant improvement, after inhalation of bronchodilator, in the patient's expiratory flow rates. The patient's obstructive airway disease is due to combined chronic bronchitis and pulmonary emphysema. The restrictive pattern is secondary to the concomitant severe kyphoscoliosis.

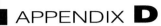

APPENDIX D

Examples of Arterial Blood Gas Data

John E. Hodgkin

Patient 1. A 56-Year-Old Woman Who, While on the Oncology Ward, Developed Shortness of Breath Is Breathing Room Air.

	ACTUAL VALUES	NORMAL VALUES
pH	7.48	7.35–7.45
PCO_2 (mmHg)	32	35–45
PO_2 (mmHg)	59	76–84
O_2 saturation (%)	91.1	>93
O_2 content (vol %)	13.4	16–20
$P(A-a)O_2$ (mmHg)	49	<23
Plasma bicarbonate (mEq/L)	24	22–26
Standard bicarbonate (mEq/L)	25	22–26
Base excess (blood) (mEq/L)	1	−2 to +2
Base excess (ECF) (mEq/L)	1	−2 to +2

Interpretation and Discussion

The PO_2 is considerably lower than the predicted normal range for this patient's age, so there is moderate hypoxemia when she is breathing room air. The PO_2 would be even lower were it not for the patient's hyperventilation, as indicated by the reduced PCO_2. The $P(A-a)O_2$ is increased, indicating the presence of ventilation–perfusion mismatch, diffusion defect, or shunt. The acid–base data are compatible with an uncompensated, mild respiratory alkalosis. A ventilation–perfusion lung scan was consistent with pulmonary embolism.

Patient 2. A 71-Year-Old Man Who Has Hypertension Is Breathing Room Air.

	ACTUAL VALUES	NORMAL VALUES
pH	7.5	7.35–7.45
PCO_2 (mmHg)	48	35–45
PO_2 (mmHg)	62	69–77
O_2 saturation (%)	92.5	>93
O_2 content (vol %)	16.7	16–20
$P(A-a)O_2$ (mmHg)	29	<30
Plasma bicarbonate (mEq/L)	37	22–26
Standard bicarbonate (mEq/L)	35	22–26
Base excess (blood) (mEq/L)	11	−2 to +2
Base excess (ECF) (mEq/L)	14	−2 to +2

Interpretation and Discussion

Moderate hypoxemia is present when breathing room air. The $P(A-a)O_2$ is normal for this patient's age, indicating that overall hypoventilation is the cause of the hypoxemia. The sum of the PO_2 and the PCO_2 while breathing room air is 110 mmHg, which would also suggest overall hypoventilation as the cause of the reduced PO_2. The acid–base data are compatible with a partially compensated metabolic alkalosis. However, this is compatible with maximal compensation based on 95% confidence limit bands. The patient is being treated with diuretics for his hypertension, which has resulted in a metabolic alkalosis, and he now is hypoventilating in an attempt to compensate for the alkalosis.

Patient 3. An 80-Year-Old Woman with a History of Chronic Renal Disease Is Breathing Room Air.

	ACTUAL VALUES	NORMAL VALUES
pH	7.36	7.35–7.45
PCO_2 (mmHg)	33	35–45
PO_2 (mmHg)	77	66–74
O_2 saturation (%)	94.4	>93
O_2 content (vol %)	7.3	16–20
$P(A-a)O_2$ (mmHg)	30	<33
Plasma bicarbonate (mEq/L)	18	22–26
Standard bicarbonate (mEq/L)	19	22–26
Base excess (blood) (mEq/L)	−6	−2 to +2
Base excess (ECF) (mEq/L)	−6	−2 to +2

Interpretation and Discussion

The PO_2 is excellent when breathing room air when compared with the predicted normal PO_2 for this patient's age. The PO_2 would be somewhat lower if the patient were not hyperventilating. The O_2 content, however, is markedly reduced, which is compatible with the patient's chronic anemia. The acid–base data are compatible with a compensated metabolic acidosis. The patient has chronic uremic acidosis. The severe anemia is due to the patient's chronic renal failure.

Patient 4. A 77-Year-Old Man Who Is Breathing Room Air.

	ACTUAL VALUES	NORMAL VALUES
pH	7.36	7.35–7.45
PCO_2 (mmHg)	25	35–45
PO_2 (mmHg)	75	67–75
O_2 saturation (%)	93.1	>93
O_2 content (vol %)	12.7	16–20
$P(A-a)O_2$ (mmHg)	43	<32
Plasma bicarbonate (mEq/L)	14	22–26
Standard bicarbonate (mEq/L)	17	22–26
Base excess (blood) (mEq/L)	−10	−2 to +2
Base excess (ECF) (mEq/L)	−10	−2 to +2

Interpretation and Discussion

The patient's PO_2 when breathing room air is excellent; however, it would be lower were it not for the hyperventilation. The $P(A-a)O_2$ difference is increased when compared with that predicted for this patient's age, which indicates the presence of ventilation–perfusion mismatch, diffusion defect, or shunt. Despite the excellent PO_2, the O_2 content is reduced because of anemia. The acid–base data are compatible with a compensated metabolic acidosis. However, 95% confidence limit bands suggest the presence of metabolic acidosis with a superimposed respiratory alkalosis. In other words, for a base excess of −10 mEq/L, one would not expect the patient to hyperventilate enough, in compensating for this acidemia, to return the pH to 7.36. This suggests that the patient has a reason for hyperventilation other than simply an attempt to compensate for the metabolic acidosis. The patient does have pneumonia in addition to diabetic ketoacidosis.

Patient 5. A 97-Year-Old Man Who Is Breathing with a 28% Ventimask Device.

	ACTUAL VALUES	NORMAL VALUES
pH	7.48	7.35–7.45
PCO_2 (mmHg)	22	35–45
PO_2 (mmHg)	51	59–67
O_2 saturation (%)	88.8	>93
O_2 content (vol %)	11.1	16–20
$P(A-a)O_2$ (mmHg)	117	<47
Plasma bicarbonate (mEq/L)	16	22–26
Standard bicarbonate (mEq/L)	20	22–26
Base excess (blood) (mEq/L)	−5	−2 to +2
Base excess (ECF) (mEq/L)	−7	−2 to +2

Interpretation and Discussion

The PO_2 is barely adequate despite 28% O_2. The $P(A-a)O_2$ is significantly increased above that predicted for this patient's age and FIO_2, indicating the presence of ventilation–perfusion mismatch, diffusion defect, or shunt. The O_2 content is markedly reduced, partly owing to the low PO_2, but also to anemia. The acid–base data are compatible with a partially compensated respiratory alkalosis. This patient has severe pneumonia that has been present for several days.

Patient 6. A 25-Year-Old Man With a Complaint of Dyspnea. His Chest X-Ray Shows Hilar Lymphadenopathy Bilaterally. He Is Breathing Spontaneously, with 3 L/min Supplemental Oxygen by Nasal Cannula.

	ACTUAL VALUES	NORMAL VALUES
pH	7.51	7.35–7.45
PCO_2 (mmHg)	33	35–45
PO_2 (mmHg)	71	89–97
O_2 saturation (%)	93.9	>93
O_2 content (vol %)	21.3	16–20
$P(A-a)O_2$ (mmHg)		
Plasma bicarbonate (mEq/L)	26	22–26
Standard bicarbonate (mEq/L)	28	22–26
Base excess (blood) (mEq/L)	4	−2 to +2
Base excess (ECF) (mEq/L)	3	−2 to +2

Interpretation and Discussion

Adequate oxygenation is present when breathing 3 L/min O_2 by nasal cannula. The $P(A-a)O_2$ cannot be calculated because the precise FiO_2 is unknown. However, the sum of the PO_2 and PCO_2 is less than 110 mmHg, indicating the presence of ventilation–perfusion mismatch, diffusion defect, or shunt. The acid–base data are compatible with a combined respiratory and metabolic alkalosis. The plasma bicarbonate is normal because of the hypocapnia; however, the standard bicarbonate and base excess values are slightly increased. Mediastinoscopy provided biopsy evidence for a noncaseating granuloma compatible with sarcoidosis. Even though in this case the patient's chest x-ray showed no evidence of lung parenchymal involvement, the diffusing capacity was 50% of predicted normal.

Patient 7. An 18-Year-Old Girl Who Presents to the Emergency Room in Coma Is Breathing Room Air.

	ACTUAL VALUES	NORMAL VALUES
pH	7.21	7.35–7.45
PCO_2 (mmHg)	12	35–45
PO_2 (mmHg)	118	92–100
O_2 saturation (%)	97.0	>93
$P(A-a)O_2$ (mmHg)	17	<6
Plasma bicarbonate (mEq/L)	5	22–26
Base excess (blood) (mEq/L)	−22	−2 to +2
Base excess (ECF) (mEq/L)	−22	−2 to +2

Interpretation and Discussion

The PO_2 is supranormal for room air. The high PO_2 is a result of the prominent hyperventilation. The PCO_2 is markedly decreased, so that, indeed, alveolar hyperventilation is present. A partially compensated metabolic acidosis is present; however, based on 95% confidence limit bands, this arterial blood gas would be compatible with a maximally compensated metabolic acidosis. The diagnosis is diabetic ketoacidosis. Even though the sum of the PO_2 and PCO_2 is between 110 and 130 when breathing room air in this young patient, the $P(A-a)O_2$ is increased, indicating the presence of $\dot{V}/\dot{Q}$ mismatch, diffusion defect, or shunt. In this case, the patient had a mild pneumonitis in addition to diabetic ketoacidosis.

Patient 8.   A 28-Year-Old Man with a 3-Day History of Fever, Cough, and Shortness of Breath Is Breathing Room Air.

	ACTUAL VALUES	NORMAL VALUES
pH	7.56	7.35–7.45
PCO_2 (mmHg)	25	35–45
PO_2 (mmHg)	30	87–95
O_2 saturation (%)	68	>93
$P(A-a)O_2$ (mmHg)	90	<11
Plasma bicarbonate (mEq/L)	23	22–26
Base excess (blood) (mEq/L)	+2	−2 to +2
Base excess (ECF) (mEq/L)	0	−2 to +2

Interpretation and Discussion

The PO_2 is markedly decreased. The $P(A-a)O_2$ is increased, and the sum of the PO_2 and PCO_2 is less than 110 mmHg, indicating the presence of $\dot{V}/\dot{Q}$ disturbance, diffusion defect, or shunt as the cause of hypoxemia. An uncompensated respiratory alkalosis is present. The diagnosis is influenzal pneumonia. Because of significant respiratory distress, the patient was intubated and placed on a volume ventilator with an FIO_2 of 1.0. Twenty minutes later, the following arterial blood gas data were obtained.

pH	7.46	7.35–7.45
PCO_2 (mmHg)	32	35–45
PO_2 (mmHg)	50	>580
O_2 saturation (%)	85.7	100
$P(A-a)O_2$ (mmHg)	631	<93
Plasma bicarbonate (mEq/L)	23	22–26
Base excess (blood) (mEq/L)	0	−2 to +2
Base excess (ECF) (mEq/L)	−1	−2 to +2

Interpretation and Discussion

Severe hypoxemia is still present. The $P(A-a)O_2$ is increased despite 100% oxygen, indicating that the cause of the hypoxemia is a right-to-left shunt. This is most likely a "physiologic shunt," rather than an anatomic shunt. A mild, uncompensated respiratory alkalosis is still present. In this patient with "adult respiratory distress syndrome," it would be appropriate to institute positive end-expiratory pressure (PEEP) in an attempt to reduce the FIO_2 and still maintain an adequate PO_2.

Patient 9. A 16-Year-Old Girl Admitted to the Emergency Room in a Comatose State Is Breathing Room Air.

	ACTUAL VALUES	NORMAL VALUES
pH	7.04	7.35–7.45
PCO_2 (mmHg)	85	35–45
PO_2 (mmHg)	45	93–101
O_2 saturation (%)	60.1	>93
$P(A–a)O_2$ (mmHg)	5	<6
Plasma bicarbonate (mEq/L)	22	22–26
Standard bicarbonate (mEq/L)	15	22–26
T_{40} bicarbonate (mEq/L)	19	22–26
Base excess (blood) (mEq/L)	−12	−2 to +2
Base excess (ECF) (mEq/L)	−7	−2 to +2

Interpretation and Discussion

Severe hypoxemia is present with room air. The $P(A–a)O_2$ is normal, and the sum of the PO_2 and PCO_2 is between 110 and 130 mmHg with room air. Therefore, the cause of the hypoxemia is overall hypoventilation. The plasma bicarbonate is normal however, the T_{40} bicarbonate is reduced. The plasma bicarbonate is normal because the PCO_2 is markedly elevated. If the PCO_2 were normal (e.g., 40 mmHg), the actual plasma bicarbonate would be 19 mEq/L. Therefore, a combined respiratory and metabolic acidosis is present. The BE_{ECF} and T_{40} bicarbonate (based on in vivo data) more accurately portray the true level of metabolic acidosis in this case than do the BE_b and standard bicarbonate (which are based on in vitro calculations). The diagnosis is drug overdose. The hypoventilation and severe respiratory acidosis are due to respiratory center depression. The metabolic acidosis is due to lactic acid accumulation secondary to inadequate tissue oxygenation resulting from the severe hypoxemia.

Patient 10. A 68-Year-Old Man with a Long History of Smoking, Cough, Sputum Production, and Shortness of Breath. Arterial Blood Gas Sample Was Reportedly Drawn with the Patient Breathing Room Air.

	ACTUAL VALUES	NORMAL VALUES
pH	7.30	7.35–7.45
PCO_2 (mmHg)	75	35–45
PO_2 (mmHg)	80	71–79
O_2 saturation (%)	93.7	>93
Plasma bicarbonate (mEq/L)	38	22–26
T_{40} bicarbonate (mEq/L)	35.7	22–26
Base excess (blood) (mEq/L)	+7	−2 to +2
Base excess (ECF) (mEq/L)	+9	−2 to +2

Interpretation and Discussion

The PO_2 is excellent. There is a partially compensated respiratory acidosis. Plasma bicarbonate is increased slightly owing to the elevated PCO_2. However, if the PCO_2 were 40 mmHg the bicarbonate would still be elevated to 35.7 mEq/L. The 95% confidence limit bands show that the data are compatible with a maximally compensated respiratory acidosis. The patient has chronic bronchitis with chronic respiratory failure. The sum of the PO_2 and PCO_2 is greater than 130 mmHg. When this happens, one should suspect that the patient is not breathing room air, but rather, breathing supplemental oxygen. The other possibility would be an error in either the PO_2 or PCO_2 measurements. Indeed, this patient was breathing 2 L/min O_2 by nasal cannula (e.g., low-flow oxygen).

Patient 11. A 56-Year-Old Man Found to Be Somnolent and Cyanotic in the Postoperative Recovery Room While Breathing Room Air.

	ACTUAL VALUES	NORMAL VALUES
pH	7.14	7.35–7.45
PCO_2 (mmHg)	85	35–45
PO_2 (mmHg)	35	76–84
O_2 saturation (%)	50	>93
O_2 content (vol %)	10.5	16–20
$P(A-a)O_2$ (mmHg)	8	<23
Plasma bicarbonate (mEq/L)	28	22–26
Standard bicarbonate (mEq/L)	21	22–26
T_{40} bicarbonate (mEq/L)	25	22–26
BB (blood) (mEq/L)	44	46–50
BE (blood) (mEq/L)	−4	−2 to +2
BE_{ECF} (mEq/L)	1.4	−2 to +2

Interpretation and Discussion

The severe hypoxemia is due to overall hypoventilation, as noted from the normal $P(A-a)O_2$ and the fact that the sum of the PO_2 and PCO_2 when breathing room air is between 110 and 130 mmHg. Respiratory acidosis is present. Plasma bicarbonate is slightly elevated; however, this is simply a result of the acute hypercapnia, as indicated by the normal T_{40} bicarbonate and normal BE_{ECF}. The standard bicarbonate, blood buffer base, and blood base excess values are low and, thus, misleading, since there is no metabolic acidosis present. This again points out the value of using calculations based on in vivo information (i.e., T_{40} bicarbonate and BE_{ECF}), rather than on those based on in vitro measurements (i.e., standard bicarbonate, BB_b, and BE_b). This patient's acute, uncompensated, respiratory acidosis and severe hypoxemia are a result of hypoventilation from respiratory center depression in a patient who has not yet recovered from the effects of his general anesthesia.

Patient 12. A 71-Year-Old Woman on the Surgery Unit Is Breathing 6 L/min Oxygen by Nasal Cannula.

	ACTUAL VALUES	NORMAL VALUES
pH	7.15	7.35–7.45
PCO_2 (mmHg)	35	35–45
PO_2 (mmHg)	95	69–77
O_2 saturation (%)	94	>93
O_2 content (vol %)	19.9	16–20
Plasma bicarbonate (mEq/L)	12	22–26
Base excess (ECF) (mEq/L)	−15	−2 to +2

Interpretation and Discussion

Oxygenation is excellent while breathing 6 L/min O_2 by nasal cannula. The arterial blood analysis shows a prominent metabolic acidosis, with the PCO_2 at the lower limits of normal. This patient, 48-hours postlaparotomy, became cyanotic and unresponsive after an injection of morphine. The patient received IV naloxone hydrochloride to reverse the respiratory center depression induced by the morphine. She now has excellent oxygenation with spontaneous breathing; however, she still has severe lactic acidosis resulting from tissue hypoxia during her period of acute hypoventilation.

APPENDIX E

Gas Laws and Certain Indispensable Conventions

George G. Burton
H. Frederic Helmholz, Jr.

Readers of this book will probably have learned, and then promptly forgotten, some of the basic physical laws and principles that undergird this profession unless they use them frequently in their day-to-day practice (e.g., in the pulmonary physiology laboratory). Accordingly, these laws and principles bear repeating, despite the caveat that their memorization (perish the thought!) can be relegated to an operative sequence of memory devices (mnemonics).[4] Detailed descriptions and discussions of this material have been published elsewhere.[1-7]

STANDARD ABBREVIATIONS AND SYMBOLS

The literature of pulmonary physiology and respiratory care requires a familiarity with scientific notation and its standard abbreviations and symbols (Table E–1).

FACTORS INFLUENCING THE BEHAVIOR OF GASES

Four basic variables affect gas volumetric relationships.

1. Temperature (T), when expressed as degrees Kelvin, indicates the level of energy of a gas sample and is referred to as absolute temperature, converted from temperature centigrade or Celsius, or Fahrenheit.
2. Pressure (P), defined as absolute or total, exerted pressure, is conventionally expressed in atmospheres, or as a given column of mercury or of water balancing the pressure (mmHg, torr, or cmH_2O), or in pascals or kilopascals in the Systeme Internationale (SI) (see under Standard Units).
3. Volume (V) is expressed in cubic units, such as cubic meters or cubic centimeters, or in liters.
4. Relative mass of gas or number of molecules (n) is expressed in gram molecules (the molecular weight of the substance in grams).

For all physiologic measurements the general ("*ideal*") *gas law* can be used without significant error (see a physical chemistry text for Van der Waals equation, which includes the factor of space taken up by molecules and intermolecular forces). The unit R is used to indicate the gas constant and perhaps should be designated R^g to differentiate it from R, which indicates exchange ratio of respired gases. The ideal gas law states that

$$PV = nR^gT$$

Table E–1 Standard Abbreviations and Symbols Used in Respiratory Care

---

PULMONARY FUNCTION TESTS

C_{st}	Static compliance; compliance measured under conditions of prolonged interruption of airflow
E	Elastance; equal to the reciprocal of compliance
G_{aw}	Airway conductance; equal to reciprocal of R_{aw}
sG_{aw}	Airway conductance at a specific lung volume
P_{aw}	Pressure in the airway; further modifiers to be specified
P_A	Alveolar pressure
P_{es}	Esophageal pressure used to estimate P_{pl}
P_L	Transpulmonary pressure
P_{pl}	Intrapleural pressure
P_{tm}	Transmural pressure, pertaining to an airway or blood vessel
PI_{max}	Maximal inspiratory pressure; this term is often symbolized as MIP
PE_{max}	Maximal expiratory pressure; this term is often symbolized as MEP
R	Resistance (i.e., pressure per unit flow)
$\bar{R}$	Mean total resistance ($[R_I + R_E] \div 2$)
R_{aw}	Airway resistance
R_E	Total expiratory resistance measured by esophageal balloon method
R_I	Total inspiratory resistance measured by esophageal balloon method
R_L	Lung resistance
WOB	Work of breathing

ARTERIAL BLOOD GAS, ACID-BASE, AND GAS EXCHANGE

pH	Symbol relating the hydrogen ion concentration or activity of a solution to that of a standard solution; approximately equal to the negative logarithm of the hydrogen ion concentration. pH is an indicator of the relative acidity or alkalinity of a solution.
P_{aO2}	Arterial oxygen tension, or partial pressure
P_{AO2}	Alveolar oxygen tension, or partial pressure
P_{aCO2}	Arterial carbon dioxide tension, or partial pressure
P_{ACO2}	Alveolar carbon dioxide tension, or partial pressure
$P_{\bar{v}O2}$	Oxygen tension of mixed venous blood
$P_{(A-a)O2}$	Alveolar-arterial oxygen tension difference. The term formerly used ($A-a\ DO_2$) is discouraged.
$P_{(a/A)O2}$	Alveolar-arterial tension ratio: $P_{aO2} : P_{AO2}$. We propose the term *oxygen exchange index* to describe this ratio.
$C_{a-\bar{v}O2}$	Arteriovenous oxygen content difference
S_{aO2}	Oxygen saturation of the hemoglobin of arterial blood
S_{pO2}	Oxygen saturation is measured by pulse oximetry
C_{aO2}	Oxygen content of arterial blood

BLOOD FLOW AND SHUNTS

Q	Blood volume
$\dot{Q}$	Blood flow (volume units and time must be specific)
Q_c	Pulmonary capillary blood volume
Q_{sp}	Physiologic shunt flow (total venous admixture)
$Q_{sp}/\dot{Q}_{tot}$	Shunt as percent of total blood flow

DIFFUSING CAPACITY

D_{LCOsb}	Diffusing capacity of the lung for carbon monoxide determined by the single-breath technique
D_m	Diffusing capacity of the alveolocapillary membrane (STPD)
D/V_A	Diffusion per unit of alveolar volume, with D at STPD and VA in liters BTPS

---

and is expressed in a conglomerate unit telling what units of pressure, volume, and temperature are used. The equation is better understood if one expresses it as follows:

$$\frac{PV}{nT} = \text{a constant,}$$

as long as energy equilibrium is obtained, when temperature is expressed on an absolute scale, pressure is absolute pressure, and uniform units are used for pressure, volume, and mass of material. Thus, as long as the amount of gas under consideration remains the same, the following powerful equation is available:

$$\frac{P_1 V_1}{T_1} = \frac{P_2 V_2}{T_2}$$

This enables one to calculate the changes produced by changing conditions for any gas volume. The general gas law is actually composed of five separate but related laws.

1. *Boyle's law* states that volume varies inversely with absolute pressure (e.g., volume is reduced as pressure is increased), other factors remaining constant.

$$V_1 P_1 = V_2 P_2,$$

where *T* and *n* are constant.

2. *Charles' law* states that volume is directly proportional to temperature when it is expressed on an absolute scale, other factors remaining constant.

$$\frac{V_1}{T_1} = \frac{V_2}{T_2},$$

where P and n are constant.

3. *Gay-Lussac's law* expresses the same relationship but is stated as follows:

$$\frac{P_1}{T_1} = \frac{P_2}{T_2},$$

where V and n are constant. Thus, the pressure of gases when volume is maintained constant is directly proportional to the absolute temperature for a constant amount of gas.

4. *Avogadro's law* states that equal volumes of gases under identical conditions contain equal numbers of molecules, or that the number of molecules is directly proportional to the volume, other factors remaining constant.

$$\frac{n_1}{V_1} = \frac{n_2}{V_2},$$

where P and T are constant.

5. *Dalton's law* states that gases in a mixture exert pressure equivalent to the pressure each would exert were it present alone in the volume of the tidal mixture, which means that each gas present in a mixture exerts a partial pressure equal to the fractional concentration (by volume) multiplied by the total pressure.

Taken together, Avogadro's law and Dalton's law indicate that in the gas phase, partial pressures will be proportional to molar concentrations, and volumetric expressions will indicate numbers of molecules if a standard is accepted.

By convention, numbers of molecules are indicated in physiology as follows: Whenever gas exchanges (uptake or utilization, or both, or elimination or production, or both) are being studied, volumes are corrected to agreed-on conditions that are standard conditions designated by the initials STPD (standard temperature is 0°C or 273K; standard pressure is 1 atmosphere or 760 mmHg or

14.69 psi; and *D* stands for a dry gas). One molecular weight of a true gas has a volume STPD (V^{stpd}) of 22.41 L.*

The number of molecules in 1 g molecular weight (mole) of a gas has been calculated at 6.06×10^{23}. This is fittingly called *Avogadro's number*.

Other conditions under which gases are often measured or in which volumes are expressed are indicated by the initials BTPS (body temperature and pressure saturated). Body temperature is 37°C or 310 K; body pressure is whatever pressure is ambient; and a gas saturated with water at body temperature contains 43.9 mg/L and has a partial pressure of water vapor of 47 mmHg. Volumes of gas (V^{btps}) at body temperature and pressure saturated are effective in washing carbon dioxide out of the pulmonary alveoli, and oxygen partial pressure under these same conditions is that which is effective at the alveolar level in causing diffusion into the blood.

ATPS refers to gas volumes at ambient temperature and pressure, saturated at ambient temperature. This would be the condition of gas in a measuring vessel in which expired air had been collected. ATP alone is used to indicate the same as the foregoing, without water vapor present. (ATPD is preferred for this condition).

Since accurate tables of water vapor pressure at various temperatures are available, it is customary to use water vapor pressure in correcting volumes from wet to dry conditions. One may conclude from the foregoing laws that the volume of a wet gas will bear the following relation to the volume of that gas when the water vapor has been removed (P_B equals total or barometric pressure).

$$V_{dry} \times P_B = V_{wet} \times (P_B - P_{H_2O}{}^T);$$

$$V_{dry} = V_{wet} \frac{P_B - P_{H_2O}{}^T}{P_B}$$

since the gas present exerts pressure in the wet gas equivalent to the total pressure minus the partial pressure of water vapor. Thus to correct a volume

---

* For CO_2, N_2O, and other gases, the critical temperatures of which are relatively high (near room temperature), this number is somewhat smaller, but it is not significantly different for purposes of respiratory therapy and, therefore, the same "molecular volume" can be used for all gases. Thus, one can calculate R^g using an expression such as

$$\frac{760 \times 22.41}{1 \times 273} = R,$$

with the notation that pressure is in mmHg, volume in liters, temperature in degrees Kelvin, and n in moles.

of gas BTPS or STPD, the following calculation can be given as an example.

$$V_{STPD} = V_{BTPS} \times \frac{P_B - 47}{760} \times \frac{273}{273 + 37}$$
$$= V_{BTPS} \times 0.8146$$

if $P_B = 760$.

OTHER RELATIONS OF IMPORTANCE IN RESPIRATORY THERAPY

Flowing fluids (gases or liquids) obey certain important laws. Fluids flow only when acted on by a force, this force being proportional to a difference in pressure. Some of the laws are given in the following:

Poiseuille's law states that the flow of a fluid or gas that escapes through a tube (V) will be proportional to the pressure difference (ΔP) across the tube, to the fourth power of the radius (r) of the tube, and to time (t), and will be inversely proportional to the length of the tube (L) and the viscosity of the fluid (n).

$$\dot{V} = \frac{\Delta P \pi r^4 t}{8Ln}$$

The density of the fluid is not involved. This law holds only as long as the fluid flows in a laminar (orderly) fashion. Note that π and 8 are constants.

In the last century, Osborn Reynolds presented the concept that a nondimensional number could characterize a system in which there was fluid flow. This number is proportional to the density of the fluid, the velocity of the fluid flow, and the size of the system and is inversely proportional to the viscosity of the fluid. When this number exceeds a certain critical value (which depends on units used in expressing the determining variables), the fluid flow will become turbulent, and Poiseuille's law will no longer describe the situation. Under such circumstances, the flow will no longer increase directly as the differential in pressure increases but will increase only as the square root of the increase of pressure. In normal breathing there is little turbulence in the airway. The formula for the *Reynold's number* is

$$N_R = \frac{\text{fluid density} \times \text{velocity} \times \text{size (of tube or particle)}}{\text{viscosity of fluid}}$$

If the density of a fluid is reduced, and since viscosity is not affected by the density changes, the increase in velocity required to raise the Reynolds' number to a critical level is increased. Thus, the less the density of the fluid, the greater the velocity it must obtain before the flow will become turbulent. The velocity at which any fluid will become turbulent will be characteristic of that fluid and is called the *critical velocity* of that fluid.

The foregoing relationships have important implications for respiratory therapy:

1. In very small tubes of any length, the velocity of the gas cannot exceed the critical velocity at any pressure differential, and thus turbulent flow is impossible (e.g., in the small bronchi and bronchioles of the lung).
2. Since turbulent flow in the airways is essential for an effective cough, low-density gases (He–O_2) will make coughing ineffective. Moreover, the cough cannot effectively move secretions in peripheral airways.
3. Helium as a diluent for oxygen will effectively increase volume flows obtainable through short, narrowed segments of the major airways in which turbulence is present. This is particularly useful when there is turbulence during resting tidal flows.
4. Because aerosol particles are very small, their carriage and deposition are determined essentially by viscosity and kinetic factors alone. Therefore, aerosols are delivered equally well by warm as by cold gases and by helium–oxygen mixtures as by oxygen or air.
5. During forced expiration, substitution of helium for nitrogen in the inhaled mixture will increase that part of the expiratory flow that was restricted by its turbulent character, which would be that in the larger airways—larynx, trachea, and the first few bronchial branchings.

Daniel Bernoulli noted that when the pressure drop across a tubing system was ignored, the total energy at points along the system remained constant. Thus, the lateral pressure energy, the kinetic energy (energy of motion), and the potential energy (energy of position) added up to a constant, when one ignored the effect of friction.*

* Of course, to maintain flow, the total pressure at one end of any system in which a fluid is flowing must be greater than that at the other end.

$$P + hdg + \tfrac{1}{2}dv^2 = \text{a constant},$$

where P = pressure; h = height above a reference plane; d = density; g = acceleration of gravity; and v = velocity. Thus decrease in pressure = $\tfrac{1}{2}dv^2$.

This theorem (*Bernoulli's principle*) explains the way jets of gas entrain materials brought to the side of a high-velocity stream, how the wings of an airplane work, and how water pumps on faucets work. When a fluid flows through a restricted portion of a tube, the velocity must increase; consequently, the energy of motion increases and the pressure energy (lateral wall pressure) decreases, so that at the edges of any high-velocity fluid stream pressures will be reduced. (*Note*: In a tube beyond the restriction, the lateral pressure again rises.) A high-velocity stream of gas escaping from a nozzle will be surrounded by an area of pressure below atmospheric, and any fluid in the area will be entrained. This explains the way a so-called venturi–oxygen dilutor system works and how jet nebulizers and the Babbington nebulizer entrain fluids at the jets of gas.

Thomas Graham described *effusion*—the process by which a gas passes through an orifice. (An *orifice* is a hole with size, or area but no length.) The relative rates at which gases can be forced through an orifice are inversely proportional to the square root of the densities of the gases. Adolph Eugen Fick also showed that the rate of diffusion of a gas into another gas was inversely proportional to the square root of the molecular weight and thus the density. The foregoing laws apply only to gas effusion and diffusion in gases. In the diffusion of a gas through other substances (in our frame of reference, an aqueous medium), the solubility of the gas in the medium directly influences the diffusion.

Orders of magnitude should be considered. The diffusion of one gas into another is very rapid and is described by coefficients of "units" per second. When one considers diffusion in an aqueous medium, the coefficients are "units" of the same order of magnitude per 24 hours. The diffusion of gases in gas is at a rate at least 86,000 times that of gases in fluids. In the alveoli and alveolar ducts of the lung, diffusion maintains mixing without any need for gas movement. The process of diffusion is limiting only in the alveolar membrane and plasma, and primarily for oxygen, because it is so much less soluble than carbon dioxide. In a gas, oxygen diffuses faster than carbon dioxide by a factor of 1.173, whereas in an aqueous medium carbon dioxide diffuses at least 20 times more rapidly than oxygen because it is more than 20 times more soluble.

STANDARD UNITS

For several years now there has been a movement to try to standardize units used in expressing laboratory data. The English, as they have converted to the metric system, have begun using the International System of Units (Systeme Internationale d'Units, or SI) (Table E–2). This involves some changes from the metric-based system used in this country. The English recommended the substitution of joules for gram calories (c) and kilocalories (C) as units of energy; the substitution of the pascal and the kilopascal for centimeters of water or millimeters of mercury (torr) as units of pressure, and the substitution of the newton for the barye (1 dyne per square centimeter) as a unit of force (1 newton equals 100,000 baryes). They also advocate the use of the mole as the unit for amount of material instead of grams, milligrams, or other weights, and the substitution of moles per liter for grams percent, milligrams percent, and grams per liter. The use of concentrations as moles per liter is difficult in some situations (e.g., for hemoglobin concentrations). Moreover, it is recommended that the very useful convention of expressing ionized materials in equivalents per liter, rather than moles per liter, be retained for physiologic and biochemical expressions. The potential use of SI in respiratory care has recently been described by Chatburn,[3] whose entire discussion bears review by the interested reader.

Some of the implications of the SI system are given in Table E–3, along with the conversion factors for units. All units, including the US units, are based on the international prototype meter and the international prototype kilogram kept at the International Bureau of Weights and Measures in Sèvres, France.

In the metric system the dyne is the unit of force equal to the force required to give a free mass

Table E–2 Units With Abbreviations

VARIABLE	UNIT	ABBREVIATION
Temperature	kelvin	K
Length	meter	m
Mass	kilogram	kg
Time	second	s
Pressure	pascal	Pa
Work, or energy	joule	J

Table E–3   Method of Converting Between Usual Units and Metric or SI Units

PHYSICAL QUANTITY	CONVENTIONAL UNIT	SI UNIT	CONVERSION FACTOR*
Length	inch (in)	meter (m)	0.025 4
	foot (ft)	m	0.304 8
Area	in^2	m^2	6.452×10^{-4}
	ft^2	m^2	0.092 90
Volume	dl (= 100 mL)	L	0.01
	ft^3	m^3	0.028 32
	ft^3	L	28.32
	fluid ounce → mL		29.57
Amount of substance	mg/dL	mmol/L	10/molecular weight
	mEq/L	mmol/L	valence
	mL of gas at STPD	mmol	0.044 62
Force (weight)	pound (lb)	newton (N)	4.448
	dyne	N	0.000 01
	kilogram-force	N	9.807
	pound → kilogram-force		0.453 6
	ounce → gram-force		28.35
Pressure	cm H$_2$O	kilopascal (kPa)	0.098 06
	mm Hg (torr)	kPa	0.133 3
	pounds/in^2 (psi)	kPa	6.895
	psi → cm H$_2$O		70.31
	cm H$_2$O → torr		0.7355
	standard atmosphere	kPa	101.3
	millibar (mbar)	kPa	0.100 0
Work, energy	kg · m	joule (J)	9.807
	L · cm H$_2$O	joule (J)	0.098 06
	calorie (cal)	joule (J)	4.185
	kilocalorie (kcal)	J	4 185
	British thermal unit (BTU)		1055
Power	kg · m min^{-1}	watt (W)	0.163 4
Surface tension	dyn/cm	N/m	0.001
Compliance	L/cm H$_2$O	L/kPa	10.20
Resistance	cm H$_2$O · s · L^{-1}	kPa · s · L^{-1}	0.098 06
	cm H$_2$O · min · L^{-1}	kPa · s · L^{-1}	5.884
Gas transport (ideal gas, STPD)†	mL · s^{-1} · cm H$_2$O^{-1}	mmol · s^{-1} · kPa^{-1}	0.455 0
Temperature	°C	°K	°K = °C + 273.15
	°F → °C		°C = (°F − 32)/1.8
	°C → °F		°F = (1.8 · °C) + 32

* To convert from convention to SI unit, multiply conventional unit by conversion factor. To convert in the opposite direction, divide by conversion factor. Examples: 10 torr = 10 × 0.133 3 kPa = 1.333 kPa, 1 L = i L/0.10 = 10 dL

† Gas transport is the same as diffusing capacity and transfer factor and should be distinguished from oxygen transport, which is defined as oxygen content of arterial blood (Ca$_{O2}$) × cardiac output (Q̇).

(Chatburn RL: Measurement, physical quantities, and le système international d'units (SI Units). Resp Care 33:861, 1988)

of 1 g an acceleration of 1 cm per second per second. In the SI system the newton is the unit of force equal to the force required to give a free mass of 1 kg an acceleration of 1 m per second per second. The pascal is suggested as the unit of pressure and is equal to a force of 1 newton acting over 1 m^2.

This, however, is a very small unit, as is the barye of the usual metric system, and, therefore, it is suggested that the kilopascal be used as a unit of pressure for physiologic data.

Examples of SI conversions are given in Table E–4.

Table E—4 Examples of Conversions Commonly Used in Respiratory Physiology and Respiratory Care

PHYSICAL QUANTITY	KNOWN UNIT	DESIRED UNIT	EXAMPLE OF CONVERSION CALCULATION
Force (or mass)	lb	kg	$150 \text{ lb} \times \dfrac{0.4536 \text{ kg}}{1 \text{ lb}} = 68 \text{ kg}$
	kg	lb	$68 \text{ kg} \times \dfrac{1 \text{ lb}}{0.4536 \text{ kg}} = 150 \text{ lb}$
Pressure	torr	kPa	$35 \text{ torr} \times \dfrac{0.1333 \text{ kPa}}{1 \text{ torr}} = 4.7 \text{ kPa}$
	kPa	torr	$4.7 \text{ kPa} \times \dfrac{1 \text{ torr}}{0.1333 \text{ kPa}} = 35 \text{ torr}$
	psi	torr	$1.0 \text{ psi} \times \dfrac{70.31 \text{ cm } H_2O}{1 \text{ psi}} \times \dfrac{0.7355 \text{ torr}}{1 \text{ cm } H_2O} = 52 \text{ torr}$
	torr	psi	$51.72 \text{ torr} \times \dfrac{1 \text{ cm } H_2O}{0.7355 \text{ torr}} \times \dfrac{1 \text{ psi}}{70.31 \text{ cm } H_2O} = 1.0 \text{ psi}$
Work	L · cm H_2O	kg · m	$20 \text{ L} \cdot \text{cm } H_2O \times \dfrac{0.09806 \text{ J}}{1 \text{ L} \cdot \text{cm } H_2O} \times \dfrac{1 \text{ kg} \cdot \text{m}}{9.807 \text{ J}} = 0.2 \text{ Kg} \cdot \text{m}$
	J	L · cm H_2O	$2 \text{ J} \times \dfrac{1 \text{ kg} \cdot \text{m}}{9.807 \text{ J}} = \dfrac{1 \text{ L} \cdot \text{cm } H_2O}{0.01 \text{ kg} \cdot \text{m}} = 20 \text{ L} \cdot \text{cm } H_2O$
Power	kg · m · min^{-1}	W	$2.5 \text{ kg} \cdot \text{m} \cdot \text{min}^{\times 1} \times \dfrac{0.1634 \text{ W}}{1 \text{ kg} \cdot \text{m} \cdot \text{min}^{-1}} = 0.41 \text{ W}$
Compliance	ml/cm H_2O	L/kPa	$100 \text{ ml} \cdot \text{cm } H_2O \times \dfrac{1 \text{ L}}{1000 \text{ mL}} \times \dfrac{10.20 \text{ L} \cdot \text{kpa}^{-1}}{1 \text{ L} \cdot \text{cm } H_2O^{-1}} = 1.02 \text{ L} \cdot \text{kPa}^{-1}$
Resistance	cm H_2O · s · L^{-1}	kPa · s · L^{-1}	$55 \text{ cm } H_2O \cdot \text{s} \cdot \text{L}^{-1} \times \dfrac{0.090806 \text{ kPa} \cdot \text{L}^{-1}}{1 \text{ cm } H_2O \cdot \text{s} \cdot \text{L}^{-1}} = 5.4 \text{ kPa} \cdot \text{s} \cdot \text{L}^{-1}$

Note: Retain all digits during computation to avoid roundoff error. However, the lest precise measurement used in a calculation determines the number of significant digits in the answer. Thus, the final product or quotient should be written with the same number of significant figures as the term with the fewest significant figures, as shown in the examples above. The least ambiguous method of indicating the number of significant figures is to write the number in scientific notation. For example, the number 30 may have either one or two significant figures, but written as 3.0×10^1, it is understood that there are two significant figures. For more information about scientific notation, significant figures, and rounding off, see Lough MD, Chatburn RI, Shrock WA: Handbook of Respiratory Care. Chicago, Year Book Medical Publishers, 1985, pp 170–173.
(Chatburn RL: Measurement, physical quantities, and le système international d'units (SI Units). Resp Care 33:861, 1988)

REFERENCES

1. Altman, PL, Dittmer DS (eds): Respiration and Circulation. Bethesda, Md, Federation of American Societies for Experimental Biology, 1971
2. Bartels H et al: Methods in Pulmonary Physiology (Workman JM, trans) London, Hafna, 1963
3. Chatburn, RL: Measurement, physical quantities, and le système international d'units (SI Units). Resp Care 33:861, 1988
4. Corrie D: Gas law mnemonics. Respir Care 20:1041, 1975
5. Handbook of Chemistry and Physics. Cleveland, Chemical Rubber Publishing Company, 1976
6. International Organization for Standardization: Units of Measurement: ISO Standards Handbook 2. Geneva, ISO, 1979
7. Lentner C (ed): Geigy Scientific Tables: Units of Measurement, Body Fluids, Composition of the Body, Nutrition. West Caldwell, NJ, Ciba-Geigy Corp, 1981
8. Standardization of definitions and symbols in respiratory physiology. Fed Proc 9:602, 1950

Terms and Symbols Used in Respiratory Physiology

John E. Hodgkin

The terms and symbols used in respiratory physiology, and their definitions, change from time to time. In an attempt to standardize these terms and symbols, the American Thoracic Society/ American College of Chest Physicians Committee on Pulmonary Nomenclature published an initial report in 1975.[1] An American Thoracic Society Pulmonary Nomenclature Subcommittee on Respiratory Physiology subsequently revised the section dealing with terms and symbols used in respiratory physiology and published a portion of their report in Spring 1978.[2] The editors and publishers have used this latest report with some minor modifications.

GENERAL

P	Pressures in general
$\overline{X}$	Dash above any symbol indicates a mean value
$\dot{X}$	Dot above any symbol indicates a time derivative
$\ddot{X}$	Two dots above any symbol indicate the second time derivative
%X	Percent sign before a symbol indicates percentage of the predicted normal value
X/Y%	Percent sign after a symbol indicates a ratio function with the ratio expressed as a percentage. Both components of the ratio must be designated (e.g., $FEV_1/FEV\% = 100 \times FEV_1/FVC$)
f	Frequency of any event in time (e.g., respiratory frequency: the number of breathing cycles per unit of time)
t	Time
anat	Anatomic
max	Maximum

GAS PHASE SYMBOLS

Primary

V	Gas volume in general. Pressure, temperature, and percentage saturation with water vapor must be stated
F	Fractional concentration in dry gas phase

Qualifying

I	Inspired
E	Expired
A	Alveolar
T	Tidal
D	Dead space
B	Barometric
STPD	Standard temperature and pressure, dry. These are the conditions of a volume of gas at 0°C, at 760 torr, without water vapor
BTPS	Body temperature (37°C), barometric pressure (at sea level = 760 torr), and saturated with water vapor
ATPD	Ambient temperature, pressure, dry
ATPS	Ambient temperature and pressure, saturated with water vapor
L	Lung

BLOOD PHASE SYMBOLS

Primary

$\dot{Q}$	Volume flow of blood
C	Concentration in blood phase
S	Saturation in blood phase

Qualifying

b	Blood in general
a	Arterial. Exact location to be specified in text when term is used
v	Venous. Exact location to be specified in text when term is used
$\bar{v}$	Mixed venous
c	Capillary. Exact location to be specified in text when term is used
c′	Pulmonary end-capillary

PULMONARY FUNCTION

Lung Volumes (Expressed as BTPS)

RV	Residual volume: volume of air remaining in the lungs after maximum exhalation
ERV	Expiratory reserve volume: maximum volume of air that can be exhaled from the end-tidal volume
V_T	Tidal volume: volume of gas inspired or expired during one ventilatory cycle
IRV	Inspiratory reserve volume: maximum volume that can be inspired from an end-tidal inspiratory level
V_L	Volume of the lung, including the conducting airways. Conditions of measurement must be stated

IC	Inspiratory capacity: volume that can be inspired from the end-tidal expiratory volume.
IVC	Inspiratory vital capacity: maximum volume measured on inspiration after a full expiration
VC	Vital capacity: volume measured on complete expiration after the deepest inspiration but without respect to the effort involved
FRC	Functional residual capacity: volume of gas remaining in the lungs and airways at the end of a resting tidal expiration
TLC	Total lung capacity: volume of gas in the lung and airways after as much as possible has been inhaled
RV/TLC%	Residual volume to total lung capacity ratio, expressed as a percentage
V_D	Physiologic dead space: calculated volume (BPTS), which accounts for the difference between the pressures of CO_2 in expired gas and arterial blood. Physiologic dead space reflects the combination of anatomic dead space and alveolar dead space, the volume of the latter increasing with the importance of the nonuniformity of the ventilation/perfusion ratio in the lung
$V_{D_{anat}}$	Volume of the anatomic dead space (BTPS)
V_{D_A}	Alveolar dead space volume (BTPS)

Forced Respiratory Maneuvers (Expressed as BTPS)

FVC	Forced vital capacity: the volume of gas expired after full inspiration, and with expiration performed as rapidly and completely as possible
FIVC	Forced inspiratory vital capacity: maximal volume of air inspired after a maximum expiration, and with inspiration performed as rapidly and completely as possible
FEV_1	Volume of gas exhaled in a given time interval during the execution of a forced vital capacity (in this case, the volume exhaled in one second)
$FEV_1/FVC\%$	Ratio of timed forced expiratory volume to forced vital capacity, expressed as a percentage (in this case, the volume exhaled in 1 second/FVC)
PEF	Peak expiratory flow (L/min or L/sec)
$\dot{V}max_{XX\%}$	Maximum expiratory flow (instantaneous) qualified by the volume at which measured, expressed as percentage of the FVC that has been exhaled. (*Example:* $\dot{V}max_{75\%}$ is the maximum expiratory flow after 75% of the FVC has been exhaled and 25% remains to be exhaled)
$\dot{V}max_{XX\%TLC}$	Maximum expiratory flow (instantaneous) qualified by the volume at which measured, expressed as percentage of the TLC that remains in the lung. (*Example:* $\dot{V}max_{40\%TLC}$ is the maximum expiratory flow when 40% of the TLC remains in the lung)
FEF_{x-y}	Forced expiratory flow between two designated volume points in the FVC. These points may be designated as absolute volumes starting from the full inspiratory point or by designating the percentage of FVC exhaled
$FEF_{0.2-1.2L}$	Forced expiratory flow between 200 mL and 1200 mL of the FVC; formerly called maximum expiratory flow
$FEF_{25\%-75\%}$	Forced expiratory flow during the middle half of the FVC; formerly called maximum midexpiratory flow
MVV	Maximal voluntary ventilation: maximum volume of air that can be breathed per minute by a subject breathing quickly and as deeply as possible. The time of measurement of this tiring lung function test is usually between 12 and 30 seconds, but the test result is given in L (BTPS)/min
FET_x	Forced expiratory time required to exhale a specified FVC (e.g., $FET_{95\%}$ is the time required to deliver the first 95% of the FVC; $FET_{25\%-75\%}$ is the time required to deliver the middle half of the FVC)
MIF_x	Maximum inspiratory flow (instantaneous). As with the FET, appropriate modifiers designate the volume at which flow is being measured. Unless otherwise specified, the volume qualifiers indicate the volume inspired from RV at the point of measurement

Measurements of Ventilation

$\dot{V}_E$	Expired volume per minute (BTPS)
$\dot{V}_I$	Inspired volume per minute (BTPS)
$\dot{V}_{CO_2}$	Carbon dioxide production per minute (STPD)
$\dot{V}_{O_2}$	Oxygen consumption per minute (STPD)
R	Respiratory exchange ratio in general. Quotient of the volume of CO_2 produced divided by the volume of O_2 consumed
$\dot{V}_A$	Alveolar ventilation: physiologic process by which alveolar gas is completely removed and replaced with fresh gas. The volume of alveolar gas actually expelled completely is equal to the tidal volume minus the volume of the dead space
$\dot{V}_D$	Ventilation per minute of the physiologic dead space, BTPS
$\dot{V}_{D_{anat}}$	Ventilation per minute of the anatomic dead space, that portion of the conducting airway in which no significant gas exchange occurs (BTPS)
$\dot{V}_{D_A}$	Ventilation of the alveolar dead space (BTPS), defined by the equation $\dot{V}_{D_A} = \dot{V}_D - \dot{V}_{D_{anat}}$

Mechanics of Breathing (All Pressures Are Expressed Relative to Ambient Pressure Unless Otherwise Specified)

Pressure terms

Paw	Pressure at any point along the airways
Pao	Pressure at the airway opening (i.e., mouth, nose, tracheal cannula)
Ppl	Pleural pressure: the pressure between the visceral and parietal pleura relative to atmospheric pressure, in cmH_2O
Palv	Alveolar pressure
P_L	Transpulmonary pressure: $P_L = Palv - Ppl$, measurement conditions to be defined
Pst_L	Static recoil pressure of the lung; transpulmonary pressure measured under static conditions
Pbs	Pressure at the body surface
Pes	Esophageal pressure used to estimate Ppl
Pw	Transthoracic pressure: pressure difference between parietal pleural surface and body surface. Transthoracic in the sense used means "across the wall." $Pw = Ppl - Pbs$
Ptm	Transmural pressure pertaining to an airway or blood vessel
Prs	Transrespiratory pressure: pressure across the respiratory system. $Prs = Palv - Pbs = P_L + Pw$

Flow–pressure relationships

R	Flow resistance: the ratio of the flow-resistive components of pressure to simultaneous flow in $cmH_2O/L/sec$
Raw	Airway resistance calculated from pressure difference between airway opening (Pao) and alveoli (Palv) divided by the airflow, $cmH_2O/L/sec$
R_L	Total pulmonary resistance includes the frictional resistance of the lungs and air passages. It equals the sum of airway resistance and lung tissue resistance. It is measured by relating flow-dependent transpulmonary pressure to airflow at the mouth
Rrs	Total respiratory resistance includes the sum of airway resistance, lung tissue resistance, and chest wall resistance. It is measured by relating flow-dependent transrespiratory pressure to airflow at the mouth
Rus	Resistance of the airways on the upstream (alveolar) side of the point in the airways at which intraluminal pressure equals Ppl (equal pressure point), measured during maximum expiratory flow

Rds	Resistance of the airways on the downstream (mouth) side of the point in the airways where intraluminal pressure equals Ppl, measured during maximum expiratory flow
Gaw	Airway conductance, reciprocal of Raw
Gaw/V_L	Specific conductance expressed per liter of lung volume at which Gaw is measured

Volume–pressure relationships

C	Compliance: the slope of a static volume–pressure curve at a point, or the linear approximation of a nearly straight portion of such a curve expressed in L/cmH_2O or mL/cmH_2O
Cdyn	Dynamic compliance: the ratio of the tidal volume to the change in intrapleural pressure between the points of zero flow at the extremes of tidal volume in L/cmH_2O or mL/cmH_2O
Cst	Static compliance, value for compliance based on measurements made during periods of cessation of airflow
C/V_L	Specific compliance: compliance divided by the lung volume at which it is determined, usually FRC
E	Elastic: the reciprocal of compliance; expressed in cmH_2O/L or cmH_2O/mL
Pst	Static components of pressure
W	Work of breathing: the energy required for breathing movements

Diffusing Capacity

D_L	Diffusing capacity of the lung: amount of gas (O_2, CO, CO_2) commonly expressed as milliliters of gas (STPD) diffusing between alveolar gas and pulmonary capillary blood per torr mean gas pressure difference per minute
	Total resistance to diffusion for oxygen $\left(\dfrac{1}{D_LO_2}\right)$ and CO $\left(\dfrac{1}{D_LCO}\right)$ includes resistance to diffusion of the gas across the alveolo–capillary membrane, through plasma in the capillary, and across the red cell membrane ($1/D_M$), and the resistance to diffusion within the red cell arising from the chemical reaction between the gas and hemoglobin, ($1/\theta V_C$), according to the formulation $\dfrac{1}{D_L} = \dfrac{1}{D_M} + \dfrac{1}{\theta V_C}$
D_M	The diffusing capacity of the pulmonary membrane
θ	The rate of gas uptake by 1 mL of normal whole blood per minute for a partial pressure of 1 torr
V_C	Average volume of blood in the capillary bed in milliliters
D_L/V_A	Diffusion per unit of alveolar volume. D_L is expressed STPD, and V_A is expressed in liters (BTPS)

Respiratory Gases

PX	Tension of gas x, torr (mmHg)
PaX	Arterial tension of gas x, torr (mmHg)
P_AX	Alveolar tension of gas x, torr (mmHg)
SaO_2	Arterial oxygen saturation (percent)
C	Concentration: e.g., CaO_2 is the concentration of oxygen in a blood sample, including both oxygen combined with hemoglobin and physically dissolved oxygen, ordinarily expressed as mLO_2 (STPD)/100 mL blood
P ($_A$ − a)	Alveolar–arterial gas pressure difference: the difference in partial pressure of a gas (e.g., O_2 or N_2) in the alveolar gas spaces and that in the systemic arterial blood, measured in torr. For oxygen, as an example, P ($_A$ − a)O_2 (Also symbolized $AaDO_2$)
C (a − v)	Arterial–venous concentration difference. For oxygen, as an example, C (a − v)O_2

Pulmonary Shunts

$\dot{Q}s$ Shunt: vascular connection between circulatory pathways so that venous blood is directed into vessels containing arterialized blood (right-to-left shunt, venous admixture) or vice versa (left-to-right shunt).

PULMONARY DYSFUNCTION

Altered Breathing

Dyspnea   An unpleasant subjective feeling of difficult or labored breathing.
Hyperventila-   An alveolar ventilation that is excessive relative to the simultaneous metabolic rate. As a
tion   result the alveolar PCO_2 is significantly reduced below normal.
Hypoventilation   An alveolar ventilation that is small relative to the simultaneous metabolic rate so that
                     the alveolar PCO_2 rises significantly above normal.

Altered blood gases

Hypoxia   Any state in which oxygen in the lung, blood, or tissues is abnormally low compared
                     with that of a normal resting person breathing air at sea level.
Hypoxemia   A state in which the oxygen pressure or concentration in arterial blood is lower than its
                     normal value at sea level. Normal oxygen pressures in arterial blood at sea level are
                     based on the patients age.
Hypocapnia   Any state in which the systemic arterial carbon dioxide pressure is below 35 torr, as in
                     hyperventilation.
Hypercapnia   Any state in which the systemic arterial carbon dioxide pressure is above 45 torr. May
                     occur when alveolar ventilation is inadequate for a given metabolic rate (hypoventila-
                     tion) or during carbon dioxide inhalation.

Altered Acid–Base Balance

Acidemia   Any state of systemic arterial plasma in which the pH is less than the normal value,
                     <7.35.
Alkalemia   Any state of systemic arterial plasma in which the pH is greater than the normal value,
                     >7.45.
Base excess   Base excess: measure of metabolic alkalosis or metabolic acidosis (negative values of
   (BE)   base excess) expressed as the mEq of strong acid or strong alkali required to titrate a
                     sample of 1 L of blood to a pH of 7.40. The titration is made with the blood sample kept
                     at 37°C, oxygenated, and equilibrated to PCO_2 of 40 torr.
Acidosis   The result of any process that by itself adds excess CO_2 or nonvolatile acids to arterial
                     blood. Acidemia does not necessarily result because compensating mechanisms (in-
                     crease of HCO_3^- in respiratory acidosis, increase of ventilation, and, consequently,
                     decrease of arterial CO_2 in metabolic acidosis) may intervene to restore pH to normal.
Alkalosis   The result of any process that, by itself, diminishes acids or increases bases in arterial
                     blood. Alkalemia does not necessarily result because compensating mechanisms may
                     intervene to restore plasma pH to normal.

Other

Pulmonary   Altered function of the lung that produces clinical symptoms usually including dys-
   insufficiency   pnea.
Acute   Rapidly occurring hypoxemia, hypercarbia, or both caused by a disorder of the respira-
   respiratory   tory system. The duration of the illness and the values of arterial oxygen tension and
   failure   arterial carbon dioxide tension used as criteria for this term should be given. The term
                     acute ventilatory failure should be used only when the arterial carbon dioxide tension

	is increased. The term pulmonary failure has been used to indicate respiratory failure specifically caused by disorders of the lung.
Chronic respiratory failure	Chronic hypoxemia or hypercapnia caused by a disorder of the respiratory system. The duration of the condition and the values of arterial oxygen tension and arterial carbon dioxide tension used as criteria for this term should be given.
Obstructive ventilatory defect	Slowing of airflow during forced ventilatory maneuvers.
Restrictive ventilatory defect	Reduction of vital capacity *not* explainable by airflow obstruction.
Impairment	A measurable degree of anatomic or functional abnormality that may or may not have clinical significance. Permanent impairment is that which persists for some time (e.g., 1 year after maximum medical rehabilitation has been achieved).
Disability	A legally or administratively determined state in which a patient's ability to engage in a specific activity under certain circumstances is reduced or absent because of physical or mental impairment. Other factors, such as age, education, and customary way of making a livelihood, are considered in evaluating disability. Permanent disability exists when no substantial improvement of the patient's ability to engage in the specific activity can be expected.

REFERENCES

1. Pulmonary terms and symbols. A report of the ACCP-ATS Joint Committee on Pulmonary Nomenclature. Chest 67:583, 1975
2. Updated nomenclature for membership reaction. Report from the ATS Pulmonary Nomenclature Subcommittee on Respiratory Physiology. ATS News 4:12, Spring 1978

■ Index

NOTE: *A t* following a page number indicates tabular material and an *f* following a page number indicates an illustration. Drugs are listed under their generic names. When a drug trade name is listed, the reader is referred to the generic name.

Cardiovascular system, mechanical ventilation affecting, 526
Carina, 139, 452
Carlens tube, 474
Carotid body, in respiratory control, 148, 149f, 903
Cartilaginous airways, 138. See also Central airways
"Cascade" humidifier, 371–372
"Cascade" II humidifier, 371f, 372t
CASP. See Catheter aspiration
Catalase, in fetal lung, 724
Catecholamines, 421
actions of, 425t
adenylate cyclase affected by, 421
epinephrine as prototype of, 423
structure of, 425t
Catheter aspiration, for traumatic pneumothorax, 838–839
Catholicism, ethical views in, 74
Cavitation (cavities), 252–254
in bacterial pneumonias, 246
physical signs in, 228t
radiographic appearance of, 252–254
CDC. See Centers for Disease Control
CDH. See Congenital diaphragmatic hernia
Cell-mediated immunity, 401
Centers for Disease Control, 114
and decontamination standards, 409
isolation procedures recommended by, 406
universal precautions and, 407
Centimist nebulizer, 385t
Central airways, anatomy and physiology of, 138–141
Central apnea of prematurity, 745
Central chemoreceptors, 903
Central cyanosis, 229–230
Centralized management, for respiratory care department, 93f
Central nervous system, mechanical ventilation in diseases of, 517
Central neurogenic hyperventilation, 905
Central neurogenic hypoventilation, 905–906
Central sleep apnea, 281, 282f, 906
Centronuclear myopathy, respiration affected in, 910
Cerebral blood flow, arterial carbon dioxide tension affecting, 904
Cerebral oxygen toxicity, 344
Cerebral resuscitation, after cardiac arrest, 901
Cerebral trauma, carbon dioxide tension and, 904
Certification, for respiratory care practitioners, 28–29
Certified Inhalation Therapy Technician, 15
Certified Respiratory Therapy Technician, 24
credentialing for, 29
Cervical spine, assessment of for endotracheal intubation, 483–484, 485f

CGA. See Compressed Gas Association
Chamber, for hyperbaric therapy. See Hyperbaric chambers
Channels of Lambert (canals of Lambert), 144
in infants and children, 761
Charles, Jacques-Alexandre-Cesar, 6
Charles' law, 972
Charting monitors, 103
Charts, patient care, computerization of, 108–109
CHD. See Congenital heart disease
Chemoreceptors, in respiratory control, 148, 149f
central, 903
medullary, 148, 149f
peripheral, 148, 149f, 903
Chest
auscultation of, 222–227
sequence for, 226f
technique for, 226–227
barrel, 221, 222f
configuration of, 221–222
expansion of, 220–221
flail, 275, 836
inspection and palpation of, 219–222
percussion of, 227–228, 229f
in common respiratory diseases, 228t
Chest cuirass, for negative-pressure ventilation in home, 679
Chest injury, sucking, 836. See also Trauma
Chest motion, in mechanically ventilated patient
asymmetric, 606
paradoxic, 606
Chest pain, 215
in pulmonary embolism, 269
Chest percussion
in assessment of respiratory patient, 227–228, 229f
in common respiratory diseases, 228t
in chest physical therapy, 640
benefits of, 642–643
hemorrhage and, 649
in infants and children, 771
in lung abscess, 647
in newborn, 753–754
in postoperative atelectasis, 831
in pulmonary rehabilitation, 661
radioaerosol clearance affected by, 642t
sputum clearance affected by, 642t
Chest physical therapy, 625–654. See also specific technique and disorder
in acute myocardial ischemia, 881
assessment of components of, 641–642
in asthma, 645–646
benefits of, 642–644
in bronchiectasis, 645
in chronic obstructive lung disease, 644
complications of, 649–650

controlled-breathing techniques (breathing training) in, 625–635
coughing as technique in, 640–641
in critically ill patients, 648–649
in cystic fibrosis, 645, 798–799
definition of techniques in, 637–641
forced expiration technique in, 641
goal of, 637
hypermetabolic response to, 648
in infants and children, 770–771
in lower airway obstruction in infants, 769
in lung abscess, 646–647
and mechanism of cough, 636–637
and mucus clearance, 635–636
abnormal, 636–637
in neuromuscular disease, 646
in newborns, 753–754
in obstructive atelectasis caused by retained airway secretions, 647–648
percussion as technique in, 640. See also Chest percussion
in infants and children, 771
in newborn, 753–754
in pneumonia, 646
in postoperative atelectasis, 831
postural drainage as technique in, 637–640
in infants and children, 771
in newborn, 753
in preoperative and postoperative care, 647
in pulmonary rehabilitation, 661–662
radioaerosol clearance affected by, 641–642
sputum clearance affected by, 641, 642t
in traumatic quadriplegia, 646
vibration as technique in, 640
in infants and children, 771
in newborn, 754
Chest roentgenography, 233–277. See also specific disorder
in AIDS patients, 273, 274t
angiography in, 238–239
anteroposterior supine chest film in, 237
in asthma, 254
in atelectasis, 250–251
basic principles of, 233–234
in bronchial obstruction, 251–252
bronchography in, 238, 240f
cavities and, 252–254
in chronic bronchitis, 255
in chylothorax, 267
in complications of mechanical ventilation, 271–272
in compromised host, 273, 274t
computed tomographic scans in, 240–241, 242f
contrast changes and, 238
cysts and, 252–254
and decreased lung volume, 251
diagnostic pneumoperitoneum in, 238
diagnostic pneumothorax in, 238
in diaphragmatic abnormalities, 268